Handbook of Competence and Motivation

Edited by
Andrew J. Elliot
Carol S. Dweck

FOREWORD BY Martin V. Covington

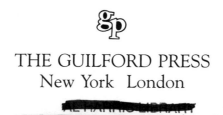

THE GUILFORD PRESS
New York London

© 2005 The Guilford Press
A Division of Guilford Publications, Inc.
72 Spring Street, New York, NY 10012
www.guilford.com

Printed in the United States of America

This book is printed on acid-free paper.

Last digit is print number: 9   8   7   6   5   4   3   2   1

Library of Congress Cataloging-in-Publication Data

Handbook of competence and motivation / edited by Andrew J. Elliot,
   Carol S. Dweck ; foreword by Martin V. Covington.
     p. cm.
   Includes bibliographical references and index.
   ISBN 1-59385-123-5 (hardcover : alk. paper)
   1. Achievement motivation. I. Elliot, Andrew J. II. Dweck, Carol
S., 1946–.
  BF504.H36 2005
  153.8—dc22

                                      2004029882

About the Editors

Andrew J. Elliot, PhD, is Professor of Psychology at the University of Rochester, and is currently an associate editor of the *Journal of Personality*. Dr. Elliot has written over 70 scholarly publicaions, has received research grants from public and private agencies, and has been awarded four different early- and mid-career awards for his research contributions. His research areas include achievement and affiliation motivation; approach–avoidance motivation; personal goals; subjective well-being; and parental, teacher, and cultural influences on motivation and self-regulation.

Carol S. Dweck, PhD, is Professor of Psychology at Stanford University, and has published significant work in the area of achievement motivation since the early 1970s. Dr. Dweck is one of the first researchers linking attributions to patterns of achievement motivation, an originator of achievement goal theory, and a pioneer in the area of self-theories of motivation. Her recent books include *Self-Theories: Their Role in Motivation, Personality, and Development* and *Motivation and Self-Regulation across the Lifespan* (coedited with Jutta Heckhausen). Her research is extensively cited in social, developmental, personality, and educational psychology.

Contributors

Sami Abuhamdeh, MA, Department of Psychology, University of Chicago, Chicago, Illinois

Phillip L. Ackerman, PhD, School of Psychology, Georgia Institute of Technology, Atlanta, Georgia

Joshua Aronson, PhD, Department of Applied Psychology, New York University, New York, New York

John A. Bargh, PhD, Department of Psychology, Yale University, New Haven, Connecticut

Jeanne Brooks-Gunn, PhD, Teachers College and College of Physicians and Surgeons, Columbia University, New York, New York

Kirk W. Brown, PhD, Department of Psychology, University of Rochester, Rochester, New York

Joachim C. Brunstein, PhD, Department of Psychology, University of Giessen, Giessen, Germany

Ruth Butler, PhD, School of Education, Hebrew University of Jerusalem, Jerusalem, Israel

Charles S. Carver, PhD, Department of Psychology, University of Miami, Coral Gables, Florida

Chi-yue Chiu, PhD, Department of Psychology, University of Illinois at Urbana–Champaign, Champaign, Illinois

Mihaly Csikszentmihalyi, PhD, Quality of Life Research Center, Claremont Graduate University, Claremont, California

Edward L. Deci, PhD, Department of Clinical and Social Sciences in Psychology, University of Rochester, Rochester, New York

Joan L. Duda, PhD, School of Sport and Exercise Sciences, University of Birmingham, Edgbaston, Birmingham, United Kingdom

Amanda M. Durik, PhD, Department of Psychology, University of Wisconsin–Madison, Madison, Wisconsin

Carol S. Dweck, PhD, Department of Psychology, Stanford University, Stanford, California

Jacquelynne S. Eccles, PhD, Institute for Research on Women and Gender and Department of Psychology, University of Michigan, Ann Arbor, Michigan

Andrew J. Elliot, PhD, Department of Clinical and Social Sciences in Psychology, University of Rochester, Rochester, New York

Rebecca C. Fauth, PhD, National Center for Children and Families, Teachers College, Columbia University, New York, New York

Peter M. Gollwitzer, PhD, Department of Psychology, New York University, New York, New York

Sandra Graham, PhD, Department of Education, University of California–Los Angeles, Los Angeles, California

Wendy S. Grolnick, PhD, Department of Psychology, Clark University, Worcester, Massachusetts

Meike Hagenah, MA, Department of Psychology, University of Hamburg, Hamburg, Germany

Jutta Heckhausen, PhD, Department of Psychology and Social Behavior, University of California–Irvine, Irvine, California

Ying-yi Hong, PhD, Department of Psychology, University of Illinois at Urbana–Champaign, Champaign, Illinois

Cynthia Hudley, PhD, Department of Education, University of California–Santa Barbara, Santa Barbara, California

Julie Hwang, PhD, Department of Psychology, University of Oregon, Eugene, Oregon

Janet Shibley Hyde, PhD, Department of Psychology, University of Wisconsin–Madison, Madison, Wisconsin

Ruth Kanfer, PhD, School of Psychology, Georgia Institute of Technology, Atlanta, Georgia

Anastasia Kitsantas, PhD, Graduate School of Education, George Mason University, Fairfax, Virginia

Michael Lewis, PhD, Institute for the Study of Child Development, Robert Wood Johnson Medical School, University of Medicine and Dentistry of New Jersey, New Brunswick, New Jersey

Miriam R. Linver, PhD, Department of Human Ecology, Montclair State University, Montclair, New Jersey

Hazel Rose Markus, PhD, Department of Psychology, Stanford University, Stanford, California

Gerald Matthews, PhD, Department of Psychology, University of Cincinnati, Cincinnati, Ohio

Daniel C. Molden, PhD, Department of Psychology, Northwestern University, Evanston, Illinois

Arlen C. Moller, MA, Department of Clinical and Social Sciences in Psychology, University of Rochester, Rochester, New York

Jeanne Nakamura, PhD, Quality of Life Research Center, Claremont Graduate University, Claremont, California

Gabriele Oettingen, PhD, Department of Psychology, New York University, New York, New York, and Department of Psychology, University of Hamburg, Hamburg, Germany

Frank Pajares, PhD, Department of Educational Studies, Emory University, Atlanta, Georgia

Victoria C. Plaut, PhD, Department of Psychology, College of the Holy Cross, Worcester, Massachusetts

Eva M. Pomerantz, PhD, Department of Psychology, University of Illinois at Urbana–Champaign, Champaign, Illinois

Carrie E. Price, MA, Department of Psychology, Clark University, Worcester, Massachusetts

Frederick Rhodewalt, PhD, Department of Psychology, University of Utah, Salt Lake City, Utah

Mary K. Rothbart, PhD, Department of Psychology, University of Oregon, Eugene, Oregon

Mark A. Runco, PhD, Department of Child and Adolescent Studies, California State University–Fullerton, Fullerton, California, and Norwegian School of Economics and Business Administration, Bergen, Norway

Richard M. Ryan, PhD, Department of Psychology, University of Rochester, Rochester, New York

Michael F. Scheier, PhD, Department of Psychology, Carnegie Mellon University, Pittsburgh, Pennsylvania

Oliver C. Schultheiss, PhD, Department of Psychology, University of Michigan, Ann Arbor, Michigan

Dale H. Schunk, PhD, School of Education, University of North Carolina at Greensboro, Greensboro, North Carolina

Claude M. Steele, PhD, Department of Psychology, Stanford University, Stanford, California

Robert J. Sternberg, PhD, Department of Psychology, Yale University, New Haven, Connecticut

Margaret Wolan Sullivan, PhD, Institute for the Study of Child Development, Robert Wood Johnson Medical School, University of Medicine and Dentistry of New Jersey, New Brunswick, New Jersey

Jerry Suls, PhD, Department of Psychology, University of Iowa, Iowa City, Iowa

Julianne C. Turner, PhD, Institute for Educational Initiatives, University of Notre Dame, Notre Dame, Indiana

Tim Urdan, PhD, Department of Psychology, Santa Clara University, Santa Clara, California

Kathleen D. Vohs, PhD, Sauder School of Business, University of British Columbia, Vancouver, British Columbia, Canada

A. Laurel Wagner, BA, Department of Human Development, University of Maryland, College Park, Maryland

Bernard Weiner, PhD, Department of Psychology, University of California–Los Angeles, Los Angeles, California

Kathryn R. Wentzel, PhD, Department of Human Development, University of Maryland, College Park, Maryland

Ladd Wheeler, PhD, Department of Psychology, Macquarie University, Sydney, New South Wales, Australia

Allan Wigfield, PhD, Department of Human Development, University of Maryland, College Park, Maryland

Moshe Zeidner, PhD, Faculty of Education, University of Haifa, Mount Carmel, Haifa, Israel

Barry J. Zimmerman, PhD, Doctoral Program in Educational Psychology, Graduate Center of the City University of New York, New York, New York

Foreword

The *Handbook of Competence and Motivation,* edited by Andrew J. Elliot and Carol S. Dweck, is intended as a comprehensive resource for researchers and theoreticians on the broad topic of achievement motivation. The *Handbook* succeeds admirably in this function. It draws together a wide range of theoretical and empirical topics brought to life by a group of world-renowned contributors. Some topics, such as evaluation anxiety and self-regulated learning, are staples in the achievement motivation tradition, while others, such as government and social policy, although having considerable relevance to this classic literature, have for too long been separated from the mainstream of research. The breadth and reach, as well as the depth of treatment, of all these topics hold special benefits for the reader. The broad encyclopedic nature of the *Handbook* will allow readers easily to place their own particular interests in this field firmly in a neighborhood of related research topics and kindred issues. This will certainly facilitate the kinds of communication among scholars that Elliot and Dweck hope to encourage. Additionally, the depth of treatment within chapters, particularly the way contributors place their observations in the context of historical trends, provides rich, detailed perspectives from which readers can cast up accounts regarding the strides made in this field over the past half century.

However, beyond being an authoritative compendium, the *Handbook* is all the more remarkable for the efforts of Elliot and Dweck to infuse the entire enterprise with a conceptual coherence that they rightly observe has been lacking in the achievement motivation literature. They seek to establish competence as the conceptual core of the achievement motivation literature, arguing that competence is an innate, pancultural, psychological need whose recognition can bring an overall coherence to the achievement-related findings from a diversity of disciplines, including, among others, social–personality psychology, industrial–organizational psychology, educational psychology, sport psychology, and developmental perspectives, all of which are well represented in the *Handbook*.

The contributors, in their turn, have responded exceedingly well to this invitation to view their own work through a conceptual lens of competence. A careful reading of the *Handbook* from this guiding perspective will provide the reader with a strong sense of the potential, evolving benefits of seeking a unifying, conceptual coherence within which to frame the field and an appreciation for the particularly astute choice of competence as the rallying point. This evaluation is based on several observations.

First, the notion of competence provides the basis for a rapprochement between the need-based traditions of achievement motivation, arising from the earlier work of Atkinson and McClelland a half century ago, and contemporary achievement goal work, with its roots in a cognitive tradition. From a competence perspective, goals can be profitably viewed as conscious, social, and cognitively derived manifestations of underlying needs. Goals organize, control, and direct actions, particularly when they are linked to the satisfaction of basic needs—in this case, according to Elliot and Dweck, the desire to experience competence and to avoid experiencing incompetence.

As these competence needs become thwarted and one's goals lapse into an avoidance mode, hopelessness and despair result. The adaptive, clinical, and medical implications of these dynamics are taken up by many of the contributors, who explore the potential linkages between successful and unsuccessful efforts at competence maintenance and feelings of well-being and illness, respectively. As a group, these investigators point to the unifying value of competence concerns as a powerful mediator of a range of adaptive and maladaptive responses to life stresses, as well as to the higher order values of creativity and intrinsic engagement.

Second, the study of self-reference processes has long remained at the periphery of research on achievement motivation. However, the enormous potential contributions of the study of self-processes to our understanding of achievement dynamics become illuminated by the operation of competence needs. For example, self-presentational concerns are likely triggered by the perennial struggle to maintain a sense of competence and evade feelings of incompetence. The contributors to the *Handbook* make clear that self-referent cognitions are not solely activated by rational, information-seeking considerations, but also serve the higher-order need of attaining acceptance of self as a competent person. In short, the *Handbook*, with its focus on competence concerns, lays the foundation for a rapprochement between the cognitive, rational world of the individual and one's self-protective, defensive tendencies.

Third, this elevation of competence underscores the critical role played by social and cultural factors in achievement dynamics. Indeed, contributors make the compelling case that competence is best defined in group contexts, and that any expression of competence is largely a social event. For example, academic competence in individuals is typically judged by making peer comparisons of performance, and a reputation for social competence is gained through behaving cooperatively and respecting group norms. Of particular interest here is the question of how social needs and goals enter into the achievement process. It is at this interface between social and intellectual competence that contributors have properly focused study, both for the sake of improving school and classroom performance, and as a window through which researchers can study the composition and effects of multiple-goal patterns.

At the same time, these contributors have made clear that contemporary thinking has moved well beyond earlier missteps in which investigators tended to equate cultural differences in achievement motivation with deficits. It is clear that new, better perspectives are unfolding, thanks in part to a renewed consideration of notions of competence, and the different ways it is construed and how its meaning is defined across a variety of cultures.

Fourth, by rallying around the topic of competence, investigators will gain a renewed appreciation for the influential role that contextual factors play in achievement dynamics, as the contributors have discovered. The rules that govern what counts as successful and failing performances in a given context also determine perceptions of competence and incompetence, with enormous motivational implications for one's willingness to continue learning. Of special interest here is the variety of contextual rules for defining competence that now beckons study (beyond the traditional distinctions of norm-based and criterion- or mastery-based rules), in particular, investigating the nature of competence-based mechanisms that operate in the pursuit of personal interests, pastimes, and hobbies. Personal interests are not simply the product of performing well at something, but of defining competence in terms of surpassing one's own idiosyncratic standards of excellence that may remain private yet nonetheless compelling. Focusing on competence invites inquiries in as yet understudied but promising areas, including the playful discovery of one's hidden talents and the motivational benefits of picking and choosing different ways of pursuing whatever invites one's attention.

For all these many reasons the *Handbook* represents a signal contribution to the field of achievement motivation, particularly in its potential for organizing thinking around competence as a common focus, or as Elliot and Dweck put it, "a conceptual North Star to help theorists navigate the achievement motivation universe."

MARTIN V. COVINGTON, PhD
University of California–Berkeley

Contents

PART I. INTRODUCTION

PART II. CENTRAL CONSTRUCTS

PART V. DEMOGRAPHICS AND CULTURE

PART VI. SELF-REGULATORY PROCESSES

PART I

❧

Introduction

CHAPTER 1

∝

Competence and Motivation

Competence as the Core of Achievement Motivation

ANDREW J. ELLIOT
CAROL S. DWECK

Why is this volume not entitled *Handbook of Achievement and Motivation* or *Handbook of Achievement Motivation*? The reason is that we are taking the occasion of this *Handbook* to propose a refocusing of the achievement motivation literature around the concept of "competence." As we describe below, our aim in doing so is to bring greater clarity and precision to the field, while emphasizing its great reach and potential to integrate important areas of psychology.

Research on achievement and motivation has a long and distinguished history. In fact, achievement motivation concepts were present at the dawn of psychology as a scientific discipline, when James (1890) offered speculation about how achievement strivings are linked to self-evaluation. Soon thereafter, an assortment of research studies appeared that focused on achievement-relevant issues such as the effect of intentions on perseverance (Ach, 1910) and the effect of increasing difficulty on task per-

formance (Hillgruber, 1912). However, truly programmatic empirical work on achievement motivation began in Kurt Lewin's laboratory with the investigation of aspiration-setting behavior (Hoppe, 1930; see Frank, 1941, for a review of this research program), and formal models of achievement motivation have been present since Lewin and colleagues (Escalona, 1940; Festinger, 1942; Lewin, Dembo, Festinger, & Sears, 1944) proposed their theory of "resultant valence" to account for aspiration processes. A decade later, the central place of research on achievement motivation in scientific psychology was solidified by McClelland, Atkinson, and colleagues' work on need for achievement (Atkinson, 1957; McClelland, Atkinson, Clark, & Lowell, 1953; McClelland, Clark, Roby, & Atkinson, 1949). From this time onward, the collective corpus of research on achievement and motivation has been referred to as "the achievement motivation literature."

An enormous amount of research has followed these seminal speculations, empirical investigations, and theoretical frameworks. Over the years, researchers have devised and tested models incorporating a variety of different constructs, such as motive dispositions, attributions, evaluation anxiety, goals, competence perceptions, values, and implicit theories. These efforts have contributed a great deal to our understanding of the nature of achievement motivation. Importantly, many working in the achievement motivation literature have applied the knowledge acquired from these efforts to real-world achievement settings, and innumerable students, employees, ballplayers, and others have benefited as a result.

Clearly, there is much to praise about the contributions of the achievement motivation literature. However, we believe that the literature has important weaknesses that limit its utility and breadth of influence. In this chapter, we articulate the nature of these weaknesses and propose that placing competence at the core of the achievement motivation literature directly addresses them.

WEAKNESSES OF THE ACHIEVEMENT MOTIVATION LITERATURE

The concept of "achievement" is not clearly defined in the achievement motivation literature. That is, there is no broadly articulated, consensually shared understanding of how "achievement" should be conceptualized. We believe that this definitional–conceptual issue lies at the root of two fundamental weaknesses of the literature.

A first weakness of the achievement motivation literature is that it lacks coherence and a clear set of structural parameters. If the precise nature of "achievement" is not clear, then the precise nature of what should and should not be included under the "achievement motivation" rubric will be unclear as well. Indeed, although psychologists across a diversity of disciplines recognize the existence of a body of research called "the achievement motivation literature," we suspect that few would be able to articulate the specific contents of this literature. This lack of coherence and clear parameters has negative implications for both empirical efforts and theory development.

On the empirical front, it is difficult to know how constructs should be operationalized without clear conceptual guidance. Any given empirical investigation may provide specific construct definitions and matching operationalizations, but these definitions and operationalizations are likely to vary considerably across investigators and investigations. The result is a cumulative body of studies that may be easy to interpret individually but are difficult to interpret as a whole. Likewise, on the theoretical front, it is difficult to build theoretical models when a solid conceptual foundation is not in place. Without such a foundation, devising a blueprint for how to fully cover the conceptual space under consideration without incorporating additional, superfluous constructs or relationships (i.e., establishing a parsimonious theoretical framework) is near impossible.

A second weakness of the achievement motivation literature is that it is too narrowly focused and limited in scope, particularly relative to its potential. Given the absence of a precise definition of "achievement" in the literature, researchers likely rely on intuition or a generic, lay understanding of the term "achievement" to guide their empirical and theoretical efforts. For example, most research in the achievement motivation literature has emerged from Western, individualistic societies that tend to conceive of achievement in terms of individual, self-defining accomplishment in the prototypical domains of school, sports, and work. As a result, more often than not, research in the achievement motivation literature has focused on individual, self-defining accomplishment in the domains of school, sports, and work.

However, "achievement" and "achievement motivation" may be conceptualized in a much broader fashion than this suggests. Interdependent achievement striving (see Fuligni, 1997; Maehr & Nicholls, 1980), cooperative achievement striving (Johnson & Johnson, 1989; Parsons & Goff, 1980), and striving for learning and task mastery (see Dweck & Elliott, 1983; Nicholls, 1984) would all seem to warrant full consideration as manifestations of achievement motivation; only the latter has begun to receive significant attention in the past several years. Furthermore, achievement motivation appears to be operative in many areas of daily life beyond the classroom, the ballfield, and the workplace. The avocational gardener seeking to grow an excellent tomato would seem to be striving for achievement, as would the infant struggling to put a peg in a hole, the adolescent trying to become a better conversationalist, and the adult committed to becoming the best parent possible. From this broader perspective, the achievement motivation literature seems applicable to many other established research literatures. Issues regarding achievement motivation pertain to research on flow, creativity, cognitive strategies, self-regulated learning, coping and disengagement, and social comparison, to name but a few important domains of inquiry. Yet given the rather narrow way that achievement has been construed, there exists little integration between the achievement motivation literature and these other bodies of work. As such, the achievement motivation literature remains relatively isolated and, we believe, is not being applied to its full potential. The landmark research on need for achievement by McClelland et al. (1953) may be used to illustrate these points.

McClelland, Atkinson, and colleagues created their need for achievement measure empirically, without a precise conceptual definition of achievement motivation to guide their efforts. Briefly, they experimentally aroused achievement motivation in some subjects but not others, and then had these subjects write stories to pictures. Any differential story content between the two groups was presumed to be indicative of achievement motivation, and the need for achievement scoring system was devised accordingly. Importantly, the subjects used in this research were predominantly male ex-GIs, whose achievement motivation was aroused by informing them that they would be administered a test of intelligence used in the selection of government and military leaders. Thus, the method of achievement arousal utilized was based on the researchers' intuitive, culturally based understanding of achievement motivation, and one may question whether these procedures, as well as the type of subjects used in the research, yielded a tool that is broadly applicable across persons and achievement situations. Furthermore, at the same time that the need for achievement construct was being estab-

lished, White (1959, 1960) offered his analysis of effectance motivation. White posited a fundamental need for individuals to be effective in negotiating their environment, the prototypical manifestation of which is the infant's curiosity and exploratory play. Although need for achievement and effectance motivation would seem to be conceptually related, the pioneers of the two constructs made almost no reference to the work of the other, and subsequent proponents of the two traditions have followed suit. To this day, although the need for achievement construct is considered a central part of the achievement motivation literature, effectance motivation is rarely mentioned (for exceptions, see Elliot & Reis, 2003; Nicholls, 1984; Veroff, 1969). The achievement motivation literature (and for that matter, research on effectance motivation) is less rich as a result.

In summary, the absence of a clear definition of "achievement" has led to some important weaknesses in the achievement motivation literature. The literature lacks coherence and a clear set of structural parameters, and the literature is too narrowly focused and limited in scope. In essence, what is commonly referred to as the "achievement motivation literature" represents a rather loose compendium of theoretical and empirical work focused on a colloquial understanding of the term "achievement." We suggest that for the achievement motivation literature to flourish, it is important to delineate its conceptual core carefully and precisely. We seek to do so by proposing that competence be considered the conceptual core of the achievement motivation literature.

COMPETENCE AND MOTIVATION

Based on *Webster's Revised Unabridged Dictionary* and the *Oxford English Dictionary*, "competence" may be defined as a condition or quality of effectiveness, ability, sufficiency, or success. Once this definition is embraced, many questions come into focus: How is competence evaluated? To what levels of action and domains of endeavor does competence apply? How are individuals motivated with regard to competence?

Competence may be evaluated in several different ways: People may use an absolute standard inherent in a task, an interpersonal standard implicating change over time, or an interpersonal standard implicating normative comparison. The way in which competence is evaluated influences the psychological meaning that competence has and the form that competence-relevant strivings take in any given situation. Competence is applicable across a broad range of levels, from concrete actions (e.g., putting a peg in a hole) to specific outcomes (e.g., a grade on a test) to identifiable patterns of skill and ability (e.g., piano playing) to overarching characteristics (e.g., intelligence) to omnibus compilations (e.g., a life).

A motivational analysis of competence must account for the ways in which individuals' behavior is energized (instigated, activated) and directed (focused, aimed). Our analysis of the *energization* of competence-relevant behavior is grounded in the premise that competence is an inherent psychological need of the human being. That is, in keeping with several theorists (Deci & Ryan, 1990; Dweck & Elliott, 1983; Elliot, McGregor, & Thrash, 2002; Skinner, 1995; see also White, 1959), we view the need for competence as a fundamental motivation that serves the evolutionary role of helping people develop and adapt to their environment.[1] This need for competence instigates and activates behavior that is oriented toward competence. Over time, individuals learn to *direct* this general motivational energy using concrete, cognitively based goals and strategies; that is, people learn to use self-regulatory tools to channel their general desire for competence toward specific outcomes and experiences that satisfy the competence need (Elliot & Church, 1997, 2002).

Importantly, competence-relevant behavior is not only motivated by the positive, appetitive possibility of competence but is also motivated by the negative, aversive possibility of incompetence. The need for competence may initially be a thoroughly appetitive motivational source that orients infants toward positive competence-relevant possibilities, but a variety of factors (e.g., temperament, socialization, experience) may reorient this natural appetitive orientation toward the avoidance of negative competence-relevant outcomes. Consequently, people may develop a general desire to avoid in-

competence and may adopt goals or strategies focused on avoiding negative possibilities in competence-relevant settings. These aversive forms of motivation may serve a self-protective function, but they may often do a poor job of providing the individual with the positive competence outcomes and experiences required for continued growth and development. As such, some competence-relevant desires and pursuits may be ineffective at facilitating, or may even interfere with, the long-term growth of competence.

We consider this distinction between approach (i.e., appetitive) and avoidance (i.e., aversive) motivation to be integral to a motivational analysis of competence (much as it has been integral to the motivational analysis of achievement per se; see Atkinson, 1957; Elliot, 1999; Hoppe, 1930; Lewin et al., 1944; McClelland et al., 1953; Weiner, 1972). Using a dictionary, "competence" may be defined in purely appetitive fashion with regard to effectiveness, ability, sufficiency, and success, but from a *motivational* standpoint, the study of competence-relevant motivation will necessarily entail consideration of ineffectiveness, inability, insufficiency, and failure as well.

WHY COMPETENCE?

Our primary contention, then, is that "achievement" in the achievement motivation literature is best viewed through the lens of competence. That is, we propose that "achievement" be conceptualized in terms of "competence," and that "achievement motivation" be characterized as "competence motivation." Competence seems an ideal core for the achievement motivation literature, because competence at once has a precise meaning and is a rich and profound psychological concept. This richness and profundity is in bold relief as one considers the central role of competence motivation in human functioning. Competence motivation is ubiquitous in daily life, it has a substantial impact on emotion and well-being, it is operative across the lifespan, and it is evident in all individuals across cultural boundaries. We elaborate on these points in the following paragraphs.

First, competence motivation is ubiquitous in daily life. Whether individuals are conscious of it or not, much of their everyday behavior is energized or directed by the possibility of competence or incompetence. Competence-relevant desires, investments, and strivings are present in mundane actions (e.g., trying to do a good job of brushing one's teeth), as well as more grand pursuits (e.g., trying to become a world-class athlete). They are present in the social domain (e.g., working to improve one's conversational skills), as well as the achievement domain (e.g., striving to do well on an exam). They are present in internally focused pursuits (e.g., seeking discipline and clarity in one's mental life), as well as public demonstrations (e.g., wanting to give an outstanding speech). Anywhere in which competence evaluation energizes or directs behavior (either appetitively or aversively), competence motivation is operative.

Second, competence motivation has a substantial impact on emotion and well-being. The affective reactions people have in response to positive and negative outcomes in competence-relevant settings clearly reflect an investment in attaining competence and avoiding incompetence. Not surprisingly, positive outcomes typically lead to affects such as joy, pride, and happiness, whereas negative outcomes lead to affects such as sadness, shame, and anxiety (Heckhausen, 1984; Lewis, Alessandri, & Sullivan, 1992; Stipek, Recchia, & McClintic, 1992). Researchers have also demonstrated that the precise nature of affective experience following positive or negative outcomes can vary as a function of approach and avoidance motivation. Approach-oriented, positive outcomes produce joy and pride, whereas avoidance-oriented, positive outcomes produce relief. Approach-oriented negative outcomes tend to produce sadness and disappointment, whereas avoidance-oriented negative outcomes tend to produce shame and distress (Higgins, Shah, & Friedman, 1997; Roseman, 1991; Stein & Levine, 1989; see also Carver & Scheier, 1998; Mowrer, 1960). The approach–avoidance nature of competence motivation has implications for overall well-being as well. For example, research has shown that the pursuit of avoidance (relative to approach)

goals leads to a decrease in life satisfaction and physical health over time (Elliot & McGregor, 2001; Elliot & Sheldon, 1997), because avoidance goals are not as effective at providing people with the competence experiences they need for continued growth and development (Elliot & Sheldon, 1998; Elliot, Sheldon, & Church, 1997).

Third, competence motivation is operative across the lifespan. It is clearly manifested differently at different ages. The initial manifestation of competence motivation, effectance motivation (White, 1959), is presumed to be present at birth; it is an appetitive desire to explore and master the environment, reflected in the infant's natural tendency toward curiosity and exploratory play. As children acquire greater representational capacities, encounter an array of socialization experiences, and are marked by positive and negative competence-relevant events, this rudimentary form of motivation develops and differentiates (See Dweck, 2002; Elliot et al., 2002). Specifically, children begin to use different standards for evaluating competence; they begin to represent competence at higher levels of abstraction, and they begin to focus on avoiding incompetence as well as on approaching competence. This process of differentiation continues into adulthood, and competence motivation often becomes increasingly intertwined with other motivational concerns commonly activated in competence-relevant settings (e.g., self-presentation concerns, affiliative concerns, self-worth concerns). In the elderly, diminishing opportunities to exercise their competencies, along with a gradual decline in their skills and abilities, may prompt a modest decline in competence motivation (Veroff, Depner, Kukla, & Douvan, 1980; or, more precisely, may increase competence-relevant motivation focused on the avoidance of incompetence, Elliot & McGregor, 2001). Nevertheless, competence motivation remains important, and competence outcomes continue to impact emotion and well-being deep into old age (Geppert & Halisch, 2001; Halisch & Geppert, 2001). Indeed, successful old age may be a function of finding newer and more appropriate competence-relevant goals to pursue. Thus, the intensity and extent of competence motivation, its specific manifestations, and the typical settings in which it is operative may change considerably over time, but a desire for competence and an investment in competence-relevant strivings remains invariant from infancy to old age (Brim, 1990; Heckhausen & Schultz, 1995).

Fourth, competence motivation is evident in all individuals across cultural boundaries. Much as competence motivation may be manifested differently at different ages, this motivation may take on different appearances in different cultures. For example, relative to the competence motivation of persons from Western cultures (e.g., Canada, the United States, Western Europe), those from Eastern cultures (e.g., China, Japan, South Korea) appears to be more group- and socially oriented (Chang, Wong, & Teo, 2000), more grounded in obligation and responsibility (Fuligni, Tseng, & Lam, 1999), more avoidance-oriented (Eaton & Dembo, 1999), and more focused on improvement (Heine et al., 2001). Furthermore, studies show that competence-relevant words such as "success," "failure," and "learn" have different connotations in different countries (Li, 2003; Maehr & Nicholls, 1980). We contend that underlying the different meanings and manifestations of competence motivation in different cultures lies a similar desire for and commitment to competence (see also Bandura, 2001; for a conceptual parallel with regard to positive self-regard, see Heine, Lehman, Markus, & Kitayama, 1999). Indeed, data indicate that competence is an important concept that is highly valued by individuals across a wide diversity of cultures (Li, 2003; Van de Vliert & Janssen, 2002), and that competence-relevant outcomes strongly influence emotion and well-being across cultures (Sheldon, Elliot, Kim, & Kasser, 2001).

In summary, we contend that competence is a construct optimally suited to serves as the conceptual core in the achievement motivation literature. Competence can be seen as a basic psychological need that has a pervasive impact on daily affect, cognition, and behavior, across age and culture. As such, competence would seem to represent not only an ideal cornerstone on which to rest the achievement motivation literature but also a foundational building block for any theory of personality, development, and well-being.

ADDRESSING THE WEAKNESSES OF THE ACHIEVEMENT MOTIVATION LITERATURE

It should now be clear how grounding the achievement motivation literature in the competence construct addresses the weaknesses of the literature. The first weakness of the achievement motivation literature that we identified is that it lacks coherence and a clear set of structural parameters. Because competence can be defined in a precise fashion, it provides a clear criterion for what should and should not be considered a part of the achievement motivation literature, and thus provides much needed guidelines for empirical and theoretical work. Empirically, grounding achievement motivation research in competence provides a benchmark for how constructs should be operationalized: They should focus on competence as directly as possible. The result is likely to be a sharpening and increased uniformity of manipulations and measures that will likely produce more comparable results that are easier to interpret. Theoretically, grounding achievement motivation models in competence provides an orienting point, a conceptual North Star to help theorists navigate the achievement motivation universe. The result is likely to be more parsimonious theoretical frameworks that allow the literature to progress more straightforwardly and rapidly.

The second weakness of the achievement motivation literature that we identified earlier is that it is too narrowly focused and limited in scope. Although competence may be defined in precise fashion, it is nevertheless a highly inclusive concept that is much more widely applicable than a colloquially based understanding of "achievement." Establishing competence as the central focus of the literature makes evident the links between standard achievement motivation foci and other explicitly competence-based constructs such as social competence (Masten & Coatsworth, 1998), emotional competence (Cherniss, 2001), cognitive competence (Bertrand, Willis, & Sayer, 2001), health competence (Marks & Lutgendorf, 1999), cultural competence (Chin, 2002), and moral competence (Haight, 2000). Links to other constructs (and, accordingly, literatures) that are grounded in competence, such as the control construct (Skinner, 1995), the power construct (Halisch & Geppert, 2001), the agency construct (Bakan, 1966), and the cognitive mastery construct (Kelley, 1967), also become clear. Indeed, many of the most central topics in the psychological literature, such as the self-concept and self-esteem, have competence at their core (Harter, 1999; James, 1890; Tafarodi & Swann, 2001), and issues regarding competence and competence motivation are often at the heart of cross-cultural and lifespan analyses of behavior. Thus, placing competence at the center of the achievement motivation literature expands its conceptual reach considerably and forges integrative links among domains of inquiry.

In summary, grounding the achievement motivation literature in competence addresses both of the weaknesses of the achievement motivation literature that we have identified. Although the provision of *any* precise definition of "achievement" would be a welcome addition to the literature, using competence as this definition is particularly appealing given its clarity and flexibility as a construct, and its broad and integrative reach. It is our hope that, over time, the term "competence motivation" will take the place of the term "achievement motivation," and that a host of both established and upcoming researchers will join us under this conceptual umbrella.

OVERVIEW OF THE *HANDBOOK OF COMPETENCE AND MOTIVATION*

It was in this spirit that we conceived the present volume. We approached scholars who have made enduring contributions to the achievement motivation literature and asked them to think about their work in terms of competence. We also brought in people who might not typically identify with the field of achievement or achievement motivation but who would resonate to the concept of competence, and we asked them to cast their area of expertise in terms of competence.

Specifically, we gave our authors the charge of bringing their area of inquiry under the umbrella of the competence construct by rethinking their basic concepts and processes in terms of competence. The first section of the volume focuses on the central constructs in the achievement motivation literature: intelligence and ability (competence itself); competence-relevant motives and goals, which shape people's competence-based strivings; the perceived causes of competence (and incompetence) and the consequences of perceived competence; the different ways in which people value competence; people's conceptions of competence and its role in motivation; and competence-relevant anxiety, an emotion that affects what people strive for and how successfully (or unsuccessfully) they do so.

Next come developmental issues. How does temperament shape competence and competence motivation? How does the development of self-conscious emotions and cognitive abilities influence competence motivation? And how do competence and competence motivation change over the lifespan? These issues are fundamental to our understanding of competence-relevant processes.

Questions of development continue as the focus turns to the impact of socialization agents and contexts. What are the roles of parents, peers, teachers, and coaches? What about schools and workplaces? How do government policies, such as high-stakes testing, affect the desire for and the acquisition of competence?

The issue of socialization and contexts is carried further as the next chapters consider the role of gender, race/ethnicity, and socioeconomic status in competence motivation. Here, the impact of stereotypes comes to the fore, as do questions regarding the critical role of culture in competence—in what it means, how it is gained, and how it is displayed.

The final section explores different facets of self-regulation. Self-regulatory processes may be seen as the means through which people pursue and attain competence, and they may also be seen as competencies in and of themselves. The chapters focus on various forms of self-regulation, such as self-regulated learning, coping, cognitive strategies, and social comparison. They examine motivational states that foster competence processes, such as intrinsic motivation, flow, and creativity. Finally, they examine conscious and deliberate self-regulation and powerful automatic processes that take place outside of awareness.

We are delighted by the many fresh and fascinating insights that our authors generated as they considered their work from the perspective of competence. We hope that our readers will find these chapters as original, thought-provoking, and enlightening as we do.

ACKNOWLEDGMENTS

Preparation of this chapter was facilitated by a grant from the William T. Grant Foundation (Grant No. 2565) and a Friedrich Wilhelm Bessel Research Award from the Alexander von Humboldt Foundation to Andrew J. Elliot, and grants from the National Science Foundation (Grant No. BCS-02-17251), the Department of Education (Grant No. R305-H-02-0031), and the William T. Grant Foundation (Grant No. 2379) to Carol S. Dweck

NOTE

1. Positing the existence of basic psychological needs such as competence or belongingness (see Baumeister & Leary, 1995) was once highly controversial (and, for some, continues to be so), but in the past few years, it has become much more widely accepted. Space considerations preclude us from reviewing the evidence supporting competence as a basic psychological need; we refer the interested reader to Deci and Ryan (1990) and Elliot et al. (2002).

REFERENCES

Ach, N. (1910). *Uber den willensakt und das temperament*. Leipzig: Quelle & Meyer.

Atkinson, J. W. (1957). Motivational determinants of risk-taking behavior. *Psychological Review, 64*, 359–372.

Bakan, D. (1966). *The duality of human existence: Isolation and communion in Western man*. Boston: Beacon Press.

Bandura, A. (2001). Social cognitive theory: An agentic perspective. *Annual Review of Psychology, 52*, 1–26.

Baumeister, R. F., & Leary, M. R. (1995). The need to belong: Desire for interpersonal attachments as a fundamental human motivation. *Psychological Bulletin, 117*, 497–529.

Bertrand, R. M., Willis, S. L., & Sayer, A. (2001). An evaluation of change over time in everyday cognitive competence among Alzheimer's patients. *Aging Neuropsychology and Cognition, 8*, 192–212.

Brim, O. G. (1990). *Ambition: How we manage success and failure throughout our lives*. New York: Basic Books.

Carver, C., & Scheier, M. (1998). *On the self-regulation of behavior*. New York: Cambridge University Press.

Chang, W., Wong, W., & Teo, G. (2000). The socially oriented and individually oriented achievement motivation of Singaporean and Chinese students. *Journal of Psychology in Chinese Societies, 1*, 39–63.

Cherniss, C. (2001). Social and emotional competence in the workplace. In R. Bar-on & J. Parker (Eds.), *The handbook of emotional intelligence: Theory, development, assessment, and applications at home, school, and in the workplace* (pp. 433–458). San Francisco: Jossey-Bass.

Chin, J. L. (2002). Assessment of cultural competence in mental health systems of care for Asian Americans. In K. Kurasaki & S. O. Kazaki (Eds.), *Asian American mental health: Assessment theories and methods* (pp. 301–314). New York: Kluwer Academic.

Deci, E., & Ryan, R. (1990). A motivational approach to the self: Integration in personality. In R. Dienstbier (Ed.), *Nebraska Symposium on Motivation* (Vol. 38, pp. 237–288). Lincoln: University of Nebraska Press.

Dweck, C. S. (2002). The development of ability conceptions. In A. Wigfield & J. Eccles (Eds.), *Development of achievement motivation* (pp. 57–88). San Diego: Academic Press.

Dweck, C. S., & Elliott, E. (1983). Achievement motivation. In E. Heatherington (Ed.), *Handbook of child psychology* (Vol. 4, pp. 643–691). New York: Wiley.

Eaton, M. J., & Dembo, M. H. (1999). Differences in the motivational beliefs of Asian and American and non-Asian students. *Journal of Educational Psychology, 89*, 433–440.

Elliot, A. J. (1999). Approach and avoidance motivation and achievement goals. *Educational Psychologist, 34*, 169–189.

Elliot, A. J., & Church, M. A. (1997). A hierarchical model of approach and avoidance achievement motivation. *Journal of Personality and Social Psychology, 72*, 218–232.

Elliot, A. J., & Church, M. A. (2002). Client-articulated avoidance goals in the therapy context. *Journal of Counseling Psychology, 49*, 243–254.

Elliot A. J., & McGregor, H. A. (2001). A 2 × 2 achievement goal framework. *Journal of Personality and Social Psychology, 80*, 501–519.

Elliot, A. J., McGregor, H. A., & Thrash, T. M. (2002). The need for competence. In E. Deci & R. Ryan (Eds.), *Handbook of self-determination theory* (pp. 361–387). Rochester, NY: University of Rochester Press.

Elliot, A. J., & Reis, H. (2003). Attachment and adult exploration. *Journal of Personality and Social Psychology, 85*, 317–331.

Elliot, A. J., & Sheldon, K. M. (1997). Avoidance achievement motivation: A personal goals analysis.

Journal of Personality and Social Psychology, 73, 171–185.

Elliot, A. J., & Sheldon, K. M. (1998). Avoidance personal goals and the personality–illness relationship. *Journal of Personality and Social Psychology, 75,* 1282–1299.

Elliot, A. J., Sheldon, K. M., & Church, M. A. (1997). Avoidance personal goals and subjective well-being. *Personality and Social Psychological Bulletin, 23,* 915–927.

Escalona, S. K. (1940). The effect of success and failure upon the level of aspiration and behavior in manic–depressive psychoses. *University of Iowa, Studies in Child Welfare, 16,* 199–302.

Festinger, L. (1942). A theoretical interpretation of shifts in level of aspiration. *Psychological Review, 49,* 235–250.

Frank, J. D. (1941). Recent studies of the level of aspiration. *Psychological Bulletin, 38,* 218–225.

Fuligni, A. J. (1997). The academic achievement of adolescents from immigrant families: The roles of family background, attitudes, and behavior. *Child Development, 68,* 351–363.

Fuligni, A. J., Tseng, V., & Lam, M. (1999). Attitudes toward family obligations among American adolescents with Asian, Latin American, and European backgrounds. *Child Development, 70,* 1030–1044.

Geppert, U., & Halisch, F. (2001). Genetic vs. environmental determinants of traits, motives, self-referential cognitions, and volitional control in old age. In A. Efklides, J. Kuhl, & R. Sorrentino (Eds.), *Trends and prospects in motivational research* (pp. 359–387). Dordrecht: Kluwer.

Haight, W. L. (2000). Moral development in context. *Human Development, 43,* 157–160.

Halisch, F., & Geppert, U. (2001). Motives, personal goals, and life satisfaction in old age. In A. Efklides, J. Kuhl, & R. Sorrentino (Eds.), *Trends and prospects in motivational research* (pp. 389–409). Dordrecht: Kluwer.

Harter, S. (1999). *The construction of the self: A developmental perspective.* New York: Guilford Press.

Heckhausen, H. (1984). Emergent achievement behavior: Some early developments. In J. Nicholls (Ed.), *Advances in achievement motivation* (pp. 1–32). Greenwich, CT: JAI Press.

Heckhausen, J., & Schultz, R. (1995). A life-span theory of control. *Psychological Review, 102,* 289–304.

Heine, S. J., Kitayama, S., Lehman, D. R., Takata, T., Ide, E., Leung, C., et al. (2001). Divergent consequences of success and failure in Japan and North America: An investigation of self-improving motivations and malleable selves. *Journal of Personality and Social Psychology, 81,* 599–615.

Heine, S. J., Lehman, D. R., Markus, H. R., & Kitayama, S. (1999). Is there a universal need for positive self-regard? *Psychological Review, 106,* 766–794.

Higgins, E. T., Shah, J., & Friedman, R. (1997). Emotional responses to goal attainment: Strength of regulatory focus as a moderator. *Journal of Personality and Social Psychology, 66,* 276–286.

Hillgruber, A. (1912). Fortlaufende Arbeit und Willensbetatigung. *Untersuchungen zur Psychologie und Philosophie, 1,* 6.

Hoppe, F. (1930). Untersuchungen zur Handlungs— und Affektpsychologie IV. *Psychologiche Forschung, 14,* 1–63.

James, W. (1890). *The principles of psychology* (Vol. I). New York: Holt.

Johnson, D. W., & Johnson, R. T. (1989). *Cooperation and competition: Theory and research.* Edina, MN: Interactive.

Kelley, H. H. (1967). Attribution theory in social psychology. In D. Levine (Ed.), *Nebraska Symposium on Motivation* (Vol. 15, pp. 192–237). Lincoln: University of Nebraska Press.

Lewin, K. Dembo, T., Festinger, L., & Sears, P. S. (1944). Level of aspiration. In J. McV. Hunt (Ed.), *Personality and the behavior disorders* (pp. 333–378). New York: Ronald.

Lewis, M., Alessandri, S., & Sullivan, M. W. (1992). Differences in shame and pride as a function of gender and task difficulty. *Child Development, 63,* 630–638.

Li, J. (2003). U.S. and Chinese cultural beliefs about learning. *Journal of Educational Psychology, 95,* 258–267.

Maehr, M. L., & Nicholls, J. G. (1980). Culture and achievement motivation: A second look. In J. Warren (Ed.), *Studies in cross-cultural context* (pp. 221–267). New York: Academic Press.

Marks, G. R., & Lutgendorf, S. K. (1999). Perceived health competence and personality factors differentially predict health behaviors in older adults. *Journal of Aging and Health, 11,* 221–239.

Masten, A. S., & Coatsworth, J. D. (1998). The development of competence in favorable and unfavorable environments: Lessons from research on successful children. *American Psychologist, 53,* 205–220.

McClelland, D. C., Atkinson, J. W., Clark, R. A., & Lowell, E. L. (1953). *The achievement motive.* New York: Appleton–Century–Crofts.

McClelland, D. C., Clark, R. A., Roby, R. A., & Atkinson, J. W. (1949). The projective expression of needs: The effect of the need for achievement on thematic apperceptions. *Journal of Experimental Psychology, 39,* 242–255.

Mowrer, O. H. (1960). *Learning theory and behavior.* New York: Wiley.

Nicholls, J. G. (1984). Achievement motivation: Conceptions of ability, subjective experience, task choice, and performance. *Psychological Review, 91,* 328–346.

Parsons, J. E., & Goff, S. B. (1980). Achievement motivation and values: An alternative perspective. In L. Fyans (Ed.), *Achievement motivation: Recent trends in theory and research* (pp. 349–373). New York: Plenum Press.

Roseman, I. J. (1991). Appraisal dimensions of discrete emotions. *Cognition and Emotion*, *5*, 161–200.

Sheldon, K. M., Elliot, A. J., Kim, Y., & Kasser, T. (2001). What is satisfying about satisfying events?: Testing 10 candidate psychological needs. *Journal of Personality and Social Psychology*, *80*, 325–339.

Skinner, E. A. (1995). *Perceived control, motivation, and coping*. Thousand Oaks, CA: Sage.

Stein, N. L., & Levine, L. (1989). The causal organization of emotional knowledge: A developmental study. *Cognition and Emotion*, *3*, 343–378.

Stipek, D. J., Recchia, S., & McClintic, S. (1992). Self-evaluation in young children. *Monographs of the Society for Research in Child Development*, *57*(1, Serial No. 226).

Tafarodi, R. W., & Swann, W. B., Jr. (2001). Two-dimensional self-esteem: Theory and measurement. *Personality and Individual Differences*, *31*, 653–673.

Van de Vliert, E., & Janssen, O. (2002). "Better than" performance motives as roots of satisfaction across more and less developed countries. *Journal of Cross-Cultural Psychology*, *33*, 380–397.

Veroff, J. (1969). Social comparison and the development of achievement motivation. In C. Smith (Ed.), *Achievement-related motives in children* (pp. 46–100). New York: Russell Sage Foundation.

Veroff, J., Depner, C., Kukla, A., & Douvan, E. (1980). Comparison of American motives: 1957 versus 1976. *Journal of Personality and Social Psychology*, *39*, 1249–1262.

Weiner, B. (1972). *Theories of motivation: From mechanism to cognition*. Chicago: Markham.

White, R. W. (1959). Motivation reconsidered: The concept of competence. *Psychological Review*, *66*, 297–333.

White, R. W. (1960). Competence and the psychosexual stages of development. In M. R. Jones (Ed.), *Nebraska Symposium on Motivation* (pp. 97–140). Lincoln: University of Nebraska Press.

PART II

☙

Central Constructs

CHAPTER 2

∽

Intelligence, Competence, and Expertise

ROBERT J. STERNBERG

For roughly 100 years, psychologists have been administering tests of intelligence. These tests are supposed to measure a construct that is (1) unified (so-called *general intelligence*), (2) relatively fixed by genetic endowment, and (3) distinct from and precedent to the competencies that schools develop (see, e.g., Carroll, 1993). All three of these assumptions are questioned in this chapter.

An alternative view, consistent with the topic of "competence" highlighted in this volume, is that intelligence represents a set of competencies in development, and that these competencies in turn represent expertise in development. Thus, intelligence tests measure developing competencies on the way toward developing expertise. Rather than intelligence (and other sets of abilities), competencies, and expertise being viewed as relatively distinct, as they tend to be in the literature of cognitive psychology, they are viewed as regions along a developmental continuum. Thus, whereas a cognition textbook might have separate chapters, say, on intellectual abilities, various kinds of competencies (e.g., memory and reasoning competencies), and expertise (e.g., Sternberg &

Ben Zeev, 2001), the three levels of skill development psychologically should not be viewed as distinct. A major goal of work under the point of view presented here is to integrate the study of intelligence and related abilities (see reviews in Sternberg, 1990, 1994, 2000) with the study of competence (Sternberg & Kolligian, 1990), and in turn to link the study of these two constructs to the study of expertise (Chi, Glaser, & Farr, 1988; Ericsson, 1996; Ericsson, Krampe, & Tesch-Römer, 1993; Ericsson & Smith, 1991; Hoffman, 1992). These literatures, typically viewed as distinct, are here viewed as ultimately involved with the same psychological mechanisms.

"Developing competence" is defined here as the ongoing process of the acquisition and consolidation of a set of skills needed for performance in one or more life domains at the journeyman-level or above. "Developing expertise" is defined here as the ongoing process of the acquisition and consolidation of a set of skills needed for a high level of mastery in one or more domains of life performance. Experts, then, are people who have developed their competencies to a high level; competent individuals are people who have developed their abilities to a high level. Abilities, competencies, and expertise are on a continuum. One moves along the continuum as one acquires a broader range of skills, a deeper level of the skills one already has, and increased efficiency in the utilization of these skills.

According to this view, good performance on intelligence tests requires certain kinds of competencies (in test-taking skills, understanding word meanings, being able to do basic arithmetic, visualizing spatial relations, etc.), and to the extent that these competencies overlap with the competencies required by schooling or by the workplace, there will be a correlation between the tests and performance in school or in the workplace. Some people are experts in taking intelligence tests and receive very high scores. Because the same skills on which they have shown expertise are also required in school and the workplace (e.g., reading, arithmetic), they will also be expert in work and on the job. Generally, there is more overlap between the kinds of competencies and expertise required on intelligence tests and in schooling than between those required on intelligence tests and in job performance. Hence, typically, intelligence test scores will show somewhat more correlation with school than with job performance. But many factors, such as range of scores and complexity of the work done in school or on the job, can affect this correlation, so it is difficult to speak in totally general terms.

According to the view of the measurement of intelligence representing the measurement of competencies in development, such correlations represent no intrinsic relation between intelligence and other kinds of performance, but rather overlap in the kinds of competencies needed to perform well under different kinds of circumstances. The greater the overlap in skills, in general, the higher the correlations.

There is nothing mystical or privileged about the intelligence tests. One could as easily use, say, academic or job performance to predict intelligence-related scores and vice versa. For example, many tests of intelligence contain items requiring memory skills, vocabulary, reading, arithmetic skills, and reasoning skills. Tests of achievement require the same skills. Both kinds of tests,

therefore, measure competencies, albeit at different levels of development. In summary, what distinguishes ability tests from other kinds of assessments is how the ability tests are used (usually predictively) rather than what they measure. There is no qualitative distinction among the various kinds of assessments.

According to this view, the main thing that distinguishes ability tests from achievement tests is not the tests themselves, but rather how psychologists, educators, and others interpret the scores on these tests. The ability tests are viewed as measuring something psychologically distinct from the achievement tests, hence the use of different labels to describe the tests. But the distinction is quantitative, not qualitative. A testing company that seems to have recognized this fact is the College Board, which originally called its test the Scholastic Aptitude Test, then changed the name to Scholastic Assessment Test, and finally just to its acronym, SAT. Indeed, items on the SAT-I (formerly the ability test) and the SAT-II (formerly the achievement tests) are often, for all intents and purposes, indistinguishable. The various kinds of assessments are of the same kind psychologically.

Conventional tests of intelligence and related abilities measure achievement that individuals should have accomplished several years back (see also Anastasi & Urbina, 1997). In other words, the tests are measuring competencies at a somewhat less developed level. Tests such as vocabulary, reading comprehension, verbal analogies, arithmetic problem solving, and the like, are all, in part, tests of achievement. Even abstract reasoning tests measure achievement in dealing with geometric symbols, skills taught in Western schools (Laboratory of Comparative Human Cognition, 1982; Serpell, 2000). One might as well use academic performance to predict ability test scores. The conventional view infers some kind of causation (abilities cause achievement) from correlation, but the inference is not justified from the correlational data.

The view of intelligence and other abilities as a set of competencies in development is not inconsistent with there being a contribution of genetic factors as a source of individual differences in who will be able to develop given amounts of competence or expertise. Many human attributes, including intelligence, reflect the covariation and inter-action of genetic and environmental factors. But the contribution of genes to an individual's intelligence cannot be directly measured or even directly estimated. Rather, what is measured is a portion of what is expressed, namely, manifestations of developing competencies and expertise.

According to this view, measures of intelligence *should* be correlated with later success, because both measures of intelligence and various measures of success require developing expertise of related types. For example, both typically require what can be referred to as *metacomponents* of thinking: recognition of problems, definition of problems, formulation of strategies to solve problems, representation of information, allocation of resources, and monitoring and evaluation of problem solutions. These skills develop as results of gene–environment covariation and interaction. If we

wish to call them *intelligence*, that is certainly fine, so long as we recognize that what we are calling intelligence is a form of developing competencies that can lead to expertise.

HOW ABILITIES DEVELOP INTO COMPETENCIES, AND COMPTENCIES INTO EXPERTISE

The specifics of a model for how abilities can develop into competencies, and competencies into expertise, are shown in Figure 2.1. At the heart of the model is the notion that individuals are constantly in a process of developing expertise when they work within a given domain. They may and do, of course, differ in rate and asymptote of development. The main constraint in achieving expertise is not some fixed prior level of capacity, but purposeful engagement involving direct instruction, active participation, role modeling, and reward.

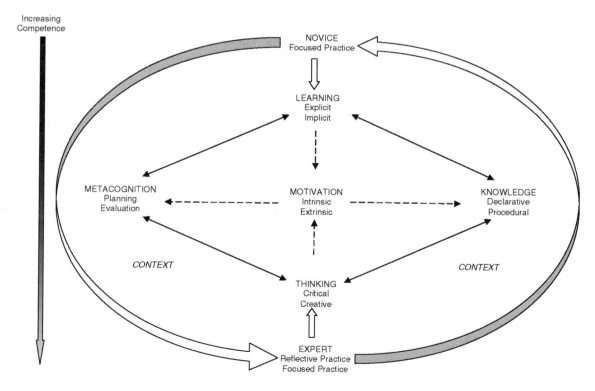

FIGURE 2.1. The development of abilities into competencies, and competencies into expertise.

Elements of the Model

The model of developing expertise has five key elements (although they certainly do not constitute an exhaustive list of elements in the ultimate development of expertise from abilities): metacognitive skills, learning skills, thinking skills, knowledge, and motivation. Although it is convenient to separate these five elements, they are fully interactive, as shown in Figure 2.1. They influence each other, both directly and indirectly. For example, learning leads to knowledge, but knowledge facilitates further learning.

These elements are, to some extent, domain specific. The development of competencies or expertise in one area does not necessarily lead to the development of competencies or expertise in another area, although there may be some transfer, depending upon the relationship of the areas, a point that has been made with regard to intelligence by others as well (e.g., Gardner, 1983, 1999; Sternberg, 1994).

In the theory of successful intelligence (Sternberg, 1985, 1997, 1999), intelligence is viewed as having three aspects: analytical, creative, and practical. Our research suggests that the development of competencies or even expertise in one creative domain (Sternberg & Lubart, 1995) or in one practical domain (Sternberg, Wagner, Williams, & Horvath, 1995) shows modest to moderate correlations with the development of competencies or expertise in other such domains. Psychometric research suggests more domain generality for the analytical domain (Jensen, 1998; Sternberg & Grigorenko, 2002b). Moreover, people can show analytical, creative, or practical expertise in one domain without showing all three of these kinds of expertise, or even two of the three.

Metacognitive Skills

Metacognitive skills (or metacomponents; Sternberg, 1985) refer to people's understanding and control of their own cognition. For example, such skills would encompass what an individual knows about writing papers or solving arithmetic word problems, both with regard to the steps that are involved and to how these steps can be executed effectively. Seven metacognitive skills are particularly important: problem recognition, problem definition, problem representation, strategy formulation, resource allocation, monitoring of problem solving, and evaluation of problem solving (Sternberg, 1985, 1986). All of these skills are modifiable (Sternberg, 1986, 1988; Sternberg & Grigorenko, 2000; Sternberg & Spear-Swerling, 1996).

Learning Skills

Learning skills (knowledge-acquisition components) are essential to the model (Sternberg, 1985, 1986), although they are certainly not the only learning skills that individuals use. Learning skills are sometimes divided into explicit and implicit ones. Explicit learning is what occurs when we make an effort to learn; implicit learning is what occurs when we pick up information incidentally, without any systematic effort. Examples of learning skills are selective encoding, which involves distinguishing relevant from irrelevant information; selective combination, which involves putting together the relevant information; and selective comparison, which involves relating new information to information already stored in memory (Sternberg, 1985).

Thinking Skills

There are three main kinds of thinking skills (or performance components) that individuals need to master (Sternberg, 1985, 1986, 1994). It is important to note that these are sets of, rather than individual, thinking skills. Critical (analytical) thinking skills include analyzing, critiquing, judging, evaluating, comparing and contrasting, and assessing. Creative thinking skills include creating, discovering, inventing, imagining, supposing, and hypothesizing. Practical thinking skills include applying, using, utilizing, and practicing (Sternberg, 1997). They are the first step in the translation of thought into real-world action.

Knowledge

Two main kinds of knowledge are relevant in academic situations. Declarative knowledge is of facts, concepts, principles, laws, and the like. It is "knowing that." Procedural knowledge is of procedures and strategies. It is "knowing how." Of particular importance is procedural tacit knowledge, which involves knowing how the system functions in which one is operating (Sternberg et al., 2000; Sternberg et al., 1995).

Motivation

One can distinguish among several different kinds of motivation. A first kind of motivation is achievement motivation (McClelland, 1985; McClelland, Atkinson, Clark, & Lowell, 1976). People who are high in achievement motivation seek moderate challenges and risks. They are attracted to tasks that are neither very easy nor very hard. They are strivers—constantly trying to better themselves and their accomplishments. A second kind of motivation is competence (self-efficacy) motivation, which refers to persons' beliefs in their own ability to solve the problem at hand (Bandura, 1977, 1996). Experts need to develop a sense of their own efficacy to solve difficult tasks in their domain of expertise. This kind of self-efficacy can result both from intrinsic and extrinsic rewards (Amabile, 1996; Sternberg & Lubart, 1996). Of course, other kinds of motivation are important too. Indeed, motivation is perhaps the indispensable element needed for school success. Without it, the student never even tries to learn. And, of course, if a test is not important to the examinee, he or she may do poorly simply through a lack of effort to perform well.

Dweck (1999, 2002; Dweck & Elliott, 1983) has shown that one of the most important sources of motivation is individuals' need to enhance their intellectual skills. What Dweck has shown is that some individuals are entity theorists with respect to intelligence: They believe that to be smart is to show oneself to be smart, and that means not making mistakes or otherwise showing intellectual weakness. Incremental theorists, in contrast, believe that to be smart is to learn and to increase one's intellectual skills. These individuals are not afraid to make mistakes and even believe that making mistakes can be useful, because it is a way to learn. Dweck and her colleagues' research suggests that, under normal conditions, en-

tity and incremental theorists perform about the same in school. But under conditions of challenge, incremental theorists do better, because they are more willing to undertake difficult challenges and to seek mastery of new, difficult material.

Context

All of the elements discussed earlier are characteristics of the learner. Returning to the issues raised at the beginning of this chapter, a problem with conventional tests is that they assume that individuals operate in a more or less decontextualized environment (see Grigorenko & Sternberg, 2001b; Sternberg, 1985, 1997; Sternberg & Grigorenko, 2001). A test score is interpreted largely in terms of the individual's internal attributes. But a test measures much more, and the assumption of a fixed or uniform context across test-takers is not realistic. Contextual factors that can affect test performance include native language, family background, emphasis of test on speedy performance, and familiarity with the kinds of material on the test, among many other things.

Interactions of Elements

The novice works toward competence and then expertise through deliberate practice (Ericsson, 1996). But this practice requires an interaction of all five of the key elements. At the center, driving the elements, is motivation. Without it, the elements remain inert. Eventually, one reaches a kind of expertise, at which one becomes a reflective practitioner of a certain set of skills. But expertise occurs at many levels. The expert first-year graduate or law student, for example, is still a far cry from the expert professional. People thus cycle through many times, on the way to successively higher levels of expertise. They do so through the elements in Figure 2.1.

Motivation drives metacognitive skills, which in turn activate learning and thinking skills, which then provide feedback to the metacognitive skills, enabling one's level of expertise to increase (see also Sternberg, 1985). The declarative and procedural knowledge acquired through the extension of the thinking and learning skills also results in these skills being used more effectively in the future.

All of these processes are affected by, and can in turn affect, the context in which they operate. For example, if a learning experience is in English but the learner has only limited English proficiency, his or her learning will be inferior to that of someone with more advanced English-language skills. Or if material is presented orally to someone who is a better visual learner, that individual's performance will be reduced.

How does this model of developing competencies and expertise relate to the construct of intelligence?

THE g FACTOR AND
THE STRUCTURE OF ABILITIES

Some intelligence theorists point to the stability of the alleged general (g) factor of human intelligence as evidence for the existence of some kind of stable and overriding structure of human intelligence (e.g., Bouchard, 1998; Kyllonen, 2002; Petrill, 2002). But the existence of a g factor may reflect little more than an interaction between whatever latent (and not directly measurable) abilities individuals may have and the kinds of competencies and expertise that are developed in school. With different forms of schooling, g could be made either stronger or weaker. In effect, Western forms and related forms of schooling may, in part, create the g phenomenon by providing a kind of schooling that teaches in conjunction the various kinds of skills measured by tests of intellectual abilities.

Suppose, for example, that children were selected from an early age to be schooled for a certain trade. Throughout most of human history, this is in fact the way most children were schooled. Boys, at least, were apprenticed at an early age to a master who would teach them a trade. There was no point in their learning skills that would be irrelevant to their lives.

To bring the example into the present, imagine that we decided, from an early age, that certain students would study English (or some other native language) to develop language expertise; other students would study mathematics to develop their mathe-

matical expertise. Still other students might specialize in developing spatial expertise to be used in flying airplanes or doing shop work, or whatever. Instead of beginning at the university level, specialization would begin from the age of first schooling.

This point of view is related to, but different from, that typically associated with the theory of crystallized and fluid intelligence (Cattell, 1971; Horn, 1994). In that theory, fluid ability is viewed as an ability to acquire and reason with information, whereas crystallized ability is viewed as the information so acquired. According to this view, schooling primarily develops crystallized ability, based in part on the fluid ability the individual brings to bear upon school-like tasks. In the theory proposed here, however, both fluid and crystallized ability are roughly equally susceptible to development through schooling or other means that societies create for developing expertise. One could argue that the greater validity of the position presented here is shown by the near-ubiquitous Flynn effect (Flynn, 1987, 1998; Neisser, 1998), which documents massive gains in IQ around the world throughout most of the 20th century. The effect must be due to environment, because large genetic changes worldwide in such a short time frame are virtually impossible. Interestingly, gains are substantially larger in fluid abilities than in crystallized abilities, suggesting that fluid abilities are likely to be as susceptible as, or probably more susceptible, than crystalloid abilities to environmental influences. Clearly, the notion of fluid abilities as some basic genetic potential one brings into the world, whose development is expressed in crystallized abilities, does not work.

These students then would be given an omnibus test of intelligence or any broad-ranging measure of intelligence. There would be no g factor, because people schooled in one form of expertise would not have been schooled in others. One can imagine even negative correlations between subscores on the so-called intelligence test. The reason for the negative correlations would be that developing expertise in one area might preclude developing expertise in another because of the form of schooling.

Lest this tale sound far-fetched, I hasten to add that it is a true tale of what is happening now in some places. In the United States and most of the developed world, of course, schooling takes a fairly standard course. But this standard course and the value placed upon it are not uniform across the world. And we should not fall into the ethnocentric trap of believing that the way Western schooling works is the way all schooling should work.

In a collaborative study among children near Kisumu, Kenya (Sternberg et al., 2001), we devised a test of practical intelligence that measures informal knowledge for an important aspect of adaptation to the environment in rural Kenya, namely, knowledge of the identities and use of natural herbal medicines that could be used to combat illnesses. The children use this informal knowledge an average of once a week in treating themselves or suggesting treatments to other children, so this knowledge is a routine part of their everyday existence. By *informal knowledge*, we are referring to kinds of knowledge not taught in schools, and not assessed on tests given in the schools.

The idea of our research was that children who knew what these medicines were, what they were used for, and how they should be dosed would be in a better position to adapt to their environments than would children without this informal knowledge. We do not know how many, if any, of these medicines actually work, but from the standpoint of measuring practical intelligence in a given culture, the important thing is that the people in Kenya believe that the medicines work. For that matter, it is not always clear how effective are the medicines used in the Western World.

We found substantial individual differences in the tacit knowledge of like-age and schooled children about these natural herbal medicines. More important, however, was the correlation between scores on this test and scores on an English-language vocabulary test (the Mill Hill), a Dholuo equivalent (Dholuo is the community and home language), and the Raven Coloured Progressive Matrices. We found significantly *negative* correlations between our test and the English-language vocabulary test. Correlations of our test with the other tests were trivial. The better children did on the test of indigenous tacit knowledge, the worse they did on the test of vocabulary used in school, and vice versa. Why might we have obtained such a finding?

Based on ethnographic observation, we believe a possible reason is that parents in the village may emphasize either a more indigenous or a more Western education. Some parents (and their children) see little value to school. They do not see how success in school connects with the future of children who will spend their whole lives in a village, where they do not believe they need the expertise the school teaches. Other parents and children seem to see Western schooling as being of value in itself or potentially as a ticket out of the confines of the village. The parents thus tend to emphasize one type of education or the other for their children, with corresponding results. The kinds of developing expertise the families value differ and so, therefore, do scores on the tests. From this point of view, the intercorrelational structure of tests tells us nothing intrinsic about the structure of intelligence per se, but rather something about the way abilities as developing forms of expertise structure themselves in interaction with the demands of the environment.

In a more recent study (Grigorenko et al., 2004), we studied the academic and practical skills of Yup'ik Eskimo children who live in the southwestern portion of Alaska. The Yup'ik generally live in geographically isolated villages along waterways that are accessible primarily by air. Most of us would have no choice in traveling from one village to another, because we would be unable to navigate the terrain using, say, a dogsled. These villages are embedded in mile after mile of frozen tundra that, to us, would all look relatively the same. The Yup'ik, however, can navigate this terrain, because they learn to find landmarks that most of us would never see. They also have extremely impressive hunting and gathering skills that almost none of us would have. Yet most of the children do quite poorly in school. Their teachers often think that they are rather hopeless students. The children thus have developed extremely impressive competencies and even expertise for surviving in a difficult environment, but because these skills often are not ones valued by teachers (who typically are not from the Yup'ik community), the children are viewed as not very competent.

Nuñes (1994) has reported related findings based on a series of studies she conducted in Brazil (see also Ceci & Roazzi, 1994). Street children's adaptive intelligence is tested to the limit by their ability to form and successfully run a street business. If they fail to run such a business successfully, they risk either starvation or death at the hands of death squads should they resort to stealing. Nuñes and her collaborators have found that the same children who are doing the mathematics needed for running a successful street business cannot do well the same types of mathematics problems presented in an abstract, paper-and-pencil format.

From a conventional abilities standpoint, this result is puzzling. From a standpoint of intelligence as developing competencies and competencies as developing expertise, it is not. Street children grow up in an environment that fosters the development of practical but not academic mathematical skills. We know that even conventional academic kinds of expertise often fail to show transfer (e.g., Gick & Holyoak, 1980). It is scarcely surprising, then, that there would be little transfer here. The street children have developed the kinds of practical arithmetical expertise they need for survival and even success, but they will get no credit for these skills when they take a conventional abilities test.

It also seems likely that if the scales were reversed, and privileged children who do well on conventional ability tests or in school were forced out on the street, many of them would not survive long. Indeed, in the ghettoes of urban America, many children and adults who for one reason or another end up on the street, in fact barely survive or do not make it at all.

Jean Lave (1989) has reported similar findings with Berkeley housewives shopping in supermarkets. There just is no correlation between their ability to do the mathematics needed for comparison shopping and their scores on conventional paper-and-pencil tests of comparable mathematical skills. And Ceci and Liker (1986) found, similarly, that expert handicappers at race tracks generally had only average IQs. There was no correlation between the complexity of the mathematical model they used in handicapping and their scores on conventional tests. In each case, important kinds of developing expertise for life were not adequately reflected by the kinds of developing expertise measured by the conventional ability tests.

One could argue that these results merely reflect the fact that the problem these studies raise is not with conventional theories of abilities, but with the tests that are loosely based on these theories: These tests do not measure street math, but more abstracted forms of mathematical thinking. But psychometric theories, I would argue, deal with a similarly abstracted g factor. The abstracted tests follow largely from the abstracted theoretical constructs. In fact, our research has shown that tests of practical intelligence generally do not correlate with scores on these abstracted tests (e.g., Sternberg et al., 1995, 2000).

The problem with the conventional model of abilities does not just apply in what to us are exotic cultures or exotic occupations. In one study (Sternberg, Ferrari, Clinkenbeard, & Grigorenko, 1996; Sternberg, Grigorenko, Ferrari, & Clinkenbeard, 1999), high school students were tested for their analytical, creative, and practical abilities via multiple-choice and essay items. The multiple-choice items were divided into three content domains: verbal, quantitative, and figural pictures. Students' scores were factor-analyzed and then later correlated with their performance in a college-level introductory psychology course.

We found that when students were tested not only for analytical abilities but also for creative and practical abilities (as follows from the model of successful intelligence; Sternberg, 1985, 1997), the strong g factor that tends to result from multiple-ability tests becomes much weaker. Of course, there is always some general factor when one factor-analyzes but does not rotate the factor solution, but the general factor was weak and, of course, disappeared with a varimax rotation. We also found that all of analytical, creative, and practical abilities predicted performance in the introductory psychology course (which itself was taught analytically, creatively, or practically, with assessments to match). Moreover, although the students who were identified as high analytical were the traditional population—primarily white, middle- to upper-middle-class, and well educated, the students who were identified as high creative or high practical were much more diverse in all of these attributes. Most importantly, students whose instruction better matched their triarchic pattern of abilities outperformed those students whose instruction more poorly matched their triarchic pattern of abilities.

Thus, conventional tests may unduly favor a small segment of the population by virtue of the narrow kind of developing expertise they measure. When one measures a broader range of developing competencies and expertise, the results look quite different. Moreover, the broader range of expertise includes kinds of skills that will be important in the world of work and in the world of the family.

Even in developed countries, practical competencies probably matter as much as or more than do academic ones for many aspects of life success. Goleman (1995), for example (see also Salovey & Mayer, 1990; Mayer, Salovey, & Caruso, 2000), has claimed that emotional competencies are more important than academic ones, although he has offered no direct evidence. In a study we did in Russia (Grigorenko & Sternberg, 2001a), although both academic and practical intelligence predicted measures of adult physical and mental health, the measures of practical intelligence were the better predictors.

Analytical, creative, and practical abilities, as measured by our tests or anyone else's, are simply forms of developing competencies and ultimately of developing expertise. All are useful in various kinds of life tasks. But conventional tests may unfairly disadvantage those students who do not do well in a fairly narrow range of kinds of expertise. By expanding the range of developing expertise we measure, we discover that many children not now identified as able have, in fact, developed important kinds of expertise. The abilities that conventional tests measure are important for school and life performance, but they are not the only abilities that are important.

Teaching in a way that departs from notions of abilities based on a g factor also pays dividends. In a recent set of studies, we have shown that generally lower socioeconomic class third-grade and generally middle-class eighth-grade students who are taught social studies (a unit in communities) or science (a unit on psychology) for successful intelligence (analytically, creative, and practically, as well as for memory) outperform students who are taught just for analytical (critical) thinking or just for memory (Sternberg, Torff, & Grigorenko, 1998a, 1998b). The students taught "triarchically" outperform the other students not only on performance assessments that look at analytical, creative, and practical kinds of achievements, but even on tests that measure straight memory (multiple-choice tests already being used in the courses). None of this is to say that analytical abilities are not important in school and life—obviously, they are. Rather, what our data suggest is that other types of abilities—creative and practical ones—are important as well, and that students need to learn how to use all three kinds of abilities together.

Thus, teaching students in a way that takes into account their more highly developed expertise and that also enables them to develop other kinds of expertise results in superior learning outcomes, regardless of how these learning outcomes are measured. The children taught in a way that enables them to use kinds of expertise other than memory actually remember better, on average, than do children taught for memory.

We have also done studies in which we have measured informal procedural knowledge in children and adults. We have done such studies with business managers, college professors, elementary school students, salespeople, college students, and general populations. This important aspect of practical intelligence, in study after study, has been found to be uncorrelated with academic intelligence, as measured by conventional tests, in a variety of populations, occupations, and at a variety of age levels (Sternberg et al., 1995, 2000). Moreover, the tests predict job performance as well as or better than do tests of IQ. The lack of correlation of the two kinds of ability tests suggests that the best prediction of job performance will result when both academic and practical intelligence tests are used as predictors. Most recently, we have developed a test of common sense for the workplace—for example, how to handle oneself in a job interview—that predicts self-ratings of common sense but not self-ratings of various kinds of academic abilities (Sternberg & Grigorenko, 1998).

Although the kinds of informal procedural expertise we measure in these tests does not correlate with academic expertise, it does correlate across work domains. For example, we found that subscores (for managing oneself, managing others, and managing tasks) on measures of informal procedural knowledge are correlated with each other, and that scores on the test for academic psychology are moderately correlated with scores on the test for business managers (Sternberg et al., 1995). So the kinds of developing expertise that matter in the world of work may show certain correlations with each other that are not shown with the kinds of developing expertise that matter in the world of the school.

It is even possible to use these kinds of tests to predict effectiveness in leadership. Studies of military leaders showed that tests of informal knowledge for military leaders predicted the effectiveness of these leaders, whereas conventional tests of intelligence did not. We also found that although the test for managers was significantly correlated with the test for military leaders, only the latter test predicted superiors' ratings of leadership effectiveness (Sternberg et al., 2000).

Both conventional academic tests and our tests of practical intelligence measure forms of developing expertise that matter in school and on the job. The two kinds of tests are not qualitatively distinct. The reason the correlations are essentially null is that the kinds of developing expertise they measure are quite different. The people who good at abstract, academic kinds of expertise are often people who have not emphasized learning practical, everyday kinds of expertise, and vice versa, as we found in our Kenya study. Indeed, children who grow up in challenging environments such as the inner city may need to develop practical over academic expertise as a matter of survival. As in Kenya, this practical expertise may better predict their survival than do academic kinds of expertise. The same applies in business, where tacit knowledge about how to perform on the job is as likely or more likely to lead to job success than is the academic expertise that in school seems so important.

The practical kinds of expertise matter in school too. In a study at Yale, Wendy Williams and I (cited in Sternberg, Wagner, & Okagaki, 1993) found that a test of tacit knowledge for college predicted grade-point average as well as did an academic ability test. But a test of tacit knowledge for college life better predicted adjustment to the college environment than did the academic test.

TAKING TESTS

One of the best ways of measuring abilities as developing competencies is through dynamic assessment (Sternberg & Grigorenko, 2002a). Dynamic assessment has been proposed as a way of uncovering this information. What is dynamic assessment? Dynamic assessment is testing plus an instructional intervention. In other words, the instructional and assessment functions, instead of being separated, are integrated. In a conventional assessment, sometimes called a *static assessment*, individuals receive a set of test items and solve these items with little or no feedback. Often, giving feedback is viewed as a source of error of measurement, and therefore as something to be avoided at all costs. In a *dynamic assessment*, individuals receive a set of test items with explicit instruction (Grigorenko & Sternberg, 1998; Lidz, 1987, 1997; Sternberg & Grigorenko, 2002b; Wiedl, Guthke, & Wingenfeld, 1995). Dynamic assessments have been found to reveal developing expertise in members of underrepresented minority groups around the world that is not revealed by conventional static tests (see, e.g., Feuerstein, Rand, & Hoffman, 1979; Lidz & Elliott, 2000; Sternberg & Grigorenko, 2002a).

Dynamic assessment is far from perfect. Scores on dynamic assessments can be influenced by many factors, such as the kinds of instruction given, the match between the kind of instruction given and the test-taker's existing pattern of skills, the relationship between the examiner and the examinee, and so on. No method of assessment gives a totally accurate picture of a person's potentials.

Why should dynamic instruction and assessment tend to benefit members of underrepresented minority groups in particular? There are at least four reasons.

1. Members of such groups may have less tacit knowledge about how to manage themselves in schools, which often reflect middle-class values. Moreover, they may have less knowledge of how to take tests (test-wiseness), due to lesser experience with tests. Dynamic instruction and assessment help make this tacit knowledge explicit.
2. The coldness and interpersonal distance characteristic of static learning and assessment situations may be more threatening to members of underrepresented minority groups than to others.
3. Members of underrepresented minority groups may have less cognitive scaffolding than do members of other groups. Dynamic instruction and assessment help provide this missing scaffolding.
4. Members of underrepresented minority groups who might disidentify with a static assessment situation may identify with the situation when they are given an opportunity not only to show what they have learned in the assessment situation but also to learn in this situation.

Member of underrepresented minority groups may actually have less developed expertise than do members of others groups. But they may have as great or greater developing expertise, or at least, capacity to develop expertise. Dynamic instruction and assessment help elucidate this developing expertise and capacity to acquire developing expertise.

There are two common formats for dynamic assessments. The first format is that the instruction may be sandwiched between a pretest and a posttest. The second format is that the instruction may be in response to the examinee's solution to each test item. Note that they are not the only possible formats, just the two most commonly used ones. Here, I use two terms of our own invention to describe the *sandwich format* and the *cake format*.

In the first format, examinees take a pretest, which is essentially equivalent to a static test. After they complete the pretest, they are given instruction in the skills measured by the pretest. The instruction may be given in an individual or a group setting. If it is in an individual setting, it may or may not be individualized to reflect a particular

examinee's strengths and weaknesses. If it is individualized, then the amount as well as the type of feedback can be individualized. If it is in a group setting, then the instruction typically is the same for all examinees. After instruction, the examinees are tested again on a posttest. The posttest is typically an alternate form of the pretest, although, less commonly, it may be exactly the same test. For convenience, this is referred to as the *sandwich format*. In individual testing settings, the exact contents of the sandwich (type of instruction), as well as its thickness (amount of instruction), can be varied to suit the individual. In group testing settings, the contents and thickness of the sandwich are typically uniform.

In the second format, which is always done individually, examinees are given instruction item by item. An examinee is given an item to solve. If he or she solves it correctly, then the next item is presented. But if the examinee does not solve the item correctly, he or she is given a graded series of hints. The hints are designed to make the solution successively more nearly apparent. The examiner then determines how many and what kinds of hints the examinee needs in order to solve the item correctly. Instruction continues until the examinee is successful, at which time the next item is presented. The successive hints are presented like successive layers of icing on a cake. For convenience, this is referred to as the *cake format*. In the cake format, the number of layers of the cake is almost always varied (i.e., the amount of feedback depends on how quickly the examinee is able to use the format to reach a correct solution). The contents of the layers, however (i.e., the type of feedback), may or may not be constant. Most often, they are constant: The number of hints varies across examinees, but not the content of them.

There are three major differences between the static and dynamic paradigms. The differences are best viewed as ones of emphasis rather than of dichotomous differences. A static test can have dynamic elements, just as a dynamic test can have static elements.

The first difference regards the respective roles of static states versus dynamic processes. *Static assessment* emphasizes products formed as a result of preexisting skills, whereas *dynamic assessment* emphasizes quantification of the psychological processes involved in learning and change. In other words, static testing taps more into a developed state, whereas dynamic testing taps more into a developing process. In both of the formats of dynamic testing described, the examiner is able to assess how the problem-solving process develops as a result of instruction. In the sandwich format of dynamic testing, the instruction is given all at once between the pretest and the posttest. In the cake format of dynamic testing, the instruction is given in graded bits after each test item, as needed. Static testing typically does not allow the examiner to draw such inferences.

The second difference regards the role of feedback. In *static assessment*, an examiner presents a graded sequence of problems and the test-taker responds to each of the problems. There is no feedback from examiner to test-taker regarding quality of performance. In *dynamic assessment*, feedback is given, either explicitly or implicitly.

The type of feedback depends on which kind of dynamic assessment is used. In the sandwich format described above, the feedback may be explicit if the testing is individual, but will probably be implicit if the testing is in a group. The instruction sandwiched between the pretest and the posttest gives each examinee an opportunity to see which skills he or she has mastered and which skills he or she has not mastered. But in a group testing situation, the examiner is not able explicitly to tell each examinee about these skills. In an individual testing situation with the sandwich format, it is possible to provide explicit feedback, should the examiner decide to give it.

In the cake format, the examiner presents a sequence of progressively more challenging tasks, but after the presentation of each task, the examiner gives the test-taker feedback, continuing with this feedback in successive iterations until the examinee either solves the problem or gives up. Testing thus joins with instruction, and the test-taker's ability to learn is quantified while he or she learns.

The third difference between static and dynamic assessment pertains to the quality of the examiner–examinee relationship. In static testing, the examiner attempts to be as neutral and as uninvolved as possible to-ward the examinee. The examiner wants to have good rapport, but nothing more. Involvement beyond good rapport risks the introduction of error of measurement. In dynamic assessment, the assessment situation and the type of examiner–examinee relationship are modified from the one-way traditional setting of the conventional psychometric approach to form a two-way, interactive relationship between the examiner and the examinee.

In individual dynamic assessment, this tester–testee interaction is individualized for each child: The conventional attitude of neutrality is thus replaced by an atmosphere of teaching and helping. In group dynamic assessment using the sandwich format, the examiner is still helpful, although at a group rather than an individual level. The examiner is giving instruction in order to help the examinees improve on the posttest. As in the individual assessment format, he or she is anything but neutral.

Thus, dynamic assessment is based on the link between testing and intervention, and examines the processes of learning, as well as its products. By embedding learning in evaluation, dynamic assessment assumes that the examinee can start at the "zero (or almost zero) point" of having certain developed skills to be assessed, and that teaching will provide all the necessary information for mastery of the assessed skills. In other words, what is assessed, in theory, is not just previously acquired skills, but the capacity to master, apply, and reapply skills taught in the dynamic assessment situation. In practice, results of dynamic assessments can be affected by many things, such as match between tester and test-taker, sensitivity of the tester to the test-taker, the tester's expectations for the child, and so forth. Thus, the tests may be less than perfect. The view of dynamic tests as measuring learning skills at the time of test underlies the use of the term *test of learning potential*, which is often applied to dynamic assessment.

In a study near Bagamoyo, Tanzania, we investigated dynamic tests administered to children. Although dynamic tests have been developed for a number of purposes (see Grigorenko & Sternberg, 1998; Sternberg & Grigorenko, 2002a), one of our particular purposes was to look at how dynamic testing affects score patterns. In particular, we developed more or less conventional measures but administered them in a dynamic format. In an experimental group, first, students took a pretest. Then they received a short period of instruction (generally no more than 10–15 minutes) on how to improve their performance in the expertise measured by these tests. Then the children took a posttest. In a control group, children took the pretest and posttest but did not receive instruction in between.

A first finding was that the correlation between pretest and posttest scores, although statistically significant, was relatively weak (about .3) in the experimental group but strong (about .8) in the control group. In other words, even a short period of instruction fairly drastically changed the rank orders of the students on the test.

We again interpret these results in terms of the model of abilities as developing competencies and expertise. The Tanzanian students had developed very little expertise in the skills required to take American-style intelligence tests. Thus, even a short intervention could have a fairly substantial effect on their scores. When the students developed somewhat more of this test-taking expertise through a short intervention, their scores changed and became more reflective of their true capabilities for cognitive work.

Sometimes the expertise children learn that is relevant for in-school tests may actually hurt them on conventional ability tests. In one example, we studied the development of children's analogical reasoning in a country day school, where teachers taught in English in the morning and in Hebrew in the afternoon (Sternberg & Rifkin, 1979). We found a number of second-grade students who got no problems right on our test. They would have seemed, on the surface, to be rather stupid. We discovered the reason why, however. We had tested in the afternoon, and in the afternoon, the children always read in Hebrew. So they read our problems from right to left, and got them all wrong. The expertise that served them so well in their normal environment utterly failed them on the test.

Our sample was of upper-middle-class children who, in a year or two, would know better. But imagine what happens with other children in less supportive environments who develop kinds of expertise that may

serve them well in their family or community lives or even school life, but not on the tests. They will appear to be stupid, rather than lacking the kinds of expertise the tests measure.

Greenfield (1997), who has done a number of studies in a variety of cultures, found that the kinds of test-taking expertise assumed to be universal in the United States and other Western countries are by no means universal. She found, for example, that children in Mayan cultures (and probably in other highly collectivist cultures as well) were puzzled when they were not allowed to collaborate with parents or others on test questions. In the United States, of course, such collaboration would be viewed as cheating. But in a collectivist culture, someone who had not developed this kind of collaborative expertise, and moreover, someone who did not use it, would be perceived as lacking important adaptive skills (see also Laboratory of Comparative Human Cognition, 1982).

CONCLUSIONS

Intelligence tests measure developing competencies, and these developing competencies can be transformed into the development of expertise. Tests can be created that favor the kinds of developing expertise formed in any kind of cultural or subcultural milieu. Those who have created conventional tests of abilities have tended to value the kinds of skills most valued by Western schools. This system of valuing is understandable, given that Binet and Simon (1905) first developed intelligence tests for the purpose of predicting school performance. Moreover, these skills are important in school and in life. But in the modern world, the conception of abilities as fixed or even as predetermined is an anachronism. Moreover, our research and that of others (reviewed more extensively in Sternberg, 1997) shows that the set of abilities assessed by conventional tests measures only a small portion of the kinds of developing expertise that are relevant for life success. It is for this reason that conventional tests predict only about 10% of individual difference variation in various measures of success in adult life (Herrnstein & Murray, 1994).

Not all cultures value equally the kinds of expertise measured by these tests. In a study comparing Latino, Asian, and Anglo subcultures in California, for example, we found that Latino parents valued social kinds of expertise as more important to intelligence than did Asian and Anglo parents, who more valued cognitive kinds of expertise (Okagaki & Sternberg, 1993). Predictably, teachers also more valued cognitive kinds of expertise, with the result that the Anglo and Asian children would be expected to do better in school, and did. Of course, cognitive expertise matters in school and in life, but so does social expertise. Both need to be taught in the school and the home to all children. This latter kind of expertise may become even more important in the workplace. Until we expand our notions of abilities and recognize that when we measure them, we are measuring developing forms of expertise, we will risk consigning many potentially excellent contributors to our society to bleak futures. We will also be potentially overvaluing students with expertise for success in a certain kind of schooling, but not necessarily with equal expertise for success later in life.

ACKNOWLEDGMENTS

Preparation of this chapter was supported under the Javits Act Program (Grant No. R206R00001) as administered by the Institute of Educational Sciences, U.S. Department of Education. Grantees undertaking such projects are encouraged to express freely their professional judgment. This chapter, therefore, does not necessarily represent the position or policies of the Institute of Educational Sciences or the U.S. Department of Education, and no official endorsement should be inferred.

REFERENCES

Amabile, T. M. (1996). *Creativity in context*. Boulder, CO: Westview.

Anastasi, A., & Urbina, S. (1997). *Psychological testing* (7th ed.). Upper Saddle River, NJ: Prentice-Hall.

Bandura, A. (1977). Self-efficacy: Toward a unifying theory of behavioral change. *Psychological Review, 84*, 181–215.

Bandura, A. (1996). *Self-efficacy: The exercise of control*. New York: Freeman.

Binet, A., & Simon, T. (1905). Méthodes nouvelles pour le diagnostic du niveau intellectuel des anormaux. [New methods for the diagnosis of the intellectual level of the abnormal]. *L'Année psychologique, 11*, 191–336.

Bouchard, T. J., Jr. (1998). Genetic and environmental influences on adult intelligence and special mental abilities. *Human Biology, 70*, 257–279.

Carroll, J. B. (1993). *Human cognitive abilities: A survey of factor-analytic studies*. New York: Cambridge University Press.

Cattell, R. B. (1971). *Abilities: Their structure, growth, and action*. Boston: Houghton Mifflin.

Ceci, S. J., & Liker, J. (1986). Academic and nonacademic intelligence: An experimental separation. In R. J. Sternberg & R. K. Wagner (Eds.), *Practical intelligence: Nature and origins of competence in the everyday world* (pp. 119–142). New York: Cambridge University Press.

Ceci, S. J., & Roazzi, A. (1994). The effects of context on cognition: Postcards from Brazil. In R. J. Sternberg & R. K. Wagner (Eds.), *Mind in context: Interactionist perspectives on human intelligence* (pp. 74–101). New York: Cambridge University Press.

Chi, M. T. H., Glaser, R., & Farr, M. J. (Eds.). (1988). *The nature of expertise*. Hillsdale, NJ: Erlbaum.

Dweck, C. S. (1999). *Self-theories: Their role in motivation, personality, and development*. Philadelphia: Psychology Press/Taylor & Francis.

Dweck, C. S. (2002). Messages that motivate: How praise molds students' beliefs, motivation, and performance (in surprising ways). In J. Aronson (Ed.), *Improving academic achievement: Impact of psychological factors on education* (pp. 37–60). San Diego: Academic Press.

Dweck, C. S., & Elliott, E. S. (1983). Achievement motivation. In P. H. Mussen (General Ed.) & E. M. Heatherington (Vol. Ed.), *Handbook of child psychology: Socialization, personality, and social development* (4th ed., Vol. 4, pp. 644–691). New York: Wiley.

Ericsson, K. A. (Ed.). (1996). *The road to excellence: The acquisition of expert performance in the arts and sciences, sports and games*. Hillsdale, NJ: Erlbaum.

Ericsson, K. A., Krampe, R. T., & Tesch-Römer, C. (1993). The role of deliberate practice in the acquisition of expert performance. *Psychological Review, 100*, 363–406.

Ericsson, K. A., & Smith, J. (Eds.). (1991). *Toward a general theory of expertise: Prospects and limits*. New York: Cambridge University Press.

Feuerstein, R., Rand, Y., & Hoffman, M. B. (1979). *The dynamic assessment of retarded performers: The learning potential assessment device: Theory, instruments, and techniques*. Baltimore: University Park Press.

Flynn, J. R. (1987). Massive IQ gains in 14 nations: What IQ tests really measure. *Psychological Bulletin, 101*, 171–191.

Flynn, J. R. (1998). WAIS-III and WISC-III gains in the United States from 1972 to 1995: How to compensate for obsolete norms. *Perceptual and Motor Skills, 86,* 1231–1239.

Gardner, H. (1983). *Frames of mind: The theory of multiple intelligences.* New York: Basic Books.

Gardner, H. (1999). *Intelligence reframed: Multiple intelligences for the 21st century.* New York: Basic Books.

Gick, M. L., & Holyoak, K. J. (1980). Analogical problem solving. *Cognitive Psychology, 12,* 306–355.

Goleman, D. (1995). *Emotional intelligence.* New York: Bantam.

Greenfield, P. M. (1997). You can't take it with you: Why assessment abilities don't cross cultures. *American Psychologist, 52,* 1115–1124.

Grigorenko, E. L., Meier, E., Lipka, J., Mohatt, G., Yanez, E., & Sternberg, R. J. (2004). The relationship between academic and practical intelligence: A case study of the tacit knowledge of Native American Yup'ik people in Alaska. *Learning and Individual Differences, 14,* 185–207.

Grigorenko, E. L., & Sternberg, R. J. (1998). Dynamic testing. *Psychological Bulletin, 124,* 75–111.

Grigorenko, E. L., & Sternberg, R. J. (2001a). Analytical, creative, and practical intelligence as predictors of self-reported adaptive functioning: A case study in Russia. *Intelligence, 29,* 57–73.

Grigorenko, E. L., & Sternberg, R. J. (Eds.). (2001b). *Family environment and intellectual functioning: A life-span perspective.* Mahwah, NJ: Erlbaum.

Herrnstein, R. J., & Murray, C. (1994). *The bell curve.* New York: Free Press.

Hoffman, R. R. (Ed.). (1992). *The psychology of expertise: Cognitive research and empirical AI.* New York: Springer-Verlag.

Horn, J. L. (1994). Fluid and crystallized intelligence, theory of. In R. J. Sternberg (Ed.), *Encyclopedia of human intelligence* (Vol. 1, pp. 443–451). New York: Macmillan.

Jensen, A. R. (1998). *The g factor: The science of mental ability.* Westport, CT: Praeger/Greenwoood.

Kyllonen, P. C. (2002). g: Knowledge, speed, strategies, or working-memory capacity?: A systems perspective. In R. J. Sternberg & E. L. Grigorenko (Eds.), *The general factor of intelligence: How general is it?* (pp. 415–445). Mahwah, NJ: Erlbaum.

Laboratory of Comparative Human Cognition. (1982). Culture and intelligence. In R. J. Sternberg (Ed.), *Handbook of human intelligence* (pp. 642–719). New York: Cambridge University Press.

Lave, J. (1989). *Cognition in practice.* New York: Cambridge University Press.

Lidz, C. S. (Ed.). (1987). *Dynamic assessment.* New York: Guilford Press.

Lidz, C. S. (1997). Dynamic assessment approaches. In D. P. Flanagan, J. L. Genshaft, & P. L. Harrison (Eds.), *Contemporary intellectual assessment: Theories, tests, and issues* (pp. 281–296). New York: Guilford Press.

Lidz, C. S., & Elliott, J. (Eds.). (2000). *Dynamic assessment: Prevailing models and applications.* Greenwich, CT: Elsevier/JAI Press.

Mayer, J. D., Salovey, P., & Caruso, D. (2000). Emotional intelligence. In R. J. Sternberg (Ed.), *Handbook of intelligence* (pp. 396–421). New York: Cambridge University Press.

McClelland, D. C. (1985). *Human motivation.* New York: Scott, Foresman.

McClelland, D. C., Atkinson, J. W., Clark, R. A., & Lowell, E. L. (1976). *The achievement motive.* New York: Irvington.

Neisser, U. (Ed.). (1998). *The rising curve.* Washington, DC: American Psychological Association.

Nuñes, T. (1994). Street intelligence. In R. J. Sternberg (Ed.), *Encyclopedia of human intelligence* (Vol. 2, pp. 1045–1049). New York: Macmillan.

Okagaki, L., & Sternberg, R. J. (1993). Parental beliefs and children's school performance. *Child Development, 64,* 36–56.

Petrill, S. A. (2002). The case for general intelligence: A behavioral genetic perspective. In R. J. Sternberg & E. L. Grigorenko (Eds.), *The general factor of intelligence: How general is it?* (pp. 281–298). Mahwah, NJ: Erlbaum.

Salovey, P., & Mayer, J. D. (1990). Emotional intelligence. *Imagination, Cognition, and Personality, 9,* 185–211.

Serpell, R. (2000). Intelligence and culture. In R. J. Sternberg (Ed.), *Handbook of intelligence* (pp. 549–580). New York: Cambridge University Press.

Sternberg, R. J. (1985). *Beyond IQ: A triarchic theory of human intelligence.* New York: Cambridge University Press.

Sternberg, R. J. (1986). *Intelligence applied.* Orlando, FL: Harcourt Brace College.

Sternberg, R. J. (1988). *The triarchic mind: A new theory of human intelligence.* New York: Viking-Penguin.

Sternberg, R. J. (1990). *Metaphors of mind.* New York: Cambridge University Press.

Sternberg, R. J. (1994). Cognitive conceptions of expertise. *International Journal of Expert Systems: Research and Application, 7,* 1–12.

Sternberg, R. J. (1997). *Successful intelligence.* New York: Plume.

Sternberg, R. J. (1999). The theory of successful intelligence. *Review of General Psychology, 3,* 292–316.

Sternberg, R. J. (Ed.). (2000). *Handbook of intelligence.* New York: Cambridge University Press.

Sternberg, R. J., & Ben-Zeev, T. (2001). *Complex cognition: The psychology of human thought.* New York: Oxford University Press.

Sternberg, R. J., Ferrari, M., Clinkenbeard, P. R., & Grigorenko, E. L. (1996). Identification, instruction, and assessment of gifted children: A construct validation of a triarchic model. *Gifted Child Quarterly, 40,* 129–137.

Sternberg, R. J., Forsythe, G. S., Hedlund, J., Horvath, J., Snook, S., Williams, W. M., Wagner, R. K., &

Grigorenko, E. L. (2000). *Practical intelligence in everyday life*. New York: Cambridge University Press.

Sternberg, R. J., & Grigorenko, E. L. (1998). *Measuring common sense for the work place*. Unpublished manuscript.

Sternberg, R. J., & Grigorenko, E. L. (2000). *Teaching for successful intelligence*. Arlington Heights, IL: Skylight Training and Publishing.

Sternberg, R. J., & Grigorenko E. L. (Eds.). (2001). *Environmental effects on cognitive abilities*. Mahwah, NJ: Erlbaum.

Sternberg, R. J., & Grigorenko, E. L. (2002a). *Dynamic testing*. New York: Cambridge University Press.

Sternberg, R. J., & Grigorenko, E. L. (Eds.). (2002b). *The general factor of intelligence: How general is it?* Mahwah, NJ: Erlbaum.

Sternberg, R. J., Grigorenko, E. L., Ferrari, M., & Clinkenbeard, P. (1999). A triarchic analysis of an aptitude–treatment interaction. *European Journal of Psychological Assessment*, 15(1), 1–11.

Sternberg, R. J., & Kolligian, J., Jr. (Eds.). (1990). *Competence considered*. New Haven, CT: Yale University Press.

Sternberg, R. J., & Lubart, T. I. (1995). *Defying the crowd: Cultivating creativity in a culture of conformity*. New York: Free Press.

Sternberg, R. J., & Lubart, T. I. (1996). Investing in creativity. *American Psychologist*, 51, 677–688.

Sternberg, R. J., Nokes, K., Geissler, P. W., Prince, R., Okatcha, F., Bundy, D. A., et al. (2001). The relationship between academic and practical intelligence: A case study in Kenya. *Intelligence*, 29, 401–418.

Sternberg, R. J., & Rifkin, B. (1979). The development of analogical reasoning processes. *Journal of Experimental Child Psychology*, 27, 195–232.

Sternberg, R. J., & Spear-Swerling, L. (1996). *Teaching for thinking*. Washington, DC: American Psychological Association Books.

Sternberg, R. J., Torff, B., & Grigorenko, E. L. (1998a). Teaching for successful intelligence raises school achievement. *Phi Delta Kappan*, 79, 667–669.

Sternberg, R. J., Torff, B., & Grigorenko, E. L. (1998b). Teaching triarchically improves school achievement. *Journal of Educational Psychology*, 90, 1–11.

Sternberg, R. J., Wagner, R. K., & Okagaki, L. (1993). Practical intelligence: The nature and role of tacit knowledge in work and at school. In H. Reese & J. Puckett (Eds.), *Advances in lifespan development* (pp. 205–227). Hillsdale, NJ: Erlbaum.

Sternberg, R. J., Wagner, R. K., Williams, W. M., & Horvath, J. A. (1995). Testing common sense. *American Psychologist*, 50, 912–927.

Wiedl, K. H., Guthke, J., & Wingenfeld, S. (1995). Dynamic assessment in Europe: Historical perspectives. In J. S. Carlson (Ed.), *Advances in cognition and educational practice* (Vol. 3, pp. 33–82). Greenwich, CT: JAI Press.

CHAPTER 3

&

An Implicit Motive Perspective on Competence

OLIVER C. SCHULTHEISS
JOACHIM C. BRUNSTEIN

In this chapter, we approach the competence construct from the perspective of a person's motive dispositions. We first provide a short review of how nonconscious (i.e., implicit) motives differ from self-attributed (i.e., explicit) motives in terms of measurement, operating characteristics, and predictive validity. We then turn to approach and avoidance aspects of implicit achievement motivation, portray some key measures of implicit achievement motivation, review how achievement motivation is formed through mastery experiences in early childhood, and discuss how implicit achievement motivation is related to the effectiveness, success, and ability aspects of competence. In closing, we make the case for the concept of motivational competence, that is, the ability to make one's explicit and implicit motives congruent.

IMPLICIT AND SELF-ATTRIBUTED MOTIVES

When examining the role of achievement motivation in the development and expression of competence, it is important to keep in mind that motives can be assessed in two fundamentally different ways that tap different constructs and predict different types of outcomes. When McClelland, Atkinson, Clark, and Lowell (1953) started their pioneering work, published as *The Achievement Motive*, their research was based on the premise that people may have no or only very limited insight into what motivates their behavior (cf. McClelland, 1984; see also LeDoux, 2002; Wilson, 2002). McClelland and colleagues (1953) therefore decided to assess motivational dispositions indirectly by analyzing fantasy stories written in response to ambiguous picture cues akin to Morgan and Murray's (1935) Thematic Apperception Test instead of asking participants directly about their level of achievement motivation. The story-coding approach (which eventually became known as the Picture Story Exercise, or PSE, technique) turned out to be a sensitive and valid measure of achievement motivation: It responded strongly to experimental arousal of achievement motivation (e.g., through success feedback, failure feedback, or a combination of both) on various performance tasks, and it predicted achievement-related behaviors such as number of anagrams solved or arithmetic operations completed. Based on their findings, McClelland et al. (1953) defined the achievement motive as a recurrent need to improve one's skills and do well according to a standard of excellence, and this need is manifested in PSE stories as themes of (1) competing with a standard of excellence, (2) unique accomplishments, and (3) long-term involvement in achievement goals. This PSE measure of achievement motivation was termed need (or n) Achievement.

Because doubts were raised about the PSE motive measure's reliability and validity (e.g., Entwisle, 1972; Lazarus, 1961; but see Atkinson, 1981) and also because picture story assessment of implicit motives is comparatively laborious, other researchers developed questionnaires aimed at tapping into the same motive dispositions as the PSE. For instance, the widely used Personality Research Form (PRF; Jackson, 1984) contains an achievement scale, with items such as "I will not be satisfied until I am the best in my field of work" or "My goal is to do at least a little bit more than anyone else has done before," which, at face value, assess a concern with excellence and achievement that is very similar to what McClelland et al. (1953) described as the core of achievement motivation. Other prominent achievement motivation questionnaires include the Mehrabian Achievement Risk Preference Scale (Mehrabian, 1968), which measures the behavioral correlates of high achievement motivation identified in work with the n Achievement measure, and Gjesme and Nygard's (1970) Achievement Motivation Scale, which gauges individuals' affective responses to achievement successes and failures.

In light of the immense care that researchers have taken to construct questionnaire measures of achievement motivation that closely correspond to the contents and correlates of the original n Achievement coding system, it is particularly striking that across hundreds of studies over the years, questionnaire and PSE motive measures have shown little to no variance overlap. For instance, Spangler (1992) found in a meta-analysis of studies using questionnaire- and PSE-based measures of achievement motivation that the former shared less than 3% variance with the latter. This means that individuals' n Achievement scores are essentially independent of their endorsement of achievement-oriented statements on questionnaire measures of achievement motivation. Common responses by proponents of either measurement approach have included glossing over the lack of overlap between questionnaires and the PSE, ignoring the "other" measure, or questioning its reliability and validity. We agree with Koestner and McClelland's (1990) view that it has been a mistake to call by the same name (i.e., "achievement motive") two measures that show no substantial overlap with each other, because this erroneously suggests that both represent the same underlying construct (for related arguments, see also Kagan, 1994), and that a more straightforward interpretation of the lacking overlap is to assume that the measures tap two qualitatively different types of motivation. This view was further elaborated by McClelland, Koestner, and Weinberger (1989), who posited that two different types of motives coexist within the person: *implicit* motives, which operate nonconsciously and are captured by the PSE, and *self-attributed* (or *explicit*) motives, which reflect facets of a person's language-based, consciously accessible self-concept and can be assessed with self-report measures.

McClelland et al. (1989) also specified the sources of implicit and explicit motives, the types of incentives implicit and explicit motives respond to, and the classes of behavior they affect most strongly. Implicit motives are hypothesized to be based on affective preferences, that is, on the capacity to experience the consummation of a motive-specific incentive as rewarding and pleasurable (cf. Brunstein, Schultheiss & Grässmann, 1998; McClelland et al., 1953). This capacity is at the core of three major functions of implicit motives: They *select*, *orient*, and *energize* behavior (McClelland, 1987). Through processes of Pavlovian, instrumental, and episodic learning, cues, behaviors, and contexts that were associated with pleasurable incentive attainment are learned and retained (selecting function; cf. Schultheiss & Rohde, 2002; Woike, 1995). Cues and contexts that have been associated with incentive attainment in turn are more likely to capture the individual's attention in the future (orienting function; cf. Atkinson & Walker, 1958) and to invigorate behaviors aimed at reinstating the rewarding goal state (energizing function; cf. McClelland et al., 1953; Schultheiss & Brunstein, 1999). Implicit motives' effect on learning, attentional orienting, and behavioral energization is automatic and neither represented in nor ruled by conscious awareness. This is why the PSE, which taps into the cues and contexts that automatically arouse motivation, as well as the behaviors that aim at incentive attainment (Heckhausen, 1991), is more suitable for assessing implicit motives than self-report instruments.

McClelland et al. (1989) hypothesized that explicit motives, in contrast, are linked to the goals and expectations that are normative for a particular group (e.g., family, peers, society) and that thus focus the individual's decisions and behaviors on what the group deems important and desirable. To some extent, explicit motives may also arise from the individual observing her or his own behavior (e.g., "I get straight As; therefore, I must be achievement-motivated") or feedback from others about their perceptions of one's own behavior (cf. Kagan, 1994; Schultheiss & Brunstein, 2002). Explicit motives are part of the individual's self-related, verbally represented knowledge and can be assessed through self-report. According to McClelland et al. (1989), explicit motives guide voluntary goal setting and thus can either channel the expression of implicit motives into certain contexts and behaviors or even override motivational impulses, which increases both the flexibility and the stability of human behavior beyond what is feasible for other species (e.g., going to the dentist despite one's knowledge of what will happen there, or learning for an exam despite the lure of a night at the movies with one's friends; cf. Muraven, Tice, & Baumeister, 1998; Schultheiss, 2001a). Thus, a crucial difference between implicit and explicit motives is that the former *motivate* and the latter *channel* (or *regulate*) goal-directed behavior.

Implicit and explicit motives also differ in the types of incentive cues to which they respond. McClelland et al. (1989) have argued that implicit motives respond to task-intrinsic (or activity) incentives, that is, to the pleasure of working on a challenging task, in the case of achievement motivation. Explicit motives, in contrast, respond to social-extrinsic incentives, that is, to salient external demands and social norms as reflected in, for instance, an experimenter's instructions or others' performance on a task. Thus, a person who scores high on a questionnaire measure of achievement motivation should be particularly sensitive to instructions highlighting the importance of excellent performance on a task (a demand) or how well others have done on a similar task (a social norm). Recent research also suggests that implicit motives, including the achievement motive, are more likely to respond to nonverbal incentive cues than to verbal–symbolic stimuli (cf. Klinger, 1967; Schultheiss, 2001a; Schultheiss & Brunstein, 1999, 2002).

Finally, implicit and explicit motives influence different types of behavior. McClelland et al. (1989) have argued that implicit motives affect operant behavior, that is, behavior that occurs spontaneously and without elicitation by any identifiable stimulus, whereas explicit motives generate respondent behavior, that is, behavior that is displayed in response to identifiable stimuli. While we are not ruling out that behavior driven by implicit motives can occur spontaneously, McClelland et al.'s distinction is, in our view, contradicted by the empirical finding that implicit motives are differentially responsive to different, clearly identifiable stimuli (as can be most clearly seen on the PSE; cf. Schultheiss & Brunstein, 2001) and is also at odds with the notion that motives operate in part by learning to associate specific cues with incentive attainment, and by orienting attention to such incentive cues. We therefore offer an alternative distinction that we deem to be more valid and heuristically fruitful. We suggest that implicit motives are particularly likely to show an effect on *procedural* measures of motivation (i.e., measures that tap a person's know-how in operating on his or her environment), whereas explicit motives and goals have a stronger influence on *declarative* measures of motivation (i.e., measures that assess a person's self-related "knowing that," or her or his attitudes, judgments, and decisions; cf. deCharms, Morrison, Reitman, & McClelland, 1955).

Let us illustrate the difference between implicit and explicit motives, the incentives they respond to, and the types of behavior they affect with a recent study by Brunstein and Hoyer (2002). In this experiment, 88 students first completed a PSE measure (implicit) and a questionnaire measure (explicit) of achievement motivation, and then worked on a mental concentration task that required them to respond as quickly as possible to various stimuli presented on a computer screen. After each block of stimulus presentations, they received graphical feedback about their performance (1) relative to their performance on a previous block (self-

referenced feedback) and (2) relative to the performance of "previous participants" (norm-referenced feedback). Direction of performance feedback (ascending or descending, relative to one's own previous performance or others' performance) was varied independently for self- and norm-referenced feedback. After the sixth block of the mental concentration task, participants could decide whether they wanted to continue or switch to a different task, unrelated to achievement. Dependent variables were participants' average response time (reflecting energization and thus representing a procedural measure of motivation) and their decision to continue the mental concentration task (a declarative measure of motivation).

Results revealed that implicit and explicit measures of achievement motivation not only had little overlap ($r = .08$), but that they also predicted different outcomes in response to different incentive cues. As depicted in Figure 3.1 (Panel A), implicit achievement motivation, in conjunction with self-referenced feedback, was a significant predictor of response speed. After baseline response speed was controlled for, high

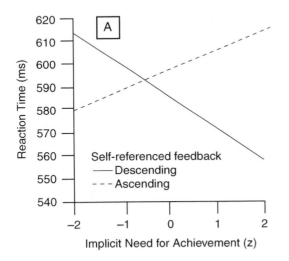 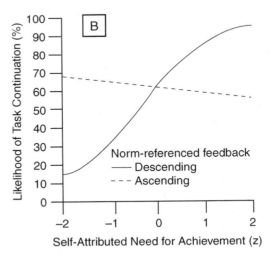

FIGURE 3.1. Effects of implicit and self-attributed achievement motives on procedural and declarative measures of motivation. Panel A: Joint effect of self-referenced feedback and *n* Achievement (PSE) on students' response speed. A descending pattern of self-referenced feedback sped up response latencies of students high in *n* Achievement. Panel B: Joint effect of norm-referenced feedback and the self-attributed achievement motive (values questionnaire) on students' task continuation. Students high in the self-attributed achievement motive were most likely to continue with the test task if they were exposed to a descending pattern of norm-referenced feedback. Adapted from Brunstein and Hoyer (2002, p. 58). Copyright 2002 by Verlag Hans Huber. Adapted by permission.

3. Implicit Motives and Competence

levels of *n* Achievement were predictive of significantly faster response times after feedback indicating performance decreases (*pr* = −.33) than after feedback indicating performance increases (*pr* = .27). However, implicit achievement motivation failed to predict, either by itself or in interaction with self-referenced or norm-referenced feedback, participants' decision to continue with the task, which depended on their explicit achievement motivation and norm-referenced feedback. As shown in Panel B of Figure 3.1, under conditions of descending norm-referenced feedback, participants who considered themselves to be achievement-motivated were much more likely to continue the task than individuals who did not place much value on achievement (*r* = .46). In the presence of ascending norm-referenced feedback, explicit achievement motivation had no detectable impact on task continuation (*r* = −.05). Importantly, explicit achievement motivation, either by itself or in interaction with the feedback variables, did not predict participants' response speed.

These findings support McClelland et al.'s (1989) basic claims: First, not only do implicit motive measures show little overlap with explicit motive measures but they also respond to different kinds of incentive cues and affect different kinds of behavior. And second, implicit motives are the primary source of motivational energy, whereas explicit motives serve a predominantly regulatory or channeling function for behavior. Note that the latter claim can only be tested in a straightforward fashion in studies that, like Brunstein and Hoyer's (2002), employ measures of both implicit and explicit motives, that vary incentive cues independently for implicit and explicit motives, and, most importantly, that allow one to distinguish between motivational and decisional aspects of behavior at the dependent-variable level. Where these conditions have been fulfilled in past research, findings very similar to those of Brunstein and Hoyer were obtained (e.g., Biernat, 1989; deCharms et al., 1955).

In the following sections dealing with the link between achievement motivation and competence, we focus our discussion on findings obtained with *implicit motive measures*, because, consistent with McClelland et al.'s (1989) model of motivation, we consider implicit motives to provide the primary

source of motivational energy for the actual development of competence, whereas explicit motives are more likely to serve a channeling role and to determine in which life domain a person seeks to become competent (cf. French & Lesser, 1964). In addition, the relationship between explicit achievement motivation and competence has received extensive coverage in recent reviews (e.g., Bong & Skaalvik, 2003; Spence, 1983; Zanobini & Usai, 2002), whereas reviews dealing specifically with implicit achievement motivation are comparatively scarce (for the most recent exception, see Koestner & McClelland, 1990) and the topic therefore deserves a fresh look.

APPROACH AND AVOIDANCE MODES OF ACHIEVEMENT MOTIVATION

As soon as the original *n* Achievement scoring system was developed, it was noted that there are two aspects to achievement motivation, hope of success (HS) and fear of failure (FF), that show up in subtle differences in achievement imagery on PSE stories, as well as in behavior observed in the laboratory and the field (Clark, Teevan, & Ricciuti, 1958; McClelland et al., 1953). However, it seems to us that researchers never fully came to grips with the double-facedness of achievement motivation and particularly with the nature of its fear-of-failure component (but see Elliot & Covington, 2001). Before we go on to describe the measures that have been developed to assess HS and FF, the problems associated with them, and some of the findings obtained with them, we therefore first take a closer look at issues of approach and avoidance within the domain of implicit achievement motivation.

We believe that it is informative to examine approach and avoidance motivation within a learning psychology framework. In the following, we consider the simplified case that an individual either does or does not display a goal-directed behavior (e.g., a rat pressing a bar or a human showing achievement-related behavior), and that the individual can either be punished (e.g., by foot shock or social disapproval) or rewarded (e.g., by food or warmth and praise) as a consequence, which yields the four motivational modes depicted in Table 3.1. With the exception of the case that an organism is rewarded for doing nothing (which rarely happens and goes against the grain of phylogenetic learning and the brain's incentive-seeking systems; cf. Panksepp, 1998), we consider each, starting with the case of active approach and moving clockwise through Table 3.1.

The most straightforward case is that a goal-directed behavior is displayed and leads to contact with a positive incentive, which will make the behavior more likely to be emitted in similar future situations. The motivational mode induced by this contingency is *active approach*, and the paradigmatic example from the learning psychologist's laboratory is the rat that learns that pressing a bar in the presence of certain discriminative stimuli (e.g., a red light) will provide access to food. After the initial association between bar pressing, discriminative stimulus, and food has been formed, the rat will press the bar more frequently and vigorously in the future, provided that the proper discriminative cues are present. In the case of a human who for the first time tackles a challenging task (the paradigmatic example from the achievement motivation literature), success-

ful mastery of the task may already provide a sense of satisfaction by itself and hence be rewarding. As we discuss later, there is also evidence that warmth and praise for a task well done can have rewarding value. In either case, the person will form a HS motive, which makes him or her more likely to seek out and try to master challenging tasks in the future. As in the animal experiment, discriminative stimuli typically come to play a pivotal role. If the original mastery experience occurred in the context of solving a puzzle, the person will be more likely to seek further mastery experiences in other puzzles; if it was learning a piece on the piano, then other piano pieces are particularly promising candidates for further mastery experiences. Over time and through stimulus generalization, the person may extend her or his HS motive to other tasks and situations. This should not blind us to the fact, however, that some activities and situations (e.g., working on a challenging task) will always be more suitable than others (e.g., watching TV) for achieving a sense of mastery and thus more likely to be included in the learning process.

It is noteworthy that the active approach mode of achievement motivation, HS, seems to be supported by what Gray (1971) has

TABLE 3.1. Comparison of Effects of Reward and Punishment on Motivation and Behavioral Changes in Animal Learning Studies and on the Development of Achievement Motivation in Humans

Behavior	Contingency	
	Reward	Punishment
Displayed	Active approach	Passive avoidance
	Behavior displayed more frequently	Behavior suppressed
	Rat presses bar to get food	Rat stops bar pressing to avoid shock
	Person works on challenging tasks to get praise, mastery satisfaction	Person stops working on challenging tasks to avoid negative consequences (e.g., ridicule, disrupted relationships)
	Achievement motive: hope of success	Achievement motive: low (fear of success)
	Mesolimbic dopamine system	Septohippocampal system
Not displayed	(passive approach)	Active avoidance
		Behavior displayed more frequently
		Rat presses bar to avoid shock
		Person works on challenging tasks to avoid negative consequences (e.g., scolding for dependency, lack of effort)
		Achievement motive: fear of failure
		Mesolimbic dopamine system

termed the Behavioral Approach System (BAS), which is rooted in the mesolimbic–mesocortical dopamine system and its structures (e.g., the nucleus accumbens), and initiates behavioral activation and approach behavior upon contact with stimuli predicting reward. Evidence for a connection between the BAS and HS comes from a study by Bäumler (1975), who administered a dopamine agonist, which increases dopamine transmission in, and thus activates, the BAS, to one group of participants, a dopamine antagonist, which decreases dopamine transmission in, and thus deactivates, the BAS, to another group, and a placebo to a third group. He then administered a PSE to all participants and analyzed their stories for HS imagery with Heckhausen's (1963) coding system, which allows separation of HS and FF imagery (see below). Bäumler found that stories written by participants in the dopamine agonist condition contained the most HS imagery, stories written by placebo condition participants contained medium levels of HS imagery, and stories written by participants in the dopamine antagonist condition contained the least HS imagery. This suggests that the approach mode of achievement motivation is mediated in part by a brain system whose role in various types of approach motivation (e.g., food, sex, affiliation) has been thoroughly studied and documented in mammals (for an overview, see Panksepp, 1998).

Moving on to the next quadrant of Table 3.1, we find the case that the display of a goal-directed specific behavior is followed by punishment, which decreases the occurrence of the behavior in the future and thus describes the motivational mode of *passive avoidance*, in which an organism tries to dodge negative incentives by inhibiting a behavior. The paradigmatic illustration from the learning laboratory is the rat that learns to stop bar pressing in the presence of specific discriminatory stimuli, because bar pressing then reliably produces foot shock. The parallel example for the domain of achievement motivation in humans would be the case of a person encountering negative consequences after successfully mastering a task (e.g., ridicule or jealousy and resentment by others). As a consequence, the person's motivation to try similar challenging tasks in the future will be reduced and he

or she may come to suppress the impulse to achieve and master, particularly when faced with achievement-related cues. Thus, the person should be motivated by a fear of success (FS). In the PSE, this fear should be evident in a peculiar absence of achievement-related imagery, particularly in response to pictures that typically elicit at least a moderate amount of achievement fantasies. In other words, FS is the antimotive of HS, and a person can either be high in one or the other, but not both. In support of this notion, Karabenick (1977) found that individuals whose PSE stories were largely devoid of achievement imagery scored high on Horner's (cf. Horner & Fleming, 1992) FS measure, which codes for a preoccupation with negative consequences of one's actions, the maintenance of harmonious relationships with others, relief from anxiety, and a general absence of any competent instrumental activity toward the attainment of a goal. Although little is known about the brain substrates associated with FS, we would tentatively identify this mode of achievement motivation with Gray's (1971) Behavioral Inhibition System, a brain network that responds with the inhibition of behavior to stimuli predicting punishment.

The third and final quadrant of theoretical interest presents the case in which the absence of a particular behavior results in punishment, which increases the likelihood that the behavior is displayed in the future. The motivational mode associated with this kind of learning is one of *active avoidance*, in which the individual tries to cope proactively with an imminent threat. To the extent that one's goal-directed behavior reliably eliminates the occurrence of the punishment, active avoidance can be a particularly stable mode of dealing with specific situations, as animal experiments show. For instance, Solomon and Wynne (1953) trained dogs to jump from one compartment to another as soon as a stimulus signaling impending foot shock appeared. Remarkably, most dogs not only learned to avoid shock by jumping to the safe compartment within very few trials but also were amazingly resistant to extinction: Some continued to traverse over to the safe compartment upon presentation of the warning signal for more than 600 trials! Equally remarkably, they quickly ceased to show any sign of fear after they had learned how to cope with the threat of shock. For these and many similar findings, Gray (1971) has offered the following explanation: The stimulus associated with nonshock (e.g., the safe compartment in Solomon and Wynne's study) takes on the meaning of a *safety signal* that has a *rewarding* effect on avoidance behavior. And as long as the safety signal remains associated with the absence of punishment, it does not lose its validity and thus retains its rewarding effects. Indeed, there is also strong, but often overlooked, evidence that the mesolimbic–mesocortical dopamine system, where Gray localizes the BAS, is activated by stressors, but only if the organism can cope with them through active behavior (i.e., behavior that helps bring about safety and relief) and not if they require suppression of behavior (i.e., passive avoidance; cf. Salamone, 1994).

What does this mean for the active avoidance mode of achievement motivation? We would argue that individuals who have been punished (e.g., through criticism or parental disapproval) for not taking on or failing to master a challenging task will learn to master the challenge in order to avoid similar punishments in the future. In the process, the successful mastery of the task acquires the properties of a rewarding safety signal, which should maintain the person's motivation to achieve as long as it remains associated with the absence of punishment. As a consequence, FF should give rise to observable achievement-oriented behavior, both in the real world and in the form of scorable achievement imagery in PSE stories. Thus, individuals high in FF should share with individuals high in HS a preference for mastery experiences, although for different reasons and through sometimes different behavioral means and strategies. It seems noteworthy in this context that Bäumler (1975) found that dopamine antagonists, which decrease BAS activation, also reduce the amount of FF imagery in participants' PSE stories relative to the placebo group, which is exactly what we would predict based on Gray's model and our suggestion that the pleasure of mastery (HS) and the relief that comes with mastery (FF) should both elicit approach motivation. Thus, unlike fear of success, FF and HS are functionally compatible, because both have as their

goal the mastery of challenging tasks, but we also predict that they should represent largely independent constructs, because different kinds of learning experiences (reward for mastery or punishment for failure to master a task) give rise to them.

In summary, then, we argue that achievement motivation has one approach mode but two fundamentally different avoidance modes (active and passive). In the remainder of this chapter, we conceive of HS as a motive to get pleasure by mastering a challenging task, FF as a motive to gain relief from punishment by mastering a challenge, and FS as a motive to avoid challenging tasks and the cues associated with them altogether. Based on the findings we have sketched out, we expect HS to produce in PSE stories imagery related to wanting, and working toward, success at challenging tasks, FF to produce imagery related to wanting and working to avoid failure at challenging tasks, and FS to be marked by the absence of achievement imagery in response to achievement-related picture cues. Thus, our view of avoidance in the context of achievement motivation is very similar to Heckhausen's (1986): "The fear-of-failure motive has turned out to have a double- or even multi-faceted nature—to say the least. One facet is coping- and approach-oriented, the other fearful and avoiding" (p. 13). In the following we provide a short review of measures of avoidance modes of achievement motivation that have been developed by researchers working in the field of implicit motives and evaluate them on the basis of our approach–avoidance framework.

MEASURES OF THE AVOIDANCE MODES OF ACHIEVEMENT MOTIVATION

One of the first systematic attempts to assess HS and achievement avoidance motivation separately was made by Atkinson and his colleagues, who used McClelland et al.'s (1953) original *n* Achievement measure to assess a person's tendency to approach success, and Mandler and Sarason's (1952) Test Anxiety Questionnaire (TAQ) to assess the person's tendency to avoid failure. Because Atkinson conceived of this avoidance tendency as passive avoidance and thus the mirror image of HS in its effects on task choice and behavior (cf. Atkinson & Birch, 1970), he often used a measure of the difference between participants' *n* Achievement scores and their TAQ scores in his research. Heckhausen (1986) had the following to say about this approach:

> Even more disquieting is the habit of American researchers to use the Test Anxiety Questionnaire (Mandler & Sarason, 1952), or one of its equivalents, as the fear-of-failure component in the resultant motive equation of hope-of-success minus fear-of-failure. Because test anxiety is indicative of self-perceived lower or inadequate ability, the fear-of-failure component in most American research is contaminated with perceived low ability, as Nicholls (1984) has rightly pointed out. This contamination might by itself devalue a large part of the risk-taking literature. (p. 13)

And Covington and Roberts (1994) remarked about the frequent use of hope–fear difference measures in Atkinson's research:

> Not only does this treatment of data disregard the possibility of conflicting tendencies, but it also renders ambiguous the meaning of the zero point midway between high avoidance and high approach. Does it represent the complete absence of motivation or simply the result of canceling two extreme motives? Obviously genuine indifference is not the same, psychologically, as apparent indifference in which placidity may mask extreme and opposite forces held in uneasy check. (p. 161)

We agree with Heckhausen's (1986) and Covington and Roberts's (1994) judgments about the problems associated with Atkinson's approach and would only add that by today's state of knowledge about the fundamental differences between implicit and explicit measures of motivation, the calculation of a difference score between a PSE measure and a questionnaire measure represents a forced marriage between incommensurable assessment instruments (see also Heckhausen, 1991).

A second approach to the assessment of fear of failure was presented by Birney, Burdick and Teevan (1969) in the form of a scoring system for Hostile Press (HP). The HP measure was developed based on arousal studies in which participants were frustrated in a variety of tasks such as public speaking,

dart throwing, or speed reading. Many of these tasks involved performance in front of a group or under the scrutiny of an "expert" and thus created a situation in which participants' performance was socially evaluated. Compared to PSE stories written under control conditions, stories written under what Birney et al. described as fear-of-failure conditions were characterized by themes of criticism for one's actions, legal or judicial retaliation for one's actions, deprivation of affiliative relationships, vague environmental threats, and assaults on one's well-being. Thus, stories written under aroused conditions did not directly express any fear of failure, but instead portrayed the environment as exerting hostile pressure and threatening a person's self-esteem. The HP measure was validated extensively (cf. Birney et al., 1969). The following findings emerged from the validation studies: First, HP correlates slightly negatively with McClelland et al.'s (1953) original *n* Achievement measure. Second, high-HP individuals avoid achievement situations if they can but work very hard to do well if they cannot avoid an achievement situation (as reflected by the consistently better grades of high-HP students at all age levels). Third, high-HP individuals are more likely to bend to group pressure and are less likely to play competitive games against other individuals. Thus, HP seems to capture both passive avoidance (shunning achievement situations; low *n* Achievement scores) and active avoidance (working hard to do well on achievement tasks) aspects of achievement motivation. Another ambiguity of the HP system results from the measure's substantial overlap with *n* Affiliation, particularly its fear-of-rejection aspect and, we suspect, its overlap with *n* Power, because many of the hostile actions of the environment against a story protagonist could also be scored as power imagery. Thus, it remains unclear to what extent the findings obtained with the HP measure represent unique effects of FF (active avoidance) or FS (passive avoidance), and to what extent they could also be explained on the basis of power and affiliation motivation.

The third major attempt to develop a fear-of-failure measure was presented by Heckhausen (1963; see Schultheiss, 2001b, for a translation). Heckhausen tried to overcome several shortcomings of McClelland et al.'s (1953) *n* Achievement measure. First, McClelland et al. noted in their original work that in addition to containing many purely success-oriented scoring categories, the *n* Achievement coding system also captures some aspects of FF (likely due to the failure feedback that these researchers used to arouse achievement motivation in some experimental groups), and that HS and FF should be assessed separately in the further development of measures of achievement motivation. Second, some of the *n* Achievement coding categories (e.g., Nurturing Press) were infrequent and often did not validly discriminate between individuals high and low in achievement motivation. Third, with hindsight, it seems that the original *n* Achievement system also captured some aspects of power motivation (e.g., by scoring imagery related to beating others; cf. Heckhausen, 1963; Winter, 1973), presumably because some of the arousal conditions stressed the importance of leadership ability, and affiliation motivation (by including a scoring category for Nurturing Press, that is, the presence of others who help a story character reach an achievement goal), and that it therefore was not a pure-bred measure of achievement motivation.

Heckhausen (1963) tried to solve these problems in his new coding system by (1) dropping invalid coding categories, (2) narrowing the focus of the coding system to achievement imagery proper and excluding imagery related to power or affiliation, and (3) making the HS–FF distinction the cornerstone of his system. Heckhausen adopted most of the original *n* Achievement scoring categories (need, instrumental activity, goal anticipation, outcome, outcome-related affect), but he defined them separately for HS (wanting to do well on a task) and FF (wanting to avoid failing at a task), and added a social evaluation category to each (praise for success and criticism for failure).

The resulting coding system yields separate scores for HS and FF, and thus allows the study of separate and conjoint effects of both components of achievement motivation on behavior. HS and FF are not substantially correlated with each other, but both are positively correlated with McClelland et al.'s (1953) original *n* Achievement measure (HS more strongly so than FF). The FF measure correlates close to zero with Birney et al.'s

(1969) HP measure, which supports the notion that FF and HP measure different types of fear motivation. Validation studies reported by Heckhausen (1963; see also Heckhausen, 1968, 1991) revealed that both HS and FF were equally predictive of the choice of difficult goals, performance increases on challenging tasks (maze learning), and higher muscle tone, both at rest and during mental activity. Differences between the two components of achievement motivation were also observed: High-FF individuals were more likely to overestimate their successes and to recall completed tasks, whereas high-HS individuals were more likely to overestimate their failures (!) and less likely to remember tasks after they were completed. Thus, Heckhausen's FF measure, which is independent of his HS measure, tends to predict some motivational markers and behaviors that reflect approach toward challenge mastery. The aforementioned results of Bäumler's (1975) pharmacological study also support this conclusion. This suggests that mastering challenging tasks is rewarding not only for high-HS individuals but to some extent also for high-FF individuals, and therefore provides some evidence that, according to our approach–avoidance framework, Heckhausen's FF measure primarily taps the active avoidance mode of achievement motivation. The differences between HS and FF in their influence on estimations of success and failure, and recall of completed tasks, may reflect a greater need for "achievement safety" among high-FF individuals, which contrasts with a greater tolerance for frustrations on the way to success among high-HS individuals. Both may echo differences in the early socialization of implicit achievement motivation, to which we turn next.

DEVELOPMENTAL PRECURSORS OF IMPLICIT ACHIEVEMENT MOTIVATION

Some of the strongest evidence for a role of achievement motivation in competence development comes from research on the developmental antecedents of this motive. Consider the case of 15-year-old Jose, which McClelland et al. (1953) presented in *The Achievement Motive*. Jose grew up with several siblings in a Spanish American family in New Mexico. The conditions of his upbringing were described by a field worker in the following way:

"All the children are going to school. They have to take care of themselves. They cook themselves, take care of each other, clean the house, and keep the place going. The children had to take care of themselves ever since they were little—since the oldest boy was about two or three. . . . They all started working—helping to take care of the cattle and the pigs, milking the cows, and doing all sorts of work such as cleaning the house and cooking—from the age of five or earlier. . . . As soon as they could sit up, which was about three months, they would sit in a chair and eat by themselves. [The mother] said they learned early to eat by themselves. Toilet training began really quite early. They would begin about four months; [she] had a special high chair for them. The oldest boy taught the younger. By five months, he would know where to go and she said it was the same with all the children. By five months they were all trained. . . . The children learned to dress themselves shortly after they were a year old. She would just put their clothes out in a little box near their bed, and they had to dress themselves or else they didn't get dressed." (McClelland et al., 1953, pp. 307–308)

The field worker also collected PSE stories from Jose that were later coded for n Achievement. It was found that Jose had n Achievement levels more than one standard deviation above the mean of his classmates in school, which led McClelland and colleagues to suggest that socialization practices emphasizing early independence, self-reliance, and mastery of skills help to build a strong need for achievement in the child. Subsequent research confirmed this prediction.

McClelland and Pilon (1983) followed up 78 participants of Sears, Maccoby, and Levin's (1957) study on the patterns of child rearing. The participants had been children when Sears and colleagues collected data on how their mothers had raised them during the first 5 years of life, and were in their early 30s when McClelland and Pilon contacted and administered PSEs to them. McClelland and Pilon found that mothers who had been particularly strict when toilet training their infants, or fed their babies on schedule instead of on demand, were consistently more likely to raise children with high n Achievement scores on the PSE than mothers who did not engage in these socialization practices (note that "strictness" referred to punishing and scolding children for mishaps in the study of Sears et al. [1957]; in their sample, the modal age of toilet-training onset was 5 to 9 months, with training usually lasting between 5 and 6 months!). This pattern of maternal strictness resembles the conditions of Jose's upbringing and suggests that the origins of a strong need for achievement and mastery lie in rigid and punitive socialization practices in early childhood.

But there is also another pathway to a strong need for achievement, one that emphasizes reward and affection for the child's mastery and independent accomplishments. Winterbottom (1958) found that mothers of school-age boys high in n Achievement are more likely to report than mothers of low-achievement boys that they use affectionate, nonverbal ways (e.g., hugging, kissing) of commending their sons when they succeed in their mastery- and independence-related efforts. They also report that they made demands for the child's independent accomplishments earlier than mothers of low-achievement boys. In contrast, mothers of boys low in n Achievement were more likely to report that they imposed restrictions on the child's ability to make decisions by himself, and that they curtailed their sons' ability to choose their own friends; in other words, they did not want their children to be independent. Winterbottom did not explicitly report whether these mothers used punishment to restrict their sons' drive toward mastery and independent decision making; but if they did, it would certainly be consistent with our claim that punishment for mastery and independence should lead to passive avoidance of achievement and thus low n Achievement scores on the PSE.

Results from a study by Rosen and D'Andrade (1959) suggest that both punitive and rewarding parenting techniques, as well as the parents' standards and expectations of excellence with regard to their children's performance, may be conducive to high levels of n Achievement in children. Rosen and D'Andrade brought forty 9- to 11-year-old boys and their parents into the lab and observed interactions between the boys and their mothers and fathers, while they were working on a number of problem-solving and performance tasks (e.g., ring-tossing games, anagrams). They found that parents of high-achievement boys were more likely than parents of low-achievement boys to set challenging goals for their sons, to have a higher regard for their problem-solving competence, and, in the case of mothers, to be directive, to reward good performance with affection, but also to punish poor performance with hostility and disapproval.

Taken together, the results from these three studies suggest that parents who emphasize early self-reliance and mastery of basic skills, and who teach their children to "reach higher" and set challenging goals for themselves, have children who are characterized by high levels of achievement motivation. It should be noted, however, that subsequent studies did not provide straightforward evidence for the notion that early independence training per se is conducive to a strong need for achievement in the child (cf. McClelland, 1987, for an overview). Rather, it is *age-appropriate* demands for mastery and independence that foster the child's achievement motivation (McClelland, 1961; Veroff, 1969). For instance, both Reif (1970) and Trudewind (1975; both cited in Heckhausen, 1980) found that children whose mothers had emphasized independence too early were high in FF (Heckhausen measure), and children whose mothers had emphasized self-reliance too late were low in overall achievement motivation (HS + FF) compared to children whose mothers' demands for independence were in tune with the child's budding abilities.

The studies by McClelland and Pilon (1983), Winterbottom (1958), and Rosen and D'Andrade (1959) also suggest that a strong need for achievement may have a dual root in affectionate reward for the mastery of challenging goals and in punishment for failing to meet the parents' (particularly the mother's) expectations for the child to be independent. It remains to be tested, though, whether a relative predominance of rewarding versus punitive parenting strategies are differentially related to the HS and FF aspects of achievement motivation. We believe that it is highly plausible that parental punishment for failure to master challenging tasks specifically enhances an active avoidance orientation of the child's achievement motivation (i.e., FF), which makes the child want to master tasks and skills primarily to avoid, or gain relief from, parental punishment for failure. Conversely, a positively challenging parenting style that uses affectionate reward for the child's mastery of difficult but age-appropriate tasks should nourish in the child a strong need to approach challenges and help the child learn to associate the effort invested in and the accomplishment of a task with satisfaction and pleasure. Some suggestive evidence for an association between parental punitiveness and FF comes from Birney et al.'s (1969) research. They found that mothers of students high in HP were more likely to report that they had punished their sons when they had failed to meet achievement-related demands but had remained neutral about their sons' achievement successes than mothers of students low in HP. However, due to HP's considerable fear-of-rejection component, it is difficult to sort out whether the former mothers had fostered high FF, high fear of rejection, or both in their sons.

MOTIVES AND COMPETENCE

Competence is a multifaceted concept. It can refer to the *skills and abilities* a person has developed, to the degree to which the person is *effective* in her or his transactions with the environment, and to how *successfully* a person performs. In the following, we review how the need for achievement (HS and FF) contributes to all three aspects of competence. Because research on implicit motives has been most prolific when it has studied the strategies that individuals use to effect rewarding changes in the situation or the environment, and when it has looked at the effects of motives on performance results (in the laboratory) and, even more so, career and life outcomes (in the field), we start with the notions of competence-as-effectiveness and competence-as-success, and then work our way back to competence-as-ability.

Competence as Effectiveness

McClelland (1987, p. 595) has argued that achievement-motivated individuals are really concerned with efficiency, that is, with figuring out ways to get more accomplished in less time or with less effort. Research has uncovered several strategies that achievement-motivated individuals use to be efficient. First and foremost, they are attracted to and choose tasks that allow them to improve their performance and skills, which are typically neither the very easy tasks (which they already master) nor the extremely difficult tasks (which overtax their skills and are thus almost impossible to master) but tasks of medium difficulty that challenge their current capabilities but are not unsolvable, and therefore provide an optimally stimulating incentive for them. Evidence for this preference for medium risks is pervasive in the achievement literature. For instance, high-achievement individuals choose intermediate distances from a target in ball-pitching games (Atkinson, Bastian, Earl, & Litwin, 1960), prefer arithmetic tasks of medium difficulty (i.e., with an approximately 50% chance of solving them; deCharms & Carpenter, 1968), and show the highest persistence on challenging tasks (Feather, 1966).

Atkinson (1966) has proposed a theoretical framework for the ∩ shape of high-achievement individuals' choice of medium task difficulty. According to his model, the positive incentive value of success (I) *increases* linearly with difficulty level but is multiplicatively linked to expectancy of success (E), which *decreases* linearly with difficulty level. The product between the two, that is, the resulting tendency to approach or choose tasks of a certain difficulty, will be maximal at medium difficulty levels (e.g., at 50%) but close to zero at minimum or maximum difficulty levels. This product score in turn is multiplicatively weighted by individuals' *n* Achievement (which Atkinson considered to be a measure of HS), and the ∩ shape resulting from I × E will therefore be steeper for high-achievement individuals and closer to a flat line for low-achievement individuals. Thus, HS amplifies a person's tendency to choose medium-difficulty tasks. Atkinson also constructed a parallel case for FF. Here, the negative incentive value of failure *decreases* linearly with difficulty level (it is more embarrassing to fail on an easy task than on a difficult task), while the expectancy of failure *increases* with task difficulty.

If both variables are multiplied, the result is a U-shaped function, in which the choice of medium levels of difficulty produces the strongest tendency to avoid the task. Again, through multiplication with individuals' FF motive, the curve is steeper for high-FF individuals and closer to a flat line for low-FF individuals. Atkinson therefore argued that FF has a dampening effect on behavior that is the exact mirror image of the augmenting effect of HS.

Atkinson's (1966) model was very useful in that it helped lift the achievement motivation construct above the level of "just another personality trait" and generated a huge body of basic and applied research. Like all good theories, however, its limitations were eventually revealed by the data it helped generate. Most crucially, there is surprisingly little evidence for a dampening effect of FF. Rather, deCharms and Dave (1965) found that individuals high in HS and FF (assessed in the PSE with a measure similar to Heckhausen's) were more likely to choose medium difficulty levels and also showed better performance on a ball-pitching game than individuals low in either component of achievement motivation, which contradicts the predictions of the Atkinson model. Moreover, there is little evidence that individuals high in FF are motivated primarily by the negative incentive of failure. In a study with 90 participants that used a carefully constructed measure of the valence of succeeding or failing on a task, Halisch and Heckhausen (1989) found that individuals high in HS *and* individuals high in FF judged succeeding on difficult tasks as more rewarding than did individuals low in these motives. By comparison, they judged failing on difficult tasks as less aversive than did individuals low in either HS or FF. Thus, this study, too, fails to support Atkinson's prediction that failure should be particularly aversive for FF-motivated individuals. Rather, it suggests that both HS and FF predispose an individual to place less emphasis on the prospect of failing at a task than on the prospect of mastering it, which is consistent with the notion that the approach (HS) and active avoidance (FF) components of achievement motivation are both geared toward rewarding–relieving mastery experiences. It is also notable that individuals low in HS or FF were the only ones who perceived the prospect of succeeding at challenging tasks as scarcely attractive, which supports our notion that the passive avoidance mode of achievement motivation is not expressed as a high level of FF, but by a conspicuous absence of achievement themes in participants' PSE stories.

So how, then, can the tendency of achievement-motivated individuals to choose challenging tasks be explained? We believe that the affective–arousal model of achievement motivation proposed by McClelland et al. (1953) provides a better account and can also integrate the FF findings that are incompatible with Atkinson's theory, particularly if their model is integrated with Gray's (1971) notion that relief from punishment and reward are often behaviorally indistinguishable. In a nutshell, the McClelland et al. (1953) model posits that a motive comes into being when a situational cue becomes predictive of a change in a situation and concomitant changes in affective state. For the case of achievement motivation, they posit that deviations from expectation, or moderate uncertainty when tackling a task, is the cue which through previous learning has become associated with the positive affect of mastery and regaining certainty and control at a higher level of complexity or quality. This knowledge (which is emotional, not declarative) inoculates achievement-motivated individuals against the initial frustrations of working on a challenging task and turns the challenge into an opportunity for reward: *per aspera ad astra*, through hardship to new heights (for related arguments, see Eisenberger, 1992). Not surprisingly, they are also better able to delay gratification (Mischel, 1961). Note that McClelland et al.'s (1953) predictions only hold for tasks of subjectively moderate difficulty; at the fringes of the difficulty continuum, high-achievement individuals find very easy tasks boring (perfect predictability, and thus no opportunity for positive affect through mastery) and very difficult tasks aversive (failure is certain; therefore, there is little hope for rewarding mastery). Also note that the association between moderate difficulty and rewarding mastery is something that, according to our previous analysis, characterizes both HS- (approach of the mastery incentive as reward) and FF-motivated individuals (approach of the mastery

incentive as relief from impending punishment) but not individuals low in achievement motivation generally, who have either never come to associate the initial difficulties of solving a challenging task with the subsequent pleasure of mastery or have been punished for mastery and therefore engage in passive avoidance.

In conjunction with Gray's (1971) suggestion that relief equals reward, McClelland et al.'s (1953) theory can therefore account for why HS- and FF-motivated individuals (as assessed with Heckhausen-type measures) both prefer medium-difficulty tasks, judge them as more satisfying, and show superior performance at this difficulty level (deCharms & Dave, 1965; Halisch & Heckhausen, 1989). It also helps explain why achievement-motivated individuals in Brunstein and Hoyer's (2002) study responded with increased effort to feedback indicating a decline in their performance, but not to feedback indicating performance increases. It is only when the cue of moderate task difficulty is present that the prospect of mastery reward comes into play and has a motivating effect on behavior, but not if everything proceeds predictably and smoothly (as in Brunstein and Hoyer's positive feedback condition). In this sense, then, achievement-motivated individuals are really more concerned with efficiency than with excellence for its own sake, as McClelland (1987) argued.

Two other strategies follow almost by necessity from achievement-motivated (HS or FF) individuals' concern with mastering challenging tasks. First, they must have some way of knowing how well they are doing and whether they are improving. In other words, they seek feedback about their performance. In the absence of feedback, individuals high in achievement motivation do not differ in their performance from individuals low in achievement motivation (McClelland, 1987). Achievement-motivated individuals are also discriminating in the type of feedback they seek: They prefer feedback that informs them about how well they are doing now, relative to their own previous performance (i.e., self-referenced feedback), but ignore for the most part feedback about how well they do relative to others' performance (i.e., norm-referenced feedback), because knowledge of others' performance usually does not help them determine whether they improved their skills on a task (Breckler & Greenwald, 1986; Brunstein & Hoyer, 2002; Halisch & Heckhausen, 1989; Horner, 1974; O'Connor, Atkinson, & Horner, 1966; Spangler, 1992; Veroff, 1969; Wendt, 1955; it is notable, however, that individuals with a strong implicit power motive or high levels of explicit achievement motivation do respond to such norm-referenced feedback; see Schultheiss & Brunstein, 1999, Study 2; Tauer & Harackiewicz, 1999). The only exception to the preference for self-referenced over norm-referenced feedback seems to be the special case in which all members of the social comparison group are highly similar in their ability to the achievement-motivated individual seeking feedback, and their performance thus becomes more diagnostic of the individual's own improvement (O'Connor et al., 1966).

Finally, achievement-motivated (HS or FF) individuals also prefer personal responsibility for performance and thus show a greater interest in, and better performance on, tasks that are under their direct control than on tasks whose outcomes depend on chance (e.g., Raynor & Smith, 1966) or other people's performances (e.g., McClelland & Boyatzis, 1982). This preference for personal responsibility is not surprising in light of the parental push for independence that achievement-motivated individuals have been exposed to in childhood and is, of course, a necessary prerequisite for the choice of medium-difficulty tasks and the search for, and availability of, self-referenced feedback. It is probably safe to say that in order to be effective, an achievement-motivated individual has to be able to do all three: choose challenging tasks, get self-referenced information about his or her performance, and have direct personal control over the task outcome. If one of these ingredients is missing, individuals high in achievement motivation will not be more effective than individuals low in achievement motivation.

Competence as Success

Reflecting a general trend in the implicit motive literature, PSE-based achievement motivation measures fared best and produced the most convincing body of data when they were used to predict real-life phenomena and outcomes. This was particularly evident in the domain of entrepreneurship and economic success. McClelland (1961, 1987) has argued that individuals high in n Achievement should do particularly well in a small business, in which all three prerequisites for mastery experiences (personal responsibility, direct feedback, liberty to set and attain challenging goals) are provided. Evidence supporting this prediction comes from research on the effects of achievement motivation on economic success at the individual and at the collective level. For instance, Wainer and Rubin (1969) found that small companies led by high-achievement entrepreneurs had a growth rate 250% higher than those led by entrepreneurs with low or medium levels of n Achievement. This type of finding has been replicated in other cultures and with different types of entrepreneurial behavior (see McClelland, 1961, for an overview). Thus, Singh and Gupta (1977) found that Indian farmers high in n Achievement had a substantially steeper increase of income-per-acre over 6 years than farmers low in n Achievement, suggesting that the former had been more successful in getting the most (or best) output from their farms than the latter.

Effects of high levels of achievement motivation can also be found in life outcome measures, such as income levels and career paths. McClelland and Franz (1992) reported that n Achievement (but not measures of explicit achievement motivation) at age 31 predicted higher annual income at age 41 for both men and women. Because this study's sample was identical with the one originally studied by McClelland and Pilon (1983), McClelland and Franz (1992) could test whether there was a direct link between early parental pressure for the child's independence and mastery, and the "child's" income level at age 41. The correlation between the two variables was positive and significant but dropped to near zero after they controlled for participants' n Achievement levels. Thus, effects of early emphasis on independence on later income were completely mediated by the achievement motivation measure. There is also evidence that achievement motivation and sociocultural values and constraints interact in shaping life outcomes. For instance, Jenkins (1987) reports that women high in *n* Achievement in college are more likely to work as teachers 14 years later. Teaching is a traditionally female career and provides some of the incentives that should be attractive to the high-achievement person: The teacher is personally responsible for creating situations and tasks conducive to student learning, controls the level of task difficulty (both for the teacher and the students), and also gives and receives performance feedback through tests and exams. Thus, just as an entrepreneurial business is a more traditional career path for high-achievement men, teaching appears to be a traditional career path for high-achievement women (see also French & Lesser, 1964).

A meta-analysis conducted by Spangler (1992) on 105 studies provides a more comprehensive evaluation of the effects of implicit achievement motivation on various outcome measures, such as farm output, occupational success, or creative achievements. He found that *n* Achievement was a strong and positive predictor of success at all kinds of tasks, but only if they contained achievement incentives (e.g., if they were challenging, provided objective feedback, and required personal responsibility) and used procedural measures of motivation (i.e., if they provided individuals with an opportunity to apply their know-how and skills). If these conditions were met, correlation coefficients for achievement motivation–outcome relationships could rise as high as .66. If, on the other hand, the criterion measures contained no achievement incentives or were declarative (e.g., measures of attitudes and opinions), correlation coefficients dropped to near zero. Notably, Spangler also found evidence that the wrong kind of incentives can drive achievement-motivated individuals away from good performance and success. In the presence of verbal instructions to do well on a task or experimenter-assigned goals, achievement motivation was a negative predictor of procedural outcome measures. Thus, it looks like achievement-motivated individuals do not like to be told what to do, which is consistent with the socialization pressure toward autonomy and self-reliance they have been exposed to in childhood.

In a very ambitious, successful, and controversial attempt to apply psychological constructs to the explanation of societal, economic, and historical processes, McClelland and colleagues (for an overview, see McClelland, 1987) have used content coding measures developed in implicit motive research to assess motivational needs at the collective level by, for instance, scoring folk tales or children's storybooks representative of a given culture at a certain historic time, and have used these scores to predict indices of economic success within and across nations. Thus, deCharms and Moeller (1962) found that in the 19th century, an increase of levels of *n* Achievement in U.S. children's books preceded an increase in the U.S. patent index by 10 to 30 years. The increase in collective *n* Achievement correlated at .79 with the increase in the patent index, suggesting that societal emphasis of achievement and mastery when a new generation is in childhood (as reflected in the readers) translates into higher innovativeness when that generation reaches adulthood and joins the workforce. Based on findings such as this, McClelland (1961) argued that collective values of self-reliance and achievement translate at the individual level into parenting practices nurturing independence and mastery, which give rise to increased achievement motivation in the next generation, and thus to the high entrepreneurial activity and innovativeness that drive the growth of national economies.

Competence as Ability

Although relatively little is known about whether and how motives are related to a person's skills and abilities, we suggest that the relationship can have two main forms: (1) Motives may have a *causal effect* on the development of skills, because mastery of a skill may put the individual in a better position to obtain a motive-specific incentive and thus satisfy her or his motivational need; (2) motives may *interact* with existing skills in shaping behavior (cf. Atkinson, Lens, & O'Malley, 1976). We primarily rely on examples taken from the literature on power and affiliation motivation to illustrate each point, because, for the most part, research on achievement motivation has not addressed the issue of motives and skills. (We acknowledge that there is a huge body of research documenting the effect of achievement motivation on performance. However, because in these studies learning proper is usually not separated from performance, and it is therefore unclear whether the performance effects are entirely due to the energizing function of motives or in part driven by their selecting function, too, no firm conclusions can be drawn about the effects of achievement motivation on skill development.)

A recent study by Schultheiss and Rohde (2002) documents how motives in conjunction with situational outcomes can help shape procedural skills. Sixty-six men participated in pairs in a speed-based dominance contest whose outcome was experimentally varied by having one participant in each dyad win, and the other lose, most contest rounds. The paper-and-pencil task participants worked on during the contest required them to track consecutive numbers arranged in a matrix as quickly as possible. On half of the forms, the numbers were arranged in a repetitive visuospatial pattern that could be learned procedurally; on the other half, the number connections did not feature any pattern. A measure of procedural learning was obtained by subtracting participants' postcontest performance on patterned forms from their performance on unpatterned forms. Power motivation and contest outcome conjointly determined how well participants learned: Among winners, the power motive correlated .68 with pattern execution and was thus predictive of enhanced procedural learning, whereas in losers, it was correlated −.58 with pattern execution and was thus predictive of impaired procedural learning (this pattern of results was predicted and obtained only for participants low in activity inhibition, a measure of motivational impulse control, and did not emerge for high-inhibition participants). Notably, participants were unable to reproduce or identify the repeating pattern on subsequent free recall and forced-choice recognition tasks, which indicates that procedural learning occurred in the complete absence of participants' awareness of the process. These findings suggest that motives may play a crucial role in procedural learning of behaviors that are instrumental for incentive attainment

(and suppression of behaviors that are associated with motivational disincentives), and thus help build a repertoire of skills that maximize the frequency of incentive contact and, thus, pleasant affective states.

Motives are not involved only in the development of skills; they can also interact with existing skills in shaping goal-directed behavior. McClelland (1987) reported on data from an unpublished study by Constantian (1981), in which a procedural measure of affiliative behavior was obtained by beeping participants randomly and having them report whether they were engaged in affiliative contact (conversing with someone or writing a letter) or not. Participants also provided a measure of perceived social skill on which they indicated how sure and confident they felt when interacting with others. Although participants' n Affiliation (assessed with a PSE) correlated close to zero with their social skill, both measures conjointly predicted the frequency of affiliative acts, such that only individuals who were high both in n Affiliation and social skills frequently interacted with others, but not individuals low in either n Affiliation or social skills. In other words, a skill will only be put to use if the person expects to attain a highly attractive incentive with it (as was the case for the affiliation incentive as perceived by high-affiliation individuals), but not if the person is not motivated to procure the incentive. The flip side of these findings is that even a strong motive will not guarantee incentive attainment (i.e., being engaged in friendly contact with others) unless the person also has the skills to get to the incentive. In the absence of the skills necessary to satisfy a motive, a frustrated motive may become expressed in impulsive, unsophisticated behavior, such as raw aggression or narcissistic fantasies induced by drinking, in the case of power-motivated individuals who have not learned more appropriate forms of having impact since their childhood days (cf. McClelland, 1987; Winter, 1973), or behavioral "short-cuts" to a motivational incentive, such as achievement-motivated individuals' tendency to cheat if they have no other way of demonstrating superior performance (Mischel & Gilligan, 1964). It remains an open question whether a strong motive disposition can survive for long in the absence of skills necessary for incentive attainment or if it will, through learning by frustration and punishment, become weaker over time (cf. McClelland, 1942). The fact, however, that motives aid in the development of instrumental skills, as suggested by Schultheiss and Rohde (2002), indicates that they not only depend on and interact with existing skills, but, in the absence of these, also readily help to build new abilities and competencies.

MOTIVATIONAL COMPETENCE

Let us conclude by returning to what we believe is one of the most interesting and important emerging issues in the field of human motivation: the independence between implicit and explicit motivational systems, their effects on well-being, and the identification of factors and processes that promote harmony between the two systems. Past research shows that implicit motive dispositions not only have little overlap with explicit motives but also seem to have only little (e.g., Elliot & Sheldon, 1997) or no influence on the types of goals individuals choose or develop in their daily lives (e.g., Brunstein et al., 1998). At the same time, however, mismatches between implicit and explicit motives spell trouble, as McClelland et al. (1989) pointed out. We have found some evidence for this prediction in our own research on the effects of motive–goal congruence on emotional well-being (Brunstein et al., 1998): People who pursue goals that match their implicit motives experience increases in emotional well-being when they make good progress in realizing their goals and thus have many opportunities to satisfy their motives, but people who pursue goals that are not backed up by their motives do not derive any emotional satisfaction from the goal's successful realization. On the contrary, they even experience decreases in their well-being, because spending time on the pursuit of motive-incongruent goals takes away time from the pursuit of motive-congruent goals, which leads to motive frustration. It does not take much speculation, then, to see a link between severe or prolonged motive–goal mismatches and clinical states of depression and other mood disorders (cf. Becker, 1960), just as it seems rea-sonable to assume that individuals whose explicit motives are well aligned with their implicit motives, and who consistently choose and pursue motive-congruent goals, are more likely to experience stable and heightened well-being. We therefore believe that it will be fruitful to study and explore motivational competence, that is, an individual's ability to bring and keep his or her implicit and explicit motives into alignment (cf. Rheinberg, 2002). We furthermore suggest that motivational competence can be promoted by flexible processes and strategies, as well as dispositional factors. We obtained considerable evidence for the former in our research on the effects of goal imagery on goal commitment and pursuit (Schultheiss & Brunstein, 1999, 2002). When participants were given a chance to explore an experimenter-assigned goal imaginatively and thus to translate it into the nonverbal format that their implicit motives could process, their willingness to adopt the goal and their efforts to realize it were directly proportional to how well the goal fit their implicit needs; without goal imagery, goal commitment and effort expenditure were independent of their motives. Other studies point to stable dispositions that promote (or inhibit) motive–goal congruence. Brunstein (2001) found that individuals with a particular self-regulatory deficit, namely, the inability to downregulate negative affect after encountering a stressor (cf. Kuhl, 1981), were particularly prone to report personal goals that did not match their motives. In contrast, individuals without this deficit were much more likely to report goals that were well-aligned with their motives. Thrash and Elliot (2002) recently reported that achievement-related implicit and explicit motives are better aligned in individuals who are high in self-determination than in individuals low in this disposition. It is clear that these scattered findings can only be the beginning, and much more work needs to be done, until we have a better sense of what the core constituents of motivational competence are and how this type of competence can be promoted. It is equally clear, though, that finding ways to increase motivational competence will help people gain greater awareness of and access to their implicit motives, and thereby promote the development of motive-specific competencies and well-being.

REFERENCES

Atkinson, J. W. (1966). Motivational determinants of risk-taking behavior. In J. W. Atkinson & N. T. Feather (Eds.), *A theory of achievement motivation* (pp. 11–30). New York: Wiley.

Atkinson, J. W. (1981). Studying personality in the context of an advanced motivational psychology. *American Psychologist, 36,* 117–128.

Atkinson, J. W., Bastian, J. R., Earl, R. W., & Litwin, G. H. (1960). The achievement motive, goal setting, and probability preferences. *Journal of Abnormal and Social Psychology, 60,* 27–36.

Atkinson, J. W., & Birch, D. (1970). *The dynamics of action.* New York: Wiley.

Atkinson, J. W., Lens, W., & O'Malley, P. M. (1976). Motivation and ability: Interactive psychological determinants of intellective performance, educational achievement, and each other. In W. H. Sewell, R. M. Hauser, & D. L. Featherman (Eds.), *Schooling and achievement in American society* (pp. 29–60). New York: Academic Press.

Atkinson, J. W., & Walker, E. L. (1958). The affiliation motive and perceptual sensitivity to faces. In J. W. Atkinson (Ed.), *Motives in fantasy, action, and society: A method of assessment and study* (pp. 360–366). Princeton, NJ: Van Nostrand.

Bäumler, G. (1975). Beeinflussung der Leistungsmotivation durch Psychopharmaka: I. Die 4 bildthematischen Hauptvariablen [The effects of psychoactive drugs on achievement motivation: I. The four motivation scales]. *Zeitschrift für Experimentelle und Angewandte Psychologie, 22,* 1–14.

Becker, J. (1960). Achievement related characteristics of manic–depressives. *Journal of Abnormal and Social Psychology, 60,* 334–339.

Biernat, M. (1989). Motives and values to achieve: Different constructs with different effects. *Journal of Personality, 57,* 69–95.

Birney, R. C., Burdick, H., & Teevan, R. C. (1969). *Fear of failure.* New York: Van Nostrand Reinhold.

Bong, M., & Skaalvik, E. M. (2003). Academic self-concept and self-efficacy: How different are they really? *Educational Psychology Review, 15,* 1–40.

Breckler, S. J., & Greenwald, A. G. (1986). Motivational facets of the self. In R. M. Sorrentino & E. T. Higgins (Eds.), *Handbook of motivation and cognition: Foundations of social behavior* (Vol. 1, pp. 145–164). New York: Guilford Press.

Brunstein, J. C. (2001). Persönliche Ziele und Handlungs- versus Lageorientierung: Wer bindet sich an realistische und bedürfniskongruente Ziele? [Personal goals and action versus state orientation: Who builds a commitment to realistic and need-congruent goals?]. *Zeitschrift für Differentielle und Diagnostische Psychologie, 22,* 1–12.

Brunstein, J. C., & Hoyer, S. (2002). Implizites und explizites Leistungsstreben: Befunde zur Unabhängigkeit zweier Motivationssysteme [Implicit versus explicit achievement strivings: Empirical evidence of the independence of two motivational systems]. *Zeitschrift für Pädagogische Psychologie, 16,* 51–62.

Brunstein, J. C., Schultheiss, O. C., & Grässmann, R. (1998). Personal goals and emotional well-being: The moderating role of motive dispositions. *Journal of Personality and Social Psychology, 75*(2), 494–508.

Clark, R. A., Teevan, R., & Ricciuti, H. N. (1958). Hope of success and fear of failure as aspects of need for achievement. In J. W. Atkinson (Ed.), *Motives in fantasy, action, and society* (pp. 586–595). Princeton, NJ: Van Nostrand.

Covington, M. V., & Roberts, B. W. (1994). Self-worth and college achievement: Motivational and personality correlates. In P. R. Pintrich, D. R. Brown, & C. E. Weinstein (Eds.), *Student motivation, cognition, and learning. Essays in honor of Wilbert J. McKeachie* (pp. 157–187). Hillsdale, NJ: Erlbaum.

deCharms, R., & Carpenter, V. (1968). Measuring motivation in culturally disadvantaged school children. In H. J. Klausmeier & G. T. O'Hearn (Eds.), *Research and development toward the improvement of education.* Madison, WI: Educational Research Services.

deCharms, R., & Dave, P. N. (1965). Hope of success, fear of failure, subjective probability, and risk-taking behavior. *Journal of Personality and Social Psychology, 1,* 558–568.

deCharms, R., & Moeller, G. H. (1962). Values expressed in American children's readers. *Journal of Abnormal and Social Psychology, 64,* 136–142.

deCharms, R., Morrison, H. W., Reitman, W., & McClelland, D. C. (1955). Behavioral correlates of directly and indirectly measured achievement motivation. In D. C. McClelland (Ed.), *Studies in motivation* (pp. 414–423). New York: Appleton–Century–Crofts.

Eisenberger, R. (1992). Learned industriousness. *Psychological Review, 99,* 248–267.

Elliot, A. J., & Covington, M. V. (2001). Approach and avoidance motivation. *Educational Psychology Review, 13,* 73–92.

Elliot, A. J., & Sheldon, K. M. (1997). Avoidance achievement motivation: A personal goals analysis. *Journal of Personality and Social Psychology, 73,* 171–185.

Entwisle, D. R. (1972). To dispel fantasies about fantasy-based measures of achievement motivation. *Psychological Bulletin, 77,* 377–391.

Feather, N. T. (1966). Effects of prior success and failure on expectations of success and subsequent performance. *Journal of Personality and Social Psychology, 3,* 287–298.

French, E. G., & Lesser, G. S. (1964). Some characteristics of the achievement motive in women. *Journal of Abnormal and Social Psychology, 68,* 119–128.

Gjesme, T., & Nygard, R. (1970). *Achievement-related motives: Theoretical considerations and construction of a measuring instrument.* Unpublished manuscript, University of Oslo.

Gray, J. A. (1971). *The psychology of fear and stress.* New York: McGraw-Hill.

Halisch, F., & Heckhausen, H. (1989). Motive-dependent versus ability-dependent valence functions for success and failure. In F. Halisch, J. H. L. van den Bercken, & S. Hazlett (Eds.), *International perspectives on achievement and task motivation* (pp. 51–67). Amsterdam: Swets & Zeitlinger.

Heckhausen, H. (1963). *Hoffnung und Furcht in der Leistungsmotivation* [Hope and fear components of achievement motivation]. Meisenheim am Glan: Anton Hain, Germany.

Heckhausen, H. (1968). Achievement motive research: Current problems and some contributions toward a general theory of motivation. In W. J. Arnold (Ed.), *Nebraska Symposium on Motivation* (Vol. 16, pp. 103–174). Lincoln: University of Nebraska Press.

Heckhausen, H. (1980). *Motivation und Handeln* [Motivation and action] (1st ed.). Berlin: Springer.

Heckhausen, H. (1986). Why some time out might benefit achievement motivation research. In J. H. L. v. d. Bercken, E. E. J. D. Bruyn, & T. C. M. Bergen (Eds.), *Achievement and task motivation* (pp. 7–39). Lisse: Swets & Zeitlinger.

Heckhausen, H. (1991). *Motivation and action.* Berlin: Springer.

Horner, M. (1974). Performance of men in noncompetitive and interpersonal competitive achievement-oriented situations. In J. W. Atkinson & J. O. Raynor (Eds.), *Motivation and achievement* (pp. 237–254). Washington, DC: Winston & Sons.

Horner, M. S., & Fleming, J. (1992). A revised scoring manual for the motive to avoid success. In C. P. Smith (Ed.), *Motivation and personality: Handbook of thematic content analysis* (pp. 190–204). New York: Cambridge University Press.

Jackson, D. N. (1984). *Personality Research Form* (3rd ed.). Port Huron, MI: Sigma Assessment Systems.

Jenkins, S. R. (1987). Need for achievement and women's careers over 14 years: Evidence for occupational structure effects. *Journal of Personality and Social Psychology, 53,* 922–932.

Kagan, J. (1994). *Galen's prophecy.* New York: Westview Press.

Karabenick, S. A. (1977). Fear of success, achievement and affiliation dispositions, and the performance of men and women under individual and competitive conditions. *Journal of Personality, 45,* 117–149.

Klinger, E. (1967). Modeling effects on achievement imagery. *Journal of Personality and Social Psychology, 7,* 49–62.

Koestner, R., & McClelland, D. C. (1990). Perspectives on competence motivation. In L. A. Pervin (Ed.), *Handbook of personality: Theory and research* (pp. 527–548). New York: Guilford Press.

Kuhl, J. (1981). Motivational and functional helplessness: The moderating effect of state versus action orientation. *Journal of Personality and Social Psychology, 40,* 155–170.

Lazarus, R. S. (1961). A substitutive–defensive conception of apperceptive fantasy. In J. Kagan & G. S. Lesser (Eds.), *Contemporary issues in thematic apperceptive methods* (pp. 51–71). Springfield, IL: Thomas.

LeDoux, J. E. (2002). *The synaptic self.* New York: Viking.

Mandler, G., & Sarason, S. B. (1952). A study of anxiety and learning. *Journal of Abnormal and Social Psychology, 47,* 166–173.

McClelland, D. C. (1942). Functional autonomy of motives as an extinction phenomenon. *Psychological Review, 49,* 272–283.

McClelland, D. C. (1961). *The achieving society.* New York: Free Press.

McClelland, D. C. (1984). *Motives, personality, and society: Selected papers.* New York: Praeger.

McClelland, D. C. (1987). *Human motivation.* New York: Cambridge University Press.

McClelland, D. C., Atkinson, J. W., Clark, R. A., & Lowell, E. L. (1953). *The achievement motive.* New York: Appleton–Century–Crofts.

McClelland, D. C., & Boyatzis, R. E. (1982). Leadership motive pattern and long-term success in management. *Journal of Applied Psychology, 67,* 737–743.

McClelland, D. C., & Franz, C. E. (1992). Motivational and other sources of work accomplishments in mid-life: A longitudinal study. *Journal of Personality, 60,* 679–707.

McClelland, D. C., Koestner, R., & Weinberger, J. (1989). How do self-attributed and implicit motives differ? *Psychological Review, 96,* 690–702.

McClelland, D. C., & Pilon, D. A. (1983). Sources of adult motives in patterns of parent behavior in early childhood. *Journal of Personality and Social Psychology, 44,* 564–574.

Mehrabian, A. (1968). Male and female scales of the tendency to achieve. *Educational and Psychological Measurement, 28,* 493–502.

Mischel, W. (1961). Delay of gratification, need for achievement, and acquiescence in another culture. *Journal of Abnormal and Social Psychology, 62,* 543–552.

Mischel, W., & Gilligan, C. (1964). Delay of gratification, motivation for the prohibited gratification, and responses to temptation. *Journal of Abnormal and Social Psychology, 69,* 411–417.

Morgan, C., & Murray, H. A. (1935). A method for investigating fantasies: The Thematic Apperception Test. *Archives of Neurology and Psychiatry, 34,* 289–306.

Muraven, M., Tice, D. M., & Baumeister, R. F. (1998). Self-control as limited resource: Regulatory depletion patterns. *Journal of Personality and Social Psychology, 74(3),* 774–789.

Nicholls, J. G. (1984). Achievement motivation: Conceptions of ability, subjective experience, task choice, and performance. *Psychological Review, 91,* 328–346.

O'Connor, P., Atkinson, J. W., & Horner, M. (1966). Motivational implications of ability grouping in school. In J. W. Atkinson & N. T. Feather (Eds.), *A theory of achievement motivation* (pp. 231–248). New York: Wiley.

Panksepp, J. (1998). *Affective neuroscience: The foundations of human and animal emotions.* New York: Oxford University Press.

Raynor, J. O., & Smith, C. P. (1966). Achievement-related motives and risk-taking in games of skill and chance. *Journal of Personality, 34*(2), 176–198.

Rheinberg, F. (2002). Freude am Kompetenzerwerb, Flow-Erleben und motivpassende Ziele [The pleasures of becoming competent, experiencing flow, and pursuing motive-congruent goals]. In M. v. Salisch (Ed.), *Emotionale Kompetenz entwickeln* [Developing emotional competence] (pp. 179–206). Stuttgart: Kohlhammer.

Rosen, B. C., & D'Andrade, R. (1959). The psychological origins of the achievement motive. *Sociometry, 22,* 185–218.

Salamone, J. D. (1994). The involvement of nucleus accumbens dopamine in appetitive and aversive motivation. *Behavioural Brain Research, 61,* 117–133.

Schultheiss, O. C. (2001a). An information processing account of implicit motive arousal. In M. L. Maehr & P. Pintrich (Eds.), *Advances in motivation and achievement: Vol. 12. New directions in measures and methods* (pp. 1–41). Greenwich, CT: JAI Press.

Schultheiss, O. C. (2001b). *Manual for the assessment of hope of success and fear of failure (English translation of Heckhausen's need Achievement measure).* Unpublished manuscript, Department of Psychology, University of Michigan, Ann Arbor.

Schultheiss, O. C., & Brunstein, J. C. (1999). Goal imagery: Bridging the gap between implicit motives and explicit goals. *Journal of Personality, 67,* 1–38.

Schultheiss, O. C., & Brunstein, J. C. (2001). Assessing implicit motives with a research version of the TAT: Picture profiles, gender differences, and relations to other personality measures. *Journal of Personality Assessment, 77*(1), 71–86.

Schultheiss, O. C., & Brunstein, J. C. (2002). Inhibited power motivation and persuasive communication: A lens model analysis. *Journal of Personality, 70,* 553–582.

Schultheiss, O. C., & Rohde, W. (2002). Implicit power motivation predicts men's testosterone changes and implicit learning in a contest situation. *Hormones and Behavior, 41,* 195–202.

Sears, R. R., Maccoby, E. E., & Levin, H. (1957). *Patterns of child rearing.* Evanston, IL: Row, Peterson & Company.

Singh, S., & Gupta, B. S. (1977). Motives and agricultural growth. *British Journal of Social and Clinical Psychology, 16,* 189–190.

Solomon, R. L., & Wynne, L. C. (1953). Traumatic avoidance learning: Acquisition in normal dogs. *Psychological Monographs, 67*(Whole No. 354).

Spangler, W. D. (1992). Validity of questionnaire and TAT measures of need for achievement: Two meta-analyses. *Psychological Bulletin, 112,* 140–154.

Spence, J. T. (Ed.). (1983). *Achievement and achievement motives.* San Francisco: Freeman.

Tauer, J. M., & Harackiewicz, J. M. (1999). Winning isn't everything: Competition, achievement orientation, and intrinsic motivation. *Journal of Experimental Social Psychology, 35,* 209–238.

Thrash, T., & Elliot, A. J. (2002). Implicit and self-attributed achievement motives: Concordance and predictive validity. *Journal of Personality, 70,* 729–756.

Veroff, J. (1969). Social comparison and the development of achievement motivation. In C. P. Smith (Ed.), *Achievement-related motives in children* (pp. 46–101). New York: Russell Sage Foundation.

Wainer, H. A., & Rubin, I. M. (1969). Motivation of research and development entrepreneurs: Determinants of company success. *Journal of Applied Psychology, 53,* 178–184.

Wendt, H.-W. (1955). Motivation, effort, and performance. In D. C. McClelland (Ed.), *Studies in motivation* (pp. 448–459). New York: Appleton–Century–Crofts.

Wilson, T. D. (2002). *Strangers to ourselves: Discovering the adaptive unconscious.* Cambridge, MA: Belknap Press.

Winter, D. G. (1973). *The power motive.* New York: Free Press.

Winterbottom, M. R. (1958). The relation of need for achievement to learning experiences in independence and mastery. In J. W. Atkinson (Ed.), *Motives in fantasy, action, and society: A method of assessment and study* (pp. 453–478). Princeton, NJ: Van Nostrand.

Woike, B. A. (1995). Most-memorable experiences: Evidence for a link between implicit and explicit motives and social cognitive processes in everyday life. *Journal of Personality and Social Psychology, 68,* 1081–1091.

Zanobini, M., & Usai, M. C. (2002). Domain-specific self-concept and achievement motivation in the transition from primary to low middle school. *Educational Psychology Review, 22,* 203–217.

CHAPTER 4

℘

A Conceptual History
of the Achievement Goal Construct

ANDREW J. ELLIOT

Many different psychological constructs have been used over the years to explain and predict the energization and direction of behavior in achievement situations, such as the classroom, the workplace, and the ballfield. Each of these constructs (e.g., the achievement motive construct, the perceived competence construct, the achievement goal construct) has focused in some way and to some degree on competence. The study of competence and how individuals are motivated with regard to competence has had an important place in many different disciplines within psychology, including developmental psychology, educational psychology, industrial–organizational psychology, social–personality psychology, and sport psychology.

Integral to a motivational analysis of competence is the issue of valence. Persons may be energized by or directed toward the positive possibility of competence per se, and/or they may be energized by or directed away from the negative possibility of incompetence. This distinction between approach motivation and avoidance motivation is a fundamental and basic aspect of competence-relevant motivation.

The construct that currently receives the most research attention in the literature on competence-relevant motivation is the achievement goal construct. In this chapter, I offer a conceptual history of the achievement goal construct, describing the emergence of the construct and noteworthy developments in the achievement goal literature from its inception to the present day. From day one, the achievement goal construct was grounded in a distinction between mastery and performance forms of competence-relevant motivation. It was not until significantly later in the development of the literature that the approach–avoidance distinction was also considered fundamental to the achievement goal construct. As such, in overviewing the achievement goal literature, I devote particular attention to the question of when and how this approach–avoidance distinction was incorporated into the achievement goal construct. I conclude my conceptual overview by offering some observations regarding the contemporary achievement goal literature.

THE EMERGENCE OF THE ACHIEVEMENT GOAL CONSTRUCT

The achievement goal construct was developed in independent and collaborative work by Carol Ames, Carol Dweck, Marty Maehr, and John Nicholls. In the mid- to late 1970s, each of these individuals conducted research programs at the University of Illinois that focused on achievement motivation. In the fall of 1977, they began meeting together in a seminar series on motivation at the Institute for Child Behavior and Development in the Children's Research Center to discuss issues regarding achievement and motivation (Roberts, 2001). The discussions in this seminar series seemed to have had an important influence on the thinking of the participants, because shortly thereafter, unpublished (e.g., Nicholls & Dweck, 1979) and published (e.g., Maehr & Nicholls, 1980) papers emerged that articulated the foundational ideas of the achievement goal approach to achievement motivation. In the ensuing years, Dweck and Nicholls proceeded to offer somewhat distinct achievement goal conceptualizations that have been particularly influential in this tradition. Therefore, their conceptual work is the central focus of the following overview (see also Ames, 1984, and Maehr, 1983, 1984).

Dweck's achievement goal conceptualization emerged from her research on helplessness in achievement settings with late grade-school-age children. In a series of studies, Dweck and her colleagues (Diener & Dweck, 1978, 1980; Dweck, 1975; Dweck & Reppucci, 1973) demonstrated that children of equal ability respond differently to failure on achievement tasks. Some children display an adaptive, "mastery" response pattern, characterized by attributing failure to insufficient effort, continued positive affect and expectancies, sustained or enhanced persistence and performance, and pursuit of subsequent challenge, whereas other children display a maladaptive, "helpless" response pattern, characterized by attributing failure to insufficient ability, the onset of negative affect and expectancies, decrements

in persistence and performance, and avoidance of subsequent challenge.

Dweck (Dweck, 1986; Dweck & Elliott, 1983) sought to explain why children of equal ability display such divergent responses to failure, and she embraced the achievement goal construct as the key explanatory variable. A person's achievement goal was said to represent his or her purpose for engaging in behavior in an achievement situation (Dweck & Leggett, 1988). Two types of goals were identified: performance goals, in which the purpose of behavior is to demonstrate one's competence (or avoid demonstrating one's incompetence), and learning goals, in which the purpose of behavior is to develop one's competence and task mastery.

Children were posited to adopt different goals in achievement settings, and these goals were presumed to lead to differential task construals and differential patterns of affect, cognition, and behavior. Performance goals were presumed to lead to the "helpless" response pattern upon failure, because failure directly implies a lack of normative ability; learning goals, on the other hand, were posited to lead to the "mastery" response pattern, because failure feedback could simply be construed as helpful information in the process of developing competence or mastering a task. Achievement goals were posited to interact with confidence in one's ability in predicting achievement-relevant affect, cognition, and behavior. Performance goals were thought to lead to the "mastery" response pattern when accompanied by high confidence in ability but were thought to lead to the "helpless" pattern when accompanied by low confidence in ability. Learning goals were viewed as leading to the "mastery" pattern regardless of level of confidence in ability.

In articulating her achievement goal construct, Dweck overviewed and highlighted the limitations of both the achievement motive and achievement attribution traditions (as well as others). She believed that the achievement motive tradition overemphasized dispositions and underemphazied the role of cognitions in predicting achievement behavior (Dweck & Wortman, 1982; Dweck & Elliott, 1983), and that the achievement attribution tradition was unable to explain why people strive for competence in the first place (Dweck & Elliott, 1983). The achievement goal construct was construed as addressing these limitations, albeit not replacing or invalidating the motive and attribution constructs. Achievement goals were viewed as amenable to situation-specific, as well as dispositional, levels of analysis, were viewed as cognitively represented, and were thought to express the specific reason why an individual engaged in achievement behavior (Dweck & Elliott, 1983; Dweck & Leggett, 1988). Implicit theories of ability were identified as separable from achievement goals and were construed as predictors of their adoption. A belief that ability is a stable entity was posited to lead to performance goal adoption, whereas a belief that ability is malleable was posited to lead to learning goal adoption (Dweck & Leggett, 1988). For Dweck, "Achievement goals must lie at the heart of any analysis of achievement motivation" (Dweck & Elliott, 1983, p. 653).

Nicholls's achievement goal conceptualization emerged from his research on the development of conceptions of ability in children. According to Nicholls (1976, 1978, 1980), children initially possess an undifferentiated conception of ability, in which they do not distinguish between ability and effort. From this perspective, high ability is essentially equated with learning and improvement through effort; the more effort expended, the more learning and improvement (and, therefore, ability) implied. By around the age of 12, children acquire a differentiated conception of ability, in which they distinguish between ability and effort, and construe ability as a fixed capacity. From this perspective, effort expenditure must be controlled for when making ability inferences; high ability is inferred when one outperforms others while expending equal effort, or performs the same as others while expending less effort.

Nicholls (1984) sought to integrate his findings on the development of conceptions of ability with existing theories of adolescent and adult achievement motivation, and it is through this process that he articulated his achievement goal construct. An achievement goal was viewed as the purpose of achievement behavior, and it was presumed that the purpose of achievement behavior is to demonstrate or develop high ability (or to avoid

demonstrating low ability). For adolescents and adults, ability may be construed in both undifferentiated and differentiated fashion, so two different types of goals may be identified on this basis. The term "task involvement" was used to refer to seeking ability in the undifferentiated sense (i.e., seeking to develop skills by learning or mastering tasks), and the term "ego involvement" was used to refer to seeking ability in the differentiated sense (i.e., seeking to demonstrate that one has capacity by outperforming others, especially with less effort expenditure).

The two types of goals were presumed to lead to different patterns of achievement-relevant processes and outcomes. Task involvement was portrayed as an intrinsically motivated state that leads to positive achievement-relevant affect, cognition, and behavior, whereas ego involvement was portrayed as a self-conscious, evaluative motivational state that leads to a negative pattern of affect, cognition, and behavior. These goal states were posited to interact with perceived ability in predicting some processes and outcomes (e.g., task choice). Ego involvement was viewed as leading to positive consequences (e.g., selecting moderately challenging tasks) when accompanied by high perceived ability, and to negative consequences (e.g., selecting very easy or very difficult tasks) when accompanied by low perceived ability. Task involvement was viewed as leading to positive consequences across levels of perceived ability.

In articulating his achievement goal construct, Nicholls overviewed the way in which both the achievement motive and achievement attribution traditions (among others) viewed the concept of ability. He noted that both of these traditions emphasized the undifferentiated conception of ability, and failed to recognize that ability may be construed in different ways (Nicholls, 1983). The achievement goal approach was said to offer a more complete portrait of achievement motivation by distinguishing between two different conceptions of ability, and by making different predictions for goals states focusing on each. Nicholls also critiqued the degree to which the achievement motive approach emphasized dispositions (Maehr & Nicholls, 1980), and focused on how achievement goals may be manifest as either situationally specific states (involvements) or dispositional preferences (orientations). Dispositional goal preferences were viewed as predictors of situationally specific goal states, and goal states were construed as cognitively based intentions. The distinction between ability as capacity and ability as something to be developed was considered an inherent aspect of ability conceptions; as such, this notion of ability as stable or changeable was construed as part of the goal per se rather than as an antecedent of goal adoption. For Nicholls (1984), the conceptions of ability that established achievement goals were "the keys to understanding achievement motivation" (p. 329).

Two additional points regarding Nicholls's theorizing on achievement goals are important to note. First, he explicitly stated that his views on achievement goals were based not only on scientific theorizing but also on his philosophical values regarding the importance of equal motivational opportunities for all individuals (Nicholls, 1979, 1984). From this standpoint alone (independent of empirical data), task involvement was to be championed over ego involvement, because only task involvement affords motivational equality. Second, it must be acknowledged that Nicholls seemed to describe goals and related constructs in different ways across his writings, and that these descriptions were not always clearly articulated. Thus, one may characterize Nicholls's goal construct differently depending on the writings on which one focuses and how one interprets various statements.

Although there are differences in the achievement goal conceptualizations proffered by Dweck and Nicholls, it is their similarities that are most striking and most important to consider in this chapter. First, both conceptualizations were articulated in the context of a literature that emphasized achievement motives and achievement attributions as explanatory constructs. From early conceptual pieces written by Dweck (Dweck & Wortman, 1982; Dweck & Elliott, 1983) and Nicholls (1983; Maehr & Nicholls, 1980), it was clear that their emerging idea of the achievement goal construct was in part a response to perceived weaknesses or limitations of the achievement motive and attribution constructs. Thus, the motive and attribution approaches

to achievement motivation clearly influenced the way in which the achievement goal approach emerged, and both Dweck and Nicholls viewed the achievement goal construct as more of an integration of new and existing concepts than as a completely novel construct created *ex nihilo*.

Second, both Dweck and Nicholls delineated their achievement goal construct in terms of the purpose of achievement behavior. The concept of "purpose" can be defined in two primary ways: as "the reason for which something is done, made, used, etc." and as "an intended or desired result, end, aim, goal" (*Random House Dictionary of the English Language*, 1993). It appears to be used by both Dweck and Nicholls in both of these senses—as the reason for behavior in an achievement situation (e.g., the development or demonstration of ability) and as the aim or outcome that is sought in an achievement situation (e.g., normative or self-referential ability).

Third, both Dweck and Nicholls viewed competence as an important component of the achievement goal construct but clearly incorporated other components as well. For example, the focus on demonstrating ability in the performance/ego involvement goal implicates approval and/or self-presentation, in addition to competence. Indeed, both Dweck (Dweck & Elliott, 1983) and Nicholls (1984) indicated that the demonstration of ability can involve demonstrating ability to others, and this approval/self-presentation aspect of performance/ego involvement goals was a key feature of both the manipulations (e.g., "although you won't learn new things, it will really show me what kids can do"; see Elliott & Dweck, 1988) and measures (e.g., "I feel that I am successful when I show people I'm good at something"; see Nicholls, 1989) used to empirically examine the effects of these goals.

Fourth, both Dweck and Nicholls proffered a comparable achievement goal dichotomy, and the hypothesized effects of each goal were presumed to be quite similar in nature. One goal (learning/task) was characterized in terms of developing ability and seeking task mastery, and was posited to lead to a wide range of positive processes and outcomes. The other goal (performance/ego) was characterized in terms of demonstrating ability and seeking normative competence, and was posited to lead to a wide range of negative processes and outcomes. In addition, for both theorists, the effects of achievement goals were expected to be moderated by perceptions of competence, at least for some processes and outcomes. Performance/ego goals were posited to exert the most negative impact when accompanied by low perceptions of competence, whereas learning/ego goals were posited to exert the same positive impact across competence perceptions.

Fifth, in articulating their views on achievement goals, both Dweck and Nicholls described the two different goals relative to each other, and Dweck, in particular, sometimes categorized individuals in terms of one type of goal or the other. This has led some to suggest that Dweck, in particular, but also Nicholls, viewed performance/ego and learning/task as opposite poles on a single goal continuum. However, neither theorist explicitly articulated a unidimensional conceptualization of achievement goals, and it seems best to conclude that neither theorist took a firm stance on the dimensionality issue in their early writings. Instead, they simply focused on which of the two goals was most salient for an individual, and this in no way necessitates a unidimensional conceptualization of goals. In their later writings, both Dweck (1989) and Nicholls (1989) explicitly construed the two goals as distinct and separate forms of regulation.

Sixth, both Dweck and Nicholls portrayed achievement goals as applicable to both situational and dispositional levels of analysis (Dweck & Leggett, 1988). In developing their achievement goal constructs, both theorists highlighted the limitations of dispositional constructs (Dweck & Elliott, 1983; Maehr & Nicholls, 1980) and conveyed the importance of attending to more situationally oriented constructs. Interestingly, in empirical work, Dweck tended to focus on situation-specific manifestations of goals (e.g., Elliott & Dweck, 1988), whereas Nicholls tended to focus on dispositional goal orientations (e.g., Nicholls, Cheung, Lauer, & Patashnick, 1989).

Seventh, neither Dweck nor Nicholls made use of the distinction between approach and avoidance motivation in articulating their achievement goal construct.

Early in their writing on achievement goals, it seems as though both theorists may have considered incorporating the approach–avoidance distinction into their work in some manner (see Dweck & Elliott, 1983; Nicholls, 1984). However, it is clear that both decided against explicitly attending to this distinction. Dweck either described both mastery and performance goals in purely appetitive terms (Dweck & Leggett, 1988) or collapsed across approach–avoidance in characterizing performance goals in terms of seeking positive and avoiding negative judgments of ability (Elliott & Dweck, 1988). Nicholls explicitly ignored avoidance motivation altogether, characterizing task and ego goals as "two forms of approach motivation" (Nicholls, Patashnick, Cheung, Thorkildsen, & Lauer, 1989, p. 188).

SUBSEQUENT RESEARCH AND DEVELOPMENTS WITHIN THE ACHIEVEMENT GOAL LITERATURE

In the mid- to late 1980s, Dweck and Nicholls began to produce empirical work that supported their ideas about achievement goals (e.g., Elliott & Dweck, 1988; Nicholls, Patashnick, & Nolen, 1985). Many other researchers joined these efforts, and helped to document the utility of the fledgling achievement goal approach (see Ames & Archer, 1988; Butler, 1988; Duda, 1988; Jagacinski & Nicholls, 1987; Koestner, Zuckerman, & Koestner, 1987; Meece, Blumenfeld, & Hoyle, 1988; Nolen, 1988; Sansone, Sachau, & Weir, 1989; Stipek & Kowalski, 1989; Thorkildsen, 1989).

In an influential set of articles, Ames and Archer (1987, 1988) laid out the rationale for an integrative achievement goal approach that brought together not only the conceptualizations of Dweck and Nicholls but also those of theorists such as Ames (1984), Covington (1984), Maehr (1983), and Ryan (1982). Ames and Archer (1987, 1988) argued that the conceptual accounts proposed by the aforementioned theorists were similar enough to justify terminological convergence in the form of a mastery/performance goal dichotomy. This integrative move brought cohesion to the extant literature on achievement and motivation, and helped to solidify the importance of the achievement goal construct.

It is important to note that in the process of integrating the work of many different researchers, Ames and Archer (1987, 1988) offered an expanded conceptualization of the achievement goal construct. Achievement goals were characterized as networks or patterns of beliefs and feelings about success, effort, ability, errors, feedback, and standards of evaluation. These various beliefs and feelings were presumed to be interrelated within each type of goal, and were thought to provide a wide-ranging framework, or schema, labeled "orientation," through which achievement situations are construed and engaged.

A final aspect of the work of Ames and Archer (1988) warrants highlighting. These researchers introduced the idea that the achievement goal construct could be applied at the classroom, as well as the individual, level of analysis. In their research, they assessed students' perceptions of their classrooms in terms of an emphasis on mastery goals and performance goals, and linked these goal perceptions to students' learning strategies, task choices, attitudes, and attributions. Furthermore, Ames and Archer examined how different combinations of mastery goal and performance goal perceptions correlated with these process and outcome variables. In similar fashion, Duda (1988) examined how different combinations of individuals' mastery and performance goals correlated with process and outcome variables in the sport context.

In the early 1990s, research on achievement goals began to proliferate. There were undoubtedly many reasons for this influx of empirical attention, including the following: The achievement goal construct was intuitively appealing; the achievement goal construct fit nicely with the widespread interest in cognitively based constructs; achievement goal ideas clearly had straightforward applied value; achievement goals were relatively easy to measure and manipulate; and Ames and Archer's (1987, 1988) integration helped generate new research ideas. By this time, empirical research on achievement goals was appearing in a broad range of disciplines, including developmental psychology (see work by Butler, Stipek), educational psychology (see work by Ames, Meece,

Nicholls, Pintrich), sport psychology (see work by Duda, Roberts), and social–personality psychology (see work by Dweck, Harackiewicz).

As previously noted, the achievement goal approach emerged, in part, from philosophical values regarding the importance of equal motivational opportunities for all individuals. In light of this metatheoretical foundation and the clear implications of achievement goal concepts for real-world achievement settings, it is not surprising that educational psychologists, in particular, began to actively utilize the achievement goal approach as a guide for intervention and reform. Ames (1990; 1992) offered an elaborate and particularly influential intervention framework labeled TARGET (Tasks, Authority, Recognition, Grouping, Evaluation, Time; see Epstein, 1988). This framework was designed to create classroom environments that would enhance mastery goal adoption and minimize performance goal adoption in students (see also Blumenfeld, 1992). Maehr and Midgley (1991) established the importance of examining achievement goal influences at the school, as well as the personal and classroom levels, and made the case for a focus on mastery goals in each instance. In sport psychology, Duda and colleagues applied the concept of "perceived motivational climate" to coaches (Seifriz, Duda, & Chi, 1992) and parents (White, Duda, & Hart, 1992), and demonstrated the benefits of mastery goals in these contexts as well. Meece (1991) went beyond measurement of the perceived motivational climate to acquire observers' ratings of goal-relevant features of the achievement environment.

In the early to mid-1990s, several reviews of achievement goal research appeared in journal articles, chapters in edited volumes, and textbooks. Nearly all of these reviews rather unequivocally stated that the extant research on mastery and performance goals provided strong support for the basic hypothesis that mastery goals lead to positive processes and outcomes, whereas performance goals lead to negative processes and outcomes. These reviews tended to focus on the main effects of achievement goals rather than the perceived competence moderator hypothesis. At this point, minimal research on this moderator hypothesis had been conducted, and the extant data had yielded mixed results (see Miller, Behrens, Greene, & Newman, 1993; Smiley & Dweck, 1994).

For some, these reviews of the literature portraying the effects of mastery goals as exclusively positive and those of performance goals as exclusively negative seemed overstated (Butler, 1992; Harackiewicz & Elliot, 1993). A closer examination of the available research seemed to indicate that mastery goals indeed tended to lead to a host of positive processes and outcomes (although evidence linking mastery goals to positive performance outcomes was conspicuously sparse), but that performance goals sometimes had negative consequences, sometimes had no consequences, and sometimes even had positive consequences. For example, performance goals were shown to have null or positive effects in certain types of achievement contexts (see Koestner et al., 1987; Miller & Hom, 1990; Sansone et al., 1989) and for persons with certain types of personality dispositions (see Elliot & Harackiewicz, 1994; Harackiewicz & Elliot, 1993). This pattern of results led Harackiewicz (Harackiewicz & Elliot, 1993; Harackiewicz & Sansone, 1991), in particular, to explicitly question the proposal that performance goals are maladaptive.

On a related note, some researchers began to posit mastery goals coupled with performance goals as the optimal achievement goal profile, rather than mastery goals coupled with the absence of performance goals (Farr, Hofmann, & Ringenbach, 1993). Research examining the predictive nature of different goal profiles lent some credence to this proposition. Several studies indicated that the "high mastery–high performance goal" combination was linked to the best pattern of processes and outcomes (Ainley, 1993; Bouffard, Boisvert, Vezeau, & Larouche, 1995; Fox, Goudas, Biddle, Duda, & Armstrong, 1994; Wentzel, 1991, 1993), although others supported the "high mastery–low performance goal" combination (Meece & Holt, 1993; Pintrich & Garcia, 1991). The Farr et al. (1993) article cited earlier is also noteworthy for a different reason: It was one of the first articles to emerge from industrial–organizational psychology that explicitly discussed achievement goals (see Kanfer, 1990, for the initial consideration of achievement goals in this discipline). Corresponding empirical work

began to appear shortly thereafter (see Sujan, Weitz, & Kumar, 1994).

Other goals besides the "big two" had been considered for inclusion in achievement goal accounts from the beginning of conceptual and empirical work in this area (see Maehr, 1983; Maehr & Nicholls, 1980; Nicholls et al., 1985). Several candidates for inclusion began to receive more extensive consideration and scrutiny in the early to mid-1990s, most notably, work avoidance goals, extrinsic goals, and social goals (see Urdan, 1997, for a review). Work avoidance goals (also labeled "academic alienation") were defined in terms of trying to get away with putting as little work or effort as possible into achievement tasks (Meece et al., 1988; Nicholls et al., 1985; Nolen, 1988). Extrinsic goals were defined in terms of striving to earn a reward or avoid a punishment (Maehr, 1983; Midgley & Urdan, 1995; Pintrich & Garcia, 1991). Social goals were defined as strivings that focus on interpersonal relationships (Maehr & Nicholls, 1980; Wentzel, 1989), and a number of different variants were delineated, including social approval goals, social responsibility goals, social status goals, prosocial goals, and affiliation goals (Urdan & Maehr, 1995). Importantly, no criteria were in place by which to judge the merit of these additional goal candidates, and this proved an impediment to deciding which, if any, warranted inclusion into a model of achievement goals. It was clear that each of the goal candidates was operative in achievement situations, but it was equally clear that none of the goals focused on a commitment to achievement per se.

The year 1994 saw the premature passing of one of the pioneers of the achievement goal construct, John Nicholls.

INCORPORATION OF THE APPROACH–AVOIDANCE DISTINCTION

The distinction between approach and avoidance motivation has deep and widespread intellectual roots. It has been a part of theorizing on motivation since the advent of psychology as a scientific discipline, and it has been utilized by proponents of all major psychological traditions (Elliot, 1999).

Within the achievement motivation literature, the approach–avoidance distinction was incorporated into the first formal model of achievement motivation (the theory of resultant valence offered by Lewin, Dembo, Festinger, & Sears, 1944), and has figured prominently in many other influential accounts of achievement behavior since that time (see Alpert & Haber, 1960; Atkinson, 1957; Covington & Beery, 1976; McClelland, Atkinson, Clark, & Lowell, 1953; Weiner, 1972). Given this history, it is surprising that as the achievement goal approach emerged in the 1990s as the predominant account of achievement behavior, the approach–avoidance distinction continued to be ignored. All researchers either followed the lead of Dweck in not attending to separable approach and avoidance forms of performance goals (Butler, 1992; Skaalvik, Valans, & Sletta, 1994) or they followed the lead of Nicholls in explicitly characterizing both mastery and performance goals as approach forms of motivation (Ames, 1992; Meece & Holt, 1993). My own work at this time focused explicitly on the approach–avoidance distinction and sought to incorporate it within the achievement goal construct.

As a social–personality psychology graduate student in the early 1990s, I read broadly and deeply in the achievement motivation literature. In my reading, I was struck by the absence of attention to the approach–avoidance distinction in achievement goal work, especially given how richly the conceptual and empirical utility of this distinction had been documented in other theoretical frameworks over the years. I was also aware of the fact that a close examination of the extant achievement goal research indicated that the performance goals were not necessarily as deleterious as hypothesized, but could have both negative and positive effects on achievement-relevant processes and outcomes. This pattern of results matched my personal experience with performance goals, perhaps in particular, my experience on the ballfield as a baseball player and coach.

Accordingly, I reexamined the existing empirical work on achievement goals to determine whether the approach–avoidance distinction could help explain the variation in results for performance goals (Elliot,

1994). I noticed that for laboratory experiments, it was possible to distinguish between performance goal manipulations that drew participants' attention to the possibility of a positive outcome (thereby presumably instantiating approach motivation) and those that drew their attention to the possibility of a negative outcome (thereby presumably instantiating avoidance motivation). In similar fashion, for field studies, it was possible to distinguish between performance goal measures comprised entirely of items focused on the possibility of a positive outcome (presumably representing approach motivation) and those that contained items focused on the possibility of a negative outcome (presumably representing avoidance motivation). Classifying the manipulations and measures from extant research on this basis seemed to bring a great deal of clarity to the empirical pattern for performance goals. In general, performance goal manipulations and measures classified as approach tended to produce a positive set of processes and outcomes, whereas those classified as avoidance tended to produce a negative set of processes and outcomes (see Rawsthorne & Elliot, 1999, for an empirically based meta-analytic validation of these observations). If, as this analysis suggested, performance goals focused on positive outcomes and performance goals focused on negative outcomes have very different effects, it seemed quite likely that combining these types of goals together under the (omnibus) performance goal rubric would produce the mixed empirical pattern observed in the extant data.

Thus, on the basis of the long-documented utility of the approach–avoidance distinction, and the apparent utility of this distinction in clarifying the extant achievement goal literature, in my dissertation work I posited that the dichotomous achievement goal framework be revised to form a trichotomous framework (Elliot, 1994; see Elliot & Harackiewicz, 1996). Specifically, I bifurcated the conventional performance goal into conceptually independent approach and avoidance goals, and posited three separate achievement goals: a mastery goal focused on the development of competence or the attainment of task mastery, a performance–approach goal focused on the attainment of normative competence, and a performance–avoidance goal focused on the avoidance of normative incompetence. Mastery and performance–approach goals were characterized as approach goals, because they focused on potential positive outcomes (improvement/mastery and normative competence, respectively), whereas performance–avoidance goals were characterized as avoidance goals, because they focused on a potential negative outcome (normative incompetence).

The focus on positive possibilities in both mastery and performance–approach goal regulation was posited to lead to a somewhat similar set of positive processes and outcomes. However, some differences in the predictive profile of these forms of approach motivation were also posited given their differential evaluative standards. For example, the external evaluative focus inherent in performance–approach goals was thought to limit the extent to which they, relative to mastery goals, produced positive phenomenological processes and outcomes. However, this same characteristic of performance–approach goals was thought to make them better facilitators of performance attainment than mastery goals, particularly in situations where such attainment depends on following externally imposed criteria rather than inherently interesting aspects of the task itself (Elliot, 1994; Elliot & Harackiewicz, 1996). The focus on negative possibilities in performance–avoidance goals was posited to lead to a broad range of negative processes and outcomes.

Rather than view perceived competence as a moderator of achievement goal effects, I posited it to be an antecedent of achievement goal adoption (Elliot, 1994; Elliot & Church, 1997). High perceived competence was posited to orient individuals to the possibility of success and to facilitate the adoption of approach goals, both mastery and performance–approach, whereas low perceived competence was posited to orient individuals to the possibility of failure and to facilitate the adoption of performance–avoidance goals. Thus, competence expectancies were presumed to exert their effects on processes and outcomes indirectly through their influence on achievement goal adoption, rather than directly in interaction with achievement goals.

Importantly, the influence of perceived competence on achievement goal adoption was thought to be of moderate magnitude. Many other factors besides perceived competence were viewed as contributing to achievement goal adoption, including achievement motives, implicit theories of ability, and characteristics of the achievement task or evaluative setting (Elliot, 1994; 1997). This is a critical point, because several theorists in the 1970s and 1980s had portrayed high–low perceptions of competence as functionally isomorphic with approach–avoidance motivational tendencies (Kukla, 1972; Meyer, 1987). Indeed, it is likely that this portrait of approach–avoidance motivation as reducible to perceived competence was a major reason that approach–avoidance constructs lay fallow during the 1970s and 1980s. That is, perceived competence constructs were quite popular as explanatory constructs during this time, and approach–avoidance motivation was presumed to be redundant with such constructs. In contrast, I portrayed achievement goals as emerging from competence perceptions (as well as other influences), but as having a direct effect on processes and outcomes independent of perceived competence.

The trichotomous achievement goal framework incorporated the distinction between approach and avoidance motivation within performance goals, but left mastery goals intact. In subsequent work (Elliot, 1999), I proposed a 2 × 2 achievement goal framework that incorporated the approach–avoidance distinction within mastery goals as well as performance goals (see also Pintrich, 2000). As I stated earlier, the extant empirical work on mastery goals had yielded a rather clear pattern of findings that indicated that these goals led to a host of positive processes and outcomes. I examined the existing research on mastery goals and concluded that the clarity of the empirical yield was due to the fact that the manipulations and measures used in this research focused uniformly on positive possibilities. That is, in contrast to the extant research on performance goals, in which approach and avoidance motivation were often mixed indiscriminantly, in the extant research on mastery goals, avoidance motivation was simply omitted altogether. As such, whereas the trichotomous framework separated omnibus performance goals into conceptually independent performance–approach and performance–avoidance goals, the 2 × 2 framework added mastery–avoidance goals as the conceptually independent complement to the mastery–approach goals that were already in place.

Mastery–avoidance goals were described as a focus on avoiding self-referential or task-referential incompetence. Whereas mastery–approach goals entail striving to develop one's skills and abilities, advance one's learning, understand material, or master a task, mastery–avoidance goals entail striving to avoid losing one's skills and abilities (or having their development stagnate), forgetting what one has learned, misunderstanding material, or leaving a task incomplete. These goals were characterized as mastery goals because of their focus on development and task mastery; they were characterized as avoidance goals because of their focus on a potential negative outcome (self- or task-referential incompetence).

Predictions for mastery–avoidance goals were proffered tentatively given the fact that the mastery component of the goal was usually viewed as facilitating positive processes and outcomes, whereas the avoidance component of the goal was usually viewed as producing negative processes and outcomes. Nothing was known about the precise way in which these two components would integrate and function together in self-regulation, so specific hypotheses were viewed as difficult to generate a priori. In general, mastery–avoidance goals were expected to produce less optimal consequences than those for mastery–approach goals, but less deleterious consequences than those for performance–avoidance goals (Elliot, 1999; Elliot & McGregor, 2001). Perceived competence was not expected to moderate the influence of mastery–avoidance goals on processes and outcomes. Rather, perceived competence was viewed as an antecedent of mastery–avoidance goals, such that low perceptions of competence were thought to orient individuals to the possibility of task- or self-referential incompetence and, therefore, to prompt the adoption of mastery–avoidance goals.

Overall, mastery–avoidance goals were presumed to be less prevalent than mastery–approach, performance–approach, and performance–avoidance goals, at least in the achievement contexts typically studied in the achievement goal literature. However, mastery–avoidance goals were viewed as quite common in some instances and for some types of individuals. For example, these goals were thought to be quite common among the elderly. Physical and mental skills and abilities gradually diminish during the aging process, and it is likely that many who experience this diminution adopt a variant of the goal "avoid losing my skills and abilities." Athletes, students, or employees who have sought to maximize their skills and abilities may at some point feel that they have fully exploited their potential ("reached their peak") and shift to a focus on "not doing worse than I have done in the past." Perfectionists may be particularly likely to adopt goals such as "avoid making any mistakes" or "not lose a single point." Mastery–avoidance goals may also be common among those who think that they have a bad memory and consequently focus on "not forgetting what I have learned" (Elliot, 1999; Elliot & Thrash, 2001). Thus, mastery–avoidance goals were construed as important forms of regulation in some instances, and attending to these goals was viewed as necessary in the interest of more fully accounting for the diverse nature of achievement strivings in real-world situations.

In addition to fully incorporating the approach–avoidance distinction into the achievement goal construct, the 2 × 2 framework sought to explicitly establish competence as the conceptual core of the achievement goal construct. Competence has always been considered an important part of the achievement goal construct, but, as noted earlier, other motivational concepts (e.g., self-presentation, self-assessment, impression management) have also been included in conceptualizing and operationalizing achievement goals. In the 2 × 2 framework, "achievement" was explicitly portrayed in terms of competence, and the achievement goal construct was explicitly grounded in competence alone. Other motivational concerns and foci were thought to commonly become associated with competence-based goals, but these other concerns and foci were portrayed as antecedents or consequences of competence-based goal adoption, rather than as part of the goal per se (Elliot & Thrash, 2001; Thrash & Elliot, 2001).

Establishing competence as the core of the achievement goal construct provided a firm foundation from which achievement goals could be clearly conceptualized, and different types of achievement goals could be straightforwardly derived. I posited that within a motivational context, the concept of competence may be differentiated in two fundamental ways, in terms of definition and in terms of valence (Elliot, 1999; Elliot & McGregor, 2001).

Competence is *defined* by the standard or referent that is used in evaluating it. Three different standards may be used: an absolute standard (the requirements of the task itself), an intrapersonal standard (one's own past attainment or maximum potential attainment), and a normative standard (the performance of others). That is, competence may be evaluated and, therefore defined, in absolute terms according to one's mastery of a task, in intrapersonal terms according to one's personal trajectory, and in interpersonal terms according to one's attainment relative to others. Absolute and intrapersonal competence share many conceptual and empirical similarities and, at present, may be considered jointly rather than separately. As such, competence may be defined in absolute–intrapersonal terms or in interpersonal terms, and two types of achievement goals may be delineated according to the type of competence that an individual commits to in an achievement situation. This definition aspect of competence has been an important (although, to reiterate, not exclusive) focus of the dichotomous achievement goal framework, with mastery goals commonly entailing commitment to an absolute–intrapersonal standard and performance goals commonly entailing commitment to an intrapersonal standard (Ames, 1984; Dweck & Elliott, 1983; Maehr, 1983; Nicholls, 1984).

Competence is *valenced* in that it can be construed in positive terms (i.e., competence or success) or in negative terms (i.e., incompetence or failure). Two types of achievement goals may be delineated according to whether the competence-relevant focus is on approaching the positive possibility of competence per se, or on avoiding the negative possibility of incompetence. This valence aspect of competence represents the approach–avoidance motivation distinction.

Both definition and valence are integral to the concept of competence in motivational contexts and are presumed to be represented in any and all forms of achievement goals. That is, definition and valence are construed as necessary features of achievement goals, because it is not possible to formulate an achievement goal that does not include, implicitly or explicitly, information as to how competence is defined and valenced. These two aspects of competence are combined to form the four different types of goals represented in the 2 × 2 framework.

Establishing competence as the core of the achievement goal construct not only delineated the precise conceptual nature of achievement goals but also provided clear, systematic guidelines for the evaluation of additional achievement goal candidates. Such candidates must be competence-based and must either extend the two central aspects of competence, definition and valence, or be grounded in an additional aspect of competence not yet identified. A 3 × 2 framework that separates the absolute and intrapersonal definitions of competence was viewed as the most plausible option (Elliot, 1999); these definitions were construed as conceptually separable, with the remaining task being to determine whether they are indeed empirically separable. The definition and valence aspects of competence were portrayed as sufficient to delineate the competence construct; therefore, these components were viewed as sufficient building blocks with which to comprehensively model competence-based strivings.

SUBSEQUENT RESEARCH AND DEVELOPMENTS WITHIN THE ACHIEVEMENT GOAL LITERATURE

In the mid- to late 1990s, my colleagues and I produced empirical work testing the trichotomous achievement goal framework (e.g., Elliot & Church, 1997; Elliot & Harackiewicz, 1996). Many other researchers did likewise (see, especially, Middleton & Midgley, 1997; Skaalvik, 1997; VandeWalle, 1997), and the resulting data base provided strong evidence for the need to attend to the approach–avoidance distinction in achievement goal research. Initially, the three goals in the trichotomous framework were manipulated in the experimental laboratory, and the importance of separating performance–approach and performance–avoidance goals was documented (Elliot & Harackiewicz, 1996). Shortly thereafter, measures of the three goals were developed, and the factor-analytic separability and differential predictive utility of the three goals was demonstrated (Elliot & Church, 1997; Middleton & Midgley, 1997; Skaalvik, 1997; VandeWalle, 1997). Additional empirical work further illustrated the benefits of the trichotomous model (Bembenutty, 1999; Brett & VandeWalle, 1999; Elliot & McGregor, 1999; Elliot, McGregor, & Gable, 1999; Halvari & Kjormo, 1999; Lopez, 1999; Midgley et al., 1998; VandeWalle & Cummings, 1997). In a few of these studies, perceived competence was examined as a moderator variable and as a possible alternative explanation for observed effects; little evidence emerged for either possibility (Elliot & Church, 1997; Elliot & Harackiewicz, 1996). Perceived competence was, however, documented as a predictor of achievement goals, as posited by the trichotomous model (Elliot & Church, 1997; Lopez, 1999).

During this time, research utilizing the dichotomous achievement goal framework proceeded apace. Most researchers utilizing the dichotomous framework either explicitly labeled their performance goal construct performance–approach, or at minimum were careful to purify their manipulations or measures of avoidance content. The proliferation in achievement goal research that was witnessed early in the 1990s continued, seemingly in linear fashion, as individuals linked goals to a variety of different antecedents and, especially, consequences. Research in educational and sport psychology, in particular, burgeoned (for reviews, see Duda, 2001; Midgley, 2002; Pintrich & Schunk, 2002; Roberts, 2001; Treasure, 2001). Work on achievement goals in industrial–organizational psychology began in earnest during this period, facilitated, in part, by the development of a dichotomous achievement

goal measure by Button, Mathieu, and Zajac (1996; for a review, see Kozlowski et al., 2001).

Of particular note during this time was an influx of important research contributions from individuals at, or trained at, the University of Michigan. These researchers focused on expanding the achievement goal nomological network, establishing interrelations among goals at different levels of analysis, supplementing perceived goal structure measures with observation-based goal structure measures, and documenting the impact of school transitions on goals and goal-related processes and outcomes (see E. Anderman & Midgley, 1997; L. Anderman, 1999; Kaplan & Midgley, 1999; Middleton & Midgley, 1997; Midgley, Arunkumar, & Urdan, 1996; Patrick et al., 1997; Roeser, Midgley, & Urdan, 1996; Ryan & Pintrich, 1997; Turner, Thorpe, & Meyer, 1998; Urdan, Midgley, & Anderman, 1998; Wolters, Yu, & Pintrich, 1996). Much of this work emerged from an unusually fruitful, large-scale longitudinal study of elementary through high school students (see Midgley, 2002). These efforts were fueled by, and fit hand in glove with, a focus on intervention and school reform, articulately expressed in Maehr and Midgley's (1996) *Transforming School Cultures*.

In addition to examining the influence of both personal and structural achievement goals on process and outcomes, researchers in sport psychology, in particular, began to examine achievement goals from an interactionist perspective. This research focused on questions regarding the fit between the goals held by the person and those emphasized in the achievement context (e.g., Can personal performance goals be adaptive in contexts with a performance goal emphasis?). Results from this research tended to support the importance of attending to issues of fit, although no single goal combination emerged as optimal for all processes and outcomes (see Treasure & Roberts, 1998; Walker, Roberts, & Nyheim, 1998; cf. Newton & Duda, 1999)

By the end of the 1990s, several studies examining the role of perceived competence as a moderator of achievement goal effects had been conducted, and the results continued to be decidedly mixed. Some studies found evidence for the hypothesized pattern of moderation (Cury, Biddle, Sarrazin, & Famose, 1997; Elliott & Dweck, 1988; Smiley & Dweck, 1994), but many did not (Elliot & Church, 1997; Elliot & Harackiewicz, 1994, 1996; Harackiewicz & Elliot, 1993; Kaplan & Midgley, 1997; Miller et al., 1993). This mixed empirical yield prompted Hong, Chiu, Dweck, Lin, and Wan (1999) to question the idea that performance goals can have positive consequences when perceived competence is high. Instead, these researchers suggested that it may be more appropriate to expect performance goals to have inimical consequences across perceptions of competence.

At the beginning of this decade, research on the 2 × 2 achievement goal framework commenced. In the initial work on this model, a measure of the four goals was developed, factor-analytic data supporting the separability of the four goals were presented, and evidence for differential nomological networks was provided (Elliot & McGregor, 2001). Subsequent experimental and field work provided additional support for the viability of the 2 × 2 framework in general, and the mastery–avoidance goal variable specifically (Conroy, in press; Conroy & Elliot, 2004; Conroy, Elliot, & Hofer, 2003; Cury, Elliot, Da Fonseca, & Moller, 2004; Elliot & Reis, 2003; Finney, Pieper, & Barron, 2004; Karabenick, 2003, 2004; Malka & Covington, in press; Van Yperen, 2003; see Moller & Elliot, in press). The available data seemed to indicate that mastery–avoidance goals have antecedents and consequences that are much more similar to performance–avoidance goals than to mastery–approach goals.

Empirical work on the trichotomous achievement goal framework continued to accumulate. By the end of 2003, over 60 studies from 12 different countries had appeared in print, the vast majority of which were published in educational, industrial–organizational, and social–personality psychology journals. This research clearly documented and illustrated the importance of separating performance–approach and performance–avoidance goals, and placed the majority of the deleterious consequences of performance-based goals on performance–avoidance goals. Mastery goals were shown to have widespread positive effects, whereas performance–approach goals were

shown to have a primarily positive but truncated set of positive consequences.

An empirical pattern that began to be acknowledged in the 1990s (see Harackiewicz, Barron, & Elliot, 1998) but became particularly salient as evidence from the 2 × 2, trichotomous, and dichotomous frameworks accumulated, was that mastery–approach goals often did not positively predict performance attainment, whereas performance–approach goals did so on a rather consistent basis. This and other positive findings for performance–approach goals elicited an engaging dialogue on the costs and benefits of these goals, and, importantly, on implications for application (see Harackiewicz, Barron, Pintrich, Elliot, & Thrash, 2002; Midgley, Kaplan, & Middleton, 2001; Kaplan & Midgley, 2002; for an equally engaging exchange on more general topics, see Harwood & Hardy, 2001; Harwood, Hardy, & Swain, 2000; Treasure, Duda, Hall, Roberts, & Ames, 2001).

As this dialogue transpired, research from the dichotomous perspective on the antecedents and consequences of mastery–approach and performance–approach goals at all levels of analysis continued to appear in journals in various disciplines, industrial–organizational and sport psychology, in particular (for reviews, see Biddle, Wang, Kavussanu, & Spray, 2003; Deshon & Carr, 2004; Duda, 2004; Sonnentag, Niessen, & Ohly, 2004). Multiple goal perspectives of various sorts became more salient as researchers developed new conceptual and empirical approaches to the study of goal combinations (Barron & Harackiewicz, 2001; Brophy, 2004; Deshon, Kozlowski, Schmidt, Milner, & Wiechmann, 2004; Pintrich, 2000).

The years 2001 and 2003 saw the premature passing of two integral contributors to the achievement goal literature, Carol Midgley and Paul Pintrich, respectively.

ISSUES CURRENTLY FACING THE ACHIEVEMENT GOAL LITERATURE

The achievement goal approach remains the predominant approach to achievement motivation in the contemporary literature. This tradition is now over 20 years old and continues to generate important basic and applied research across a host of psychological disciplines. However, several basic questions continue to demand attention in achievement goal work, and I close this chapter by briefly making note of what I view to be some important conceptual (and associated operational) issues facing the literature today.

1. There is surprisingly little consensus in the achievement goal literature on whether "goal" in "achievement goal" is best represented as aim (Elliot & Thrash, 2001), a combination of reason and aim (Dweck, 1986), or overarching orientation (Ames & Archer, 1988). My perspective is that the term "goal" is best conceptualized as aim, because this use is consistent with the prototypical use of the term in the broader motivational literature, and it affords conceptual precision without, ultimately, sacrificing conceptual breadth. In any given achievement context, an aim (e.g., to do well relative to others) is always undergirded by a more general reason (e.g., to show others I have ability, to feel the satisfaction of success, to avoid the shame of failure, to get the reward my mother promised me), so clearly both aim and reason are important in accounting for achievement behavior. However, as illustrated by the preceding examples, a single aim may be undergirded by many different reasons, and I think it is optimal to keep the aim and reason constructs conceptually separate, and to explore the implications of an assortment of different aim–reason combinations (i.e., "goal complexes"; Elliot & Thrash, 2001; see Grant and Dweck, 2003, for what may be viewed as a step in this direction). With regard to the conception of goals as overarching orientations, I think it is best to keep aims conceptually separate from the many different dispositions, tendencies, processes, and outcomes to which aims are associated, and to empirically examine the links between the antecedents of aims and their affective, cognitive, and behavioral consequences (for more on this issue, see Elliot & Thrash, 2001; Thrash & Elliot, 2001).

2. The way in which the aforementioned conceptual issue is addressed has direct implications for measurement and manipulation. If "goal" is conceptualized as aim, goal measures/manipulations should focus on the appetitive or aversive standard of evaluation, but if "goal" is conceptualized as a combination of reason and aim, measures/manipulations should focus on both the standard of evaluation and the reason(s) for commitment to that standard, and if "goal" is conceptualized as an overarching orientation, measures/manipulations should include the many different dispositions, tendencies, processes, and outcomes associated with the aim (see Elliot & Thrash, 2001; Thrash & Elliot, 2001). On a related note, it should be acknowledged that the same labels are commonly used to refer to measures/manipulations of great diversity. For example, some performance–avoidance goal measures focus on incompetence, whereas others focus on self-presentation concerns. This poses problems not only across different measures/manipulations but also within individual measures/manipulations. To continue the preceding example, in some achievement goal measures, the performance–avoidance items focus on self-presentation concerns, whereas the performance–approach items focus on normative competence, with little or no focus on self-presentation (thereby confounding approach–avoidance and competence–self-presentation). Operationalization problems of this nature impede interpretational clarity and, ultimately, impede progress in the literature.

3. Some researchers, and indeed some entire disciplines, have largely adopted Ames and Archer's (1987, 1988) terminological recommendation of "mastery" and "performance" goals. Other researchers, and indeed other entire disciplines, have continued to use an assortment of different labels or, in the case of sport psychology, have continued to utilize Nicholls's original task–ego labels. The move toward uniform labels paid substantial dividends in the 1990s, and it seems that the more the achievement goal literature can move in this unified direction, the better. There may be important reasons to gravitate to labels other than mastery and performance in some instances, and as the aforementioned conceptual and operational issues become clarified, it may even be necessary for entirely new terminology to emerge. However, in the main, it seems that a continued movement toward uniform labels would help facilitate interdisciplinary cross talk and cross-fertilization, which

would undoubtedly move the literature toward greater integration and maturity. Importantly, Ames and Archer's terminological recommendation is separable from their conceptual expansion of the achievement goal construct; one may be embraced without the other.

4. The term "orientation" is used by achievement goal researchers not only to refer to a broad network of beliefs and feelings, but also to refer to a dispositional goal adoption tendency. Indeed, many, if not most, researchers in this area utilize the achievement goal construct in a dispositional manner in their empirical work. This strong dispositional focus is surprising from both conceptual and empirical standpoints. Conceptually, the achievement goal approach originated, in part, as a critique of dispositional constructs (especially the need for achievement), and as a move toward a more specific, contextual level of analysis (see Maehr & Nicholls, 1980; Dweck & Wortman, 1982). In addition, when construed as a disposition, it is difficult to see how the achievement goal construct differs from the self-attributed achievement motive construct that has been articulated within the classic achievement motive tradition (McClelland, 1985; see Spence & Helmreich's [1983] distinction between work–mastery and competitiveness in the self-attributed need for achievement). Furthermore, if achievement goal orientations are portrayed as general tendencies to adopt particular achievement goals in specific situations, and achievement goals in specific situations are viewed as the direct regulators of achievement behavior, then it seems that achievement goal orientations merely serve a descriptive, and not an explanatory function (see McAdams, 2001, for an analogous statement regarding the Big Five traits). From an empirical standpoint, it is well established that the predictive utility of an independent variable is maximized when it is operationalized at the same level as the dependent variable of interest (see Ajzen & Fishbein, 1977). This correspondence between independent variable and dependent variables is violated in achievement goal research that seeks to predict affect, cognition, or behavior in a specific achievement situation with a dispositional achievement goal measure. When dispositional achievement goal measures are associated with self-reports of general affective, cognitive, or behavioral tendencies in achievement situations, it is difficult to know precisely what has been learned about actual, real-world achievement motivation. Thus, although the achievement goal construct can be utilized at both dispositional and situation-specific levels of analysis, conceptual and empirical considerations seem to suggest that it may be best suited for the situation-specific level.

5. Conceptual and empirical work on achievement goals is commonly referred to using the term "theory," as in "achievement goal theory" or "goal orientation theory." An important question to ask is what is being referred to when this "theory" moniker is utilized. On one hand, it seems as though there are (a) several different ways to conceptualize mastery and performance goals (e.g., aim, combination of aim and reason, overarching orientation), (b) several different conceptual frameworks that delineate different types of achievement goals (e.g., the dichotomous, trichotomous, and 2×2 frameworks), and (c) several different models that explicate links between achievement goals and their antecedents and consequences (e.g., the social-cognitive model, the hierarchical model). In each instance, it would seem that "theories" would be a more accurate descriptor than "theory." On the other hand, it may be the case that "theory" is most often used in general fashion to refer to the differentiation of achievement goals in terms of the mastery–performance distinction. In this case, a legitimate question to ask is whether this distinction alone (construed at this general level) warrants the "theory" designation. It is for the aforementioned reasons that I recommend the term "achievement goal approach" to refer to this most generative and fruitful of achievement motivation traditions.

6. Finally, since its inception, theoretical and empirical work on achievement goals has emerged from two desires: a desire to scientifically account for motivated achievement behavior, and a desire to help individuals (especially children) be optimally motivated in achievement settings. These desires are not incompatible or antagonistic and, on the contrary, it may be argued that these

dual foundations are part of what makes the achievement goal approach so generative and achievement goal research so invigorating and satisfying to conduct. However, disagreements in the achievement goal literature seem to arise when one desire takes precedent over the other—when theoretical work begins to lose its tether to real-world considerations, or when real-world considerations alone begin to drive data interpretation and summary. Importantly, theoretically derived empirical work can tell us how achievement goals operate in the present social–psychological context; this work is mute regarding whether the social–psychological context optimally should be this way, whether the social–psychological context can be changed, and whether achievement goals operate the same way across different social–psychological contexts (see Elliot & Moller, 2003). Simply stated, theory-based description and explanation is altogether different from real-world prescription. Theory begets application, and application informs theory, and I believe it is in drawing deeply from both that the achievement goal approach will develop to its full potential.

ACKNOWLEDGMENTS

Preparation of this chapter was facilitated by support from the William T. Grant Foundation (Grant No. 2565) and a Friedrich Wilhelm Bessel Research Award from the Alexander von Humboldt Foundation. Thanks are extended to Martin Maehr for his comments on an earlier draft of this chapter.

REFERENCES

Ainley, M. D. (1993). Styles of engagement with learning: Multidimensional assessment of their relationship with strategy use and school achievement. *Journal of Educational Psychology, 85,* 395–405.

Ajzen, I., & Fishbein, M. (1977). Attitude–behavior relations: A theoretical analysis and review of empirical research. *Psychological Bulletin, 84,* 888–918.

Alpert, R., & Haber, R. N. (1960). Anxiety in academic achievement situations. *Journal of Abnormal and Social Psychology, 61,* 207–215.

Ames, C. (1984). Competitive, cooperative, and individualistic goal structures: A cognitive–motivational analysis. In C. Ames & R. Ames (Eds.), *Research on motivation in education* (Vol. 3, pp. 177–207). New York: Academic Press.

Ames, C. (1990). Motivation: What teachers need to know. *Teachers College Record, 91,* 409–421.

Ames, C. (1992). Achievement goals, motivational climate, and motivational processes. In G. Roberts (Ed.), *Motivation in sports and exercise* (pp. 161–176). Champaign, IL: Human Kinetics.

Ames, C., & Archer, J. (1987). Mothers' belief about the role of ability and effort in school learning. *Journal of Educational Psychology, 79,* 409–414.

Ames, C., & Archer, J. (1988). Achievement goals in the classroom: Students' learning strategies and motivation processes. *Journal of Educational Psychology, 80,* 260–267.

Anderman, E., & Midgley, C. (1997). Changes in achievement goal orientations, perceivedacademic competence, and grades across the transition to middle level schools. *Contemporary Educational Psychology, 22,* 269–298.

Anderman, L. (1999). Classroom goal orientation, school belonging, and social goals as predictors of students' positive and negative affect following the transition to middle school: Schools can make a difference. *Journal of Research and Development in Education, 32,* 131–147.

Atkinson, J. W. (1957). Motivational determinants of risk-taking behavior. *Psychological Review, 64,* 359–372.

Barron, K. E., & Harackiewicz, J. M. (2001). Achievement goals and optimal motivation: Testing multiple goal models. *Journal of Personality and Social Psychology, 80,* 706–722.

Bembenutty, H. (1999). Sustaining motivation and academic goals: The role of academic delay of gratification. *Learning and Individual Differences, 11,* 233–259.

Biddle, S. J., Wang, C. K., Kavussanu, M., & Spray, C. M. (2003). Correlates of achievement goal orientations in physical activity: A systematic review of research. *European Journal of Sport Science, 3,* 1–20.

Blumenfeld, P. (1992). Classroom learning and motivation: Clarifying and expanding goal theory. *Journal of Educational Psychology, 84,* 272–281.

Bouffard, T., Boisvert, J., Vezeau, C., & Larouche, C. (1995). The impact of goal orientation of self-regulation and performance among college students. *British Journal of Educational Psychology, 65,* 317–329.

Brett, J. F., & VandeWalle, D. (1999). Goal orientation and goal content as predictors of performance in a training program. *Journal of Applied Psychology, 84,* 863–873.

Brophy, J. (2004). *Motivating students to learn* (2nd ed.). Mahwah, NJ: Erlbaum.

Butler, R. (1988). Task-involving and ego-involving properties of evaluation: Effects of different feedback conditions on motivational perceptions, interest, and performance. *Journal of Educational Psychology, 79,* 474–482.

Butler, R. (1992). What young people want to know when: Effects of mastery and ability goals on interest in different kinds of social comparisons. *Journal of Personality and Social Psychology, 62,* 934–943.

Button, S. B., Mathieu, J. E., & Zajac, D. M. (1996). Goal orientation in organizational research: A conceptual and empirical foundation. *Organizational Behavior and Human Decision Processes, 67,* 26–48.

Conroy, D. E. (in press). The unique psychological meanings of multidimensional fears of failing. *Journal of Sport and Exercise Psychology.*

Conroy, D. E., & Elliot, A. J. (2004). Fear of failure and achievement goals in sport: Addressing the issue of the chicken and the egg. *Anxiety, Stress, and Coping, 17,* 271–285.

Conroy, D. E., Elliot, A. J., & Hofer, S. M. (2003). A 2 × 2 achievement goals questionnaire for sport. *Journal of Sport and Exercise Psychology, 25,* 456–476.

Covington, M. V. (1984). Strategic thinking and the fear of failure. In J. Segal, S. Chipman, & R. Glaser (Eds.), *Thinking and learning skills: Relating instruction to basic research* (pp. 389–416). Hillsdale, NJ: Erlbaum.

Covington, M., & Beery, R. (1976). *Self-worth and school learning.* New York: Holt, Rinehart & Winston.

Cury, F., Biddle, S., Sarrazin, P., & Famose, J. (1997). Achievement goals and perceived ability predict investment in learning a sport task. *British Journal of Educational Psychology, 67,* 293–309.

Cury, F., Elliot, A. J., Da Fonseca, D., & Moller, A. C. (2004). *The social-cognitive model of achievement motivation and the 2 × 2 achievement goal framework.* Manuscript submitted for publication.

Deshon, R. P., & Carr, J. Z. (2004). *A motivated action theory account of goal oriented behavior.* Manuscript submitted for publication.

Deshon, R. P., Kozlowski, S. W. J., Schmidt, A. M., Milner, K. R., & Wiechmann, D. (2004). A multiple goal, multilevel model of feedback effects on the regulation of individual and team performance in training. *Journal of Applied Psychology, 89,* 1035–1056.

Diener, C. I., & Dweck, C. S. (1978). An analysis of learned helplessness: Continuous changes in performance, strategy, and achievement cognitions following failure. *Journal of Personality and Social Psychology, 36,* 451–462.

Diener, C. I., & Dweck, C. S. (1980). An analysis of learned helplessness: II. The processing of success. *Journal of Personality and Social Psychology, 39,* 940–952.

Duda, J. L. (1988). The relationship between goal perspectives, persistence and behavioral intensity among male and female recreational sport participants. *Leisure Studies, 10,* 95–106.

Duda, J. L. (2001). Achievement goal research in sport: Pushing the boundaries and clarifying some misunderstandings. In G. Roberts (Ed.), *Advances in motivation in sport and exercise* (pp. 129–182). Champaign, IL: Human Kinetics.

Duda, J. L. (2004). Goal setting and achievement motivation in sport. In C. Spielberger (Ed.), *Encyclopedia of applied psychology.* San Diego: Academic Press.

Dweck, C. S. (1975). The role of expectations and attributions in the alleviation of learned helplessness. *Journal of Personality and Social Psychology, 31,* 674–685.

Dweck, C. S. (1986). Motivational processes affecting learning. *American Psychologist, 41,* 1040–1048.

Dweck, C. S. (1989). Motivation. In A. Lesgold & R. Glaser (Eds.), *Foundations for a psychology of education* (pp. 87–136). Hillsdale, NJ: Erlbaum.

Dweck, C. S., & Elliott, E. S. (1983). Achievement motivation. In E. M. Heatherington (Ed.), *Handbook of child psychology: Socialization, personality, and social development* (Vol. 4, pp. 643–691). New York: Wiley.

Dweck, C. S., & Leggett, E. L. (1988). A social cognitive approach to motivation and personality. *Psychological Review, 95,* 256–273.

Dweck, C. S., & Reppucci, N. D. (1973). Learned helplessness and reinforcement responsibility in children. *Journal of Personality and Social Psychology, 25,* 109–116.

Dweck, C., & Wortman, C. (1982). Learned helplessness, anxiety, and achievement motivation: Neglected parallels in cognitive, affective, and coping responses. In H. Krohne & L. Laux (Eds.), *Achievement, stress, and anxiety* (pp. 92–126). Washington, DC: Hemisphere.

Elliot, A. J. (1994). *Approach and avoidance achievement goals: An intrinsic motivation analysis.* Unpublished doctoral dissertation. University of Wisconsin, Madison.

Elliot, A. J. (1997). Integrating "classic" and "contemporary" approaches to achievement motivation: A hierarchical model of approach and avoidance achievement motivation. In P. Pintrich & M. Maehr (Eds.), *Advances in motivation and achievement* (Vol. 10, pp. 143–179). Greenwich, CT: JAI Press.

Elliot, A. J. (1999). Approach and avoidance motivation and achievement goals. *Educational Psychologist, 34,* 149–169.

Elliot, A. J., & Church, M. A. (1997). A hierarchical model of approach and avoidance achievement motivation. *Journal of Personality and Social Psychology, 72,* 218–232.

Elliot, A. J., & Covington, M. V. (2001). Approach and avoidance motivation. *Educational Psychology Review, 12,* 73–92.

Elliot, A. J., & Harackiewicz, J. M. (1994). Goal setting, achievement orientation, and intrinsic motivation: A mediational analysis. *Journal of Personality and Social Psychology, 66,* 968–980.

Elliot, A. J., & Harackiewicz, J. M. (1996). Approach

and avoidance achievement goals and intrinsic motivation: A mediational analysis. *Journal of Personality and Social Psychology, 70,* 968–980.

Elliot, A. J., & McGregor, H. A. (1999). Test anxiety and the hierarchical model of approach and avoidance achievement motivation. *Journal of Personality and Social Psychology, 76,* 626–644.

Elliot, A. J., & McGregor, H. A. (2001). A 2 × 2 achievement goal framework. *Journal of Personality and Social Psychology, 80,* 501–519.

Elliot, A. J., McGregor, H. A., & Gable, S. (1999). Achievement goals, study strategies, and exam performance: A mediational analysis. *Journal of Educational Psychology, 91,* 549–563.

Elliot, A. J., & Moller, A. (2003). Performance–approach goals: Good or bad forms of regulation? *International Journal of Educational Research, 39,* 339–356.

Elliot, A. J., & Reis, H. (2003). Attachment and exploration in adulthood. *Journal of Personality and Social Psychology, 85,* 317–331.

Elliot, A. J., & Thrash, T. M. (2001). Achievement goals and the hierarchical model of achievement motivation. *Educational Psychology Review, 12,* 139–156.

Elliott, E. S., & Dweck, C. S. (1988). Goals: An approach to motivation and achievement. *Journal of Personality and Social Psychology, 54,* 5–12.

Epstein, J. L. (1988). Effective schools or effective students: Dealing with diversity. In R. Haskins & D. MacRae (Eds.), *Policies for America's public schools: Teacher quality indicators* (pp. 89–126). New York: Academic Press.

Farr, J. L., Hofmann, D. A., & Ringenbach, K. L. (1993). Goal orientation and action control theory: Implications for industrial and organizational psychology. *International Journal of Organizational Psychology, 8,* 193–232.

Finney, S. J., Pieper, S. L., & Barron, K. E. (2004). Examining the psychometric properties of the achievement goal questionnaire in a general academic context. *Educational and Psychological Measurement, 64,* 365–382.

Fox, K., Goudas, M., Biddle, S., Duda, J. L., & Armstrong, N. (1994). Children's task and ego profiles in sport. *British Journal of Educational Psychology, 64,* 253–261.

Grant, H., & Dweck, C. S. (2003). Clarifying achievement goals and their impact. *Journal of Personality and Social Psychology, 85,* 541–553.

Halvari, H., & Kjormo, O. (1999). A structural model of achievement motives, performance approach and avoidance goals, and performance among Norwegian Olympic athletes. *Perceptual and Motor Skills, 89,* 997–1022.

Harackiewicz, J., Barron, K., & Elliot, A. (1998). Rethinking achievement goals: When are they adaptive for college students and why? *Educational Psychologist, 33,* 1–21.

Harackiewicz, J. M., Barron, K. E., Pintrich, P. R., Elliot, A. J., & Thrash, T. M. (2002). Revision of achievement goal theory: Necessary and illuminating. *Journal of Educational Psychology, 94,* 638–645.

Harackiewicz, J. M., & Elliot, A. J. (1993). Achievement goals and intrinsic motivation. *Journal of Personality and Social Psychology, 65,* 904–915.

Harackiewicz, J. M., & Sansone, C. (1991). Goals and intrinsic motivation: You *can* get there from here. In M. Maehr & P. Pintrich (Eds.), *Advances in motivation and achievement* (Vol. 7, pp. 21–49). Greenwich, CT: JAI Press.

Harwood, C., & Hardy, L. (2001). Persistence and effort in moving achievement goal research forward: A response to Treasure and colleagues. *Journal of Sport and Exercise Psychology, 23,* 330–345.

Harwood, C., Hardy, L., & Swain, A. (2000). Achievement goals in sport: A critique of conceptual and measurement issues. *Journal of Sport and Exercise Psychology, 22,* 235–255.

Hong, Y., Chiu, C., Dweck, C. S., Lin, D., & Wan, W. (1999). Implicit theories, attributions, and coping: A meanings system approach. *Journal of Personality and Social Psychology, 77,* 588–599.

Jagacinski, C. M., & Nicholls, J. G. (1987). Competence and affect in task involvement and ego involvement: The impact of social comparison information. *Journal of Educational Psychology, 79,* 107–114.

Kanfer, R. (1990). Motivation theory and industrial and organizational psychology. In M. Dunnette & L. Hough (Eds.), *Handbook of industrial and organizational psychology* (Vol. 1, 2nd ed., pp. 75–170). Palo Alto, CA: Consulting Psychologists Press.

Kaplan, A., & Midgley, C. (1997). The effect of achievement goals: Does level of perceived competence make a difference? *Contemporary Educational Psychology, 22,* 415–435.

Kaplan, A., & Midgley, C. (1999). The relationship between perceptions of the classroom goal structure and early adolescents' affect in school: The mediating role of coping strategies. *Learning and Individual Differences, 11,* 187–212.

Kaplan, A., & Midgley, C. (2002). Should childhood be a journey or a race?: Response to Harackiewicz et al. (2002). *Journal of Educational Psychology, 94,* 646–648.

Karabenick, S. A. (2003). Seeking help in large college classes: A person-centered approach. *Contemporary Educational Psychology, 28,* 37–58.

Karabenick, S. A. (2004). Perceived achievement goal structure and college student help seeking. *Journal of Educational Psychology, 96,* 569–581.

Koesnter, R., Zuckerman, M., & Koestner, J. (1987). Praise, involvement, and intrinsic motivation. *Journal of Personality and Social Psychology, 53,* 383–390.

Kozlowski, S. W., Gully, S. M., Brown, S. G., Salas, E., Smith, E. M., & Nason, E. (2001). Effects of training goals and goal orientation traits on multidimensional training outcomes and performance adaptability. *Organizational Behavior and Human Decision Processes, 85,* 1–31.

Kukla, A. (1972). Attributional determinants of achievement-related behavior. *Journal of Personality and Social Psychology, 21,* 166–174.

Lewin, K., Dembo, T., Festinger, L., & Sears, R. (1944). Level of aspiration. In J. McV. Hunt (Ed.), *Personality and the behavioral disorders* (pp. 333–378). New York: Ronald Press.

Lopez, D. F. (1999). Social cognitive influences on self-regulated learning: The impact of action–control beliefs and academic goals on achievement-related outcomes. *Learning and Individual Differences, 11,* 301–319.

Maehr, M. L. (1983). On doing well in science: Why Johnny no longer excels, why Sarah never did. In S. Paris, G. Olson, & H. Stevenson (Eds.), *Learning and motivation in the classroom* (pp. 179–210). Hillsdale, NJ: Erlbaum.

Maehr, M. L. (1984). Meaning and motivation. In R. Ames & C. Ames (Eds.), *Research on motivation in education: Student motivation* (Vol. 1, pp. 115–144). New York: Academic Press.

Maehr, M. L., & Midgley, C. (1991). Enhancing student motivation: A schoolwide approach. *Educational Psychologist, 26,* 399–427.

Maehr, M. L., & Midgley, C. (1996). *Transforming school cultures.* Boulder, CO: Westview Press.

Maehr, M. L., & Nicholls, J. G. (1980). Culture and achievement motivation: A second look. In N. Warren (Ed.), *Studies in cross cultural psychology* (Vol. 3, pp. 221–267). New York: Academic Press.

Malka, A., & Covington, M. V. (in press). Perceiving school performance as instrumental to future goal attainment: Effects on graded performance. *Contemporary Educational Psychology.*

McAdams, D. (2001). *The person: An integrated introduction to personality psychology* (3rd ed.). New York: International Thomson.

McClelland, D. C. (1985). *Human motivation.* Cambridge, UK: Cambridge University Press.

McClelland, D. C., Atkinson, J. W., Clark, R. A., & Lowell, E. L. (1953). *The achievement motive.* New York: Appleton–Century–Crofts.

Meece, J. L. (1991). The classroom context and students' motivational goals. In M. Maehr & P. Pintrich (Eds.), *Advances in motivation and achievement* (Vol. 7, pp. 261–285). Greenwich, CT: JAI Press.

Meece, J. L., Blumenfeld, P. C., & Hoyle, R. H. (1988). Students' goal orientations and cognitive engagement in classroom activities. *Journal of Educational Psychology, 80,* 514–523.

Meece, J. L., & Holt, K. (1993). A pattern analysis of students' achievement goals. *Journal of Educational Psychology, 85,* 582–590.

Meyer, W. (1987). Perceived ability and achievement-related behavior. In F. Halisch & J. Kuhl (Eds.), *Motivation, intention, and volition* (pp. 73–86). New York: Springer-Verlag.

Middleton, M., & Midgley, C. (1997). Avoiding the demonstration of lack of ability: An underexplored aspect of goal theory. *Journal of Educational Psychology, 89,* 710–718.

Midgley, C. (Ed.). (2002). *Goals, structures, and patterns of adaptive learning.* Mahwah, NJ: Erlbaum.

Midgley, C., Arunkumar, R., & Urdan, T. (1996). If I don't do well tomorrow, there's a reason: Predictors of adolescents' use of academic self-handicapping behavior. *Journal of Educational Psychology, 88,* 423–434.

Midgley, C., Kaplan, A., & Middleton, M. (2001). Performance–approach goals: Good for what, for whom, under what circumstances, and at what cost? *Journal of Educational Psychology, 93,* 77–86.

Midgley, C., Kaplan, A., Middleton, M., Maehr, M., Urdan, T., Hicks, L., Anderman, L., et al. (1998). The development and validation of scales assessing students' achievement goal orientations. *Contemporary Educational Psychology, 23,* 113–131.

Midgley, C., & Urdan, T. (1995). Predictors of middle school students= use of self-handicapping strategies. *Journal of Early Adolescence, 15,* 389–411.

Miller, R. B., Behrens, J. T., Greene, B. A., & Newman, D. (1993). Goals and perceived ability: Impact on student valuing, self-regulation, and persistence. *Contemporary Educational Psychology, 18,* 2–14.

Miller, A., & Hom, H. L. (1990). Influence of extrinsic and ego incentive value on persistence after failure and continuing motivation. *Journal of Educational Psychology, 82,* 539–545.

Moller, A. C., & Elliot, A. J. (in press). The 2 × 2 achievement goal framework: An overview of empirical research. *Progress in Educational Research.*

Newton, M. L., & Duda, J. L. (1998). The interaction between motivational climate, dispositional goal orientation, and perceived ability in predicting indices of motivation. *International Journal of Sport Psychology, 29,* 1–20.

Nicholls, J. G. (1976). Effort is virtuous, but it's better to have ability: Evaluative responses to perceptions of effort and ability. *Journal of Personality and Social Psychology, 31,* 306–315.

Nicholls, J. G. (1978). The development of concepts of effort and ability, perception of own attainment, and the understanding that difficult tasks require more ability. *Child Development, 49,* 800–814.

Nicholls, J. G. (1979). Quality and equality in intellectual development. *American Psychologist, 34,* 1071–1084.

Nicholls, J. G. (1980). The development of the concept of difficulty. *Merrill–Palmer Quarterly, 26,* 271–281.

Nicholls, J. G. (1983). Conceptions of ability and achievement motivation. In R. Ames & C. Ames (Eds.), *Research on motivation in education* (Vol. 3, pp. 185–218). New York: Academic Press.

Nicholls, J. G. (1984). Achievement motivation: Conceptions of ability, subjective experience, task choice, and performance. *Psychological Review, 91,* 328–346.

Nicholls, J. G. (1989). *The competitive ethos and democratic education.* Cambridge, MA: Harvard University Press.

Nicholls, J. G., Cheung, P., Lauer, J., & Patashnick, M. (1989). Individual differences in academic motivation: Perceived ability, goals, beliefs, and values. *Learning and Individual Differences, 1,* 63–84.

Nicholls, J. G., & Dweck, C. S. (1979). *A definition of achievement motivation.* Unpublished manuscript, University of Illinois.

Nicholls, J. G., Patashnick, M., Cheung, P., Thorkildsen, T., & Lauer, J. (1989). Can achievement motivation succeed with only one conception of success? In F. Halisch & J. Van den Beroken (Eds.), *Competence considered* (pp. 187–204). Lisse, The Netherlands: Swets & Zeitlinger.

Nicholls, J. G., Patashnick, M., & Nolen, S. (1985). Adolescents' theories of education. *Journal of Educational Psychology, 77,* 683–692.

Nolen, S. B. (1988). Reasons for studying: Motivational orientations and study strategies. *Cognition and Instruction, 5,* 269–287.

Patrick, H., Ryan, A. M., Anderman, L. H., Middleton, M., Linnenbrink, L., Hruda, L. Z., et al. (1997). *Manual for observing patterns of adaptive learning (OPAL): A protocol for classroom observations.* Ann Arbor: University of Michigan Press.

Pintrich, P. (2000). An achievement goal theory perspective on issues in motivation terminology, theory, and research. *Contemporary Educational Psychology, 25,* 92–104.

Pintrich, P., & Garcia, T. (1991). Student goal orientation and self-regulation in the college classroom. In M. Maehr & P. Pintrich (Eds.) *Advances in motivation and achievement* (Vol. 7, pp. 371–402). Greenwich, CT: JAI Press.

Pintrich, P. R., & Schunk, D. (2002). *Motivation in education: Theory, research, and applications* (2nd ed.). Englewood Cliffs, NJ: Prentice-Hall.

Rawsthorne, L. J., & Elliot, A. J. (1999). Achievement goals and intrinsic motivation: A meta-analytic review. *Personality and Social Psychology Review, 3,* 326–344.

Roberts, G. C. (2001). Understanding the dynamics of motivation in physical activity: The influence of achievement goals on motivational processes. In G. Roberts (Ed.), *Advances in motivation in sport and exercise* (pp. 1–50). Champaign, IL: Human Kinetics.

Roeser, R. W., Midgley, C., & Urdan, T. C. (1996). Perceptions of the school psychological environment and early adolescents' psychological and behavioral functioning in school: The mediating role of goals and belonging. *Journal of Educational Psychology, 88,* 408–422.

Ryan, A., & Pintrich, P. (1997). Should I ask for help?: The role of motivation and attitudes in adolescents' help-seeking in math class. *Journal of Educational Psychology, 89,* 329–341.

Ryan, R. M. (1982). Control and information in the interpersonal sphere: An extension of cognitive evaluation theory. *Journal of Personality and Social Psychology, 43,* 450–461.

Sansone, C., Sachau, D. A., & Weir, C. (1989). Effects of instruction on intrinsic interest: The importance of context. *Journal of Personality and Social Psychology, 57,* 819–829.

Seifriz, J. J., Duda, J. L., & Chi, L. (1992). The relationship of perceived motivational climate to intrinsic motivation and beliefs about success in basketball. *Journal of Sport and Exercise Psychology, 14,* 375–391.

Skaalvik, E. M. (1997). Self-enhancing and self-defeating ego orientation: Relations with task and avoidance orientation, achievement, self-perceptions, and anxiety. *Journal of Educational Psychology, 89,* 71–81.

Skaalvik, E. M., Valans, H., & Sletta, O. (1994). Task involvement and ego involvement: Relations with academic achievement, academic self-concept, and self-esteem. *Scandanavian Journal of Educational Research, 38,* 231–243.

Smiley, P. A., & Dweck, C. S. (1994). Individual differences in achievement goals among young children. *Child Development, 65,* 1723–1743.

Sonnentag, S., Niessen, C., & Ohly, S. (2004). Learning at work: Training and development. In C. Cooper & I. Robertson (Eds.), *International review of industrial and organizational psychology* (Vol. 19, pp. 255–289). New York: Wiley.

Spence, J. T., & Helmreich, R. L. (1983). Achievement-related motives and behavior. In J. T. Spence (Ed.), *Achievement and achievement motives: Psychological and sociological approaches* (pp. 10–74). San Francisco: Freeman.

Stipek, D. J., & Kowalski, P. S. (1989). Learned helplessness in task-orienting versus performance-orienting test conditions. *Journal of Educational Psychology, 81,* 384–391.

Sujan, H., Weitz, B., & Kumar, N. (1994). Learning orientation, working smart, and effective selling. *Journal of Marketing, 58,* 39–52.

Thorkildsen, T. A. (1989). Pluralism in children's reasoning about social justice. *Child Development, 60,* 965–972.

Thrash, T. M., & Elliot, A. J. (2001). Delimiting and integrating achievement motive and goal constructs. In A. Efklides, J. Kuhl, & R. Sorrentino (Eds.), *Trends and prospects in motivational research* (pp. 1–19). Dordrecht, The Netherlands: Kluwer Academic.

Treasure, D. C. (2001). Enhancing young people's motivation in youth sport: An achievement goal approach. In G. Roberts (Ed.), *Advances in motivation in sport and exercise* (pp. 79–100). Champaign, IL: Human Kinetics.

Treasure, D. C., Duda, J. L., Hall, H. K., Roberts, G. C., & Ames, C. (2001). Clarifying misconceptions and misrepresentations in achievement goal research in sport: A response to Harwood, Hardy, and Swain. *Journal of Sport and Exercise Psychology, 23,* 317–329.

Treasure, D. C., & Roberts, G. C. (1998). Relationship between female adolescents' achievement goal orientations, perceptions of the motivational climate, belief about success and sources of satisfaction in basketball. *International Journal of Sport Psychology*, 29, 211–230.

Turner, J., Thorpe, P., & Meyer, D. (1998). Students' reports of motivation and negative affect: A theoretical and empirical analysis. *Journal of Educational Psychology*, 90, 758–771.

Urdan, T. C. (1997). Achievement goal theory: Past results, future directions. In M. Maehr & P. Pintrich (Eds.), *Advances in motivation and achievement* (Vol. 10, pp. 243–269). Greenwich, CT: JAI Press.

Urdan, T. C., & Maehr, M. (1995). Beyond a two-goal theory of motivation and achievement: A case for social goals. *Review of Educational Research*, 65, 213–243.

Urdan, T. C., Midgley, C., & Anderman, E. (1998). The role of classroom goal structure in students' use of self-handicapping. *American Educational Research Journal*, 35, 101–122.

VandeWalle, D. (1997). Development and validation of a work domain goal orientation instrument. *Educational and Psychological Measurement*, 57, 995–1015.

VandeWalle, D., & Cummings, L. L. (1997). A test of the influence of goal orientation on the feedback-seeking process. *Journal of Applied Psychology*, 82, 390–400.

Van Yperen, N. W. (2003). Task interest and actual performance: The moderating effects of assigned and adopted purpose goals. *Journal of Personality and Social Psychology*, 85, 1006–1015.

Walker, B. W., Roberts, G. C., & Nyheim, M. (1998). Predicting enjoyment and beliefs about success in sport: An interactional perspective. *Journal of Sport and Exercise Psychology*, 20(Suppl.), S59.

Weiner, B. (1972). *Theories of motivation: From mechanism to cognition*. Chicago: Rand McNally.

Wentzel, K. R. (1989). Adolescent classroom goals, standards for performance, academic achievement: An interactionist perspective. *Journal of Educational Psychology*, 81, 131–142.

Wentzel, K. R. (1991). Social and academic goals at school: Motivation and achievement in context. In M. Maehr & P. Pintrich (Eds.), *Advances in motivation and achievement* (Vol. 7, pp. 185–212). Greenwich, CT: JAI Press.

Wentzel, K. R. (1993). Motivation and achievement in early adolescence: The role of multiple classroom goals. *Journal of Early Adolescence*, 13, 4–10.

White, S. A., Duda, J. L., & Hart, S. (1992). An exploratory examination of the Parent Initiated Motivational Climate Questionnaire. *Perceptual and Motor Skills*, 75, 875–880.

Wolters, C., Yu, S., & Pintrich, P. (1996). The relation between goal orientation and students' motivational beliefs and self-regulated learning. *Learning and Individual Differences*, 8, 211–238.

CHAPTER 5

Motivation from an Attribution
Perspective and the Social Psychology
of Perceived Competence

BERNARD WEINER

Discussions of competence, which I view as synonymous with ability and "can," often regard it a structure—a whole, with parts or components, that is measured and used above all to predict learning and performance. As an attribution theorist, rather than considering competence a structure, I construe it as a subjective inference or a social construction that can pertain to the self and to others. Competence as defined here is not a "thing" or an "it" but is a perception, or an inference, often about others, and usually implicating causality. Perception of competence, along with its underlying causal determinants, then gives rise to additional social inferences about the self and others, as well as influencing affects and social behaviors. Furthermore, in contrast to the structural approach, "more of" competence is not necessarily equated with "better." Quite the contrary, competence is not only linked with positive outcomes but also is associated with a number of undesired consequences.

These include, for example, being labeled a "nerd"; being the target of envy, and hence dislike, by others; and proneness to being regarded as arrogant. These adverse consequences are elaborated on later in this chapter. Hence, for the psychologist, the richness of the concept of competence does not merely lie in answers to questions such as "How can someone get more of it?" or "How many are there?" and the usual list of suspects when addressed from a structural viewpoint.

In the present discussion of competence, I contrast the ability to perform a task that implies high aptitude with competence attained because of effort expenditure. Typically, this is not a distinction that is articulated, for researchers also tend to be remiss in regarding competence from an ahistorical perspective as something one has or does not have, irrespective of its history. But it makes a great deal of difference whether one was competent and lost it, or

73

never had it; or worked hard to gain it as opposed to always having it. Of particular importance in this chapter is the path to attaining competence—via aptitude versus expended effort. I believe if the distinction between aptitude and effort expenditure as antecedents of competence were fully understood, then a great deal of psychological insight would be gained. I borrow from many titles in the psychological literature by stating that, in this chapter, I move toward that end. To address this distinction, I first present my version of attribution theory (or, I should say, attribution theories, for I have proposed both an intrapersonal and an interpersonal conceptual framework, see Weiner, 2000). Then, I more fully turn to competence.

ATTRIBUTION THEORY

Imagine, for example, that a student has just received a poor grade on an exam and we, as psychologists and educators, want to predict whether she will continue in school or drop out. Among the likely predictors I identify are the subjective expectancy of future success, as well as emotions related to self-esteem, guilt, and shame. These self-directed thoughts and feelings comprise what I label an *intrapersonal* theory of motivation.

Now consider that, following the poor exam performance, significant others, including peers, teachers, and parents, evaluate or judge this person. They consider her good or bad, responsible or not responsible for the low test score, moral or immoral, and she is the target of emotions including anger and sympathy. These thoughts and emotions, in turn, arouse help or neglect, positive or negative feedback, and the like. These other-directed thoughts and feelings comprise what I label an *interpersonal* theory of motivation. A distinction between intrapersonal versus interpersonal perspectives is particularly important in the examination of competence. This is because, from an intrapersonal perspective, being competent usually (but not always) facilitates motivation. On the other hand, from an interpersonal perspective, competence also is associated with motivational inhibitors; that is, it is tied to some factors that decrease personal motivation.

Intrapersonal Motivation from the Attributional Perspective

My views on intrapersonal motivation are guided by the metaphor that people are scientists trying to understand themselves and their environment, and they act on the basis of this knowledge (see Weiner, 1992). This approach begins with a completed event, such as success or failure at an exam (see Figure 5.1). At the end of this sequence is a behavioral reaction, which might be dropping out of school. In between is the remainder of the motivation process, guided by attribution inferences and their consequences, which fill the gap between the stimulus (the exam outcome) and the response (dropping out).

In the far left of Figure 5.1, it can be seen that, in achievement contexts, the motivation process begins with the exam outcome. Following this is an affective reaction: One feels happy following goal attainment and unhappy when there is nonattainment of a goal. These general affective reactions are not mediated by a great deal of cognitive work and are labeled "outcome-dependent" emotions. Then, individuals ask: "Why did this happen? What caused this outcome?" Because of cognitive limits, search is not undertaken following all events and is particularly likely when the outcome is negative, unexpected, and/or important. Thus, if one expects to succeed at something trivial and does, then *why* questions are not likely to follow. In contrast, unexpected failure at an important exam surely will evoke attributional processes (see Gendolla & Koller, 2001; Weiner, 1986).

The answer to this *why* question, which is a causal attribution, is influenced by many sources of evidence (see Figure 5.1). These are not further examined given the goals of this chapter. Guided by these sources of information, a cause is selected, such as lack of ability, lack of effort or bad luck given failure. Similarly, if one is rejected for a date, then again as shown in Figure 5.1, an array of causes is possible, including unattractive physical characteristics, poor personality, and so forth. Assume for purposes of clarity that there is only one phenomenological cause, although we all recognize life is not that simple. This sets the stage for the next step in the process, which concerns the un-

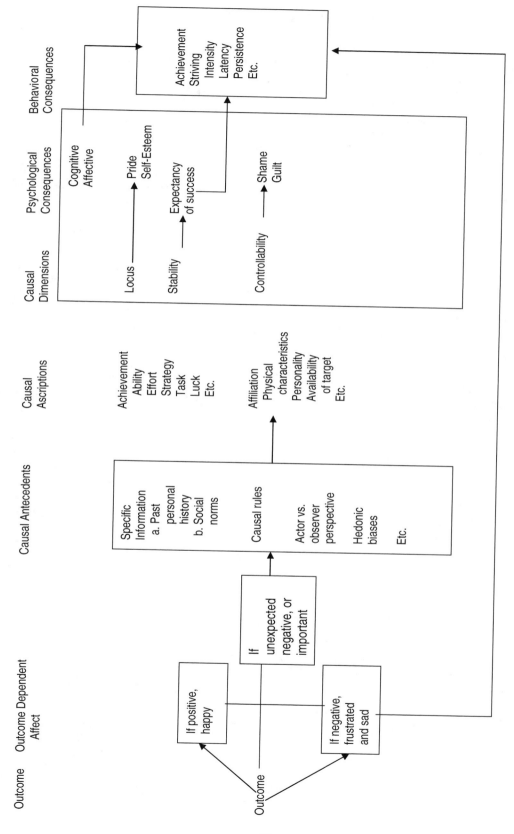

FIGURE 5.1. An intrapersonal attributional theory of motivation.

derlying characteristics or properties of that cause. These so-called causal dimensions are the very heart and soul of my attributional approach to motivation.

To understand the motivational consequences of causal beliefs, it is necessary that qualitative differences between causes such as effort and ability are altered to quantitative differences, and for this to occur, the causes must be comparable on some psychological dimensions. A great deal of research has documented that there are three, and I think only three, underlying causal properties that have cross-situational generality (see Weiner, 1986). These properties are labeled locus, stability, and controllability. Locus refers to the location of a cause, which is either within or outside of the actor. For example, ability and effort are considered internal causes of success, whereas chance and help from others are construed external causes. Causal stability refers to the duration of a cause. Some causes, such as math aptitude, are perceived as constant, whereas causes such as chance are regarded unstable or temporary. Finally, a cause such as effort is subject to volitional alteration and is personally controllable, whereas other causes cannot be willfully changed and are regarded uncontrollable. Luck and aptitudes have this property.

All causes can be located within this three-dimensional causal space. Although there may be disagreements regarding how a cause is dimensionalized because this depends on "how it seems to me," there also is a great deal of agreement that, for example, aptitude is internal, stable, and uncontrollable, whereas chance, while also uncontrollable, is external to the actor and unstable.

The significance of these causal properties is that they map onto what are considered by some to be the two main determinants of motivated action, namely, expectancy and value. Expectancy refers to the subjective likelihood of future success, while value, in this context, is considered the emotional consequences of goal attainment or nonattainment (see Atkinson, 1964). I turn first to expectancy. It has been documented that if a cause is regarded as stable, then the same outcome is anticipated again following a success or a failure. Hence, if failure is perceived as being due to lack of aptitude, then taking another exam is expected to result in

another failure. To the contrary, failure perceived as being due to unstable factors, such as bad luck or lack of preparation because of the flu, is not an indicator that there will be further failure (see review in Weiner, 1992).

Locus and controllability relate to feeling states, or to the "value" of achievement outcomes. I do not use the concept locus *of* control but rather differentiate locus *and* control. These are two independent dimensions. A cause may be internal to the person but quite uncontrollable, such as lack of height as the cause of not being selected for the basketball team.

Locus influences feelings of pride in accomplishment and self-esteem. Pride and increments in self-esteem require internal causality for success. One might be happy following a high grade on an exam (an outcome-dependent feeling), but one would not experience pride if he or she believed the teacher gave only high grades. Controllability, in conjunction with locus, influences whether guilt or shame is experienced following nonattainment of a goal (although, in research, these two affects are highly correlated, so I have somewhat shaky confidence in the presumptions that follow). If one assumes a desire to succeed, attribution of failure to insufficient effort, which is internal and controllable, often elicits guilt. On the other hand, an ascription of failure to lack of aptitude, which is internal but uncontrollable, tends to evoke feelings of shame, embarrassment, and humiliation. The controllability dimension influences other affects as well, including regret, but these are not considered here. Finally, expectancy of success and the emotions of pride, guilt, and shame are believed to determine subsequent behavior; that is, behavior is a function of thoughts and feelings.

Let me illustrate the logic of this analysis and show why it is motivationally dysfunctional for one to believe that he or she is not competent. Assume that Bill failed an exam. We now want to correctly predict whether this results in an increment or decrement in his motivation to achieve. The attribution framework contends to accurately make this prediction, Bill's perceived cause for failure must be determined (which may or may not be the "real" cause). Assume that Bill believes he failed because he lacks scholastic aptitude. This aspect of the self refers to an internal, stable, and uncontrollable cause. Hence, Bill should suffer a decrement in self-esteem (mediated by personal causality); he will expect to fail again (mediated by causal stability); and feel ashamed, humiliated, and embarrassed (mediated by internal causality that is uncontrollable). This analysis leads to the hypothesis that his motivation will be severely dampened and he might drop out of school.

Conversely, suppose Bill believes he is competent and ascribes his failure to lack of effort—he did not put in enough study time. Inasmuch as this also is an internal cause, self-esteem is lowered (but perhaps not to the same extent as given an aptitude ascription, which may be perceived as more internal than effort). Since effort expenditure is unstable, expectancy of success is not reduced; and given that effort is under volitional control, Bill may be experiencing guilt (which motivates one to make reparations). Hence, his total motivation increases and Bill is predicted to display heightened motivation to do well (assuming that success is one of his goals).

In summary, the prior analysis provides the conceptual foundation for why high competence is a favorable self-perception from a motivation standpoint. I have focused here only on failure, although a similar logic applies when the prior achievement was a success.

Interpersonal Motivation from the Attributional Perspective

I now turn to the social world and to other-perception of competence, where I contend that inferences of high competence in others do not always have favorable consequences. The interpersonal conception of motivation from an attributional perspective is shown in Figure 5.2 (for a history of this development, see Weiner, 1996). For the moment, concentrate on the top row of Figure 5.2. It can be seen the motivation sequence again is initiated by an achievement outcome, exam failure. Once more, there is a causal search (not shown in Figure 5.2), in this case, not by the actor but by an involved observer, such as a teacher or parent. And again, based on a variety of factors not included in

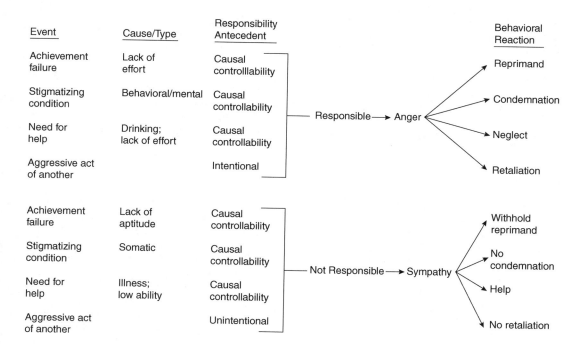

FIGURE 5.2. An interpersonal attributional theory of motivation.

Figure 5.2, a causal explanation is reached. This may or may not be the same inference made by the failing student.

This cause is then placed in the previously described dimensional space, with the dimension of causal controllability being of prime importance. As shown in the top row of Figure 5.2, failure is ascribed to a lack of effort, which is subject to volitional change and therefore regarded a controllable cause. Recall that this was an adaptive causal belief from a self-perspective framework. If a cause (and also the linked negative event) "could have been otherwise," then the actor is perceived as responsible for the outcome (for greater detail regarding the link between controllability and responsibility, and a discussion of mitigating factors, see Weiner, 1995). Hence, the motivation process is proposed to proceed from a causal decision to an inference about the responsibility of the person. Perceived other-responsibility for a negative event, in turn, gives rise to anger. One is mad when one's child fails an exam because of not studying, just as one is angry with a roommate for leaving the kitchen dirty following a meal. Anger, in turn, evokes a variety of antisocial responses, including punishment and reprimand. Thus, while lack of effort is a "positive" or functional ascription in the context of intrapersonal motivation, it has negative consequences in social settings.

Now consider the sequence when achievement failure is caused by lack of ability, depicted a few lines lower in Figure 5.2. Recall how detrimental this causal belief was in the context of self-perception. Ability, conceived here as akin to aptitude, is an uncontrollable cause. Because the cause (and the linked exam outcome) cannot be volitionally altered, the failing student is not responsible (able to respond) or accountable for what happened. Lack of responsibility for a negative achievement outcome tends to elicit sympathy (but see a later discussion for some negative emotional reactions as well). We feel sorry for the mentally handicapped person who cannot perform cognitive tasks and for the physically handicapped person who cannot perform motor tasks. Sympathy, in turn, evokes prosocial reactions. In an interpersonal context, the absence of ability has positive consequences, particularly when compared with an attribution to lack of effort.

This interpersonal approach to classroom experience is not confined to an explanation of achievement-related behaviors. A number of other phenomena can be examined within the same conceptual framework. Figure 5.2 shows that, in addition to achievement-related evaluation, reactions to the stigmatized, help giving, and aggression also are subject to a responsibility-mediated analysis. If a person is responsible for being in a stigmatized state (e.g., having cancer because of smoking), for needing financial help (e.g., because of failure to appear at work), or for a hostile act (the aggression was intentional), then anger is experienced and the behavioral reaction of the observer is negative. This is regarded as the "appropriate" or deserved reaction to "sin" and moral failure (see Forsterling & Rudolph, 1988). On the other hand, stigmatizations because of noncontrollable causes such as being blind at birth, needing help because of missing school when ill, and perhaps even aggression against someone by accident (e.g., stepping on toes in a crowded subway) elicit sympathy and prosocial behaviors. These are conceptually similar to lacking ability in achievement contexts inasmuch as one "cannot"; that is, they represent "sickness" rather than sin.

In summary, rules regarding the morality of "can" and "cannot" are linked to interpersonal behavior in achievement and other social contexts. The metaphor guiding this theory is that people are judges and life is a courtroom where interpersonal dramas related to innocence and guilt are played out! Hence, the foundation for this theory is in theology and law.

Interrelations of the Theories

The two motivational systems have been presented as though they are quite separate. In fact, they are closely intertwined and interactive, with rather paradoxical results. Consider, for example, a student whom others believe performed poorly because of lack of aptitude. Inasmuch as aptitude is construed as an uncontrollable cause, some involved observers may communicate sympathy and pity to this pupil following failure. These are positive "moral" emotions. The affective communications then provide evidence to the person that he or she "cannot," which increase the likelihood of personal feelings of shame and humiliation. These affects dampen motivation. Thus, what appears positive in the interpersonal context has negative consequences for personal motivation. On the other hand, if the student is thought by others (e.g., the teacher) to have failed because of lack of effort, then the teacher is likely to communicate anger. Inasmuch as expressed anger is used to infer personal causality and responsibility (see review in Weiner, 1995), the student is more likely to ascribe his or her personal failure to lack of effort. This, in turn, increases guilt and motivation. Thus, what appears negative in the interpersonal context (expression of an antisocial emotion) has (some) positive consequences for personal motivation.

Or consider the following example: Teachers, of course, provide help to their students. Help is particularly likely to be offered if the student tries but fails, inasmuch as the determinants of help giving are perceptions of uncontrollability and the linked emotional reactions of sympathy and compassion (see Graham & Barker, 1990). But help may therefore communicate to the recipient that he or she "cannot." If the student uses help to form personal attributions for his or her need, then motivation is weakened. Hence, a positive and well-intentioned behavior of the teacher may have negative consequences for the student. In summary, as illustrated in these examples, the two motivation theories overlap and are involved in the thoughts, feelings, and actions of both the actor and the observer, within the same behavioral episode.

ATTRIBUTION THEORY AND COMPETENCE

Now I consider in greater detail inferences of competence and incompetence. In keeping with the prior distinction between intrapersonal and interpersonal theories of motivation, one can ask about the meaning and significance of self- or of other-perception of competence. I examine here primarily other-perception of competence (some aspects of self-perception are included in the prior discussion). I chose this direction because the social psychology of competence receives far less attention in these *Handbook* chapters and in the general psychological literature than do the self-construal and measurement

of competence. I also do not distinguish between competence as a trait-like quality as opposed to a specific ability to complete a specific task. This differentiation, while important in many contexts, is not essential here.

The starting point for my analysis concerns inferred causal characteristics that constitute antecedents of the perceived competence of others. There are (at least) two roads or paths to gaining competence, reflecting the nature–nurture controversy (see Dweck, 1991; Dweck & Leggett, 1988). And here I shift from the competence label to constructs used by attribution theorists (see Figures 5.1 and 5.2), as well as by laypeople. On the one hand, competence or ability to complete a task may be considered to be attained because of "aptitude." Aptitudes are perceived as being not only internal to the person but also as stable and uncontrollable; that is, they remain the same over time, and one cannot do anything about them. For example, math aptitude is typically construed as an inborn characteristic; it does not radically (if at all) change over time, and one cannot willfully make it stronger (or weaker). Others often are regarded as competent at math because of high math aptitude or competent at music because of inborn talent. In this sense, competence is a structure.

The second path to being able more involves learning and effort expenditure. In this case, the causes of competence are conceived as controllable. For example, a competent car mechanic is usually perceived as having a learning history that includes expending effort or practicing to reach a competent state. Over time, as new challenges or more difficult tasks arise, competence may decrease. Someone with high math aptitude is rarely considered as having lost this trait (disease or old age may cause a decrease in competence). However, a competent mechanic may readily become an incompetent one if new technological advances are not mastered.

In summary, the meaning or definition of competence (ability to perform a task) as discussed in this chapter includes its causes—genetics versus effort, and its placement in the three-dimensional causal space earlier described. Both aptitude- and effort-linked competence are properties of the person. But when associated with aptitude, the concept of competence is conceived as mainly uncontrollable, whereas when associated with effort expended, the attainment of competence is conceived as controllable. Recognizing differences in perceptions of control, as previously revealed in Figure 5.2, is essential when considering the consequences of the success and failure of others.

Social and Emotional Implications of Being Perceived as Competent or Incompetent Because of Aptitude

There are many social benefits to being perceived as competent, particularly when it is due to aptitude. If a person is competent in school-related activities, others want him or her as their work partner; they will seek the person out for help, and so on. Similarly, the individual regarded as competent in sports is among the first selected when teams are formed. Competence is therefore associated with choice and popularity. Indeed, so positive are judgments of competence that one flatters others and ingratiates oneself by relaying how smart and capable others are (see Hareli & Weiner, 2002).

Contempt and Sympathy

It logically also follows that being perceived as incompetent at academics results in a person being shunned as a laboratory partner, just as those considered incompetent at sports are often selected last when teams are formed for athletic competitions. And like the behavioral responses, the emotional reactions to failure because of lack of aptitude-linked competence also may be negative, with failure accompanied by social emotions such as scorn and contempt (emotions neglected in the earlier discussion of help giving). Contempt is elicited when observers feel (or are satisfied by feeling) better than others, such as having beliefs of greater intelligence, strength, and so on (Izard, 1977). Feelings of contempt indicate a devaluing of others and elicit antisocial behaviors, including social rejection.

However, as previously reasoned, reactions to incompetence also include positive and prosocial emotions, including sympathy, pity, and compassion, when the incompetence is linked to uncontrollable deficits. Nonetheless, sympathetic reactions may not necessarily change overt social behavior toward the incompetent person (as opposed to evoking helping tendencies, as emphasized in Figure 5.2). For example, although children can be taught that obesity is uncontrollable, they do not increase their social interactions with overweight others (Anesbury & Tiggemann, 2000). In a similar manner, although one may feel sorry for a person with a mental handicap, this person will not be a desired laboratory partner when achievement goals are linked.

It would seem, then, that aptitude-based competence has only positive associates, such as popularity and peer bonding, whereas reactions to incompetence are more complex and embrace both negative (contempt and rejection) and positive (sympathy and help giving) social emotions and behaviors. But that oversimplifies social life. In social settings, there also are some negatively linked social and emotional consequences associated with high competence in others, social outcomes typically overlooked in discussions that depict only the positive value of competence. Reactions of envy and beliefs that those having competence are arrogant are among the subtle negative social products of being able.

Envy

Envy is aroused when a person desires the advantages of another. These advantages are often materialistic, such as a new car or an expensive vacation. But envy also is targeted toward qualities others have, such as being beautiful, strong, and smart. When the target of envy is a characteristic of another, then it tends to be an uncontrollable quality, something the other is "given" or "has" (see Smith, Parrott, Diener, Hoyle, & Kim, 1999). Aptitudes, such as mathematical and artistic talents, are prime desires of the envious.

Envy is related to feelings of inferiority, which are brought about by unfavorable social comparisons and can contribute to negative self-evaluations. For example, students assess their ability by comparing their performance with peers, and they may conclude that others have higher ability than they do. This has negative affective consequences. Even when one achieves an identical level of success by investing more effort than another, the individual who works harder may experience negative affect inasmuch as self-perceptions of ability are reduced (Jagacinski & Nicholls, 1987; also see Tesser, 1988).

Among students, believing that another is more competent than oneself can evoke negative feelings toward that envied individual. This is consistent with balance theory, as formulated by Heider (1958), in that a system is in balance if one dislikes another for causing personal harm, even if this harm was not intended. The hypothesis that we dislike those we envy finds support in the psychological literature (see Brigham, Kelso, Jackson, & Smith, 1997; Smith, Parrott, Ozer, & Moniz, 1994). Hence, envy is one potentially negative consequence of being able, especially in a competitive classroom, where social comparisons abound.

One indication of the social costs of being competent is implied by the label of "nerd." These individuals are perceived as high in academic competence (but low in social competence). They elicit negative reactions that may include envy as one of their sources. Other peer group labels also are linked to behavioral competence in complex ways. For example, "jocks" are perceived as high in athletic competence but low in academic skills. These and other classifications (e.g., "geeks") on the basis of competencies, or patterns of competencies, reveal that these labels can have unwanted negative associates.

Arrogance and Modesty

Observers of an achievement often form attitudes about the character and personality of the achiever. Two such personality inferences in achievement-related contexts are arrogance and modesty. Arrogance and modesty are linked to actual causes of success, as well as to self-presentations of the achiever. Arrogant communications by the achiever emphasize that one's quality or worth is superior to that of others. Hence, impressions of arrogance are formed if unique personal qualities are highlighted by that individual in connection with attainment of an achievement-related goal (Ben-Ze'ev, 1993). In support of this, it has been documented that accounts of success are more arrogant if they describe internal rather than external causes (Carlston & Shovar, 1983; Wosinska, Dabul, Whetstone-Dion, & Cialdini, 1996). However, the most arrogant accounts are

not only internal to the person but also uncontrollable, such as beauty and intelligence, for these are desirable qualities that not many persons can attain (Hareli & Weiner, 2000). The difficulty of an accomplishment or the degree of success does not influence judgments of arrogance. If one publicly attributes success to high aptitude, then that individual is regarded as arrogant whether the accomplishment is winning a Nobel Prize or completing a trivial task (Hareli & Weiner, 2000). Einstein is arrogant if he states: "I am an Einstein."

People attempt to vary their self-presentations in an optimal fashion to create a favorable impression on their audience (Carlson & Shovar, 1983; Schlenker & Leary, 1982). Individuals who respond to achievements boastfully are not well liked (see Stebbins, 1976; Wosinska, et al., 1996), so arrogant communications are undesirable obstacles to important social benefits (Carlston & Shovar, 1983). It therefore would be anticipated that arrogant communications are less frequent than are expressions of modesty.

However, it also is the case that individuals prefer honest communications (Schlenker, 1975). Hence, a dilemma is created for those succeeding because of high aptitude. If the truth is communicated, then both the positive consequences of perceived honesty and the negative consequences of perceived arrogance might follow. In one study examining causal revelations, we (Hareli, Weiner, & Yee, 2004) provided respondents with true, as well as communicated, causes of success (with aptitude, effort, luck, and help from others being the manipulated causes). For example, respondents read that a person succeeded because of aptitude but stated to others that the cause of success was good luck, or success was due to luck but high aptitude was communicated. Our participants reported that, even when truthful, persons stating that they succeed because of high ability are arrogant and not modest. This was not the case for any other cause.

In a subsequent study, we found that, in spite of the costs of being perceived as arrogant, individuals often are truthful when communicating the reason for their success. When persons succeed because of high aptitude, they may convey this cause. Certainly "hiding one's light" could have unintended negative outcomes, for others may not recognize one's talents, and personal goals could be hindered. Yet, as already indicated, a truthful communication also places the competent person at risk for being regarded as arrogant. There are subtle and socially acceptable ways to convey high aptitude, but not all individuals have the social skills to communicate this in a manner not regarded as arrogant.

In summary, experiences of envy and inferences of arrogance are both linked with high competence. If another succeeds because of high aptitude, then envy may be aroused, perhaps producing disliking, and if this cause for success is communicated, then arrogance is inferred, which has adverse social effects. An emotional reaction of envy does not require the successful achiever to disclose aptitude ascriptions, whereas an inference of arrogance does assume an implicit or explicit expression of internal causes, and especially of aptitude.

Although the high-aptitude individual is at special risk for displaying arrogance if there also is a desire for honesty, those who are incompetent also are at risk, for any person claiming success because of high aptitude is regarded as arrogant. Arrogance is a claim and is inferred whether the other truthfully or falsely conveys high aptitude a cause of success.

On the other hand, those doing well because of high aptitude have a special advantage over those low in aptitude: They can appear modest. If people who succeed because of aptitude communicate other causes, such as good luck or hard work, then they are regarded as modest. But modesty is only weakly inferred when the other succeeds because of external reasons, such as luck or help from others, and conveys these reasons; that is, to be modest, one must lie in a "good" way (i.e., mask aptitude and communicate an external cause) (see Hareli & Weiner, 2000; Hareli et al., 2004). Someone who is incompetent is therefore excluded from the potential benefit of being regarded as modest. This is unfortunate for the incompetent person, inasmuch as modesty evokes admiration, liking, and positive social actions. In summary, competent individuals are disadvantaged in that they are more likely to be regarded as arrogant than are incompetent individuals, but are advantaged in that they may be considered modest, whereas incompetent individuals do not have this opportunity.

In conclusion, aptitude-related competence and incompetence are linked to a variety of affects (e.g., contempt, envy, scorn, sympathy), to group-based labels (e.g., nerd, jock) and to affect-laden personality inferences (e.g., arrogance and modesty). And these are just some examples of the many positive and negative social aspects of competence attained or not attained because of given abilities. As intimated earlier, there are varied consequences of being perceived as competent. The mere measurement of structure does not address the psychological meaning or significance of this inference.

Social and Emotional Consequences of Being Perceived as Competent or Incompetent Because of Effort Expenditure

The second path to the attainment or nonattainment of competence is by means of expending or failing to expend effort; that is, the cause of success or failure is whether or not one "tries." As is the case when the path to competence is aptitude, individuals competent because of effort expenditure may reap the benefits of work-partner and sport-partner choice. But there are additional affective and inferential results that are the product of effort attributions.

Admiration and Dislike

One's success and the attainment of competence ascribed to high effort and hard work are not anticipated to evoke envy because others also may work hard; that is, high effort, unlike high aptitude, is an advantage that can be attained. Competence or the fact that one "can" due to high effort is considered to be deserved and results in admiration (see Feather, 1999; Frijda, 1986; Hareli & Weiner, 2000; Ortony, Clore, & Collins, 1988). Admiration elicits rewards and prosocial behavior from others; individuals tend to praise those who succeed because of hard work.

Competence and the success it produces because of hard work, however, also are not without social costs. In addition to admiration, extra effort as a cause of success may result in rejection and dislike, in part because this behavior indicates acceptance of values that adolescents and others of school age may reject (see Juvonen & Murdock, 1993, 1995).

In general, success and competence ascribed by peers to hard work may provoke mixed emotions. For example, one stereotype of Asian Americans is that they obtain competence and success because they are always working (they are "drudges"). This is a negative stereotype, although I just indicated that competence attained because of hard work promotes admiration. Think about a physically handicapped person completing a marathon race! Yet this heartfelt admiration does not seem to describe an emotion that students experience when they observe their Asian American peers overcoming language and cultural barriers to attain competence through extra effort. Expending effort and gaining competence, then, evoke varied and conflicting reactions.

Anger

There is high agreement among emotion theorists that anger is generated by judgments of responsibility for nonattainment of a goal (see Averill, 1982). Anger is an accusation or a value judgment that follows from the belief that another "could and should have done otherwise." Anger, then, communicates that one "ought to have" attained competence and succeeded. Failure because of lack of effort evokes not only anger but also punishment and other antisocial responses elicited by this feeling. Yet just as one may dislike another who has attained competence because of hard work, a peer may like another student because of effortless incompetence; that is, rejection of adult (or organizational) values and norms, as revealed in a refusal to seriously try, may be positively viewed in some situations (see Juvonen & Murdock, 1995). Hence, there also are mixed consequences associated with incompetence because of low effort.

A CONCLUDING STATEMENT

Assume that I ask the following question of experts in the area of competence: "What can be predicted from knowledge of a person's competence?" I suspect that most answers would be something like "actual success rate," "the subjective likelihood or expec-tancy of success," "degree of achievement motivation," "self-esteem," "desire to undertake tasks," "persistence in the face of failure," and the like. I have not undertaken such a survey, but I believe I have reasonably captured the type of answers that would be provided. And they are very important answers pertaining to intrapersonal psychology; that is, competence is automatically considered from the perspective of what it means to the one who possesses (or does not possess) it.

In this chapter, I have played a different game and introduced a different theme, one capturing not the psychology of the competent or incompetent person, but rather the psychology of others viewing that individual. My answers to the question of what competence predicts, as suggested in this chapter, are whether others are envious of this individual; whether he or she elicits sympathy, contempt, anger and/or admiration when succeeding or failing; whether he or she is regarded as arrogant or modest; whether the individual is liked or disliked; and so on; that is, I have presented a social psychology of perceived competence.

This position does not conceive competence as a structure, but rather as a socially constructed perception that influences interpersonal dynamics. The focus of attention is not the competent or incompetent person but the reactor to that individual and the dyad. The emotions considered are not confined to self-directed pride, self-esteem, guilt, and shame, but rather are other-directed admiration, anger, contempt, envy, liking, sympathy, and so forth. And thoughts are not only about expectancy of success and the likelihood of goal attainment but also concern the meaning and significance of competence to the observer and the personality inferences that are elicited.

In achievement contexts, reactions of others often prove more important to the achiever than objective success or failure. For example, I may be more concerned with how this chapter is regarded by my peers than with the quality of my work. Of course, these perceptions or judgments influence one another, which further underscores the point being made. If one reasonably assumes that the social world impacts the achievement world (see Juvonen & Wentzel, 1996), then understanding the reactions of others is a major psychological issue in the study of competence.

REFERENCES

Anesbury, T., & Tiggemann, M. (2000). An attempt to reduce negative stereotyping of obesity in children by changing controllability beliefs. *Health Education Research, 15*, 145–152.

Atkinson, J. W. (1964). *An introduction to motivation.* Princeton, NJ: Van Nostrand.

Averill, J. R. (1982). *Anger and aggression; An essay on emotion.* New York: Springer-Verlag.

Ben-Ze'ev, A. (1993). On the virtue of modesty. *American Philosophical Quarterly, 30*, 235–246.

Brigham, N. L., Kelso, K. A., Jackson, M. A., & Smith, R. H. (1997). The roles of invidious comparisons and deservingness in sympathy and Schadenfreude. *Basic and Applied Psychology, 19*, 363–380.

Carlston, D. E., & Shovar, N. (1993). Effects of performance attributions on other's perception of the attributor. *Journal of Personality and Social Psychology, 44*, 515–525.

Dweck, C. S. (1991). Self-theories and goals: Their role in motivation, personality, and development. In R. A. Dienstbier (Ed.), *Nebraska Symposium on Motivation* (Vol. 38, pp. 195–235). Lincoln: University of Nebraska Press.

Dweck, C. S., & Leggett, E. L. (1988). A social-cognitive approach to motivation and personality. *Psychological Review, 95*, 256–273.

Feather, N. T. (1999). *Values, achievement, and justice.* New York: Kluwer Academic.

Forsterling, F., & Rudolph, U. (1988). Situations, attributions, and evaluation of reactions. *Journal of Personality and Social Psychology, 54*, 225–232.

Frijda, N. H. (1986). *The emotions.* Cambridge, UK: Cambridge University Press.

Gendolla, G. H. E., & Koller, M. (2001). Surprise and causal search: How are they affected by outcome valence and importance? *Motivation and Emotion, 25*, 237–250.

Graham, S., & Barker, G. (1990). The downside of help: An attributional–developmental analysis of helping behavior as a low ability cue. *Journal of Educational Psychology, 82*, 7–14.

Hareli, S., & Weiner, B. (2000). Accounts for success as determinants of perceived arrogance and modesty. *Motivation and Emotion, 24*, 215–236.

Hareli, S., & Weiner, B. (2002). Social emotions and personality inferences: A scaffold for a new direction in the study of achievement motivation. *Education Psychologist, 37*, 183–193.

Hareli, S., Weiner, B., & Yee, J. (2004). *Perceived arrogance and modesty as a function of the true and communicated causes of success.* Unpublished manuscript, University of California, Los Angeles.

Heider, F. (1958). *The psychology of interpersonal relations.* New York: Wiley.

Izard, C. E. (1977). *Human emotions.* New York: Plenum Press.

Jagacinski, C. M., & Nicholls, J. G. (1987). Competence and affect in task involvement and ego involvement: The impact of social comparison information. *Journal of Educational Psychology, 79*, 107–114.

Juvonen, J., & Murdock, T. B. (1993). How to promote social approval: Effects of audience and outcome on publicly communicated attributions. *Journal of Educational Psychology, 85*, 365–376.

Juvonen, J., & Murdock, T. B. (1995). Grade-level differences in the social value of effort: Implications for self-presentation tactics in early adolescents. *Child Development, 66*, 1694–1705.

Juvonen, J., & Wentzel, K. R. (Eds.). (1996). *Social motivation: Understanding children's school adjustment.* New York: Cambridge University Press.

Ortony, A., Clore, G. L., & Collins, A. (1988). *The cognitive structure of emotions.* Cambridge, UK: Cambridge University Press.

Schlenker, B. R. (1975). Self-presentation: Managing the impression of consistency when reality interferes with self-enhancement. *Journal of Personality and Social Psychology, 32*, 1030–1037.

Schlenker, B. R., & Leary, M. R. (1982). Audiences' reactions to self-enhancing, self-denigrating and accurate self-presentations. *Journal of Experimental Social Psychology, 18*, 89–104.

Smith, R., Parrott, W., Diener, E., Hoyle, R., & Kim, S. H. (1999). Dispositional envy. *Personality and Social Psychology Bulletin, 25*, 1007–1020.

Smith, R., Parrott, W. G., Ozer, D., & Moniz, A. (1994). Subjective injustice and inferiority as predictors of hostile and depressive feelings in envy. *Personality and Social Psychology Bulletin, 20*, 705–711.

Stebbins, R. A. (1976). Conceited talk: A test of hypothesis. *Psychological Reports, 39*, 1111–1116.

Tesser, A. (1988). Toward a self-evaluation maintenance model of social behavior. In L. Berkowitz (Ed.), *Advances in experimental social psychology* (Vol. 21, pp. 181–222). New York: Academic Press.

Weiner, B. (1986). *An attributional theory of motivation and emotion.* New York: Springer-Verlag.

Weiner, B. (1992). *Human motivation: Metaphors, theories, and research.* Newbury Park, CA: Sage.

Weiner, B. (1995). *Judgments of responsibility: A foundation for a theory of social conduct.* New York: Guilford Press.

Weiner, B. (1996). Searching for order in social motivation. *Psychological Inquiry, 7*, 197–214.

Weiner, B. (2000). Intrapersonal and interpersonal theories of motivation from an attributional perspective. *Educational Psychology Review, 12*, 1–14.

Wosinka, W., Dabul, A. J., Whetstone-Dion, R., & Cialdini, R. B. (1996). Self-presentation responses to success in the organization: The costs and benefits of modesty. *Basic and Applied Social Psychology, 18*, 229–242.

CHAPTER 6

ℭ℞

Competence Perceptions and Academic Functioning

DALE H. SCHUNK
FRANK PAJARES

There is an increasing emphasis in education and other fields on the study of the self (Graham & Weiner, 1996). The current interest in self-beliefs is grounded on the assumption that individuals' perceptions of themselves and their capabilities are vital forces in their success or failure in achievement settings.

In this chapter, we acquaint readers with self-constructs that have received extensive attention in academic motivation research; specifically, perceptions of competence. Although competence perceptions are central to many theories of motivation, we focus our chapter on *perceived self-efficacy*—one's perceived capabilities to learn or perform behaviors at designated levels (Bandura, 1986, 1997).

This focus seems prudent for various reasons. For one, the literature on competence perceptions is too vast to be covered in one chapter. For another, self-efficacy is well grounded theoretically; it is a key mecha-

nism in Bandura's (1986) social cognitive theory of human functioning. Third, since Bandura's (1977a, 1977b) original writings on self-efficacy, researchers have demonstrated the generality of its operation across various fields including education, health, business, sports, and interpersonal relations (Bandura, 1997). And finally, self-efficacy research findings are representative of the larger research literature on perceived competence constructs.

We begin by providing a brief overview of Bandura's (1986) social cognitive theory. We then identify other competence beliefs prominent in motivation research today, describe the defining characteristics of each construct, and distinguish these conceptions from self-efficacy. We provide empirical results that speak to the relation between self-efficacy and motivation and achievement outcomes. We also address the difficulty of comparing findings across studies of competence perceptions when definitions and methodological practices have differed so markedly in investigations. We trace the cultural, social, familial, and educational influences on self-efficacy, and we close the chapter by offering recommendations for further study.

SOCIAL COGNITIVE THEORY

Bandura (1986) advanced a view of human functioning that accords a central role to cognitive, vicarious, self-regulatory, and self-reflective processes in human adaptation and change. People are viewed as self-organizing, proactive, self-reflecting, and self-regulating rather than as reactive organisms shaped and shepherded by environmental forces or driven by inner impulses. From this theoretical perspective, human functioning is the product of a dynamic interplay of personal, behavioral, and environmental influences. How people interpret the results of their behavior informs and alters their environments and the personal factors, they possess, which, in turn, inform and alter subsequent behavior. This is the foundation of Bandura's conception of *reciprocal determinism*, the view that (1) personal factors in the form of cognition, affect, and biological events, (2) behavior, and (3) environmental influences, interact in reciprocal fashion.

Social cognitive theory is rooted in a view of human agency in which individuals are agents proactively engaged in their own development. Key to this sense of agency is the fact that individuals possess self-beliefs that enable them to exercise a measure of control over their thoughts, feelings, and actions (Bandura, 1986). Thus, individuals are viewed both as products and as producers of their own environments and of their social systems. Because human lives are not lived in isolation, Bandura expanded the conception of human agency to include collective agency. People work together on shared beliefs about their capabilities and common aspirations to better their lives. This conceptual extension makes the theory applicable to human adaptation and change in collectively oriented societies, as well as individually oriented ones.

Rooted within Bandura's (1986) social cognitive theory is the understanding that individuals are imbued with capabilities that define what it is to be human. Primary among these are the capabilities to symbolize, to plan alternative strategies, to learn through vicarious experience, to self-regulate, and to self-reflect. These capabilities provide human beings with the cognitive means by which they are influential in determining their own destiny. For Bandura, a key capability is *self-reflection*, through which people make sense of their experiences, explore their own cognitions and self-beliefs, engage in self-evaluation, and alter their thinking and behavior.

SELF-EFFICACY

According to Bandura (1986), human motivation, well-being, and personal accomplishment are based more on what an individual believes than on what is objectively true. Unless people believe that their actions can produce the outcomes they desire, they have little incentive to act or to persevere in the face of obstacles. For this reason, how people behave can often be better predicted by the beliefs they hold about their capabilities than by what they are actually capable of accomplishing, for these self-efficacy perceptions help determine what individuals do with the knowledge and skills they have. This helps explain why people's behaviors are sometimes disjoined from their actual capabilities, and why their behaviors may differ widely even when they have similar knowledge and skills. Many individuals suffer frequent and sometimes debilitating self-doubts about capabilities they clearly possess, just as many others are sometimes confident about what they can accomplish despite possessing modest skills.

Because individuals operate collectively as well as individually, self-efficacy is both a personal and a social construct. Groups develop a sense of collective efficacy—a shared belief in the group's capability to attain goals and accomplish tasks. Schools develop collective beliefs about the capability of their students to learn, of their teachers to teach and otherwise enhance the lives of their students, and of their administrators and policymakers to create environments conducive to these tasks. Organizations with a strong sense of efficacy empower and vitalize their constituents.

Effects of Self-Efficacy

Positive self-efficacy beliefs enhance human accomplishment and well-being in countless ways. They influence the *choices* people make and the courses of action they pursue (Bandura, 1997). Individuals select tasks and activities in which they feel competent and avoid those in which they do not. Unless people believe that their actions will have the desired consequences, they have little incentive to engage in those actions.

Self-efficacy beliefs also help determine how much *effort* people will expend on an activity, how long they will *persevere* when confronting obstacles, and how *resilient* they will be in the face of adverse situations (Pajares, 1996b; Schunk, 1995). The higher the sense of efficacy, the greater the effort, persistence, and resilience (Bandura, 1997). People with a strong sense of personal competence approach difficult tasks as challenges to be mastered rather than as threats to be avoided. They have greater intrinsic interest and deep engrossment in activities, set challenging goals and maintain strong commitment to them, and heighten and sustain their efforts in the face of failure. They quickly recover their self-efficacy after failures or setbacks and attribute failure to insufficient effort or deficient knowledge and skills that are acquirable.

Self-efficacy also influences an individual's *thought patterns* and *emotional reactions* (Bandura, 1997). High self-efficacy helps create feelings of serenity in approaching difficult tasks and activities. Conversely, people with low self-efficacy may believe that things are tougher than they really are, a belief that fosters anxiety, stress, depression, and a narrow vision of how best to solve a problem.

We do not mean to suggest from this discussion that self-efficacy is the only, or even the most important, influence on achievement outcomes. No amount of self-efficacy will produce a competent performance when requisite skills are lacking (Schunk, 1995). Similarly, high self-efficacy will not influence behavior when people do not value the outcomes or take pride in their accomplishment (Schunk, 1995). Individuals with high self-efficacy will not attempt an activity if they expect negative outcomes (outcome expectations are discussed later). A vast amount of

goal research shows that goals motivate and direct behavior (Locke & Latham, 2002). People may pursue a valued goal even when they have low self-efficacy for attaining it. These other factors notwithstanding, a wealth of research shows that self-efficacy can affect individuals' choice of activities, motivation, and achievement outcomes (Bandura, 1997; Pajares, 1996b; Schunk, 1995).

Sources of Self-Efficacy

Individuals form perceptions of self-efficacy by interpreting information primarily from four sources (Bandura, 1997). The most influential source is the interpreted result of one's previous performance, or *mastery experience*. Individuals engage in tasks and activities, interpret the results of their actions, use the interpretations to develop perceptions of their capability to engage in subsequent tasks or activities, and act in concert with the beliefs created. Outcomes interpreted as successful raise self-efficacy, whereas those interpreted as failures lower it, although an occasional failure after many successes will not have much effect.

People form self-efficacy perceptions through the *vicarious experience* of observing others perform tasks. This source of information has weaker effects on self-efficacy than do mastery experiences, but when people are uncertain about their own abilities, or when they have limited prior experience, they become more sensitive to what others do. The effects of modeling are particularly relevant. Vicarious experience is particularly powerful when observers see similarities in some attribute and then assume that the model's performance is diagnostic of their own capability. Conversely, watching models with perceived similar attributes fail can undermine observers' beliefs about their own capabilities. It bears noting that people seek out models who possess qualities they admire and capabilities to which they aspire. A significant model in one's life can help instill self-beliefs that will influence the course and direction that life takes.

Individuals also create and develop self-efficacy as a result of the *social persuasions* and verbal judgments they receive from others. Persuaders play an important role. But social persuasions should not be confused with knee-jerk praise or empty inspirational homilies. Effective persuaders must cultivate people's beliefs in their capabilities, while at the same time ensuring that the envisioned success is attainable. Just as positive persuasions may work to encourage and empower, negative persuasions can work to defeat and weaken self-efficacy.

Somatic and emotional states such as anxiety, stress, arousal, and mood states also provide information about self-efficacy. People can gauge their confidence by the emotional state they experience as they contemplate an action. Strong emotional reactions to a task provide cues about the anticipated success or failure. When people experience negative thoughts and fears about their capabilities, those affective reactions can lower self-efficacy perceptions and trigger additional stress and agitation that help to ensure the inadequate performance feared. One way to raise self-efficacy is to improve physical and emotional well-being and reduce negative emotional states. Because individuals have the capability to alter their own thinking and feeling, enhanced self-efficacy can, in turn, powerfully influence the physiological states. People live in psychical environments that are primarily of their own making (Bandura, 1997).

RELATED VIEWS OF PERCEIVED COMPETENCE

As we noted earlier, competence perceptions are important components of other theories of achievement motivation. In this section, we identify other competence beliefs prominent in motivation research, describe the defining characteristics of each construct, and distinguish these self-beliefs from self-efficacy perceptions.

Self-Concept

Self-concept refers to one's collective self-perceptions formed through experiences with and interpretations of the environment, and heavily influenced by reinforcements and evaluations by significant other persons (Shavelson & Bolus, 1982). No single theorist is credited with formulating the construct of self-concept and outlining its basic tenets, as Bandura has done for self-efficacy.

Because of its varied parentage, researchers have not agreed on a name or operational definition. In any particular study, self-concept may travel under the guise of self-esteem, self-awareness, self-image, self-perception, self-appraisal, self-schema, self-worth, self-evaluation, or even the self itself. Wylie (1974) addressed this problem when she argued that the basic constructs as defined and used by self-concept researchers typically pointed to no clear empirical referents. Small wonder, she wrote, that "a wide array of operational definitions of some of these constructs has been devised by various experimenters" (p. 8).

Theorists have often drawn a distinction between self-concept and self-esteem—the evaluative component of self-concept. However, various researchers have concluded that descriptive and evaluative perceptions of self have not been empirically separated in research studies and may not be empirically separable (Hattie, 1992; Shavelson & Bolus, 1982). For this reason, researchers typically use the terms interchangeably, although most prefer the term "self-concept."

During the 1980s, researchers identified seven features critical to a definition of self-concept: organized, multifaceted, hierarchical, stable, developmental, evaluative, and differentiable (Shavelson & Marsh, 1986). The hierarchical feature has received the most attention. Marsh and Shavelson (1985) differentiated between the self-perceptions that one has about oneself as an individual, and that involve the totality of one's self-knowledge, and the self-perceptions that one has in regards to specific areas or domains in one's life. General self-perceptions comprise the global self-concept, whereas the more discrete self-perception can comprise self-concepts about academic, social, emotional, or physical facets of the self. The hierarchy progressively narrows into even more discrete self-concepts. Academic self-concepts can be subject-specific (e.g., language arts, mathematics, science); social self-concepts can include self-perceptions regarding family, peers, or significant others. People become increasingly aware of their differing domain-specific self-concepts as they grow older, and it is the self-views in discrete and specific areas of one's life that are most likely to guide and inform behavior in those areas. Researchers have found support for this hierarchical model (Bong & Clark, 1999; Hattie, 1992; Marsh, 1993).

After a thorough examination of their empirical properties, Bong and Skaalvik (2003) concluded that self-efficacy and self-concept differ in important ways. Self-efficacy comprises cognitive, goal-referenced, relatively context-specific, and future-oriented judgments of competence that are relatively malleable due to their task dependence. Self-concept beliefs, on the other hand, are primarily affective, heavily normative, typically aggregated, hierarchically structured, and past-oriented self-perceptions that are relatively stable due to their generality. According to Bong and Skaalvik, self-efficacy acts as an active precursor of self-concept development.

Self-efficacy and self-concept theorists have emphasized the need to keep the contextual nature of these self-perceptions in mind when conducting investigations. Bandura (1997) argued that to predict academic outcomes from students' efficacy beliefs, "self-efficacy beliefs should be measured in terms of particularized judgments of capability that may vary across realms of activity, different levels of task demands within a given activity domain, and under different situational circumstances" (p. 6). In a similar vein, Marsh (1993) cautioned that "research clearly demonstrates that self-concept and its relation to other variables cannot be adequately understood if its multidimensional, domain-specific nature is ignored" (p. 92). And both have cautioned that the self-beliefs assessed should always correspond with the achievement index with which they are compared.

Despite their differences, self-efficacy and self-concept are related (Pajares & Schunk, 2002). Students with high academic self-efficacy are apt to hold favorable self-concepts, and a positive self-concept can lead students to approach new tasks with self-efficacy for learning. At the same time, however, there is no automatic relationship between one's perceptions about what one can or cannot do and whether one feels positively or negatively about oneself. Some students may approach mathematics with confidence but without the corresponding positive self-concept, in part because self-efficacy for mathematics is only one contributor to overall self-concept. One could sur-

mise that skilled soldiers in war may possess strong efficacy beliefs about their professional capabilities but not view themselves more favorably for performing them well, plagued as they may be by the emotional distress that accompanies warfare. Conversely, students may readily admit to dismal self-efficacy when it comes to mathematics but suffer no loss of self-concept on that account, in part because they do not invest their self-concept in this activity. There are many things that individuals do poorly but that have little influence on how they feel about themselves.

Outcome Expectations

Self-efficacy should not be confused with *outcome expectations*, or judgments of the likely consequences of behavior (Bandura, 1977b). Self-efficacy often helps to determine the outcomes one expects. Confident individuals anticipate successful outcomes. Students confident in their social skills anticipate successful social encounters. Those confident in their academic skills expect high marks on exams and expect the quality of their work to reap personal and professional benefits. The opposite is true of those who lack confidence. Students who doubt their social skills often envision rejection or ridicule even before they establish social contact. Those who lack confidence in their academic skills envision a low grade before they begin an examination or enroll in a course.

Although self-efficacy and outcome expectations often are related, mismatches can occur. High perceptions of self-efficacy may not result in consistent behavior when individuals believe that the outcome of engaging in that behavior will have undesired effects. Students who are highly self-efficacious in their academic capabilities may elect not to apply to a particular university whose selective entrance requirements make a negative admission decision likely. Students may realize that strong mathematics skills are essential for a good Graduate Record Examination (GRE) score and eligibility for graduate school, but low self-efficacy in mathematics may lead them to shun challenging courses, the GRE, and graduate school. Conversely, if students expect positive outcomes from a certain action and value those outcomes, they may engage in the activity even if they have low self-efficacy for success. Thus, both self-efficacy and outcome expectations often are useful in explaining achievement outcomes.

Expectancy Beliefs in Expectancy–Value Theory

Expectancy–value theories of motivation stress two key cognitive influences: people's judgments about the likelihood of success at a task (*expectancies*) and their reasons for engaging in the task (*values*). The historical impetus derives from work by Lewin, Dembo, Festinger, and Sears (1944), who proposed that *level of aspiration*, or the goal that people set in a task, was a function of expectancy and value components. The results of much research showed that level of aspiration depended on prior experiences— successes raised and failures lowered it, that people felt more successful when they met the goals they set for themselves than with an objective level of attainment, and that level of aspiration reflected individual and group differences (Weiner, 1992).

Based on level of aspiration and other motivation research, Atkinson (1957, 1964) developed a comprehensive theory of motivation that included achievement motives, probabilities for success, and incentive values of success. Key achievement motives were the motive to approach success and the motive to avoid failure. Probability for success reflected expectancy, and incentive value referred to how much individuals valued success. Performance, persistence, and choice of behavior are linked directly to the beliefs that individuals hold about their expectancy and the value of the task. Individuals will be motivated to engage in tasks when they value the outcome they expect to attain.

Modern expectancy–value theories differ from earlier conceptions (Eccles & Wigfield, 2002). Current theories define expectancy and value beliefs more specifically and link them to many psychological and sociocultural factors. Atkinson (1964) had posited that expectancy and value beliefs can interact in such a way that they can be inversely related, in the sense that success at difficult tasks is valued more than success at easy tasks. Today, theorists contend that expec-

tancy and value are positively related. They also define expectancies for success as "individuals' beliefs about how well they will do on upcoming tasks, either in the immediate or longer-term future" (Eccles & Wigfield, 2002, p. 119), and they assess them in a manner similar to that used by self-efficacy researchers.

Eccles and her colleagues (1983) formulated an expectancy–value model in which human behavior is viewed as influenced both by the positive and negative features of a particular task or activity, and in which the choices that people make have costs associated with them, because one choice can eliminate others. In this model, the relative value and probability of success of various options are key determinants of choice, and individuals' expectancies for success are influenced by self-perceptions such as self-efficacy. The expectancies themselves directly influence performance, persistence, and task choice. Competence beliefs are construed as domain-specific judgments of competence, in contrast to expectancies, which are operationalized as relatively specific expectations to succeed on a specific upcoming task. Expectancy–value theorists contend that, even though the two constructs are conceptually distinct, they are not empirically separable, and they report that children and adolescents do not easily distinguish between domain- and task-specific competence beliefs (Eccles & Wigfield, 2002).

Research shows that, even after controlling for previous performance, competence beliefs and expectancies predict academic performance in various academic areas, whereas task values predict course plans and enrollment decisions, as well as involvement in sport activities (Eccles, 1987; Eccles, Adler, & Meece, 1984; Eccles et al., 1983; Meece, Wigfield, & Eccles, 1990). Expectancies and values also predict career choices (Wigfield & Eccles, 1992).

Expectancy–value theories bear much similarity to self-efficacy theory. Both stress the role of personal expectations as cognitive motivators of behavior. Although the expectancy construct in Atkinson's theory seems more akin to outcome expectancy than to self-efficacy, the Eccles and Wigfield model differentiates different types of expectancies. Expectancy–value theories emphasize the role of personal values in the direction of behavior. Self-efficacy theory also claims their importance as one of several factors that influence achievement strivings in addition to self-efficacy. However, Bandura (1986) also notes that efficacy judgments can affect perceived value. Individuals who expect success in a particular enterprise tend to value those enterprises. Bandura argued that because the outcomes that people value and expect are largely dependent on their judgments of what they can accomplish, beliefs such as perceived value may not contribute significantly to predictions of behavior when self-efficacy perceptions are controlled.

Perceived Control

The notion of perceived control is also related to competence beliefs. For example, according to locus of control theory (Rotter, 1966), people expect success to the degree that they feel in control of their behavior, often referred to as internal locus of control. Research supports this contention (Findley & Cooper, 1983). Connell and Wellborn (1991) proposed that internal locus of control is related to competence beliefs. People who believe they can control what they learn and perform are more apt to initiate and sustain behaviors directed toward those ends than are those with a low sense of control over their capabilities (Schunk, 1995). Deci and Ryan's (1985) *self-determination* theory stresses the need for autonomy and control of one's life.

In Bandura's (1986) system of triadic reciprocality, a sense of control over the significant outcomes of one's life is a key motivator of behavior in addition to self-efficacy. In fact, it is demoralizing to believe that one has the capabilities to succeed but that environmental barriers (e.g., discrimination) preclude one from doing so. Self-efficacy is apt to be most influential in predicting behavior when the environment is responsive and allows one to exercise one's capabilities without restraint.

Assessment of Self-Efficacy and Competence Beliefs

The events over which personal influence is exercised vary (Bandura, 1986). Depending on what is being managed, it may entail reg-ulation of one's motivation, thought processes, affective states and actions, or changing environmental conditions. Self-efficacy beliefs are sensitive to these contextual factors. As such, they differ from other competence beliefs in that self-efficacy judgments are typically more task- and situation-specific, and individuals make use of these judgments in reference to some goal (Pintrich & Schunk, 2002). Consequently, self-efficacy is generally assessed at a more microanalytic level than are other competence beliefs.

Researchers assess self-efficacy beliefs by asking individuals to report the level, generality, and strength of their confidence to accomplish a task or succeed in a certain situation. Assessors of other competence beliefs do not ask individuals to make these level, strength, and generality judgments. Rather, such assessment includes asking students to report how well they expect to do in an academic subject (e.g., performance expectancies; Meece et al., 1990), whether they understand what they read (e.g., perceptions of competence; Harter, 1996), or whether they are good in an academic subject (e.g., ability perceptions; Meece et al., 1990). It is a testament to the field's inability to agree on the nature and conceptualization of perceived competence that several constructs are found in the literature. Beyond those we have identified, these include task-specific self-concept, self-concept of ability, perceptions of task difficulty, self-perceptions of ability, perceived ability, self-appraisals of ability, subjective competence, and, of course, self-confidence.

Theorists do not have to conceptualize competence beliefs in identical fashion or agree, without clear empirical evidence, that one conceptualization is superior to others. Rather, differing conceptualizations must be subjected to empirical scrutiny, so that the most useful and explanatory ones emerge. It also may be that conceptualizations play differing roles; thus, constructs can provide alternative insights. Such progress in the evolution of competence beliefs conceptions currently in use would be possible if they reasonably differed from each other, but that presently is not the case. For example, Boekaerts's (1991) definition of subjective competence as "a person's knowledge, beliefs, and feelings about his capabilities and skills" (p. 2) is remarkably similar to Byrne's (1984) definition of self-concept as the self-perceptions that individuals have about their academic abilities, specifically, their "feelings and knowledge about [these] abilities [and] skills" (p. 428). Also, competence beliefs are assessed with questions that, although similar, are just different enough to make comparing findings a difficult task. Contrast a perceived ability item, "I can do well on this exam," (Greene & Miller, 1996) with one from math ability perceptions, "How have you been doing in math this year?" (Meece et al., 1990), or one from self-appraisal of ability, "How do you rate yourself in school ability compared with those in your grade at school?" (Felson, 1984). When these similarly conceptualized but differently operationalized competence beliefs are used to suit specific research agendas, researchers must sift through various competence beliefs, determining their decisive characteristics (Bong, 1996), evaluating whether findings are consistent or inconsistent with theoretical tenets and prior research, and planning follow-up investigations.

RELATIONSHIP BETWEEN SELF-EFFICACY AND ACHIEVEMENT OUTCOMES

There is ample empirical evidence showing that self-efficacy relates to and influences numerous academic outcomes. Researchers also have shown that self-efficacy mediates the effect of skills, previous experience, mental ability, and other self-beliefs on subsequent achievement, which is to say that it acts as a filter between these prior determinants and academic indexes. Bandura (1997) provides extensive evidence to suggest that percepts of self-efficacy are powerful determinants of achievement outcomes in varied fields. In a meta-analysis, Stajkovic and Luthans (1998) found that the average weighted correlation between self-efficacy and work-related performance was $(G)r = .38$, which transforms to an impressive 28% gain in task performance.

In education, a meta-analysis of studies published between 1977 and 1988 revealed that self-efficacy beliefs were positively related to academic achievement (Multon,

Brown, & Lent, 1991). Self-efficacy related to academic outcomes ($r_\mu = .38$) and accounted for approximately 14% of the variance. Effects were stronger for high school and college students than for elementary students. Effect sizes also depended on characteristics of the studies, such as the types of self-efficacy and performance measures used. Stronger effects were obtained by researchers who compared specific efficacy judgments with cognitive skills measures of performance or classroom-based indexes such as grades than with global, standardized achievement tests. Effect sizes also were stronger in studies in which researchers developed highly concordant self-efficacy/performance indexes and administered them at the same time.

Correlations between self-efficacy and academic performances in investigations in which self-efficacy is analyzed at the item- or task-specific level and corresponds to the criterial task have ranged from .49 to .70; direct effects in path-analytic studies have ranged from beta = .349 to .545 (Pajares, 1996b, 1997). Results tend to be higher in studies of mathematics than of other academic areas such as language arts, but even in these areas, relationships are considerably higher if the criteria by which students judge self-efficacy are used as the criteria for scoring essays or assessing reading comprehension (Pajares, 2003).

Self-efficacy also is related to self-regulated learning variables and use of learning strategies. Zimmerman and his associates have traced the relationships among self-efficacy perceptions, academic self-regulatory processes, and academic achievement. This line of inquiry has demonstrated that self-efficacy influences self-regulatory processes such as goal setting, self-monitoring, self-evaluation, and strategy use (Zimmerman, 1989, 1990, 1994, 2000; Zimmerman & Bandura, 1994; Zimmerman & Martinez-Pons, 1990). Confident students embrace more challenging goals (Zimmerman, Bandura, & Martinez-Pons, 1992), and they engage in more effective self-regulatory strategies to include enhanced memory performance through increased persistence (Bouffard-Bouchard, Parent, & Larivée, 1991). In studies of college students who pursue science and engineering courses, high self-efficacy influences the academic persistence necessary to maintain high academic achievement (Hackett, 1995; Lent, Brown, & Larkin, 1984; Lent & Hackett, 1987). Students who believe they are capable of performing tasks use more cognitive and metacognitive strategies, and persist longer at those tasks than those who do not. Academic self-efficacy influences cognitive strategy use and self-regulation through use of metacognitive strategies, and it is correlated with in-class seatwork and homework, exams and quizzes, and essays and reports. Pintrich and De Groot (1990) suggested that self-efficacy facilitates cognitive engagement such that raising self-efficacy likely leads to higher achievement by increasing use of cognitive strategies.

Students with similar previous achievement and cognitive skills may differ in subsequent achievement as a result of differing self-efficacy perceptions, because these perceptions mediate between prior attainments and academic achievement. As a consequence, performances often are better predicted by self-efficacy than by prior attainments. Collins (1982) identified children of low, middle, and high mathematics ability who had, within each ability level, either high or low mathematics self-efficacy. After instruction, the children were given new problems to solve and could rework those they missed. Collins reported that ability was related to performance but that, regardless of ability level, children with high self-efficacy completed more problems correctly and reworked more of the ones they missed. Pajares and Kranzler (1995) tested the joint contribution of self-efficacy and mental ability (the variable typically acknowledged as the most powerful predictor of academic outcomes) to mathematics performance and found that, despite the influence of mental ability, self-efficacy beliefs made a powerful and independent contribution to the prediction of performance.

Studies of goal setting have demonstrated that self-efficacy and skill development are stronger in students who set proximal goals than in those who set distal goals, in part because proximal attainments provide evidence of growing expertise (Bandura & Schunk, 1981; Locke & Latham, 2002). In addition, students who have been verbally encouraged to set their own goals experience increases in confidence, competence, and

commitment to attain those goals (Schunk, 1995). Self-efficacy also is increased when students are provided with frequent and immediate feedback while working on a task (Schunk, 1983b), and when students are taught to attribute this feedback to their own effort, they work harder, experience stronger motivation, and report greater efficacy for further learning (Schunk, 1987). Self-efficacy explains approximately 25% of the variance in the prediction of academic outcomes beyond that of instructional influences. Self-efficacy is responsive to changes in instructional experiences and plays a causal role in students' development and use of academic competencies (Schunk, 1995).

A growing number of findings support Bandura's contention that self-efficacy mediates the effect of possessed skills or other self-beliefs on subsequent performance by influencing effort, persistence, and perseverance. Schunk (1981) used path analysis to show that modeling treatments increased persistence and accuracy on division problems by raising children's self-efficacy, which had a direct effect on skill (.46). He later demonstrated that effort attributional feedback for prior performance (e.g., "You've been working hard") raised children's self-efficacy, and this increase was, in part, responsible for increased skill in performance of subtraction problems (Schunk, 1982a). In subsequent experiments, he found that ability feedback (e.g., "You're good at this") had an even stronger effect on self-efficacy and subsequent performance (Schunk, 1983b; Schunk & Gunn, 1986).

Not only do children learn from the actions of models, but much research shows that modeling practices also affect self-perceptions (Schunk, 1981, 1987, 1999; Schunk & Gunn, 1985; Schunk, Hanson, & Cox, 1987; Zimmerman & Ringle, 1981). When peer models make errors, engage in coping behaviors in front of students, and verbalize emotive statements reflecting low confidence and achievement, low-achieving students perceive the models as more similar to themselves and develop greater skills and self-efficacy. Social cognitive theorists recommend that teachers engage in effective modeling practices, and that they select peers for classroom models judiciously so as to ensure that students view themselves as comparable in learning ability to the models.

Of course, academic achievement is too complex to reduce to the conclusion that it is due to differences in any competence belief. Such beliefs are neither the *prima causa* of achievement in all cases nor a magic elixir that can make all learners work to their full potential. Students perform differently in school because of differences in aptitudes, general mental abilities, interests, perceived values, effort, perseverance, use of self-regulatory strategies, teaching and instruction, and availability of materials (Gustafson & Undheim, 1996; Keogh & MacMillan, 1996; Snow, Corno, & Jackson, 1996). Social and familial variables such as peer influence, family income, and parental expectations also play a hand in students' academic outcomes (Steinberg, Brown, & Dornbusch, 1996). And no amount of confidence can produce success when requisite skills and knowledge are absent. As we have illustrated, however, there is good reason to believe that many differences in achievement can be better explained by students' perceptions of their academic capabilities than by constructs often thought to be the key determinants of achievement.

The causal influence of self-efficacy on students' academic achievement-related behaviors has been effectively demonstrated in a series of studies (Schunk, 1982a, 1982b, 1983a, 1983b, 1984a, 1984b; Schunk & Swartz, 1993; Schunk et al., 1987). Students' self-efficacy beliefs were raised by providing them with instructional strategies designed to enhance their competence, such as modeling, strategy training, goal setting, rewards for progress, attributional feedback, and progress feedback. The increase in self-efficacy also resulted in improved performance. Research also shows that self-efficacy for learning new skills predicts subsequent motivation and achievement during instruction.

Gender, Race/Ethnicity, and Competence Beliefs

Research on gender differences in self-efficacy and related competence beliefs typically shows that girls hold lower competence beliefs than do boys on tasks perceived as masculine (Meece, 1991). Boys and girls report similar confidence in their mathematics ability during the elementary years, but reliable differences begin to emerge following children's transition to middle or junior high school (Eccles & Midgley, 1989; Midgley, Feldlaufer, & Eccles, 1989; Pajares & Valiante, 2002). By high school, boys are more confident and girls more likely to underestimate their capability (Pajares & Kranzler, 1995; Pajares & Miller, 1994, 1997; Pajares, Miller, & Johnson, 1999; Pajares & Valiante, 1999, 2001). Gifted girls are especially likely to be underconfident about their capabilities (Pajares, 1996a).

Among adolescents, gender differences in self-efficacy should not be expected when students are able to derive clear performance information about their capabilities or progress in learning. Schunk and Lilly (1984) had middle school students judge their self-efficacy for learning a novel mathematical task, after which students received instruction and opportunities to practice. Students received performance feedback by checking answers to alternate problems. Although girls initially judged their self-efficacy for learning lower than boys, following the instructional program, girls and boys did not differ in achievement or self-efficacy. The performance feedback conveyed to students that they were learning and raised girls' self-efficacy to that of boys.

Other research shows that gender differences in self-efficacy can arise from the linkage of skills to contexts (Bandura, 1997). Women typically judge self-efficacy for scientific occupations lower than do men, but gender differences disappear when women judge self-efficacy for performing the same skills in everyday activities (Matsui & Tsukamoto, 1991). Women also typically judge self-efficacy lower than men for occupations requiring quantitative skills, but differences disappear when self-efficacy judgments for the quantitative activities are made in stereotypically feminine tasks (Junge & Dretzke, 1995). Gender differences can arise as a function of home, cultural, educational, and mass media influences. Developmental research shows that parents often underestimate their daughters' academic competence and hold lower expectations for daughters (Phillips & Zimmerman, 1990). Parents also act differentially with respect to mathematics and science, often portraying them as male domains

(Meece & Courtney, 1992). As girls enter junior and senior high, the perception of mathematics as a masculine domain may further weaken their interest in it.

Fewer studies have been conducted on differences as a function of race or ethnicity. Some findings show that minority students hold lower competence beliefs than do nonminority students, but studies often confound ethnicity with social class by comparing middle-class white children with lower class minority children (Pintrich & Schunk, 2002). Graham's (1994) summary of the literature on the motivation of African American students revealed that they "maintain undaunted optimism and positive self-regard even in the face of achievement failure" (p. 103). She found little support for the notion that African Americans have lower competence beliefs than do white students once socioeconomic status is controlled. Similar findings have been reported with Hispanic American students (Stevenson, Hanson, & Uttal, 1990). These findings have resulted primarily from studies of global or domain-specific self-concept. In studies in which task-specific self-efficacy perceptions are assessed, African American students and Hispanic American students' self-efficacy tends to be lower than that of whites. Despite differences in self-efficacy, minority students report positive self-concepts (Pajares & Johnson, 1996; Pajares & Kranzler, 1995). Beliefs at differing levels of specificity may perform different functions for minority students.

DEVELOPMENT OF SELF-EFFICACY

Beginning in early infancy, parents and other caregivers provide experiences that differentially influence self-efficacy. Home variables that help children interact effectively with the environment influence cognitive development and self-efficacy (Bandura, 1997). Initial self-efficacy sources are centered in the family, but the influence is bidirectional. Parents who provide an environment that stimulates curiosity and allows for mastery experiences help build children's self-beliefs. In turn, children who display more curiosity and exploratory activities promote parental responsiveness. When environments are rich in interesting activities that arouse children's cu-

riosity and offer moderate challenges, children are motivated to work on the activities and learn new information and skills. Home environments vary greatly. Some contain many resources that stimulate children's thinking; parents may be heavily invested in their children's cognitive development and spend time with them on learning. Other homes do not have these resources, and adults may devote little time to children's education.

Parents who provide a warm, responsive, and supportive home environment, encourage exploration, stimulate curiosity, and provide play and learning materials, accelerate their children's intellectual development (Meece, 1997). Parents also are key providers of self-efficacy information. Parents who arrange for varied mastery experiences develop more self-efficacious youngsters than do parents who arrange fewer opportunities (Bandura, 1997). Such experiences occur in homes enriched with activities and in which children have freedom to explore.

With respect to vicarious sources, parents who teach children ways to cope with difficulties and model persistence and effort strengthen children's efficacy. With development, the role of peers becomes increasingly important. Parents who steer their children toward efficacious peers provide vicarious boosts in self-efficacy. Homes also are prime sources of persuasive information. Parents who encourage their youngsters to try different activities and support their efforts help to develop children who feel more capable of meeting challenges (Bandura, 1997). Self-efficacy suffers in homes where new activities are not encouraged.

Peers influence children's self-efficacy in various ways. Observing similar others succeed can raise observers' self-efficacy and motivate them to perform the task if they believe that they too will succeed (Schunk, 1987). Observing others fail can lead students to believe that they lack the competence to succeed and may dissuade them from attempting the task. Similarity is most influential for students who are uncertain about their performance capabilities, such as those lacking task familiarity and information to use in judging self-efficacy or those who have experienced difficulties and hold doubts (Bandura, 1986; Schunk, 1987). Model similarity is potent among children and adolescents, because peers are similar in many ways, and students at these developmental levels are unfamiliar with many tasks.

Peer influence also operates through *peer networks*, or large groups of peers with whom students associate. Students in networks tend to be similar to each other (Cairns, Cairns, & Neckerman, 1989), which enhances the likelihood of influence by modeling. Networks help define students' opportunities for interactions and observations of others' interactions, as well as their access to activities (Dweck & Goetz, 1978). Over time, network members become more similar to one another. Discussions between friends influence their choices of activities, and friends often make similar choices (Berndt & Keefe, 1992). Furthermore, peer groups promote motivational socialization. Changes in children's motivational engagement across the school year are predicted by their peer group membership at the start of the year (Kindermann, McCollam, & Gibson, 1996). Children affiliated with motivated groups change positively across the school year; those in less-motivated groups change negatively. It seems that peer group socialization influences the group's academic self-efficacy, which affects academic motivation.

Added support for these points comes from research by Steinberg et al. (1996), who tracked students from high school entrance until their senior year and found developmental patterns in the influence of peer pressure on many activities, including academic motivation and performance. Peer pressure rises during childhood and peaks around grades 8 or 9 but then declines through high school. A key time of influence is roughly between ages 12 and 16, a period during which parental involvement in children's activities declines. Steinberg et al. found that students who begin high school with similar grades but who become affiliated with academically oriented crowds achieve better during high school than do students who become affiliated with less academically oriented crowds.

Research often shows that competence beliefs and motivation decline as students advance in school (Pintrich & Schunk, 2002). This decline has been attributed to factors such as greater competition, more norm-referenced grading, less teacher attention to

individual student progress, and stresses associated with school transitions. These and other school practices can retard the development of academic efficacy, especially among students who are poorly prepared to cope with ascending academic challenges. Lockstep sequences of instruction frustrate some students, who fail to grasp skills and increasingly fall behind their peers (Bandura, 1997). Ability groupings can hurt self-efficacy among those relegated to lower groups. Classrooms that allow for much social comparison tend to lower self-efficacy for students who find their performances deficient compared to those of peers.

Also important is students' sense of relatedness to the school environment. Students' involvement and participation in school depend in part on how much the school environment contributes to their perceptions of autonomy and relatedness, which in turn influence self-efficacy and academic achievement (Hymel, Comfort, Schonert-Reichl, & McDougall, 1996). Although parents and teachers contribute to feelings of autonomy and relatedness, peers become highly significant during adolescence. The peer group can enhance or diminish students' feelings of belonging and affiliation.

Periods of transition in schooling bring additional factors into play that affect self-efficacy. Eccles and her colleagues have investigated the transition from elementary (grades K–6) to junior high (grades 7–9) school (Eccles & Midgley, 1989; Eccles, Midgley, & Adler, 1984). Elementary school students remain with the same teacher and peers for much of the school day, children receive much attention, and individual progress is stressed. The transition brings several changes. Because many elementary schools typically feed into the same junior high, and because students change classes, they are exposed to peers whom they do not know. Most evaluation is normative, and there is less teacher attention to individual progress. The widely expanded social reference group, coupled with the shift in evaluation standards, necessitates that students reassess their academic capabilities. Compared with grade 6, competence beliefs typically decline by grade 7 (Harter, 1996). We might expect a comparable decline between grades 5 and 6 in school systems in which middle school begins at grade 6.

As do other cognitive capabilities, self-appraisal skill improves with development. Most children overestimate their academic capabilities (Pajares, 1997). Even feedback indicating low performance may not decrease self-efficacy (Schunk, 1995). Less frequently, children underestimate their capabilities and believe that they cannot acquire basic skills.

The incongruence between self-efficacy and actual performances may be due to various causes. Children often lack task familiarity and do not fully understand what is required to execute a task successfully. As they gain experience, their judgmental accuracy improves. Children may be unduly swayed by certain task features and decide based on these that they can or cannot perform the task, while ignoring many other features. In subtraction, for example, children may focus on how many numbers the problems contain and judge longer problems more difficult than those with fewer numbers, even when the longer ones are conceptually simpler. As their cognitive capability to focus on multiple features improves, so does their accuracy.

Another influence is children's faulty knowledge about their performance capabilities. In writing, for example, it is difficult for children to know how clearly they can express themselves or whether their writing skills are improving (Schunk & Swartz, 1993). Teacher feedback—especially at the elementary level—is intended to encourage and stress what children do well. They may believe they can write well when in fact their writing is far below normal. With development, children gain task experience and peer social comparisons, which improve self-assessments.

FUTURE DIRECTIONS IN THE STUDY OF ACADEMIC SELF-EFFICACY

As we have illustrated, the empirical connection between self-efficacy and other competence beliefs, and academic performances and achievement has been reasonably shown. In this section, we suggest some directions that we find especially appropriate for uncovering additional insights about the role played by self-efficacy and other competence beliefs.

Research is required on the extent to which self-efficacy beliefs generalize from one domain to another and whether such generalization varies as a function of development. Self-efficacy refers to perceived capabilities within specific domains. Although most researchers have not investigated whether self-efficacy generalizes beyond specific domains, there is evidence for a generalized sense of self-efficacy (Smith, 1989). Students' initial self-efficacy for learning is affected by their aptitudes, prior experiences, and social supports (Schunk, 1995). Children who perform well in mathematics should have higher self-efficacy for learning new content than those who have had learning difficulties. Self-efficacy might generalize when the new domain builds on prior skills (e.g., self-efficacy for subtracting and multiplying may transfer to long division).

Bandura (1997) identified conditions under which competence judgments can generalize across performance tasks or domains. When differing tasks require similar subskills, capability perceptions for demonstrating the requisite subskills should predict the differing outcomes. Generality can also occur when the skills required to accomplish dissimilar activities are acquired together. In school, students' mathematics and verbal self-efficacy may generalize if the skills for each subject have been adequately taught and developed by a competent teacher. Subskills required to organize a course of action are themselves governed by broader self-regulatory skills, such as knowing how to diagnose task demands, or constructing and evaluating alternative strategies. Possessing these self-regulatory skills allows students to improve their performances across varied academic activities (Zimmerman, 1989). Coping skills work in similar fashion by reducing stress and promoting effective functioning across domains. Self-efficacy also should generalize when commonalities are cognitively structured across activities. For instance, if students realize that increased effort and persistence result in academic progress and greater understanding in mathematics, they may make similar connections with other subject areas.

The hypothesized conditions under which competence perceptions should generalize across domains provide rich opportunity for empirical investigation that would help trace the genesis and interconnections of self-perceptions. These insights might also shed light on findings from cognitive psychology, demonstrating that students often have difficulty transferring strategies and knowledge across academic domains (Pressley et al., 1990). It is possible that although strategies or knowledge functions may not so easily transfer, the beliefs that accompany these cognitive processes may travel more easily. Thus, cognitive, knowledge-based components required to carry out an activity or task may make the voyage from one activity to another with greater difficulty than the perceptions that provide the effort and persistence necessary to attack the related or novel activity. It will be interesting to discover to what degree the process of transferring perceptions resembles the transfer of other cognitive processes.

Researchers should also investigate how self-efficacy relates to its outcomes as a consequence of development. In academic settings, the influence of self-efficacy on choice of activities, effort, and persistence is complex. The early school grades are skills oriented, and teachers assign tasks they expect all students to master. Children's self-efficacy generally is high, and they often overestimate their capabilities (Pajares, 1996b). Choice of activities is not a good index, because students rarely get to choose learning activities in which they engage.

Persistence also presents problems. Students typically persist on activities not necessarily because of high self-efficacy but rather because the teacher keeps them on task. Educational research has yielded inconsistent results on the relation of self-efficacy to persistence (Schunk, 1995). A positive relation may be found in the early stages of learning, when persistence leads to better performance. As skills develop, students should require less time to complete a task, which means that self-efficacy will relate negatively to persistence. With development, children are better able to determine how much persistence may be necessary to succeed. Thus, self-efficacy may predict persistence better at the higher grades. The same concerns apply to effort. Although learning problems begin to appear in the early grades, most children master the basic skills. Effort should be a more reliable outcome of self-efficacy with development, but academic learning research is needed.

Bandura (1986) argued that successful functioning is best served by reasonably accurate efficacy appraisals, although the most functional efficacy judgments are those that slightly exceed what one can accomplish, because overestimation increases effort and persistence. Indeed, most students are overconfident about their academic capabilities. But how much confidence is too much confidence? When should overconfidence be characterized as excessive and maladaptive? What factors create inaccurate self-perceptions, and what are the likely effects of inaccuracy? Researchers should determine to what degree high self-efficacy demonstrated in the face of incongruent performance attainments ultimately results in greater motivation and achievement (Stone, 1994). Efforts to lower students' efficacy percepts or interventions designed to raise already overconfident beliefs should be discouraged, but improving students' calibration (the accuracy of their self-perceptions) will require helping them understand what they know and do not know, so that they may effectively deploy appropriate strategies to perform a task.

With the explosion of technology in schools, research is also needed on how students develop self-efficacy for learning to use technology. Although children and adolescents are more technologically competent now than ever before, there remains wide variability among students.

As with other skills, we should expect that academic attainments, vicarious experiences, and persuasive communications would influence self-efficacy in the context of sound instruction. Some questions need to be addressed: Do children benefit more from mastery experiences than from teacher encouragement and observing peers succeed? Does exposure to technologically competent peer models enhance adolescents' self-efficacy? How can technology be integrated across the curriculum to promote self-efficacy at different developmental levels?

The sensitivity to context of self-efficacy makes it an ideal vehicle with which to explore the difference in perceptions of competence as a function of developmental factors. It seems likely that self-perceptions of competence take on different meanings and are weighed differently as a function of development (Wigfield & Karpathian, 1991). For example, Nicholls (1984) suggested that young children view effort and ability as complementary; with age and schooling, they come to view them as contradictory. A better understanding of the development of academic self-efficacy, familial and schooling influences, and developmental factors that contribute to changes in self-efficacy will require longitudinal investigations. More information also is required about how students at various ages, academic levels, or grades use the diverse sources of efficacy information in developing their perceptions. Because children judge their capabilities partly by comparing their performances with those of others, future studies should also explore the influence of peers on the development of self-efficacy, as well as the social comparative information that students find most useful.

Researchers have reported that teachers' beliefs of personal efficacy affect their instructional activities and their orientation toward the educational process. For example, preservice teachers' sense of efficacy is related to their beliefs about controlling students. Teachers with a low sense of efficacy tend to hold a custodial orientation that pessimistically views students' motivation, emphasizes rigid control of classroom behavior, and relies on extrinsic inducements and negative sanctions to get students to study (Woolfolk & Hoy, 1990). Teachers with high self-efficacy create mastery experiences for students, whereas teachers with low instructional efficacy undermine students' cognitive development, as well as judgments of their capabilities (Ashton & Webb, 1986). Teacher self-efficacy also predicts student achievement and students' achievement beliefs across various areas and levels (Ashton & Webb, 1986; Midgley et al., 1989). There is a need to discover additional correlates of teacher self-efficacy, as well as to understand how it influences educational outcome variables, such as instructional practices and student achievement.

Educators should continue to explore how teacher self-efficacy develops, what factors contribute to strong and positive teaching self-efficacy in varied domains, and how teacher education programs can help preservice teachers develop high efficacy. Beliefs act as a filter through which new phenomena are interpreted and subsequent behavior is mediated, but information can be filtered such that similar beliefs can have differing outcomes. For example, high teacher self-efficacy can promote or inhibit conceptual change (Guskey, 1986); that is, teachers who are highly confident in their instruction may be highly resistant to changing any facet of it because of the confidence they have in themselves, or they may also be confident enough in themselves to attempt conceptual change. It should prove insightful to discover how teachers make the connection between belief and action, and under what conditions similar teacher self-efficacy perceptions result in differing performances. Also, if beliefs are difficult to alter (Pajares, 1992), how can low teacher self-efficacy be raised? And if self-efficacy is critical to the process of teaching, how can it be made an explicit focus of teacher education programs?

We also recommend research on how to structure teacher preparation programs so that preservice teachers acquire competencies to work effectively with students at different developmental levels. The rise of inclusion has further diversified classrooms. Teachers must know how to tailor instruction to developmental differences within classrooms. Research should explore how to enhance preservice teachers' self-efficacy for helping diverse students learn. Research is especially needed on how field experiences in diverse settings and exposure to models affect preservice teachers' self-efficacy.

Bandura (1986) observed that there are a number of conditions under which self-efficacy beliefs do not perform their influential, predictive, or mediational role in human functioning. In prejudicially structured systems, for example, students may find that no amount of skillful effort will bring about desired outcomes. Although they may possess the necessary skill and high self-efficacy required to achieve, they may choose not to, because they lack the necessary incentives. Self-efficacy also will have no bearing on performance if schools lack the effective teachers, necessary equipment, or resources required to aid students in the adequate performance of academic tasks. Bandura suggested that when social constraints and inadequate resources impede academic performances, self-efficacy may exceed actual performance, because learners are unable to perform what they know. This observation may be insightful in light of findings regarding self-beliefs of minority students in some contexts. There is need to explore the role that schools play as social systems for developing and cultivating self-efficacy, as well as the roles that the various incentives and disincentives such systems create play in the development of students' self-efficacy.

As the world shrinks, attempting to understand to what degree the effects of self-efficacy are universal across cultures seems critical. Cross-cultural research will help clarify how efficacy beliefs are created and develop as a result of different cultural practices, as well as how these differing practices influence children's self-efficacy about their schooling. Although there is already evidence to suggest that self-efficacy has similar effects across cultures (Bandura, 1995), the link between culture and belief has yet to be made empirically. Moreover, the relationship between cultural differences and the effects of the cultural practices of institutions such as the family, community, and workplace on children's self-efficacy has yet to be determined (Oettingen, 1995).

Bandura (1986) observed that confidence is a personal and a social construct. Collective systems such as classrooms, teams of teachers, schools, and school districts develop a sense of *collective efficacy*—a group's shared belief in its capability to attain their goals and accomplish desired tasks. Students, teachers, and school administrators operate collectively and individually. As a result, schools develop collective beliefs about the capabilities of their students to learn, of their teachers to teach and enhance the lives of their students, and of their administrators and policymakers to create environments conducive to those tasks.

Schools with a strong sense of collective efficacy exercise empowering and vitalizing influences on their constituents, and these effects are palpable and in evidence (Bandura, 1997). Collective efficacy mediates the influence of students' socioeconomic status, prior academic achievement, and teachers' longevity on the academic achievement of middle school students. There is evidence to suggest that the collective efficacy of teachers is related to personal teaching efficacy and satisfaction with the school administration (Fuller & Izu, 1986). We might ask, what role does a student's or teacher's sense of efficacy play in the creation of a

school's collective efficacy, and vice versa? What role does the collective efficacy in place at a school play in the creation and development of novice teachers' and new students' entering sense of efficacy? Can collective efficacy undermine–enhance students' and teachers' sense of efficacy? Is collective efficacy contagious?

Researchers have made noteworthy contributions to the understanding of competence perceptions, self-regulatory practices, and academic motivation, but the connection from theory and findings to practice has been slow. Classroom teachers and policymakers may well be impressed by the force of research findings arguing that self-efficacy perceptions are important determinants of performance and mediators of other variables, but they are apt to be more interested in useful educational implications, sensible intervention strategies, and practical ways to alter self-efficacy when it is inaccurate and debilitating to children (or to teachers and school administrators).

We have shown that theory and research strengthen the claim of social cognitive theorists that competence beliefs play an influential role in human agency, and they support the work of investigators reporting a significant relationship between students' perceptions of their competence in academic areas and their subsequent performance in these areas. The clear implication is that researchers and school practitioners should continue to look to students' beliefs about their academic capabilities as important predictors and determinants of academic achievement, for they are critical components of motivation and behavior.

REFERENCES

Ashton, P. T., & Webb, R. B. (1986). *Making a difference: Teachers' sense of efficacy and student achievement.* New York: Longman.

Atkinson, J. W. (1957). Motivational determinants of risk-taking behavior. *Psychological Review, 64,* 359–372.

Atkinson, J. W. (1964). *An introduction to motivation.* Princeton, NJ: Van Nostrand.

Bandura, A. (1977a). Self-efficacy: Toward a unifying theory of behavioral change. *Psychological Review, 84,* 191–215.

Bandura, A. (1977b). *Social learning theory.* Englewood Cliffs, NJ: Prentice-Hall.

Bandura, A. (1986). *Social foundations of thought and action: A social cognitive theory.* Englewood Cliffs, NJ: Prentice-Hall.

Bandura, A. (Ed.). (1995). *Self-efficacy in changing societies.* New York: Cambridge University Press.

Bandura, A. (1997). *Self-efficacy: The exercise of control.* New York: Freeman.

Bandura, A., & Schunk, D. H. (1981). Cultivating competence, self-efficacy, and intrinsic interest through proximal self-motivation. *Journal of Personality and Social Psychology, 41,* 586–598.

Berndt, T. J., & Keefe, K. (1992). Friends' influence on adolescents' perceptions of themselves at school. In D. H. Schunk & J. L. Meece (Eds.), *Student perceptions in the classroom* (pp. 51–73). Hillsdale, NJ: Erlbaum.

Boekaerts, M. (1991). Subjective competence: Appraisals and self-assessments. *Learning and Instruction, 1,* 1–17.

Bong, M. (1996). Problems in academic motivation research and advantages and disadvantages of solutions. *Contemporary Educational Psychology, 21,* 149–165.

Bong, M., & Clark, R. (1999). Comparisons between self-concept and self-efficacy in academic motivation research. *Educational Psychologist, 34,* 139–154.

Bong, M., & Skaalvik, E. M. (2003). Academic self-concept and self-efficacy: How different are they really? *Educational Psychology Review, 15,* 1–40.

Bouffard-Bouchard, T., Parent, S., & Larivée, S. (1991). Influence of self-efficacy on self-regulation and performance among junior and senior high-school aged students. *International Journal of Behavioral Development, 14,* 153–164.

Byrne, B. M. (1984). The general/academic self-concept nomological network: A review of construct validation research. *Review of Educational Research, 54,* 427–456.

Cairns, R. B., Cairns, B. D., & Neckerman, J. J. (1989). Early school dropout: Configurations and determinants. *Child Development, 60,* 1437–1452.

Collins, J. L. (1982, March). *Self-efficacy and ability in achievement behavior.* Paper presented at the meeting of the American Educational Research Association, New York.

Connell, J. P., & Wellborn, J. G. (1991). Competence, autonomy, and relatedness: A motivational analysis of self-system processes. In M. Gunnar & L. A. Sroufe (Eds.), *Minnesota Symposia on Child Psychology* (Vol. 23, pp. 43–77). Hillsdale, NJ: Erlbaum.

Deci, E. L., & Ryan, R. M. (1985). *Intrinsic motivation and self-determination in human behavior.* New York: Plenum Press.

Dweck, C. S., & Goetz, T. (1978). Attributions and learned helplessness. In J. Harvey, W. Ickes, & R. Kidd (Eds.), *New directions in attribution research* (pp. 157–179). Hillsdale, NJ: Erlbaum.

Eccles, J. S. (1987). Gender roles and women's achievement-related decisions. *Psychology of Women Quarterly, 11,* 135–172.

Eccles, J., Adler, T. F., Futterman, R., Goff, S. B., Kaczala, C. M., Meece, J. L., & Midgley, C. (1983). Expectancies, values, and academic behaviors. In J. E. Spence (Ed.), *Achievement and achievement motivation* (pp. 75–146). San Francisco: Freeman.

Eccles, J. S., Adler, T., & Meece, J. L. (1984). Sex differences in achievement: A test of alternate theories. *Journal of Personality and Social Psychology, 46,* 26–43.

Eccles, J. S., & Midgley, C. (1989). Stage–environment fit: Developmentally appropriate classrooms for young adolescents. In C. Ames & R. Ames (Eds.), *Research on motivation in education* (Vol. 3, pp. 139–186). San Diego: Academic Press.

Eccles, J. S., Midgley, C., & Adler, T. (1984). Grade-related changes in the school environment: Effects on achievement motivation. In J. Nicholls (Ed.), *Advances in motivation and achievement: The development of achievement motivation* (Vol. 3, pp. 283–331). Greenwich, CT: JAI Press.

Eccles, J. S., & Wigfield, A. (2002). Motivational beliefs, values, and goals. *Annual Review of Psychology, 53,* 109–132.

Felson, R. B. (1984). The effect of self-appraisals of ability on academic performance. *Journal of Personality and Social Psychology, 47,* 944–952.

Findley, M. J., & Cooper, H. M. (1983). Locus of control and academic achievement: A literature review. *Journal of Personality and Social Psychology, 44,* 419–427.

Fuller, B., & Izu, J. (1986). Explaining school cohesion: What shapes the organizational beliefs of teachers. *American Journal of Education, 94,* 501–535.

Graham, S. (1994). Motivation in African Americans. *Review of Educational Research, 64,* 55–117.

Graham, S., & Weiner, B. (1996). Theories and principles of motivation. In D. C. Berliner & R. C. Calfee (Eds.), *Handbook of educational psychology* (pp. 63–84). New York: Macmillan.

Greene, B. A., & Miller, R. B. (1996). Influences on achievement: goals, perceived ability, and cognitive engagement. *Contemporary Educational Psychology, 21,* 181–192.

Guskey, T. R. (1986). Staff development and the process of teacher change. *Educational Researcher, 15*(5), 5–12.

Gustafson, J., & Undheim, J. O. (1996). Individual differences in cognitive functions. In R. C. Calfee & D. C. Berliner (Eds.), *Handbook of educational psychology* (pp. 186–242). New York: Macmillan.

Hackett, G. (1995). Self-efficacy in career choice and development. In A. Bandura (Ed.), *Self-efficacy in changing societies* (pp. 232–258). New York: Cambridge University Press.

Harter, S. (1996). Teacher and classmate influences on scholastic motivation, self-esteem, and level of voice in adolescents. In J. Juvonen & K. R. Wentzel (Eds.), *Social motivation: Understanding children's school adjustment* (pp. 11–42). Cambridge, UK: Cambridge University Press.

Hattie, J. (1992). *Self-concept.* Hillsdale, NJ: Erlbaum.

Hymel, S., Comfort, C., Schonert-Reichl, K., & McDougall, P. (1996). Academic failure and school dropout: The influence of peers. In J. Juvonen & K. R. Wentzel (Eds.), *Social motivation: Understanding children's school adjustment* (pp. 313–345). Cambridge, UK: Cambridge University Press.

Junge, M. E., & Dretzke, B. J. (1995). Mathematical self-efficacy gender differences in gifted/talented adolescents. *Gifted Child Quarterly, 39,* 22–26.

Keogh, B. K., & MacMillan, D. J. (1996). Exceptionality. In R. C. Calfee & D. C. Berliner (Eds.), *Handbook of educational psychology* (pp. 311–330). New York: Macmillan.

Kindermann, T. A., McCollam, T. L., & Gibson, E., Jr. (1996). Peer networks and students' classroom engagement during childhood and adolescence. In J. Juvonen & K. R. Wentzel (Eds.), *Social motivation: Understanding children's school adjustment* (pp. 279–312). Cambridge, UK: Cambridge University Press.

Lent, R. W., Brown, S. D., & Larkin, K. C. (1984). Relation of self-efficacy expectations to academic achievement and persistence. *Journal of Counseling Psychology, 31,* 356–362.

Lent, R. W., & Hackett, G. (1987). Career self-efficacy: Empirical status and future directions. *Journal of Vocational Behavior, 30,* 347–382.

Lewin, K., Dembo, T., Festinger, L., & Sears, P. (1944). Level of aspiration. In J. McV. Hunt, (Ed.), *Personality and the behavioral disorders* (Vol. 1, pp. 333–378). New York: Ronald Press.

Locke, E. A., & Latham, G. P. (2002). Building a practically useful theory of goal setting and task motivation: A 35-year odyssey. *American Psychologist, 57,* 705–717.

Marsh, H. W. (1993). Academic self-concept: Theory, measurement, and research. In J. Suls (Ed.), *Psychological perspectives on the self* (Vol. 4, pp. 59–98). Hillsdale, NJ: Erlbaum.

Marsh, H. W., & Shavelson, R. J. (1985). Self-concept: Its multifaceted, hierarchical structure. *Educational Psychologist, 20,* 107–125.

Matsui, T., & Tsukamoto, S. (1991). Relation between career self-efficacy measures based on occupational titles and Holland codes and model environments: A methodological contribution. *Journal of Vocational Behavior, 38,* 78–91.

Meece, J. L. (1991). The classroom context and students' motivational goals. In M. L. Maehr & P. R. Pintrich (Eds.), *Advances in motivation and achievement* (Vol. 7, pp. 261–285). Greenwich, CT: JAI Press.

Meece, J. L. (1997). *Child and adolescent development for educators.* New York: McGraw-Hill.

Meece, J. L., & Courtney, D. P. (1992). Gender differences in students' perceptions: Consequences for achievement-related choices. In D. H. Schunk & J. L.

Meece (Eds.), *Student perceptions in the classroom* (pp. 209–228). Hillsdale, NJ: Erlbaum.

Meece, J. L., Wigfield, A., & Eccles, J. S. (1990). Predictors of math anxiety and its consequences for young adolescents' course enrollment intentions and performances in mathematics. *Journal of Educational Psychology, 82,* 60–70.

Midgley, C., Feldlaufer, H., & Eccles, J. S. (1989). Change in teacher efficacy and student self- and task-related beliefs in mathematics during the transition to junior high school. *Journal of Educational Psychology, 81,* 247–258.

Multon, K. D., Brown, S. D., & Lent, R. W. (1991). Relation of self-efficacy beliefs to academic outcomes: A meta-analytic investigation. *Journal of Counseling Psychology, 38,* 30–38.

Nicholls, J. (1984). Achievement motivation: Conceptions of ability, subjective experience, task choice, and performance. *Psychological Review, 91,* 328–346.

Oettingen, G. (1995). Cross-cultural perspectives on self-efficacy. In A. Bandura (Ed.), *Self-efficacy in changing societies* (pp. 149–176). New York: Cambridge University Press.

Pajares, F. (1992). Teachers' beliefs and educational research: Cleaning up a messy construct. *Review of Educational Research, 62,* 307–332.

Pajares, F. (1996a). Self-efficacy beliefs and mathematical problem solving of gifted students. *Contemporary Educational Psychology, 21,* 325–344.

Pajares, F. (1996b). Self-efficacy beliefs in achievement settings. *Review of Educational Research, 66,* 543–578.

Pajares, F. (1997). Current directions in self-efficacy research. In M. Maehr & P. R. Pintrich (Eds.), *Advances in motivation and achievement* (Vol. 10, pp. 1–49). Greenwich, CT: JAI Press.

Pajares, F. (2003). Self-efficacy beliefs, motivation, and achievement in writing: A review of the literature. *Reading and Writing Quarterly, 19,* 139–158.

Pajares, F., & Johnson, M. J. (1996). Self-efficacy beliefs and the writing performance of high school students. *Psychology in the Schools, 33,* 163–175.

Pajares, F., & Kranzler, J. (1995). Self-efficacy beliefs and general mental ability in mathematical problem-solving. *Contemporary Educational Psychology, 20,* 426–443.

Pajares, F., & Miller, M. D. (1994). The role of self-efficacy and self-concept beliefs in mathematical problem-solving: A path analysis. *Journal of Educational Psychology, 86,* 193–203.

Pajares, F., & Miller, M. D. (1997). Mathematics self-efficacy and mathematical problem-solving: Implications of using varying forms of assessment. *Journal of Experimental Education, 65,* 213–228.

Pajares, F., Miller, M. D., & Johnson, M. J. (1999). Gender differences in writing self-beliefs of elementary school students. *Journal of Educational Psychology, 91,* 50–61.

Pajares, F., & Schunk, D. H. (2002). Self and self-belief

in psychology and education: A historical perspective. In. J. Aronson (Ed.), *Improving academic achievement: Impact of psychological factors on education* (pp. 3–21). San Diego: Academic Press.

Pajares, F., & Valiante, G. (1999). Grade level and gender differences in the writing self-beliefs of middle school students. *Contemporary Educational Psychology, 24,* 390–405.

Pajares, F., & Valiante, G. (2001). Gender differences in writing motivation and achievement of middle school students: A function of gender orientation? *Contemporary Educational Psychology, 26,* 366–381.

Pajares, F., & Valiante, G. (2002). Students' self-efficacy in their self-regulated learning strategies: A developmental perspective. *Psychologia, 45,* 211–221.

Phillips, D. A., & Zimmerman, M. (1990). The developmental course of perceived competence and incompetence among competent children. In R. J. Sternberg & J. Kolligian, Jr. (Eds.), *Competence considered* (pp. 41–66). New Haven, CT: Yale University Press.

Pintrich, P. R., & De Groot, E. V. (1990). Motivational and self-regulated learning components of classroom academic performance. *Journal of Educational Psychology, 82,* 33–40.

Pintrich, P. R., & Schunk, D. H. (2002). *Motivation in education: Theory, research, and applications* (2nd ed.). Upper Saddle River, NJ: Merrill/Prentice-Hall.

Pressley, M., Woloshyn, V., Lysynchuk, I. M., Martin, V., Wood, E., & Willoughby, T. (1990). A primer of research on cognitive strategy instruction: The important issues and how to address them. *Educational Psychology Review, 2,* 1–58.

Rotter, J. B. (1966). Generalized expectancies for internal versus external control of reinforcement. *Psychological Monographs, 80,* 1–28.

Schunk, D. H. (1981). Modeling and attributional effects on children's achievement: A self-efficacy analysis. *Journal of Educational Psychology, 73,* 93–105.

Schunk, D. H. (1982a). Effects of effort attributional feedback on children's perceived self-efficacy and achievement. *Journal of Educational Psychology, 74,* 548–556.

Schunk, D. H. (1982b). Verbal self-regulation as a facilitator of children's achievement and self-efficacy. *Human Learning, 1,* 265–277.

Schunk, D. H. (1983a). Developing children's self-efficacy and skills: The roles of social comparative information and goal setting. *Contemporary Educational Psychology, 8,* 76–86.

Schunk, D. H. (1983b). Reward contingencies and the development of children's skills and self-efficacy. *Journal of Educational Psychology, 75,* 511–518.

Schunk, D. H. (1984a). Enhancing self-efficacy and achievement through rewards and goals: Motivational and informational effects. *Journal of Educational Research, 78,* 29–34.

Schunk, D. H. (1984b). Sequential attributional feedback and children's achievement behaviors. *Journal of Educational Psychology, 76,* 1159–1169.

Schunk, D. H. (1987). Peer models and children's behavioral change. *Review of Educational Research, 57,* 149–174.

Schunk, D. H. (1995). Self-efficacy and education and instruction. In J. E. Maddux (Ed.), *Self-efficacy, adaptation, and adjustment: Theory, research, and application* (pp. 281–303). New York: Plenum Press.

Schunk, D. H. (1999). Social-self interaction and achievement behavior. *Educational Psychologist, 34,* 219–228.

Schunk, D. H., & Gunn, T. P. (1985). Modeled importance of task strategies and achievement beliefs: Effects on self-efficacy and skill development. *Journal of Early Adolescence, 5,* 247–258.

Schunk, D. H., & Gunn, T. P. (1986). Self-efficacy and skill development: Influence of task strategies and attributions. *Journal of Educational Research, 79,* 238–244.

Schunk, D. H., Hanson, A. R., & Cox, P. D. (1987). Peer-model attributes and children's achievement behaviors. *Journal of Educational Psychology, 79,* 54–61.

Schunk, D. H., & Lilly, M. W. (1984). Sex differences in self-efficacy and attributions: Influence of performance feedback. *Journal of Early Adolescence, 4,* 203–213.

Schunk, D. H., & Swartz, C. W. (1993). Goals and progress feedback: Effects on self-efficacy and writing achievement. *Contemporary Educational Psychology, 18,* 337–354.

Shavelson, R. J., & Bolus, R. (1982). Self-concept: The interplay of theory and models. *Journal of Educational Psychology, 74,* 3–17.

Shavelson, R. J., & Marsh, H. W. (1986). On the structure of self-concept. In R. Schwarzer (Ed.), *Self-related cognition in anxiety and motivation* (pp. 79–95). Hillsdale, NJ: Erlbaum.

Smith, R. E. (1989). Effects of coping skills training on generalized self-efficacy and locus of control. *Journal of Personality and Social Psychology, 56,* 228–233.

Snow, R. E., Corno, L., & Jackson, D., III. (1996). Individual differences in affective and conative functions. In R. C. Calfee & D. C. Berliner (Eds.), *Handbook of educational psychology* (pp. 243–310). New York: Macmillan.

Stajkovic, A. D., & Luthans, F. (1998). Self-efficacy and work-related performance: A meta-analysis. *Psychological Bulletin, 124,* 240–261.

Steinberg, L., Brown, B. B., & Dornbusch, S. M. (1996). *Beyond the classroom: Why school reform has failed and what parents need to do.* New York: Simon & Schuster.

Stevenson, H. W., Hanson, A. R., & Uttal, D. H. (1990). Beliefs and achievement: A study of Black, White, and Hispanic children. *Child Development, 61,* 508–523.

Stone, D. N. (1994). Overconfidence in initial self-efficacy judgments: Effects on decision-processes and performance. *Organizational Behavior and Human Decision Processes, 59,* 452–474.

Weiner, B. (1992). *Human motivation: Metaphors, theories, and research.* Newbury Park, CA: Sage.

Wigfield, A., & Eccles, J. S. (1992). The development of achievement task values: A theoretical analysis. *Developmental Review, 12,* 265–310.

Wigfield, A., & Karpathian, M. (1991). Who am I and what can I do?: Children's self-concepts and motivation in achievement situations. *Educational Psychologist, 26,* 233–261.

Woolfolk, A. E., & Hoy, W. K. (1990). Prospective teachers' sense of efficacy and beliefs about control. *Journal of Educational Psychology, 82,* 81–91.

Wylie, R. C. (1974). *The self-concept: A review of methodological considerations and measuring instruments.* Lincoln: University of Nebraska Press.

Zimmerman, B. J. (1989). A social cognitive view of self-regulated academic learning. *Journal of Educational Psychology, 81,* 329–339.

Zimmerman, B. J. (1990). Self-regulating academic learning and achievement: The emergence of a social cognitive perspective. *Educational Psychology Review, 2,* 173–201.

Zimmerman, B. J. (1994). Dimensions of academic self-regulation: A conceptual framework for education.
In D. H. Schunk & B. J. Zimmerman (Eds.), *Self-regulation of learning and performance: Issues and educational implications* (pp. 3–21). Hillsdale, NJ: Erlbaum.

Zimmerman, B. J. (2000). Attaining self-regulation: A social cognitive perspective. In M. Boekaerts, P. R. Pintrich, & M. Zeidner (Eds.), *Handbook of self-regulation* (pp.13–39). San Diego: Academic Press.

Zimmerman, B. J., & Bandura, A. (1994). Impact of self-regulatory influences on writing course attainment. *American Educational Research Journal, 31,* 845–862.

Zimmerman, B. J., Bandura, A., & Martinez-Pons, M. (1992). Self-motivation for academic attainment: The role of self-efficacy beliefs and personal goal setting. *American Educational Research Journal, 29,* 663–676.

Zimmerman, B. J., & Martinez-Pons, M. (1990). Student differences in self-regulated learning: Relating grade, sex, and giftedness to self-efficacy and strategy use. *Journal of Educational Psychology, 82,* 51–59.

Zimmerman, B., & Ringle, J. (1981). Effects of model persistence and statement of confidence on children's self-efficacy and problem-solving. *Journal of Educational Psychology, 73,* 485–493.

CHAPTER 7

ભ

Subjective Task Value
and the Eccles et al. Model
of Achievement-Related Choices

JACQUELYNNE S. ECCLES

Over the past 25 years, my colleagues and I have studied the motivational and social factors influencing such long- and short-range achievement goals and behaviors as career aspirations, vocational and avocational choices, course selections, persistence on difficult tasks, and the allocation of effort across various achievement-related activities. Given the striking differences in the educational, vocational, and avocational patterns of males and females, we began this work with a particular interest in the motivational factors that might underlie the gender differences in such achievement-related choices. Frustrated with the number of seemingly disconnected theories proliferating to explain gender differences in these achievement patterns, we developed a comprehensive theoretical model of achievement-related choices that could be used to guide our subsequent research efforts (see Figure 7.1 for most recent version). Drawing on the theoretical and empirical work associated with decision making, achievement

theory, and attribution theory (see Crandall, 1969; Weiner, 1992), we proposed that educational, vocational, and other achievement-related choices are most directly related to two sets of beliefs: the individual's expectations for success, and the importance or value the individual attaches to the various options perceived by the individual as available. In this model, we also specified the relation of these beliefs to cultural norms, experiences, aptitudes, and to those personal beliefs and attitudes that are commonly assumed to be associated with achievement-related activities (see Eccles, 1987; Eccles, Wigfield, & Schiefele, 1998).

For example, let us consider course enrollment decisions. The model predicts that people will be most likely to enroll in courses that they think they can master and that have high task value for them. Expectations for success (alternatively, a sense of domain-specific personal efficacy) depend on the confidence the individual has in his or her intellectual abilities and on the individual's

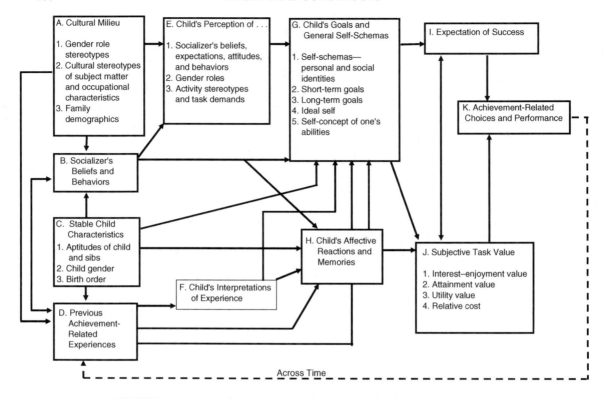

FIGURE 7.1. General expectancy–value model of achievement choices.

estimations of the difficulty of the course. These beliefs are shaped over time by the individual's experiences with the subject matter and by his or her subjective interpretation of those experiences (e.g., Does the person think that his or her successes are a consequence of high ability or lots of hard work?). Likewise, the value of a particular course to the individual is influenced by several factors. For example, does the person enjoy doing the subject material? Is the course required? Is the course seen as instrumental in meeting one of the individual's long- or short-range goals? Have the individual's parents or counselors insisted that the course be taken or, conversely, have other people tried to discourage the individual from taking the course? Is the person afraid of the material to be covered in the course? Does the person think that the course is appropriate for people like him or her? Finally, does taking the course interfere with other more valued options?

Four features of our approach that are not well captured by the static model depicted in Figure 7.1 are particularly important for understanding individual, as well as gender and other group, differences in achievement-related choices: First, we focus on achievement-related behaviors that involve both conscious and nonconscious choices. Although the language we use to describe the various components makes it seem that we are talking about quite conscious processes, this is not our intention. Please bear in mind that this is a problem with the language rather than the theory. We believe that the conscious and nonconscious choices people make about how to spend time and effort lead, over time, to marked differences between groups and individuals in lifelong achievement-related patterns. For example, many of the most interesting gender differences (e.g., educational and vocational aspirations, and educational, vocational, and avocational activity choice/involvement) occur on achievement-related behaviors, aspirations, or involve the element of choice, even if the outcome of that choice is heavily influenced by socialization pressures and cultural norms.

Focusing attention on achievement-related choices reflects a second important aspect of our perspective, namely, the issue of what becomes part of an individual's field of possible choices. Although individuals choose from among several options, they do not actively, or consciously, consider the full range of objectively available options. Many options are never considered, because the individual is unaware of their existence. Other options are not seriously considered, because the individual has inaccurate information regarding either the option itself or the individual's possibility of achieving the option. For example, young people often have inaccurate information regarding the full range of activities associated with various career choices or the financial assistance available for advanced educational training. Yet they make decisions about which occupations to pursue, and they select courses in high school that they believe are important for getting into college and majoring in the subject most directly linked to their career aspirations. Too often, these choices are based on either inaccurate or insufficient information. In addition, many options may not be seriously considered, because the individual does not believe that a particular choice fits well with his or her gender-role or other social-role schemas. Again, inaccurate information about what occupations are actually like can lead to premature elimination of quite viable career options. For example, a young woman with excellent math skills may reject the possibility of becoming an engineer, because she has a limited view of what engineers actually do. She may stereotype engineers as nerds or as folks who focus on mechanical tasks, with little direct human relevance, when, in fact, many engineers work directly on problems related to pressing human needs.

A third important feature of our perspective is the explicit assumption that achievement-related decisions, such as the decision to enroll in an accelerated math program or to major in education rather than law or engineering, or to devote a lot of energy to school achievement rather than social activities, are made within the context of a complex social reality that presents each individual with a wide variety of choices, each of which has both long-range and immediate consequences. Furthermore, the choice is often between two or more positive options, or between two or more options that each have both positive and negative components. For example, the decision to enroll in an advanced math course is typically made in the context of other important decisions, such as whether to take advanced English or a second foreign language, whether to take a course with one's best friend or not, or whether it is more important to spend one's senior year working hard or having fun, and so on. The critical issue in our view is the relative personal value of each option. Given high likelihood of success, we assume that people will then choose those tasks or behaviors that have relatively higher personal value. Thus, it is the hierarchy of subjective task values that matter, rather than the absolute values attached to the various options under consideration. This feature of our approach makes within-person comparisons much more relevant than between-group, mean-level comparisons.

Consider, as an example, two junior high school students: Mary and Barbara. Both young women enjoy mathematics and have always done very well. Both have been identified as gifted in mathematics and have been offered the opportunity to participate in an accelerated math program at the local college during the next school year. Barbara hopes to major in communications when she gets to college and has also been offered the opportunity to work part-time at the local television news station doing odd jobs and some copyediting. Mary hopes to major in chemistry in college and plans a career as a research scientist. Taking the accelerated math course involves driving to and from the college. Since the course is scheduled for the last period of the day, it will take the last two periods of the day, as well as 1 hour of afterschool time to take the course. What will the young women do? In all likelihood, Mary will enroll in the program, because she likes math and thinks that the effort required to both take the class and master the material is worthwhile and important for her long-range career goals. Barbara's decision is more complex. She may want to take the class but may also think that the time required is too costly, especially given her alternative opportunity at the local television station. Whether she takes the college course or not will depend, in part, on the advice she gets at home and from her counselors. If they stress the importance of the math course, then its subjective worth to her is likely to increase. If its subjective worth increases sufficiently to outweigh its subjective cost, then Barbara will probably take the course despite its cost in time and effort.

A true-life experience with my daughter provides another example. In the third grade, she did not do very well on her report card. I asked her why she was doing so poorly. In her first reply, she said other children also were doing poorly. I reacted by saying I really did not care how the other children were doing. I was only concerned with her poor performance, to which she replied, "But I would have to work harder to do better." I agreed and asked why she was not working harder. She replied, "What do you want me to do? Waste my childhood doing schoolwork?" Clearly, she had no problems with her sense of personal efficacy. Instead, she just did not value doing schoolwork as much as she valued other ways of spending her time. These two examples point to the importance of the value component of the Eccles et al. expectancy–value model. I focus on this component in this chapter.

Finally, we assume that the processes summarized in Figure 7.1 are both developmental and dynamic. The model provides a snapshot of both the processes at one point in time and a global view of the developmental sequence linking exogenous and sociocultural influences to the emergence of the psychological processes depicted on the right side of Figure 7.1. But the relations within the entire system are quite dynamic both moment-to-moment and across developmental history. Like many researchers interested in self-processes, we assume that both personal states and situational characteristics will make the various components of the self-system more or less salient at different times. As such, the immediate subjective task value of various options and behaviors will fluctuate depending on the salience of different components of the self-system. We also assume that the components of the self-system change across developmental time in response to experience with specific

tasks, changing cognitive abilities and interpretative beliefs, changing socialization pressures, and changing sociocultural influences. Finally, we assume the relative salience of the subcomponents of subjective task value will change developmentally and across situations. Like Deci and Ryan (1985), we believe that the relative importance of different aspects of a task for behavioral choices will vary across developmental time due to such developmental processes as internalization, maturation, and life stage. For example, the relative salience of intrinsic enjoyment of a task may be particularly salient to young children and to people primarily interested in leisure pursuits (Wigfield & Eccles, 1992). In contrast, the utility value of a task for fulfilling one's goals may be particularly salient during those periods in life when one is most engaged in striving to achieve these goals. For example, the utility value of particular school courses for one's career goals is likely to be a particularly salient influence on choices during adolescence, when one is preparing oneself for a particular occupation.

In summary, as outlined in Figure 7.1, my colleagues and I assume that achievement-related choices (e.g., educational, occupational, and leisure-time choices), whether made consciously or nonconsciously, are guided by the following: (1) one's expectations for success on, and sense of personal efficacy for, the various options, as well as one's sense of competence for various tasks; (2) the relation of the options both to one's short- and long range goals and one's core personal and social identities, and basic psychological needs; (3) the individual's culturally based role schemas, such as those linked to gender, social class, religious group, and ethnic group; and (4) the potential cost of investing time in one activity rather than another. We assume that all of these psychological variables are influenced by one's experiences and interpretation of these experiences, by cultural norms, and by the behaviors and goals of one's socializers and peers.

In this chapter, I focus on the subjective task value (STV) component of the Eccles et al. expectancy–value model. As the example of the two young women given earlier illustrates, I am particularly interested in the role that STV plays in shaping individuals' achievement-related decisions about activity choice, participation, and degree of engagement. Because the Eccles et al. model was originally designed to explain a sociocultural phenomenon—gender differences in achievement-related choices, I believe it is particularly well suited for a sociocultural analysis of motivation and activity choices. I predict that sociocultural differences in a wide array of activity and behavioral choices, particularly in the achievement domain, reflect cultural differences in success expectations and STV-related beliefs, which, in turn, likely result from sociocultural differences in the wide range of social experiences that shape human development. The work my colleagues and I have done on gender within the United States provides comprehensive examples of just how these sociocultural processes can work. I summarize some of this work in this chapter, paying particular attention to our gender work on STV.

OVERVIEW OF THE COMPONENTS OF SUBJECTIVE TASK VALUE

Our initial theorizing about STV was heavily influenced by the work of Norm Feather (1988, 1992). Like Feather, we assume that task value is a quality of the task that contributes to the increasing or decreasing probability that an individual will select it (see Eccles, 1987; Eccles et al., 1983; Wigfield & Eccles, 1992). We define this quality of tasks in terms of four components: (1) attainment value, or the value an activity has because engaging in it is consistent with one's self-image; (2) intrinsic or interest value—expected enjoyment of engaging in the task; (3) the utility value of the task for facilitating one's long-range goals or helping the individual obtain immediate or long-range external rewards; and (4) the cost of engaging in the activity.

Attainment Value

Building on Battle's (1966) work on "attainment value," we define it in terms of the personal importance attached to doing well on, or participating in, a given task. Our notion of attainment value is closely linked to work on identity: We predict that tasks will be seen as important when individuals view engaging in the task as central to their own sense of themselves (i.e., their core social and personal identities), because such tasks provide the opportunity for the individual to express or confirm important aspects of the self. In this sense, our notion of attainment value is similar to ideas proposed by Connell and Wellborn (1991) and Deci and Ryan (1985) linking motivation and engagement to the extent to which tasks and activities fulfill the basic human needs of autonomy, competence, and relatedness. Connell and Wellborn (1991) argued that people's motivation to engage in a task is influenced by the extent to which the task provides opportunities to fulfill their basic needs for autonomy, social relatedness, and a sense of competence. In this sense, their theory is a variant on more basic person–environment fit theories that stress the importance of a good fit between the opportunities provided by the environment and the needs of the individuals for optimal motivation. Our notion of attainment value represents our operationalization of this same principle. In addition, however, I would add the following basic needs and values to the list proposed by Connell and Wellborn: (1) the need to feel that what one does matters in a fundamentally important way to one's social group, and (2) the need to feel respected and valued by one's social group.

Other theorists (e.g., Harter, 1983; White, 1959) have also pointed out the importance of effectance, competence, and social relatedness needs. The importance of competence needs, in particular, has received a great deal of attention in the achievement literature. For example, in her model of mastery or effectance motivation, Harter (1983) described the effects of both success and failure experiences on mastery motivation. She proposed that successful mastery attempts that are positively reinforced lead to internalization of the reward system. They also enhance perceptions of competence and perceived internal control over outcomes, give the individual pleasure, and ultimately increase mastery motivation. In contrast, when mastery attempts fail, the need for approval by others persists, with a corresponding increase in external control beliefs, lower competence beliefs, higher anxiety in mastery situations, and ultimately, lower mastery motivation. This perspective is important, because it links success and failure experiences to subsequent general motivational orientations, which, we believe, in turn influence the attainment values attached to whole categories of activities (e.g., activities that provide opportunities to demonstrate mastery and competence).

A similar analysis applies to the success and failure on particular tasks. If one has had a history of success on particular tasks, then, through the processes associated with both self-knowledge and identity formation, and classical conditioning, the individual will come to see him- or herself in terms of these particular competencies and to feel good when anticipating engaging in tasks that provide the opportunity to demonstrate these specific competencies. In contrast, if the individual has failed at mastery attempts on particular tasks and feels incompetent at those tasks, then he or she is likely to lower the value attached to being competent at these particular types of tasks because he or she will not see such tasks as providing the opportunity to feel competent (see Bandura, 1986, for similar discussion of the relation between prior success and failure and current task value).

We believe that the attainment value of various tasks is influenced by the affordances provided by these tasks to fulfill a whole array of individual needs and personal values. As we grow up, we develop images of who we are and what we would like to be. These image are made up of many component parts, including (1) our conceptions of our own personality and capabilities; (2) our long-range goals and plans; (3) our schema regarding the proper roles of people "like us" (e.g., men vs. women, Jews vs. Gentiles, Italians vs. Englishmen, young people vs. older people, Goths vs. Preppies), as well as our more general social scripts regarding proper behavior in a variety of situations; (4) our instrumental and terminal values (Rokeach, 1973); (5) our motivational sets or goal orientations; and (6) our images of our ideal or hoped-for selves. Together, the most central parts of these images and schemas comprise our personal and social identities. These social and personal identities should have the most powerful influence on the value each individual attaches to various educational and vocational op-

tions; these differential values, in turn, should influence the individual's achievement-related choices (Eccles, 1984, 1987). For example, if helping other people is a central part of an individual's personal identity, then that person should place higher value on "helping" than on "nonhelping" occupations. Essentially, I am arguing that individuals perceive tasks in terms of certain characteristics that can be related to their needs and values. In turn, tasks that fit well with one's values, goals or needs, will be seen as having high STV; tasks that do not fit well, or that actually are in opposition to one's values, goals, or needs, will be seen as having low or even negative STV.

Recent work by scholars interested in goal orientations (Ames & Ames, 1989; Dweck & Elliott, 1983; Elliot & McGregor, 2001; Midgley, Anderman, & Hicks, 1995; Nicholls, 1984; see also Pintrich & Schunk, 2002) provides a good example of these processes. Initially, goal orientation theorists hypothesized that achievement tasks vary along two dimensions: (1) the extent to which mastery or improvement is stressed, and (2) the extent to which doing better than others is stressed. They also hypothesized that individuals differ in the salience and importance of these two dimensions: Some are oriented primarily to the mastery component; others, primarily to the competitive component; and still others, to both or neither of these aspects of achievement tasks. To the extent that these individual differences in goal orientation are a central part of one's core self, achievement tasks or situations that emphasis one or the other of these two components will have different STV to individuals, depending on their goal orientation. People who think of themselves as very competitive, or who have a highly competitive temperament or motivational need, will attach greater STV to competitive achievement tasks than individuals who do not value competitiveness as a personal characteristic, or who do not want to seen by others as a competitive person. In contrast, if individuals place great importance on the mastery component of achievement tasks, they should place high value on mastery-based achievement tasks and may avoid achievement tasks that stress comparing one's performance to others rather than to one's own past performance.

Tasks may be also perceived in terms of nurturance, power, aesthetic pleasure, and so on. Participating in particular tasks requires the demonstration of the characteristics associated with the task. Whether this requirement is seen as an opportunity or a burden will depend on the individual's needs, motives, and personal values, and on his or her desire to demonstrate these characteristics both to him- or herself and to others.

In summary, we assume the following: (1) Individuals seek to confirm their possession of those characteristics central to their self-image; (2) various tasks provide differential opportunities for such confirmation; (3) individuals place more value on those tasks that either provide the opportunity to fulfill their self-image or are consistent with their self-image and long-range goals; and (4) individuals are more likely to select tasks with high subjective value than tasks with lower subjective value. To the extent that groups of people, such as males and females, come to have different self-images, needs, goals, and personal values through the processes associated with sociocultural learning, various activities will come to have different subjective value for males and females.

Intrinsic and Interest Value

I reserve the term "intrinsic value" for either the enjoyment one gains from doing the task or the anticipated enjoyment one expects to experience while doing the task. In this sense, my notion of intrinsic value is similar to the idea of flow, as proposed by Csikszentmihalyi (1988), who discussed intrinsically motivated behavior in terms of the immediate subjective experience that occurs when people are engaged in the activity. Interviews with climbers, dancers, chess players, basketball players, and composers revealed that these activities yield a specific form of experience, labeled "flow," characterized by (1) holistic feelings of being immersed in, and of being carried by, an activity; (2) merging of action and awareness; (3) focus of attention on a limited stimulus field; (4) lack of self-consciousness; and (5) feeling in control of one's actions and the environment. Flow is only possible when people feel that the opportunities for action in a given situation match their ability to master the challenges. The challenge of an activity may be something concrete or physical, such as the peak of a mountain to be scaled, or it can be something abstract and symbolic, such as a set of musical notes to be performed, a story to be written, or a puzzle to be solved. Research has shown that both the challenges and skills must be relatively high before a flow experience becomes possible (Massimini & Carli, 1988).

Our notion of intrinsic task value is also related to the idea of interest value used by Hidi (1990), Renninger, Hidi, and Krapp (1992), Schiefele (1991), and Tobias (1994). These researchers differentiate between individual and situational interest. Individual interest is a relatively stable evaluative orientation toward certain domains; situational interest is an emotional state aroused by specific features of an activity or a task. Two aspects or components of individual interest are distinguishable (Schiefele, 1991, 1996): feeling-related and value-related interest. "Feeling-related interest" refers to the feelings that are associated with an object or an activity itself—feelings such as involvement, stimulation, or flow. "Value-related interest" refers to the attribution of personal significance or importance to an object. In addition, both feeling-related and value-related valences are directly related to the object rather than to the relation of this object to other objects or events. For example, if students associate mathematics with high personal significance because mathematics can help them get prestigious jobs, then we would describe this aspect as utility value rather than interest value.

We know little about the origins of either within-individual or between-individual differences in interest. In some ways, individual differences in patterns of interest are related to issues discussed under attainment value: The attraction to, or enjoyment of, particular types of activities are undoubtedly linked to core aspects of the self, such as temperament, personality, motivational orientations. It is also likely to be linked to both genetic propensities and to classical learning associated with either positive or negative emotional experiences during initial encounters with particular activities.

In the last 30 years, educational psychologists have become interested in individual differences in a more general, individual interest pattern, namely, one associated with trait-like individual differences in what might be referred to as the desire to learn (see Amabile, Hill, Hennessey, & Tighe, 1994; Gottfried, 1990; Harter, 1981; Midgley, 2002; Nicholls, 1984; Schiefele, 1996). These researchers define this enduring learning orientation in terms of three components: (1) preference for hard or challenging tasks, (2) learning that is driven by curiosity or interest, and (3) striving for competence and mastery. The second component is most central to the idea of intrinsic task value. Both preference for hard tasks and striving for competence are linked more closely with what we call "attainment value." Nonetheless, empirical findings suggest that these three components are highly correlated, and that high levels of a trait-like desire to learn facilitates positive emotional experience (Matsumoto & Sanders, 1988), self-esteem (Ryan, Connell, & Deci, 1985), mastery-oriented coping with failure and high academic achievement (Benware & Deci, 1984), and use of appropriate learning strategies (Pintrich & Schrauben, 1992).

We know much more about the task characteristics linked to situational interest in part because the research on school-related situational interest has focused on the characteristics of academic tasks that create interest (e.g., Hidi, 1990). Among others, the following text features arouse situational interest: personal relevance, both familiarity and novelty, activity level, and comprehensibility (Hidi & Baird, 1986). We also know that there is strong empirical support for the relation of both individual and situational interest with text comprehension and recall, and with deep-level learning (see Renninger et al., 1992; Schiefele, 1996).

Before leaving this discussion of intrinsic–interest value, it is important to note that we do not see it is as the same as intrinsic motivation. Certainly doing something because one loves the experience of doing it is an example of intrinsic motivation. But, as I discuss later, intrinsic motivation has more to do with the origin of the decision to exchange in the activity than with the source of the activities value. Extrinsic rewards can undermine an individual's intrinsic motivation to engage in tasks that the individual finds intrinsically interesting.

Utility Value

"Utility value," or usefulness, refers to how a task fits into an individual's future plans, for instance, taking a math class to fulfill a requirement for a science degree. In certain respects, utility value is similar to extrinsic motivation, because when doing an activity out of utility value, the activity is a means to an end rather than an end in itself (see Ryan & Deci, 2000). However, the activity can relate also to some important personal goals, such as attaining a certain occupation. In this sense, utility value is also related to personal goals and one's sense of self. This aspect of utility value makes this component of task value somewhat similar to Deci and Ryan's (1985) idea of introjected value. The relation between utility value and attainment value is also quite close to the distinction Deci and Ryan make between introjected behavioral regulation and integrated behavioral regulation. To the extent that one's short- and long-range goals become an integral part of one's identity and needs, then tasks that fulfill these goals have both utility and attainment value. In this sense, the distinction also relates to Harter's (1998) notion of the authentic self and to the distinction Higgins (1987) makes between the ought, ideal, and actual selves.

Perceived Cost

According to the Eccles et al. model, the value of a task should also depend on a set of beliefs that can best be characterized as the cost of participating in the activity. Cost is influenced by many factors, such as anticipated anxiety, fear of failure, fear of the social consequences of success, such as rejection by peers, or anticipated sexual harassment or discrimination, or anger from one's parents or other key people, and fear of loss of a sense of self-worth (Covington, 1992).

The last conceptualization of cost is similar to the kinds of dynamics discussed by Covington in his self-worth theory. Covington (1992) defined the motive for self-worth as the desire to establish and maintain a positive self-image, or sense of self-worth. Because children spend so much time in classrooms and are evaluated so frequently there, Covington argued that protecting one's sense of academic competence is likely to be critical for maintaining a positive sense of self-worth. However, school evaluation, competition, and social comparison can make it difficult for some children to maintain the belief that they are competent academically. Covington outlined various strategies children develop to avoid appearing to lack ability, including procrastination, making excuses, avoiding challenging tasks, and not trying. The last two strategies are particularly interesting. Covington and Omelich (1979) referred to effort as a "double-edged sword," because although trying is important for success (and is encouraged by both teachers and parents), if children try and fail, then it is difficult to escape the conclusion that they lack ability. Therefore, if failure seems likely, some children will not try, precisely because trying and failing threatens their ability self-concepts. Avoiding challenging tasks is a good way to avoid or minimize failure experiences that is used by even high-achieving students who are failure avoidant. Rather than responding to a challenging task with greater effort, these students try to avoid the task altogether, in order to maintain both their own sense of competence and others' perceptions of their competence.

Cost can also be conceptualized in terms of the loss of time and energy for other activities. People have limited time and energy. They cannot do everything they would like to do. They must choose among activities. To the extent that one loses time for Activity B by engaging in Activity A, and to the extent that Activity B is high in one's hierarchy of importance, then the subjective cost of engaging in A increases. Alternatively, even if the attainment value of A is high, the value of engaging in A will be reduced to the extent that the attainment value of B is higher, and to the extent that engaging in A jeopardizes the probability of successfully engaging in B (see Kerr, 1985, for good examples of this process in action in gifted women's lives).

Thus, cost refers to what the individual has to give up to do a task (e.g., "Do I do my math homework or call my friend?"), as well as the anticipated effort one will need to put into task completion. Is working this hard to get an A in math worth it? My col-

leagues and I have emphasized that cost is especially important to choice, and that sociocultural processes linked to gender and cultural socialization should have a big influence on the perceived cost of various activities precisely because the goal of these socialization practices is to teach which activities should be given the highest priority (e.g., see Eccles, 1984, 1987, 1989).

The examples provided earlier illustrate this idea of cost very concretely. Choices are influenced by both negative and positive task characteristics, and all choices are assumed to have costs associated with them, because one choice often eliminates other options. If Mary, from the earlier example, follows her inclinations and chooses to major in chemistry in college, she will not be able to pursue other possible majors. In addition, because chemistry is a particularly demanding major with lots of requirements, she will not even be able to take very many nonscience courses. Thus, she will have to forgo the opportunity to take courses in many other fields and on many other topics. She will also have to spend a great deal of time on her course work. How she reacts to these inherent costs in majoring in chemistry will impact on her decision to complete this major.

RELATION OF SUBJECTIVE TASK VALUE THEORY TO TWO OTHER MOTIVATIONAL THEORIES: INTRINSIC MOTIVATION AND GOAL THEORIES

In the previous sections, I related the specific components of my STV theory to other motivational theories. There are, however, two more global theories of motivation that relate to various aspects of STV in a more holistic way.

Self-Determination Theory

Several motivational theorists have focused attention on the distinction between *intrinsic* motivation and *extrinsic* motivation (e.g., Deci & Ryan, 1985; Harter, 1983; Lepper, 1988; Ryan & Deci, 2000). When individuals are intrinsically motivated, they do activities for their own sake and out of interest in the activity. When extrinsically motivated, individuals do activities for instrumental or other reasons, such as receiving a reward. Typically, these theorists assume that intrinsic motivation is better than extrinsic motivation. In general, evidence supports this assumption. For example, many studies have documented the debilitating effects of extrinsic incentives and pressures on the motivation to perform even inherently interesting activities and the facilitative effects of intrinsic motivation on many aspects of learning and task engagement (e.g., see Deci & Ryan, 1985; Harter, 1983; Lepper, 1988). But what determines intrinsic motivation? Most theorists believe that instrinsic motivation derives from human beings' basic needs for competence and effectance (Harter, 1983; White, 1959) and their basic need for personal causation and self-determination (deCharms, 1968). Deci and Ryan (1985) argued that the basic needs for both competence and self-determination are the major reason why people seek out optimal stimulation and challenging activities, and that intrinsic motivation is maintained only when actors feel both competent and self-determined.

Deci and Ryan (1985) also argued that the basic needs for competence and self-determination play a role in more extrinsically motivated behavior. Consider, for example, a student who consciously, and without any external pressure, selects a specific major because it will help him or her earn a lot of money. This student is guided by basic needs for competence and self-determination, but his or her choice of major is based on reasons totally extrinsic to the major itself. Thus, although this student's choice of major is intrinsically motivated in that it is self-determined, it is not intrinsically motivated in the sense that the activity itself is intrinsically interesting. In our terms, the major has utility value rather than intrinsic value.

By introducing the idea of self-determination, Deci and Ryan (e.g., Ryan, 1992; Ryan & Deci, 2000) went beyond the extrinsic–intrinsic motivation dichotomy common in most discussions of intrinsic versus extrinsic motivation. Key to their perspective is not whether the task has intrinsic or extrinsic value, but whether or not engagement in the task is self-determined. They do, however, also argue that optimal motivation and performance is linked to both self-determination and valuing the task itself.

Deci and Ryan (1985) also elaborated a developmental theory associated with internalization to explain the process of transferring the regulation of behavior from outside to inside the individual. They postulated that a basic need for interpersonal relatedness explains why people turn external regulation into internal regulation through the process of internalization. Furthermore, they argued that internalization takes place through a series of developmental steps. At the beginning, behavior is primarily under *external regulation*. Later, behavior comes under the *introjected regulation processes* associated with feelings that one should do the behavior. This step is followed by the *identified regulation processes* associated with the utility of that behavior to meet internalized goals (e.g., studying hard to get grades to get into college) and then by the *integrated regulation processes* associated with what the individual thinks is valuable and important to the self. Even at the integrated regulation level, however, behavior is not fully internalized and self-determined; for the behaviors to be full internalized and self-determined, the individual must also be highly interested in the behavior. Although this theory of internalization has sequential properties inherent in its structure, Deci and Ryan also measure all aspects of behavioral regulation at the same time and sometimes assume that individuals can be motivated by all aspects of regulation at the same time— an assumption with which I agree. In this way, these forms of behavioral regulation have some similarity to the different aspects of STV discussed earlier: Attainment value comes closest to Deci and Ryan's notion of integrated regulation; intrinsic/interest value comes closest to Deci and Ryan's notion of internalized regulation; utility value comes closest to Deci and Ryan's notion of identified regulation, but it also shares some similarity with both introjected and external regulation.

There are several differences in the emphases in these two approaches. In my approach to STV theory, these various aspects of task value cumulate to determine the final STV. In addition, I stress the role of cost in determining each task's or activity's STV.

Thus, I stress the fact that the same activity can have multiple sources of STV simultaneously, that more sources can yield higher levels of STV, and that it is this cumulative STV that is key to predicting behavioral choice. I also avoid privileging internal regulation over the other forms of task value. Finally, I do not conceptualize the developmental sequence in such a linear way. Some activities are intrinsically interesting from the start and have high value because the young child finds them inherently interesting, fun, and rewarding. Similarly, although I do believe that some aspects of behavioral regulation do follow the type of internalization sequence proposed by Deci and Ryan, I also believe that other aspects of the values underlying behavioral choices do not follow such a linear sequence. Attainment value is a good example. I believe that many of the self-system dynamics underlying attainment value are discovered through the processes of self-socialization and identity formation, rather than the processes associated with internalization. In addition, I believe that life stages will lead the various subcomponents of STV to have different salience at different points in one's life.

Goal Theories

Recently researchers have become interested in children's achievement goals and their relation to achievement behavior (see Ames & Ames, 1989; Dweck & Elliott, 1983; Elliot & MacGregor, 2001; Ford, 1992; Harackiewicz & Elliot, 1993; Meece, 1991, 1994; Midgley, 2002; Midgley et al., 1995; Nicholls, 1984). Earlier, I discussed the relation of some aspects of achievement goal orientation work to our idea of attainment value. In this section, I say more about the link between goal theories and STV.

Achievement goal orientation theories are currently the most popular form of goal theory. Proponents of this approach focus broadly on two basic goals: mastery or task-involved goals and performance or ego-involved goals. For example, Nicholls and his colleagues (e.g., Nicholls, Cobb, Wood, Yackel, & Patashnick, 1990) defined two major goal patterns or orientations: ego-involved goals and task-involved goals. Individuals with ego-involved goals seek to maximize favorable evaluations of their competence and minimize negative evaluations of competence. Questions such as "Will I look smart?" and "Can I outperform others?" reflect ego-involved goals. In contrast, individuals with task-involved goals focus on mastering tasks and increasing their competence. Questions such as "How can I do this task?" and "What will I learn?" reflect task-involved goals. Nicholls also discussed a third type of goal orientation, work avoidance.

Dweck and her colleagues (e.g., Dweck & Elliott, 1983), Ames (1992), and Midgley and her colleagues (see Midgley, 2002) provide complementary analyses distinguishing between performance goals (e.g., ego-involved goals), and mastery goals (e.g., task-involved goals). Most recently, Elliot and MacGregor (2001) made the distinction between approach and avoidance goals, and suggested a 2×2 matrix of achievement goals that crossed approach and avoidance goals with performance and mastery goals. To the extent that these goals represent core aspects of the self or trait-like motivational orientations, these goals should relate to STV through their impact on attainment value and perceived cost.

Other researchers (e.g., Ford, 1992; Wentzel, 1991) have adopted a broader perspective on goals and motivation, arguing that there are many different kinds of goals that individuals can have in achievement settings. For example, Ford defined "goals" as desired end states that people try to attain through the cognitive, affective, and biochemical regulation of their behavior. Ford (1992) outlined an extensive taxonomy of goals that distinguished most broadly between *within-person* goals, which concern desired within-person consequences, and *person–environment* goals, which concern the relation between the person and his or her environment. The within-person goals include affective goals (e.g., happiness, physical well-being), cognitive goals (e.g., exploration, intellectual creativity), and subjective organization goals (e.g., unity, transcendence). The person–environment goals include self-assertive goals, such as self-determination and individuality, integrative social relationship goals, such as belongingness and social responsibility, and task goals, such as mastery, material gain, and safety. In many respects, both of these clusters of goals are similar to the types of goals that, I argue, influence the attainment value of various tasks, because the tasks provide an opportunity to enact and demonstrate one's goals.

Wentzel, a student of Ford, has examined the role of multiple goals in adolescents in achievement settings (e.g., Wentzel 1991, 1993). She focuses on the way in which the *content* of children's goals guides and directs behavior. In this sense, Wentzel's goals are like the goals and self-schema that relate to our notion of attainment value hierarchies. For instance, Wentzel found that the goals such as seeing oneself as successful, dependable, wanting to learn new things, and wanting to get things done, predict school achievement. In order to understand students' engagement in school achievement-related activities, one would need to measure these various goals and the extent to which various activities were perceived by the students as providing opportunities or barriers to their fulfillment of these goals. Wentzel has begun this work by demonstrating that both social and academic goals predict adolescents' school performance and behavior (see Juvonen & Wentzel, 1996).

BUT DO SUBJECTIVE TASK VALUES ACTUALLY INFLUENCE ACHIEVEMENT-RELATED CHOICES?

Is there any evidence to support the importance of these aspects of STV for predicting behavioral choices? *Yes* (see Eccles et al., 1998, for review). In this chapter, I focus on only one aspect of the question: Do individual differences in relative perceived value of a variety of occupations influence individual differences in occupational choice? Several studies provide support for the hypothesized link of personal values to a variety of achievement-related choices, including course enrollment decisions, occupational choices, college major, and involvement in sports (see Eccles et al., 1998). Given space limitations, I focus only on the findings from our longitudinal study of approximately 1,000 adolescents from southeastern Michigan (Michigan Study of Adolescent Life Transitions, MSALT). When these adolescents were seniors in high school, we assessed the following constructs: their occupational aspirations, the value and impor-

tance they attached to a wide array of both occupations and occupational characteristics (e.g., work that allows one to help other people, work that allows one to earn a lot of money, etc.), and their personal efficacy for success in the same array of occupations. We then used discriminant analysis to determine the strongest predictors of occupational choice within rather than across genders (Eccles, Barber, & Jozefowicz, 1999; Eccles & Vida, 2003; Jozefowicz, Barber, & Eccles, 1993).

As predicted, the relevant dimension of personal efficacy/expectations for success was an important predictor for every occupational category (e.g., efficacy for health-related occupations was a strong predictor only of plans to enter a health-related profession; efficacy for working with people was a strong predictor only of plans to enter a human service occupation). In addition, as predicted, the values attached to relevant job characteristics were significant predictors of occupational aspirations. But the findings for values were more complex, in that values had both positive and negative predictive power. As predicted in our model, for any given occupational category, the extent to which the individual valued characteristics associated with the occupation predicted plans to enter that occupational category (e.g., valuing creativity predicted women's plans to become artists or writers, valuing helping others predicted women's plans to enter either human service or health-related professions). In addition, however, and consistent with the notion that the individual hierarchy of values matters, valuing helping others predicted *not aspiring* to either a physical science–related profession or a business/law-related profession, as well as not majoring in these fields and not being employed in these fields as a young adult. Similarly, valuing occupational prestige predicted *not aspiring* to a human service occupation.

SUBJECTIVE TASK VALUE AND BOTH CULTURAL AND GENDER DIFFERENCES IN ACHIEVEMENT-RELATED CHOICES

As noted in the introduction to this chapter, I believe that the sociocultural processes associated with gender-role and cultural socialization should influence the ways in which members of different culturally based groups come to see themselves, as well as the goals and values they develop for their lives. In addition, experiences in different types of learning environments should influence the emotional experiences associated with different activities. Finally, cultures and countries should vary in the opportunities provided to try different types of activities, as well as in the range of activities made available and salient to various individuals living within the group. Each of these processes should lead to both cultural group differences and within-culture individual differences in STVs. I discuss this more later.

At an even more basic level, cultures differ in the extent to which individuals have "choice" over such achievement-related behaviors as educational focus, careers, and leisure activities. Western cultures pride themselves on allowing individuals to make these choices for themselves, even though choice still continues to be heavily socialized in these Western cultures. Other cultures place less emphasis on individual choice, particularly individual choice based on maximizing self-fulfillment and self-actualization. For example, in interviews with young professionals in China, I found that career choices were based much more on the needs of the community for particular types of skills than on the needs of the individual to find a job that maximized the fit of one's occupation with one's talents and interests. In most cases, the students think that their occupation was determined for them by their community, or by the State. Similarly, in interviews with Japanese students, I found that choices about future occupations were based more on the quality of the company than on the fit of the particular job category with the individual's talents and interests. In this case, the individuals were given more power to select their future occupation; but the criteria for their choice were quite different from the criteria advocated in vocational counseling in the United States.

Does this mean that the Eccles et al. expectancy–value model is not a useful theoretical tool for such cultures? I think not. It does mean that we need to consider the cultural and social, as well as the psychological components, of the Eccles et al. model. For

this chapter, we need to pay particular attention to the sociocultural forces that underlie individual differences in STV. In both the Chinese and Japanese cases discussed earlier, the STV of various occupational categories was based on more communial considerations than is typical for European American adolescents. In addition, the relevance of ability self-concepts for choice should be less than it is for European American adolescents. These hypotheses need to be tested.

Equally important, cultures will differ in the range of options provided. Individuals are only exposed to narrow range of options available to them in any achievement domain. Cultures differ greatly in the kinds of day-to-day activities to which their children are exposed. For example, urban children in the United States are not likely to be exposed to playing cricket, African drums, or Balinese dancing for a leisure activity, or to farming as an occupational choice. Consequently, it is not surprising that American children are unlikely to choose these activities.

Sociocultural processes are also likely to produce cultural differences in expectancies, ability self-concepts, and all components of STV. For example, cultures likely differ in the stereotypes of different abilities. Some cultures believe that individual differences in math and sport ability reflect individual differences in practice and learning. Others believe these individual differences are due primarily to innate aptitude. It is likely that the conclusions the children in these different types of cultures draw about their abilities from their success and failure experiences in math and sports will differ—leading to culture differences in ability self-concepts for different academic domains.

The potential impact of sociocultural processes on the various components of STV is even clearer. Attainment value, for example, should be very culturally embedded. The value of various identity components, activities, and behaviors is a central component of culture. To the extent that individuals within a culture internalize the culturally proscribed identity components, these individuals will place greater importance (attainment value) on those behaviors and activities that are consistent with these identity components. Similarly, to the extent that individuals have internalized the culturally proscribed identity components, the lower value, and the higher cost, they will attach to activities and behaviors that are inconsistent or antithetical with the culturally proscribed identity components.

The impact of sociocultural processes on utility and cost can be analyzed in a similar manner. If various adult roles are valued differently across cultures, then the utility value of those activities and behaviors likely to be instrumental to achieving these adult roles will also vary across cultures and subcultural groups. Similarly, the cost of engaging in activities or behaviors that reduce the likelihood of achieving these adult roles will vary across cultures. In addition, cultures will vary in their tolerance and encouragement of nontraditional and nonnormative behavioral choices. As the tolerance and encouragement go down, the cost of non-normative and nontraditional choices goes up—in some cases, to the point of death.

Finally, females and males in all cultures, as well as other cultural subgroups within a culture, engage in quite different activities both as children and adults. In part, these differences are likely to reflect differences in the choices to which females and males are exposed; in part, these differences reflect the impact of sociocultural processes on the development of females' and males' ability self-perceptions and STVs.

In summary, there are many ways in which culture might relate to the Eccles et al. expectancy–value model of achievement-related choices. In this section, I have stressed the relation between culture and the various components underlying STV. In the next section, I explore these links more fully, drawing upon our work in the area of gender.

DO GENDER DIFFERENCES IN SUBJECTIVE TASK VALUES HELP US UNDERSTAND GENDER DIFFERENCES IN ACHIEVEMENT-RELATED CHOICES?

Given the probable impact of gender-role socialization on the variables associated with STV, gender differences in the STV attached to various achievement-related options should be important mediators of gender differences in educational and occupational choices in both typical and gifted populations. Our research supports this hypothesis. In a longitudinal study of the math course enrollment decisions of intellectually able, college-bound high school students, gender differences in students' decisions to enroll in advanced mathematics were mediated primarily by gender differences in the value that the students' attached to mathematics (Eccles, Adler, & Meece, 1984). More specifically, the young women were less likely than the young men to enroll in advanced mathematics, primarily because they felt that math was less important, less useful, and less enjoyable than did the young men. We also found clear evidence of gender differences in the value attached to various school subjects and activities in our study of elementary school-age children enrolled in a gifted program (Eccles & Harold, 1992). Even though there was no gender difference in expectations for success in mathematics, these girls reported liking math less than did the boys and rated math as less useful than did the boys. In addition, the boys also attached greater importance to sports than did the girls. Not surprisingly, the boys were much more likely to be engaged in sports activities throughout their elementary school years than the girls. Other studies of both gifted and more typical populations have yielded similar findings (Dauber & Benbow, 1990; see Eccles & Harold, 1992).

In summary, there is substantial evidence of gender differences in the valuing of various educational and occupational options. But do these differences explain gender differences in educational occupational choice? As noted earlier, I have found evidence that the answer is yes (see Eccles, 1987). Additional support for this hypothesis comes from the work of Benbow (1988; Benbow & Minor, 1986). Gifted girls in their study were less likely than gifted boys to take advanced mathematics, in part because they liked language-related courses more than they liked mathematics courses. In addition, they found weak but consistent positive relations in their gifted samples between liking of biology, chemistry, and physics, and subsequent plans to major in biology, chemistry, and physics. Finally, students' interest predicted course taking in high school and college.

CONCLUDING REMARKS

I had several goals for this chapter. First I wanted to outline in some detail my perspective of STV as a part of the Eccles et al. expectancy–value theory of achievement-related behavioral choices. The general outline of a theory of STV was developed by myself and my colleagues during the 1970s and 1980s. The basic elements were first discussed in Eccles (Parsons) et al. (1983) and in my 1984 Nebraska Symposium on Motivation chapter. These basic elements included an articulation of four critical subcomponents or influences on STV: attainment value, intrinsic interest value, utility value, and perceived cost. More recent accounts of these basic elements, along with a developmental analysis and an attempt to relate the basis elements to other motivational theories, appeared in a 1992 article by Wigfield and Eccles and a 1998 chapter by Eccles, Wigfield, and Schefiele. In this chapter, I have tried to articulate more fully my own perspective on each of the four basic elements, focusing most intensively on attainment value. This focus reflects my current interest in both social and personal identities.

I also wanted to articulate the relation of this perspective to other related motivational theories. This proved to be quite a challenge for two reasons: (1) The complexity of current theories of motivation made clear, unidimensional links difficult, and (2) all currently popular theories are dynamic and changing as the theorists talk more with each other. I found both of these challenges intrinsically interesting and important for the field. As each of the theories become more complex, they also become more similar. Being an integrative optimist, I want to interpret these theoretical shifts in terms of a developmental progression toward convergence on a comprehensive and predictively powerful set of principles of behavioral choice and motivation. We are not there yet, but we are getting closer.

Finally, I wanted to lay out the power of the STV perspective to analyze the sociocultural processes underlying group differences in behavioral choices. As the world becomes closer and globalization becomes more common, we are forced to think about group differences in behavioral choice. We need to understand the motivations of people who are culturally quite different from us. The fundamental question of motivation is why people do what they do. But can we develop theories that are sufficiently powerful to help us understand behavioral differences across various socioculturally defined groups? The final sections of this chapter represent my attempt to address this question. Again, I found this a quite challenging task, in part due to my own culturally and genetically based cognitive limitations, and in part due to the complexity of the task itself. But again, my optimism was reinforced. Many very smart people are trying to address this task, and I think our motivational theories are getting more powerful as we share our ideas with each other.

ACKNOWLEDGMENTS

I wish to thank all of my colleagues and former students who have worked with me in developing the studies summarized in this chapter. These include Judith Meece, Carol Kaczala, Allan Wigfield, Janis Jacobs, Constance Flanagan, Rena Harold, Bonnie Barber, and Deborah Jozefowicz. This work was supported by grants from the National Institute of Mental Health, the National Institute of Child Health and Human Development, and the National Science Foundation.

REFERENCES

Amabile, T. M., Hill, K. G., Hennessey, B. A., & Tighe, E. M. (1994). The Work Preference Inventory: Assessing intrinsic and extrinsic motivational orientations. *Journal of Personality and Social Psychology, 66,* 950–967.

Ames, C. (1992). Classrooms: Goals, structures, and student motivation. *Journal of Educational Psychology, 84,* 261–271.

Ames, C., & Ames, R. (Eds.). (1989). *Research on motivation in education: Goals and cognition.* San Diego: Academic Press.

Bandura, A. (1986). *Social foundations of thought and action: A social cognitive theory.* Englewood Cliffs, NJ: Prentice-Hall.

Battle, E. S. (1966). Motivational determinants of academic competence. *Journal of Personality and Social Psychology, 4,* 634–642.

Benbow, C. P. (1988). Sex differences in mathematical reasoning ability in intellectually talented preadolescents: Their nature, effects, and possible causes. *Behavioral and Brain Sciences, 11,* 169–232.

Benbow, C. P., & Minor, L. L. (1986). Mathematically

talented males and females and achievement in the high school sciences. *American Educational Research Journal, 23,* 425–436.

Benware, C. A., & Deci, E. L. (1984). Quality of learning with an active versus passive motivational set. *American Educational Research Journal, 21,* 755–765.

Connell, J. P., & Wellborn, J. (1991). Competence, autonomy, and relatedness: A motivational analysis of self-system processes. In M. R. Gunnar (Ed.), *Self processes and development* (pp. 43–77). Hillsdale, NJ: Erlbaum.

Covington, M. V. (1992). *Making the grade: A self-worth perspective on motivation and school reform.* New York: Cambridge University Press.

Covington, M. V., & Omelich, C. L. (1979). Effort: The double-edged sword in school achievement. *Journal of Educational Psychology, 71,* 169–182.

Crandall, V. C. (1969). Sex differences in expectancy of intellectual and academic reinforcement. In C. P. Smith (Ed.), *Achievement-related behaviors in children* (pp. 11–45). New York: Russell Sage Foundation.

Csikszentmihalyi, M. (1988). The flow experience and its significance for human psychology. In M. Csikszentmihalyi & I. S. Csikszentmihalyi (Eds.), *Optimal experience* (pp. 15–35).Cambridge, MA: Cambridge University Press.

Dauber, S. L., & Benbow, C. P. (1990). Aspects of personality and peer relations of extremely talented adolescents. *Gifted Child Quarterly, 34,* 10–15.

deCharms, R. (1968). *Personal causation: The internal affective determinants of behavior.* New York: Academic Press.

Deci, E. L., & Ryan, R. M. (1985). The general causality orientations scale: Self-determination in personality. *Journal of Research in Personality, 19,* 109–134.

Dweck, C. S., & Elliott, E. S. (1983). Achievement motivation. In P. H. Mussen, *Handbook of child psychology* (Vol. IV, 3rd ed., pp. 643–691). New York: Wiley.

Eccles, J. S. (1984). Sex differences in achievement patterns. In T. Sonderegger (Ed.), *Nebraska Symposium on Motivation* (Vol. 32, pp. 97–132). Lincoln: University of Nebraska Press.

Eccles, J. S. (1987). Gender roles and women's achievement-related decisions. *Psychology of Women Quarterly, 11,* 135–172.

Eccles, J. S. (1989). Bringing young women to math and science. In M. Crawford & M. Gentry (Eds.), *Gender and thought: Psychological perspectives* (pp. 36–57). New York: Springer-Verlag.

Eccles, J. S., Adler, T. F., & Meece, J. L. (1984). Sex differences in achievement: A test of alternate theories. *Journal of Personality and Social Psychology, 46*(1), 26–43.

Eccles, J. S., Barber, B., & Jozefowicz, D. (1999). Linking gender to education, occupation, and recreational choices: Applying the Eccles et al. model of achievement-related choices. In W. B. Swann, J. H.

Langlois, & L. A. Gilbert (Eds.), *Sexism and stereotypes in modern society: The gender science of Janet Taylor Spence* (pp. 153–192). Washington, DC: American Psychological Association Press.

Eccles, J. S., & Harold, R. D. (1992). Gender differences in educational and occupational patterns among the gifted. In N. Colangelo, S. G. Assouline, & D. L. Amronson (Eds.), *Talent development: Proceedings from the 1991 Henry B. and Jocelyn Wallace National Research Symposium on Talent Development* (pp. 3–29). Unionville, NY: Trillium Press.

Eccles, J. S., & Vida, M. (2003, April). *Predicting mathematics-related educational and career choices.* Paper presented at the Biennial Meeting of the Society of Research on Child Development, Tampa, FL.

Eccles, J. S., Wigfield, A., & Schiefele, U. (1998). Motivation. In N. Eisenberg (Ed.), *Handbook of child psychology* (Vol. 3, 5th ed., pp. 1017–1095). New York: Wiley.

Eccles (Parsons), J., Adler, T. F., Futterman, R., Goff, S. B., Kaczala, C. M., Meece, J. L., et al. (1983). Expectations, values and academic behaviors. In J. T. Spence (Ed.), *Perspective on achievement and achievement motivation* (pp. 75–146). San Francisco: Freeman.

Elliot, A. J., & McGregor, H. (2001). A 2 × 2 achievement goal framework. *Journal of Personality and Social Psychology, 80,* 501–519.

Feather, N. T. (1988). Values, valences, and course enrollment: Testing the role of personal values within an expectancy–value framework. *Journal of Educational Psychology, 8,* 381–391.

Feather, N. T. (1992). Values, valences, expectations, and actions. *Journal of Social Issues, 48,* 109–124.

Ford, M. E. (1992). *Human motivation: Goals, emotions, and personal agency beliefs.* Newbury Park, CA: Sage.

Gottfried, A. E. (1990). Academic intrinsic motivation in young elementary school children. *Journal of Educational Psychology, 82,* 525–538.

Harackiewicz, J. M., & Elliot, A. J. (1993). Achievement goals and intrinsic motivation. *Journal of Personality and Social Psychology, 65,* 904–915.

Harter, S. (1981). A new self-report scale of intrinsic versus extrinsic orientation in the classroom: Motivational and informational components. *Developmental Psychology, 17,* 300–312.

Harter, S. (1983). Developmental perspectives on the self-system. In P. H. Mussen (Ed.), *Handbook of child psychology* (pp. 275–385). New York: Wiley.

Harter, S. (1998). The development of self-representations. In W. Damon & N. Eisenberg (Eds.), *Handbook of child psychology: Vol. 3. Social, emotional, and personality development* (5th ed., pp. 553–618). New York: Wiley.

Hidi, S. (1990). Interest and its contribution as a mental resource for learning. *Review of Educational Research, 60,* 549–571.

Hidi, S., & Baird, W. (1986). Interestingness—a neglected variable in discourse processing. *Cognitive Science*, *10*, 179–194.

Higgins, E. (1987). Self-discrepancy: A theory relating self and affect. *Psychological Review*, *94*, 319–340.

Jozefowicz, D. M., Barber, B. L., & Eccles, J. S. (1993, March). *Adolescent work-related values and beliefs: Gender differences and relation to occupational aspirations*. Paper presented at the Biennial Meeting of the Society for Research in Child Development, New Orleans, LA.

Juvonen, J., & Wentzel, K. R. (1996). *Social motivation: Understanding children's school adjustment*. New York: Cambridge University Press.

Kerr, B. A. (1985). *Smart girls, gifted women*. Dayton, OH: Ohio Psychology Publishing.

Lepper, M. R. (1988). Motivational considerations in the study of instruction. *Cognition and Instruction*, *5*, 289–309.

Massimini, F., & Carli, M. (1988). The systematic assessment of flow in daily experience. In M. Csikszentmihalyi (Ed.), *Optimal experience: Psychological studies of flow in consciousness* (pp. 266–287). New York: Cambridge University Press.

Matsumoto, D., & Sanders, M. (1988). Emotional experiences during engagement in intrinsically and extrinsically motivated tasks. *Motivation and Emotion*, *12*, 353–369.

Meece, J. L. (1991). The classroom context and students' motivational goals. In M. Maehr & P. Pintrich (Eds.), *Advances in motivation and achievement* (pp. 261–286). Greenwich, CT: JAI Press.

Meece, J. L. (1994). The role of motivation in self-regulated learning. In D. H. Schunk (Ed.), *Self-regulation of learning and performance: Issues and educational applications* (pp. 25–44). Hillsdale, NJ: Erlbaum.

Midgley, C. (Ed.). (2002). *Goals, goal structures, and patterns of adaptive learning*. Mahwah, NJ: Erlbaum.

Midgley, C., Anderman, E., & Hicks, L. (1995). Differences between elementary and middle school teachers and students: A goal theory approach. *Journal of Early Adolescence*, *15*, 90–133.

Nicholls, J. G. (1984). Achievement motivation: Conceptions of ability, subjective experience, task choice, and performance. *Psychological Review*, *91*, 328–346.

Nicholls, J. G., Cobb, P., Wood, T., Yackel, E., & Patashnick, M. (1990). Assessing students' theories of success in mathematics: Individual and classroom differences. *Journal for Research in Mathematics Education*, *21*, 109–122.

Pintrich, P. R., & Schrauben, B. (1992). Students' motivational beliefs and their cognitive engagement in classroom academic tasks. In D. H. Schunk (Ed.), *Student perceptions in the classroom* (pp. 149–183). Hillsdale, NJ: Erlbaum.

Pintrich, P. R., & Schunk, D. H. (2002). *Motivation in education: Theory, research and applications* (2nd ed.). Upper Saddle River, NJ: Merrill/Prentice-Hall.

Renninger, K. A., Hidi, S., & Krapp, A. (Eds.). (1992). *The role of interest in learning and development*. Hillsdale, NJ: Erlbaum.

Rokeach, M. (1973). *The nature of human values*. New York: Free Press.

Ryan, R. M. (1992). Agency and organization: Intrinsic motivation, autonomy, and the self in psychological development. In J. Jacobs (Ed.), *Nebraska Symposium on Motivation* (pp. 1–56). Lincoln: University of Nebraska Press.

Ryan, R. M., Connell, J. P., & Deci, E. L. (1985). A motivational analysis of self-determination and self-regulation in education. In C. Ames & R. Ames (Eds.), *Research on motivation in education: Vol. 2. The classroom milieu* (pp. 13–51). London: Academic Press.

Ryan, R. M., & Deci, E. L. (2000). Intrinsic and extrinsic motivations: Classic definitions and new directions. *Contemporary Educational Journal*, *25*, 54–67.

Schiefele, U. (1991). Interest, learning, and motivation. *Educational Psychologist*, *26*, 299–323.

Schiefele, U. (1996). Topic interest, text representation, and quality of experience. *Contemporary Educational Psychology*, *21*, 3–18.

Tobias, S. (1994). Interest, prior knowledge, and learning. *Review of Educational Research*, *64*, 37–54.

Weiner, B. (1992). *Human motivation: Metaphors, theories, and research*. Newbury Park, CA: Sage.

Wentzel, K. R. (1991). Social competence at school: Relation between social responsibility and academic achievement. *Review of Educational Research*, *61*, 1–24.

Wentzel, K. R. (1993). Motivation and achievement in early adolescence: The role of multiple classroom goals. *Journal of Early Adolescence*, *13*, 4–20.

White, R. H. (1959). Motivation reconsidered: The concept of competence. *Psychological Review*, *66*, 297–333.

Wigfield, A., & Eccles, J. S. (1992). The development of achievement task values: A theoretical analysis. *Developmental Review*, *12*, 265–310.

CHAPTER 8

☞

Self-Theories

Their Impact on Competence Motivation and Acquisition

CAROL S. DWECK
DANIEL C. MOLDEN

Achievement motivation is about striving for competence. Thus, a major part of understanding achievement motivation is understanding people's theories about competence—what competence is and what it means about the self.

Why do people want competence? First, there appears to be an inborn desire to acquire and exercise competence. From the beginning, its acquisition is readily initiated, inherently sustained, and intrinsically rewarded. This is simply part of our survival. Later, this can become a more conscious valuing of learning and growth. A second reason that people want competence is that it becomes part of the self-concept, part of what people measure themselves by, and part of what other people esteem them for. Thus, achievement motivation is powered by a valuing of both competence acquisition (learning goals) and competence validation (performance goals).

Self-theories help us understand which of these two faces of competence—the competence acquisition or the competence validation—becomes most valued. This is important, for we show how an overemphasis on competence validation can drive out learning. By illuminating the valuing of different competence goals, self-theories can also give us entrée into the "meaning systems" people use to construct meaning in competence-relevant situations. Often, motivational variables are considered in isolation. Rarely do researchers look at a network of beliefs and goals *that work together* to produce important behaviors and outcomes; that is, rarely do they look at the meaning systems that give rise to the behaviors and outcomes we care about.

In this chapter, we begin by showing how self-theories create meaning systems—how they attract or highlight certain competence goals and certain attributions, which go on to foster particular strategies (see also Dweck, 1999; Dweck & Molden, 2004; Grant & Dweck, 2003). These strategies, in turn, result in different levels of self-esteem, interest, and competence, especially in the face of challenge or threat. We show how these theory-based meaning systems operate in the arenas of academic achievement, sports, relationships, and organizations. We also describe how socialization practices can foster different self-theories, and how altering people's self-theories has a cascade of effects, altering their meaning systems and their academic outcomes. Finally, we close by showing how thinking in terms of self-theories and the meaning systems they engender can link competence and motivation to other important areas of psychology.

SELF-THEORIES

The self-theories we focus on in this chapter are people's beliefs about the fixedness or malleability of their personal qualities, such as their intelligence: Do people believe that their intelligence is a fixed trait ("You have it or you don't") or a malleable quality that they can cultivate through learning and effort? These theories are typically measured by asking people to agree or disagree with a series of statements, such as "Your intelligence is something basic about you that you can't really change" or "No matter who you are, you can substantially change your level of intelligence." Agreement with statements like the first one reflects an "entity" theory, that is, the idea that intelligence is a fixed entity. In contrast, agreement with statements like the second one reflects a malleable or "incremental" theory, that is, the idea that intellectual ability can be increased through one's efforts.

Although many people think the entity theory is the dominant one in our society, it turns out that both theories are equally popular. When self-theories are assessed in children or adults, about 40% of people tend to endorse the entity theory, about 40% tend to endorse the incremental theory, and about 20% are undecided.

Self-theories can also be induced experimentally. That is, although these theories are relatively stable beliefs that individuals hold (see, e.g., Robins & Pals, 2002), they can also be taught or primed. In many studies, researchers have taught their participants an entity or an incremental theory, often by means of persuasive articles (e.g., Niiya,

Crocker, & Bartmess, 2004). These articles depict the attribute in question, such as intelligence or personality, as a relatively inborn trait that is resistant to change or, alternatively, as a quality that can be developed throughout one's life. Researchers have also manipulated self-theories by portraying the task that people are about to embark on as one that measures (or requires) either inherent abilities or, alternatively, skills that can be acquired through practice. This has been done for such diverse abilities as intellectual skills (e.g., Aronson, 1998; Martocchio, 1994), physical skills (e.g., Jourden, Bandura, & Banfield, 1991), and managerial skills (e.g., Wood & Bandura, 1989). Finally, as we will see, people's self-theories can be changed in a more long-term way through targeted interventions (Aronson, Fried, & Good, 2002; Blackwell, Dweck, & Trzesniewski, 2003; Good, Aronson, & Inzlicht, 2003).

Can people hold different theories about different attributes? Can they believe that their intelligence is fixed but their personality is malleable? Yes, people can and often do hold different theories about different personal qualities (Dweck, Chiu, & Hong, 1995). They can even hold different theories about different intellectual skills, for example, believing that their math ability is fixed but their verbal abilities can be developed.

Which theory is correct? Historically, psychologists have heatedly argued both sides of the issue, and they are still at it today. As with most issues, the answer probably lies somewhere in between, but evidence increasingly suggests that important parts of many abilities can be acquired (see Brown, 1997; Nickerson, Perkins, & Smith, 1985; Sternberg, 1985; Chapter 2, this volume). This trend is clear not only in the research literature but also in the popular literature, where we see more and more documented cases of disadvantaged, failing, or "backward" children learning calculus (Mathews, 1988) or reading and discussing Shakespeare (Collins, 1992; Esquith, 2003; Levin, 1987). In Marva Collins's inner-city Chicago school, all 4-year-olds who entered in September were reading by Christmas. These were the same children who might typically reach high school without knowing how to read.

In this context, it is interesting to note that even Alfred Binet the inventor of the IQ test, was a strong proponent of the incremental theory of intelligence. Although his test was later used to measure the "entity" of intelligence, that was far from his intention. His life's work was devoted, not to pigeonholing failing students, but to devising educational programs that would help them become smarter:

> A few modern philosophers . . . assert that an individual's intelligence is a fixed quantity which cannot be increased. We must protest and react against this brutal pessimism. . . . With practice, training, and above all method, we manage to increase our attention, our memory, our judgment, and literally to become more intelligent than we were before. (Binet, 1909/1973, pp. 105–106)

However, this is not simply an intellectual issue of interest to psychologists. In the sections that follow, we see the profound consequences for people of believing in one theory or the other. We see the way in which believing in fixed attributes leads people to become highly concerned (sometimes overconcerned) with measuring those attributes, often to the detriment of their learning. It leads people to interpret setbacks as a reflection of their underlying competence and to show defensive or ineffective self-regulatory strategies in the face of threat. In contrast, we see how believing in malleable attributes leads people to place a priority on learning and self-development, to interpret setbacks as a reflection of their effort or learning strategies, and to mobilize effective self-regulatory strategies in the face of threat.

SELF-THEORIES AND MEANING SYSTEMS

In this section, we describe three longitudinal studies (Blackwell et al., 2003; Robins & Pals, 2002; Trzesniewski & Robins, 2003) that show how self-theories of intelligence form the core of motivationally important meaning systems. These studies, all of which trace students across difficult transitions, are in striking agreement. As they follow students who are coping with challenge, these studies find basically the same constellation of factors working together to affect self-esteem and/or achievement.

Self-Theories and Achievement

In the first study, Blackwell et al. (2003) followed several hundred seventh graders across the transition to junior high school. At the beginning of 7th grade, we assessed the students' theories of intelligence, along with a host of other motivational variables, and we monitored their math grades over the next 2 years. Math is perhaps the subject that poses the greatest difficulty for many students as they find themselves in new conceptual realms during these years. In many studies, students show a sharp decline in grades as they go from grade school to junior high, and this decline continues throughout junior high.

Effects on Goals

What did we find? First, we found that students' theories of intelligence were significant predictors of other key motivational variables. Specifically, holding an incremental theory of intelligence (vs. an entity theory of intelligence) was associated with holding strong learning goals. Students with an incremental theory more strongly endorsed statements such as "It is much more important for me to learn things in my classes than it is to get the best grades." That is, when students believed their intelligence could be developed, they sought learning as a means to do so. When they believed their intelligence was fixed, they were diverted from learning by their need to validate their intelligence through their performance.

Another study, examining students making the transition to college, also highlighted the ways in which theories of intelligence orient students toward different goals. Hong, Chiu, Dweck, Lin, and Wan (1999) questioned students who were entering the University of Hong Kong, where all of the classes are conducted in English, but not all of the entering students are proficient in English. We knew students' English proficiency scores and, as the students filled out their registration materials, they were asked whether they would take a remedial English course if the faculty were to offer it. Students who held an incremental theory of intelligence replied with a resounding yes— they wanted to learn, but students with an entity theory of intelligence were not at all enthusiastic. They perhaps preferred to live with their deficiency, even if it put their college career in jeopardy, rather than expose it, for in that framework a deficiency can reflect a permanent inadequacy.

Effects on Effort Beliefs

In the junior high school sample, students' theories of intelligence also strongly predicted their beliefs about effort. For those with an incremental theory, effort was a positive thing, a means to becoming smarter: "The harder you work at something, the better you'll be at it." However, for those with an entity theory, effort was negative: "To tell the truth, when I work hard at my schoolwork, it makes me feel like I'm not very smart." In this fixed intelligence framework, effort reflected deficient ability. Since effort is the path to achievement, you can see how such a belief could set up roadblocks.

Effects on Attributions

Beyond goals and effort beliefs, theory of intelligence was a significant predictor of students' attributions for their difficulties as well. Students with an incremental theory took setbacks to mean that "I didn't study hard enough" or "I didn't go about studying in the right way." When you're oriented toward learning, mistakes are signals of what you did wrong and what you should do differently in the future. In contrast, students with the entity theory, saw setbacks (like effort) as a sign of deficient ability: "I wasn't smart enough" or "I'm just not good at this subject." When you're oriented toward performance, mistakes signal failure and inadequacy.

Effects on Strategies

What would they do after a setback? What were their strategies? In line with the belief that they could develop their competence through effort, those students with an incremental theory said (significantly more than the entity theorists) that after a failure on a test, "I would work harder in this class from now on" and "I would spend more time studying for the tests." Perfectly sensible. However, those with an entity theory—with

their lack-of-ability attributions and their concern over exposing deficiencies—said (significantly more than the incremental theorists), "I would spend less time on this subject from now on," "I would try not to take this subject ever again," and "I would try to cheat on the next test." The entity theory leaves students with no good recipe for success. If you lack ability and if further effort will just confirm it, there are few constructive strategies left at your disposal.

Effects on Grades

Did students' theories of intelligence predict their math grades? The performance of two groups, who entered junior high with equivalent math achievement, increasingly pulled apart over the 2-year period. Entity theorists were performing markedly worse after only one term, and this gap grew larger over time. Moreover, despite the often-reported tendency for all students' grades to decline over this period, the grades of the incremental theorists actually rose every semester.

Meaning System Analysis

The most important question from a meaning system perspective, however, is how the motivational variables worked in concert to produce differences in achievement. Path analyses showed that the incremental theory, by encouraging learning goals, positive effort beliefs, and effort attributions, gave rise to positive, "mastery-oriented" strategies. These strategies, in turn, predicted increasing math scores across the junior high years. Interestingly, students' entering achievement test scores did not predict increasing or decreasing grades. Only the motivational variables did that.[1]

The question then becomes whether other studies measuring similar variables yield evidence for the same meaning system. Trzesniewski and Robins (2003) conducted a similar study, following children from their last semester of grade school (in this case, grade 5) through three semesters of middle school. They assessed students' theories of intelligence, as well as other motivational variable, and then monitored their math grades during middle school. Aside from the fact that Trzesniewski and Robins did not measure effort beliefs or mastery-oriented strategies, the path analysis looked highly similar to that of Blackwell et al. (2003). The incremental theory, by orienting students toward learning goals rather than performance goals, led to effort attributions for setbacks, and from there to increasing math grades. Despite the fact that math grades were declining for the sample as a whole, the incremental students showed a rise in grades over the course of the study.

Self-Theories and Self-Esteem

In addition to scholastic achievement, can self-theories and their allied meaning systems predict the course of other important outcomes? Robins and Pals (2002) used a similar set of variables to predict changes in self-esteem. They followed 363 students at the University of California at Berkeley across their college years, another challenging time. Students' theories of intelligence were assessed and used to predict other motivational variables, as well as students' increasing or decreasing self-esteem. Would the same meaning system that predicted students' grade trajectories predict their self-esteem trajectories?

Relation to Motivational Variables

First, students' theories of intelligence were significant predictors of other important variables. Incremental theorists were more focused on learning goals, whereas entity theorists were more focused on performance goals. Further, incremental theorists made more attributions to effort and study skills, while entity theorists made more attributions to lack of ability when they explained setbacks.[2] Looking at responses to challenge, the incremental theory was highly predictive of the positive, mastery-oriented responses ("When something I am studying is difficult, I try harder"), while the entity theory was highly predictive of the more "helpless" responses to setbacks ("When I fail to understand something, I become discouraged to the point of wanting to give up"). Finally, entity theorists were on a downward self-esteem trajectory relative to incremental theorists, and this tendency was independent of any differences in their average level of self-esteem. This difference was also independent of their grades. Thus, self-theories were able

to predict self-esteem trajectories in addition to the grade trajectories found in the previous studies.

Meaning System Analysis

Importantly, the self-theories and related motivational variables again hung together into a coherent meaning system. The incremental theory was again related (positively) to learning goals and (negatively) to performance goals, which were each related to the effort versus ability attributions for failure. The goals and the attributions led to mastery-oriented versus helpless strategies, and these strategies, in turn, predicted the changes in self-esteem.[3]

Implications

In effect, a very similar meaning system to the one found to govern grade changes was found to predict self-esteem changes. Motivational variables, rather than working in isolation, were repeatedly seen to work together to create favorable or unfavorable outcomes—self-theories leading to goals, goals (sometimes together with the self-theories) leading to attributions and strategies, and attributions and strategies leading to self-esteem and achievement outcomes. These findings raise several important issues. For example, attributions have long been known to be important predictors of self-related affect and coping in the face of setbacks (Abramson, Seligman, & Teasdale, 1978; Dweck & Reppucci, 1973; Weiner, 1986; Weiner & Kukla, 1970), and this was found in each of the studies reviewed as well. Thus, the importance of attributional processes was confirmed. However, the attributions in each case were predicted by the self-theories and goals. Thus, the attributions appear to grow out of the meaning systems in which people are operating. When people believe in fixed intelligence and are oriented toward competence validation, negative outcomes speak to a lack of ability. When, instead, people believe in developable intelligence and are oriented toward competence acquisition, negative outcomes speak to effort and strategy. Therefore, it becomes important to understand the origins and impact of attributions in terms of the meaning systems that appear to give rise to them.

In a related vein, much research has been directed toward styles of coping, for example, coping through active problem solving versus avoidance coping. Most typically, these styles are not seen in the context of people's beliefs and goals, but rather as styles that have somehow been learned over time. However, the research reviewed in this chapter suggests that some of the very coping styles in which researchers have been most interested may stem from the meaning systems we have been describing. Meaning systems built around an incremental theory appear to promote active, direct, and constructive coping, whereas those built around an entity theory appear to foster more avoidant, indirect, and defensive coping. As with attributions, then, a full understanding of coping styles should include an examination of the core beliefs that lead people to cope in characteristic ways.

Thus, this analysis has the potential to illuminate some of the key processes of interest to psychologists, and to bring these processes, such as coping processes, into the realm of motivation.

WHAT IS COMPETENCE?

We have shown how self-theories affect whether people are primarily focused on competence validation or competence acquisition. Yet, beyond these effects, self-theories set up different meanings to the point that the very idea of competence is quite different within the two frameworks (see Molden & Dweck, 2000). Butler (2000) examined the issue of what constitutes competence with a sample of junior high school students and their math teachers. For some of the participants, Butler simply measured their existing theories of intelligence; for others, she induced an entity or incremental theory of math ability. Those in the entity condition were told, "People differ in mathematical ability. Studies show that people's mathematical ability does not change much throughout life." In contrast, those in the incremental condition were told, "Studies show that people acquire math ability through learning and practice; people who learn as they work develop higher ability." All were then shown the performance of a student on math problems over a series of days, and asked to judge his ability.

Specifically, half were shown the performance of a student whose performance declined over the time period (i.e., he started high and dropped off), whereas the other half were shown a student whose performance increased (he started lower, but rose over time), and were asked to rate his ability. Those with an entity theory thought the student with declining performance had higher ability. He had the competence right away, without working; no matter that he slacked off later on. However, those with the incremental theory thought the student with ascending performance had higher ability. He presumably had worked hard and acquired competence.

Even when people were shown both patterns at the same time and asked which student was smarter, entity theorists chose the declining student and incremental theorists chose the ascending student. Moreover, it did not matter whether the students' and teachers' theories of intelligence were their natural, preexisting theories or theories that had been experimentally induced. The results were the same.

These findings are important, because educators or employers are often in the position of judging people's competence. If they have an entity theory, they will make an immediate judgment based on initial performance. If they have an incremental theory, they will instead value what people can learn over time. In other words, they will value and recognize growth. In fact, Rheinberg (1980) found that teachers with entity-like beliefs ("According to my experience, students' achievement mostly keeps constant in the course of a year" and "As a teacher I have no influence on students' intellectual ability") did not produce maximal growth in students who came into their classroom with lower achievement. These students remained low achievers. In contrast, teachers with more incremental beliefs promoted growth in achievement among those who were initially behind, to the point that many of them caught up to the higher achievers.

A second study by Butler (2000) showed that people's self-theories not only affect their definitions of competence when they observe others but also influence their definition of competence for themselves. Students worked on a task and were given feedback that indicated either a decline in their performance over time or an improvement over time. Butler then assessed their intrinsic motivation by asking them: "How interesting did you find the problems? How interested are you in receiving more problems like the ones you worked on? How interested would you be in working on extra problems during recess?" Incremental theorists displayed higher interest when their performance had improved rather than declined, but entity theorists showed a trend in the opposite direction.

These findings are important, because they suggest that entity theorists may not enjoy something fully unless they are good at it right away, whereas incremental theorists can take pleasure in things they have worked hard to master over time. This is supported by research that monitored people's affect and enjoyment as they learned a variety of difficult tasks (e.g., a perceptual–motor task: Jourden et al., 1991; computer skills: Martocchio, 1994; managerial skills: Tabernero & Wood, 1999). For example, in a study by Jourden et al. (1991), people learned a challenging perceptual–motor skill. For half of them, an entity theory was induced by telling them that their performance reflected inherent aptitude; for the other half, an incremental theory was induced by telling them that their performance reflected an acquirable skill.

On this difficult task, people in the entity theory condition showed no growth in confidence over learning trials, negative reactions to their performance, and low interest in the activity. Since they were not good at it right away, they could not enjoy the task or any progress they were making on it. As a result, their final skill level was limited as well. In contrast, those in the incremental condition showed growth in confidence, positive reactions to their performance, and widespread interest in the activity. Since an incremental theory orients people toward learning, their progress was a source of pride and enjoyment. In line with this, they displayed a high level of skill acquisition.

In summary, self-theories change the very meaning of competence. In one system, the entity system, competence is something people simply have and display right away. If it does not emerge at once, they lose interest or become distressed. In the other, the incre-

mental system, competence is something that grows over time through effort. That growth of competence over time is the occasion for growing confidence, pride, and interest.

IMPLICATIONS OF MEANING SYSTEMS

Handling Threats to Competence

We have already seen how the different self-theories and the meaning systems that grow up around them affect people's self-esteem and performance as they grapple with the threat of difficult tasks and difficult transitions. Here, we see how these same theories affect the self-esteem and performance of people who may be particularly prone to threat—either because their self-esteem is based on their academic performance or because their race or gender makes them the target of negative stereotypes.

Contingent Self-Esteem

Niiya et al. (2004) studied the impact of failure (and success) on students' self-esteem, with particular attention to students who reported that their self-esteem was highly contingent on their academic performance; that is, it typically increased when they succeeded but decreased when they failed. In this study, Niiya et al. gave college students a Graduate Record Examination (GRE) test assessing verbal, quantitative, and analytical reasoning skills. They embedded a self-theories manipulation in the reading comprehension passages. Half of the students read that intelligence is largely hereditary and cannot really increase. The other half read that intelligence can be substantially increased. After the test, half of the students received failure feedback (i.e., that they had scored in the 45th percentile) and half received success feedback (97th percentile), and all students filled out a self-esteem scale indicating how they felt about themselves at that point.

Looking at students whose self-esteem was highly contingent on their academic performance, Niiya et al. (2004) found that those who had received the entity theory priming showed significantly lower self-esteem after failure than after success. Their fixed intelligence had been measured, and they felt bad or good about themselves depending on whether it had been measured unfavorably or favorably. In striking contrast, those who had received the incremental message showed no difference in self-esteem as a function of the feedback they had received. Their self-esteem remained relatively high in the face of failure. The idea that their intelligence was in their control and could be developed over time protected them against the threatening message that failure carried and allowed them to continue to feel good about themselves.

Looking at students' emotional reactions to failure, Niiya et al. (2004) found that when these highly contingent students had been primed with an entity theory, their anxiety and depression were significantly higher after failure than after success. This was not true for those primed with an incremental theory. Failure did not increase their feelings of anxiety or depression, presumably because no permanent verdict about their ability had been rendered.

Stereotype Threat

Several studies have now shown that an incremental theory can protect students from the debilitating effects of negative stereotypes on performance (Steele & Aronson, 1995). As Steele and Aronson point out, the presence of a negative stereotype about a group's ability poses a threat, because it calls the competence of group members into question and makes them concerned about confirming the stereotype of low ability. It makes sense that some of the sting of that stereotype would be removed when people believe that the ability in question is one that they can develop.

The first study to suggest this was by Aronson et al. (2002). In this research, African American and Caucasian college students were taught different theories of intelligence. One group was taught the incremental theory that intelligence was expandable, and that every time they learned new things, their brain formed new connections. They saw a film on this, they discussed it, and, in order to stamp in the message, they went on to mentor a younger student using the incremental message. Another group was

taught the theory of multiple intelligences, with the message being not to worry if they lack intelligence in one area, they may still have it in another area. They, too, mentored younger children in terms of this theory. Finally, a third group was a no-treatment control.

At the end of the semester, Aronson et al. (2002) looked at the students' grade point averages and assessed both their valuing of academics and their enjoyment of academic work. They found that those students who had received the incremental theory had earned significantly higher grades than the students in the other two groups, and that this difference was even more significant for the African American students. They also found that the incremental message led to a significant increase in students' valuing of academics (with these students reporting that, in the larger scheme of things, their academic work was more important to them) and a significant increase in their enjoyment of their academic work (e.g., doing homework assignments, studying for tests, writing papers). Interestingly, the African American students in the incremental theory condition did not report any less exposure to negative stereotypes in their academic environment than the African Americans in other groups. The incremental theory simply armed them to deal with these experiences without harm to their academic attitudes and performance.

This analysis received support from an experimental study performed by Aronson (1998), in which he found that information fostering an entity theory of intelligence before a difficult test heightened the debilitating effects of stereotype threat on the performance of African American students. In contrast, information that highlighted an incremental theory wiped out the effects of the same threat. In this condition, African American students performed well even when negative stereotype about their ability were evoked.

Extending these studies, Good and Dweck (2004) went on to study the impact of holding an entity versus incremental theory on female college students' sense of belonging in mathematics (i.e., the feeling that they were valuable and accepted members in their math environment). They asked: Which students would be most susceptible to stereotyped messages of lower ability in females? As they followed female students through their calculus course, they found that those who held an entity theory of math ability and perceived a high degree of stereotyping in their environment showed a decline over the course of the semester in their sense of belonging in math, their confidence in their math ability, and their enjoyment of math. This was true despite the fact that their entering math Scholastic Aptitude Test scores were as high as those of any of the other groups.

In contrast, when female students held an incremental theory, even a high degree of negative stereotyping in their environment did not lead them to question their membership in the math community, to lose their confidence in their math abilities, or to suffer a decline in their interest in math. As in the Aronson et al. (2002) study, holding an incremental theory appeared to buffer students against the negative effects of stereotypes. It did not blind them to the fact that these stereotypes exist, but it allowed them to function more effectively in the face of them.

Learning and Self-Regulatory Strategies

Let us now look at how self-theories and the meaning systems that grow up around them affect more fine-grained attentional, learning, and self-regulatory strategies, for it is through these strategies that they come to affect performance.

Event-Related Potentials and Attentional Strategies

The first study we examine (Mangels and Dweck, see Dweck, Mangels, & Good, 2004) used ERPs (event-related potentials) to track people's attentional strategies as they worked on a task. On this task, college students, who wore a cap covered with electrodes, were asked a series of difficult questions, one at a time, on the computer. They were given time to type in their answer, and shortly thereafter were told whether they were right or wrong (ability-oriented feedback). Then, a short time later, they were told the correct answer (learning-oriented feedback). By tracking their brain activity during the different stages of the task, we could tell what their

attentional strategies were and, more specifically, whether and when they were entering a state of attentional vigilance to receive their feedback.

We found that regardless of whether students held an entity or an incremental theory of intelligence, their ERPs showed that they all entered a state of vigilance to receive the initial feedback about whether their answer was right or wrong. This information is important for entity theorists, who want to validate their ability, but it is also important to incremental theorists, who put a premium on learning. However, entity theorists did not enter a state of vigilance in preparation for the right answer. Even when their original answer was incorrect, they did not mobilize their resources to learn about the correct answer. Apparently, once they learned whether they had been right or wrong, their job was over. This is clearly not a stance that fosters learning.

In contrast, the incremental theorists entered a state of vigilance to receive the right answer—whether they had been right or wrong. They were apparently interested in seeing and mentally elaborating the correct answer, even when they had been correct. Thus, the impact of self-theories can be seen at the most basic attentional level in the brain activity that prepares people to learn.

Strategies of Self-Esteem Repair

Much has been written about how people repair their self-esteem after a threat or a failure, but most typically, it is assumed that everyone does it in roughly the same way (Gollwitzer & Wicklund, 1985; Tesser, 2000). For example, Tesser (2000) has shown that, after a failure, people want to compare themselves to or associate with people who are less competent than they are. Gollwitzer and Wicklund (1985), in their program of research on symbolic self-completion, also show the humiliating lengths to which people will go after a failure to restore their sense of self.

However, it stands to reason that people will use different strategies of self-repair when the self that has been undermined consists of fixed versus expandable qualities. When the traits are perceived as fixed and, therefore, there is nothing people can do to truly enhance them, they have to turn to defensive strategies: They must expose themselves to information, even distorted information, that will make them feel good about themselves again. However, when the trait in question can be developed, the most sensible strategy for repairing the failure and the blow to self-esteem is rededicate oneself to such development. In this framework, it is basically a waste of time to artificially prop yourself up when you could be remedying the deficit.

In two studies, Nussbaum and Dweck (2004) showed that students working in entity versus incremental frameworks repair their self-esteem in very different ways. In the first study, students first read articles that primed either an entity or an incremental theory of intelligence. They then worked on a very difficult task on which they initially failed and, before the next trial, were given the option of examining strategies of previous students. They could examine strategies of students who had done better than they had on the task or of students who had done as poorly or worse than they had done. To repair their self-esteem, students primed with an entity theory looked at the strategies of students who had also done extremely poorly on the task. However, students primed with an incremental theory looked at strategies of students who had done substantially better than they had, presumably in an effort to remedy their deficit and do better on the next trial.

In the second study, engineering students were given a difficult test of engineering ability, with four subtests. They were given feedback that they had done well on three tests and poorly on one. Which did they want to work further on? Those who had been primed with an entity theory wanted to keep on working on the things they were good at, presumably in order to avoid the threat to their identity that was posed by the test on which they failed. Although it seems counterproductive to avoid the skills one lacks in the very area that is central to one's identity, that is just what the entity theory encourages as a balm to self-esteem. However, students who had been primed with an incremental theory had no such need. They overwhelmingly chose to go back to the test they failed, presumably to try to master the skills they lacked.

Similarly Rhodewalt (1994) has shown

that entity theorist will act to protect their self-esteem even before failure occurs, by using self-handicapping strategies. These are strategies, such as not studying until the last minute, that make any subsequent failure less diagnostic of ability. Although it makes failure more likely, it leaves people the option of saying, "I could have done well if I had studied earlier." Specifically, Rhodewalt found that students who believed that ability was more innately determined and fixed (and who were more focused on performance goals) were more likely to engage in self-handicapping than students who held an incremental theory of intelligence (and pursued learning goals). Once again, the fixed view fosters strategies that are inimical to learning and oriented more toward self-esteem protection, whereas the malleable view fosters strategies that are conducive to the growth of competence.

Self-Regulatory Strategies

Grant (2004) examined the relation between students' goal orientations and their study strategies in a premed chemistry course, a course that is of great importance to students, since it serves as the gateway to the premed curriculum. Although she focused on goals and not self-theories in this study, she contrasted the two goals that are typically associated with self-theories: performance goals that center on competence validation versus learning goals that center on competence acquisition. Grant found that learning goals predicted knowledge *and* use of all the self-regulatory strategies that predicted success in the course. These included deep-level study strategies and time management, as well as self-regulation of emotion and motivation. Students with strong learning goals took responsibility for keeping up their interest in chemistry, regulating their level of stress, and maintaining their motivation to study. They did not leave things to fixed ability or to chance. Moreover, the use of such strategies mediated the superior performance of those with strong learning goals in the course. In contrast, ability-focused performance goals predicted little knowledge of effective strategies and little use of them. Although these students fervently wished to do well in this course, their focus on ability did not lead them to think in terms of the regulatory strategies that would help them do so.

In summary, a focus on fixed ability leads to attentional strategies, self-esteem regulation strategies, self-handicapping strategies (see Rhodewalt & Vohs, Chapter 29, this volume), and poor knowledge of self-regulated learning strategies (see Zimmerman & Kitsantas, Chapter 27, this volume), all of which can impede the acquisition of competence. A focus on malleable ability on the other hand leads to the self-regulation of attention, of self-esteem, of motivation, and of study strategies in ways that enhance the acquisition of competence.

BEYOND ACADEMIC COMPETENCE: MEANING SYSTEMS ACROSS MULTIPLE SKILLS DOMAINS

Most of the work reviewed thus far has dealt with motivation and competence in students facing challenging academic tasks. Although academic competence is of great interest and importance to many people, the impact of self-theories and their attendant meaning systems is not limited to this domain. In this section, therefore, we present work that shows the generality of our conceptualization and its utility for understanding other skills areas.

Computer Skills

In a study that is close to what we have examined, Martocchio (1994) studied employees who had enrolled in a computer training course. Half of them were given instructions that oriented them toward an entity theory of computer skills (the idea that learning computer skills depends on their existing, underlying ability), whereas the other half were oriented toward an incremental theory of ability (the idea that the more you practice, the more capable you become). As they learned, trainees in the incremental condition reported diminished anxiety and a heightened sense of efficacy, and they displayed superior learning. However, as those in the entity condition learned, their anxiety remained high and their sense of efficacy actually diminished. Since the task remained challenging and mistakes were still made, their confidence eroded.

Sports

Biddle and his colleagues (Biddle, Wang, Chatzisaray, & Spray, 2003; Sarrazin et al., 1996) studied the impact of theories of sports ability on young people's motivation for sports and physical activity. They devised a questionnaire to assess self-theories, containing questions such as "You have a certain level of ability in sport and you cannot really do much to change that level" (entity belief) and "How good you are at sport will *always* improve if you work harder at it" (incremental belief). Biddle and his colleagues found that the incremental theory was associated with feeling successful when learning goals were achieved ("when I improve and master new things") and with greater enjoyment of sports. In contrast, the entity theory was linked to feeling successful when performance goals were achieved ("when I beat out others") and to "amotivation" (the belief that sports is a waste of time).

Following up on this work, Ommundsen (2001, 2003) showed that an incremental theory predicted effective self-regulatory strategies in sports, such as generalizing effective strategies across activities, varying learning strategies when necessary, and being willing to ask for help when necessary. Entity beliefs predicted not taking an analytical stance toward one's learning strategies, not asking for help, and giving up when the activities were difficult. They also predicted increased levels of anxiety and reduced enjoyment of physical activity. In addition, as in the academic domain, the entity beliefs predicted a tendency to use self-handicapping strategies. Thus, in the domain of sports, self-theories have been linked to many of the same variables as in the academic domain: learning versus performance goals, mastery-oriented versus helpless learning strategies, and intrinsic motivation versus amotivation or anxiety.

Organizational Behavior

Wood and his colleagues (Tabernero & Wood, 1999; Wood & Bandura, 1989; Wood, Philips, & Tabernero, 2002) have taken self-theories into the realm of organizational behavior (see also Maurer, Wrenn, Pierce, Tross, & Collins, 2003), examining the acquisition of managerial skills on a complex task. They have tracked this process in people working individually on the task and people working in groups. In all of these studies, self-theories of managerial ability were either measured or experimentally induced. Then, participants worked on a managerial decision-making task in which they had to match employee attributes to the different jobs in the organization and, over trials, learn how best to guide and motivate each employee so as to reach the production quota. To discover the best solutions, they had to continue testing hypotheses and revising their decisions as a function of the feedback.

Wood and Bandura (1989) had participants in their study work individually, and induced their self-theories by telling them either that the required skills reflected their underlying cognitive capacities (entity induction) or that the skills were developed through practice (incremental induction). Although both groups confronted the task with a relatively strong sense of managerial efficacy, the people in the entity group showed a progressive decrease in self-efficacy across trials as they continued to try to meet the challenging production quota. In addition, they set less and less challenging goals across trials, became less and less efficient in their use of analytic strategies, and showed a steady decline in performance. Those in the incremental group, in contrast, were able to maintain their sense of efficacy, became increasingly systematic in use of strategies, and sustained a high level of organizational performance.

In the study by Wood et al. (2002, study 2), people's theories of managerial ability were assessed and work groups were formed, consisting of three incremental theorist or three entity theorists. The groups, which had worked together for some weeks, were given the same managerial decision-making task described earlier. Although the two groups started out with similar attributions, group efficacy, and group goals, they diverged over the course of the task. The entity groups blamed the task, their ability, and their luck—all uncontrollable factors—when they experienced difficulty, whereas the incremental groups remained committed to strategy attributions when they encountered difficulty. The incremental groups also

gained in efficacy over trials compared to the entity groups, and set higher goals for themselves than did the entity groups on the later trials.

The group processes in the two types of groups were found to differ in important ways, with members of the incremental groups being more likely to openly state their opinions and express disagreements. They were also, as a group, more focused on the task and able to use their time more effectively. This greater focus on the task, along with the more challenging group goals and the strategy attributions, mediated the effects of people's entity or incremental theories on group performance. Not only did the incremental groups show superior performance, but this superiority emerged early and became even more pronounced over time. Thus, the entity theorists, concerned about their fixed managerial ability, appear to have fallen prey to a "groupthink" process (Janis, 1972), in which frank discussions are not held and disagreements are not aired, and in which valuable task time is wasted in activities that do not further the goal of reaching the best solution.

In summary, many of the same factors that mediate the effects of self-theories on performance in other settings—goals, attributions, and mastery-oriented versus helpless learning strategies—appear to be at play in organizational decision making as well.

Social Relationships

A number of studies have now examined the role of self-theories in social relationships, both intimate relationships (Knee, 1998; Knee, Nanayakkara, Vietor, Neighbors, & Patrick, 2001; Knee, Patrick, Vietor, & Neighbors, 2004; Ruvolo & Rotondo, 1998) and in peers relationships in children (Erdley, Cain, Loomis, Dumas-Hines, & Dweck, 1997) and adults (Beer, 2002). Here, too, many of the same patterns have been found, with the goals, attributions, affective responses, and coping strategies echoing those found in other areas. We describe the Beer (2002) studies, since they beautifully illustrate the role of self-theories in moderating people's response to threat and speak to the impact of threat of social competence. In her studies, Beer measured people's self-theories of shyness, with items such as "My shyness is something about me that I can't change very much" (entity theory) and "I can change aspects of my shyness if I want to" (incremental theory). She also had people report on their level of shyness by rating the extent to which they exhibited the physiological (e.g., racing pulse), observable (e.g., reduced eye contact), and cognitive–emotional (feelings of anxiety) components of shyness. In three studies, Beer found that holding an incremental versus entity theory of shyness led to many of the same effects we have been seeing in other realms and mitigated the negative effects of shyness on both the shy person's sense of well-being and the interactions in which the person participated.

First, Beer (2002) pitted the opportunity to pursue learning goals (an opportunity to learn some social skills that might help people master their shyness, although they might appear awkward on the videotape) against the opportunity to pursue a performance goal (the chance to be paired with people of lesser social ability, so that the shy person's social skills would be shown to advantage). The results showed that shy incremental theorists were indeed more likely than shy entity theorists to opt for the learning goals. In line with this approach to challenge, shy incrementals also reported more approach tendencies than shy entity theorists (agreeing more that "If the chance comes to meet new people, I often take it") and fewer avoidance tendencies (such as avoiding social situations, avoiding eye contact, or preventing the conversation from focusing on them).

Then participants engaged in an actual dyadic interaction. During this interaction, they rated themselves over three 5-minute time periods and were also rated by observers. In the first 5-minute period, entity and incremental theorists reported similar levels of avoidant strategies and were rated by observers as exhibiting similar, high levels of avoidant behavior. However, clear differences emerged in the second and third periods, with shy entity theorists now reporting and showing significantly higher levels of avoidant behavior than shy incrementals. Moreover, although all shy people were perceived by observers as experiencing shyness and nervousness throughout the entire interaction, observers rated shy incrementals as

having fewer undesirable social consequences of their shyness. Specifically, in the second and third periods, they were rated as more socially skilled, likeable, and more enjoyable to be with than their entity theorist counterparts.

Thus, in this arena as well, people's self-theories are linked to other motivational variables, such as goals (Beer, 2002; Erdley et al., 1997; Knee, 1998), attributions (Erdley et al., 1997), and mastery-oriented versus helpless responses to threat (Beer, 2002; Knee et al., 2004), and lead to more or less favorable outcomes.

SOCIALIZATION OF MEANING SYSTEMS

Where do self-theories come from? How are self-theories and their associated meaning systems socialized? One way is through the praise and criticism children receive (Kamins & Dweck, 1999; Mueller & Dweck, 1998). In a series of studies, we have shown that feedback that focuses on and judges the child's traits (whether in a positive or negative way) fosters an entity theory and the whole entity-oriented meaning system, whereas feedback that focuses on the child's process (e.g., effort or strategy) fosters an incremental theory and its meaning system. A series of six studies by Mueller and Dweck (1998) reveals this process. In these studies, late grade-school-age children worked on a nonverbal IQ test and succeeded on the first trial. They were then praised. One-third of the children were praised for their intelligence ("You must be smart at this"), one-third were praised for their effort ("You must have worked really hard"), and one-third were simply praised for their performance ("That's a really good score"). (This last group typically fell in between the other two, and we do not focus on it.)

The results showed that the intelligence praise indeed fostered an entity theory in children—the idea that their fixed ability was captured by their performance, whereas the effort praise fostered a more dynamic, malleable view of intelligence. Along with the self-theories came different goals. When given a choice between pursuing a learning goal that would challenge and allow them to grow, and a performance goal that would allow them to look smart, children given the intelligence praise chose the performance goal, whereas those given the effort praise overwhelmingly chose the learning goal.

Although the problems in the first set were moderately difficult, children next received a far more difficult set of problems and, consequently, received much lower scores on this trials. What attributions did they make for their poor score? Those who had received intelligence praise now made *lack* of ability attributions. If success meant they were smart, then failure meant they were not. The effort-praised children instead attributed their failure to lack of effort. If effort is the way to success, it is also the way to overcome failure. What happened to children's intrinsic motivation? After the success, all groups thought the task was great fun and interesting, but after the failure, the intelligence-praised group showed a sharp decline in intrinsic motivation, whereas the effort-praised group showed no decline at all.

Finally, all children were given a third set of problems, comparable in difficulty to the first set. How did they do on these? The intelligence-praised children showed a significant decrease in performance from the first trial to the third, and showed the lowest performance of the three groups. The effort-praised children, in contrast, showed a clear increase in performance, and displayed the best performance of any group. In short, praise that judged intelligence and praise that focused on effort evoked not only different theories of intelligence but also the meaning systems that surround these self-theories (e.g., the performance vs. learning goals and the ability vs. effort attributions), as well as their characteristic impact of intrinsic motivation and performance in the face of difficulty.

These studies demonstrated the direct causal effect of different types of praise on children's self-theories and the meaning systems that accompany them. We are also investigating the real-world parallels. For example, we are examining the extent to which parents who tend to judge their children's traits, as opposed to parents who tend to foster their children's learning processes, will have children with entity theories. In a preliminary study (Dweck & Lennon, 2001), we have seen that students who hold an en-

tity theory of intelligence report more trait judgments from their parents than do children who hold an incremental theory, who report relatively more process feedback. In ongoing studies with parents, Eva Pomerantz and the first author are attempting to determine whether parents' beliefs and behaviors do in fact accord with their children's reports.

In a relevant study, Grolnick (2001) examined mothers' controlling behaviors (e.g., giving directives to her child on a task without the child's requesting them, telling the child the answers, or writing for the child instead of letting the child do it) as opposed to their autonomy supportive behaviors (e.g., providing feedback or hints when the child is stuck). The controlling behaviors could be construed as sending the child an ability message, whereas helpful hints could be seen as supporting the child's own learning process. In line with this, in a sample of seventh-grade children and their mothers, Grolnick found a correlation of .44 between mothers' controlling behavior and the children's entity theories. These intriguing findings suggest that there is much fertile ground yet to be plowed with respect to these issues.

Moreover, Smiley, Coulson, and Van Ocker (2000) have shown in a study of 4-year-olds and their parents that parents' theories of intelligence already predict the achievement tasks they prefer for their children, with incremental parents much more strongly than entity parents preferring challenging tasks for their child, even if it means the child might not succeed. Next, incremental parents are already emphasizing effort, in that they think effort is the reason children succeed. In contrast, entity parents are already emphasizing ability, in that they attribute children's success to talent, and they (the mothers) are more interested in knowing from teachers how their children compare to other children. And, finally, fathers' implicit theories are already predicting children's task persistence, with incremental fathers having more persistent children.

Recently, we have lamented the lack of attention to mental representations—to children's beliefs—in the study of social development and socialization (Dweck & London, 2004). Certainly children build up beliefs about themselves and the world as they develop, and certainly these beliefs play a critical role in their behavior and adjustment. Yet social developmental psychologists, with the exception of attachment researchers, have paid scant attention to such beliefs. Given the impact of self-theories, the study of self-theories and their development could be a fruitful place to correct this deficit.

ALTERING MEANING SYSTEMS: SMALL INTERVENTION, BIG CHANGE

One important implication of a meaning system approach is that merely altering people's self-theories should produce widespread effects on their meaning systems, and should lead to changes in learning and achievement. It is often difficult for people to believe that simply changing a belief will have much impact given the many things that affect students' learning. However, if this belief is at the heart of students' motivation, it can have more impact than one would expect. We have already seen how the relatively short intervention by Aronson et al. (2002) that taught an incremental theory succeeded in changing students' valuing of their schoolwork, enjoyment of their schoolwork, and grade point averages. Two other studies, both with junior high school students, have now yielded similarly encouraging findings.

In one, by Blackwell et al. (2003, study 2), seventh graders were given an eight-session workshop. All of the students in the workshop were given lessons on study skills, the danger of negative labels, and a variety of useful skills and ideas. Half of the children were also taught an incremental theory of intelligence and how to apply it to their schoolwork. As in the Aronson et al. (2002) study, students were taught that the brain grows new connections every time they learn and that, in this sense, they are in charge of how smart they become. Students' math grades were monitored over the course of the semester and, at the end of the semester, teacher reports on the students in the workshop were solicited.

First, after this relatively short intervention, students in the incremental intervention earned significantly higher math grades than children in the other workshop. Second, the teachers, who had no idea which group the different children were in, singled

out significantly more of the children in the incremental group as showing positive motivational change. Moreover, what the teachers reported about these students was precisely in line with our meaning system analysis. Teachers pinpointed changes in the valuing of learning and improvement, and in the belief in effort, the very factors that were found to lead to enhanced achievement in the studies described at the outset (e.g., Blackwell et al., 2003, study 1).

In another study with junior high school students, Good et al. (2003) taught students an incremental theory of intelligence as part of a course in computer skills. As part of the course, students were mentored by college students, who delivered the incremental message and helped them design a Web page that conveyed the incremental message. The message was reinforced throughout the year through e-mail correspondence between the mentors and the students. The control group also received a constructive message (an antidrug message) and engaged in similar activities with respect to this message. At the end of the year, the groups were compared on their performance on standardized, statewide reading and math achievement tests. The incremental group showed significantly higher performance than the control group on both tests. Another interesting result emerged. Although the incremental intervention was beneficial to all, it was particularly beneficial to females in math. Although there was a gender gap in math achievement in the control group, this gap virtually disappeared in the incremental group. Once again, the incremental theory seems to have helped students combat stereotypes.

Thus, in three studies, a relatively modest intervention yielded encouraging changes. The Blackwell et al. (2003) study suggests that these changes came about by boosting students valuing of learning and improvement, and their belief in the efficacy of their efforts.

SUMMARY AND CONCLUSIONS

We have seen that self-theories form the core of meaning systems, attracting goals and beliefs (attributions, effort beliefs) that work in concert to produce patterns of behavior and outcomes across important realms: school, work, sports, and relationships. An entity theory creates a meaning system focused on the goal of measuring and validating competence, and is thus associated with ability-oriented performance goals, ability attributions for setbacks, and the belief that effort indicates low ability. These goals and beliefs lead, in turn, to helpless or defensive reactions to difficulty and to lowered self-esteem, intrinsic motivation, and learning in the face of difficulty. An incremental theory, in contrast, creates a meaning system built around the acquisition of competence and is thus linked to learning goals, effort and strategy attributions for setbacks, and the belief that effort increases ability. These goals and beliefs then promote mastery-oriented strategies in the face of challenge, which lead to enhanced self-esteem, intrinsic motivation, and learning. We have also seen that changing people's self-theories can lead to a cascade of changes in their motivation, behavior, and outcomes. Thus, the self-theories provide powerful frames for situations, ones that influence what people try to accomplish in those situations, how they go about it, and how successful they are likely to be.

The fact that self-theories can be induced experimentally and altered through interventions suggests a dynamic view of these theory-based motivational systems. Although, as noted at the outset, self-theories can be relatively stable over long periods of time (e.g., Robins and Pals, 2002), they are knowledge structures and, as such, their accessibility can be changed by powerful situations and interventions. The malleability of the self-theories also suggests that people may be familiar with both theories and can apply either one to a task or domain when faced with potent cues. This dynamic view may provide a window into how personality often operates: People may have relatively stable tendencies based on their more chronic beliefs and goals, but they are attuned to cues from the environment that shape the beliefs and goals they will apply to a given situation (cf. Grant & Dweck, 1999; Dweck & Leggett, 1988; Mischel & Shoda, 1995; see Hong & Chiu, 2001; Chiu & Hong, Chapter 26, this volume, for a discussion of how a similar analysis can be applied to cultural differences and similarities).

This view, as noted earlier, can also link the study of motivation and competence to the literature on coping, since coping styles, it is clear, can grow from self-theories. Indeed, interventions to aid coping would profit from altering the theories from which maladaptive coping may arise rather than simply attempting to alter the strategies directly. For example, rather than trying to discourage the avoidant or defensive coping we have seen in entity theorists and teaching more direct, problem-focused coping, one might, in conjunction with this, encourage a more incremental theory in the relevant domains.

In the same vein, this approach may hold promise of giving insight into emotion and emotion regulation. As we saw, different emotions seem to arise more readily within particular meaning systems (see Lewis & Sullivan, Chapter 11, this volume). For example, anxiety seems to arise more quickly and subside more slowly within the entity-based system, whereas interest and enjoyment seem to be hardier and longer lasting within the incremental system. As we also saw, people appear to be using different self-regulatory strategies to deal with their negative emotions, for example, following blows to their self-esteem. Although the idea of cognitive appraisal processes leading to emotions has received much attention (e.g., Lazarus & Folkman, 1984), less attention has been paid to the meaning systems that may facilitate these emotions and that may, in addition, affect their regulation (but see Park & Folkman, 1997). This would be a fascinating line of future research, and one that would strengthen the much-needed link between the study of emotion and the study of motivation.

In conclusion, the study of self-theories has shed light on the ways in which people strive for competence and the degree to which they attain it across a variety of domains. The study of self-theories also holds promise for linking the study of motivation and competence to other key areas of psychology.

ACKNOWLEDGMENTS

Preparation of this chapter was supported in part by grants from the National Science Foundation (Grant No. BCS-02-17251), the Department of

Education (Grant No. R305-H-02-0031), and the William T. Grant Foundation (Grant No. 2379) to Carol S. Dweck.

NOTES

1. An elegant set of new studies by Cury, Elliot, Da Fonseca, and Moller (2004) lends support to our analysis. In their first study, Cury et al. showed that theories of intelligence predicted adolescents' math grades, and that this was mediated through students' achievement goals. In their second study, they showed that manipulating adolescents' theories of intelligence affected their IQ scores, through their achievement goals and mastery-oriented strategies.

2. Robins and Pals (2002) also measured affective responses to failure (which were not assessed in the previous studies), and found that, even equating for grades, incremental theorists more often felt determined and enthusiastic, whereas entity theorists more often felt distressed or ashamed.

3. Trzesniewski and Robins (2003) also measured self-esteem. They found that the same meaning system that predicted change in math grades predicted change in self-esteem, and that the change in self-esteem mediated the change in grades.

REFERENCES

Abramson, L. Y., Seligman, M. E., & Teasdale, J. D. (1978). Learned helplessness in humans: Critique and reformulation. *Journal of Abnormal Psychology*, 87, 49–74.

Aronson, J. (1998). *The effects of conceiving ability as fixed or improvable on responses to stereotype threat*. Unpublished manuscript, University of Texas, Austin.

Aronson, J., Fried, C., & Good, C. (2002). Reducing the effects of stereotype threat on African American college students by shaping theories of intelligence. *Journal of Experimental Social Psychology, 38*, 113–125.

Beer, J. S. (2002). Implicit self-theories of shyness. *Journal of Personality and Social Psychology, 83*, 1009–1024.

Biddle, S., Wang, J., Chatzisaray, N., & Spray, C. M. (2003). Motivation for physical activity in young people: Entity and incremental beliefs about athletic ability. *Journal of Sports Sciences, 21*, 973–989.

Binet, A. (1973). *Les idees modernes sur les enfants* [Modern ideas on children]. Paris: Flamarion. (Original work published in 1909)

Blackwell, L. S., Dweck, C. S., & Trzesniewski, K. (2003). *Implicit theories of intelligence predict achievement across an adolescent transition: A longi-*

tudinal study and an intervention. Unpublished manuscript, Columbia University, New York.

Brown, A. L. (1997). Transforming schools in to communities of thinking and learning about serious matters. *American Psychologist, 52*, 399–413.

Butler, R. (2000). Making judgments about ability: The role of implicit theories of ability in moderating inferences from temporal and social comparison information. *Journal of Personality and Social Psychology, 78*, 965–978.

Collins, M. (1992). *Ordinary children, extraordinary teachers*. Charlottesville, VA: Hampton Roads.

Cury, F., Elliot, A. J., Da Fonseca, D., & Moller, A. C. (2004). *The social-cognitive model of achievement motivation and the 2 × 2 achievement goal framework*. Manuscript submitted for publication.

Dweck, C. S. (1999). *Self-theories: Their role in motivation, personality, and development*. Philadelphia: Psychology Press.

Dweck, C. S., Chiu, C., & Hong, Y. (1995). Implicit theories and their role in judgments and reactions: A world from two perspectives. *Psychological Inquiry, 6*, 267–285.

Dweck, C. S., & Leggett, E. L. (1988). A social-cognitive approach to motivation and personality. *Psychological Review, 95*, 256–273.

Dweck, C. S., & Lennon, C. (2001, April). *Person vs. process-focused parenting styles*. Symposium paper presented at the Meeting of the Society for Research in Child Development, Minneapolis, MN.

Dweck, C. S., & London, B. E. (2004). The role of mental representation in social development. *Merrill–Palmer Quarterly* (50th Anniversary Issue), 50, 428–444.

Dweck, C. S., Mangels, J., & Good, C. (2004). Motivational effects on attention, cognition, and performance. In D. Y. Dai & R. J. Sternberg (Eds.), *Motivation, emotion, and cognition: Integrated perspectives on intellectual functioning* (pp. 41–56). Mahwah, NJ: Erlbaum.

Dweck, C. S., & Molden, D. C. (2004). *Meaning systems in psychology*. Manuscript submitted for publication.

Dweck, C. S., & Reppucci, N. D. (1973). Learned helplessness and reinforcement responsibility in children. *Journal of Personality and Social Psychology, 25*, 109–116.

Erdley, C., Cain, K., Loomis, C., Dumas-Hines, F., & Dweck, C. S. (1997). The relations among children's social goals, implicit personality theories and response to social failure. *Developmental Psychology, 33*, 263–272.

Esquith, R. (2003). *There are no shortcuts*. New York: Pantheon.

Gollwitzer, P. M., & Wicklund, R. A. (1985). The pursuit of self-defining goals. In J. Kuhl & J. Beckmann (Eds.), *Action control: From cognition to behavior* (pp. 61–85). Heidelberg: Springer-Verlag.

Good, C., Aronson, J., & Inzlicht, M. (2003). Improving adolescents' standardized test performance:

An intervention to reduce the effects of stereotype threat. *Journal of Applied Developmental Psychology, 24*, 645–662.

Good, C., & Dweck, C. S. (2004). *An incremental theory decreases vulnerability to stereotypes about math ability in college females.* Unpublished data, Columbia University, New York.

Grant, H. (2004). *Goal orientations influence both knowledge and use of self-regulated learning strategies.* Unpublished data, New York University, New York.

Grant, H., & Dweck, C. S. (1999). A goal analysis of personality and personality coherence. In D. Cervone & Y. Shoda (Eds.), *The coherence of personality: Social-cognitive bases of consistency, variability, and organization coherence* (pp. 345–371). New York: Guilford Press.

Grant, H., & Dweck, C. S. (2003). Clarifying achievement goals and their impact. *Journal of Personality and Social Psychology, 85*, 541–553.

Grolnick, W. (2001, April). *Discussant's comments: Symposium on Influences on Children's Motivation: New concepts and new findings.* Presented at the Meeting of the Society for Research in Child Development, Minneapolis, MN.

Hong, Y. Y., & Chiu, C. Y. (2001). Toward a paradigm shift: From cross-cultural differences in social-cognition to social-cognitive mediation of cultural differences. *Social Cognition, 19*, 181–196.

Hong, Y. Y., Chiu, C., Dweck, C. S., Lin, D., & Wan, W. (1999). Implicit theories, attributions, and coping: A meaning system approach. *Journal of Personality and Social Psychology, 77*, 588–599.

Janis, I. L. (1972). *Groupthink: A psychological study of foreign-policy decisions and fiascoes.* Boston: Houghton Mifflin.

Jourden, F. J., Bandura, A., & Banfield, J. T. (1991). The impact of conceptions of ability on self-regulatory factors and motor skill acquisition. *Journal of Sport and Exercise Psychology, 13*, 213–226.

Kamins, M., & Dweck, C. S. (1999). Person vs. process praise and criticism: Implications for contingent self-worth and coping. *Developmental Psychology, 35*, 835–847.

Knee, C. R. (1998). Implicit theories of relationships: Assessment and prediction of romantic relationship initiation, coping, and longevity. *Journal of Personality and Social Psychology, 74*, 360–370.

Knee, C. R., Nanayakkara, A., Vietor, N. A., Neighbors, C., & Patrick, H. (2001). Implicit theories of relationships: Who cares if romantic partners are less than ideal? *Personality and Social Psychology Bulletin, 27*, 808–819.

Knee, C. R., Patrick, H., Vietor, N. A., & Neighbors, C. (2004). Implicit theories of relationships: Moderators of the link between conflict and commitment. *Personality and Social Psychology Bulletin, 30*, 617–628.

Lazarus, R., & Folkman, S. (1984). *Stress, appraisal, and coping.* New York: Springer-Verlag.

Levin, H. M. (1987). New schools for the disadvantaged. *Teacher Education Quarterly, 14*, 60–83.

Martocchio, J. J. (1994). Effects of conceptions of ability on anxiety, self-efficacy, and learning in training. *Journal of Applied Psychology, 79*, 819–825.

Mathews, J. (1988). *Escalante: The best teacher in America.* New York: Holt.

Maurer, T. J., Wrenn, K. A., Pierce, H. R., Tross, S. A., & Collins, W. C. (2003). Beliefs about improvability of career-relevant skills: Relevance to job/task analysis, competency modeling, and learning orientaion. *Journal of Organizational Behavior, 24*, 107–131.

Mischel, W., & Shoda, Y. (1995). A cognitive-affective systems theory of personality: Reconceptualizing the invariances in personality and the role of situations. *Psychological Review, 102*, 246–268.

Molden, D., & Dweck, C. S. (2000). Meaning and motivation. In C. Sansone & J. Harackiewicz (Eds.), *Intrinsic motivation.* San Diego: Academic Press.

Mueller, C. M., & Dweck, C. S. (1998). Intelligence praise can undermine motivation and performance. *Journal of Personality and Social Psychology, 75*, 33–52.

Nickerson, R. S., Perkins, D. N., & Smith, E. E. (1985). *Teaching thinking.* Hillsdale, NJ: Erlbaum.

Niiya, Y., Crocker, J., & Bartmess, E. N. (2004). From vulnerability to resilience: Learning orientations buffer contingent self-esteem from failure. *Psychological Science, 15*, 801–805.

Nussbaum, D., & Dweck, C. S. (2004). [*Self-theories and modes of self-esteem maintenance.*] Unpublished raw data, Columbia University, New York.

Ommundsen, Y. (2001). Pupils' affective responses in physical education classes: The association of implicit theories of the nature of ability and achievement goals. *European Physical Education Review, 7*, 219–242.

Ommundsen, Y. (2003). Implicit theories of ability and self-regulation strategies in physical education classes. *Educational Psychology, 23*, 141–157.

Park, C. L., & Folkman, S. (1997). Meaning in the context of stress and coping. *Review of General Psychology, 1*, 115–144.

Rheinberg, F. (1980). *Leistungsbewertung und Lernmotivation* [Achievement evaluation and motivation to learn]. Göttingen, Germany: Hogrefe.

Rhodewalt, F. (1994). Conceptions of ability, achievement goals, and individual differences in self-handicapping behavior: On the application of implicit theories. *Journal of Personality, 62*, 67–85.

Robins, R. W., & Pals, J. L. (2002). Implicit self-theories in the academic domain: Implications for goal orientation, attributions, affect, and self-esteem change. *Self and Identity, 1*, 313–336.

Ruvolo, A. P., & Rotondo, J. L. (1998). Diamonds in the rough: Implicit personality theories and views of partner and self. *Personality and Social Psychology Bulletin, 24*, 750–758.

Sarrazin, P., Biddle, S., Famose, J. P., Cury, F., Fox, K.,

& Durand, M. (1966). Goal orientation and conceptions of the nature of sport ability in children: A social cognitive approach. *British Journal of Social Psychology, 35,* 399–414.

Smiley, P. A., Coulson, S. L., & Van Ocker, J. C. (2000, April). *Beliefs about learning in mothers and fathers of preschoolers.* Paper presented at the meeting of the American Educational Research Association, New Orleans, LA.

Steele, C. M., & Aronson, J. (1995). Stereotype threat and the intellectual test performance of African-Americans. *Journal of Personality and Social Psychology, 68,* 797–811.

Sternberg, R. J. (1985). *Beyond IQ.* New York: Cambridge University Press.

Tabernero, C., & Wood, R. E. (1999). Implicit theories versus the social construal of ability in self-regulation and performance on a complex task. *Organizational Behavior and Human Decision Processes, 78*(2), 104–127.

Tesser, A. (2000). On the confluence of self-esteem maintenance mechanisms. *Personality and Social Psychology Review, 4,* 290–299.

Trzesniewski, K., & Robins, R. (2003, April). *Integrating self-esteem into a process model of academic achievement.* Symposium paper presented at the Biennial Meeting of the Society for Research in Child Development, Tampa, FL.

Weiner, B. (1986). *An attributional theory of motivation and emotion.* New York: Springer-Verlag.

Weiner, B., & Kukla, A. (1970). An attributional analysis of achievement motivation. *Journal of Personality and Social Psychology, 15,* 1–20.

Wood, R., & Bandura, A. (1989). Impact of conceptions of ability on self-regulatory mechanisms and complex decision making. *Journal of Personality and Social Psychology, 56,* 407–415.

Wood, R. E., Phillips, K. W., & Tabernero, C. (2002). *Implicit theories of ability, processing dynamics and performance in decision-making groups.* Unpublished manuscript, University of New South Wales, Sydney, Australia.

CHAPTER 9

☙

Evaluation Anxiety

Current Theory and Research

MOSHE ZEIDNER
GERALD MATTHEWS

The second part of the 20th century has been variously designated as the "age of stress," or "age of anxiety." While stress and anxiety are universal human experiences, intrinsic to the human condition, the nature of the specific environmental stimuli evoking stress and anxiety emotions has changed remarkably over the years. Whereas in ancient times it may have been natural catastrophes, wild beasts, hostilities among rival tribes or clans, and the like, that served as major sources of apprehension and anxiety, in our modern technological and achievement-oriented society, stress and anxiety are frequently evoked by evaluative environmental situations and events. The various forms of evaluation anxiety (e.g., test anxiety, math anxiety, sports anxiety, social anxiety) share the prospect of personal evaluation in real or imagined social situations, particularly when a person perceives a low likelihood of obtaining satisfactory evaluations from others (Leitenberg, 1990). All types are quite common, with prevalence estimates in adults ranging from 20–50% for math and computer anxiety (e.g., Bozionelos, 2001) to 60% or more for social anxiety (Crozier & Alden, 2001). Evaluation anxiety has frequently been linked to performance decrements in real-world situations such as test taking.

We demonstrate in this chapter that although the different forms are distinguished by the antecedent conditions and contexts evoking the anxiety (e.g., tests, computers, athletic contests, social situations), they have important structural similarities, and are governed by similar cognitive and motivational processes. Transactional and interactional models of stress and anxiety (Endler & Parker, 1992; Lazarus, 1999) view anxiety as being cognitively mediated, emphasizing the role of cognitive appraisals and coping processes in mediating the effects of evaluation stress on anxiety reactions. Such models also assume that situation-specific forms of anxiety and their behavioral concomitants are determined by the reciprocal interaction of personal traits and the characteristics of situations. State anxiety will be experienced in an evaluation situation when there is a congruency or fit between the nature of a person's vulnerability (i.e., high evaluative trait anxiety) and the nature of the situation (evaluation/ego-threatening). The *differential hypothesis* of the interactional model (cf. Endler & Parker, 1992) claims that individuals high on evaluation anxiety will show a higher increase in state anxiety than subjects low on evaluation anxiety, primarily in a social evaluation situation (as opposed to, say, a physical threat). Thus, theory must capture how stable individual differences in cognitive structures moderate the processing of situational demands, threats, and affordances to generate variability in emotional and behavioral response.

We note briefly that experience of evaluative anxiety is also near-universal across people differing in age, gender, and culture. A meta-analysis of test anxiety data from 14 national sites (Seipp & Schwarzer, 1996) showed that although mean test anxiety levels varied somewhat across cultures, test anxiety was a prevalent and relatively homogenous cross-cultural phenomenon. Women tend to report higher levels of test, math, and computer anxiety than men, but the gender difference often does not translate into objective performance differences (Cassady & Johnson, 2002; Zeidner, 1998). Gender differences are attributable to differential exposure and learning experiences (Rosen & Maguire, 1990). Appraisal processes may also be important: Males may be more likely than females to be socialized to perceive a test situation as a personal challenge rather than as a threat (Cassady & Johnson, 2002).

We begin this chapter with an introductory overview of some different forms of evaluation anxiety: test anxiety, math and computer anxiety, social anxiety, and sports anxiety. Next, we describe some features of anxiety that appear to generalize across the different forms, including the state–trait distinction and different facets of the anxiety response. In the section that follows, we review empirical studies of evaluative anxiety and performance. Finally, we examine more theoretically driven studies that seek to uncover cognitive and motivational bases for performance impairment. These studies include both those that follow the traditional cognitive-psychological approach of discriminating "stages" of processing that are especially sensitive to anxiety, as well as studies that adopt a self-regulative perspective, aiming to link processing impairments to the person's strategies and goals for managing evaluative threats.

BASIC ISSUES AND CONCEPTUALIZATIONS OF EVALUATION ANXIETY

Test Anxiety

The term "test anxiety" refers to the set of phenomenological, physiological, and behavioral responses that accompany concern about possible negative consequences or poor performance on an exam or similar evaluative situation (Zeidner, 1998). Test anxious behavior is typically evoked when a person believes that his or her intellectual, motivational, and social capabilities are taxed or exceeded by demands stemming from the test situation. Test anxiety figures prominently in the literature as one of the key villains in the ongoing drama surrounding psychoeducational testing (Zeidner, 1990). Thus, test anxiety is frequently cited among the factors at play in determining a wide array of unfavorable outcomes and contingencies, including poor cognitive performance, scholastic underachievement, and psychological distress and ill health (Hembree, 1988; Zeidner, 1990). Indeed, many students are competent enough to do well on exams but perform poorly because of their debilitating levels of anxiety. Consequently, test anxiety may limit educational or vocational development, as test scores and grades influence entrance to many educational training programs in modern society.

Test anxiety has taken on a variety of different meanings throughout its relatively brief history as a scientific construct (Zeidner, 1998). In the early days of research, the construct was defined in *motivational* terms, either as drive level, goal interruption, or need to avoid failure. Subsequently, it was conceptualized as a relatively stable *personality disposition* linked to *cognitive–attentional* phenomena. Accordingly, the highly anxious person is one who attends excessively to evaluative cues concerning personal competence, and to feelings of physiological arousal. Test anxiety may also be a concomitant of *self-handicapping* employed to preserve one's self-merit in the face of potential failure. Cybernetic *self-regulative models* have seen test anxiety as resulting from a conflict between competing reference values.

Recent theorizing (Zeidner, 1998) emphasizes the distinction between test anxiety as an attribute of the person, and as a dynamic process. From the first perspective, dispositional test anxiety may be construed as a *contextualized personality trait*.[1] Accordingly, test anxiety refers to the individual's disposition to react with extensive worry, intrusive thoughts, mental disorganization, tension, and physiological arousal when exposed to evaluative contexts or situations (Spielberger, Anton, & Bedell, 1976). The more transient state expressions of anxiety may be assessed separately from the more stable trait. From the second, process-oriented perspective, test anxiety depends on the reciprocal interaction of a number of distinct elements at play in the ongoing stressful encounter between a person and an evaluative situation (Zeidner, 1998). These elements include the evaluative context, individual differences in vulnerability (trait anxiety), threat perceptions, appraisals and reappraisals, state anxiety, coping patterns, and adaptive outcomes. Events that elicit test anxiety consist of a number of distinct temporal phases, including preparation, confrontation, anticipation, and resolution (Carver & Scheier, 1989; Zeidner, 1998). Accordingly, threat appraisals, state anxiety levels, and levels of task performance may change at different stages.

Math and Computer Anxiety

Both math and computer anxieties are conceptually related to test anxiety through a common theme of concerns about evaluation (e.g., Rosen & Maguire, 1990). *Math anxiety* is defined by feelings of tension, helplessness, mental disorganization, and associated bodily symptoms that are evoked in mathematical problem-solving situations (Ashcraft, 2002; Richardson & Woolfolk, 1980). Math anxiety is claimed to interfere with the manipulation of numbers and the solving of complex mathematical problems in a wide variety of ordinary life and aca-

demic situations. Statistics anxiety, referring to the feeling of anxiety encountered when taking a statistics course or doing statistical analysis, has frequently been construed as a subset of math anxiety (cf. Zeidner, 1991). Math anxiety, coupled with objective cognitive difficulties experienced in learning math, may lead people to reject goals for which studying math is instrumental, such as scientific career choices.

Computer anxiety (sometimes termed "computerphobia," "technophobia," or "cyberphobia") may be decomposed into (1) anxiety about present or future interactions with computers or computer-related technologies; (2) specific negative cognitions or self-critical internal dialogues when interacting with the computer, or when contemplating future computer interaction; and (3) negative global attitudes about computers, their operation, or their societal impact (Weil, Rosen, & Wugalter, 1990). Effects of computer anxiety on utilization of computer-based technology may incur serious economic costs estimated at the level of billions of dollars per year (Bozionelos, 2001).

Math and computer anxiety may relate not only to the obvious stimulus attributes of math/numbers and computers but also to deeper personal concerns. Math anxiety focuses not only on the evaluative nature of math tests but also concerns mathematical content, its distinctive features as an intellectual activity, and its meanings for many persons in our society (Richardson & Woolfolk, 1980). Similarly, computer anxiety is evoked by the consideration of the broader implications of computer use for perception of the self, society, and culture (Worthington & Zhao, 1999). Computer-anxious persons may also suffer from a more generalized "technophobia," which itself is evident before adulthood (Weil et al., 1990).

Social Anxiety

Social anxiety refers to feelings of apprehension, self-consciousness, and emotional distress that are triggered in anticipated or social situations (Crozier & Alden, 2001). Social anxiety may occur in response to immediate, "real" social encounters in which the individual is presently engaged (e.g., meeting new people, performing before an audience, making a date) or to "imagined" encounters in which the individual contemplates an upcoming social interaction. Moderate social anxiety may have an adaptive function in that a realistic and proportionate concern about others' opinions and evaluations can inhibit behavior that is socially unacceptable. However, high levels of anxiety are liable to interfere with social competence and may be a concomitant of clinical conditions such as social phobia.

There is uncertainty over the centrality of evaluative concerns to social anxiety. Some authors (e.g., Leitenberg, 1990) explicitly define social anxiety in social–evaluative terms. From this perspective, the essence of social anxiety is that the person is motivated to make a favorable impression on others but fears that he or she will be found to be deficient or inadequate by others and will therefore be rejected (Leary, 2001). Socially anxious persons are typically self-devaluing of themselves and worry often quite unrealistically about appearing physically unattractive, foolish, or boring. By contrast, Crozier and Alden (2001) indicate that some forms of social anxiety, such as fear of strangers, are not evaluative in nature. Psychometric studies have found distinct traits related to anxieties concerning evaluation, separation from significant others, and self-disclosure (Endler et al., 2002). In this chapter, we focus on those aspects of social anxiety that relate to concerns about personal social competence, although the role of evaluative concerns in research studies is not always clear.

The literature differentiates various affective constructs that are closely related to social anxiety, including speech anxiety, audience anxiety, stage fright, dating anxiety, shyness, shame, communication apprehension, social embarrassment, and so on (e.g., Bippus & Daly, 1999). Although these constructs are conceptually distinct from one another, social anxiety is seen as a central element of each one: For example, Bruch (2001, p. 197) defines "dispositional shyness" as "anxious preoccupation and behavioral inhibition in various contexts due to the prospect of interpersonal evaluation." Schlenker and Leary (1982) differentiated between "interaction anxiety" and "audience anxiety" as two broad classes of social anxiety. On the one hand, shyness and dating anxiety occur in *contingent interactions*,

in which people must be continually responsive to the actions of others. On the other hand, stage fright and speech anxiety occur in *noncontingent interactions*, in which people are performing some preplanned material before others. *Shyness* and *embarrassment* may relate to separate types of social interaction anxiety (Schlenker & Leary, 1982). Accordingly, shyness characterizes a person who desires to make a favorable impression on others but expects to fall short in impressing others. Embarrassment, by contrast, is said to occur when something actually happens that repudiates the intended impression management.

A number of alternative theoretical perspectives on social anxiety have been proposed over the years (see Crozier & Alden, 2001; Schlenker & Leary, 1982). The *individual differences perspective* sees social anxiety as a personality trait emerging from the interaction between biological and environmental factors, whereas the *learning perspective* attributes anxiety to the pairing of neutral stimuli (public presentation, asking a person out for a date, oral exam, etc.) with aversive social consequences (e.g., rejection, ridicule, criticism). The *self-presentational* perspective maintains that people are typically motivated to make a positive impression on a relevant audience. Socially anxious individuals perceive a discrepancy between their relatively high social standards and their actual levels of social performances or expected outcomes. An alternative, but complementary perspective, the *skills deficit* perspective, assumes that anxiety experienced in social situations is due to an inadequate or inappropriate repertoire of social skills. The *cognitive self-evaluation model* views social anxiety as resulting from the individual's often unrealistic perception of personal inadequacies, such as social incompetence. Finally, the *self-handicapping* perspective claims that people strategically use their anxiety as a handicap in order to reduce people's expectations of them and provide an explanation for failure, which will protect them from negative self-evaluation.

Sports Anxiety

The sports environment has a number of advantages for the scientific study of the antecedents, phenomenology, and consequences of evaluative anxiety within a meaningful real-life context. Various sources of threat reside in the competitive sports situation, including the possibility of both short-term and permanent physical injury, but perhaps the most salient sources of perceived threat are psychological in nature (see Woodman & Hardy, 2001, for a review). These include the possibility of failure and of disapproval by significant others who are evaluating the athlete's performance in relation to some standard of excellence, including coaches, teammates, other competitors, and spectators. As with other forms of evaluative anxiety, sports anxiety reflects the interaction of personal vulnerability and the potentially stressful evaluative situation. High levels of anxiety in a particular sports context may affect a variety of important outcomes, including the athlete's level of performance, degree of enjoyment of and satisfaction with the competitive situation, interactions with opponents, teammates, coaches, officials, and injury proneness, as well as monetary gain.

The Uniformity Myth

One of the most difficult problems for the field is gauging the degree of similarity between the different anxieties. A minimalist approach would focus on the positive correlations between scales for the different forms of anxiety, and on their substantial correlations with broad personality traits such as anxiety or neuroticism. The bulk of studies have not been overly concerned with the issue of discriminant validity of the evaluative anxiety traits as predictors of performance outcomes with general personality traits controlled. Possibly, neuroticism, trait anxiety or negative affectivity provide a common element to the specialized anxiety traits (cf. Matthews, Deary, & Whiteman, 2003). However, test anxiety scales tend to be more predictive of reduced performance than general anxiety scales (Gaudry & Spielberger, 1971), and a few studies (e.g., Ferrando, Varea, & Lorenzo, 1999) have shown discriminant validity for test anxiety measures with related general personality traits controlled. Although scales for math, computer, and test anxiety, for example, are positively correlated, the correlations are too low for the constructs to be considered interchange-

able (e.g., Dew, Galassi, & Galassi, 1984). Similarly, test and social anxiety correlate at about .30 (Mueller & Thompson, 1984).

A general difficulty is that current research is only as good as the particular tests and operationalizations that have been used. There is a lack of multivariate research establishing the latent generic and context-specific traits to which the various anxiety scales may relate. However, research so far suggests that each anxiety trait may be a rather heterogeneous category. In the domain of test anxiety research, Zeidner (1998) has sketched some distinct yet potentially overlapping categories of subjects with test anxiety, which we present informally for illustrative purposes.

1. *Examinees with deficient study and test-taking skills.* One type of test-anxious student is characterized by a major deficiency in study and test-taking skills (Naveh-Benjamin, 1991). Their poor exam performance results from deficits that include problems in acquisition (encoding), organization–rehearsal (study skills), and retrieval–application during a test.

2. *Examinees experiencing anxiety blockage and retrieval problems.* A second type of test-anxious student includes those who have efficient study skills but suffer from anxiety blockage and, consequently, have problems retrieving information during the exam (Covington, 1992). These anxious students study effectively but cannot handle the stresses and pressures of evaluative situations.

3. *Failure-accepting examinees.* These students are characterized by a personal history of repeated test failures. They come to accept low ability as the primary explanation of their failures. As a consequence, they become accepting of failure, exhibiting apathy, resignation and a sense of defeat, not unlike those reactions traditionally associated with learned helplessness.

4. *Failure-avoiding examinees.* Failure-avoiding students are those driven to achieve primarily as a means of protecting themselves against beliefs that they lack ability. For these students, effort is truly a "double-edged sword" (Covington, 1992). They may strive for success through meticulous preparation, yet failure despite high efforts increases the probability that their ability will

be considered low, thus inducing anxiety reactions.

5. *Self-handicappers.* Self-handicapping students avoid diagnostic information about intellectual tasks by reducing effort or avoiding the test situation. Accordingly, if a low score is obtained, the student can rely on the debilitating effects of anxiety as an excuse to escape responsibility for actions, thus reducing otherwise burdensome expectations others hold for that person.

6. *Perfectionistic overstrivers.* Overstriving high-test-anxious perfectionists are characterized by high personal standards of academic success, perception of high or even exaggerated expectations, perceived doubt regarding quality of academic performance, and a need for order and organization in their academic work (Covington, 1992). No effort is ever sufficient as the perfectionistic examinee seeks approval and acceptance, and tries to avoid errors and failure through an endless cycle of self-defeating overstriving.

Thus, discussions of evaluative anxiety in the literature are commonly guilty of a "uniformity myth," conveying the impression that evaluative anxiety is a rather homogeneous category. In fact, as Zeidner's tentative typology of test-anxious students demonstrates, test anxiety has a variety of sources and, similarly, its behavioral consequences vary with contextual and personal factors. Other forms of evaluative anxiety may be similarly multifaceted. For example, the socially anxious person may respond either with behavioral withdrawal, or alternatively, affiliative behaviors such as seeking reassurance from others: Affect and behavior are only loosely coupled (Leary, 2001). Theoretical accounts must identify common elements, while leaving room for these individual differences.

CRITICAL FACETS AND COMPONENTS OF EVALUATION ANXIETY

The anxiety construct was dramatically advanced by a number of important conceptual distinctions. First, the interactionist perspective distinguishes anxiety as a personality *trait* from anxiety as a transient *state*, influenced by the situation, as well as by dispositional characteristics (Spielberger et al., 1976). Second, Liebert and Morris (1967) advanced the critical differentiation between a cognitive (worry) and an affective (emotionality) component. This distinction proved to be instrumental in shifting evaluative anxiety theory and research toward a more cognitive orientation. Current anxiety research often finds it useful to further distinguish a *behavioral facet* (deficient study skills, procrastination, avoidance behaviors, etc.), from *cognitive* (worry, irrelevant thinking, etc.), and *affective–physiological* facets (tension, bodily reaction, perceived arousal) of evaluative anxiety. In this section, we discuss the applicability of these distinctions across the different forms of evaluative anxiety.

Trait versus State Anxiety

Test anxiety is conceptualized as a contextualized form of trait anxiety that interacts with situational evaluative threat to provoke state anxiety (Spielberger et al., 1976; Zohar & Brandt, 2002). Similarly, trait math anxiety reflects relatively stable individual differences in the tendency to perceive situations involving the manipulation of numbers, and the use of mathematical concepts and data as threatening or harmful. Persons high in trait math anxiety respond to these situations with elevations in state anxiety, involving both heightened emotion and interfering worry responses (Anton & Klisch, 1995). Likewise, state computer anxiety is aroused by specific objects (personal computer) or situations (computer error), and individuals high in trait computer anxiety are especially vulnerable to state anxiety responses (Gaudron & Vignoli, 2002). "Trait sports anxiety" is defined as a relatively stable disposition to view sports competition situations as threatening and to respond with elevated cognitive and/or somatic state anxiety in actual competition (Hanton, Mellalieu, & Hall, 2002). Crozier and Alden (2001) identify unfamiliar social situations, power and status differences, and large numbers of people as situational factors that elicit state anxiety in those individuals high in trait social anxiety—although some forms of social anxiety may be nonevaluative in nature.

Facets of Anxiety:
Cognition, Emotion, and Behavior

Liebert and Morris (1967) viewed "worry" primarily as cognitive concern about the consequences of failure, whereas "emotionality" was defined as consisting of perceptions of autonomic reactions evoked by evaluative stress. At the state level, worry refers to intrusive, self-evaluative cognitions, whereas emotion is experienced as nervousness and tension, along with bodily disturbances such as racing heart and gastric discomfort. Liebert and Morris demonstrated that the two components are empirically distinct, though correlated, and that worry relates more strongly to performance decrements than does emotionality. On the basis of extensive research evidence, Irwin Sarason and his coworkers (e.g., Sarason, Sarason, & Pierce, 1990, 1995) demonstrated that, in evaluative situations, high test-anxious examinees are indeed more self-centered and self-critical than those who are low in test anxiety, and are also more likely to emit personalized, derogatory responses during testing that interfere with their task performance. The distinction between affective and cognitive components of the anxiety state has also been applied to computer anxiety (McInerney, Marsh, & McInerney, 1999), social anxiety (Sarason et al., 1990) and sports anxiety (Dunn, Dunn, Wilson, & Syrotuik, 2000). Emotion and cognitive facets are sometimes further subdivided. Sarason et al. (1995) describe two "emotion" factors for trait test anxiety—tension and bodily symptoms, along with two cognitive factors—worry and test-irrelevant thinking. McInerney et al. (1999) found four similar factors for computer anxiety, based on factor and content analyses of interview data.

Avoidance of the feared situation or stimulus is a common theme across the various types of evaluative anxiety, together with loss of motivation to perform (e.g., Hancock, 2001). Elliot (e.g., 1999) distinguishes approach and avoidance motivations in performance settings. His research shows that state test anxiety appears to relate to performance-avoidance goals (i.e., avoidance of incompetence with reference to some norm) but not to approach-related goals. However, behavioral expressions of avoidance show some specificity to different sources of anxiety. For example, the test-anxious student may specifically avoid study or learning situations. By contrast, in social anxiety, the instrumental (or action) component refers to awkwardness, reticence, inhibition of gestures and speech, and the disorganization or absence of social behavior.

Sports anxiety has both cognitive and affective components, which may interact in affecting performance (Dunn et al., 2000; Woodman & Hardy, 2001). Cognitive expressions of anxiety in sports situations include attentional deficits, such as distraction, negative self-statements, and mental disorganization. The physiological manifestations of anxiety, such as autonomic nervous system arousal designed to prepare the body for fight or flight, are not very conducive to maximal athletic performance—except for those tasks that require a burst of adrenalized energy (e.g., weightlifting and sprinting). Much recent work distinguishes between cognitive anxiety, somatic anxiety, and confidence as key aspects of state, measured by the Competitive State Anxiety Inventory–2 (CSAI-2; Martens et al., 1990), with high cognitive anxiety and low confidence predicted to be the strongest predictors of performance impairment.

ANXIETY AND COMPETENCE

In this section, we review studies of evaluative anxiety and competence from an empirical standpoint, focusing on the moderator factors that influence the direction and magnitude of the associations. Although anxiety is predominantly harmful to task performance, it may sometimes have a positive effect: Alpert and Haber (1960) differentiated between *facilitating* and *debilitating* anxiety. One of the factors that may especially tip the scales toward debilitating effects is the presence of worry, because of its tendency to produce distracting cognitive interference. The nature of the task may also play an important moderating role. Generally, evaluative anxiety is more detrimental to attentionally demanding tasks, and may even facilitate performance on easy tasks (Zeidner, 1998). There may also be more subtle effects related to the qualitative nature of the task.

Test Anxiety

Hundreds of studies have investigated the complex pattern of relations between anxiety and different kinds of performance (see Zeidner, 1998, for a full review). Test anxiety has been found to interfere with cognitive performance both in laboratory settings and in true-to-life testing situations in school or collegiate settings (e.g., Zeidner, Klingman, & Papko, 1988; Zeidner & Nevo, 1992). Processing deficits that relate to test anxiety including general impairments of attention and working memory, together with more subtle performance changes, such as failure to organize semantic information effectively. The performance-avoidance goals associated with test anxiety have also been linked to loss of intrinsic motivation (Elliot, 1999).

Studies also identify moderator variables that accentuate or reduce deficits in performance. For example, negative feedback appears to be especially detrimental to test-anxious subjects, whereas providing reassurance and social support may eliminate the deficit. However, there have been sufficient instances of nonconfirmation of predicted deficits to suggest that high anxiety does not automatically generate lower achievement outcomes.

A meta-analytic study (Hembree, 1988), based on 562 North American studies, demonstrated that test anxiety correlated negatively, though modestly, with a wide array of conventional measures of school achievement and ability at both high school and college levels. Data collected on students from upper elementary school level through high school show that test anxiety scores were significantly related to grades in various subjects, although the correlation was typically about −.2. Cognitive measures (i.e., aptitude and achievement measures combined) correlated more strongly with the worry than emotionality component of test anxiety ($r = -.31$ vs. −.15). Similarly, worry was slightly more strongly correlated with course grades than emotionality ($r = -.26$ vs. −.19). Higher effects sizes were reported for low- than for high-ability students and for tasks perceived as difficult than those perceived as being easy. Furthermore, test anxiety correlated inversely with performance on laboratory cognitive tasks such as problem solving ($r = -.20$) and memory ($r = -.28$). Another meta-analysis (Ackerman & Heggestad, 1997) showed a mean r of −.33 between test anxiety and general intelligence test performance. Test anxiety was also correlated in the −.20–.30 range with other broad intellectual abilities, including fluid and crystallized intelligence, learning and memory, visual perception, and math ability.

The nature of the anxiety–performance relationship is best viewed as reciprocal in nature (Zeidner, 1998). Thus, high levels of test anxiety produce certain aversive patterns of motivation, coping, and task strategies that interfere with learning and performance. The result is that performance suffers, thus leading to further anxiety over time, and generating a vicious circle of increasing anxiety and degrading performance (Wells & Matthews, 1994). Future research would profit from employing nonrecursive process models in order to better capture the dynamic and cyclical nature of the anxiety–competence relationship.

Math and Computer Anxiety

Probably the most reliable estimate of the strength of the math anxiety–performance relationship is provided by a meta-analytic study (Schwarzer, Seipp, & Schwarzer, 1989) based on 28 studies published from 1975 to 1986 (total N of 9,140). The population estimate, from 47 effect sizes (correlation coefficients), was $r = -.23$. Contrary to prior research on test anxiety, the worry component ($r = -.20$) was not found to be a significantly better predictor of poor math performance than the emotionality component ($r = -.19$). Overall, the relation between math anxiety and performance appears to be very much like the relation between test anxiety and performance—a low-to-moderate but not overwhelmingly strong one.

The little amount of data that is currently available suggests that computer anxiety bears a negative impact on competence in using computers. Heinssen, Glass, and Knight (1987) reported that computer anxiety was related to lower expectations and poorer performance during computer interaction, possibly mediated by attention to bodily sensations and debilitating thoughts. As for test anxiety, the detrimental effects of math and computer anxieties are typically attributed to cognitive interference associated with loss of working memory capacity (Ashcraft & Kirk, 2001) or negative self-evaluations and off-task thoughts (Smith & Caputi, 2001). Math anxiety may lower math performance, because paying attention to intrusive thoughts during testing acts like a secondary task, distracting attention from the math task (Ashcraft, 2002). However, we cannot assume that a direct causal effect of state anxiety on performance is the only factor contributing to correlations between trait anxiety and performance. Trait anxiety may also signal lack of interest, preparation, and experience.

Social Anxiety

Anxiety may play as important a role in the social realm as in the domain of intellectual or sports performance. For example, social anxiety relates to various difficulties in occupational adjustment (Bruch, Fallon, & Heimberg, 2003). However, a major problem is that the criteria for adequate performance in social settings are less clear than is the case for other forms of evaluation anxiety. In spite of the criterion problem, various relationships between self-reports of social anxiety and deficits in social behaviors or skills have been documented in the literature. Scores on social anxiety measures tend to correlate with peer rating of social skills and with observational behavioral measures (Arkowitz, Lichtenstein, McGovern, & Hines, 1975). Specific deficits described by Bruch (2001) include inaccurate decoding of nonverbal cues and difficulties in communication, such as lack of fluency and expressiveness in conversational speech. In addition, in a recent longitudinal study, Strahan (2003) found that detrimental effects of social anxiety may predict (self-reported) skill deficits relating to effective verbal discourse, self-presentation, and decoding nonverbal information, but not measures of academic performance such as grade point average (GPA).

Task-irrelevant thinking appears to play a detrimental role in social behavior, much as it does in test-taking situations (Sarason et al., 1990). As with other forms of evaluative anxiety, social anxiety may impair social performance via diversion of limited attentional resources to self-related

processing. Excessive self-focusing may be especially problematic, since competence in social settings is linked to attending to other people in the environment. Bruch (2001) claims that at least some social skills deficits may reflect inadequate skills learning rather than disruption of performance by states of cognitive interference. Overall, however, the relationship between self-reported levels of social anxiety and measures of social competence is not as well understood as in the cases of other forms of evaluative anxiety.

Sports Anxiety

Traditionally, sports psychologists conceptualized anxiety in terms of arousal, said to be related to performance by an inverted-U curve. It was assumed that both under- and overarousal were detrimental to performance, with a lower optimal level of arousal for more difficult tasks, so that anxiety should be especially damaging to sports requiring complex skills (Tenenbaum & Bar-Eli, 1995). Inverted-U relationships between anxiety and sports performance are occasionally reported, but, in general, studies of psychomotor performance fail to support the validity of the inverted-U hypothesis (Neiss, 1988).Contemporary studies are more likely to adopt a multidimensional view of anxiety. Kleine's (1990) meta-analysis of the anxiety–performance relationship in sports included 50 studies published from 1970 to 1988. On the basis of 77 independent effect sizes (total $N = 589$), the population effect size was estimated at $r = -.19$, converging with prior meta-analytic results on test and math anxiety. Separate effect sizes calculated for the emotionality and worry components of sports anxiety yielded estimates of $-.08$ and $-.33$, respectively, underscoring the overall importance of the cognitive component. Craft, Magyar, Becker, and Feltz's (2003) meta-analysis focused on 29 studies ($N = 2,905$) that used the Martens et al. (1990) CSAI-2 scale. Mean effect sizes for cognitive anxiety, somatic anxiety, and confidence were .01, $-.03$, and .25, respectively. The failure to find the predicted negative correlation between cognitive anxiety and performance is surprising. It may be a product of psychometric deficiencies in the scale, discussed by Craft et al. (2003), or worry may be less damaging in the sports context than in other evaluative settings.

Other research has built upon Alpert and Haber's (1960) distinction between debilitating and facilitating anxiety. Many athletes perform best when experiencing very high levels of anxiety, whereas others perform optimally at lower levels of anxiety. Based on work with Soviet athletes, Hanin (see Raglin & Hanin, 2000) found that each athlete has an optimal anxiety level prior to competition, which may be low, moderate, or high, depending on the individual. Thus, a moderate level of precompetition anxiety can actually worsen rather than optimize the performance of some athletes. In fact, anxiety may have different consequences for different athletes: Superior performers may be better at interpreting their anxiety state as being facilitative to performance than nonelite performers (Jones, Hanston, & Swain, 1993). In the next section, we discuss recent work that explores why anxiety may be facilitative to some athletes but debilitating to others.

THEORETICAL PERSPECTIVES: COGNITION, MOTIVATION, AND SELF-REGULATION

We have seen that cognition and motivation are central to most contemporary theories of evaluation anxiety and competence. Table 9.1 lists some of the dominant theoretical approaches in work on evaluation anxiety. Although there are numerous theories of the various types of anxiety, we aim here to pick out those ideas that have been most influential. Most of these theories have some demonstrable validity as a basis for predicting correlates of anxiety, including loss of competence. Indeed, different mechanisms for anxiety may be interrelated; for example, a skills deficit might lead to avoidance motivation (or vice versa). However, it is often difficult to see how these differing theoretical insights might be integrated into some overarching conceptual framework. Furthermore, especially in recent theorizing, the causal status of anxiety is ambiguous. For

TABLE 9.1. Some Focal Theoretical Concepts in Evaluation Anxiety Research

Theory	Central assumptions	Status
Drive/arousal	Excessive drive or arousal leads to potentially debilitating levels of emotion.	Out of favor due to failure to differentiate emotionality and worry
Negative self-beliefs and self-preoccupation	Explicit and implicit negative self-beliefs generate worry, negative emotion and avoidance goals.	A central element of most theories of evaluative anxiety
Skills deficit	Anxiety reflects inadequate learning of performance skills that leads to failure to accomplish tasks.	Prominent in contemporary accounts of both test and social anxiety
Avoidance motivation	Anxiety is linked to motives to avoid the feared situation.	Prominent in contemporary accounts of both test and social anxiety
Metacognition	Behavioral consequences of anxiety reflect meaning attributed to anxiety.	Best known from sports anxiety but of general relevance
Self-regulative strategies	Anxiety is a concomitant of strategies for dealing with discrepancy between preferred and actual self-status.	Specific strategies of interest, including self-handicapping, procrastination, and some forms of social impression management
Maladaptive stress processes	Anxiety is a concomitant of generally maladaptive appraisal and coping in evaluatively demanding situations.	Consistent with contemporary stress research; developed mainly in the context of test anxiety

example, we could see anxiety as a cause of self-protective coping strategies, such as self-handicapping and procrastination, or as a consequence of use of these strategies, given that they are likely to be ineffective in dealing with evaluative threats, or as linked to coping through some more complex causal network.

Thus, in providing a theoretical overview, it is useful to distinguish two complementary perspectives that may put together some of the theoretical pieces. *Performance deficit* theories are concerned with the processes that mediate the detrimental effects of anxiety. Such theories typically have an "open-loop" quality, in that they describe how individual differences in cognition and motivation feed forward into loss of competence in evaluative settings. By contrast, *self-regulative* theories are concerned with the dynamic interplay between personal characteristics and external demands over periods of time ranging from minutes to years. These theories also assume that cognitions and motivations control situational competence, but they are also concerned with how feedback from these encounters reshapes cognition and motivation over time. In this section, we first outline theories that seek to identify the cognitive–motivational sources and consequences of anxiety. Next, we seek to place anxiety–performance associations within a wider account of self-regulation in threatening environments. The self-regulative framework addresses the dynamic interplay between environmental stressors and the cognitions that support attempts at coping with those stressors. A key process operating over extended time periods is the acquisition of skills for coping with the demands of evaluative situations, a process that depends not just on effective attention but also on motivation and engagement with learning. The dynamic perspective is required to understand the reciprocal nature of the anxiety–performance relationship (Zeidner, 1998).

Performance-Deficit Theories

Theories that focus on performance deficits have two essential aspects. The first aspect concerns the sources of anxiety in evaluative situations. What are the personal characteristics that lead to elevated or reduced levels of the various facets of anxiety? Data in Table 9.1 suggest that these may include negative content of self-referent cognitions, such as low self-esteem and underestimation of personal competence, skill deficits, and potentially dysfunctional processes, such as appraising evaluative situations as threatening, and coping through rumination or self-deprecation. Data in Table 9.1 also discriminate strategic styles that may promote anxiety, such as use of self-handicapping as a means of maintaining self-worth. The second aspect concerns the consequences of anxiety for competence. In contemporary theory, anxiety is seen as a proxy for concomitant cognitive and motivational processes that directly influence performance. We may be able to discriminate key elementary processing components that contribute to performance in evaluative settings, and mediate effects of anxiety. Next, we discuss, first, evidence on cognitive–motivational antecedents of anxiety, and, second, evidence on the key processes that mediate anxiety effects on performance.

Antecedents of Evaluation Anxiety

Research identifies a number of common antecedent correlates of the various forms of evaluation anxiety. Thus, perceptions, appraisals, and expectancies tend to be powerful predictors across various forms of anxiety, with those individuals with lower expectancies of performance and greater perceived importance tending to be more anxious (Matthews, Schwean, Campbell, Saklofske, & Mohamed, 2000). Furthermore, low personal ability, self-efficacy, and self-confidence are among the best personal predictors of anxiety in a variety of domains. These cognitive antecedents of anxiety may overlap with motivational antecedents, such as adoption of performance-avoidance goals that focus on avoiding performance failure (Elliot, 1999). A meta-analytic study of 36 different studies reported a substantial inverse mean population effect size ($r = -.42$) between self-esteem and test anxiety (Hembree, 1988; cf. Zeidner & Schleyer, 1999). Test anxiety and self-esteem are expected to be mutually intertwined and reciprocally impact upon each other during the course of development and behavior in evaluative situations (Zeidner, 1998). Indeed, both positive self-concept and high self-esteem are related to higher academic ability and attainment, whereas negative beliefs about the self are associated with lower ability, scholastic underachievement, and failure (Covington, 1992). Test anxiety relates to a range of failure outcome appraisals, suggesting that anxiety relates to fairly broad social–evaluative concerns (Hagtvet, Man, & Sharma, 2001).

There is also abundant evidence showing that socially anxious persons have a low self-concept and lack social self-esteem, perhaps because they feel tense and awkward with others, or because they feel inhibited and uncomfortable socially. The highly socially anxious individual appears to have a stable set of self-devaluing cognitions readily elicited in social–evaluation situations that degrade social performance (Sarason et al., 1990). In sports anxiety, low basic self-esteem also relates to higher levels of cognitive anxiety, lower levels of self-confidence, and maladaptive perfectionism (Koivula, Hassmen, & Fallby, 2002). Self-esteem, as a global sense of self-worth, should be distinguished from self-efficacy and outcome expectancies. Whereas efficacy expectancy is the conviction that one can execute behavior required to produce an outcome, outcome expectancy refers to a person's estimate that a given behavior will lead to certain outcomes. In general, self-efficacy is more strongly related to successful performance than is self-esteem (Caprara & Cervone, 2000). In educational contexts, academic self-efficacy measures are more predictive of performance than closely related constructs, including outcome expectancies, positive self-concept (similar to self-esteem), and perceived control (Zimmerman, 2000). Effects of self-efficacy may be mediated by motivational variables such as activity choice and persistence, together with more effective study skills.

It is no surprise that both self-efficacy and outcome expectancies have been conceptualized as key precursors of test anxiety. Using data generated through testing via the Internet on a sample of 1,413 respondents, a moderate correlation of $r = -.40$ was observed between test anxiety and self-efficacy (Schwarzer, Mueller, & Greenglass, 1999). Furthermore, data collected in Germany in nine different studies showed correlations ranging from $-.30$ to $-.66$ between self-efficacy and anxiety (Schwarzer & Jerusalem, 1992). Smith, Arnkoff, and Wright (1990) demonstrated that self-efficacy for test success contributed to the prediction of test anxiety, above and beyond the contribution of cognitive interference and poor study skills, in a sample of 178 college students. Likewise, a number of studies (e.g., Betz & Hackett, 1983) indicated that perceived math-related efficacy was a stronger predictor of college students' math anxiety relative to even prior achievement test scores in mathematics. In a study among 111 volunteers (Coffin & MacIntyre, 1999), computer anxiety correlated negatively with attitudes ($r = -.71$), computer self-efficacy ($r = -.70$), experience ($r = -.53$), control beliefs ($r = -.52$), and expectancy for success ($r = -.60$). Low self-efficacy relates also to social anxiety (Leary, 2001) and to sports anxiety (Gaudreau & Blondin, 2002).

Optimism–pessimism is a personality trait that refers to generalized individual differences in outcome expectancy. Test-anxious individuals have been conceptualized as pessimists with respect to test outcomes, that is, those whose expectations for successful test outcomes are not very favorable (Carver & Scheier, 1989). Meta-analytic work by Hembree (1988) suggests that the expectations of high-test-anxious students for success on the exam were more pessimistic, by the order of half a standard deviation, than their low-anxious counterparts. Comparably, Kleijn, Van der Ploeg, and Topman (1994) reported strong inverse correlations between optimism and both the worry ($r = -.51$) and emotionality ($r = -.44$) measures of test anxiety in a sample of 129 first-year students in the medical sciences.

Anxiety and Deficits in Competence: Mediating Processes

There is a large literature on test anxiety as a predictor of information processing in laboratory studies that overlaps with studies of general anxiety (see Zeidner, 1998, for a review). Zeidner classifies the information-processing components sensitive to test anxiety as relating to input (encoding and acquisition of information), central processing (e.g., memory, language processing, conceptual organization, judgement, and decision making), and output (e.g., information retrieval, response selection and execution). Deficits related to test anxiety have been identified at various stages of processing, suggesting some general impairment in attention and/or working memory. As previously discussed, these various performance deficits are often attributed to high levels of worry and cognitive interference (Cassady & Johnson, 2002; Sarason et al., 1995), or to loss of functional working memory (Ashcraft & Kirk, 2001). Cognitive interference has also been implicated in detrimental effects of computer anxiety (Rosen & Maguire, 1990), social anxiety (Sarason et al., 1990), and sports anxiety (Smith, 1996).

The "classic" test anxiety research of authors such as Sarason and Spielberger focused on general deficits in performance attributed to cognitive interference and loss of functional resources for processing. More recently, work focuses on *cognitive bias*, using paradigms, such as the emotional Stroop, that demonstrate bias in selective attention to threat (Matthews et al., 2003). Vasey, El-Hag, and Daleiden (1996) tested for attentional bias in 20 high- and 20 low-test-anxious sixth and eighth graders, using a task in which visual attention was indexed by latency for probes presented following neutral and threatening words. High-test-anxious children tended to allocate attention toward the threat stimuli. Biases related to test anxiety have been found at later stages of processing also. In several studies, Calvo (e.g., Calvo, Eysenck & Castillo, 1997) has shown that when subjects read ambiguous sentences, high-test-anxious persons show a bias toward inferring threatening meanings. Careful analyses of the time course of reading suggest that bias in inference operates relatively late in processing, following lexical access. Biasing effects of anxiety on memory are generally less robust than those for selective attention. However, Ingram, Kendall, Smith, Donnell, and Ronan (1987) demonstrated that high test anxiety facilitated incidental recall for threat-related trait adjectives. In a recent study of math anxiety, Hopko, McNeil, Gleason, and Rabalais (2002) failed to demonstrate any bias associated with a "Stroop" test that required naming the ink color of math-related words. The study did show that math-anxious undergraduates were impaired on a Stroop-like task that required counting of numerals printed on cards. Bias in math anxiety may be expressed in attention to the structure of numerical stimuli, rather than to words.

Emotional Stroop effects in social anxiety have been replicated several times, although these studies typically use social anxiety patients, rather than nonclinical samples. Typically, social anxiety slows speed of color-naming words such as boring, foolish, and inferior (see Roth, Fresco, & Heimberg, in press, for a review). Bias has also been demonstrated using other techniques for studying selective attention, and for lexical processes such as interpreting ambiguous homographs. Social anxiety also tends to enhance access to negative material in memory (Roth et al., in press; Wells & Matthews, 1994).

Both cognitive interference and cognitive bias appear to be pervasive in evaluative anxiety, influencing various stages of information processing. In general, these mechanisms appear to operate much as they do in general anxiety, although evidence is rather lacking on cognitive bias and evaluative anxiety (with the exception of social anxiety). Eysenck's (1992) hypervigilance theory plausibly suggests that anxiety leads to scanning of the environment for threat (generating distractibility and attentional impairment), followed by focusing of attention on sources of threat (generating attentional bias). In addition, performance deficits may also be a consequence of poor skills acquisition. For example, deleterious effects of test anxiety may reflect not only cognitive interference but also deficits in study habits and test-taking skills (Naveh-Benjamin, 1991; Zeidner, 1998). Similarly, socially anxious individuals display objective skills deficits, such as difficulties in decoding the meanings of social interaction and in maintaining eye contact (see Bruch, 2001, for a review). However, objective skills deficits may not be directly related to subjective appraisals of competence, as elaborated next.

Self-Regulative Theory of Evaluation Anxiety

Deficit theories of anxiety and competence are limited by their neglect of the interplay between the person's handling of environmental threats and their dispositional vulnerability. Next, we discuss the dynamic interaction between person and situational demands, with reference to the S-REF (self-referent executive function) theory of emotional distress (Matthews & Wells, 1999; Wells & Matthews, 1994; Wells & Matthews, in press). The theory builds on earlier work on transactional stress processes (Lazarus, 1999) and cybernetic models of self-regulation (Carver & Scheier, 1989), to specify how anxiety and worry are generated by executive processing of self-referent information. This processing is shaped by declarative and procedural self-knowledge held in long-term memory. Dispositional or trait influences on anxiety are controlled by individual differences in the content of self-knowledge (Matthews et al., 2000), consistent with evidence previously reviewed.

Figure 9.1 shows the application of the model to test anxiety (Matthews, Hillyard, & Campbell, 1999; Wells & Matthews, 1994). Self-referent processing is generated initially by intrusions of threatening cognitions or images generated by external stimuli or internal cycles of processing: in the case of test anxiety, thoughts of failure.

The intrusions activate executive processing that seeks to initiate appropriate coping. Choice of a coping strategy is influenced by retrieval from long-term memory of self-referent knowledge and schematic plans for action. In the short term, acute distress and worry are generated by accessing negative self-beliefs, that one lacks personal competence, for example, and by choosing counterproductive coping strategies, such as self-blame and avoidance, that focus attention on personal shortcomings. Of special importance are metacognitive beliefs that maintain negative self-referent thinking, for example, that it is important to monitor one's worries (Wells, 2000). In the longer term, distress may be maintained by dysfunctional styles of person–situation interaction. The well-adjusted person modifies self-knowledge to accommodate reality and learning of more effective coping strategies, such as resolving to study harder after a poor examination performance. However, perseverative worry appears to strengthen and elaborate negative self-beliefs, such as being unable to cope with examinations. In addition, avoidant coping strategies lead to lack of exposure to situations that might enhance task-relevant

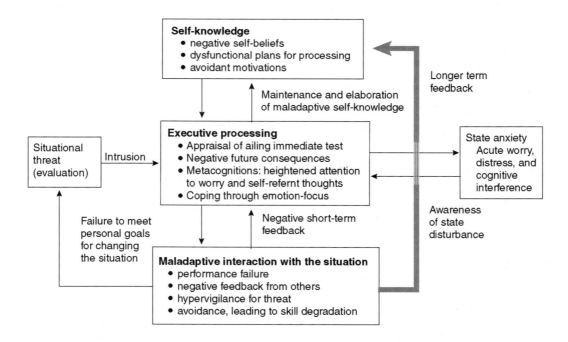

FIGURE 9.1. A prototypical self-regulative model for evaluation anxiety.

skills. The test-anxious person may be reluctant to study, because the study situation focuses attention on the feared event.

The extension of the model to the various forms of evaluative anxiety is straightforward. In each case, dysfunctional self-beliefs about the context concerned (tests, sports, etc.) generate maladaptive self-focused attention that interferes with immediate performance and also blocks longer term skills acquisition. The case of social anxiety has been elaborated by Clark and Wells (1995) in a clinical context. Social anxiety is characterized by excessive concerns about presenting a favorable impression to others. Thus, on entering feared social situations, the person builds a representation of how he or she appears to others that exaggerates visible anxiety symptoms, such as blushing and other signs of social incompetence. In addition to acute anxiety, coping with self-representation generates dysfunctional cycles of social behavior. The person may avoid social interaction as much as possible, preventing him or her from enhancing his or her social skills, and from gaining confidence from easily managed encounters.

The S-REF model predicts that evaluative anxiety should relate not only to the content of cognition, in the form of negative self-knowledge, but also to bias in self-regulative processing and the patterns of person–situation interaction that follow from these biases. Next, we review evidence on associations between anxiety and (1) dysfunctional self-referent executive processing, such as maladaptive metacognitions and coping, and (2) maladaptive dynamic interaction with the external environment, operating over longer durations.

Coping and Metacognition

Zeidner's (1998) review of coping and test anxiety concludes that text anxiety relates to higher emotion focus (e.g., trying to control anxiety symptoms) and avoidance (e.g., trying not to think of the test), but to lower task focus (e.g., focusing effort on task performance). Emotion-focused coping and avoidance both appear to predict state anxiety in evaluative situations. Perhaps surprisingly, task-focused coping also relates to higher pretest anxiety (Bolger, 1990): Exam preparations may inevitably lead to elevated

anxiety. It is often difficult to categorize coping strategies as exclusively adaptive or maladaptive, but task-focused coping tends to lead to higher grades than avoidance, although the data are mixed (Zeidner, 1998).

Matthews et al. (1999) investigated relationships between coping, metacognition, and test anxiety in a sample of students preparing for an examination. Trait test anxiety was independently related to a maladaptive coping factor, defined by a preference for self-critical, emotion-focused, and avoidant strategies in place of task-focused coping, and to metacognitive tendencies, such as preoccupation with worries and concerns about the uncontrollability of thoughts. Data on subjective states experienced during the exam showed that dispositional maladaptive coping predicted situational coping, higher perceived workload, low confidence, and emotional distress. Conversely, excessive metacognition was the strongest predictor of cognitive interference. The role of metacognition is consistent with the view that test-anxious individuals are highly self-focused; that is, they direct attention inward toward their thoughts and feelings about the test (Carver & Scheier, 1989). Kurosawa and Harackiewicz (1995) found that cognitive interference impaired performance of test-anxious students mainly when self-focused attention was induced experimentally (e.g., through being videotaped).

Most accounts of social anxiety and shyness (e.g., Leary, 2001) emphasize the predominance of avoidance coping, although anxious persons may also use strategies of blaming themselves and others. Not surprisingly, those high in social anxiety find it difficult to cope by seeking social support, an association that may be mediated by perceptions of low interpersonal competence (Jackson, Fritch, Nagasaka, & Gunderson, 2002). As with test anxiety, socially anxious persons may be negatively self-absorbed during their social interactions, and this negative self-focus may detrimentally affect their performances (Spurr & Stopa, 2002). However, *public self-consciousness* (awareness of the self as a social object) correlates strongly with social anxiety, especially with worry, whereas *private self-consciousness* (awareness of thoughts and feelings) appears to be minimally related to social anxiety (Schwarzer & Jerusalem, 1992).

Test anxiety may also motivate coping through *self-handicapping* behaviors, that is reducing effort, so that the person can attribute failure to lack of effort rather than lack of personal ability (Covington, 1992). Self-handicappers make more use of withdrawal coping strategies and tend to possess poorer study skills, which leads in turn to poor academic performance (Zuckerman, Kieffer & Knee, 1998). In this longitudinal study, self-handicapping was ineffective, in that it led to poorer adjustment and self-esteem over time, which in turn fed back into increased self-handicapping. Similarly, in social anxiety, when a person is frozen in a self-focused and uncomfortable state in which he or she is unable to create a favorable image, the person may begin to use social anxiety or shyness as an excuse (Snyder & Smith, 1986). Self-handicapping should be distinguished from *defensive pessimism*, in which the person lowers expectations to reduce the likelihood of later disappointment but remains motivated and engaged with the task. By contrast with true pessimism, defensive pessimism may lead to elevated anxiety but no performance deficit (Wilson, Raglin, & Pritchard, 2002).

A somewhat different perspective is offered from studies of sports anxiety. Some features of these studies correspond to modal evaluative anxiety findings. For example, coping through disengagement is associated with high levels of cognitive anxiety (Gaudreau & Blondin, 2002); high levels of cognitive interference are frequently detrimental to performance (Smith, 1996), and vigilance for threat-relevant information relates to higher levels of anxiety (Krohne & Hindel, 1988). However, much recent work on assessment of sports anxiety has required respondents not only to rate intensity of symptoms but also to provide a rating of whether each symptom is believed to be detrimental or facilitative to performance (Hanton et al., 2002). In other words, the athletes rate their metacognitions of anxiety. Although empirical findings are somewhat varied, the results of the Butt, Weinberg, and Horn (2003) study of field hockey performance are fairly typical. Intensity of cognitive anxiety (worry), and perceptions that both somatic and cognitive anxiety were debilitative, independently predicted poorer performance. However, high levels of cognitive anxiety were associated with a greater tendency to rate anxiety as being debilitative. The moderating effect of metacognition may have a motivational basis. Hatzigeorgiadis and Biddle (2001) showed that among volleyball players, performance worries related to increases in effort for athletes holding higher goal-attainment expectancies but decreases in effort for those holding lower goal-attainment expectancies. Thus, high levels of worry often lead performance decrements but do not necessarily do so, depending on how worry is interpreted and channeled into greater or lesser task-directed effort.

Dynamic Aspects of Maladaptive Self-Regulation

The S-REF model describes several dynamic processes that maintain dysfunctional levels of distress over time (Wells & Matthews, 1994). These processes may be internalized, such as perseverative worry driven by metacognitions that maintain the focus of attention on self-referent thoughts. They also refer to ongoing interaction with the outside world. In the case of evaluative anxiety, a common theme is concern about performance competencies and skills that must be learned over extended periods of time. It is uncertain whether evaluative anxiety relates simply to *perceptions* of lack of skill or to actual skill deficits. A dynamic perspective suggests how perceptions and actuality may be related.

Behavioral avoidance, generated in part by performance–avoidance goals (Elliot, 1999), plays a key role in maintenance of evaluative anxiety and concomitant skill degradation. Test anxiety leads to procrastination, motivated by the aversiveness of the test material or fear of failure on the test (e.g., Ferrari & Tice, 2000). Procrastination, such as failure to complete homework assignments or study for the test, leads to failure to acquire the knowledge required. In turn, this lack of preparation leads to poor performance and anxiety in the test situation (cf., Naveh-Benjamin, 1991), increasing subsequent test anxiety and avoidance of study. A similar cycle may link self-handicapping to deteriorating adjustment and performance (Zuckerman et al., 1998). Similarly, mathematics anxiety and avoidance tend to have a circular relationship: Math anxiety leads to avoidance of math; avoidance leads to greater anxiety because of poor preparation, thus leading to further avoidance, and so on (Richardson & Woolfolk, 1980). Similarly, the cognitive biases of the socially anxious person, such as expectancies of social failure, promote avoidance of interaction with others, generating a vicious cycle that prevents acquisition of social skills (Clark & Wells, 1995; Roth et al., in press). Thus, lack of actual competence expressed in skills deficits and irrational subjective biases in cognition that exaggerate personal incompetence may feed off each other over time.

TOWARD AN INTEGRATED THEORY OF EVALUATION ANXIETY AND COMPETENCE

The evidence shows that there is no single cognitive process that generates evaluation anxiety and performance impairment. Instead, evaluation anxiety is distributed across various stages of processing and representations of self-knowledge (Matthews et al., 2000). Although the sources of threat differ across the different types of anxiety, the key processes show considerable commonality, along with a few differences, such as the special role of public self-consciousness in social anxiety and the ability of some elite athletes to use worry as an effective motivator. The traditional view of evaluation anxiety as generating performance decrements via cognitive interference and worry contains some truth but is oversimplified. The impact of worry is moderated by factors such as self-focus of attention (Kurosawa & Harackiewicz, 1995), and, at least in sports, by metacognitions of whether worry is facilitative or debilitating (Butt et al., 2003), and outcome expectancies (Hatzigeorgiadis & Biddle, 2001). A more sophisticated understanding of cognitive interference requires its effects to be placed within a motivational context. Very often, cognitive interference appears to be accompanied by loss of task motivation and dysfunctional coping that directs attention away from task processing, but some individuals appear to

be able to process worries so as to maintain motivation and task-directed attention.

The self-regulative model potentially offers the most complete account of the detrimental effects of anxiety. The source of anxiety is dysfunctional self-knowledge (both declarative and procedural), but its expression as maladaptive situational coping, and its perpetuation over time, require the dynamic perspective of the transactional model of stress and emotion (Lazarus, 1999; Matthews et al., 2000). The actions of the anxious person, such as behavioral avoidance and self-denigration to others, lead to environmental exposures that confirm negative cognitive biases, and block adaptive skill learning and restructuring of self-knowledge. Among the various consequences of these processes are the disruptions in information processing seen in acute states of anxiety and worry. Self-referent processing driven by metacognitive goals initiates dysfunctional coping strategies (emotion focus, avoidance, self-handicapping) that draw attentional resources, working memory, and effort away from the task at hand, leading to impairments if the task is demanding. Vigilant monitoring for potential threats leads to potentially distracting attentional biases: Although such biases are often seen as "automatic," evidence shows that they are typically sensitive to contextual factors, implying strategic influence (Matthews & Wells, 1999). The dynamic perspective also suggests that performance deficits may reflect not only acute cognitive interference but also actual skills deficits resulting from avoidance coping. The self-regulative model also highlights the interplay among motivation, cognition, and emotion in anxiety. Effects of anxiety on behavior are the product of not only disruptive thoughts and feelings but also the anxious person's goals for coping with perceived evaluative threats.

A final comment is that self-regulative models allow an appropriate balance to be found between typical and atypical aspects of evaluative anxiety. The prototypical model shown in Figure 9.1 explains the short- and long-term detrimental effects of evaluative anxiety—effects that are common but not universal. We can also describe other, more adaptive modes of self-regulation seen in states of anxiety, such as defensive pessimism and the use of anxiety to drive compensatory effort. Specification of different contents of self-knowledge in Figure 9.1, such as beliefs in the efficacy of task-directed effort, feed into individual differences in executive processing and adaptive outcomes. Finally, the model also supports idiographic clinical case conceptualizations (Wells, 2000) that describe the specific cognitions and situational triggers for the individual anxiety patient. Thus, dynamic self-regulative models may be variously applied to the prototypical, debilitating anxiety state, to the role of moderator factors that influence the motivational concomitants of anxiety, and to individual cases of anxiety.

CONCLUSIONS

In this chapter, we describe a number of types of evaluative anxiety that are distinguished by the stimulus properties of situations considered personally threatening. In addition to the generic threat of negative evaluation, the various types also involve anxiety about the specific content under consideration (i.e., manipulation of numbers, computer technology, athletic performance, and social interaction). Evaluative anxieties are quite prevalent in contemporary society, generalizing across culture, gender, and age, although relatively minor group differences are sometimes reported. The different forms of anxiety show various forms of psychological commonality, sum-

TABLE 9.2. Some Common Features of Evaluation Anxieties

Dimensions	Description
Conceptualizations	State versus trait distinctions (proposed for test, math, computer, and sport anxiety)
Facets	Three key facets: *cognitive* (worry, irrelevant thinking, negative self-referential thoughts, etc.), *affective* (tension, bodily reaction, perceived arousal), and *behavioral* (deficient skills, procrastination, avoidance behaviors, etc.)
Temporal stages	Anxiety viewed as process unfolding over time, with distinct stages (e.g., anticipation, confrontation, resolution)
Prevalent frameworks	Transactional or interactional that link processing of situational demands to both stable personal dispositions and situational cues
Situational determinants	Demands and constraints of specific situation, evaluative/competitive atmosphere, task complexity
Subjective/personal antecedents	Appraisal of task difficulty, personal competence, and future outcomes, subjective importance of situation, aptitudes and skills, self-concept, self-efficacy, metacognition, trait anxiety, personal domain-relevant experience, and skills
Anxiety and performance	Meta-analytic studies showing correlations of about −.2 between anxiety and performance, typically higher for worry typically than for emotionality; limited data for social anxiety
Causal models and mechanisms underlying anxiety-related performance deficits	Cognitive–attentional deficit, limited working memory capacity, attentional bias, self-handicapping, avoidance coping leading to skill deficits, dysfunctional self-regulation
Group differences	Females evidencing higher levels of anxiety; some cross-cultural and age differences also reported

marized in Table 9.2. Specifically, cognitive, affective–physiological, and behavioral facets are evident in each form discussed. Cognitive aspects of evaluative anxiety may be fundamental; in each case, anxious persons fear that they will not be able to meet accepted performance standards and will be found deficient or inadequate by others, thus resulting in negative social consequences or sanctions.

The trait–state distinction is fundamental to understanding evaluative anxiety within the dynamic interactionist model proposed by Endler and Parker (1992). Over shorter time spans, the state response is a product of dispositional anxiety and situational cues that are congruent with the person's specific vulnerabilities. Over longer time spans, the dynamic unfolding of the anxiety process depends on both the individual's social learning history and basic temperament, influenced by biological factors. Space limitations have prevented discussion of developmental processes here, but in the case of test anxiety (Zeidner, 1998), it seems that dispositional evaluative anxiety feeds back into the social learning process, with potentially malign results if the child becomes avoidant of academic environments.

The massive body of empirical research on the anxiety–performance relationship points to a rather modest inverse relationship between test anxiety and cognitive performance, typically converging at a population correlation at about –.20 in meta-analytic studies. The anxiety spectrum of effects is observed to range from significant degrees of immobilization, through mild discomfort and minor performance deficit, to enhancing effects. Significant progress has been made in understanding the cognitive bases of evaluation anxiety and its effects on information processing and performance. Thus, for all types of anxiety, negative self-appraisals and outcome expectancies generate cognitive interference associated with worry that leads to acute performance deficit. However, such deficits are embedded within maladaptive modes of self-regulation operating over longer timescales.

Self-regulative models suggest that anxiety traits are shaped by stable dysfunctional knowledge (Matthews et al., 2000). This knowledge shapes the self-referent executive processing initiated by external threats and intrusive thoughts congruent with the person's specific concerns about personal competence. When such processing is characterized by excessive self-focus, self-denigration, an intense metacognitive focus, and use of emotion-focused and avoidant coping strategies, states of distress and perseverative worry ensue (Wells & Matthews, 1994). Such states block adaptive restructuring of dysfunctional self-knowledge and promote avoidant behaviors that may interfere with task-relevant skill acquisition. Consequences of test anxiety, including cognitive interference and selective attention to threat, may follow from this strategy for self-regulation. Thus, although anxiety appears to be a major cause of performance deficits, there is undoubtedly feedback from perceived and actual performance to anxiety states. Future research would profit from employing process models in order to capture better the dynamic and cyclical nature of the anxiety–performance relationship (Zeidner, 1998).

At the same time, this protypical account of evaluative anxiety leaves various open questions for future research to address. A fundamental issue is the measurement of test anxiety. Although fractionating the different response components (worry, emotion, behavior) has proved productive, more work is needed to identify the circumstances under which responses are concordant, indicating an integrated, multisystem response (Calvo & Miguel-Tobal, 1998). More work should also be done to assess the specifically motivational elements of anxiety, such as the urge to escape or avoid the evaluation situation. Recent work on the assessment of subjective states suggests that the different modes of self-regulation elicited in stressful environments may relate to well-defined complexes of affect, motivation, and cognition. Evaluation anxiety should also be understood within the context of a person's life and social milieu, certainly at the clinical case level. Thus, standardized testing may be complemented with assessment of the subject's past affective and academic history, and current social, emotional, and economic adjustments, as well as behavior when assessed.

More work is also needed to integrate studies of evaluation anxiety with those of other forms of anxiety, motivated, for example, by perceived threats to physical safety or health. In fact, it seems like the styles of self-regulation typically elicited in other forms of anxiety, including generalized anxiety, are similar to those described here, leading to dysfunctional metacognitions, counterproductive coping, cognitive impairment, and attentional bias (Matthews & Wells, 1999). Indeed, some other forms of anxiety may have hidden evaluative components. Studies of driving anxiety, for example (see Matthews, 2002, for a review), suggest that it is as much concerns about competence as a driver as immediate fear of injury that elicit anxiety, cognitive interference, and performance deficit. It remains to be determined how some generic self-regulative syndromes for anxiety may be differentiated from processes specific to evaluation threats.

A final point is that evaluation anxiety is heterogeneous with respect to its causes and consequences. We have argued that there is a prototypical experience of evaluation anxiety that can be accommodated by self-regulative models. However, such a theory needs to take into consideration accounts of individual differences in evaluation anxiety. Most obviously, such accounts may refer to the different cognitive contents and behavioral choices associated with the different forms of evaluation anxiety. In addition, the self-regulative model emphasizes the diversity of self-knowledge, and its motivational concomitants, that may accompany anxiety. Some anxious individuals may have access to more positive self-representations that counter negative self-beliefs, for example, that anxiety may be overcome by increased task focus, self-knowledge that may drive effective compensatory effort. Individuals may vary in the specific executive processing initiated by negative self-referent thoughts: Although heightened metacognition and emotion focus are common, they are not inevitable. Finally, anxious people differ in the behavioral skills that influence objective outcomes, changing the course of person–situation interaction over time. Thus, future progress requires better theories and research tools for integrating various sources of data and assimilating them into an exposition that describes the person's functioning, detailing specific strengths and weaknesses, and predicting the specific behavioral

manifestations expected under different environmental conditions.

NOTE

1. As defined by Gordon Allport (1966) traits are stable neuropsychic structures that guide response to multiple stimuli within the class of situation relevant to the trait. Some traits, such as the "Big Five," generalize across many classes of situation, but other traits, such as the evaluative anxieties, are relevant only to a limited range of situations or contexts (Matthews, Deary, & Whiteman, 2003).

REFERENCES

Ackerman, P. L., & Heggestad, E. D. (1997). Intelligence, personality and interests: Evidence for overlapping traits. *Psychological Bulletin, 121*, 219–245.

Allport, G. (1966). Traits revisited. *American Psychologist, 21*, 1–10.

Alpert, R., & Haber, R. N. (1960). Anxiety in academic achievement situations. *Journal of Abnormal and Social Psychology, 61*, 207–215.

Anton, W. D., & Klisch, M. C. (1995). Perspectives on mathematics anxiety and test anxiety. In C. D. Spielberger & P. R. Vagg (Eds.), *Test anxiety: Theory, assessment, and treatment* (pp. 93–106). Series in clinical and community psychology. Philadelphia: Taylor & Francis.

Arkowitz, H., Lichtenstein, E., McGovern, K. B., & Hines, P. (1975). Assessment of social skills. In A. R. Ciminero, K. S. Calhoun, & H. E. Adams (Eds.), *Handbook of behavioral assessment*. New York: Wiley.

Ashcraft, M. H. (2002). Math anxiety: Personal, educational, and cognitive consequences. *Current Directions in Psychological Science, 11*, 181–185.

Ashcraft, M. H., & Kirk, E. P. (2001). The relationship among working memory, math anxiety, and performance. *Journal of Experimental Psychology, 130*, 224–237.

Betz, N. E., & Hackett, G. (1983). The relationship of mathematics self-efficacy expectations to the selection of science-based college majors. *Journal of Vocational Behavior, 23*, 329–345.

Bippus, A. M., & Daly, J. A. (1999). What do people think causes stage fright?: Naive attributions about the reasons for public speaking anxiety. *Communication Education, 48*, 63–72.

Bolger, N. (1990). Coping as a personality process: A prospective study. *Journal of Personality and Social Psychology, 59*, 525–537.

Bozionelos, N. (2001). Computer anxiety: Relationship with computer experience and prevalence. *Computers in Human Behavior, 17*, 213–224.

Bruch, M. A. (2001). Shyness and social interaction. In

W. R. Crozier & L. E. Alden (Eds.), *International handbook of social anxiety: Concepts, research and interventions relating to the self and shyness* (pp. 195–295). New York: Wiley

Bruch, M. A., Fallon, M., & Heimberg, R. G. (2003). Social phobia and difficulties in occupational adjustment. *Journal of Counseling Psychology, 50,* 109–117.

Butt, J., Weinberg, R., & Horn, T. (2003). The intensity and directional interpretation of anxiety: Fluctuations throughout competition and relationship to performance. *Sport Psychologist, 17,* 35–54.

Calvo, M. G., Eysenck, M. W., & Castillo, M. D. (1997). Interpretation bias in test anxiety: The time course of predictive inferences. *Cognition and Emotion, 11,* 43–63.

Calvo, M. G., & Miguel-Tobal, J. J. (1998). The anxiety response: Concordance among components. *Motivation and Emotion, 22,* 211–230.

Caprara, G. V., & Cervone, D. (2000). *Personality: determinants, dynamics, and potentials.* Cambridge, UK: Cambridge University Press.

Carver, C. S., & Scheier, M. F. (1989). Expectancies and coping: From test anxiety to pessimism. In R. Schwarzer, H. M. Van der Ploeg, & C. D. Spielberger (Eds.), *Advances in test anxiety research* (Vol. 6, pp. 3–11). Lisse: Swets & Zeitlinger.

Cassady, J. C., & Johnson, R. E. (2002). Cognitive test anxiety and academic performance. *Contemporary Educational Psychology, 27,* 270–295.

Clark, D. M., & Wells, A. (1995). A cognitive model of social phobia. In R. Heimberg, M. Liebowitz, D. A. Hope, & F. R. Schneier (Eds.), *Social phobia: Diagnosis, assessment and treatment.* New York: Guilford Press.

Coffin, R. J., & MacIntyre, P. D. (1999). Motivational influences on computer-related affective states. *Computers in Human Behavior, 15,* 549–569.

Covington, M. V. (1992). *Making the grade.* New York: Cambridge University Press.

Craft, L. L., Magyar, T. M., Becker, B. J., & Feltz, D. L. (2003). The relationship between the Competitive State Anxiety Inventory–2 and sport performance: A meta-analysis. *Journal of Sport and Exercise Psychology, 25,* 44–65.

Crozier, W. R., & Alden, L. E. (2001). The social nature of social anxiety. In W. R. Crozier & L. E. Alden (Eds.), *International handbook of social anxiety: Concepts, research and interventions relating to the self and shyness* (pp. 1–20). New York: Wiley.

Dew, K. M. H., Galassi, J. P., & Galassi, M. D. (1984). Math anxiety: Relation with situational test anxiety, performance, physiological arousal, and math avoidance behavior. *Journal of Counseling Psychology, 31,* 581–584.

Dunn, J. D. H., Dunn, J., Wilson, P., & Syrotuik, D. G. (2000). Reexamining the factorial composition and factor structure of the Sport Anxiety Scale. *Journal of Sport and Exercise Psychology, 22,* 183–193.

Elliot, A. J. (1999). Approach and avoidance motivation and achievement goals. *Educational Psychologist, 34,* 169–189.

Endler, N. S., Flett, G. L., Macrodimitris, S. D., Corace, K. M., & Kocovski, N. L. (2002). Separation, self-disclosure, and social evaluation anxiety as facets of trait social anxiety. *European Journal of Personality, 16,* 239–269.

Endler, N. S., & Parker, J. (1992). Interactionism revisited: Reflections on the continuing crisis in the personality area. *European Journal of Personality, 6,* 177–198.

Eysenck, M. W. (1992). *Anxiety: The cognitive perspective.* Hove, UK: Erlbaum.

Ferrando, P. J., Varea, M. D., & Lorenzo, U. (1999). A psychometric study of the Test Anxiety Scale for Children in a Spanish sample. *Personality and Individual Differences, 27,* 37–44.

Ferrari, J. R., & Tice, D. M. (2000). Procrastination as a self-handicap for men and women: A task-avoidance strategy in a laboratory setting. *Journal of Research in Personality, 34,* 73–83.

Gaudreau, P., & Blondin, J.-P. (2002). Development of a questionnaire for the assessment of coping strategies employed by athletes in competitive sport settings. *Psychology of Sport and Exercise, 3,* 1–34.

Gaudron, J. P., & Vignoli, E. (2002). Assessing computer anxiety with the interaction model of anxiety: Development and validation of the computer anxiety trait subscale. *Computers in Human Behavior, 18,* 315–325.

Gaudry, E., & Spiellberger, C. D. (1971). *Anxiety and educational achievement.* New York: Wiley.

Hagtvet, K. A., Man, F., & Sharma, S. (2001). Generalizability of self-related cognitions in test anxiety. *Personality and Individual Differences, 31,* 1147–1171.

Hancock, D. R. (2001). Effects of test anxiety and evaluative threat on students' achievement and motivation. *Journal of Educational Research, 94,* 284–290.

Hanton, S., Mellalieu, S., & Hall, R. (2002). Re-examining the competitive anxiety trait–state relationship. *Personality and Individual Differences, 33,* 1125–1136.

Hatzigeorgiadis, A., & Biddle, S. J. H. (2001). Athletes' perceptions of how cognitive interference during competition influences concentration and effort. *Anxiety, Stress and Coping: An International Journal, 14,* 411–429.

Heinssen, R. K., Glass, C. R., & Knight, L. A. (1987). Assessing computer anxiety: Development and validation of the Computer Anxiety Rating Scale. *Computers in Human Behavior, 3,* 49–59.

Hembree, R. (1988). Correlates, causes and treatment of test anxiety. *Review of Educational Research, 58,* 47–77.

Hopko, D. R., McNeil, D. W., Gleason, P. J., & Rabalais, A. E. (2002). The emotional Stroop paradigm: Performance as a function of stimulus properties and self-reported mathematics anxiety. *Cognitive Therapy and Research, 26,* 157–166.

Ingram, R. E., Kendall, P. C., Smith, T. W., Donnell, C., & Ronan, K. (1987). Cognitive specificity in emotional distress. *Journal of Personality and Social Psychology, 53,* 734–742.

Jackson, T., Fritch, A., Nagasaka, T., & Gunderson, J. (2002). Towards explaining the association between shyness and loneliness: A path analysis with American college students. *Social Behavior and Personality, 30,* 263–270.

Jones, J., Hanston, S., & Swain, A. (1993). Intensity and direction dimensions of competitive state anxiety and relationships with performance. *Journal of Sports Sciences, 11,* 533–542.

Kleijn, W. C., Van der Ploeg, H., & Topman, R. M. (1994). Cognition, study habits, test anxiety, and academic performance. *Psychological Reports, 75,* 1219–1226.

Kleine, D. (1990). Anxiety and sport performance: A meta-analysis. *Anxiety Research: An International Journal, 2,* 113–131.

Koivula, N., Hassmen, P., & Fallby, J. (2002). Self-esteem and perfectionism in elite athletes: Effects on competitive anxiety and self-confidence. *Personality and Individual Differences, 32,* 865–875.

Krohne, H. W., & Hindel, C. (1988). Trait anxiety, state anxiety, and coping behavior as predictors of athletic performance. *Anxiety Research: An International Journal, 1,* 225–234.

Kurosawa, K., & Harackiewicz, J. M. (1995). Test anxiety, self-awareness, and cognitive interference: A process analysis. *Journal of Personality, 63,* 931–951.

Lazarus, R. S. (1999). *Stress and emotion: A new synthesis.* New York: Springer.

Leary, M. R. (2001). Shyness and the self: Attentional, motivational, and cognitive self-processes in social anxiety and inhibition. In W. R. Crozier & L. E. Alden (Eds.), *International handbook of social anxiety: Concepts, research and interventions relating to the self and shyness* (pp. 217–234). New York: Wiley.

Leitenberg, H. (1990). Introduction. In H. Leitenberg (Ed.), *Handbook of social and evaluative anxiety* (pp. 1–6). New York: Plenum Press.

Liebert, R. M., & Morris, L. W. (1967). Cognitive and emotional components of test anxiety: A distinction and some initial data. *Psychological Reports, 20(3),* 975–978.

Martens, R., Burton, D., Vealey, R. S., Bump, L. A., & Smith, D. E. (1990). Development and validation of the Competitive State Anxiety Inventory–2 (CSAI-2). In R. Martens, R. S. Vealey, & D. Burton (Eds.), *Competitive anxiety in sport* (pp. 193–208). Champaign, IL: Human Kinetics.

Matthews, G. (2002). Towards a transactional ergonomics for driver stress and fatigue. *Theoretical Issues in Ergonomics Science, 3,* 195–211.

Matthews, G., Deary, I. J., & Whiteman, M. C. (2003). *Personality traits* (2nd ed.). Cambridge, UK: Cambridge University Press.

Matthews, G., Hillyard, E. J., & Campbell, S. E. (1999). Metacognition and maladaptive coping as components of test anxiety. *Clinical Psychology and Psychotherapy, 6,* 111–125.

Matthews, G., Schwean, V. L., Campbell, S. E., Saklofske, D. H., & Mohamed, A. A. R. (2000). Personality, self-regulation and adaptation: A cognitive-social framework. In M. Boekarts, P. R. Pintrich, & M. Zeidner (Eds.), *Handbook of self-regulation* (pp. 171–207). New York: Academic Press.

Matthews, G., & Wells, A. (1999). The cognitive science of attention and emotion. In T. Dalgleish & M. Power (Eds.), *Handbook of cognition and emotion* (pp. 171–192). New York: Wiley.

McInerney, V., Marsh, H. W., & McInerney, D. M. (1999). The designing of the computer anxiety and learning measure (CALM): Validation of scores on a multidimensional measure of anxiety and cognitions relating to adult learning. *Educational and Psychological Measurement, 59,* 451–470.

Mueller, J. H., & Thompson, W. B. (1984). Test anxiety and distinctiveness of personal information. In H. M. Van der Ploeg, R. Schwarzer, & C. D. Spielberger (Eds.), *Advances in test anxiety research* (Vol. 3, pp. 21–38). Lisse: Swets & Zeitlinger.

Naveh-Benjamin, M. (1991). A comparison of training programs intended for different types of test-anxious students: Further support for an information-processing model. *Journal of Educational Psychology, 83,* 134–139.

Neiss, R. (1988). Reconceptualizing arousal: Psychobiological states in motor performance. *Psychological Bulletin, 103,* 345–366.

Raglin, J. S., & Hanin, Y. (2000). Competitive anxiety. In Y. Hanin (Ed.), *Emotions in sport* (pp. 93–111). Champaign, IL: Human Kinetics.

Richardson, F. C., & Woolfolk, R. L. (1980). Mathematics anxiety. In I.G. Sarason (Ed.), *Test anxiety: Theory, research, and applications* (pp. 271–287). Hillsdale, NJ: Erlbaum.

Rosen, L. D., & Maguire, P. (1990). Myths and realities of computer phobia: A meta-analysis. *Anxiety Research, 3,* 175–191.

Roth, D. A., Fresco, D. M., & Heimberg, R. G. (in press). Cognitive phenomena in social anxiety disorder. In L. B. Alloy & J. H. Riskind (Eds.), *Cognitive vulnerability to emotional disorders.* Hillsdale, NJ: Erlbaum.

Sarason, I. G., Sarason, B. R., & Pierce, G. R. (1990). Anxiety, cognitive interference, and performance. *Journal of Social Behavior and Personality, 5,* 1–18.

Sarason, I. G., Sarason, B. R., & Pierce, G. R. (1995). Cognitive interference: At the intelligence–personality crossroads. In D. Saklofske & M. Zeidner (Eds.), *International handbook of personality and intelligence* (pp. 285–296). New York: Plenum Press.

Schlenker, B. R., & Leary, M. R. (1982). Social anxiety and self presentation: A conceptualization model. *Psychological Bulletin, 92,* 641–669.

Schwarzer, R., & Jerusalem, M. (1992). Advances in

anxiety theory: A cognitive process approach. In K. A. Hagtvet & T. B. Johnsen (Eds.), *Advances in test anxiety research* (Vol. 7, pp. 2–31). Lisse: Swets & Zeitlinger.

Schwarzer, R., Mueller, J., & Greenglass, E. (1999). Assessment of perceived general self-efficacy on the internet: Data collection in cyberspace. *Anxiety, Stress and Coping: An International Journal, 12*, 145–161.

Schwarzer, R., Seipp, B., & Schwarzer, C. (1989). Mathematics performance and anxiety: A meta analysis. In R. Schwarzer, H. M. Van der Ploeg, & C. D. Spielberger (Eds.), *Advances in test anxiety research* (Vol. 6, pp. 105–119). Lisse: Swets & Zeitlinger.

Seipp, B., & Schwarzer, C. (1996). Cross-cultural anxiety research: A review. In C. Schwarzer & M. Zeidner (Eds.), *Stress, anxiety, and coping in academic settings* (pp. 13–68). Tubingen: Francke-Verlag.

Smith, B., & Caputi, P. (2001). Cognitive interference in computer anxiety. *Behavior and Information Technology, 20*, 265–273.

Smith, R. E. (1996). Performance anxiety, cognitive interference, and concentration enhancement strategies in sports. In I. G. Sarason, G. R. Pierce, & B. R. Sarason (Eds.), *Cognitive interference: Theories, methods, and findings* (pp. 261–283). Hillsdale, NJ: Erlbaum.

Smith, R. J., Arnkoff, D. B., & Wright, T. L. (1990). Test anxiety and academic competence: A comparison of alternative models. *Journal of Counseling Psychology, 37*, 313–321.

Snyder, C. R., & Smith, T. W. (1986). On being "shy like a fox." In W. H. Jones, J. M. Cheek, & S. R. Briggs (Eds.), *Shyness: Perspectives on research and treatment* (pp. 161–172). New York: Plenum Press.

Spielberger, C. D., Anton, W. D., & Bedell, J. (1976). The nature and treatment of test anxiety. In M. Zuckerman & C. D. Spielberger (Eds.), *Emotions and anxiety: New concepts, methods, and applications* (pp. 317–344). Oxford: Erlbaum.

Spurr, J. M., & Stopa, L. (2002). Self-focused attention in social phobia and social anxiety. *Clinical Psychology Review, 22*, 947–975.

Strahan, E. Y. (2003). The effects of social anxiety and social skills on academic performance. *Personality and Individual Differences, 34*, 347–366.

Tenenbaum, G., & Bar-Eli, M. (1995). Contemporary issues in exercise and sport psychology research. In S. J. H. Biddle (Eds.), *European perspective on exercise and sport psychology* (pp. 292–323). Champaign, IL: Human Kinetics.

Vasey, M. W., El-Hag, N., & Daleiden, E. L. (1996). Anxiety and the processing of emotionally threatening stimuli: Distinctive patterns of selective attention among high- and low-test-anxious children. *Child Development, 67*, 1173–1185.

Weil, M. M., Rosen, L. D., & Wugalter, S. (1990). The etiology of computer phobia. *Computers in Human Behavior, 6*, 361–379.

Wells, A. (2000). *Emotional disorders and metacognition: Innovative cognitive therapy*. Chichester, UK: Wiley.

Wells, A., & Matthews, G. (1994). *Attention and emotion: A clinical perspective*. Hove, UK: Erlbaum.

Wells, A., & Matthews, G. (in press). Cognitive vulnerability to anxiety: An integrative approach. In L. B. Alloy & J. H. Riskind (Eds.), *Cognitive vulnerability to emotional disorders*. Hillsdale, NJ: Erlbaum.

Wilson, G. S., Raglin, J. S., & Pritchard, M. E. (2002). Optimism, pessimism, and precompetition anxiety in college athletes. *Personality and Individual Differences, 32*, 893–902.

Woodman, T., & Hardy, L. (2001). Stress and anxiety. In R. Singer, H. A. Hausenblas, & C. M. Janelle (Eds.), *Handbook of research on sport psychology* (pp. 290–318). New York: Wiley.

Worthington, V. L., & Zhao, Y. (1999). Existential computer anxiety and changes in computer technology: What past research on computer anxiety has missed. *Journal of Educational Computing Research, 20*, 299–315.

Zeidner, M. (1990). Does test anxiety bias scholastic aptitude test performance by gender and sociocultural group? *Journal of Personality Assessment, 55*, 145–160.

Zeidner, M. (1991). Statistics and mathematics anxiety in social science studies: Some interesting parallels. *British Journal of Educational Psychology, 61*, 319–328.

Zeidner, M. (1998). *Test anxiety: The state of the art*. New York: Plenum Press.

Zeidner, M., Klingman, A., & Papko, O. (1988). Enhancing students' test coping skills: Report of a psychological health education program. *Journal of Educational Psychology, 80*, 95–101.

Zeidner, M., & Nevo, B. (1992). Test anxiety in examinees in a college admission testing situation: Incidence, dimensionality, and cognitive correlates. In K. A. Hagtvet & B. Johnsen (Eds.), *Advances in test anxiety research* (Vol. 7, pp. 288–303). Lisse: Zeitlinger.

Zeidner, M., & Schleyer, E. (1999). The big-fish-little-pond effect for academic self-concept, test anxiety, and school grades in gifted children. *Contemporary Educational Psychology, 24*, 305–329.

Zimmerman, B. J. (2000). Self-efficacy: An essential motive to learn. *Contemporary Educational Psychology, 25*, 82–91.

Zohar, D., & Brandt, Y. (2002). Relationships between appraisal factors during stressful encounters: A test of alternative models. *Anxiety, Stress, and Coping, 15*, 149–161.

Zuckerman, M., Kieffer, S. C., & Knee, C. R. (1998). Consequences of self-handicapping: Effects on coping, academic performance, and adjustment. *Journal of Personality and Social Psychology, 74*, 1619–1628.

PART III

&

Developmental Issues

CHAPTER 10

ભ

Temperament and the Development of Competence and Motivation

MARY K. ROTHBART
JULIE HWANG

The earliest mark of extraversion in a child is his quick adaptation to the environment, and the extraordinary attention he gives to objects, especially to his effect upon them. Shyness in regard to objects is very slight; the child moves and lives among them with trust. He makes quick perceptions, but in a haphazard way. . . . Apparently, too, he feels no barrier between himself and objects, and hence he can play with them freely and learn through them. He gladly pushes his undertakings to an extreme, and risks himself in the attempt. Everything unknown seems alluring.

—JUNG (1928, p. 303)

Basic temperamental dispositions influence motivation and competence from the earliest days. Individual differences in the affective–motivational systems of positive affect and approach, fear, frustration, sadness, and discomfort, along with attentional self-regulative controls on behavior, thought, and emotion, are all included within the temperament domain. Temperamental dispositions can be seen early in life, reflected in orientations toward or away from objects, people, and challenging events, as depicted in the

opening passage from Jung. They form the building blocks for personality development. In the course of early development, temperament comes also to include individual differences in attentional effortful control, allowing flexibility in interaction with objects and persons, and pursuit of more distant goals.

In this chapter, we define temperament and describe some early theoretical approaches to relating temperament to motivation. We then describe dimensions of temperament that have recently emerged from

167

developmental research and relate them to the development of mastery motivation and competence. Finally, we describe directions for future research in this area.

DEFINING TEMPERAMENT

We have defined *temperament* as constitutionally based individual differences in reactivity and self-regulation, displayed in the domains of emotion, activity, and attention (Rothbart & Bates, 1998; Rothbart & Derryberry, 1981). By *constitutional*, we mean that temperament systems are biologically based and influenced over time by genes, environment, and experience. By *reactivity*, we mean the onset, intensity, and duration of emotional, motor, and orienting reactions. The term reactivity can be used to describe broad behavioral dimensions, such as positive or negative emotional reactivity, as well as more specific physiological reactions, such as heart rate reactivity or fear-induced startle. Temperament also includes *self-regulation*, that is, processes that serve to modulate reactivity.

Temperament involves evolutionarily conserved systems seen in humans and other animals (Panksepp, 1998; Strelau, 1983). These systems are present in all humans, but individuals differ in the strength and sensitivity of their temperamental dispositions and the efficiency of their attentional capacities. Temperament is part of the broader domain of individual differences in personality, with *personality* defined as patterns of thought and behavior showing general consistency across situations and stability over time, and affecting the person's adaptation to the internal and external environment. In addition to the constitutionally based temperament dispositions, personality includes the content of a person's thoughts: perceptions of the self and others, personal values, morals, expectations, defenses, coping strategies, secondary motivations, attitudes, and beliefs. Both temperament and other personality characteristics influence competence, motivation, and performance. Temperament refers to the individual differences in personality that characterize the infant and young child, before many of the more cognitive and highly socialized aspects of personality have developed. It is therefore a useful place to

begin in thinking about the development of motivation and competence.

THEORETICAL APPROACHES TO TEMPERAMENT AND MOTIVATION

Theoretical approaches to temperament have often included motivational components, with these usually seen as driven by individual differences in arousability or emotional reactivity. Eysenck (1976), for example, identified three major dimensions of temperament. The first, Extraversion versus Introversion, was tied to motivation through a theory of arousability. Eysenck postulated that introverts are more sensitive and arousable to stimulation than extraverts. As stimulation increases in quantity, intensity, or duration, the introvert more rapidly reaches a level of pleasurable experience. Introverts thus enjoy low-intensity pleasures to a greater extent than do extraverts, who are likely to be bored with low levels of stimulation and require higher levels of stimulation for pleasure. Introverts, however, will reach and then exceed their optimal levels of stimulation at a lower intensity than extraverts, experiencing distress to overstimulation. Motivationally, extraverts will tend to be stimulation seekers, whereas introverts will seek to avoid overstimulation. Eysenck's dimension of Neuroticism versus Emotional Stability, seen as orthogonal to Extraversion–Introversion, was originally less closely tied to aspects of self-regulation. His third broad dimension of Psychoticism, however, includes aspects of psychopathy or disinhibition and is thus related to the ability to inhibit action (Watson & Clark, 1993).

Eysenck's (1976) model of introversion–extraversion is similar to that of Strelau (1975, 1983) and his colleagues, whose model is also based on individual arousability or reactivity. In Poland, Strelau (1983) and his associates studied reactive, motivational, and motor–tempo aspects of temperament, and related them to adults' performance in work situations. For example, Eliasz (2001) described the degree to which individuals differing in reactivity displayed differences in their motivation to control the work environment, with more reactive workers more likely to seek control.

He also found that more reactive workers were less likely to be able to adjust their motives and goals to changing situations than were less reactive workers.

Jeffrey Gray (1981) followed in Eysenck's tradition, but his model modified Eysenck's original structure: He rotated the axes of Eysenck's orthogonal Extraversion and Neuroticism dimensions, and postulated an approach system, which he labeled Impulsivity. Impulsivity was seen as low for persons low in Extraversion and Neuroticism, high for individuals high in Extraversion and Neuroticism. A second, Behavioral Inhibition System (BIS) was labeled Anxiety, and seen as low for individuals low in Extraversion and Neuroticism, and high for persons low in Extraversion and high in Neuroticism. More impulsive individuals were seen as having a more reactive approach system, with underlying brain circuits involving the medial forebrain bundle and the lateral hypothalamus, and a greater sensitivity to reward or nonpunishment. Individuals high on the BIS or Anxiety were hypothesized to have a more reactive orbital frontal cortex, medial septal area, and hippocampus, and to be more sensitive to punishment or nonreward.

Gray (1981) postulated that when a mismatch between an expectation and an outcome is detected, the BIS comes into play, interrupting the current execution of behavioral programs to allow identification of stimuli to resolve the mismatch. Gray further postulated a fight versus flight system that is clearly motivational in quality. Gray's dimensions, like Eysenck's, are reactive, although they include aspects of attention. Similar models, all based on reactive systems and a postulated underlying physiology, have been developed by Zuckerman (1991), Depue and his associates (Depue & Collins, 1999; Depue & Iacono, 1989), Panksepp (1998), and Davidson and Irwin (1999). More developmental approaches to temperament, such as our own (Rothbart, Derryberry, & Posner, 1994) and that of Thomas and Chess (1977), however, have included more self-regulatory dimensions of temperament involving attention. Thomas and Chess, for example, postulated individual differences in distractibility and attention span–persistence, and in our approach, behavior is not always under the control of

under- or overstimulation but can also be controlled through a system of executive attention or effortful control (Rothbart & Bates, 1998).

The models of Eysenck, Strelau, and Gray provide an important link to motivation, linking temperament to what people like and dislike, and what they choose to do. Their constructs suggest that introverts do not like and tend to avoid high levels of stimulation; extraverts like and tend to approach exciting situations. Temperament systems of approach and extraversion are related to the initial orientation of a person to objects. Systems of fear are related to caution, hesitation, or avoidance. Fight reactions involve approach, and flight reactions involve avoidance. When we consider developmental approaches to temperament, we add individual differences in effortful control that allow the sustained pursuit of goals (Thomas & Chess's [1977] attention span–persistence), the regulation of emotion, and flexible shifting of actions from one goal to another.

TEMPERAMENT IN EARLY DEVELOPMENT

Thomas and Chess's (1977) pioneering work in the New York Longitudinal Study (NYLS) described individual differences in temperament during infancy. Parents were interviewed about their infants' reactions to a number of situations, and content analysis of the interviews yielded nine temperament dimensions: Activity Level, Approach–Withdrawal, Mood, Attention Span–Persistence, Intensity, Distractibility, Adaptability, Threshold, and Rhythmicity (Thomas, Chess, Birch, Hertzig, & Korn, 1963). Although Thomas and Chess (1977) described temperament as style, or the "how" rather than the "what" or "why" of behavior, it should be clear that dimensions such as Approach–Withdrawal and Mood, ranging from positive to negative, specify both content and motivation.

In later research, several scales assessing Thomas and Chess's (1977) nine dimensions proved to be highly intercorrelated, and others did not demonstrate high internal reliability. Item-level factor analyses of NYLS-based questionnaires have therefore been carried out. Other approaches have used construct-based scale development to assess temperament dimensions and study the early structure of temperament. A review of infancy research using both approaches yielded a smaller number of temperament dimensions than Thomas and Chess's (1977) nine (Rothbart & Mauro, 1990). These included dimensions of Activity Level, Positive Affect and Approach, Fear, Frustration or Irritability, and Attentional Persistence. These dimensions were important for our view of temperament because they did not support "style" temperament dimensions such as Intensity or Rhythmicity. Instead, they described emotional and attentional systems that, as early as infancy, demonstrate motivational and self-regulative qualities (the "what" and "why" of development). They also stress the affectively based quality of early individual differences, as in Positive Affect–Approach, Frustration, and Fear.

Gartstein and Rothbart (2003) have more recently carried out an expanded study on the factor structure of parent-reported infant temperament, assessing a number of dimensions derived from research on temperament in childhood. In factor analysis of a large data set describing 3- to 12-month-old children, three broad dimensions were revealed: Surgency–Extraversion, with loadings for scales measuring approach, vocal reactivity, high-intensity pleasure (stimulation seeking), smiling and laughter, activity level, and perceptual sensitivity; Negative Affectivity, with loadings for sadness, frustration, fear, and negatively, falling reactivity scales; and Orienting–Regulation, with loadings for low-intensity pleasure, cuddliness, duration of orienting, and soothability, and a secondary loading for smiling and laughter. As early as infancy, there is thus evidence for broad dimensions of Surgency–Extraversion, Negative Affectivity, and Orienting–Regulation.

At Oregon, we have also developed a comprehensive and highly differentiated parent report instrument called the Children's Behavior Questionnaire, or CBQ, for children 3–7 years of age (Ahadi, Rothbart, & Ye, 1993; Rothbart, Ahadi, Hershey, & Fisher, 2001). In studies across several laboratories, three broad factors of children's temperament using the CBQ have emerged, with similarities in dimensions to those found by other researchers (Rothbart

& Bates, 1998). The first factor is called Surgency–Extraversion, defined by scales assessing positive emotionality and approach, including positive anticipation, high-intensity pleasure (sensation seeking), impulsivity, activity level, and a negative loading from shyness. This factor is very similar to the first factor found in the infancy research, and we examine motivation and competence in relation to this factor later in the chapter. The second broad factor, called Negative Affectivity, is defined by discomfort, fear, anger–frustration, and sadness, with a secondary loading for shyness, and a negative loading for soothability–falling reactivity. This factor is similar to the Negative Affectivity factor in infancy. We extract from this broad factor the dimension of fear, and relate this more narrow dimension to motivation and competence. The third broad factor, Effortful Control, is defined by inhibitory control, attentional focusing, low-intensity pleasure, and perceptual sensitivity. We also relate Effortful Control to motivation and competence.

In the United States, and in both child and adult samples, Effortful Control was found to be inversely related to Negative Affectivity, and independent of Surgency–Extraversion (Ahadi et al., 1993). In a Chinese sample of children, however, Effortful Control was negatively related to measures of Surgency–Extraversion and independent of Negative Affectivity, suggesting that Effortful Control might serve to enhance or suppress reactive behavior, in keeping with the values of the culture. In this way, temperament can be seen to provide the building blocks of personality. Cultural values and challenges shape the goals of the child's adaptations and the competencies and/or the pathologies that he or she thereby develops.

TEMPERAMENT, MOTIVATION, AND THE DEVELOPMENT OF COMPETENCE

How is temperament related to the development of motivation and competence? Following Elliot and Dweck in Chapter 1, this volume, we define *motivation* as "the energization (instigation, activation) and direction (focus, aim) of behavior," and *competence* as "effectiveness, ability, or success." We suggest that temperament dimensions of Surgency–Extraversion and Negative Affectivity are directly linked to motivation. These temperament systems are related to the child's approach, avoidance, interest, and persistence in pursuing designated outcomes, and to frustration, anger, and sadness, when the goals of a given motivation are not met. Effortful Control also has links to persistence, planning, flexibility of thought, and control of emotion, all of which support competence, and allow motivations to be extended in time.

Effortful Control does not in itself constitute motivation, however. Indeed, as in the example of U.S. and Chinese comparisons, the capacities involved in Effortful Control can serve various motivational masters. Given effective socialization, Effortful Control is likely to be related to positive adjustment and favorable outcomes, and will thus be important in the development of competence, as noted in our review below. However, the competencies sought will be influenced by the values of the culture. In addition, competencies are specified by institutions, such as home and school, and by others who are significant to the child, including parents, teachers, and peers. Finally, many competencies will become internally motivated, either directly, through early intrinsic processes influenced by temperament, or more indirectly, through internalization of the desires of significant others and the development of secondary motivations or ego structures, to be described later.

We now consider dimensions of temperament in connection with motivation and competence. We begin with aspects of emotional reactivity, including individual differences in Surgency–Extraversion, or approach, and the negative effect of fear, which is a subcomponent of the broad factor of Negative Affectivity, discussing their links to effectance, mastery motivation, and competence. Although we could also explore links between motivation and the Negative Affectivity subcomponents of anger–frustration, sensory discomfort, and sadness, we have chosen, given limitations of length, to concentrate on the broad temperamental reactivity factor of Surgency–Extraversion and the more narrow dimension of fear. Our discussion of emotional reactivity is followed by a consideration of Effortful Control.

EMOTIONAL REACTIVITY

Surgency–Extraversion and Approach

This broad temperament construct includes positive affect and the rapid approach of potentially rewarding stimuli. We have studied approach, activity level, and positive affect in the laboratory and via parent report. We used infant laboratory measures in a longitudinal study of children at the ages of 3, 6.5, 10, and 13.5 months (Rothbart, Derryberry, & Hershey, 2000). Infants' reactions were videotaped during presentation of nonsocial and social stimuli designed to elicit specific emotions or attention. For example, smiling and laughter to visual and auditory stimuli, such as a chirping mechanical bird, were coded for latency, intensity, and duration, and then aggregated into positive affect measures. Approach was assessed in infants' latency to grasp low-intensity toys, such as small squeeze toys, blocks, and a cup, and activity level was assessed in children's movement among toys distributed across a grid-lined floor. When the children reached 7 years of age, parents of a subset of the infants filled out the CBQ (Rothbart et al., 2001) describing the children's temperamental tendencies in childhood.

Smiling and laughter in infancy predicted both concurrent infant approach and 7-year-old approach tendencies as reported by parents. Infant approach at 6, 10, and 13 months also predicted mothers' later reports of high impulsivity, anger and aggression, and low sadness in the children at age 7. These findings suggest that approach tendencies may contribute to aspects of negative emotions directed against others, as well as to positive emotionality (Derryberry & Reed, 1994; Rothbart, Ahadi, & Hershey, 1994). The findings are also consonant with the idea that more active children may become more frequently frustrated, and indeed, positive correlations between anger and activity level are found throughout infancy (Rothbart, 1981, 1986; Rothbart et al., 2001).

Questionnaire measures of approach have also shown stability from the toddler to early childhood years (Pedlow, Sanson, Prior, & Oberklaid, 1993), and both approach and activity level have demonstrated stability from 2 to 12 years (Guerin & Gottfried, 1994). Caspi and Silva (1995) found that children high on confidence or approach at age 3–4 years were high on social potency and impulsiveness at age 18.

Surgency, Effectance, and Mastery Motivation

Models of effectance and mastery motivation have been directly related to positive affect and approach. White defined *effectance motivation* as the tendency to engage actively in effort with the goal of influencing the environment (White, 1959, 1963). White's model (1978) went beyond earlier learning models based on reward and punishment, and attempted to account for observations of animals and young children displaying curiosity and engaging in exploratory behavior toward objects. White also proposed a definition of *mastery* as adaptation to problems that have a "certain cognitive or manipulative complexity but which at the same time are not heavily freighted with anxiety" (p. 29). It is interesting that White attempted to remove the influence of anxiety in mastery attempts. By inference, fear or anxiety can be seen to limit attempts at problem solution.

The power of interest or positive involvement in influencing competence and achievement is suggested by a meta-analysis of studies involving children in grades 5–12 (Schiefele, Krapp, & Winteler, 1992). In a review of 121 studies conducted in 18 different countries, Schiefele et al. found that interest accounted for 10% of the variability in children's achievement. Interest also was more strongly related to achievement in boys than in girls. In our self-report research with college students, we have found that higher Surgency–Extraversion is related to higher scores on the personality dimension of openness to experience, an indicator of interest in a broad array of topics (Evans & Rothbart, 1998). Those who are high in approach and low in fear may readily launch into new situations; this behavior can be useful when one is exposed to situations with the potential for reward, but lack of fear controls can lead to impulsive behavior in situations signaling punishment. On the other hand, strong fear and/or weak approach can lead to overregulation of approach; children may avoid novel situations, resulting in missed opportunities for the positive experiences of mastery. In the Blocks'

view of personality, rigid overregulation of impulses is designated Overcontrol. Unrestrained pursuit of impulses is designated Undercontrol (Block, 2002; Block & Block, 1980).

Morgan, Harmon, and Maslin-Cole (1990) defined *mastery motivation* as a "psychological force that stimulates an individual to attempt independently, in a focused and persistent manner, to solve a problem or master a skill or task that is moderately challenging to him or her" (p. 319). One common measure of mastery motivation has been the infant's or child's persistence at challenging tasks, such as examining and manipulating interesting objects, working on puzzles, and appropriately using cause-and-effect materials. Challenging toys or situations are presented to infants and young children, and persistence of action toward making the objects "work" is taken as the sign of motivated action. Barrett and Morgan (1995) categorized mastery motivation into two types: instrumental and expressive. *Instrumental* mastery motivation refers to the tendency to persist at challenging tasks, and *expressive* mastery motivation includes affective responses such as facial, vocal, and behavioral communication of positive and negative emotions, such as pride, frustration, sadness, and shame. Measures are thus sometimes also made of children's reactions of pleasure to the task, although correlations between persistence and positive affect scores tend to be low (Barrett, Morgan, & Maslin-Cole, 1993; Redding, Morgan, & Harmon, 1988).

Because definitions of mastery motivation are often complex and include multiple processes, there have been problems in clearly conceptualizing and measuring mastery motivation (McCall, 1995). Messer (1995) suggested that these problems may be overcome by studying the processes that contribute to selection, engagement, and sustained interest in activity with an object. Children can be seen to differ in their *choice* of objects or activities, in how readily they *engage* in the task, and in how long they *remain focused* on the activity. In our section on historical temperament models, we have discussed how individuals' selection of activities can be related to their preference for different degrees of stimulation, so that introverts would select and obtain pleasure from low-intensity activities, and extraverts, from

high-intensity activities. We would also expect latency to engagement to be related to
temperamental approach and fearful inhibition systems, and have evidence of this in developmental studies (Rothbart, 1988).

Positive affect is also related to young
children's sustained engagement. Spangler
(1989) studied 24-month-old toddlers' play,
and reported that the emotional quality of
the child's play experience was related to the
child's persistence. When children showed
expressions of positive affect, either alone or
with their mother, they remained engaged in
an activity for longer periods of time. In our
laboratory, Denise Chu found that 13-
month-olds who smiled more than other infants also sustained interest in a toy for a
longer period; infants who showed more distress during play maintained interest in a toy
for a shorter time. We gauged interest
through the amount of time the child maintained attention in a small toy, before pushing the object away or discarding it on two
occasions. These findings suggested that
positive and negative affect are also related
to sustaining and terminating engagement.

In a replication sample, we found that, after adding criteria for termination of engagement to include the child's attempting to
give the toy to the parent or experimenter,
hiding the toy, or visually disengaging from
the toy for more than 10 seconds, 13-
month-old infants who were engaged with
the toy longer once again smiled more
(Hwang, 1999). Smiling was related to active involvement, that is, the duration of
time spent manipulating the toy while looking at it, and not to the duration of visual
orientation toward the toy without manipulation. These children showed little negative
affect, so we were unable to relate it to their
engagement with toys.

Ruff (1986) noted that manipulative play
can be decomposed into exploratory and
nonexploratory activity, and found that only
during exploration is the infant gathering information about an object, its properties,
and functions. She defined exploratory activity as focused visual inspection of an object, accompanied by its manual exploration, and nonexploratory activity as looking
or manipulation alone. Only visual–manipulative activity, which we found to be linked
to positive affect, was found to reflect active
intake of information and learning, while
other types of behaviors were not (Ruff &

Dubiner, 1987; Ruff & Saltarelli, 1993;
Ruff, Saltarelli, Capozzoli, & Dubiner,
1992).

Shiner (1998) defined mastery motivation
as a disposition to be "motivated by curiosity or interest, take great pleasure in mastering their environments, and prefer challenging tasks to easy ones" (p. 323). Shiner notes
that mastery motivation may be seen as an
effectance–motivational aspect of Tellegen's
(1985) positive emotionality system:

> . . . tapping a person's tendency to approach
> situations and tasks with enthusiasm and zest.
> From this perspective, achievement is distin-
> guished from behavioral control and discipline
> (Watson & Clark, 1992). . . . Persistence and
> mastery motivation may represent two distinc-
> tive but related personality dimensions, with
> persistence primarily tapping behavioral con-
> trol and mastery motivation primarily tapping
> positive emotionality. (Shiner, 1998, p. 324)

We would argue, however, that Surgency–
Extraversion as reflected in positive affect,
also makes a contribution to sustained attention.

Positive moods have also been related to
mastery motivation in adult subjects. Erez
and Isen (2002) manipulated mood state to
create positive and neutral conditions, and
found that positive affect facilitated motivation and performance on an anagrams task,
with participants in the positive mood state
performing better, showing more persistence, and reporting higher levels of motivation. A second study suggested that positive
affect may influence motivation through the
participants' expectancies and evaluations.
Participants in the positive affect condition
were more likely to have high levels of expectancy for and higher evaluations of reward. The conclusion from these studies is
that participants in a positive affect state
have enhanced expectations about goals, the
factors instrumental in reaching those goals,
and the probability of achieving those goals,
that differ from participants in a neutral affect state. Surgent–Extraverted individuals,
who are more prone to experience positive
moods (Tellegen, 1985), might be more
likely to experience these enhanced evaluations.

Mastery motivation can be sustained by
children's experiences of reward or
nonpunishment in achievement situations
(Harter, 1980), and there is also likely to be

intrinsic pleasure in performance of challenging tasks. With age, however, children's responses move from simply taking direct pleasure in mastering tasks to experiencing concerns about the results of their efforts and the evaluation of others based on those results. Goals of significant others may become internalized. Affect is still critically important to mastery motivation, but it is now at least partially mediated by children's views of how others evaluate their performance, and by children's related ego-involvement, self-evaluation, and sense of competence (Harter, 1980).

Shiner (2000) studied a sample of third-through sixth-grade children (8–12 years old) who were later seen at 15–19 years and 17–23 years. She found that parent-reported extraversion predicted social competence both concurrently and late in adolescence. Academic achievement in childhood was also predicted positively from the child's concurrent surgent–extraversion, but the correlation did not hold when IQ was controlled. High school and college academic achievement, on the other hand, was negatively related to earlier surgent–extraversion. Shiner suggests that more surgent individuals may have more impulses that require restraint during later but possibly not earlier schooling. These results are very interesting because they suggest that Surgency–Extraversion may be more of a liability for school competence in later educational settings.

Summary

From infancy, positive affect is related to the approach motivation of young children, including selection of high stimulus intensity, activity, engagement, and sustained involvement in activities. The relation between interest and involvement will continue, but as development proceeds, children will be less affected by their reactivity to the immediate situation, and more affected by long-term rewards and ego-related goals influenced strongly by socialization.

Fear, Effectance, and Mastery Motivation

One subcomponent of temperamental Negative Affectivity is fear. The fear system is related to avoidance or inhibition of action in settings that are novel, threaten punishment,

or are evolutionarily prepared, as in fear of snakes or the dark (Gray, 1971). Because individual differences in temperament include fear or behavioral inhibition, as well as approach or incentive motivation, fear, too, is likely to form an early building block for the development of effectance and mastery motivation. Although excellent models have been put forward for thinking about the development of effectance through social learning, such as that of Susan Harter (1978), they tend to stress the influence of reward and punishment in accounting for the approach to problems, whereas dispositions to approach and avoid activities can also be related to individual differences in temperament.

Late in the first year, some infants begin to demonstrate fear in their inhibited approach to unfamiliar and intense stimuli (Rothbart, 1988; Schaffer, 1974), and later behavioral inhibition can be predicted by a measure of crying and motor reactivity to stimulation at 4 months (Calkins, Fox, & Marshall, 1996; Kagan, 1994). Fearful inhibition developing within the first year of life allows inhibitory control of behavior. In mastery situations, this can not only be seen as nonapproach or avoidance of challenge, but it also can provide the time necessary to analyze a problem or challenge and plan the next steps of action.

Behavioral inhibition shows considerable stability across childhood and into adolescence (Kagan, 1998). Stability of fearful inhibition has been found in children ages 2–4 years (Lemery, Goldsmith, Klinnert, & Mrazek, 1999), 2–8 years (Kagan, Reznick, & Snidman, 1988), 3–4 years to age 18 (Caspi & Silva, 1995), and 8–12 years to early adulthood (17–24) (Gest, 1997). In our longitudinal work, infant fear in the laboratory predicted fear, sadness, and shyness, as well as low-intensity pleasure at 7 years (Rothbart et al., 2001). Fear did not predict later frustration–anger but was negatively related to later approach, impulsivity, and aggression, suggesting that fear may be involved in the control and regulation of surgent and aggressive tendencies (Gray & McNaughton, 1996).

More fearful infants also showed greater empathy, guilt, and shame in childhood (Rothbart, Ahadi et al., 1994). These findings suggest that fear might be involved in the early development of social motivation, and in our recent work linking personality to temperament, James Victor and I have found links among fear, sadness, and dependency-related behavior. Kochanska (1995, 1997) has also found that temperamental fearfulness predicts emerging conscience development in preschool-age children. Fearful children whose mothers made use of gentle socialization techniques developed particularly highly internalized conscience, demonstrating an interaction between temperament and socialization in the development of internal control. Later in development, attentionally based effortful control becomes more influential in the operation of children's conscience (Kochanska, Murray, & Harlan, 2000).

Children who show strong approach tendencies and are also fearful can inhibit approach tendencies when they might lead to negative outcomes. Because anxiety is linked to enhanced attention to threats (Derryberry & Reed, 1994, 1996; Vasey, Daleiden, Williams, & Brown, 1995), fear may enhance sensitivity to potential negative events and allow the child to avoid problems. On the other hand, extreme fear may lead to problems with rigid overcontrol of behavior, as reflected in the Blocks' description of overcontrolled patterns that can limit positive experiences (Block & Block, 1980; Kremen & Block, 1998). Thus, the dimension of fearfulness within the first year of life allows the first major control system of behavior, a reactive one.

Blair (2003) developed a parent report version of a Behavioral Activation System (BAS) and the Behavioral Inhibition System (BIS) questionnaire to use in assessing 4-year-olds in Head Start programs. He found that BIS scores were positively related to teacher reports of social competence in the children; both BIS and BAS scores were related to less behavior on-task. In this instance, the BIS was related to both a social competence variable and the tendency to disengage from an activity. It would be interesting to determine whether BIS and BAS tendencies are related to disengagement in possibly different ways. According to Gray's (1971) fear = frustration hypothesis, children high in the BIS may become discouraged more easily, whereas children high in the BAS may simply find other activities more tempting.

Elliot and Harackiewicz (1996) separated performance goals into two independent components—approach and avoidance orientations, distinguishing between an orientation toward attaining competence and an orientation toward avoiding incompetence. Two experiments were designed to compare performance between adults in approach versus avoidance conditions. Participants were asked to solve a puzzle, with instructions stressing the possibility of either success or failure. Those in the performance-avoidance condition (failure) instruction performed less well and were less cognitively involved in the task than those in the approach (reward) condition. It was concluded that performance goals aimed at avoiding incompetence can undermine intrinsic motivation.

In a second set of studies, Elliot and Thrash (2002) used a variety of approach-related and avoidance-related temperament measures in a factor-analytic investigation. Measures of positive emotionality, the BAS, and extraversion loaded on an Approach Temperament factor, and a measure of negative emotionality, the BIS, and neuroticism loaded on an Avoidance Temperament factor. Approach temperament measures were related to mastery goals (e.g., "I desire to completely master the material presented in this class") and to performance approach (e.g., "It is important for me to do well, compared to others in this class") Avoidance temperament measures were related to both performance approach and performance avoidance (e.g., "I just want to avoid doing poorly in this class"). Thus, approach temperament was related to approach goals, but avoidance temperament was related to both approach and avoidance. The authors referred to the latter as a "valence override" process, in which avoidant individuals approach normative performance, presumably to avoid failure. This is an important point, because in this instance, avoidant motivation is related to approach. Thus, similar behaviors may be differently motivated. The development of effortful control will increasingly allow this kind of flexible application of motivation.

Fear and Ego-Related Anxiety

As the child's perception of self develops during infancy and the preschool years, it is useful to distinguish between early-appearing temperamental fearfulness–shyness and ego-related anxiety. Temperamental dispositions toward fear are seen in children's inhibition of excitement and approach toward new situations and challenges. In addition, however, low and vulnerable evaluation of the self can lead children with a wide range of temperamental endowments to become anxious about the possibility of failure and/ or to resist evidence that they have failed (cf. Ausubel, 1996; Ausubel, Sullivan, & Ives, 1980). Evaluative reactions may be potentiated by temperamental fearfulness. Harter (1980), for example, reported rudimentary signs of fearful children's decreased interest in challenging tasks and behavioral withdrawal when scrutinized and evaluated by others. Longitudinal studies of the development of avoidant styles that take temperament into account will be very helpful for the future.

Values of autonomous achievement, forthrightness, and consistency between public and private selves are reported by adults in the United States (Harter, 1998). These ego values have traditionally varied for girls and boys, with individual success being more important for boys, and social approval and physical attractiveness being more important for girls, although these may be changing. As children develop representations of self, their vulnerability and anxiety about failure in these valued areas increases (Harter, 1998). Children's temperamental susceptibility to fear would be likely to potentiate these reactions, but at least equally important will be societal pressures for successful performance as perceived by the child, and socially based, as well as personally based, evaluations of the child's behavior.

This brings us to socialization-based secondary motivations. In addition to the primary motivations that are related to temperament and to bodily needs, such as thirst and hunger, these secondary motivations come to organize the life of the developing individual. The goals valued by the parent and society (e.g., attractiveness, wealth, or achievement) become part of the structure of self in the socialized child. In addition, the child develops attempts at self-defense when these are threatened. These systems have motivational properties and sometimes become functionally autonomous (Allport, 1937, 1961). Children whose feelings of

self-worth are strongly linked to their individual performance, in part because they view their parents' love and acceptance as contingent on it, will be more anxious about the possibility of failure than children who achieve satisfaction more directly from parental acceptance (Ausubel, 1996). In addition, feelings of inferiority, based on social and personal evaluations, may lead to defensive positions of vanity, envy, avarice, hate, seclusiveness, and timidity (Adler, 1946).

Ryan, Connell, and Grolnick (1992) developed a theory relating internalization to self-regulation. Internalization occurs through the development of internal regulation, redirecting or suppressing behavioral urges. "Internalization processes are thus relevant to all behavior and regulations whose occurrence initially depended upon extrinsic incentives" (p. 172). The role of internalization is important in school adjustment and societal achievement, because these areas involve many situations that are not intrinsically motivating. The authors described three types of self-regulatory styles: external regulation, introjected regulation, and identification. Identifications are interesting, because they can serve a self-protective function and can motivate the child to emulate the identification figure. Teachers and parents play critical roles in the development of self-regulation and internalization, through supporting autonomy, and providing structure and positive involvement.

Temperamental tendencies to fearfulness will contribute to ego-related anxiety reactions, but under social pressures, even a temperamentally positive and approaching child can become vulnerable to anxiety about the possibility of failure, and reactions to feelings of inferiority may be displayed in actions that seem to be their opposite (e.g., arrogance and self-importance). The goals (and related rewards and threats) with which the self is organized may be seen as personality or ego structures. In Block's (2002) terms, "Personality structures are marshaled to give priority to avoidance of immediate threats to the viability of the individual. With that constraint, the system is further disposed to gratify the individual and enhance long term viability" (p. 183). In addition, ego-involved children will be subject to the frustration, avoidance, and depression related to decreased self-evaluations (Harter, 1998).

Going beyond temperament, individuals will differ in their degree of commitment to higher order ego-related structures, including self-concepts, goals, identifications, and investments in others, creating opportunities for both rewards and anxiety (Block, 2002). In the development of these processes, temperament will be one of several influences, and longitudinal study of the development of these personality processes is needed.

Important longitudinal research has been done relating early temperament and peer experience to developmental outcomes. In Asendorpf's (1990) research on children's shyness and behavioral inhibition in the classroom, children who, at time of school entry, showed fear of strangers (in our terms, early-appearing shyness) were behaviorally inhibited in the classroom early in the year, but by the end of the year were likely to have made an adjustment to the class setting. Other children, however, who were not initially inhibited, became more inhibited during the course of the school year and increasingly isolated from others (secondary shyness). Asendorpf suggests that this later developing shyness is likely to develop in children who have behaved in ways that led to rejection from their peers. In Asendorpf and van Aken's (1994) follow-up of these children, early-appearing shyness (stranger fear) was not the major predictor of later self-esteem; the children likely to develop lower self-esteem were those with the later developing or secondary shyness.

It is important to note, however, that Asendorpf's research was conducted in German schools. Cross-cultural research suggests that the value of outgoing versus shy behavior differs from one cultural group to another, and in the United States, early-appearing shyness may create more problems of adjustment than it would in Germany. However, Asendorpf's findings suggest that punishment from peers and others that discourages the child's attempts at acceptance may be at least as important as initial temperament in the development of problems with self-esteem and general adjustment.

Summary

Temperamental fear, developing late in the first year, is related to inhibited approach and to a tendency to avoid or withdraw from exciting or potentially punishing situations. As the child's perception of self develops, however, new vulnerabilities to threat become available, so that even children who are not temperamentally inhibited may show ego-related anxiety. In turn, this anxiety may promote paradoxical approach or defensive activity.

EFFORTFUL CONTROL AND SELF-REGULATION

Approach-related motivation and fear are both reactive dispositions, yet we know that we can also sometimes approach the things we fear and avoid the things that can reward us. How does this come about? In Elliot and Thrash's (2002) model, cognitive goals are posited to provide this possibility. However, these authors do not identify psychological processes that would support the pursuit of longer term goals in overcoming reactive temperament. We (Posner & Rothbart, 1998; Rothbart & Bates, 1998) have proposed that individual differences in effortful control, based on development of the executive attention system, provide one important kind of flexibility for the developing child.

In the view we have developed in this chapter, early approach versus avoidance or disengagement will be shaped by the infants' surgent–extraverted and fearful dispositions. During the second year, language and increasing impulse control become available to the child. There is also increasing understanding of the self as a separate entity in potential control of events, and the 2-year-old often forcibly attempts to influence objects and others. Attempts to exercise control in a world that often does not allow it will be a lifelong enterprise (Adler, 1946). However, children of this age have few self-regulatory skills and little patience. When their expectations are not met, they frequently respond with anger and may cry or show temper tantrums (Kopp, 1992). Bronson (2000) notes the toddler's increasing awareness of the possibility of control; the actual skill of consciously controlling one's behavior will be developing during the preschool and school years, with the capacities of effortful control. We have suggested that these changes will be related to development of the executive attention system and demonstrated in the child's exercise of effortful control (Rothbart & Posner, 2001).

The broad dimension of Effortful Control was identified in parent report measures of temperament in childhood, including inhibitory control, attentional focusing and shifting, perceptual sensitivity, and low-intensity pleasure (Rothbart & Bates, 1998), and in a review of the literature on temperament and development (Rothbart, 1989). There is evidence that effortful control is related to the efficiency of executive attention, including the ability to perform effectively in a conflict situation that requires the child to inhibit a dominant response and/or activate a subdominant response, to plan, and to detect errors (Posner & Rothbart, 1998; Rothbart, Derryberry, et al., 1994). Kochanska et al. (2000) have characterized the construct of effortful control as being "situated at the intersection of the temperament and behavioral regulation literatures" (p. 220).

Effortful Control and Executive Attention

Our hypothesis that executive attention might underlie effortful control was initially supported by correlations among attentional focusing, attentional shifting, and inhibitory control in self-reports of adults (Derryberry & Rothbart, 1988). We then investigated the early development of attentional control under conflict conditions (Gerardi-Caulton, 2000; Posner & Rothbart, 1998, 2000). A basic measure of executive attention is the Stroop task, in which subjects report the color of ink in which a word is written, when the color word (e.g., red) might conflict with the ink color (e.g., blue). Adult brain-imaging studies have found a variety of Stroop-like tasks to activate a midline brain structure in the anterior cingulate gyrus, which has been associated with other executive attention activities (Bush, Luu, & Posner, 2000). Because young children do not read, we developed a marker task to assess executive attention in young children by creating a conflict between the identity of an object and its location. Performance on this task demonstrated considerable improvement between 27 and 36 months of age (Gerardi-Caulton, 2000). Children who performed well on the task were also described by their parents as more skilled at atten-

tional control, less impulsive, and less prone to frustration, and adults given this task showed increased cingulate activation (Fan, Flombaum, McCandliss, Thomas, & Posner, 2003).

We also developed and tested a children's version of the Attention Network Test (Rueda, Posner, & Rothbart, 2004). Employing this measure, we found that executive attention skills developed strongly between 4 and 7 years of age. Diamond and Taylor (1996) had previously evaluated performance of children between 3½ and 7 years old in a tapping test developed by Luria (1961). They found steady improvement in both accuracy and speed on the tapping test over the ages 3½–7. Most of the improvement occurred by age 6 years, with the 7-year-old group showing an accuracy rate close to 100%.

We recently assessed toddlers at 24, 30, and 36 months of age, using the spatial conflict task that we had used to mark development of executive attention (Rothbart, Ellis, Rueda, & Posner, 2003). We replicated a significant improvement on the task with increasing age. Children who showed greater skill at the task were also rated by their parents as having relatively higher levels of effortful control and lower levels of negative affectivity. In an as-yet-unpublished analysis, the children completed a block tower-building task and a nested cup-stacking task, both of which involve skills such as task orientation, error detection and correction, and goal completion. Scores for the two tasks were combined to form a composite measure of volitional skills and compared to parent-report temperament scores within each age group.

At age 24 months, scores on the volitional skills composite were positively related to parent-reported effortful control, and negatively related to both surgency and negative affect. At 30 months, composite scores were negatively related to impulsivity and, at a trend level, negatively related to surgency. At 36 months, composite scores showed a tendency to be positively related to attention focusing. These results suggest that emerging self-regulation may play an important role in the development of volitional skills, allowing a child greater control, as he or she waits or searches for appropriate opportunities to act, resists distractions, detects and corrects errors, overcomes obstacles, and completes a goal. As these skills become practiced with age, however, they may occur more automatically, making their combination with other skills directed toward goal-related competencies possible.

Kochanska et al. (2000) developed a battery of laboratory-based effortful control tasks for children between ages 22 months and 5 years. Beginning at age 2½, children's performance showed considerable consistency across tasks, indicating that they were measuring a common underlying capacity. Children showed improvement in their performance on the battery but were also remarkably stable in their individual performance over time, with correlations ranging from .44 for the youngest children (22–33 months) to .59 from 32 to 46 months, to .65 from 46 to 66 months.

Olson, Bates, Sandy, and Schilling (2002) found that parent–child interaction, child temperament, and cognitive competence in toddlerhood all significantly predicted variations in children's later self-regulatory capabilities. Olson et al. tested for individual differences in children's self-regulatory competence using laboratory tests and observations. The toddler temperament predictor of later lower competence was the measure of disengagement, "a behavioral index of unoccupied 'wandering' during a two-hour home visit" (p. 443). The authors speculate that "toddlers who manifest high levels of behavioral disengagement may be showing early difficulties with the organization and deployment of attention, a construct labeled 'effortful control' by Rothbart and her associates (Rothbart & Bates, 1998)" (p. 443).

Additional evidence for stability of effortful control has been found in research by Mischel and his colleagues (Mischel, Shoda, & Peake, 1988; Shoda, Mischel, & Peake, 1990). Preschoolers were measured on their ability to wait for a delayed treat that was preferable to a readily accessible but less preferred treat. Delay of gratification in seconds predicted later parent-reported attentiveness, concentration, competence, planfullness, and intelligence, when the children had become adolescents. Preschoolers better able to delay gratification were also later seen as having better self-control and an increased ability to deal with stress, frustration, and temptation. Seconds

of preschool delay also predicted academic competence in Scholastic Aptitude Test (SAT) scores, even when controlling for intelligence. In follow-up studies, preschool delay behavior predicted goal-setting and self-regulatory abilities when the participants reached their early 30s (Ayduk et al., 2000), suggesting remarkable continuity in self-regulatory tendencies.

Effortful control plays an important role in the development of conscience, with greater internalized conscience in children high in effortful control (Kochanska, Murray, & Coy, 1997; Kochanska, Murray, Jacques, Koenig, & Vandegeest, 1996; Kochanska et al., 2000). Thus, both the reactive temperamental control system of fear and the attentionally based system of effortful control appear to regulate the development of conscientious thought and behavior, with the influence of fear found earlier in development. At Oregon, we found that 6- to 7-year-old children high in effortful control were high in empathy and guilt–shame, and low in aggressiveness (Rothbart, Ahadi, et al., 1994). Effortful control may support empathy by allowing children to attend to the other person's condition instead of focusing only on their own sympathetic distress. Eisenberg, Fabes, Nyman, Bernzweig, and Pinulas (1994) found that 4- to 6-year-old boys with good attentional control dealt with anger using nonhostile verbal methods rather than overt aggression.

Although effortful control is a fairly recent addition to the conceptual domain of temperament, it is proving to be a fundamental one. Eisenberg and Fabes (1992), for example, proposed a model in which emotionality and regulation combine or interact to affect social behavior. The model distinguishes between emotion regulation, in which attention and cognition act to regulate internal states and processes, and behavioral regulation, involving inhibition or activation of emotion-related behavior. Eisenberg et al. (1996) examined K–3 children, measuring both negative emotionality and a composite measure of attentional regulation. Eisenberg et al. (1997) also examined socially competent (socially appropriate and prosocial) behaviors in the same sample. At all levels of emotional intensity, children high in regulation exhibited higher levels of social competence. However, this relationship was strongest for children higher in general emotional intensity. In addition, attentional control was related to resiliency but was particularly important for children prone to negative affect.

Another aspect of effortful control is the ability to persist at a task. Bramlett, Scott, and Rowell (2000) looked at relationships among temperament, social skills, academic competence, and reading and math achievement in first-grade children. Teacher ratings of persistence and approach–withdrawal and parent ratings of activity on the Temperament Assessment Battery (Martin, Drew, Gaddis, & Moseley, 1988) were used to predict academic competence. Teachers also completed the Social Skills Rating System (Gresham & Elliott, 1990) as a measure of children's social skills in school. The children's temperament, particularly their persistence, predicted academic competence, and teacher ratings of behavior were better predictors of classroom behavior and academic status than parent ratings.

Effortful control adds an important self-regulatory dimension to the domain of temperament. Going beyond the historical models described earlier that find us moved chiefly by affect or arousal, effortful control allows us to resist the immediate influence of affect. Effortful control allows us to either *approach* situations we fear or *resist* actions we desire in a flexible way. We expect, however, that the efficiency of effortful control will depend on the strength of the dominant response. Our only predictor of effortful control from infancy, given that we could not directly measure this system during the early months, was the speed with which children grasped high-intensity toys in the laboratory (Rothbart et al., 2000). Those who grasped the toys quickly showed higher impulsivity, anger–frustration, and aggression at 7 years, and tended to be lower in attentional and inhibitory control. We have suggested that strong approach tendencies may constrain the application of effortful control (Rothbart et al., 2000). If we use an analogy of approach tendencies as the "accelerator," and inhibition tendencies, both fear and inhibiting aspects of effortful control, as the "brakes" on behavior and emotional expression, stronger acceleration would be expected to weaken the braking influence of fear and effortful inhibitory control.

Effortful control can support both the internalization of competence-related goals and their achievement. Effortful control is also involved in the inhibition of immediate approach, with the goal of a larger reward later, in Block's (2002) "hedonism of the future." It is also related to the activation of behavior that would otherwise not be performed due to threatened punishment. In general, it allows the person to act "on principle." In this and most cases, effortful control is not a basic motivation, but rather the means to effectively satisfying desired ends. It is similar to the attentional capacities underlying Block's construct of ego resiliency, which allows for the flexible ability to shift levels of control depending on the situation. In Block's view, "The problem of psychological development is to move toward resiliency, or, less optimally, to find a life recess wherein resiliency is not seriously or continuously required" (p. 185).

Summary

Effortful control, based upon the development of executive attention in the preschool and early school years, provides both a basis for competent action and the ability to act or withhold action now, in the pursuit of future outcomes. Effortful control may be viewed as a means to motivationally appropriate ends. It also likely contributes to the development of differentiated ego structures creating additional, secondary sources of motivation.

DIRECTIONS FOR FUTURE RESEARCH

As in many areas of temperament research, making links between early individual differences and the development of competence and motivation has only just begun. As suggested in this chapter, research tracing approach, fear, and effortful control, as well as anger, sadness, and overstimulation, in the development of personality, will be essential in our coming to understand children's adaptation. In addition, we need to come to understand how temperamentally based motivation develops into ego structures and secondary motivation, as well as the defenses that support them. This developmental research will, of necessity, employ temperament measures. Temperament controls will also be important additions to intervention studies. Overall, we wish to support the development of competence in all children, realizing that some adaptations that are helpful to children in the short term may not be adaptive in later development. Additional longitudinal research on the development of ego structures in relation to temperament can make essential contributions toward our understanding in this area.

ACKNOWLEDGMENTS

The writing and research reported in this chapter has been supported by National Institutes of Health Grant Nos. MH01471 and MH43361 to Mary K. Rothbart. Sincere thanks to Myron Rothbart and Michael Posner for their comments on an earlier draft.

REFERENCES

Adler, A. (1946). *Understanding human nature* (W. B. Wolfe, Trans.). New York: Greenberg.

Ahadi, S. A., Rothbart, M. K., & Ye, R. (1993). Children's temperament in the U.S. and China: Similarities and differences. *European Journal of Personality, 7,* 359–377.

Allport, G. W. (1937). *Personality: A psychological interpretation.* New York: Holt.

Allport, G. W. (1961). *Patterns and growth in personality.* New York: Holt, Rinehart, & Winston.

Asendorpf, J. B. (1990). Development of inhibition during childhood: Evidence for situational specificity and a two-factor model. *Developmental Psychology, 26,* 721–730.

Asendorpf, J. B., & van Aken, M. A. G. (1994). Traits and relationship status: Stranger versus peer group inhibition and test intelligence versus peer group competence as early predictors of later self-esteem. *Child Development, 65,* 1786–1798.

Ausubel, D. P. (1996). *Ego development and psychopathology.* New Brunswick, NJ: Transaction.

Ausubel, D. P., Sullivan, E. V., & Ives, S. W. (1980). *Theory and problems of child development.* New York: Grune & Sutton.

Ayduk, O., Mendoza-Denton, R., Mischel, W., Downey, G., Peake, P. K., & Rodriguez, M. (2000). Regulating the interpersonal self: Strategic self-regulation for coping with rejection sensitivity. *Journal of Personality and Social Psychology, 79,* 776–792.

Barrett, K. C., & Morgan, G. A. (1995). Continuities and discontinuities in mastery motivation during infancy and toddlerhood: A conceptualization and re-

view. In R. H. MacTurk & G. A. Morgan (Eds.), *Advances in applied developmental psychology: Vol. 12, Mastery motivation: Origins, conceptualizations, and applications* (pp. 57–93). Norwood, NJ: Ablex.

Barrett, K. C., Morgan, G. A., & Maslin-Cole, C. A. (1993). Three studies on the development of mastery motivation in infancy and toddlerhood. In D. Messer (Ed.), *Mastery motivation in early childhood: Development, measurement, and social processes* (pp. 83–108). London: Routledge.

Blair, C. (2003). Behavioral inhibition and behavioral activation in young children: Relations with self-regulation and adaptation to preschool in children attending Head Start. *Developmental Psychobiology, 42,* 301–311.

Block, J. (2002). *Personality as an affect-processing system: Toward an integrative theory.* Mahwah, NJ: Erlbaum.

Block, J. H., & Block, J. (1980). The role of ego-control and ego-resiliency in the organization of behavior. In W. A. Collins (Ed.), *Minnesota Symposium on Child Psychology* (Vol. 13, pp. 39–101). Hillsdale, NJ: Erlbaum.

Bramlett, R. K., Scott, P. L., & Rowell, R. K. (2000). A comparison of temperament and social skills in predicting academic performance in first graders. *Special Services in Schools, 16,* 147–158.

Bronson, M. B. (2000). *Self-regulation in early childhood: Nature and nurture.* New York: Guilford Press.

Bush, G., Luu, P., & Posner, M. I. (2000). Cognitive and emotional influences in anterior cingulate cortex. *Trends in Cognitive Sciences, 4,* 215–222.

Calkins, S. D., Fox, N. A., & Marshall, T. R. (1996). Behavioral and psychological antecedents of inhibition in infancy. *Child Development, 67,* 523–540.

Caspi, A., & Silva, P. A. (1995). Temperamental qualities at age three predict personality traits in young adulthood: Longitudinal evidence from a birth cohort. *Child Development, 66,* 486–498.

Davidson, R. J., & Irwin, W. (1999). The functional neuroanatomy of emotion and affective style. *Trends in Cognitive Science, 3,* 11–21.

Depue, R. A., & Collins, P. F. (1999). Neurobiology of the structure of personality: Dopamine, facilitation of incentive motivation, and extraversion. *Behavioral and Brain Sciences, 22,* 491–569.

Depue, R. A., & Iacono, W. G. (1989). Neurobehavioral aspects of affective disorders. In M. R. Rosenzweig & L. Y. Porter (Eds.), *Annual review of psychology* (Vol. 40, pp. 457–492). Palo Alto, CA: Annual Reviews.

Derryberry, D., & Reed, M. A. (1994). Temperament and the self-organization of personality. *Development and Psychopathology, 6,* 653–676.

Derryberry, D., & Reed, M. A. (1996). Regulatory processes and the development of cognitive representations. *Development and Psychopathology, 8,* 215–234.

Derryberry, D., & Rothbart, M. K. (1988). Arousal, affect, and attention as components of temperament. *Journal of Personality and Social Psychology, 55,* 958–966.

Diamond, A., & Taylor, C. (1996). Development of an aspect of executive control: Development of the abilities to remember what I said and to "Do as I say, not as I do." *Developmental Psychobiology, 29,* 315–334.

Eisenberg, N., & Fabes, R. A. (1992). Emotion, regulation, and the development of social competence. In M. S. Clark (Ed.), *Review of personality and social psychology: Vol. 14. Emotion and social behavior* (pp. 119–150). Newbury Park, CA: Sage.

Eisenberg, N., Fabes, R. A., Guthrie, I. K., Murphy, B. C., Maszk, P., Holgren, R., et al. (1996). The relations of regulation and emotionality to problem behavior in elementary school children. *Development and Psychopathology, 8,* 141–162.

Eisenberg, N., Fabes, R. A., Nyman, M., Bernzweig, J., & Pinulas, A. (1994). The relations of emotionality and regulation to children's anger-related reactions. *Child Development, 65,* 109–128.

Eisenberg, N., Guthrie, I. K., Fabes, R. A., Reiser, M., Murphy, B. C., Holgren, R., et al. (1997). The relations of regulation and emotionality to resiliency and competent social functioning in elementary school children. *Child Development, 68,* 295–311.

Eliasz, A. (2001). Temperament, type A, and motives: A time sampling study. In H. Brandstatter & A. Eliasz (Eds.), *Persons, situations, and emotions: An ecological approach* (pp. 55–73). New York: Oxford University Press.

Elliot, A. J., & Harackiewicz, J. M. (1996). Approach and avoidance achievement goals and intrinsic motivation: A mediational analysis. *Journal of Personality and Social Psychology, 70,* 461–475.

Elliot, A. J., & Thrash, T. M. (2002). Approach–avoidance motivation in personality: Approach and avoidance temperaments and goals. *Journal of Personality and Social Psychology, 82,* 804–818.

Erez, A., & Isen, A. M. (2002). The influence of positive affect on the components of expectancy motivation. *Journal of Applied Psychology, 87,* 1055–1067.

Evans, D., & Rothbart, M. K. (1998). *Relationships between self-report temperament measures and personality.* Unpublished manuscript.

Eysenck, N. (1976). *The measurement of personality.* Baltimore: University Park Press.

Fan, J., Flombaum, J. I., McCandliss, B. D., Thomas, K. M., & Posner, M. I. (2003). Cognitive and brain consequences of conflict. *NeuroImage, 18,* 42–57.

Gartstein, M. A., & Rothbart, M. K. (2003). Studying infant temperament via the revised Infant Behavior Questionnaire. *Infant Behavior and Development, 26,* 64–86.

Gerardi-Caulton, G. (2000). Sensitivity to spatial conflict and the development of self-regulation in children 24–36 months of age. *Developmental Science, 3,* 397–404.

Gest, S. D. (1997). Behavioral inhibition: Stability and associations with adaptation from childhood to early adulthood. *Journal of Personality and Social Psychology, 72,* 467–475.

Gray, J. A. (1971). *The psychology of fear and stress.* London: Weidenfeld & Nicholson.

Gray, J. A. (1981). A critique of Eysenck's theory of personality. In H. J. Eysenck (Ed.), *A model for personality* (pp. 246–276). Berlin: Springer-Verlag.

Gray, J. A., & McNaughton, N. (1996). The neuropsychology of anxiety: Reprise. In D. A. Hope (Ed.), *Nebraska Symposium on Motivation: Vol. 43. Perspectives on anxiety, panic, and fear* (pp. 61–134). Lincoln: University of Nebraska Press.

Gresham, F. M., & Elliott, S. N. (1990). *Social skills rating system.* Circle Pines, MN: American Guidance Service.

Guerin, D. W., & Gottfried, A. W. (1994). Developmental stability and change in parent reports of temperament: A ten-year longitudinal investigation from infancy through preadolescence. *Merrill–Palmer Quarterly, 40,* 334–355.

Harter, S. (1978). Effectance motivation reconsidered: Toward a developmental model. *Human Development, 21,* 34–64.

Harter, S. (1980). The development of competence motivation in the mastery of cognitive and physical skills: Is there still a place for joy? In G. C. Roberts & D. M. Landers (Eds.), *Psychology of motor behavior and sport* (pp. 3–20). Champaign, IL: Human Kinetics.

Harter, S. (1998). The development of self-representations. In W. Damon (Series Ed.) & N. Eisenberg (Vol. Ed.), *Handbook of child psychology: Vol. 3. Social, emotional and personality development* (5th ed., pp. 105–176). New York: Wiley.

Hwang, J. (1999). *Affect and sustained engagement in infancy.* Unpublished manuscript, University of Oregon, Eugene, OR.

Jung, C. G. (1928). *Contributions to analytic psychology.* New York: Harcourt Brace.

Kagan, J. (1994). *Galen's prophecy: Temperament in human nature.* New York: Basic Books.

Kagan, J. (1998). Biology and the child. In W. Damon (Series Ed.) & N. Eisenberg (Vol. Ed.), *Handbook of child psychology: Vol. 3. Social, emotional, and personality development* (5th ed., pp. 177–235). New York: Wiley.

Kagan, J., Reznick, J. S., & Snidman, N. (1988). Biological bases of childhood shyness. *Science, 240,* 167–171.

Kochanska, G. (1995). Children's temperament, mothers' discipline, and security of attachment: Multiple pathways to emerging internalization. *Child Development, 66,* 597–615.

Kochanska, G. (1997). Multiple pathways to conscience for children with different temperaments from toddlerhood to age 5. *Developmental Psychology, 3,* 228–240.

Kochanska, G., Murray, K., & Coy, K. C. (1997). Inhibitory control as a contributor to conscience in childhood: From toddler to early school age. *Child Development*, 68, 263–277.

Kochanska, G., Murray, K. T., & Harlan, E. T. (2000). Effortful control in early childhood: Continuity and change, antecedents, and implications for social development. *Developmental Psychology*, 36, 220–232.

Kochanska, G., Murray, K., Jacques, T. Y., Koenig, A. L., & Vandegeest, K. (1996). Inhibitory control in young children and its role in emerging internalization. *Child Development*, 67, 490–507.

Kopp, C. B. (1992). Emotional distress and control in young children. In N. Eisenberg & R. A. Fabes (Eds.), *Emotion and its regulation in early development: New directions for child development, No. 55* (pp. 41–56). San Francisco: Jossey-Bass.

Kremen, A. M., & Block, J. (1998). The roots of ego-control in young adulthood: Links with parenting in early childhood. *Journal of Personality and Social Psychology*, 75, 1062–1075.

Lemery, K. S., Goldsmith, H. H., Klinnert, M. D., & Mrazek, D. A. (1999). Developmental models of infant and childhood temperament. *Developmental Psychology*, 35, 189–204.

Luria, A. R. (1961). *The role of speech in the regulation of normal and abnormal behavior*. New York: Liveright.

Martin, R. P., Drew, K. D., Gaddis, L. R., & Moseley, M. (1988). Prediction of elementary school achievement from preschool temperament: Three studies. *School Psychology Review*, 17, 125–137.

McCall, R. B. (1995). On definitions and measures of mastery motivation. In R. H. MacTurk & G. A. Morgan (Eds.), *Advances in applied developmental psychology: Vol. 12. Mastery motivation: Origins, conceptualizations, and applications* (pp. 273–292). Norwood, NJ: Ablex.

Messer, D. J. (1995). Mastery motivation: Past, present, and future. In R. H. MacTurk & G. A. Morgan (Eds.), *Advances in applied developmental psychology: Vol. 12. Mastery motivation: Origins, conceptualizations, and applications* (pp. 293–316). Norwood, NJ: Ablex.

Mischel, W., Shoda, Y., & Peake, P. K. (1988). The nature of adolescent competencies predicted by preschool delay of gratification. *Journal of Personality and Social Psychology*, 54, 687–696.

Morgan, G. A., Harmon, R. J., & Maslin-Cole, P. M. (1990). Mastery motivation: Its definition and measurement. *Early Education and Development*, 1, 318–339.

Olson, S. L., Bates, J. E., Sandy, J. M., & Schilling, E. M. (2002). Early developmental precursors of impulsive and inattentive behavior: From infancy to middle childhood. *Journal of Child Psychology and Psychiatry*, 43, 435–447.

Panksepp, J. (1998). *Affective neuroscience: The foundations of human and animal emotions*. New York: Oxford University Press.

Pedlow, R., Sanson, A. V., Prior, M., & Oberklaid, F.

(1993). The stability of temperament from infancy to eight years. *Developmental Psychology*, 29, 998–1007.

Posner, M. I., & Rothbart, M. K. (1998). Attention, self-regulation, and consciousness. *Philosophical Transactions of the Royal Society of London B*, 353, 1915–1927.

Posner, M. I., & Rothbart, M. K. (2000). Developing mechanisms of self regulation. *Development and Psychopathology*, 12, 427–441.

Redding, R. E., Morgan, G. A., & Harmon, R. J. (1988). Mastery motivation in infants and toddlers: Is it greatest when tasks are moderately challenging? *Infant Behavior and Development*, 11, 419–430.

Rothbart, M. K. (1981). Measurement of temperament in infancy. *Child Development*, 52, 569–578.

Rothbart, M. K. (1986). Longitudinal observation of infant temperament. *Developmental Psychology*, 22, 356–365.

Rothbart, M. K. (1988). Temperament and the development of inhibited approach. *Child Development*, 59, 1241–1250.

Rothbart, M. K. (1989). Temperament and development. In G. Kohnstamm, J. Bates, & M. K. Rothbart (Eds.), *Temperament in childhood* (pp. 187–248). Chichester, UK: Wiley.

Rothbart, M. K., Ahadi, S. A., & Hershey, K. L. (1994). Temperament and social behavior in childhood. *Merrill–Palmer Quarterly*, 40, 21–39.

Rothbart, M. K., Ahadi, S. A., & Hershey, K. L., & Fisher, P. (2001). Investigations of temperament at three to seven years: The Children's Behavior Questionnaire. *Child Development*, 72, 1394–1408.

Rothbart, M. K., & Bates, J. E. (1998). Temperament. In W. Damon (Series Ed.) & N. Eisenberg (Vol. Ed.), *Handbook of child psychology: Vol. 3. Social, emotional and personality development* (5th ed., pp. 105–176). New York: Wiley.

Rothbart, M. K., & Derryberry, D. (1981). Development of individual differences in temperament. In M. E. Lamb & A. L. Brown (Eds.), *Advances in developmental psychology* (Vol. l, pp. 37–86). Hillsdale, NJ: Erlbaum.

Rothbart, M. K., Derryberry, D., & Hershey, K. (2000). Stability of temperament in childhood: Laboratory infant assessment to parent report at seven years. In V. J. Molfese & D. L. Molfese (Eds.), *Temperament and personality development across the life span* (pp. 85–119). Hillsdale, NJ: Erlbaum.

Rothbart, M. K., Derryberry, D., & Posner, M. I. (1994). A psychobiological approach to the development of temperament. In J. E. Bates & T. D. Wachs (Eds.), *Temperament: Individual differences at the interface of biology and behavior* (pp. 83–116). Washington, DC: American Psychological Association.

Rothbart, M. K., Ellis, L.K., Rueda, M. R., & Posner, M. I. (2003). Developing mechanisms of temperamental effortful control. *Journal of Personality*, 71, 1113–1143.

Rothbart, M. K., & Mauro, J. A. (1990). Questionnaire measures of infant temperament. In J. W. Fagen & J. Colombo (Eds.), *Individual differences in infancy: Reliability, stability and prediction* (pp. 411–429). Hillsdale, NJ: Erlbaum.

Rothbart, M. K., & Posner, M. I. (2001). Mechanism and variation in the development of attentional networks. In C. A. Nelson & M. Luciana (Eds.), *Handbook of developmental cognitive neuroscience* (pp. 353–363). Cambridge, MA: MIT Press.

Rueda, M. R., Posner, M. I., & Rothbart, M. K. (2004). Attentional control and self regulation. In R. F. Baumeister & K. D. Vohs (Eds.), *Handbook of self-regulation: Research, theory, and applications* (pp. 283–300). New York: Guilford Press.

Ruff, H. A. (1986). Components of attention during infants' manipulative exploration. *Child Development, 52,* 105–114.

Ruff, H. A., & Dubiner, K. (1987). Stability of individual differences in infants' manipulation and exploration of objects. *Perceptual and Motor Skills, 64,* 1095–1101.

Ruff, H. A., & Saltarelli, L. M. (1993). Exploratory play with objects: Basic cognitive processes and individual differences. In M. H. Bornstein & A. W. O'Reilly (Eds.), *The role of play in the development of thought: New directions for child development, No. 59* (pp. 5–16). San Francisco: Jossey-Bass.

Ruff, H. A., Saltarelli, L. M., Capozzoli, M., & Dubiner, K. (1992). The differentiation of activity in infants' exploration of objects. *Developmental Psychology, 28,* 851–861.

Ryan, R. M., Connell, J. P., & Grolnick, W. S. (1992). When achievement is not intrinsically motivated: A theory of internalization and self-regulation in school. In A. K. Boggiano & T. S. Pittman (Eds.), *Achievement and motivation: A social-developmental perspective* (pp. 167–188). New York: Cambridge University Press.

Schaffer, H. R. (1974). Cognitive components of the infant's response to strangeness. In M. Lewis & L. A. Rosenblum (Eds.), *The origins of fear* (pp. 11–24). New York: Wiley.

Schiefele, U., Krapp, A., & Winteler, A. (1992). Interest as a predictor of academic achievement: A recta-analysis of research. In K. A. Renninger, S. Hidi, & A. Krapp (Eds.), *The role of interest learning and development* (pp. 183–212). Hillsdale, NJ: Erlbaum.

Shiner, R. L. (1998). How shall we speak of children's personalities in middle childhood?: A preliminary taxonomy. *Psychological Bulletin, 124,* 308–332.

Shiner, R. L. (2000). Linking childhood personality with adaptation: Evidence for continuity and change across time into late adolescence. *Journal of Personality and Social Psychology, 78,* 310–325.

Shoda, Y., Mischel, W., & Peake, P. K. (1990). Predicting adolescent cognitive and self-regulatory competencies from preschool delay of gratification: Identifying diagnostic conditions. *Developmental Psychology, 26,* 978–986.

Spangler, G. (1989). Toddlers' everyday experiences as related to preceding mental and emotional disposition and their relationship to subsequent mental and motivational development: A short-term longitudinal study. *International Journal of Behavioral Development, 12,* 258–303.

Strelau, J. (1975). Reactivity and activity style in selected occupations. *Polish Psychological Bulletin, 6,* 199–206.

Strelau, J. (1983). *Temperament personality activity.* New York: Academic Press.

Tellegen, A. (1985). Structures of mood and personality and their relevance to assessing anxiety, with an emphasis on self-report. In A. H. Tuma & J. Maser (Eds.), *Anxiety and the anxiety disorders* (pp. 681–706). Hillsdale, NJ: Erlbaum.

Thomas, A., & Chess, S. (1977). *Temperament and development.* New York: Brunner/Mazel.

Thomas, A., Chess, S., Birch, H. G., Hertzig, M. E., & Korn, S. (1963). *Behavioral individuality in early childhood.* New York: New York University Press.

Vasey, M. W., Daleiden, E. L., Williams, L. L., & Brown, L. M. (1995). Biased attention in childhood anxiety disorders: A preliminary study. *Journal of Abnormal Child Psychology, 23,* 267–279.

Watson, D., & Clark, L. A. (1993). Behavioral disinhibition versus constraint: A dispositional perspective. In D. M. Wegner & J. W. Pennebaker (Eds.), *Handbook of mental control* (pp. 506–527). Englewood Cliffs, NJ: Prentice-Hall.

White, R. W. (1959). Motivation reconsidered: The concept of competence. *Psychological Review, 66,* 297–333.

White, R. W. (1963). Ego and reality in psychoanalytic theory. *Psychological Issues, 3,* 1–210.

White, R. W. (1978). Strategies of adaptation: An attempt at systematic description. In L. R. Allman & D. T. Jaffe (Eds.), *Readings in adult psychology: Contemporary perspectives* (pp. 28–40). New York: Harper & Row.

Zuckerman, M. (1991). *Psychobiology of personality.* New York: Cambridge University Press.

CHAPTER 11

ℭℛ

The Development
of Self-Conscious Emotions

MICHAEL LEWIS
MARGARET WOLAN SULLIVAN

By the second and third years of life, young children show a wide range of emotional behaviors and facial expressions. From these observable surface changes in face, gaze, body, voice, and activity, children's emotions can be inferred. Because emotional behavior, including facial expressions, is present from birth or shortly thereafter, and because young children may not spontaneously or easily mask or inhibit their emotional behaviors and expressions, observable behaviors provide important clues to children's emotional state and, therefore, their motivation. Based on these expressions and behaviors, as well as on children's cognitive development, we have suggested that by 3 years of age, the full complement of human emotions exists, although emotional experience, and possibly emotional state, is likely to become more elaborated throughout life (Lewis, 1992; Lewis & Michalson, 1983).

In this chapter, we are concerned with young children's emotional development with regard to the self-conscious evaluative emotions, in particular, of shame, embarrassment, and pride. Individual differences in these particular emotions are related to individual differences in children's self-cognitions, including their beliefs about themselves, their performance, and ultimately, their competence. While the self-conscious evaluative emotions may not be unique to the human species, in humans, these self-conscious evaluative emotions have an important role in children's motivation, social competence, and adjustment. The chapter begins with our working model of emotional development, followed by a discussion of some sources of individual variation in the self-conscious evaluative emotions. Finally, we present some data on the relation of self-conscious evaluative emotions to self-cognitions related to performance appraisals, including attributions about personal success and failure.

A MODEL OF
EMOTIONAL DEVELOPMENT

In the model we have articulated, the human emotions emerge by age 3 (see Figure 11.1). The initial emotions, sometimes referred to

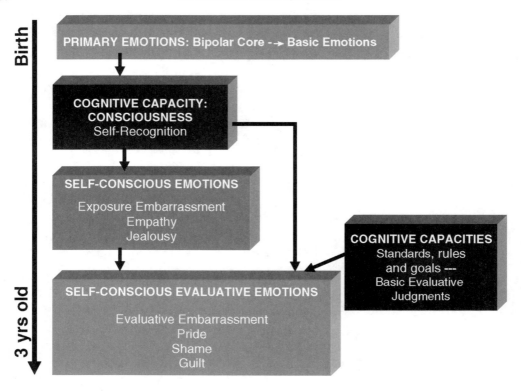

FIGURE 11.1. A model of the development of human emotions from birth to age 3, showing the influence of cognitive capacities on the development of self-conscious emotions.

as primary or basic emotions, either exist at birth or appear within the first half-year of life. With the emergence of consciousness, the first class of self-conscious emotions appear; we have labeled them the "self-conscious exposure emotions." These include empathy, jealousy, and exposure embarrassment. Following further cognitive growth, the second class of self-conscious evaluative emotions appears. These evaluative emotions include shame, guilt, and pride. This sequence in emotional development is supported by the development of a variety of emerging cognitive capacities.

The Primary Emotions

Since there is no language in this period, emotion expressions and behaviors, observed in context, are used to infer emotional states (Lewis, 1992; Lewis & Michalson, 1983). Following Bridges (1932), Lewis and Michalson (1983) assumed that the newborn has a bipolar emo-

tional life. At one extreme, there is generalized negative affect or distress, marked by crying, a variety of negative facial expressions, irritability, and nonresponsiveness to environmental stimulation. At the other extreme, there is contentment, marked by satiation and responsiveness to the environment. From the beginning of life, quiet attention—or receptivity to stimulation of low-to-moderate intensity—is present when the infant is awake. Interest expressions are the most common expressions of infants and adults, because the central nervous system appears to rest or "idle" in this mildly positive, awake, and potentially receptive state (Cacioppo & Gardner, 1999). We choose to separate this interest state from the positive and negative states, resulting in a tripartite division, with pleasure, distress, and interest as separate dimensions. From this core set comes the set of early emotions called primary or basic by Izard (1978) and Tomkins (1962, 1963). These include joy, sadness, surprise, anger, and fear. Each of these emotions has a characteristic set of facial movements, which are displayed early in life.

In most, if not all, of the basic emotions, cognitive processes have a role, although the amount and level of processing is limited. In the case of joy, sadness, and surprise, the recognition of the familiar versus the novel, or at least change from the expected, seems to be required. Since the time of Darwin (1872/1965), anger has been associated with unique action patterns designed to overcome an obstacle to a goal (Lewis, Alessandri, & Sullivan, 1990). This implies that anger requires the ability to perceive some relation between an action and a goal, a skill described as means–ends understanding (Piaget, 1952). Fear, as previously discussed, requires memory, the ability to make comparisons, and possibly prior experience of threat, although some fears may be innate (Ohman & Mineka, 2003). Thus, while some cognitive processes play a role in eliciting basic emotions, they will play a major and critical role in the class of emotions that we have called the self-conscious emotions (Lewis, 1992; Lewis & Michalson, 1983; Lewis, Sullivan, Stanger, & Weiss, 1989).

The Self-Conscious Emotions

The critical cognitive development underpinning the emergence of all self-conscious emotions is objective self-awareness, or explicit consciousness. The emergence of this skill relies on a new cognitive capacity, one that Lewis (1992, 2003) calls "explicit consciousness," or the mental state of "me." The emergence of explicit consciousness is indexed by self-referential behavior, such as the use of the personal pronouns "my," "me," or "mine," mirror self-recognition, and pretend play (Lewis & Ramsay, 1999). Self-referential capacity emerges sometime in the second half of the second year of life, typically between 15 and 24 months of age (Lewis & Brooks-Gunn, 1979). Explicit consciousness gives rise to a new class of emotions, which is called the "self-conscious emotions." These include self-conscious exposure emotions such as embarrassment, envy, and empathy, as well as the class of self-conscious evaluative emotions (Lewis, 1992). Although there is limited work on the development of the self-conscious emotions, Lewis et al. (1989) have shown that this

class of emotions emerges only after self-recognition appears. The observation of self-conscious emotions requires the presence of not only a facial expression but also bodily and vocal behavior. In Darwin's analysis, blushing was a species-specific physiological response indicating self-consciousness. Blushing, however, may occur with any of these self-conscious emotions; conversely, these emotions may occur without blushing. Whereas the primary emotions can be observed in unique facial configurations, none of the self-conscious emotions has a unique facial expression. For example, exposure embarrassment, the earliest self-conscious emotion, is indexed by partially suppressed or tense smiling or giggling, indirect or recursive eye contact, and anxious touching of the face and body (Lewis et al., 1989; Lewis & Ramsay, 1999).

Thus, by 3 years of age, the emotional life of the child has become highly differentiated, complex, and includes the self-conscious emotions (Lewis, 1992). While the emotional life of the 3-year-old will continue to grow and be sculpted by further socialization, the basic elements of human emotional life are in place. In particular, the self-conscious evaluative emotions, reflecting the child's self-appraisals of competence, are important motivators of behavior.

Self-Conscious Exposure Emotions

When consciousness emerges, emotions related to attending to oneself become possible. Emotions that require this cognitive capacity, but not self-evaluation, constitute this class of self-conscious emotions. For example, *embarrassment* emerges and can be seen as early as 15 months. However, there are two forms of embarrassment: exposure and evaluative embarrassment (Lewis, 1992; Lewis & Ramsay, 2002). Exposure embarrassment emerges first, while evaluative embarrassment appears later. Exposure embarrassment occurs only after self-recognition and appears in contexts characterized by being the object of others' attention (Lewis, Stanger, Sullivan, & Barone, 1991; Lewis et al., 1989). Lewis et al. (1991) have shown that being praised lavishly, pointed at, or asked to perform for others all elicit exposure embarrassment provided that self-recognition has emerged. Interestingly, exposure embarrassment does not lead to increases in stress. Evaluative embarrassment, however, does. Cortisol, a stress-related hormone, increases when children show embarrassment caused by the evaluation of their behavior. Evaluative embarrassment may be a mild form of shame (Lewis, 2000; Lewis & Ramsay, 2002).

Empathy, too, emerges only after objective self-recognition (Bischof-Kohler, 1991; Halperin, 1989). What appears to be empathy earlier may be only the eliciting of an emotion through contagion; for example, the sound of an infant crying prompts another infant also to cry. Only after children achieve consciousness can they understand how another is feeling, because they can put themselves in the role of the other. Jealousy has not been studied extensively, but it appears to emerge at about the time of self-recognition (Lewis & Michalson, 1983).

Self-Conscious Evaluative Emotions

Figure 11.1 shows that a second class of self-conscious emotions emerges between ages 24 and 30 months. These later emerging self-conscious emotions require additional, more elaborate sets of cognitive capacities, all of which involve evaluation of one's behavior, thus the name, self-conscious *evaluative* emotions. These emotions require capacities that include the ability to acquire and remember standards, rules, and goals (SRGs) to evaluate one's actions and behavior with reference to them, and to make judgments about personal responsibility for success and failure. This new set of skills has profound implications for not only emotional development but also competence, since these skills provide the emotional backdrop for learning, achievement, and making one's way in the world (Stipek, Recchia, & McClintic, 1992). The capacity to evaluate one's own behavior against a standard gives rise to the self-evaluative emotions, including pride, shame, guilt, and others. These emotions serve to motivate children's subsequent behavior, thus promoting further competence. For example, the ability to feel pride motivates the child to work harder to reexperience this emotion. In contrast, shame, guilt, and embarrassment motivate the child to alter his or her behavior and possibly to become avoidant of peo-

ple and situations that may elicit this emotion. Because the nature of the child's evaluation is critical to the emotion elicited, we must consider the nature of these processes.

The self-conscious evaluative emotions require a set of cognitive capacities, including the ability to evaluate one's behavior positively or negatively in regard to learned SRGs, to attribute responsibility for an outcome, and to focus attention on global versus specific aspects of the self. We define each of these evaluative processes briefly, ending with our model of how they are related to the four major evaluative emotions.

SRGs are the information children acquire about expected behavior through their socialization in a particular society. They will vary even within societies, among families and social groups, across time, and among individuals of different ages. By the second year of life, children show rudimentary understanding about "good" and "bad" behaviors, suggesting that learning of SRGs is under way (Heckhausen, 1984; Kagan, 1981; Stipek et al., 1992). SRGs may be learned in many ways, such as observation of others' behavior, or more directly by explicit statements that parents or others make about what they expect of the child in a certain context. When children compare their behavior to a learned standard, rule, or goal, there are two possibilities: success (i.e., positive relative to SRGs) or failure (i.e., negative relative to SRGs). If the child evaluates his or her behavior relative to a standard and finds that it equals or exceeds the standard, he or she judges the behavior as successful. Likewise, if the behavior is less than the standard, the child judges him- or herself as failing.

Another determination is whether the child believes that he or she is responsible for the success or failure. In the adult attribution literature, perceptions of personal responsibility for events are thought of as either internal or external attributions (Weiner, 1986). Similarly, among young children, internal attributions are those by which the child "owns" and feels responsible, whereas external attributions are those by which the child does not feel responsible.

The child can also focus on whether the outcome is due to global or specific features of the self (Beck, 1979; Lewis, 1992). Dweck (1996) has referred to this dimension as motivational dispositions of "performance" as opposed to "learning orientation." Global attributions refer to the tendency of an individual to focus on the total, unchanging self when making an evaluative judgment. Thus, for any behavior, some individuals, some of the time, are likely to focus on the self and to make trait-like statements such as "I did this because I am bad (or good)." On such occasions, the focus of the judgment is on the total self, both as object and subject. This type of total self-focus is particularly damaging, because there is no way out. The focus is not on the individual's behavior in a particular place and time (a specific, unstable attribution), but on the self's global worth. In contrast, specific attributions refer to the tendency of some individuals, some of the time, to focus on the particular actions that led to success or failure in that place and time. Specific attributions usually make reference to unstable factors. In this case, it is not the total self that has done something wrong or wonderful; instead, particular behaviors in a particular situation are blamed (Janoff-Bulman, 1979). At such times, individuals will make such statements as "What I did was wrong, and I must not do it again." The focus in such a statement is on the self's specific behavior with objects or persons and the effect of these actions.

Thus, to express self-evaluative emotions the child must have the ability to evaluate behavior in relation to SRGs, the ability to assume responsibility for success or failure, and to assess whether their success or failure is likely to be due to global, stable aspects of the self, or specific, changeable circumstances. The nature of these three evaluative judgments is the critical elicitor of self-conscious evaluative emotions.

A STRUCTURAL MODEL OF FOUR SELF-CONSCIOUS EVALUATIVE EMOTIONS

Figure 11.2 presents our structural model, identifying the judgments that serve as the elicitor for each of the four self-evaluative states (Lewis, 1992). We emphasize that this model is symmetrical with regard to positive and negative self-evaluative emotions, in that it accounts for not only shame and guilt

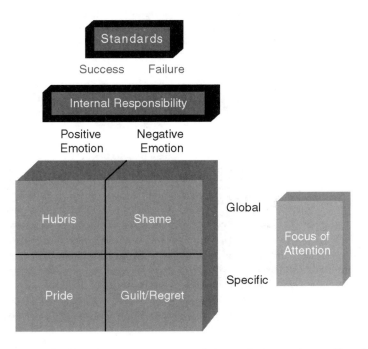

FIGURE 11.2. A model of self-evaluative processes and their relation to four self-evaluative emotions: hubris, shame, pride, and guilt.

in response to failure but also pride and hubris, sometimes called alpha and beta pride (Tangney, Wagner, & Gramzow, 1992) in response to success. It also proposes that the immediate elicitors of specific self-evaluative emotions are the quality of self-related attributions. Given the three sets of judgments shown in Figure 11.2, the model accounts for and distinguishes among four self-conscious evaluative emotional states. The immediate elicitors of these emotions are the cognitive, self-evaluative processes described. A detailed description of the four emotions and how their phenomenology and action patterns are related to each of the judgments in the structural model follows.

Shame is the product of the self's evaluation of its actions in regard to SRGs and a global attribution. This emotion is a consequence of a failure when the person accepts responsibility for failure and there is a global focus on the self. Shame can occur in response to either failed moral actions or poor achievement (Lewis, 1992). The phenomenological experience of a shamed person is a desire to hide, disappear, or die. It is a highly negative, painful state that results in the disruption of ongoing behavior, confusion in thought, and inability to speak (H. B. Lewis, 1971). This is because it is a global indictment of the self. The action tendency accompanying shame is a shrinking of the body, as though to hide oneself from the view of others, and the lowering of head and gaze, away from social contact. Because of the intensity of this emotional state and the global negative evaluation of the self, all that someone can do when shamed is attempt somehow to be rid of it. However, people have great difficulty dissipating this emotion, and such attempts often will result in maladaptive behavior (see Lewis, 1992).

Guilt/regret also occurs in response to accepting personal responsibility for a failure, but it is not as intensely negative as shame, because, with guilt, the focus of attention is on the individual's specific actions that resulted in the failure. Because the focus of attention in guilt is on specific behaviors, individuals can rid themselves of this emotion through reparative action. Rectification of the failure and prevention of a future reoccurrence are the two possible corrective paths that individuals can choose. Thus, guilt is not the self-destroying emotion that

shame is. From a phenomenological view, individuals are distressed by the failure, but this feeling is directed to the specific cause or object of the harm. The facial and gaze behaviors may be similar to shame, but guilt is not associated with withdrawal or avoidance. It does not lead to confusion and to loss of action. In fact, guilt is associated with corrective action that the individual might (but may not necessarily) take. Whereas in shame, the body is hunched over itself and immobilized, in guilt, individuals typically increase their movements, as if trying to repair the action (Cole, Barrett, & Zahn-Waxler, 1992). The marked postural differences that accompany guilt and shame are helpful both in distinguishing these emotions and in measuring individual differences.

A parallel set of processes exists for positive self-conscious evaluative emotions. When success is perceived and the child assumes internal responsibility for it, a global focus on the self leads to hubris, or arrogant pridefulness. Hubris is a highly positive and self-rewarding state; that is, the person feels extremely good about him- or herself. In this emotion, individuals are often described as "puffed-up," "full of themselves," or even conceited, insolent, or contemptuous. In extreme cases, hubris is associated with grandiosity or with narcissism (Morrison, 1989). Although hubris constitutes high reward for the person experiencing it, this emotion is unpleasant for others and, therefore, socially undesirable. Hubristic people have difficulty in their interpersonal relations, since their hubris is likely to interfere with the wishes, needs, and desires of others, leading to interpersonal conflict and possibly performance deficits. For example, too much praise of children, and the resulting overly high self-esteem, can lead to negative performance (Baumeister, Campbell, Kreuger, & Vohs, 2003; Kamins & Dweck, 1999; Mueller & Dweck, 1998). The presumed mechanism in this case might be that excessive pride leads to less effort due to an enhancement of hubris in children so treated. Three problems associated with hubris are that (1) it is a transient but addictive emotion; (2) it is unrelated to any specific action and, thus, requires altering goals or reinterpretation of what constitutes success; and (3) it interferes with interpersonal relationships because of its insolent and contemptuous nature.

Pride is the consequence of accepting responsibility for a specific, successful action. The phenomenological experience is joy about an action, thought, or feeling well done. The focus of pleasure is specific and related to a particular behavior. In pride, the self and object are separated, as in guilt, and the person focuses attention on the behavior leading to success. Some investigators have likened this state to achievement motivation (Heckhausen, 1984; Stipek et al., 1992), an association that seems particularly apt. This form of pride should be related to achievement constructs, such as "efficacy" or "mastery" feelings, and "personal satisfaction." Because positive self-evaluative emotion is associated with a particular action, individuals can identify the means by which they can recreate this rewarding state at a future date.

OTHER ATTRIBUTION–EMOTION MODELS

The idea that beliefs and attributions about personal behaviors are related to emotion has been proposed by others, although, in the past, models have been developed primarily for adults and older children, typically with regard to achievement behavior and emotion (see, e.g., Nolen-Hoeksema, Girgus, & Seligman, 1992). We briefly consider two of these other models, pointing out similarities to our structural model of self-conscious evaluative emotion.

Attribution Models of Emotion

Attributions refer to the specific causal thoughts people have about why a success or failure occurred (Weiner, 1972, 1986). Emotions, including those we have called self-conscious, as well as others, are elicited because adults and older children ascribe success or failure to causes with certain properties or dimensions. Causes vary along at least three major, orthogonal dimensions: locus of responsibility, stability, and controllability (Weiner & Graham, 1989). The locus of responsibility dimension is similar to our responsibility dimension. It refers to whether the cause of an event is internal or external to the self. Ability and effort are the

classic internal attributions, whereas task difficulty and luck are considered external to the individual. The stability dimension makes reference to whether a cause varies over time. Ability, for example, is considered in Weiner's (1986) model to be a constant and, therefore, stable factor. Likewise, task difficulty is thought to be a stable feature of any given task. In contrast, effort and luck are unstable and vary with place and time. Controllability has to do with whether the individual can personally affect the outcome. Effort attributions are unstable and under personal control, whereas luck attributions are unstable and generally perceived by most adults as something that they cannot personally influence. Other attribution dimensions, for example, the global or specific nature of a cause, have also been proposed and studied, particularly in relation to depression (Beck, 1979; Nolen-Hoeksema, Wolfson, Mumme, & Guskin, 1995; Seligman, 1975). Global attributions imply that the cause of success or failure is pervasive and catastrophic; thus, global attributions tend to be self-perpetuating and maladaptive (H. B. Lewis, 1987).

In the attribution model, as in our own, each attribution is uniquely related to a particular set of emotions and behaviors. The emotions studied in relation to attributions include achievement-related emotions, especially pride and guilt, but anger, gratitude, and sympathy are also elicited by specific causal attributions in adults. In particular, internal locus has been shown to be important to pride, and controllability to be important to guilt (Weiner & Graham, 1989). Although the model is quite broad, it has not been tested extensively with regard to young children's self-conscious emotions, in part, because traditional methods for assessing attribution are highly verbal and inappropriate for young children, and because the model ascribes no special status to these emotions.

Dweck's Motivational Model

In very young children, perceptions of ability have been studied as motivational dispositions and self-beliefs (Dweck, 1991). Children's evaluative judgments in achievement and social behavior have been studied as reflecting individual differences in an orientation toward performance or situational factors when making evaluations (i.e., performance vs. learning orientation) (Dweck, 1991; Dweck, Chiu, & Hong, 1995; Smiley & Dweck, 1995). In this work, young children's beliefs about the nature of ability result in tendencies to judge themselves in particular ways. Performance-oriented children, those who focus on "how I did," tend to blame themselves for doing badly; believe that ability is a stable, unchanging trait; experience more negative affect; and are less confident that they can succeed at challenging tasks in the future. In other words, performance-oriented children view failure as the result of an incompetent, stable self. In contrast, children with a learning orientation, those who focus on "what I did," tend to not experience failures so negatively, do not blame themselves, and are more confident that they can succeed at similar tasks in the future. They are more likely to believe that ability is "what you learn" with time and experience. Thus, these motivational dispositions appear to capture the responsibility dimension, as well as the focus of attention, described in our model.

Like our model, Dweck's rests on the idea that what children think about their performance determines their responses rather than the success or failure per se. An interesting developmental difference is highlighted by Dweck, in contrast to adult attribution models. While Weiner's (1986) model holds that an ability attribution is both internal and stable, Dweck has shown that children can perceive ability as either stable or modifiable. According to Dweck, it is individual differences in the quality of these beliefs about ability that produce individual differences in children's goals and behaviors in achievement contexts. We would argue that the nature of emotion is also affected.

Children who believe that ability is a fixed, stable quality are more likely to adopt a performance-oriented motivational style, characterized by a concern about how others evaluate them, and a strong desire to perform successfully and to avoid failure; that is, they have a global focus. On the other hand, children who believe that ability can be increased are more likely to adopt a learning-oriented motivational style. They will strive to increase their competence through experience and effort, will focus on

task mastery, and will be less concerned with immediate performance outcomes.

In our view, a performance orientation is consistent with, and perhaps an early form of, a stable and global attribution. Thus, Dweck's (1996) motivational constructs may measure one or more aspects of emerging attribution processes important to the expression of shame and pride. Performance versus learning orientation appears to index whether children focus globally on their performance and make global trait-like judgments about themselves as opposed to situational or task factors. Consequently, performance-orientation should be related to shame, whereas learning orientation (or what we have called a task focus) should not.

SOURCES OF INDIVIDUAL DIFFERENCES IN SELF-CONSCIOUS EVALUATIVE EMOTIONS

Individual differences in self-conscious emotions appear as early as objective awareness and self-referential behavior emerge. There are at least two major sources of individual differences in self-evaluative emotions. The first is constitutional and has to do with temperament, while the second source of difference is in the socialization process.

Temperament

Temperament involves biological tendencies to regulate the latency, duration, and intensity of emotional responses (Lewis, 1989; Rothbart & Goldsmith, 1985). Investigators differ regarding the number of temperament dimensions, with some suggesting as few as three (Buss & Plomin, 1984), and others as many as nine (Thomas & Chess, 1977). There is evidence that differences in temperament are related to various self-conscious emotions in children (Kochanska, 1995; Kochanska, Coy, & Murray, 2001; Kochanska, DeVet, Goldman, Murray, & Putnam, 1994). Recent analyses suggest that temperament involves individual differences in the tendency to express positive, as well as negative, emotion and differences in reactivity level (Ramsay & Lewis, 2001; Rothbart, Ahadi, & Hershey, 1994). These aspects of temperament are related to self-consciousness and evaluative emotions. For example, higher anger and fearfulness are associated with later guilt (Rothbart et al., 1994). Exposure embarrassment at 13 months is related to having a difficult or more negative temperament in infancy (Lewis & Ramsay, 1997).

Reactivity to stress is an important aspect of temperament that is related to negative self-evaluation, such that higher cortisol responses to stress are associated with greater expression of evaluative embarrassment and shame (Lewis & Ramsay, 1997, 2002). Collectively, these findings suggest that greater stress reactivity is related to greater levels of self-evaluative emotion generally, and evaluative embarrassment and shame in particular, through its relation to self-focus. Individual differences in self-focus may arise in part because of a lower threshold for pain and an inability to gate or block such internal physiological signals. The result is more attention directed toward the self and, thus, more consciousness (Csikszentmihalyi, 1990). Lewis and Ramsay (1997) have proposed that greater stress reactivity leads to greater self-awareness and attention to the self. Following failures, this greater self-focus increases the likelihood that children will attribute negative outcomes internally to the self, rather than externally to the task or situation, thereby increasing the tendency toward shame and/or evaluative embarrassment. Thus, aspects of temperament influence the tendency toward self-focus, which in turn promotes self-conscious evaluative emotion.

Socialization

Socialization can influence individual differences in the self-conscious emotions in many different ways, including influences on the acquisition of SRGs, internal focus of responsibility, and global versus specific focus of attention. The methods used to teach SRGs, how children are rewarded and punished, influence children's style of self-evaluation and, therefore, their proneness to self-conscious evaluative emotion.

Learning Standards, Rules, and Goals

The nature of SRGs themselves—and what constitutes success or failure—varies with

individuals. Exactly how one comes to evaluate an action, thought, or feeling as a success or a failure is not well understood. Yet this aspect of self-evaluation is particularly important, because the same SRG can result in radically different emotions, depending on whether success or failure is perceived and attributed to the self. Differences in SRGs within a societal group and between cultures will occur, because groups within a society and different cultures value some SRGs more than others. The initial evaluation of one's behavior in terms of success and failure is also a very important aspect of the organization of plans and the determination of new goals and future expectations of success and failure. Many factors are involved in producing idiosyncratic, unrealistic evaluations of performance relative to SRGs. High standards, however, may not themselves necessarily be bad. Instead, extremes of punishment and the quality of the discipline produce individual differences. Harsh socialization experiences, especially high levels of physical punishment for failure and the use of scorn, humiliation, or contempt as discipline techniques, may also affect the quality of SRGs and how behaviors that meet or violate them are viewed (Lewis, 1992).

Acquiring an Attribution Style

Among adults, as well as children, people may differ in the tendency to attribute failure or success to themselves. Instead, they may explain their performance in terms of chance or the actions of others (Seligman et al., 1984; Weiner, 1972). The tendency to make internal as opposed to external attribution is a function of both learning and individual characteristics. Certain inductive parenting styles are related to greater internal attributions (Ferguson & Stegge, 1995). However, some individuals are more likely to blame themselves for failure (or, alternatively, to take credit for success), no matter what happens. Dweck and Leggett (1988) found that many children attributed their academic successes and failures to external forces, although some were likely to evaluate their success and failure in terms of their own personal actions, even at young ages. In fact, the tendency to make internal attributions may be greater in young children generally, due to their greater egocentrism.

Individual differences in evaluative style can be observed even in young children. Dweck et al. (1995) showed that somewhere between ages 3 and 6, differences in perceptions of personal performance emerge and are consistent. Once learned, these early motivational dispositions eventually may become entrenched as a personality or attribution style, especially in response to negative events (Kaslow, Rehm, Pollack, & Segal, 1988). Strong negative events occurring early in children's lives seem to push children toward a global attribution style in a kind of one-trial learning; that is, children exposed to such events will more consistently make global attributions than others under most conditions of failure. Their attributions made in response to success are less likely to be predictable. The intensity and power of negative events acting on a child with still-limited coping skills may promote this development. Strong negative emotion swamps any cognitive processing that might override the child's egocentric perceptions about the event. Because the child cannot separate him- or herself from the failure, the child internalizes blame and focuses on the global self. The range of negative life events that leads to global attributions is in need of further investigation. These may include negative experiences with parents, with others in the immediate social environment, or with general calamities that impact on the self, family, or others. However, a reasonable working hypothesis is that the global attribution style of failure is created in the cauldron of stress (Lewis, 1992).

Sex differences have been widely reported in internal, global attribution styles for negative events. Our own study of parental response to children's performance on academic tasks reveals that both mothers and fathers make significantly more specific positive attributions to boys than to girls (Alessandri & Lewis, 1993). Specific positive feedback (e.g., "That's a good way of getting the piece [of the puzzle] into the box") was higher for 3-year-old boys than for 3-year-old girls. Conversely, specific negative feedback (e.g., "You didn't look for the biggest piece first") was higher for girls. Fathers made more specific attributions than

mothers. Mothers and fathers both made more specific attributions to boys than girls. Similar sex differences have been reported by others (c.f., Deaux, 1976; Dweck & Leggett, 1988; Nicholls, 1984). These findings support the notion that a major cause of the attribution style differences observed in boys and girls is such socialization patterns.

The tendency toward a particular attribution style for failure can also be learned or further consolidated at school (Graham, 1991). During the elementary school years, teachers are likely to exert considerable influence on children's attribution styles, particularly around achievement. How teachers describe and react to children's actions contribute to their emerging styles and likely influences many of the sex differences observed in achievement-related attributions in later childhood. Most of the criticism that teachers direct at elementary school boys refers to specific instances of misbehavior or lack of effort, task-specific factors, rather than to negative personality traits or lack of ability. Such feedback patterns promote specific and controllable as opposed to nonglobal or uncontrollable attributions. In girls, the opposite pattern is observed. Despite the fact that girls, on average, do better in elementary school than boys, girls are more likely to attribute failures to their lack of ability, a global factor. Dweck and Leggett (1988) viewed the teachers' use of evaluative feedback as a direct cause of learned helplessness or mastery orientation in children. They report that teachers' criticisms of girls, in contrast to boys, almost always indicated that they lacked general competence or did not understand the work, both global attributions. Thus, there is ample reason to expect sex differences in attribution styles based on the consistent pattern of sex differences observed during early socialization and the school years.

Although information on sex differences constitutes much of what we know about the socialization of attribution styles at home and in school, biological factors that covary with sex cannot be completely ruled out in accounting for some of these differences. For example, some have linked a global attribution style to the perceptual/cognitive style of field dependence. Field independence–dependence refers to the ability to separate a perceived object from the context in which it is embedded (H. B. Lewis, 1976; Witkin, 1965). Sex differences in the tendency to ruminate or engage in recursive self-refection have also been reported and are related to a depression-prone attribution style (Nolen-Hoeksema et al., 1995). In general, as noted earlier, females are more likely to make self-blaming, global attributions for their failures and to attribute their success to external causes, whereas men are more likely to show the opposite attribution style.

PRESCHOOLERS' ATTRIBUTIONS AND THEIR RELATION TO SELF-CONSCIOUS EVALUATIVE EMOTIONS

Our model suggests that particular evaluative patterns have an impact on children's emotional life, and it has been shown that children's beliefs influence their achievement behaviors and motivation, even though they may not yet make adult-like attributions. How, then, can young children's emerging evaluative emotions or attribution styles be assessed? Paper-and-pencil methods developed for older children and adults are inappropriate with young children. In the following section, we describe measurement procedures useful in obtaining individual differences in children's focus of attention (performance vs. task focus) and how such differences are related to other kinds of evaluative judgments, and, finally, their relation to some self-conscious evaluative emotions.

Measuring Performance versus Task Focus

Dweck et al. (1995) obtained performance orientation by asking children to work on both solvable and unsolvable tasks. Afterward, she assessed their choice to avoid or return to the unsolved task. Children who choose to avoid the unsolved task and choose a task on which they know they have succeeded are considered performance-oriented. Their choice of a "sure success" suggests a motive to avoid "a display of incompetence." We have developed another method that works well and can be used

with children as young as 3 years old (Lewis, Alessandri, & Sullivan, 1992). In our own work, we present children with easy and difficult tasks. "Easy" and "difficult" are defined by the number of pieces in the problem that children are given to work on in a given time period. We also vary whether they succeed or fail on these tasks by manipulating the time they are given to complete them. In this way, children get easy and difficult tasks on which they succeed or fail. After each task, we ask children whether the task was easy or difficult. Our interest is in the easy task on which they fail. Their response of "easy" or "hard" in the easy, failed task informs us about whether they are making a performance- or a task-based evaluation. If they state that it was "hard" (even though in reality it was easy), they are focusing on their performance, which was a failure. If they say "easy," they are focusing on the task despite their own performance. Thus, the easy, failed task presents the child with a discrepancy between what he or she expects (to do well when it is easy) and the outcome. The response reveals whether the child focuses attention globally on personal performance or specifically on the quality of the task. Our hypothesis is that these judgments in response to the easy, failed task should predict other self-related evaluations, as well as the expression of self-conscious evaluative emotions.

Task versus Performance Focus and Their Relation to Other Responses to Failure

If children's task versus performance focus, as measured here, is related to other self-evaluations on our achievement tasks, it will support the validity of this new measure. We used a number of methods to test how task- versus performance-focused children viewed failure. To obtain other self-evaluations, after each task, we asked children (1) whether they had done "good or not so good," and (2) whether they would be willing to do the task again. Performance-focused children were twice as likely as task-focused children to say that they had not done well (see Figure 11.3a). We have replicated this result in several studies of 4- to 6-year-old children.

Figure 11.3b shows how children re-

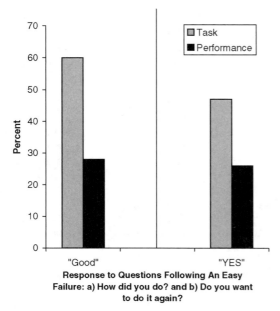

FIGURE 11.3. Children's responses to evaluative questions by task versus performance focus: (a) percentage stating their performance following failure was "good," and (b) percentage of "yes" responses expressing a desire to repeat the failed task.

sponded when asked whether they would like to do the task again. As can be seen, task-focused children were more likely to want to try the task again. Conversely, performance-focused children did not want to try again, replicating Dweck's findings that these children are motivated to avoid failure. To examine the consistency of self-related judgments to task versus performance focus, we combined responses to these two questions to produce four groups of children: those who said "good" and "yes" when asked to do the task again; those who said "good" and "no"; those who said "not good" and "yes"; and those who said "not good" and "no." Those who said both that they had done badly and that they did not want to do the task again were more likely to be performance-focused compared to all other groups (see Figure 11.4). Collectively, these findings show that a performance focus following the easy failed task is related to a variety of negative self-judgments following failure and to a motive for task avoidance.

Are these self-reported evaluations related to how children feel following failure? If performance focus reflects an internalized negative and global focus of attention, we would expect performance-focused children to say they feel unhappy. To assess children's verbal report of their feelings, we used a version of Dweck's Happy Face Scale. The pictorial scale has five schematic faces representing high positive emotion on one end and negative feelings on the other. The size of the smile or inverted U-frown allows children to point out the degree of happiness or unhappiness, ranging from very happy, a little happy, OK, in the middle, a little unhappy, to very unhappy. We asked the children to rate "how you feel right now" using this scale. The children's self-reports of unhappiness following the easy failed task were related to their performance focus. Children who were performance- as opposed to task-focused were significantly more likely to report greater sadness ($p < .01$). Collectively, these findings parallel a number of the features of the performance-oriented motivational style described by Dweck and colleagues (1995), supporting the view that performance focus is a negative self-evaluation related to global trait-like judgments following failure.

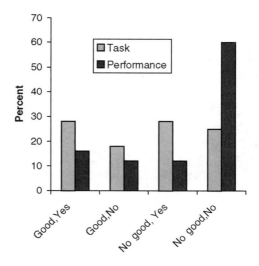

FIGURE 11.4. Children's "good vs. not good" evaluations in combination with desire to repeat the easy, failed task as a function of task versus performance focus.

Performance Focus and Self-Conscious Evaluative Emotions

We believe certain self-attributions or self-references lead to certain classes of self-conscious emotions. We have studied preschool children's behavioral expression of emotion following success and failure, relating it to their tendency to be task- or performance-focused. We expected that performance-focused children would show more shame than task-focused children. They also might show more pride following success, although this prediction was more tentative, because it is not possible to distinguish between hubris and more appropriate pride behaviorally at this age. The effect of performance focus on self-conscious evaluative emotions observed in two studies is shown in Figure 11.5. A greater percentage of performance- as opposed to task-focused children showed the negative self-evaluative emotions of shame and evaluative embarrassment following failure in both studies. Performance-focused children also showed more pride following success, especially in Study 2. There was no difference in the percentage or mean level of children expressing simple enjoyment and sadness in these studies. Collectively, the findings show that performance focus is related to more negative emotions in response to failure and somewhat more positive responses to success than is task focus.

This set of studies shows that children's task versus performance focus following failure at an easy task is related to other simple, evaluative judgments about their personal performance and to their self-conscious evaluative emotions. The consistency of children's answers to simple questions about an easy failed task can be examined to determine the degree to which they focus on the self when thinking about the failure. A performance focus, or attending to performance as opposed to task features following failure, is related to thinking poorly of oneself and being unwilling to try again, feeling badly, and to being more likely to show shame and evaluative embarrassment following failure. This pattern of negative self-judgments might represent the early precursors of the internal, stable, global attribution styles observed in older children and adults.

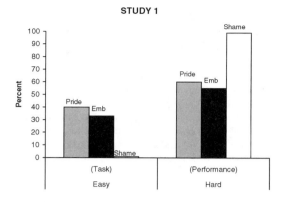

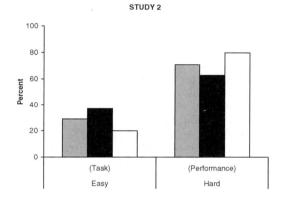

FIGURE 11.5. Self-conscious emotions as a function of task judgments of preschoolers following a "failed" easy task in two studies. The percentage of children showing pride, evaluative embarrassment, and shame is shown for those who said the task was "easy" despite the failure (task focus) and for those who said the task was hard, congruent with their failure (performance focus).

Such attribution styles for negative events promote shame, thus constituting a risk factor for subsequent maladjustment.

SELF-CONSCIOUS EVALUATIVE EMOTIONS AND ADJUSTMENT

Recently, we have begun to study the relation of the negative self-evaluative emotions of shame and embarrassment to maladjustment and competence. Such work addresses children's competence, in that self-evaluative emotions impact on psychopathology and the lack of competence that children may display in dealing with their worlds. Poor management of self-evaluative emotions can cause children a variety of social and interactional difficulties. In our work, we are especially concerned with how traumatic events impact on negative self-evaluative emotions and how shame, in particular, then impacts on psychological adjustment and competence. Figure 11.6 presents the model, which proposes that shame and negative ways of thinking about the self act as mediators of adjustment outcomes. On the far left is a traumatic event. Sexual abuse and other forms of maltreatment are examples of traumatic events that we have considered in our work. We propose that trauma leads to shame and negative thoughts about the self around the event (a), and that shame and these negative thoughts in turn lead to poor adjustment (b). This model allows for the traumatic event to directly influence shame (a), as well as adjustment (c), although our hypothesis is that adjustment is mediated by how the child feels and thinks about the event (a through b). Preliminary support for this model comes from research suggesting that individuals who are shame-prone are more likely to evidence depression and disassociation (H. B. Lewis, 1987; Lewis, 1992; Ross, 1989; Tangney et al., 1992).

Shame and Sexual Abuse

The experience of shame as a consequence of sexual abuse is related to subsequent behavioral problems leading to poor performance in a number of areas of psychological functioning (Lewis, 1992). Feiring, Taska, and Lewis (1998) measured self-evaluative emotions and attributions, especially those made regarding the cause of abuse. If an attribution is made to an internal, global cause, the resulting emotion is shame. Thus, how the victim evaluates the abusive event is critical and likely to mediate subsequent long-lasting effects of the abuse on behavior as feelings of worthlessness and self-blame are generalized to other areas of behavioral functioning (Conte, 1985; Janoff-Bulman, 1979; Wyatt & Mickey, 1988). We have been able to show relations between sexual abuse, shame, and adjustment in a longitudinal study of sexually abused children ages 8–15 years. Our findings indicate that within 6 months of the reported abuse, both severity of abuse and shame were related directly to depressive symptoms. However, 1 year after report of the abusive incidents, only the amount of shame and self-blaming attributions was related to depressive symptoms. The trauma was no longer related. Even so, changes in shame and negative attributions contributed to adjustment. Children whose shame decreased actually showed decreases in depression, and, therefore, increased social competence, compared to those whose shame stayed the same or increased (Feiring, Taska, & Lewis, 2002).

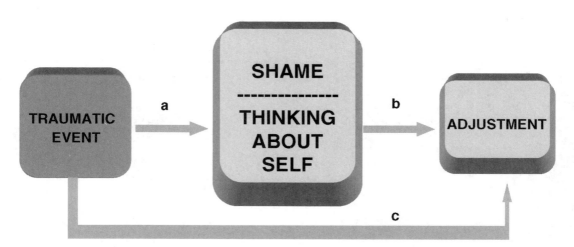

FIGURE 11.6. A model of trauma and adjustment. Shame and ways of thinking about the self are hypothesized to mediate the relation between trauma and adjustment.

Maltreatment and Shame

We have also applied our model to maltreatment, including physically abused and neglected children. The nature of parenting in maltreating families, often severely physically punitive and/or psychologically aggressive and rejecting, is likely to promote shame and perceived incompetence in children (Lewis, 1992). Maltreatment may result in more shame and less pride relative to non-maltreatment. The results of this study and more recent work indicate that maltreated children show less pride when they succeed and more shame when they fail relative to children from the same social background who have not been maltreated (Alessandri & Lewis, 1996; Sullivan, Bennett, & Lewis, 1999). Moreover, important sex differences appear. Maltreated girls show more shame when they fail a task and less pride when they succeed compared to nonmaltreated girls. Boys, on the other hand, show a suppression of both shame and pride. These sex differences have important implications for behavioral therapy with these children. For girls, maltreatment may result in depression, whereas, for boys, maltreatment may result in a suppression of emotion in general and potentially an increase in aggression, because they are not constrained by feelings of shame, guilt, or regret. Observations of these boys do indicate higher amounts of behaviors such as throwing or roughly pushing the test materials away, verbally aggressive statements, and occasionally angry faces.

CONCLUSIONS

Once the basic emotions emerge, young children's emotional lives undergo an important change during the preschool years. Objective self-awareness, marking the onset of self-conscious emotions, sets the stage for further cognitive and emotional development. The ability of children to learn standards, rules, and goals, and to assess their behavior with reference to them, makes self-conscious evaluative emotions possible. It is these emotions, along with the attributions related to them, that are primary motivators in many areas of social and academic competence.

REFERENCES

Alessandri, S. M., & Lewis, M. (1993). Parental evaluation and its relation to shame and pride in young children. *Sex Roles, 29,* 335–343.

Alessandri, S. M., & Lewis, M. (1996). Development of the self-conscious emotions in maltreated children. In M. Lewis & M. W. Sullivan (Eds.), *Emotional development in atypical children* (pp. 185–202). Mahwah, NJ: Erlbaum.

Baumeister, R. F., Campbell, J., Kreuger, J., & Vohs, K. D. (2003). Does high self-esteem cause better performance, interpersonal success, happiness, or healthier lifestyles? *Psychological Science in the Public Interest, 4*(1), 1–44.

Beck, A. T. (1979). *Cognitive therapy and emotional disorders.* New York: Times Mirror.

Bischof-Kohler, D. (1991). The development of empathy in infants. In M. E. Lamb & H. Keller (Eds.), *Infant development: Perspectives from German-speaking countries* (pp. 245–273). Hillsdale, NJ: Erlbaum.

Bridges, K. M. B. (1932). Emotional development in infancy. *Child Development, 3,* 324–334.

Buss, A., & Plomin, R. (1984). *Temperament: Early developing personality traits.* Hillsdale, NJ: Erlbaum.

Cacioppo, J. T., & Gardner, W. L. (1999). Emotion. *Annual Review of Psychology, 50,* 191–214.

Cole, P. M., Barrett, K. C., & Zahn-Waxler, C. (1992). Emotion displays in two-year-olds. *Child Development, 63,* 314–324.

Conte, J. (1985). The effects of sexual abuse on children: A critique and suggestions for future research. *Victimology: An International Journal, 10,* 110–130.

Csikszentmihalyi, M. (1990). *Flow: The psychology of optimal experience.* San Francisco: Jossey-Bass.

Darwin, C. (1965). *The expression of the emotions in man and animals.* Chicago: University of Chicago Press. (Original published in 1872)

Deaux, K. (1976). Sex: A perspective on the attribution process. In J. Harvey, W. Iches, & R. Kidd (Eds.), *New directions in attributional research* (Vol. 1, pp. 333–352). Hillsdale, NJ: Erlbaum.

Dweck, C. S. (1991). Self-theories and goals: Their role in motivation, personality and development. In R. Dienstbeir (Ed.), *Nebraska Symposium on Motivation* (Vol. 36, pp. 199–236). Lincoln: University of Nebraska Press.

Dweck, C. S. (1996). Social motivation: Goals and social-cognitive processes. In J. Juvonen & K. R. Wentzel (Eds.), *Social motivation: Understanding children's school adjustment* (pp. 181–195). New York: Cambridge University Press.

Dweck, C. S., & Chiu, C., & Hong, Y. (1995). Implicit theories and their role in judgments and reactions: A world from two perspectives. *Psychological Inquiry, 6,* 267–285.

Dweck, C. S., & Leggett, E. L. (1988). A social-cognitive approach to motivation and personality. *Psychological Review, 95,* 256–273.

Feiring, C., Taska, L., & Lewis, M. (1998). The role of

shame and attribution style in children's and adolescents' adaptation to sexual abuse. *Child Maltreatment, 3*(2), 129–142.

Feiring, C., Taska, L., & Lewis, M. (2002). Adjustment following sexual abuse discovery: The role of shame and attributional style. *Developmental Psychology, 38*(1), 79–92. [Won the APSAC (American Professional Society on the Abuse of Children) research award]

Ferguson, T. J., & Stegge, H. (1995). Emotional states and traits in children: The case of guilt and shame. In J. P. Tangney & K. W. Fischer (Eds.), *Self-conscious emotions: Shame, guilt, embarrassment and pride* (pp. 174–197). New York: Guilford Press.

Graham, S. (1991). A review of attribution theory in achievement contexts. *Educational Psychology Review, 3*, 5–39.

Halperin, M. (1989, April). *Empathy and self-awareness*. Paper presented at the meeting of Society for Research in Child Development, Kansas City, MO.

Heckhausen, H. (1984). Emergent achievement behavior: Some early developments. In J. Nicholls (Ed.), *The development of achievement motivation* (pp. 1–32). Greenwich, CT: JAI Press.

Izard, C. E. (1978). Emotions and emotion–cognition relationships. In M. Lewis & L. A. Rosenblum (Eds.), *The development of affect: The genesis of behavior* (Vol. 1, pp. 389–414). New York: Plenum Press.

Janoff-Bulman, R. (1979). Characterological versus behavioral self-blame: Inquiries into depression and rape. *Journal of Personality and Social Psychology, 37*, 1798–1809.

Kagan, J. (1981). *The second year*. Cambridge, MA: Harvard University Press.

Kamins, M. L., & Dweck, C. S. (1999). Person versus process praise and criticism: Implications for contingent self-worth and coping. *Developmental Psychology, 35*, 835–847.

Kaslow, N. S., Rehm, L. P., Pollack, S. L., & Segal, S. W. (1988). Attributional style and self-control behavior in depressed and nondepressed children and their parents. *Journal of Abnormal Child Psychology, 16*, 162–175.

Kochanska, G. (1995). Children's temperament, mothers' discipline, and security of attachment: Multiple pathways to emerging internalization. *Child Development, 65*, 852–868.

Kochanska, G., Coy, K. C., & Murray, K. T. (2001). The development of self-regulation in the first 4 years of life. *Child Development, 72*, 1091–1111.

Kochanska, G., DeVet, K., Goldman, M., Murray, K., & Putnam, S. P. (1994). Maternal reports of conscience development and temperament in young children. *Child Development, 65*, 852–868.

Lewis, H. B. (1971). *Shame and guilt in neurosis*. New York: International Universities Press.

Lewis, H. B. (1976). *Psychic war in men and women*. New York: New York University Press.

Lewis, H. B. (1987). Shame: The "sleeper" in psychopathology. In H. B. Lewis (Ed.), *The role of shame in symptom formation* (pp. 1–28). Hillsdale, NJ: Erlbaum.

Lewis, M. (1989). Culture and biology: The role of temperament. In P. Zelazo & R. Barr (Eds.), *Challenges to developmental paradigms* (pp. 203–226). Hillsdale, NJ: Erlbaum.

Lewis, M. (1992). *Shame, the exposed self*. New York: Free Press.

Lewis, M. (2000). The self-conscious emotions. In M. Lewis & J. Haviland (Eds.), *Handbook of emotions* (2nd ed., pp. 623–636). New York: Guilford Press.

Lewis, M. (2003). The development of self-consciousness. In J. Roessler & N. Eilan (Eds.), *Agency and self-awareness: Issues in philosophy and psychology* (pp. 275–295). New York: Oxford University Press.

Lewis, M., Alessandri, S. M., & Sullivan, M. W. (1990). Violation, loss of control, and anger in young infants. *Developmental Psychology, 26*, 745–751.

Lewis, M., Alessandri, S., & Sullivan, M. W. (1992). Differences in shame and pride as a function of children's gender and task difficulty. *Child Development, 63*, 630–638.

Lewis, M., & Brooks-Gunn, J. (1979). *Social cognition and the acquisition of self*. New York: Plenum Press.

Lewis, M., & Michalson, L. (1983). *Children's emotions and moods: Developmental theory and measurement*. New York: Plenum Press.

Lewis, M., & Ramsay, D. S. (1997). Stress reactivity and self-recognition. *Child Development, 68*, 621–629.

Lewis, M., & Ramsay, D. (1999). Intentions, consciousness, and pretend play. In P. D. Zelazo, J W. Astington, & D. R. Olson (Eds.), *Developing theories of intention* (pp. 77–94). Mahwah, NJ: Erlbaum.

Lewis, M., & Ramsay, D. (2002). Cortisol response to embarrassment and shame. *Child Development, 73*, 1034–1045.

Lewis, M., Stanger, C., Sullivan, M. W., & Barone, P. (1991). Changes in embarrassment as a function of age, sex and situation. *British Journal of Developmental Psychology, 9*, 485–492.

Lewis, M., Sullivan, M. W., Stanger, C., & Weiss, M. (1989). Self-development and self-conscious emotions. *Child Development, 60*, 146–156.

Morrison, A. P. (1989). *Shame: The underside of narcissism*. Hillsdale, NJ: Analytic Press.

Mueller, C. M., & Dweck, C. S. (1998). Praise for intelligence can undermine children's motivation and performance. *Journal of Personality and Social Psychology, 75*, 33–52.

Nicholls, J. G. (1984). Achievement motivation: Conception of ability, subjective experience, task choice, and performance. *Psychological Bulletin, 91*, 328–348.

Nolen-Hoeksema, S., Girgus, J. S., & Seligman, M. E. P. (1992). Predictors and consequences of childhood depressive symptoms: A 5-year longitudinal study. *Journal of Abnormal Psychology, 101,* 405–422.

Nolen-Hoeksema, W., Wolfson, A. , Mumme, D., & Guskin, K. (1995). Helplessness in children of depressed and nondepressed mothers. *Developmental Psychology, 31,* 377–387.

Ohman, A., & Mineka, S. (2003). The malicious serpent: Snakes as a prototypical stimulus for an evolved module of fear. *Current Directions in Psychological Science, 12*(1), 5–8.

Piaget, J. (1952). *The origins of intelligence in children* (M. Cook, Trans.). New York: International Universities Press.

Ramsay, D., & Lewis, M. (2001). Temperament, stress, and soothing. In T. D. Wachs & G. A. Kohnstamm (Eds.), *Temperament in context* (pp. 23–41). Mahwah, NJ: Erlbaum.

Ross, C. A. (1989). *Multiple personality disorder: Diagnosis, clinical features, and treatment.* New York: Wiley.

Rothbart, M. K., Ahadi, S., & Hershey, K. L. (1994). Temperament and social behavior in childhood. *Merrill–Palmer Quarterly, 40,* 21–39.

Rothbart, M. K., & Goldsmith, H. H. (1985). Three approaches to the study of infant temperament. *Developmental Review, 5,* 237–260.

Seligman, M.E. P. (1975). *Helplessness: On depression, development, and death.* San Francisco: Freeman.

Seligman, M. E. P., Peterson, C., Kaslow, N., Tannenbaum, R., Alloy, L., & Abramson, L. (1984). Attributional style and depressive symptoms among children. *Journal of Abnormal Psychology, 39,* 235–238.

Smiley, P. A., & Dweck, C. S. (1995). Individual differences in achievement goals among young children. *Child Development, 65,* 1723–1743.

Stipek, D., Recchia, S., & McClintic, S. (1992). Self-evaluation in young children. *Monographs of the Society for Research in Child Development, 57*(1, Serial No. 226).

Sullivan, M. W., Bennett, D., & Lewis, M. (1999, April). *The emotions of maltreated children in response to success and failure.* Paper presented at the biennial meeting of the Society for Research in Child Development, Albuquerque, NM.

Tangney, J., Wagner, P., & Gramzow, R. (1992). Proneness to shame, proneness to guilt, and psychopathology. *Journal of Abnormal Psychology, 101,* 469–478.

Thomas, A., & Chess. S. (1977). *Temperament and development.* New York: Brunner/Mazel.

Tomkins, S. (1962). *Affect, imagery, and consciousness* (Vol. 1). New York: Springer.

Tomkins, S. (1963). *Affect, imagery, and consciousness* (Vol. 2). New York: Springer.

Weiner, B. (1972). *Theories of motivation: From mechanism to cognition.* Chicago: Rand McNally.

Weiner, B. (1986). *An attributional theory of motivation and emotion.* New York: Springer-Verlag.

Weiner, B., & Graham, S. (1989). Understanding the motivational role of affect: Life-span research from an attributional perspective. *Cognition and Emotion, 3,* 401–419.

Witkin, H. (1965). Psychological differentiation and forms of pathology. *Journal of Abnormal Psychology, 70,* 317–336.

Wyatt, G. E., & Mickey, M. R. (1988). The support of parents and others as it mediates the effects of child sexual abuse: An exploratory study. In G. E. Wyatt & G. J. Powell (Eds.), *Lasting effects of child sexual abuse* (pp. 211–226). Newbury Park, CA: Sage.

CHAPTER 12

☙

Competence Assessment, Competence, and Motivation between Early and Middle Childhood

RUTH BUTLER

Contemporary theories of achievement motivation emphasize the influence of people's sense of competence on their achievement-related strivings and behaviors throughout the lifespan (Dweck, 1986; Nicholls, 1989). In this chapter, I focus on the early development of self-evaluation and on implications for children's motivation and behavior in achievement settings. This endeavor is intriguing, because, in many respects, the history of theory and research on the development of self-evaluative judgments and understandings corresponds to that on cognitive development in general. On the one hand, early studies revealed systematic age-related advances in the ways in which children construed achievement-related concepts, evaluated their competence, and set goals or formed expectations for the future. Moreover, these seemed to reflect qualitative transformations in thought and judgment that corresponded rather closely to major Piagetian shifts from preoperational to concrete operational to formal operational thought at about ages 7 and 11, respectively. In keeping with the centrality of strivings for and conceptions of competence in cognitively based theories of motivation, several researchers then proposed equivalent developmental transformations also in children's achievement motivation and behavior. On the other hand, in keeping with theoretical and empirical challenges to the strong structural assumptions of cognitive developmental theory, and to its conceptualization of the limitations of preschool thought in particular, studies began to reveal significant variability in achievement-related cognitions and motives between individuals and across contexts already in the early years.

In the first section of this chapter, I review "structural deficit" approaches to the early development of achievement-related cognitions and motives, and the relations between them. In the second and third sections, I discuss how alternative approaches that emphasize the ways in which children construct knowledge, strategies, and motives, within the contexts of their daily lives, challenge earlier assumptions and generate a different picture of young children's self-evaluative capacities and motives, and of the factors that influence competence and motivation throughout childhood. In the final section, I address some implications of this review and suggest guidelines for promoting adaptive self-evaluation, self-regulation, and motivation in both younger and older children.

STRUCTURAL DEFICIT APPROACHES TO THE DEVELOPMENT OF SELF-EVALUATION AND MOTIVATION BETWEEN EARLY AND MIDDLE CHILDHOOD

Competence Assessment

Both the earlier and some more recent reviews of the development of competence-related perceptions, judgments, and understandings reached similar conclusions that these aspects are unrealistically high, undifferentiated, and relatively unaffected by experience and relevant information during the preschool years, and become lower, more realistic, more differentiated, and more responsive to various kinds of information during middle childhood (Harter, 1999; Nicholls, 1990; Stipek, 1984). These conclusions were based on findings from several kinds of empirical designs and data. One tradition, notably represented by the research of Susan Harter and her associates, has examined age trends in children's perceptions of their own competence. In general, studies yielded four main groups of findings (see Harter, 1990, 1999, for reviews). First, they indicated that perceived competence tended to be high during the preschool years and to decline with age, with relatively marked decreases between about ages 7 and 9, and again between about ages 11 and 13. Second, perceptions tended to become more differentiated and domain-specific with age, as reflected in both the factor structure of self-reports and intercorrelations between factors. For example, Harter and Pike (1984) found that 4- to 7-year-olds could make judgments about their cognitive competence, physical competence, social acceptance, and behavioral conduct, but judgments loaded on only two, cognitive–physical versus social–behavioral,

factors. The number of distinct domains then increased steadily with age from at least five in middle childhood to at least 11 among adults (Harter, 1990). Third, perceptions also seemed to become more integrated with age. Thus, Harter and her associates found that the more general concept of global self-worth did not emerge before middle childhood (Harter, 1990). In a similar vein, children's spontaneous self-descriptions emphasized concrete actions and skills during the preschool years and did not begin to incorporate reference to traits before middle childhood (Damon & Hart, 1988). Fourth, as one would expect if perceptions become more differentiated and integrated with age, correlations between children's perceived and actual cognitive competence, as reflected in test scores or teacher ratings, were low before about age 8 and increased thereafter (Eshel & Klein, 1981; Wigfield et al., 1997).

Another research tradition has used experimental designs to examine age trends in children's self-evaluative responses to success or failure. Typically, children received information about their performance on one or more trials of some task and were then asked to (1) indicate how well they expected to do on subsequent trial; or (2) asked to evaluate their performance, ability, or affect; or (3) were observed on behavioral measures such as expression of affect or persistence, or performance on a subsequent trial or different task. Here too, studies documented rather similar and converging developmental patterns across measures. Regarding expectations, the general finding was that they were equally high after both success and failure before about age 5–6. In one representative study, Stipek and Hoffman (1980) found that expectations among 3- to 4-year-olds were close to the maximum, regardless of whether they had received perfect scores, low but improving scores, or uniformly low scores on four previous trials. Expectations after failure then declined steadily between ages 5 and 8. Moreover, Rholes, Blackwell, Jordan, and Walters (1980) documented a corresponding decline between ages 5 and 11 in children's willingness to persist after failing on a series of hidden figures problems.

Perhaps most attention has been addressed to the development of self-appraisal, using a basic paradigm in which children perform a task in a setting that provides some evaluative standard and then rate their performance or ability. Studies revealed age trends similar to those for general perceptions of competence, whereby self-appraisal was very positive during the preschool years and declined during the early elementary school years (e.g., Ruble, Grosovsky, Frey, & Cohen, 1992). Experimental procedures also added the significant information, consistent with data yielded by studies of expectancy, that young children's evaluation of their performance or ability was relatively unaffected by relevant information. In most studies, this consisted of social comparison information indicating superior or inferior performance relative to others. Such information did not reliably influence performance–appraisal before about age 7, and did not influence ability–appraisal until even later (Aboud, 1985; Ruble, Boggiano, Feldman, & Loebl, 1980).

Interpretation of these rather consistent age-related changes, coinciding as they did with the transition from preoperational to concrete operational thought at about age 6, rather naturally tended to emphasize the role of structural changes in children's cognitive capacities and understandings. Specifically, interpretations tended to focus on how one or another feature of young children's thinking about their competence reflected one or another general limitation of preschool thought. In this case, a brief description of these limitations is in order.

Most generally, Piaget (1926/1928; 1926/1930) claimed that young children's lack of operations renders it difficult for them to distinguish and coordinate between different aspects of events and phenomena, and between phenomena and their perceptions of them. As a result, preoperational children do not form coherent concepts. Instead, their thought is intuitive or transductive rather than logical, as reflected in the dominance of reasoning by perceptions and appearances, in the tendency to reason from particular to particular, and in the instability and incoherence of successive judgments. It is also egocentric, a property most generally defined as confusion of self with nonself and typically examined in terms of the capacity to consider other perspectives or points of view. For example, in the famous three-mountain

problem, preoperational children initially did not understand that a topographical scene would look different from another spatial location (Piaget, Inhelder, & Szaminska, 1948/1960). In a similar vein, Piaget maintained that preoperational thought is centered, such that young children cannot simultaneously consider more than one dimension, or variable, and do not, for example, consider both rows and columns in multiple-classification tasks (Odom, Astor, & Cunningham, 1975).

Against this background, it seemed that one could interpret young children's competence-related cognitions and judgments as particular cases of their general difficulties in differentiating and coordinating between perceptions, representations, and reality, between successive judgments, and between multiple dimensions, perspectives, or causes. For example, Veroff (1969) attributed the apparent failure of young children to use social comparison information for self-appraisal to their difficulty in distinguishing and coordinating between self–other perspectives and their corresponding tendency to focus on their own outcome alone. In a similar vein, the relatively late emergence of global self-worth and of appropriate ability, as compared with performance–appraisal, has been attributed to the role of operational thought in overcoming earlier tendencies to judge from particular to particular and corresponding limitations in integrating successive events and perceptions (Harter, 1999).

Such analyses do not, however, explain why young children's judgments seemed to be not only unrealistic but also consistently positive. Moreover, this seemed to be the case also when children performed poorly relative to prior trials or to some objective standard (Ruble et al., 1992; Stipek & Hoffman, 1980), even though some researchers have proposed that standards that do not require coordination of self–other perspectives might be more accessible to preoperational children (Dweck & Elliot, 1983; Nicholls & Miller, 1983; Stipek & Mac Iver, 1989; Suls & Mullen, 1982). To address this problem, Stipek (1984) returned to Piaget's theory and proposed a "wishful thinking" interpretation of young children's unrealistically high expectations as reflecting a particular case of their difficulty in distinguishing between reality and desire. According to Piaget (1926/1930), one consequence of this failure of differentiation is that young children have a highly exaggerated and overgeneralized sense of personal efficacy that makes its own contribution to their limited understanding of causality. Stipek reasoned that, in this case, positive biases in young children's self-related judgments may reflect their general tendency to confuse what they can do with what they want to do, and to focus mainly on the latter.

To summarize, children's inferences and judgments about their own competence seemed to accord well with their reasoning in other domains. It is, however, important to remember that Piaget's main focus was on the intensive examination of children's reasoning. Thus, identifying underlying cognitive structures and developmental transformations does not itself explicate the features and dynamics of children's reasoning about specific concepts. The development of achievement-related concepts has been studied most systematically by John Nicholls and his colleagues. In a series of studies, they applied Piaget's clinical method and assumption that concept formation progresses through a series of age-related differentiations between related concepts to examine the development of children's understanding of ability. They found that before about age 5–6, most children did not differentiate between skill and luck, and expected effort to be similarly efficacious in improving performance on both skill and luck (guessing) tasks (Nicholls & Miller, 1985). In addition, children did not understand that puzzles that fewer, rather than more, peers can solve are more difficult and require more ability before about age 6–7 (Nicholls & Miller, 1983). The authors concluded that younger children had not acquired the "normative conception of ability," defined as the understanding that others' outcomes are diagnostic of ability. In a similar vein, Nicholls (1978) found that preschool children did not differentiate between effort, ability, and outcome, and tended to center on a single factor, typically, effort. Thus, they judged children who tried harder than others to be smarter, even if they performed less well, and inferred that children who performed better must also have tried harder, even if they did not appear to be trying at all. This study also demonstrated further develop-

ments in children's differentiation of ability and related concepts. Thus, what Nicholls termed the "mature conception of ability," which rests on the understanding that individual differences in ability influence the efficacy of effort, emerged only at about age 11–12.

This research program provided a conceptual bridge, which is actually rather rare in developmental research, between cognitive structures and cognitive behaviors, or judgments. If young children do not distinguish between outcomes over which they have more or less control, and do not understand that task difficulty and personal ability place limits on the efficacy of effort, it makes sense that they expect to do very well in the future, regardless of current outcomes, if they try really hard (see also Stipek & Mac Iver, 1989). In a similar vein, if young children do not understand that others' outcomes are diagnostic of ability, it makes sense that they do not use social comparison information to evaluate their current capacities or regulate effort. Moreover, if they do not actually have any conception of ability as distinct, for example, from luck and effort, it is not surprising that their perceptions of their own competence are poorly differentiated, are not organized into general traits, including ability, and are poorly correlated with objective criteria.

Ignorance Is Bliss: Achievement-Related Behavior and Motivation in Early Childhood

The evidence and analyses just reviewed seemed to have some rather clear implications for understanding how not only concepts and judgments but also competence-related motives and behaviors should change between early and middle childhood. The prevailing assumption, well-captured in Nicholls and Miller's (1984) witty chapter title, "Development and Its Discontents," was that the immature reasoning and conceptions of young children may actually be associated with more adaptive behaviors and motivation than are the more adequate understandings of older children and adults (see also Butler, 1989a, 1989b; Dweck & Elliot; 1983; Stipek, 1984). First, researchers reasoned that younger children should be less vulnerable to the negative effects of failure. Thus, their apparent failure to consider negative information should render them less aware of deficiencies in their performance. Moreover, even when they realize that they have performed poorly, their belief in the primacy of effort, high perceived competence, and failure to understand that current outcomes have implications for their ability should converge in maintaining expectations that greater effort will ensure future success. Thus, Dweck and Elliot (1983) proposed that young children are inclined to respond to failure by increasing effort, persistence, and strategic search or, in short, with adaptive attempts to overcome difficulty and attain mastery. Moreover, they should not as yet be developmentally capable of displaying the alternative, helpless pattern identified in studies with older children, which is characterized by decrements in performance and persistence, and negative affect and self-perceptions (Diener & Dweck, 1978).

Second, researchers reasoned that the limitations of preschool children's thought have adaptive consequences for their achievement motivation. Achievement goal theorists distinguish between task (Nicholls, 1989) or learning goals (Dweck, 1986) that orient people to strive to learn and acquire worthwhile skills and understandings, and ego, or performance, goals, that orient them to strive to demonstrate superior, or disguise inferior, ability. On the whole, task involvement seems to be associated with more adaptive processes and outcomes than ego involvement, and especially with more constructive responses to challenge and difficulty (see reviews by Ames, 1992; Butler, 2000). Adults may display either kind of motivational involvement as a function of both their personal task versus ego orientations and contextual emphases on the importance of learning versus normative success (Dweck, 1986, Nicholls, 1989). In contrast, Nicholls and Miller (1984) reasoned that young children, who do not have even a partially differentiated or trait-like conception of ability, can strive to learn and acquire competence but are incapable of organizing achievement strivings around concerns with their ability. Although acquisition of the normative concept of ability by about age 7 may orient children to seek satisfac-

tion from outperforming others, Nicholls and Miller reasoned that only with the acquisition of the mature conception of ability do young adolescents understand that failing to do so has implications for their ability and future performance. Thus, only at this point can they also exhibit the maladaptive responses to failure typically associated with ego involvement.

On the one hand, proposals that young children's cognitive limitations also "limit" them to more, rather than less, adaptive patterns of motivation and behavior accorded well with the empirical evidence of their buoyant optimism and positive self-appraisals and expectations reviewed earlier. On the other hand, there are grounds for questioning whether young children are really such incompetent self-evaluators as the opening review implies, and whether they are necessarily invulnerable to failure. First, young children do not seem to behave in daily life as if they are quite so obtuse about their capacities. Left to their own devices, they do not usually attempt tasks that they cannot do, and there would be far more playground accidents if they always overestimated their abilities. In addition, young children often respond to difficulty with distress and frequently abandon challenging activities. More generally, it is not clear how they can select activities conducive to developing skills and effective interactions with the environment, without some sense of their present capacities and some interest in evaluating them. Second, the picture of young children as consistently incompetent self-evaluators across different measures, tasks, domains, and contexts is somewhat strange in view of converging evidence that their thought in other domains is both more variable and less limited than Piaget claimed. Third, developmental analyses that emphasize young children's inflated judgments have not always considered that adults also tend to overestimate their abilities and performance in ways that cannot be attributed to structural cognitive deficits.

In the next sections, I extrapolate from developments in theory and research on early cognitive development to identify other, nonstructural factors that might both account for the age-related trends in children's knowledge about their own competence reviewed earlier and indicate when young children might be quite knowledgeable about their capacities and skillful at evaluating them. I then examine motivational influences on the early development of self-evaluative strategies and judgments.

THE DEVELOPMENT
OF COMPETENCE AND COMPETENCE
ASSESSMENT REVISITED:
FROM INTERNAL STRUCTURES TO
THE ACQUISITION OF KNOWLEDGE
AND STRATEGIES IN CONTEXT

It is interesting that the cognitive-developmental analyses reviewed earlier were formulated during a period marked by serious theoretical and empirical challenges to Piaget's basic assumptions regarding the primacy of structure over content, strategy, and context, the internal consistency of thought, and the existence of universal stages of cognitive development. In brief, studies began to yield converging evidence of substantial variability in reasoning across tasks, domains, contexts, and, thus, within stages. Interpretations of the unevenness of thought range from neo-Piagetian emphases on stage-like transformations within, but not necessarily between, domains (Fischer, 1980) or for tasks that share the same logical structure and require equivalent levels of knowledge (Case, 1985), to approaches that reject the notion of stages and emphasize continuous advances in thought, information-processing capacities, and strategies within domains and contexts (Siegler, 1996). Most, however, understand the basic constructivist assumption that cognition develops through action as implying that children address the challenges and dilemmas of daily life by developing understandings and strategies that are, at most, weakly restricted by cognitive structures. Thus, theoretical analyses increasingly emphasized processing capacities, strategies, and domains rather than structures and stages, and research increasingly focused on the ways in which children acquire and use knowledge in specific domains, during specific interactions, and in specific contexts.

Before reviewing how researchers have applied these ideas to reexamining early competence assessment, it is relevant to ask how they have affected our understanding of young children in general. Although criticisms of cognitive-developmental theory apply at all ages, there is particular consensus that Piaget overestimated the limitations of the preschool mind and the degree to which these constrain concept formation and strategy acquisition. In brief, studies repeatedly indicated that young children displayed sophisticated, and apparently operational, thought in domains in which they had more, rather then less, knowledge, in contexts that were familiar, rather than novel or artificial, and for tasks that placed less, rather than more, load on memory or attentional capacities (see Flavell, 1985, 1999, and Siegler, 1996, for relevant reviews). Particularly pertinent in view of early assumptions that young children cannot coordinate self–other perspectives, children appear to be far less egocentric than Piaget maintained (Gelman, 1979). In daily life, they engage in extended dialogues and cooperative activity with peers, and adopt, maintain, and coordinate roles in sociodramatic play. They also develop a theory of mind and the understanding that others have knowledge, desires, and intentions that may differ from their own, and are able to adapt their own behavior and communications accordingly, at least to some extent.

These discrepancies between the Piagetian and post-Piagetian young child can be explained in terms of two main kinds of factors. First, the latter, and, incidentally, the apparently less egocentric young Soviet children described at about the same time by Vygotsky (1934/1978), typically have earlier and more intensive peer experience. The role of experience in the development of social cognition was confirmed in an early study in which Hollos and Cowan (1973) found that children growing up on isolated Norwegian farms demonstrated poorer social perspective taking, but not conservation, relative to their urban counterparts. These findings accorded well with other evidence that the level of children's thinking varies widely across domains, depending in large part on their knowledge base. Domain-specific knowledge and strategies for applying this knowledge vary in keeping with individual differences in experience and interests (Chi

& Koeske, 1983), but is more consistently influenced by the challenges, strategies, and solutions provided or scaffolded by young children's typical environments. For example, both age trends and cultural differences in children's verbal recall have been attributed to the influence of formal schooling on the acquisition of verbal rehearsal strategies (Rogoff & Mistry, 1990). Moreover, specific training in such strategies did indeed result in superior recall (Keeney, Canizzo, & Flavell, 1967). Second, Piaget's emphasis on the formal properties of logic and reasoning frequently led researchers to present young children with unfamiliar problems that were also rather demanding in terms of the amount and kinds of information that children needed to process as a prerequisite for engaging with the problem itself. Thus, in domains as diverse as causal reasoning (Bullock & Gelman, 1979) and perspective taking (Borke, 1975), young children consistently displayed higher levels of understanding when tasks, dilemmas, and procedures were less, rather than more, complex.

Regarding competence assessment, one implication is that self-appraisal may indeed become more accurate, differentiated, and responsive to relevant information with age, in large part, however, because of age-related changes in children's typical experiences and contexts, rather than their internal cognitive structures. Another implication is that researchers may have used methodologies that led them to underestimate the self-evaluative capacities of young children. In this case, it is important to analyze both the contexts within which younger and older children develop self-evaluative knowledge and strategies, and the contexts in which these have been studied. Moreover, one would expect variations in both to influence children's self-evaluative competence, as they do their competence in other domains.

Contexts for Developing Knowledge about Competence

An ethnographic study that followed Israeli children during the transition from kindergarten to elementary school indicated that these provided very different contexts for the development of competence and competence assessment (Baumer, 1998). In brief, in K1, children spent most of their time engaging in unstructured, expressive, and creative activities such as free play and arts and crafts. They also had considerable freedom to choose activities, to engage in them however they liked, and to abandon them whenever they wanted. As a result, they were rarely required to meet performance standards or persist until they did so. In contrast, in grade 1, they spent most of the day working on structured assignments with clearly defined procedures and solutions, which they were required to complete. Other parts of the day were devoted to direct instruction in math and reading in small ability groups. In addition, K1 teachers rarely commented on children's work and tended to praise children indiscriminately when they did so. Indeed, Baumer documented cases in which children themselves expressed dissatisfaction with, for example, a painting, and asked for new materials, so that they could try again, but their teachers responded by trying to persuade them that their work was fine as it was. In contrast, grade 1 teachers frequently evaluated children's work and were increasingly likely, as the year progressed, to compare children's work with that of peers and to require them to repeat unsatisfactory work. Thus, entrance into first grade exposed children for the first time to an environment in which they were required to acquire and demonstrate specific skills, procedures, and understandings as they and their classmates worked on the same structured tasks, at the same time, with differing degrees of proficiency.

Cognitive-developmental theorists were not oblivious to such age-related changes in children's learning environments, but they tended to emphasize the degree to which these converged with and reinforced transformations in the structure of children's thought. Thus, Nicholls (1989) proposed that increasing emphases on normative evaluation and interpersonal competition in elementary school reinforce the concerns with outperforming others that are enabled by children's acquisition of the normative concept of ability, but do not play a major role in their acquisition of this concept. Others assigned typical changes in the structure and social context of activity a more direct role in the development of self-evaluative knowledge and strategies (Higgins & Parsons, 1983; Stipek & Mac Iver, 1989). These researchers noted that it is both difficult and rather inappropriate to evaluate competence for unstructured, free-flowing activities, such as play or painting, that do not have clear and agreed outcomes or standards for evaluating them. In contrast, when children work on identical, structured assignments that focus on clearly defined skills, it is both feasible and functional to monitor and evaluate performance relative to task requirements, prior work, or others' outcomes, especially when such evaluative standards, strategies, and judgments are also modeled by significant adults. In this case, it is not surprising that children's knowledge about performance standards and their sense that they could judge their own work independently increased during middle childhood (Harter, 1981). Finally, intensive experience with different school domains, such as reading, math, music, sports, and so on, should enable children both to develop stable perceptions of competence within each domain and to distinguish between competencies in different domains.

If age-related changes in contexts can explain, at least in part, why perceptions of competence become more realistic and differentiated, and more stable, integrated, and trait-like with age, such perceptions should also be sensitive to within-age variations in context. Few studies have directly examined the influence of relevant natural variations in early childhood environments. In one exception, Stipek and Daniels (1988) examined the perceived scholastic competence of two groups of 5- to 6-year-olds, who attended either a "developmental" kindergarten, similar to that described by Baumer (1998), or an "academic" kindergarten, similar to typical elementary school classrooms. Results confirmed that perceptions were less positive and more highly correlated with teacher ratings in the academic than in the developmental kindergarten or in most other studies. Another study, in which we examined acquisition of the normative concept of ability among children at ages 4–8, who lived either in Israeli towns or on kibbutzim, indicated that experience in context also affected concept development (Butler &

Ruzany, 1993). A unique feature of kibbutz child rearing at the time was that it took place mainly in the peer group rather than the family. From the age of 3 months, children lived with a small group of same-age peers whom they could observe as they acquired physical and cognitive skills, and learned to dress, eat alone, participate in household chores, and so on. We reasoned that this intensive experience might result in relatively early appreciation of the relevance of individual differences for evaluating competence. As expected, kibbutz children acquired the normative concept about a year earlier than did urban children.

To summarize, school environments do seem to change such that, compared with older children, younger children typically have less knowledge about the meaning and nature of competence and ability across different activities and contexts, are less familiar with evaluative standards, and have less reason to acquire strategies for assessing their competence. It seems likely that even young children, however, have at least some relevant experience. Parents demand competence in different domains and respond to children's mastery attempts with various kinds of feedback (Kelley, Brownell, & Campbell, 2000); children are also often very frank about their younger siblings' competence, or lack thereof. In addition, many of the common activities of early childhood, at school and at home, from inserting shapes into holes to puzzles and coloring, do provide clear and concrete performance standards. Children also often engage in such activities alongside others. In this case, if they are less limited to their own perspective than early analyses assumed, it is unlikely that they fail to attend to differences between their own and others' performance.

Some studies have indeed indicated that 3- to 4-year-olds already behaved "as if" they attended to discrepancies between their own performance and task requirements or another's outcome, and displayed negative affect after performing poorly relative to one or the other standard (Schneider, 1984; Stipek, Recchia, & McClintic, 1992). Stipek and her colleagues also concluded that they had some sense of the valence of their outcomes for others, anticipating that adults would respond positively to their success, and attempting to avoid negative reactions to failure by avoiding eye contact. In other studies, children at age 4–5 inserted themselves appropriately into hierarchies of relative standing in meaningful and familiar domains, such as running speed (Morris & Nemcek, 1982) or social dominance (Strayer, Chapeskie, & Strayer, 1979), made spontaneous social comparison statements in classroom settings (Mosatche & Bragonier, 1981), and used information appropriately to make judgments about another child (Ruble et al., 1992; Stipek, 1984). Finally, Marsh, Ellis, and Craven (2002) recently reported evidence indicating the existence of a multidimensional self-concept already among 4-year-olds. Thus, in contrast with earlier findings (Harter & Pike, 1984), they found that perceptions of physical, verbal, and number competence, of physical appearance, and of relations with peers and parents loaded on distinct and fairly reliable factors.

To summarize, there are grounds for venturing that the cognitive capacities and typical experiences of young children suffice to enable the acquisition of at least some self-evaluative knowledge and skills. In this case, their rather consistent failure to use one or another kind of information to assess their competence in controlled studies merits further examination.

Contexts for Studying the Development of Competence Assessment

Many studies of young children's judgments can be faulted, as could many of Piaget's tasks, for requiring children to make rather complex judgments for rather meaningless activities (see also Butler, 1998; Dweck, 1999). In the interests of experimental control, many researchers deliberately used unfamiliar tasks with ambiguous outcomes, such that children could not compare outcomes directly but had to rely instead on complex, symbolic information, such as rates of success represented by numerical scores (Ruble et al., 1980; Ruble, Eisenberg, & Higgins, 1994). Such designs also differ from natural settings, in which children typically see for themselves how they are doing relative to the task or to someone else. Some studies also presented children with multiple standards, such as the outcomes of several

peers, or their own rates of success on several trials (Butler & Ruzany, 1993; Ruble et al., 1992; Stipek & Hoffman, 1980). In contrast, research on young children's thought implies that if one is interested in the emergence of the understanding that a particular standard is relevant for evaluating competence and of the capacity to use it appropriately, one should use simple, rather than complex, evaluative tasks and standards.

Analyzing different kinds of self-evaluative comparisons in terms of the specific knowledge and strategies they require can provide a framework for analyzing their relative complexity, and for predicting whether the capacity to use them for self-appraisal should develop concurrently or at different points (Case, 1985). For example, in the simplest two-instance case, self-evaluative social comparison involves a comparison between two concrete outcomes (for self and other), a task that seems formally equivalent to comparing an outcome (e.g., one's attempt to solve a puzzle) with an objective standard (e.g., the picture on the box). Thus, one might expect both to emerge at about the same time. In contrast, temporal comparison typically involves a more complex comparison between a concrete outcome (current performance) and a mental representation (past performance). In this case, young children may actually be quite proficient in using simple objective and social, but not necessarily temporal, self-evaluative standards in their daily lives, and thus also in appropriate controlled settings.

I tested this reasoning in two studies (Butler, 1998) in which children between the ages of 4 and 8 evaluated their performance on a familiar activity (tracing a winding path between a child and a house) in the presence of a simple, concrete social standard (the work of one other child who had traced either more or less of the path) or temporal standard (their performance on a prior trial in which they had completed either less or more of the path). Results confirmed that given a simple, two-instance comparison and concrete outcome information, children at age 4–5 evaluated their performance more positively when they completed more, compared with less, of the path than the other child. Indeed, the discrepancy between self-appraisals in success and failure conditions was no smaller than at age 7–8. The youngest and oldest children also used similar self-evaluative strategies. Most explained their ratings by comparing their performance appropriately with either the objective standard ("I only got halfway to the house") or the social standard ("I did more–less than him"). Moreover, about 40% of both the youngest and the oldest children explained their ratings in terms of explicit and appropriate social comparison.

In contrast, children in the youngest group did not rate their current performance differently when they performed better, rather than worse, than on a previous trial, and children did not explain their ratings in terms of temporal comparison before age 7–8, even when they were shown both their outcomes. The youngest children did not, however, evaluate themselves more favorably than did the oldest ones, even in temporal comparison conditions. Instead, they attended to the concrete standard that was accessible to them—how much of the path they had completed—and rated their performance higher when they completed more, rather than less, of the path. Thus, to summarize, already by age 4–5, children were capable of veridical self-appraisal as long as the information available to them was meaningful, accessible, and easy to process. The findings for social comparison accord well with the evidence reviewed earlier regarding early social comparison activity and interest, and suggest that the failure of young children to use social comparison appropriately in prior studies was indeed influenced by methodological factors. Analyzing evaluative standards in terms of their complexity can also explain why Ruble and her colleagues also found that young children did not use temporal comparison information for self-appraisal (Ruble et al., 1992, 1994).

Research on early cognitive development has also alerted us to the possibility that children sometimes fail to understand the question, or the researcher's intentions, rather than the concept. Findings that appropriate use of information emerged later, when children were asked to evaluate their ability, than when they were asked to evaluate their performance have been attributed to their limited understanding of traits (Ruble et al., 1992). Young children do, however, seem to form general perceptions of their competence. They also display more sophisticated reasoning about traits than we used to think (Ruble & Dweck, 1995). Moreover, given that ability is best evaluated by integrating information over different times and situations, one can ask how people at any age do so on the basis of their performance on one, or even several, experimental trials. Thus, another possibility is that young children tend to interpret questions about their ability literally, to believe that the experimenter really is interested in how good they are at solving puzzles or tracing paths, and to respond, rather appropriately from this point of view, in terms of their general experience in similar domains. In contrast, older children may be more likely to understand that the experimenter is really asking about their ability to use relevant information.

One way to examine this possibility is to ask children to explain their ratings. In one relevant study, children rated their ability at finding hidden chickens after they saw how many chickens they and two peers had found in a hidden figures task (Butler & Ruzany, 1993). Several young children in kibbutzim, which are agricultural communities, justified their high ratings by explaining that "I always find lots of chickens in the incubator"; other young children referred to their experience with similar puzzles. In contrast, most of the older children referred to the social comparison standards provided. School experience may well play a role here, as seems to be the case for strategies such as verbal rehearsal. Thus, school tasks are not only structured but are also structured in ways that scaffold understanding that school problems differ from those of daily life, and should be solved using only the information provided.

Evidence that young children can use self-evaluative standards appropriately does not necessarily imply that they are always motivated either to evaluate their competence or to do so accurately. Moreover, analyses that emphasize the acquisition and application of self-evaluative knowledge and strategies in context do not, as yet, resolve the puzzle addressed by Stipek (1984). Thus, we still need to explain why, when young children do not evaluate themselves accurately, they over- rather than underestimate their capacities. I address these issues in the next section.

DEVELOPMENTAL INFLUENCES ON SELF-EVALUATIVE MOTIVES

Are Young Children Motivated to Evaluate Their Competence?

There are grounds for venturing that self-evaluative motivation increases with age (Ruble, 1983), at least in part because preschools of the kind described earlier are less likely than typical elementary schools to convey that levels of relative competence are important. Thus, young children may be motivated mainly to seek and attend to information relevant to acquiring competence, and interest in evaluating competence should increase during middle childhood (Butler, 1989b). Ruble and Frey (1991) reached a similar conclusion on the basis of their analysis of the implications of stages of skill acquisition for self-evaluative strategies. They reasoned that young children tend to be at early stages of skill acquisition, when it is most functional to seek information relevant to clarifying task requirements and acquiring initial proficiency. With age, however, children are more likely to be at later stages of skill acquisition, when it is appropriate to seek information relevant also to evaluating their competence.

In a series of studies, we examined motives for attending to peers' work during arts-and-crafts activities. Results from the first of these studies indicated that children's interest in peers' work, as reflected in the frequency with which they looked at others' work, did not change between ages 4 and 10, but their explanations for doing so changed dramatically (Butler, 1989b). Before grade 1, almost all children explained their glances in terms of strivings to learn from others, and said, for example, "My flower came out funny so I wanted to see how he did his" or "I couldn't get the ground right." Thereafter, increasing numbers of children explained their glances in terms of strivings for self-evaluation, and by age 10, over 80% explained that "I wanted to see if my design was good" or "I wanted to see who made the best flower."

Subsequent studies were designed to clarify the roles of context, concept acquisition, and stages of skill acquisition by comparing motives for looking at peers' work among 4- to 10-year-old urban and kibbutz children at different levels of acquisition of the norma-

tive concept of ability (Butler & Ruzany, 1993) and during earlier versus later stages of task engagement (Butler, 1996). Urban preschools differed from elementary schools, as described by Baumer (1998). In keeping with the collectivist kibbutz ideology, kibbutz schools were, however, characterized throughout by an explicit commitment to cooperative and child-centered learning for mastery, and teachers refrained from normative evaluation also in elementary school. As expected, the results for urban children replicated those of the first study, and the shift from mastery to self-appraisal motives was associated with both the transition to elementary school and acquisition of the normative concept of ability. In contrast, most kibbutz children cited mastery reasons for attending to peers' work in both preschool and elementary school, and both before and after acquisition of the normative concept of ability. In both environments, however, children were more likely to cite learning reasons during early stages of task engagement, and self-appraisal reasons at later stages (Butler, 1996).

These findings confirm the extent to which not only self-evaluative knowledge and competence but also motivation to evaluate the self are constructed in context, and suggest that in typical Western environments, this does indeed increase with age-related changes in the school environment. No studies have examined the further implication that children who attend more academic preschools will display earlier interest in evaluating, and not just in acquiring, competence. Experimental studies have, however, confirmed that even 5-year-olds understood that it was more appropriate to evaluate their work relative to social, rather than objective, standards when told that they were participating in a competition to see who did the best work (Butler, 1990). They were also more likely to explain their glances in terms of self-appraisal in a competitive than in a noncompetitive condition (Butler, 1996).

In all events, even if young children typically use the informational environment mainly to acquire competence, we have seen that they also evaluate their competence in both controlled and natural settings. Indeed, explaining that one looked at someone else's work because "My flower came out funny and I wanted to see how he did his" also implies some appreciation of deficiencies in one's own work. I now turn to the second question: Do positive biases decrease between early and middle childhood?

Motivation for Accurate versus Positive Self-Evaluation

Analyses of early self-appraisal have not always considered the fact that adults also tend to overestimate their abilities and performance. Moreover, Taylor and Brown (1988) concluded that self-enhancing biases are associated with a pattern of positive adjustment and high self-esteem, reminiscent of the confident and resilient young child described in earlier sections. Overoptimistic appraisals may, however, also impair effective coping by limiting possibilities of monitoring, evaluating, and improving outcomes and capacities, of identifying and overcoming deficiencies, and of setting and working toward attainable goals. Thus, much recent research on self-evaluative strategies and judgments has been guided by the assumption that these reflect conflicting strivings for positive and veridical self-appraisal, and by attempts to identify when one or the other is more salient (Butler, 2000; Frey & Ruble, 1985), or when people are more or less likely to constrain positive biases (Sedikides, Herbst, Hardin, & Dardis, 2002).

In brief, the more important it is for people to view and present themselves in a positive light, the more likely are they to do so. Positive biases in adults increase as a function of the personal, contextual, or cultural importance of the attribute evaluated (Sedikides, Gaertner, & Toguchi, 2003). Self-presentation concerns may, however, also constrain positive biases, because people on occasion pay a price for presenting themselves as superior to others, or as self-aggrandizing and immodest self-appraisers (Brickman & Bulman, 1977). Self-serving biases also decrease as a function of the importance of veridical self-appraisal. For example, I have proposed that they are enhanced by performance goals and constrained by learning goals (Butler, 1993, 2000). I reasoned that people who strive to demonstrate superior ability or avoid the demonstration of inferior ability should be interested mainly in information that reflects favorably on their ability. In contrast, veridical self-appraisal is more adaptive when people strive to learn and acquire competence, because one cannot know whether there is room for improvement without some sense of one's current proficiency. Positive biases are also constrained when people have more, rather then less, relevant knowledge and expertise (Kruger & Dunning, 1999), and when their cognitive resources are more, rather than less, adequate for processing available information (Trope & Neter, 1993).

Integrating this, albeit schematic, review with the foregoing analysis of the development of self-evaluative competence and motivation suggests the existence of two conflicting, age-related trends. On the one hand, motivation to evaluate the self favorably may actually increase rather than decline with age, in keeping with increases in the pursuit of personal performance goals and in contextual emphases on the importance of demonstrating superior ability. On the other hand, constraints on positive biases should also increase as children acquire more domain-specific knowledge, greater capacity to process complex information, and greater social understanding of the costs of inflated self-appraisal.

This analysis can account for unexpected findings from two studies in which, instead of decreasing steadily with age, self-appraisals were most positive at age 5–6, and were less favorable not only at ages 7–9 but also at age 4–5 (Butler, 1990; 1998). Similarity between appraisals after success and failure, which is usually interpreted as evidence of motivated bias, was also greatest at age 5–6, mainly because self-appraisal in failure conditions were particularly positive in this age group. Moreover, although, as described earlier, both the youngest and the oldest children tended to evaluate themselves appropriately relative to simple and accessible standards, the evaluative strategies of 5- to 6-year-olds were quite self-serving. Thus, they were more likely to explain their ratings in terms of social comparison when they performed better, rather than worse, than another child (Butler, 1998).

The differences between children in K1 and grade 3 cannot be interpreted solely in terms of age-related decreases in wishful thinking and advances in operational thought, because the appraisals and explanations of preschool children were less self-serving. Rather, I offered the tentative explanation that the K1 children, who were about to enter elementary school, were both more motivated than the younger children to present themselves as highly competent and less capable than the older children of constraining positive biases (Butler, 1998). A recent study (Kinsborn, 2002) provided a more direct test of this analysis. We examined self-evaluative judgments when children in preschool, K1, grade 1, and grades 3–4 saw either that their performance on the tracing task described earlier was both better than that of another child and worse than that on a prior trial, or that they had performed worse than the other child but better than before. For this more complex, multistandard, evaluative task, 4- to 5-year-olds were more likely than in the earlier study (Butler, 1998) to base their appraisals on comparison with the objective rather than the social standard, but in both cases, they evaluated their performance realistically. In contrast, self-enhancing biases were marked both in K1 and in grade 1. In K1, these took the form of selective, self-enhancing comparisons with the less demanding social comparison standard. In grade 1, when children were able to attend also to the temporal information, they attended selectively to the standard that reflected more favorably on their performance. Only at age 9–10 did most children again evaluate their performance appropriately, usually by integrating information from more than one of the available objective, temporal, and social standards.

Another factor that may have constrained self-serving biases in the older children, as in adults, is their increasing awareness of the social costs of self-aggrandizing appraisals. Indeed, in two interesting studies of social comparison behaviors in K1 through grade 5 classrooms, overt, self-enhancing social comparisons were most frequent in K1 and grade 1, but more subtle comparisons, such as inquiries about peer progress, increased during middle childhood (Frey & Ruble, 1985; Pomerantz, Ruble, Frey, & Greulich, 1995). Older children were also more likely than younger children to express disapproval of public declarations of superior competence.

Further research is necessary to confirm whether children initially tend to be veridical rather than self-enhancing self-evaluators. This proposal differs markedly from most prior analyses, but many of these were based on findings from studies in which the youngest participants were already in kindergarten. In one exception, Stipek and Hoffman (1980) found that 3- to 4-year-olds were more likely than were 5- to 6-year-olds to make more favorable judgments after failure for the self than for another child. In another study, however, 4-year-old children's expectations for the self were modified by relevant information except when an anticipated reward was made contingent on success (Stipek, Roberts, & Sanborn, 1984). Thus, positive bias increased among young children, as among older children and adults, with the incentive value of success. In a similar vein, 4-year-olds in another study evaluated their work appropriately (and less favorably than did 7-year-olds) when they were instructed to copy a drawing of a flower as exactly as they could, but overestimated their performance when they were told that they were participating in a competition to see who could make the best copy (Butler, 1990). They also adopted different self-evaluative strategies in the two conditions. Thus, they explained their ratings in terms of appropriate comparisons with the original drawing in the "match-the-standard" condition, but in terms of self-serving comparisons with peers' work in the competitive condition. For example, a child in the former condition explained that his copy was not very good, because he had done too many petals, but a child in the competitive condition, who had also drawn too many petals, explained that his work was excellent, because he had drawn more petals than his friend! In this case, one can venture that if young children are indeed less prone to motivated, self-enhancing biases than are older ones, this, too, may have something to do with their typical schools, which are less likely than are elementary schools to emphasize competitive success.

Analysis in terms of increasing motivation to evaluate the self favorably alongside increasing capacity to constrain positive biases can also provide a perspective for understanding why studies tend to find that average levels of perceived competence in various academic domains were similar and high before about age 8 and declined steadily thereafter (Marsh, Craven, & Debus, 1998; Wigfield et al., 1997). As noted earlier, evaluating one's competence in one or another domain is a complex endeavor that requires systematic consideration and integration of outcomes across time and situations. Even though young children seem more capable than we once thought of forming general perceptions of their cognitive competence, they also find it difficult to integrate multiple sources of information. Thus, one would expect their perceptions to be based on a rather unsystematic sampling of relevant events and information, in keeping with their relatively limited, domain-specific experience and information-processing capacities (see also Marsh et al., 1998). These constraints can also account for their rather positive perceptions, because, as described earlier, young children typically have little reason to feel incompetent, and are rarely required to put their positive appraisals and expectations to the test. Although this changes, at least for the less able, with the transition to elementary school, so should all children's appreciation of the importance of success and their motivation to evaluate themselves favorably. Thus, even though sampling may become more systematic, motivated biases should initially maintain perceived competence at rather high levels, in real life as in controlled studies. Finally, declines after the early elementary school grades are consistent with the notion of continuous, rather than qualitative, increments in children's domain-specific experience, proficiency in integrating relevant information from different sources, awareness of the costs of self-aggrandizement, and, thus, in the capacity to constrain motivated biases.

In this context, it is important to note that theory and research with older children and adults has examined not only how people integrate experiences and information to form general perceptions of their competencies and abilities, but also how individual differences in these general perceptions influence self-evaluative strategies, inferences, and consequences. Thus, for example, high self-esteem is associated with positive self-evaluative biases, and with more resilient responses in the event of failure and adversity (Taylor & Brown, 1988). As long as re-

searchers assumed that young children uniformly overestimate their abilities and do not have a sense of global self-worth, they had little reason to consider the possibility or role of early individual differences in self-esteem. There may, however, be grounds for reconsidering this assumption as well.

Research on affective development has documented early individual differences in the degree to which children behave "as if" they have higher or lower levels of self-worth or confidence, respond to novel events with enthusiasm or fear and react to difficulty with persistence or shame (Lewis, 1998). In the most comprehensive research program to date, Dweck and her associates (e.g., Cain & Dweck, 1995; Dweck,1999; Smiley & Dweck, 1994) have documented individual differences by age 4 in children's preferences to repeat a task on which they had attained only partial success versus one that they had previously completed successfully. Moreover, in contrast with prior findings of uniformly high expectations and continuing behavioral persistence after failure, this was the case for children who preferred the challenging task, but not for those who preferred the easy one. The latter, but not the former, also displayed negative affect, self-blame, and impaired strategies. Thus, some quite young children displayed the helpless responses to challenge and failure that were once thought to emerge only in middle childhood.

Dweck (1999) has attributed this pattern to the early development of a sense of contingent self-worth, which in her view is rooted in the belief that outcomes reflect on one's worth and goodness rather than one's competence or ability. In support, she cited findings that helpless responses were not related to children's actual or perceived competence for the target activity, but when children role-played situations in which they erred on a task, 53% of the "helpless" children agreed they would feel that they were not good children. However, a higher and striking 62% made competence-related inferences and said that they would feel they were not good at the task or not smart (Heyman, Dweck, & Cain, 1992). Thus, one cannot discount the possibility that young children's early "idea of me" (Lewis, 1991) incorporates representations of the self not only as more or less worthy but also as more or less competent or efficacious. If so, one can also venture that individual differences in such representations may moderate achievement-related judgments and behaviors much earlier than previously thought.

CONCLUSIONS AND IMPLICATIONS FOR PROMOTING ADAPTIVE SELF-ASSESSMENT, SELF-REGULATION, AND MOTIVATION

To summarize, there are theoretical and empirical grounds for making several general claims about young children's self-evaluative knowledge, competence, and motivation, and how these evolve during early and middle childhood. First, early (and some later) descriptions of young children as consistently inaccurate and incompetent self-evaluators are themselves inaccurate. Already during their third year, if not before, children display differential affect and behavior in the event of more versus less successful mastery attempts, and seem to anticipate differential evaluative responses from adults. Certainly by age 4, and possibly even earlier, questions of competence are meaningful and play a role in regulating activity. Quite young children display practical understanding of the diagnosticity of various informational standards and strategies, including social comparison, and use them appropriately to evaluate their competence in controlled settings. They also form quite reliable perceptions of their competence in everyday domains. They do, however, have difficulty with some kinds of standards, such as information about prior outcomes, and cannot integrate information from multiple sources or standards. However, there is some evidence that even in such cases, they tend to evaluate themselves rather appropriately relative to that information that is accessible to them.

Second, there seems to be considerable similarity in the factors that influence younger and older children's competence-related strategies, inferences and behaviors, and, thus, in the ways in which they evaluate or misevaluate themselves. Thus, appraisals of specific outcomes and self-evaluative strategies seem to be influenced in rather similar ways by relevant experience and the complexity of relevant information. Moreover,

the level of complexity that is "too difficult" seems to change incrementally, rather than dramatically, between early and middle childhood. In a similar vein, there are grounds for attributing increasing differentiation in the self-concept to increasing experience with different domains, including school subjects, more than to qualitative differences in differentiation per se. Most generally, examination of the self-evaluative capacities and limitations of younger children, and comparisons with those of older children, serve to challenge "structural deficit" analyses of the development of competence-related judgments and concepts. Rather, I have suggested that this is better explained by parallel analyses of the typical contexts of early and middle childhood, on the one hand, and of the complexity of various self-evaluative tasks and challenges, on the other. Thus, in competence assessment, as in other domains, children seem to acquire and apply those skills, strategies, and concepts that are functional to and scaffolded by their everyday experience and commensurate with their current knowledge and processing capacities.

Third, there do seem to be age-related differences in children's motivation to evaluate themselves. Younger children seem to be more oriented to acquiring than evaluating competence, and motivation to evaluate competence does seem to increase between early and middle childhood, as other researchers have suggested (Ruble, 1983; Ruble & Frey, 1991). However, older children behaved much like younger ones in experimental and natural contexts that emphasized learning and competence acquisition, and there is some evidence that younger children behaved much like older ones in contexts that emphasized the importance of relative achievement. Thus, from an early age, children also learn what kinds of competence are important, how each is best evaluated, when it is important to demonstrate superior ability, and what price one might pay for doing so. In this context, I have ventured that younger children may actually be less inclined to motivated, self-enhancing biases than prior analyses have suggested, and have cited evidence consistent with the notion that both motivation to overestimate one's capacities and constraints on positive biases increase after early childhood.

These conclusions cast doubt on prior claims that there are clear age-related transformations in achievement-related behaviors and motivation. First, this review is consistent with other challenges to descriptions of young children as necessarily optimistic and confident about their capacities, even when they encounter difficulty (Dweck, 1999). The research program of Dweck and her associates has confirmed that at least some young children respond negatively to difficulty and challenge, and do so in ways that do not seem to change much with age. Moreover, if quite young children can attend to relevant information to evaluate their outcomes, anticipate the evaluative responses of others, and form general perceptions of their competence in familiar domains, one might also wonder whether, as a group, they are as invulnerable to failure as early analyses assumed. As noted earlier, there is very little relevant empirical evidence, possibly because, until recently, there seemed to be little reason to anticipate nonresilient responses. But even 4- to 5-year-olds displayed less intrinsic motivation for an activity after they performed worse, as compared with better, than another (Butler, 1998). Further research might examine the additional possibility that decrements in confidence and interest will be even more marked when young children experience recurring failures in one or other domain in their daily lives.

Second, this review has implications for the development of children's achievement motivation. Interestingly, the effects of age, context, and individual differences on children's self-evaluative motivations and responses to challenge reviewed in this chapter are similar to those associated with approach versus avoidance motivational orientations (Elliot & Thrash, 2002) or task versus ego-involving settings (Butler, 1993) among adults. On the one hand, analysis of the typical contexts of early versus middle childhood and findings from many empirical studies are consistent with proposals that young children typically pursue task, or learning, goals in achievement settings (Nicholls & Miller, 1984). On the other hand, I have cited evidence that even quite young children were sensitive to contextual cues regarding the importance of different kinds of success or competence. In this case,

one can ask whether their motivational strivings change as dramatically with age as some researchers have suggested. Put another way, are young children "developmentally constrained" to pursue task goals, or can they also be guided by strivings to demonstrate superior, or disguise inferior, performance or ability?

Few studies have examined the effects of different goal cues on young children's motivation and behavior, possibly because researchers tended to believe that young children are incapable of pursuing performance, or ego, goals. Consistent with this belief, competitive conditions, which present a strong performance–goal manipulation, did not undermine children's intrinsic motivation before about age 9–10 (Butler, 1989a, 1990). They did, however, undermine performance on a creative task (Butler, 1989b), motivation to learn from others (Butler, 1996) and veridical self-appraisal (Butler, 1990) among 4- to 5-year-olds, as among older children and adults. Thus, young children sometimes behaved as if they were guided by performance goals, and did so, moreover, in contexts that evoke such goals at later ages. In this case, a cautious working hypothesis that could be examined in future research is that consistent exposure to such conditions at home or at school might well create a more general orientation to pursue performance, rather than learning, goals, even in the preschool years.

Before I address some applied implications of this review, it is important to note some issues it did not address. Most significantly, in view of my emphasis on experience in context, in this review I discussed educational contexts at length but barely touched on those of the home and family. My emphasis on general processes, strategies, and concerns, and, thus, on "children in general" is also problematic in view of the role of factors such as class, ethnicity, and culture in shaping children's constructions of themselves and the world, at home, at school, and in the transition between them. In a similar vein, I did not address possible gender influences in the development of self-relevant judgments and achievement motivation and behavior.

Despite these limitations, one clear applied implication of this review is that parents and teachers should be aware that young children may display at least some of the maladaptive responses to challenge, difficulty, and contextual emphases on relative ability that have been documented at later ages. The present emphasis on the construction of self-evaluative knowledge and achievement motivation in context also suggests some more specific guides as to behaviors and contexts that are likely to promote more or less constructive responses. Providing children with supportive and informative feedback about task requirements and effective strategies in settings that emphasize the value of acquiring knowledge and understanding of the world and the self should maintain and promote tendencies to evaluate the self appropriately, and to use self-knowledge constructively to promote competence acquisition. It is questionable whether the kinds of preschool environments described by Baumer (1998) provide such scaffolds, but at least they do not seem to undermine children's sense of competence. In contrast, parents and teachers who dismiss or criticize children's mastery attempts, set unreasonable standards, or compare them with more successful siblings, neighbors, and classmates should convey both that it is more important to succeed than to learn, and that the child is incompetent and unworthy (see also Dweck, 1999; Kelley et al., 2000). Adults who respond in these ways should also be less likely to provide environments in which children can correct negative self-conceptions and behaviors, and derive satisfaction from acquiring competence.

With the transition to elementary school, children are more likely to encounter critical evaluations, tasks that they find difficult, and cues that convey the importance of demonstrating superior ability. In this case, it is not surprising that the frequency of helpless responses and the level of performance goal orientation increases during middle childhood. However, there is converging evidence that supportive settings and constructive feedback of the kinds described earlier are effective in promoting constructive self-evaluation and adaptive self-regulation, and achievement strivings at all ages (Ames, 1992; Butler, 2000).

To summarize, the evolvement of children's self-evaluative competencies, strategies, and motivations, described here and by some other researchers (Dweck, 1999; Ruble & Frey, 1991), presents a rather different picture of young children's strengths and vulnerabilities than that depicted in many earlier analyses. On the one hand, young children seem to be more competent than we once thought in evaluating their outcomes and capacities, and should, thus, also be less limited in using self-knowledge and the informational environment to monitor and regulate activity, to set goals, and to acquire strategies for attaining them. On the other hand, these very competencies may also render them more vulnerable than we once thought to developing maladaptive patterns of self-doubt and helplessness, and the belief that it is more important to succeed, or avoid failure, than it is to learn and acquire competence.

REFERENCES

Aboud, F. E. (1985). Children's application of attribution principles to social comparisons. *Child Development*, 56, 682–688.

Ames, C. (1992). Goals, structures and student motivation. *Journal of Educational Psychology*, 84, 261–271.

Baumer, S. (1998). *Self-regulation processes in preschool and school children*. Unpublished doctoral dissertation, Hebrew University, Jerusalem.

Borke, H. (1975). Piaget's mountains revisited: Changes in the egocentric landscape. *Developmental Psychology*, 11, 240–243.

Brickman, P., & Bulman, R. J. (1977). Pleasure and pain in social comparison. In J. M. Suls & R. L. Miller (Eds.), *Social comparison processes* (pp. 149–176). Washington, DC: Hemisphere.

Bullock, M., & Gelman, R. (1979). Preschool children's assumptions about cause and effect: Temporal ordering. *Child Development*, 50, 89–96.

Butler, R. (1989a). Interest in the task and interest in peer's work in competitive and non-competitive conditions: A developmental study. *Child Development*, 60, 562–570.

Butler R. (1989b). Mastery versus ability-appraisal: A developmental study of children's observations of peers' work. *Child Development*, 60, 1350–1361.

Butler, R. (1990). The effects of mastery and competitive conditions on self-assessment at different ages. *Child Development*, 61, 201–210.

Butler, R. (1993). Effects of task- and ego-achievement goals on information seeking during task-engagement. *Journal of Personality and Social Psychology*, 65, 18–31.

Butler, R. (1996). Effects of age and achievement goals on children's motives for attending to peers' work.

British Journal of Developmental Psychology, 14, 1–18.

Butler, R. (1998). Age trends in the use of social and temporal comparison for self-evaluation: Examination of a novel developmental hypothesis. *Child Development, 69,* 1054–1073.

Butler, R. (2000). What learners want to know: The role of achievement goals in shaping information-seeking, performance and interest. In C. Sansone & J. Harackiewicz (Eds.), *Intrinsic and extrinsic motivation: The search for optimal motivation and performance* (pp. 161–194). New York: Academic Press.

Butler, R., & Ruzany, N. (1993). Age and socialization effects on the development of social comparison motives and normative ability assessment in kibbutz and urban children. *Child Development, 64,* 532–543.

Cain, K. M., & Dweck, C. S. (1995). The development of children's achievement motivation patterns and conceptions of intelligence. *Merrill–Palmer Quarterly, 41,* 25–52.

Case, R. (1985). *Intellectual development: Birth to adulthood.* Orlando: Academic Press.

Chi, M. T., & Koeske, R. D. (1983). Network representations of a child's dinosaur knowledge. *Developmental Psychology, 19,* 29–39.

Damon, W., & Hart, D. (1988). *Self-understanding in childhood and adolescence.* Cambridge, UK: Cambridge University Press.

Diener, C. I., & Dweck, C. S. (1978). An analysis of learned helplessness: Continuous changes in performance, strategy and achievement cognitions following failure. *Journal of Personality and Social Psychology, 36,* 451–462.

Dweck, C. S. (1986). Motivational processes affecting learning. *American Psychologist, 41,* 1040–1048.

Dweck, C. S. (1999). *Self-theories: Their role in motivation, personality and development.* Philadelphia: Psychology Press.

Dweck, C. S., & Elliot, E. S. (1983). Achievement motivation. In E. M. Hetherington (Ed.), *Handbook of child psychology: Vol. 4. Social and personality development* (pp. 643–691). New York: Wiley.

Elliot, A. J., & Thrash, T. M. (2002). Approach–avoidance motivation in personality: Approach and avoidance temperaments and goals. *Journal of Personality and Social Psychology, 82,* 804–818.

Eshel, Y., & Klein, Z. (1981). Development of academic self-concept of lower-class and middle-class primary school children. *Journal of Educational Psychology, 73,* 287–293.

Fischer, K. W. (1980). A theory of cognitive development: The control and construction of hierarchies of skills. *Psychological Review, 87,* 477–531.

Flavell, J. H. (1985). *Cognitive development* (2nd ed.). Englewood Cliffs, NJ: Prentice-Hall.

Flavell, J. H. (1999). Cognitive development: Children's knowledge about the mind. *Annual Review of Psychology, 50,* 21–45.

Frey, K. S., & Ruble, D. N. (1985). What children say when the teacher's not around: Conflicting goals in social comparison and performance assessment in the classroom. *Journal of Personality and Social Psychology, 48,* 18–30.

Gelman, R. (1979). Preschool thought. *American Psychologist, 34,* 900–905.

Harter, S. (1981). A new self-report scale of intrinsic versus extrinsic orientation in the classroom: Motivational and informational components. *Developmental Psychology, 17,* 300–312.

Harter, S. (1990). Cause, correlates, and the functional role of global self-worth: A life-span perspective. In R. J. Sternberg & J. Kolligan Jr. (Eds.), *Competence considered* (pp. 67–97). New Haven, CT: Yale University Press.

Harter, S. (1999). *The construction of the self: A developmental perspective.* New York: Guilford Press.

Harter, S., & Pike, R. (1984). The pictorial scale of perceived competence and social acceptance for young children. *Child Development, 55,* 1969–1982.

Heyman, G., Dweck, C. S., & Cain, K. (1992). Young children's vulnerability to self-blame and helplessness: Relationship to beliefs about goodness. *Child Development, 63,* 401–415.

Higgins, E. T., & Parsons, J. E. (1983). Stages as subcultures: Social-cognitive development and the social life of the child. In E. T. Higgins, D. N. Ruble, & W. W. Hartup (Eds.), *Social cognition and social behavior* (pp. 15–62). New York: Cambridge University Press.

Hollos, M., & Cowan, P. A. (1973). Social isolation and cognitive development: Logical operations and role taking abilities in three Norwegian social settings. *Child Development, 44,* 630–641.

Keeney, T. J., Cannizzo, S. R., & Flavell, J. H. (1967). Spontaneous and induced verbal rehearsal in a recall task. *Child Development, 38,* 953–966.

Kelley, S. A., Brownell, C. A., & Campbell, S. B. (2000). Mastery motivation and self-evaluative affect in toddlers: Longitudinal relations with maternal behavior. *Child Development, 71,* 1061–1071.

Kinsborn, Y. (2002). *The development of motivation to engage in social and temporal comparison.* Unpublished master's thesis, Hebrew University, Jerusalem, Israel.

Kruger, J., & Dunning, D. (1999). Unskilled and unaware of it: How difficulties in recognizing one's own incompetencies lead to inflated self-assessments. *Journal of Personality and Social Psychology, 77,* 1121–1134.

Lewis, M. (1991). Ways of knowing: Objective self-awareness and consciousness. *Developmental Review, 11,* 231–243.

Lewis, M. (1998). Emotional competence and development. In D. Pushkar, W. M. Bukowski, A. E. Schwartzman, D. M. Stack, & D. R. White (Eds.), *Improving competence across the lifespan: Building interventions based in theory and research* (pp. 27–36). New York: Plenum Press.

Marsh, H. W., Craven, R. G., & Debus, R. (1998). Structure, stability, and development of young children's self-concepts: A multicohort–multioccasion study. *Child Development, 69,* 1030–1053.

Marsh, H. W., Ellis, L. A., & Craven, R. G. (2002). How do preschool children feel about themselves?: Unraveling measurement and multidimensional self-concept structure. *Developmental Psychology, 38,* 376–393.

Morris, W. N., & Nemcek, D. (1982). The development of social comparison motivation among preschoolers: Evidence of a stepwise progression. *Merrill–Palmer Quarterly, 28,* 413–425.

Mosatche, H. S., & Bragonier, P. (1981). An observational study of social comparison in preschoolers. *Child Development, 52,* 376–378.

Nicholls, J. G. (1978). The development of the concepts of effort and ability, perception of academic attainment, and the understanding that difficult tasks require more ability. *Child Development, 49,* 800–814.

Nicholls, J. G. (1989). *The competitive ethos and democratic education.* Cambridge, MA: Harvard University Press.

Nicholls, J. G. (1990). What is ability and why are we mindful of it?: A developmental perspective. In R. J. Sternberg & J. Kolligan Jr. (Eds.), *Competence considered* (pp. 11–40). New Haven, CT: Yale University Press.

Nicholls, J. G., & Miller, A. T. (1983). The differentiation of the concepts of difficulty and ability. *Child Development, 54,* 951–959.

Nicholls, J. G., & Miller, A. T. (1984). Development and its discontents: The differentiation of the concept of ability. In J. G. Nicholls (Ed.), *Advances in motivation and achievement: Vol. 3: The development of achievement motivation* (pp. 185–218). Greenwich, CT: JAI Press.

Nicholls, J. G., & Miller, A. T. (1985). Differentiation of the concepts of luck and skill. *Developmental Psychology, 21,* 76–82.

Odom, R. D., Astor, E. C., & Cunningham, J. (1975). Effects of perceptual salience on the matrix task performance of four- and six-year-old children. *Child Development, 46,* 758–762.

Piaget, J. (1928). *Judgment and reasoning of the child.* New York: Harcourt, Brace & World. (Original published in 1926)

Piaget, J. (1930). *The child's conception of the world.* New York: Harcourt, Brace & World. (Original published in 1926)

Piaget, J., Inhelder, B., & Szeminska, A. (1960). *The child's conception of geometry.* New York: Basic Books. (Original published in 1948)

Pomerantz, E. M., Ruble, D. N., Frey, K. S., & Greulich, F. (1995). Meeting goals and confronting conflict: Children's changing perceptions of social comparison. *Child Development, 66,* 723–738.

Rholes, W. S., Blackwell, J., Jordan, C., & Walters, C. (1980). A developmental study of learned helplessness. *Developmental Psychology, 16,* 616–624.

Rogoff, B., & Mistry, J. (1990). The social and functional context of children's remembering. In R. Fivush & J. A. Hudson (Eds.), *Knowing and remembering in young children: Emory Symposia in Cognition* (Vol. 3, pp. 197–222). New York: Cambridge University Press.

Ruble, D. N. (1983). The development of social comparison processes and their role in achievement-related self-socialization. In E. T. Higgins, D. N. Ruble, & W. W. Hartup (Eds.), *Social cognition and social behavior* (pp. 134–157). New York: Cambridge University Press.

Ruble, D. N., Boggiano, A. K., Feldman, N., & Loebl, J. (1980). A developmental analysis of the role of social comparison in self-evaluation. *Developmental Psychology, 16,* 105–115.

Ruble, D. N., & Dweck, C. S. (1995). Self-conceptions, person conceptions, and their development. In N. Eisenberg (Ed.), *Review of personality and social psychology* (Vol. 15, pp. 109–139). Thousand Oaks, CA: Sage.

Ruble, D. N., Eisenberg, R., & Higgins, E. T. (1994). Developmental changes in achievement evaluation: Motivational implications of self-other differences. *Child Development, 65,* 1091–1106.

Ruble, D. N., & Frey, K. S. (1991). Changing patterns of comparative behavior as skills are acquired: A functional model of self-evaluation. In J. Suls & T. A. Wills (Eds.), *Social comparison: Contemporary theory and research* (pp. 79–113). Hillsdale, NJ: Erlbaum.

Ruble, D. N., Grosovsky, E. H., Frey, K. S., & Cohen, R. (1992). Developmental changes in competence assessment. In A. K. Boggiano & T. S. Pittman (Eds.), *Achievement and motivation: A social-developmental perspective* (pp. 138–164). Cambridge, UK: Cambridge University Press.

Schneider, K. (1984). The cognitive basis of task choice in preschool children. In J. G. Nicholls (Ed.), *Advances in motivation and achievement: Vol. 3. The development of achievement motivation* (pp. 57–72). Greenwich, CT: JAI Press.

Sedikides, C., Gaertner, L., & Toguchi, Y. (2003). Pancultural self-enhancement. *Journal of Personality and Social Psychology, 84,* 60–79.

Sedikides, C., Herbst, K. C., Hardin, D. P., & Dardis, G. J. (2002). Accountability as a deterrent to self-enhancement: The search for mechanisms. *Journal of Personality and Social Psychology, 83,* 592–605.

Siegler, R. S. (1996). *Emerging minds: The process of change in children's thinking.* London: Oxford University Press.

Smiley, P. A., & Dweck, C. S. (1994). Individual differences in achievement goals among young children. *Child Development, 65,* 1723–1743.

Stipek, D. J. (1984). Young children's performance expectations: Logical analysis or wishful thinking? In J. G. Nicholls (Ed.), *Advances in motivation and achievement: Vol. 3. The development of achieve-*

ment motivation (pp. 33–56). Greenwich, CT: JAI Press.

Stipek, D. J., & Daniels, D. (1988). Declining perceptions of competence: A consequence of changes in the child or the educational environment? *Journal of Educational Psychology, 80,* 352–356.

Stipek, D. J., & Hoffman, J. (1980). Development of children's performance-related judgments. *Child Development, 51,* 912–914.

Stipek, D. J., & Mac Iver, D. (1989). Developmental changes in children's assessment of intellectual competence. *Child Development, 60,* 521–538.

Stipek, D. J., Recchia, S., & McClintic, S. (1992). Self-evaluation in young children. *Monographs of the Society for Research in Child Development, 57.*

Stipek, D. J., Roberts, T., & Sanborn, M. (1984). Preschool-age children's performance expectations for themselves and another child as a function of the incentive value of success and the salience of past performance. *Child Development, 59,* 1983–1989.

Strayer, F. F., Chapeskie, T. R., & Strayer, J. (1979). The perception of preschool social dominance. *Aggressive Behavior, 4,* 183–192.

Suls, J., & Mullen, B. (1982). From the cradle to the grave: Comparison and self-evaluation across the life-span. In J. M. Suls (Ed.), *Social psychological perspectives on the self* (Vol. 1, pp. 97–125). Hillsdale, NJ: Erlbaum.

Taylor, S. E., & Brown, J. D. (1988). Illusion and well-being: A social-psychological perspective on mental health. *Psychological Bulletin, 103,* 193–210.

Trope, Y., & Neter, E. (1993). Reconciling competing motives in self-evaluation: The role of self-control in feedback. *Journal of Personality and Social Psychology, 66,* 646–657.

Veroff, J. (1969). Social comparison and the development of achievement motivation. In C. P. Smith (Ed.), *Achievement-related motives in children* (pp. 46–101). New York: Russell Sage Foundation.

Vygotsky, L. S. (1978). *Thought and language* (rev. and edited by A. Kozulin). Cambridge, MA: MIT Press. (Original published in 1934)

Wigfield, A., Eccles, J. S., Yoon, K. S., Harold, R. D., Arbreton, A. J., Freedman-Doan, C., et al. (1997). Changes in children's competence beliefs and subjective task values across the elementary school years: A three-year study. *Journal of Educational Psychology, 89,* 451–469.

CHAPTER 13

☞

Competence, Motivation, and Identity Development during Adolescence

ALLAN WIGFIELD
A. LAUREL WAGNER

Adolescents experience many important changes in their lives and circumstances that impact the development of their competence and motivation. These include the biological changes associated with puberty, changes in relations with family and peers, increasing concern about their identities and roles, and the social and educational changes resulting from school transitions (see Eccles & Wigfield, 1997; Midgley & Edelin, 1998; Wigfield & Eccles, 2002). Adolescents also face many crucial decisions that can affect them over the course of their lives, such as decisions about their education, possible occupations, which social relationships to pursue, and whether or not to engage in a variety of risky behaviors. Many adolescents cope well with these changes and decisions, and make choices that lead to positive developmental outcomes for them in a variety of areas. Others, however, have difficulty with one or another of these changes and choices, and as a result are at risk for various negative outcomes.

What is the role of competence beliefs and motivation during adolescence? Motivation

theorists posit that individuals' competence beliefs, values, goals, and other motivational variables relate to their performance on different activities, effort exerted in them, and choices of which activities to pursue, and which to avoid (Eccles, Wigfield, & Schiefele, 1998; Wigfield, Eccles, Schiefele, Roeser, & Davis-Kean, in press). Adolescents with strong beliefs in their competence, and positive achievement values and goals, thus should perform more capably, be more likely to exert the effort needed to accomplish different activities, and make appropriate decisions about activities to do, as well as other, more complex choices. Thus, healthy competence beliefs and motivation are central to healthy development during adolescence.

We focus in this chapter on change during adolescence in children's beliefs about their competencies and motivation, with a primary focus on competence and motivation in academic settings. We also discuss the development of broader self-representation processes, with a special focus on identity formation. We discuss identity development, because adolescence is the time in which identities begin to take shape, and adolescents' identity development has important implications for the development of their competence and motivation, and for the kinds of decisions they make about what to do with their lives. We begin with a brief overview of the major changes adolescents experience to provide a context for our discussion of the development of adolescents' perceived competencies, motivation, and identity. Our focus primarily is on the experiences of American adolescents; the developmental course of adolescents' competence and motivation in other cultures may be quite different.

CHANGES DURING ADOLESCENCE

Puberty

The biological changes associated with puberty are among the most dramatic ones that individuals experience during their lifetimes. In part because of these dramatic biological changes, historically, different theorists portrayed the early adolescent period as a period of "storm and stress," where there is a great deal of conflict between children, parents, and teachers (e.g., Blos, 1979; Hall, 1904). Such views often are presented in the media, and in other forums as well, leading many to believe that adolescence is necessarily a turbulent time (see Buchanan, 2002). While it is undeniable that major physical changes occur during early adolescence, many researchers now believe that the characterization of this time period as one of storm and stress is an overstatement (see, e.g., Arnett, 1999; Dornbusch, Petersen, & Hetherington, 1991). However, the biological changes adolescents go through do have many influences on their thinking and behavior, posing challenges for many adolescents (Arnett, 1999).

Cognitive Changes

Children's thinking also changes during the adolescent years (e.g., see Byrnes, 1988; Keating, 1990; Moshman, 2004). For our purposes, the most important changes are the increasing propensity to think abstractly, to consider the hypothetical, as well as the real, to engage in more sophisticated and

elaborate information-processing strategies, to consider multiple dimensions of a problem at once, and to reflect on oneself and on complicated problems (see Keating, 1990, and Moshman, 2004, for more complete discussion). Such changes have potentially important influences on children's learning. They also have implications for individuals' motivation, competence beliefs, and identities. Theorists such as Erikson (1968) and Harter (1990) view the adolescent years as a time of change in children's self-beliefs, as young people consider what possibilities are available to them and try to come to a deeper understanding of themselves. These sorts of self-reflections require the kinds of higher order cognitive processes just discussed.

Along with these changes in cognitive processes, children's skills increase in many ways as they move from childhood into adolescence. Through schooling and participation in sports and other activities, adolescents gain a variety of increasingly sophisticated skills. Of course, there are great individual differences in the extent to which these skills are acquired, but all adolescents' skills do grow. Similarly, adolescents also learn to control and regulate their behavior, so that they can manage their daily routines more efficiently and independently (see Pintrich, 2003; Zimmerman, 2000). Again, some adolescents develop these regulatory skills more completely than do others, but most adolescents do develop them. These changes also have implications for adolescents' developing perceptions of their competence, motivation, and sense of themselves. Adolescents who can regulate their behavior efficiently likely develop a stronger sense of competence in different areas, as well as motivation to participate in these activities.

Changes in Social Relations

Children's social relations change in important ways as they go through adolescence (see Rubin, Bukowski, & Parker, 1998). We only have space here to make several general points about these changes. Parents obviously continue to have a strong influence on their adolescents' development, and many parents remain very involved in their adolescents' lives. They continue to provide opportunities for their children to develop their competencies, and feedback that influences adolescents' sense of competence and motivation (see Eccles et al., 1998; Jacobs & Eccles, 2000). But compared to earlier developmental periods, parental influences likely wane, at least in comparison to the influence of peers, for various reasons. One clear example of this is that parents' involvement in their children's schooling often declines during adolescence (see Epstein & Connors, 1995). Also, parents and adolescents often experience more conflict in their relations as adolescents assert their independence and spend more time away from home. Peer relations take on more importance in adolescence, both in terms of the amount of time adolescents spend with peers and the influence they have on one another (see Berndt & Keefe, 1995). In general, children and adolescents who are accepted by their peers and have good social skills do better in school and have more positive academic achievement motivation. In contrast, socially rejected and highly aggressive children are at risk for numerous negative outcomes, including competence and motivational outcomes (e.g., Parker & Asher, 1987).

Although peer influence often is portrayed in negative terms, research indicates that peers often gravitate to similar others, and strengthen each others' motivational orientations and achievement patterns (Berndt & Keefe, 1995; Kindermann, 1993; Kindermann, McCollam, & Gibson, 1996). Whether such effects are positive or negative depends on the nature of the peer groups' motivational orientations. High-achieving children who have other high achievers as friends can develop even more positive academic motivation over time. In contrast, low achievers who join a low-achieving peer group can become even less motivated to do school work and instead become motivated to engage in other activities valued by this peer group. Some of these activities may enhance adolescents' competence, and some may not (see Kindermann, 1993; Kindermann et al., 1996).

School Transitions

Most adolescents go through two school transitions, one from elementary to middle school, and one from middle to high school. The environments in these settings are quite different from one another, so students have to adjust to them in many ways. These transitions, particularly the middle school transition, have a strong impact on many students' competence beliefs and motivation, and this impact often is negative (see Anderman & Maehr, 1994; Eccles & Wigfield, 1997; Wigfield & Eccles, 2002). Students must cope with disruptions to their social networks, larger and more impersonal school bureaucracies, relations with teachers that often are less personal, and more extensive tracking and ability grouping, among other things. These changes can substantially influence adolescents' competence, identities, and motivation; we now turn to how these develop.

CHANGES IN ADOLESCENTS' ACHIEVEMENT MOTIVATION

Work on the development of motivation and achievement-related beliefs, values, and goals has flourished in the last 30 years (see Eccles et al., 1998; Pintrich & Schunk, 2002; Wigfield et al., in press). Eccles et al. (1998) categorized these belief, values, and goal constructs in terms of questions students can ask themselves that have implications for their motivation. One question is "Can I succeed on this task or activity?" Constructs related to this question include students' competence-related beliefs and self-efficacy (Bandura, 1997), their attributions for success and failure (Weiner, 1985), and their perceptions of control over outcomes (Skinner, Zimmer-Gembeck, & Connell, 1998). In general, when students have high self-efficacy, the belief that they can control their achievement outcomes, and internal attributions for their success, they tend to be more positively motivated and perform better on different achievement tasks and activities (see Eccles et al., 1998, for a complete review). The second question—"Why do I want to do this activity?"—has to do with the purposes for which students engage in academic activities. This question is crucial to motivation. Even if individuals believe they can succeed on a task or activity, they may not engage in it if they have no clear purpose for doing so. Constructs related to this question include students' valuing of achievement (Wigfield & Eccles, 2000), goals for achievement

(Ames, 1992; Pintrich, 2000), and intrinsic and extrinsic motivation (Gottfried, Fleming, & Gottfried, 2001; Ryan & Deci, 2000). When students value achievement, have clear goals for achievement, and are intrinsically motivated, they tend to be more engaged in academic activities and perform better.

Researchers have studied how these motivational constructs change across age in different ways. Some researchers have examined whether children's motivation becomes more stable over time, and they find that, indeed, it does. Adolescents' perceptions of competence, valuing of achievement, and intrinsic motivation all become more stable across age and in comparison to elementary school students' competence beliefs, values, and intrinsic motivation (e.g., Eccles et al., 1989; Gottfried et al., 2001; Wigfield et al., 1997). For instance, Gottfried et al. (2001) measured children's intrinsic motivation for verbal and math activities when children were ages 9, 10, 13, 16, and 17. In both domains, children's intrinsic motivation became more stable over time, particularly during the adolescent years, with the stability correlations reaching .86 for intrinsic motivation for verbal activities and .63 for math intrinsic motivation, when students were 16 and 17 years old. Researchers also have examined mean-level change in these constructs; we review the findings from this work next.

Changes in Competence-Related Beliefs

A consistent finding with respect to certain kinds of competence-related beliefs is that they decline during early adolescence and adolescence (for reviews, see Anderman & Maehr, 1994; Eccles et al., 1998). Specifically, early adolescents have lower perceptions of their competence for different school subjects and other activities than do their younger peers (Eccles et al., 1989; Jacobs, Lanza, Osgood, Eccles, & Wigfield, 2002; Marsh, 1989; Wigfield, Eccles, Mac Iver, Reuman, & Midgley, 1991). Jacobs et al. (2002) examined change in children's competence for math, language arts, and sports across grades 1–12. The overall pattern of change was a decline in each domain. There were some differences across domains with respect to when the strongest changes occurred, particularly in language arts and

math. In language arts, the strongest declines occurred during elementary school, and little change was observed after that. In sports, the change accelerated during the high school years. The decline in math competence beliefs was steady over time.

This same pattern does not appear to hold for self-efficacy beliefs, likely because of differences in how competence beliefs and self-efficacy are defined and measured. Bandura (1997) defined "self-efficacy" as individuals' beliefs about their *own* capabilities to accomplish a task or activities. Therefore, researchers most often measure self-efficacy by asking individuals how confident they are that they can do a given task (see Pajares, 1996). Because children's skills increase with age, adolescents should be more confident in their ability to do more complex tasks than are younger children, which indeed has been found to be the case (Shell, Colvin, & Bruning, 1995; Zimmerman & Martinez-Pons, 1990). In contrast, researchers measuring perceptions of competence often include questions asking children to compare their ability to that of others, and to assess how good they are at a more general activity, such as math. It is on these latter kinds of measures, when students compare themselves to others and provide broader evaluations of their competence, that the declines are observed.

Competence beliefs also become more accurate in the sense of relating more closely to children's performance (Assor & Connell, 1992). Indeed, competence-related beliefs relate strongly to children's performance on different academic, social, and sport activities, even when previous performance levels on the activities are controlled (for reviews, see Bandura, 1997; Wigfield & Eccles, 2002).

Changes in Adolescents' Perceived Value of Achievement, Intrinsic Motivation, and Goal Orientations

Students' valuing of different school subjects also declines as they move through school, with the declines especially marked across the transition to middle school (Eccles et al., 1989; Wigfield et al., 1991). Jacobs et al. (2002), in the study just described, found that children's valuing of the domains of math, language arts, and sports declined. As was the case for competence beliefs, children's valuing of language arts declined most during elementary school and then leveled off. By contrast, children's valuing of math declined most during high school. Researchers also have found decreases in children's intrinsic motivation to learn, in both cross-sectional and longitudinal studies (Gottfried et al., 2001; Harter, 1981). Harter measured intrinsic motivation generally, and Gottfried et al. (2001) measured intrinsic motivation for different subject areas (math, reading, social studies, science), as well as general school intrinsic motivation. Gottfried et al. found declines across ages 9–16 in all these aspects of intrinsic motivation except social studies. These findings point to the importance of measuring motivation constructs in domain-specific ways.

What about students' goals for achievement? Researchers studying children's goals often focus on achievement goal orientations, and have defined and studied several different goal orientations (see Pintrich, 2003). One goal orientation concerns individuals' desire to learn new things and master material; this orientation has been called a "task mastery" or "learning goal orientation" by different researchers (Ames, 1992; Dweck & Leggett, 1988; Maehr & Midgley, 1996; Nicholls, 1984). Another orientation concerns individuals' desires to outperform others and receive favorable evaluations of their performance; this orientation is termed "ego orientation" or "performance goal orientation." The early work on these goal orientations suggested that mastery goal orientations were associated with a variety of positive developmental outcomes, and performance goal orientations, with negative outcomes.

Researchers have explored dual aspects of both the performance and mastery orientations, dividing them into approach and avoidance goals (see Elliot, 1999; Pintrich, 2000). An example of a performance–approach goal is wanting to do better than others, whereas an example of a performance–avoid goal is not wanting to appear stupid. Mastery–avoid goals include working to avoid misunderstanding, or desiring not to be wrong when doing achievement activities. Performance–approach goals relate positively to performance and some aspects of motivation, whereas performance–avoid goals have a number of negative consequences for students. Mastery–avoid goals

have a mixture of positive and negative consequences (see Elliot & McGregor, 2001).

There has not been a lot of work on the development of goal orientations during adolescence. Extant work shows that students tend to focus more on performance goals as they get older, at the expense of task mastery goals (see Anderman, Austin, & Johnson, 2002, for review). School reform efforts designed to enhance students' mastery goal orientations have had some benefits for students' motivational outcomes (Anderman, Maehr, & Midgley, 1999).

EXPLAINING CHANGE IN ADOLESCENTS' MOTIVATION

We just discussed how adolescents' intrinsic motivation and perceptions of competence become more stable but also show a decline over time. In certain respects, these findings seem paradoxical, but they actually are not. The stability findings indicate that adolescents high in intrinsic motivation one year are more likely to be (relatively) high in intrinsic motivation the next year than are younger students; younger students' motivation is more variable year to year. But across the entire group of adolescents, intrinsic motivation is going down. The adolescent high in intrinsic motivation one year may still be intrinsically motivated the next year, but perhaps to a lesser extent. So individuals show stability, but the overall group shows a decline.

How has the mean-level decline in motivation been explained? Researchers have explained these changes in two major ways. One explanation focuses on cognitive and other changes within the individual. As children mature cognitively and receive increasing amounts of evaluative feedback, they come to understand more clearly their relative level of performance, and what the evaluative feedback means (for further discussion, see Eccles et al., 1998; Stipek & Mac Iver, 1989; Wigfield et al., in press). During their school years, children and adolescents receive a great deal of evaluative information about their school performance and also about other activities that they do. They become better at processing and understanding this information, and so become more realistic in their assessments, as noted earlier. Children and adolescents also use social comparative information more as they get older, and also understand better the implications of that information. A child might believe she is a very good reader, because she can recognize letters in books. However, when she begins school and sees other children already reading chapter books, she begins to understand that perhaps she is not such a good reader. Social comparison can lead many children to doubt their capabilities. These changes in beliefs about competence can lead to a decrease in students' motivation, especially for students doing less well in school.

The second explanation focuses on ways in which the experiences children have in school can contribute to the decline in students' motivation. As noted earlier, children receive more evaluative information as they go through school, and due to the current climate emphasizing assessment and evaluation of students and teachers, the amount of evaluative information children receive is increasing. When this information focuses children on their ability relative to others, many children find it difficult to maintain a strong sense of their competence, which can deflate their academic motivation. Furthermore, schools also often promote practices that accentuate children's tendency to compare themselves to others, which, once again, can contribute to a decline in many children's sense of competence and, ultimately, their motivation (see Wigfield & Eccles, 2002). Such practices can lead students to focus more on performance goals at the expense of mastery goals (see Anderman et al., 2002).

There has been a great deal written about how such practices (and others) become increasingly likely after students enter junior high or middle school (see Anderman & Maehr, 1994; Eccles & Midgley, 1989; Wigfield & Eccles, 2002). Students' friendship networks can be interrupted when they move to a new school; they may not have any classes with friends from their elementary school. Teachers teach a large number of students and may not get to know their students very well, and likely interact with them almost exclusively around the academic subject they teach. Family involvement in school often declines during the middle school years. All of these things can disrupt early adolescents' social relations, making the school transition more difficult.

Instructional practices change in important ways as well. There often is an increase in the use of between-classroom ability-grouping practices, and more rigorous evaluation and testing increases students' focus on their ability. These practices could contribute to the decline in competence-related beliefs experienced by many students. Such practices also lead students to focus more on performance goals, often at the expense of mastery goals (Anderman et al., 2002). Because of the larger size of the schools, administrators and teachers often feel the need to control students more closely, thus giving students fewer opportunities for choice and autonomy.

Eccles and Midgley (1989) argued that a main reason these kinds of changes in both social relations and instructional practices have a negative impact on students' motivation is that they are developmentally inappropriate for early adolescents. At a time when the children are growing cognitively and emotionally, desiring greater freedom and autonomy, and focusing on social relations, they experience school environments that do not promote these things. Therefore, for many early adolescents, these practices contribute to the negative change in motivation and achievement-related beliefs. Many of these practices continue into high school.

We have focused primarily on how changes in instructional practices influence how adolescents' competence-related beliefs and goal orientations change. With respect to intrinsic motivation and valuing of achievement, the observed decreases may occur because the materials and topics studied during middle and even high school may not hold students' interest. This likely is due in part to the nature of the topics studied, but also to adolescents' growing interests in activities outside of school, especially social activities. Adolescents have a wider range of activities from which to choose, and activities with peers take on increased importance for many adolescents. If adolescents focus too much on social activities, their academic motivation and performance can suffer. Second, some researchers have argued that children's sense of competence partially drives their intrinsic motivation for a given activity, particularly achievement-related activities (see Harter & Connell, 1984; Wigfield, 1994). The results of Jacobs et al.'s (2002) longitudinal study of the development of children's competence beliefs and valuing of achievement provides support for this view. In this study, changes in children's competence beliefs appeared to drive changes in their valuing of school (a construct related to intrinsic motivation) rather than the reverse, and, as described earlier, both competence beliefs and values declined.

Based in part on concern about the declines in student motivation, there have been a variety of middle school reform efforts designed to change school environments and instructional practices in ways that facilitate rather than debilitate students' motivation. A number of these efforts have been successful, but such reforms are not as widespread as they should be (for reviews, see Mac Iver, Young, & Washburn, 2002; Wigfield & Eccles, 2002). Such reforms are less prevalent at the high school level, but they are beginning to occur (National Research Council, 2004).

In summary, during the early adolescent and adolescent years, children's competence-related beliefs, intrinsic motivation, and goal orientations for achievement change, often in negative ways. These changes occur because of changes in children's understandings and interpretation of their achievement outcomes, and also because of changes in the instructional practices they experience in secondary schools. How individuals' broader self-representations change at adolescence is the topic in the next section.

SELF-CONCEPT AND IDENTITY FORMATION AT ADOLESCENCE

Identity formation is a fundamental process in adolescence. A discussion of competence and motivation in adolescence would be incomplete without consideration of the effects that identity development processes may have on these constructs. Furthermore, in recognition of the complex nature of individuals' identities, gender and ethnicity must be considered. We begin this section with an overview of identity development, continue with an examination of identity in relation to academic competence and motivation, and end with discussions of gender and ethnic identity in relation to academic competence and motivation.

Researchers in self-concept and identity often have not clearly defined the constructs they studied, or have defined them ambiguously (for discussion of definitional problems in this area, see Harter, 1998; Marsh, 1990b). Thus, definitions for the purposes of this chapter are in order. "Self-concept" refers to one's perception of oneself, made up of beliefs about many different aspects of self and evaluations of performance in different areas (Harter, 1990; Shavelson, Hubner, & Stanton, 1976; Wigfield & Karpathian, 1991). "Self-esteem" refers to one's judgment of one's worth or value as a person (Harter, 1990; Wigfield & Karpathian, 1991). "Identity" refers to an overall sense of who one is; it is a broader construct than other self-system components, inclusive of self-concept and self-esteem (Erikson, 1968; Spencer & Markstrom-Adams, 1990).

In his well-known psychosocial theory of the development of the self-system, Erikson (1968) identified adolescence as a period focused on identity formation. Adolescents are characterized as having to negotiate a series of developmental tasks in order to form a coherent identity; particularly relevant to our discussion is the exploration of educational and occupational options and aspirations. The process of identity formation involves an exploration of opportunities and different roles, and a synthesis into a coherent sense of self. If individuals are unable to develop a coherent identity, they may fall into role confusion.

Marcia (1980) extended Erikson's discussion of identity development by postulating four identity statuses. Adolescents who have neither explored alternatives nor made a commitment are said to be in *identity diffusion*. If commitment is made without exploration, the status is *identity foreclosure*. *Identity moratorium* describes adolescents in the midst of exploration, and *identity achievement* describes adolescents who have undergone exploration and developed a coherent identity.

These models of identity formation were all developed for the purpose of universal generalizability; however, attention has recently focused on gender and ethnicity as salient factors that may have important implications for identity development (e.g., Eisenberg, Martin, & Fabes, 1996; Phinney, 1990; Root, 1998). These factors and how they relate to academics are addressed further in later sections.

IDENTITY AND ACADEMIC COMPETENCE AND MOTIVATION

In the context of academic achievement research, identity formation has been conceptualized as the process by which individuals (1) develop a more accurate sense of their relative competencies, (2) come to understand what their values are, and (3) conceive self-esteem as grounded in these valued areas (Eccles et al., 1989). This definition emphasizes the development of academic competence and motivation as an integral part of identity formation. Researchers interested in identity and academics have approached these issues a variety of ways, which include examining relations of academic variables with identity statuses or, more frequently, exploring the development of academic self-concepts.

Identity Status and Academic Outcomes

There is a dearth of research connecting Erikson's and Marcia's identity theories with academic outcome variables, and much is unknown about the academic implications of different identity statuses. Preliminary work in this area has examined the relation between identity status classification and academic achievement in high school and college students (Berzonsky, 1985). These students were interviewed and classified by Marcia's identity statuses, and categorized as overachievers or underachievers based on the difference between predicted grade point average (as indicated by Scholastic Aptitude Test scores) and actual grade point average. It was anticipated that students in identity diffusion would display problem behaviors indicative of maladjustment and underachievement; however, this was not the case. In the high school sample, individuals with identity diffusion showed expected achievement, and in the sample of college freshman, individuals with identity diffusion displayed overachievement. Students who were categorized by identity foreclosure in high school showed overachievement, whereas individuals with identity foreclosure in college displayed underachievement. Generally, these findings suggest that the relations of identity status to competence and motivation are complex, and more research is necessary to elucidate the relationship between identity status and variables such as academic achievement, competence, and motivation.

Self as Student

The development of conceptions of the self as a student is a particular aspect of adolescent identity that has been of interest to educational researchers (Roeser & Lau, 2002). Researchers have attempted to understand and describe various aspects of students' conceptions of themselves academically, the contributions and implications of which we now discuss.

Student identities have been conceptualized as schemas derived from school experiences and academic performance that incite and direct either competent or problematic behaviors in school settings (Roeser & Lau, 2002). According to Roeser and Lau, *positive student identities* characterize adolescents who have histories of positive academic performance and relationships with classmates, positive emotions related to academic goals, high academic efficacy, positive conceptions of themselves as students, and a commitment to learning. *Negative student identities* characterize adolescents who have histories of academic failure and difficulties with peers, negative emotions associated with academic goals, poor academic efficacy, frustration with themselves as students, and diminishing aspirations for educational attainment. Roeser and Lau argue that school environments play an important role in the development of student identities, and certain practices, such as providing challenging and meaningful work, encouraging cooperative learning, and fostering motivation, may foster the development of positive student identities. Roeser and Lau's analysis of positive and negative student identities is intriguing; however, the applicability of these identity descriptors needs to be assessed with groups diverse in gender, ethnicity, and socioeconomic status.

The future-oriented components of the self-system, notably, possible selves, have been emphasized as critical for motivating different behaviors, including achievement behaviors (e.g., Markus, Cross, & Wurf, 1990; Oyserman, Gant, & Ager, 1995; Oyserman & Markus, 1990). These selves develop from past experiences and messages about what to attain and what to avoid. Academic possible selves function to organize and direct adolescents' behaviors for attaining their educational goals. A task of adolescence is to create balance in possible selves, meaning a construal of both positive selves to be attained and negative selves to be avoided in a specific content domain. This balance may provide motivation and perseverance in attaining the positive self and avoiding the negative self. In a high-poverty sample of African American middle school students, balance in possible selves predicted school persistence and achievement, with an even stronger effect for males than females (Oyserman et al., 1995).

There is some evidence of ethnic group differences in strategies used to attain achievement-related possible selves. In a study of undergraduate students, Oyserman et al. (1995) found that for European American students, the generation of achievement-related strategies was predicted by individualism, the Protestant work ethic, and balance in possible selves, whereas collectivism, low endorsement of individualism, and ethnic identity predicted strategy generation in African American students. Further research is needed to examine the role of possible selves in academic achievement with other ethnic and socioeconomic groups; available research on the relation between ethnic identity and academic outcome is reviewed in the last section of this chapter.

Recent research on academic self-concepts has emphasized the importance of domain-specificity of these beliefs. Marsh and his colleagues (Marsh, 1990a; Marsh, Byrne, & Shavelson, 1988; Marsh, Craven, & Debus, 1998) have argued that researchers studying academic self-concept need to use domain-specific measures rather than a single, general measure of academic self-concept, particularly when they are looking at relations of self-concept and achievement, because these relations often are complex. For instance, verbal and math self-concepts have been found to be nearly uncorrelated, even though reading and math achievement are significantly correlated (Marsh, Smith, & Barnes, 1985; Marsh et al., 1988). Furthermore, verbal achievement relates positively to verbal self-concept but negatively to math self-concept, and math achievement relates positively to math self-concept but negatively to verbal self-concept (Marsh et al., 1988). The implications of these findings are

somewhat troubling given gender differences in math and verbal self-concepts, which are discussed in more detail in the section on gender, identity, and academics.

The causal ordering of academic self-concept and academic achievement has been of great interest to educational researchers. Research has contrasted two models posited by Calsyn and Kenny (1977). The self-enhancement model supposes that self-concept is a determinant of academic achievement. According to this model, if students develop positive self-concepts, they will achieve better. By contrast, the skill-developmental model views academic self-concept as a consequence of academic achievement. Recently, Marsh and his colleagues proposed an integration of these models, termed the "reciprocal-effects model" (Guay, Marsh, & Boivin, 2003; Marsh & Yeung, 1997). According to the reciprocal-effects model, prior academic self-concept affects subsequent academic achievement, and past achievement affects later self-concept. There is growing research support for this model, and it should be noted that Bandura (1997) proposed similar reciprocal effects in the relation of achievement to academic self-efficacy. Interestingly, research has indicated no clear developmental pattern in the causal ordering of academic self-concept and achievement, supporting the generalizability of the reciprocal-effects model across age groups (Guay et al., 2003). Despite the growing support for this model, there still is debate in the field about the directionality of the relations of academic self-concept and achievement.

GENDER, IDENTITY, AND ACADEMICS

Because gender remains a salient factor that can influence beliefs, aspirations, and experiences in this society, a discussion of academic experiences must necessarily emphasize gender. In this section, we focus on the relation between gender identity and academics in adolescence, as well as gender differences in competence and motivation in adolescence; for a more complete consideration of gendered experiences, see Ruble and Martin (1998). Broadly, "gender identity" has been used to refer to identification of one's gender group and an understanding of what being a female or male means (Eisenberg et al., 1996). More specifically, in educational research, "gender identity" has been defined as one's gender-related attitudes, meanings, and expectations for oneself (Burke, 1989). The related but distinct construct of gender roles has been frequently studied, and refers generally to characteristics and behaviors that are culturally defined as feminine or masculine (Eisenberg et al., 1996; Huston, 1983).

Gender Identity and Academic Outcomes

An ethnographic study of early adolescent (10- to 11-year-olds) experiences revealed challenges in the negotiation of gender identities and academic self-concepts, particularly for high achievers (Renold, 2001b). Many girls, especially high achievers, had difficulty talking confidently and positively about their academic successes. They expressed tension between wanting to be academically successful and not wanting to be labeled as a high achiever, because this was not seen as "feminine" or as characteristic of a "normal" girl. These findings concur with earlier findings (e.g., Bell, 1989; Orenstein, 1994) that girls fear stigmatization if they appear too intelligent. The girls in Bell's study (1989) expressed concern about social rejection for appearing to be braggarts if they took pride in their accomplishments, and for seeming aggressive if they tried to attract their teachers' attention. Orenstein (1994) found that smart girls feared alienation from male peers who did not value intellectual abilities in girls, and from female peers who might view them as too academically competitive.

Other work indicates that some girls become less willing to express their opinions at adolescence in part because of concerns that such expressions may damage their relations with others (Gilligan, 1993). However, Harter, Waters, and Whitesell (1997) found that this phenomenon is limited to public expressions (e.g., in school) of opinions by girls with a strong feminine orientation. Thus it appears to be gender orientation rather than gender that is the key factor here.

Renold (2001a) found that high achievement was not solely a problem for girls; high-achieving boys were likewise marginalized, because studiousness and academic achievement were viewed by peers as conflicting with conventional masculinity. Many of the boys employed techniques to disguise their academic motivation and achievements, including behaving disruptively in the classroom, playing down their academic successes, teasing and bullying studious boys, investing in sports to maintain their "masculinity," and devaluing girls' schoolwork. Other researchers have similarly claimed that male students learn to equate academics with femininity, because teachers reward "feminine" behavior, such as sitting quietly and cooperating, while punishing "masculine" behaviors, such as rebellion against authority and independence (see Eisenberg et al., 1996). These studies emphasize the devaluing of academic achievement in both female and male peer cultures, and indicate the challenges of negotiating one's gender identity with peer conceptions of academic orientations.

Researchers have begun to explore links between gender identity and variables such as academic achievement, motivation, and subject choice (see also Eccles, 1987, 1994). A study of high school students measured the use of stereotyped sex-traits in self-descriptions, perceptions of school subjects as feminine or masculine, academic motivation, and subject choice (Whitehead, 1996). Results indicated that boys with strongly sex-stereotyped views of academic subjects were more likely to choose to enroll in "masculine" subjects (e.g., math, physical sciences, economics, woodworking), whereas this was not the case for girls. Interestingly, this study also found that intrinsic motivation in both girls and boys was associated with choosing "feminine subjects," and extrinsic motivation (particularly for a highly paid job in the future) was associated with choosing "masculine" subjects. We explore further research into gender differences in the areas of motivation, competence, and values next.

Gender Differences in Competence Beliefs and Values

Eccles (1987) asserted that identity formation is influenced by self-perceptions of abilities, achievement goals, motivations, and gender-role schemas, among other things.

Through gender-role socialization, females and males acquire different self-concepts, different patterns of expectations for success, and different task values and goals (Eccles, 1994). This is of particular importance to our present discussion, because adolescence has been noted as a time of increased pressure to conform to gender stereotypes and expectations (e.g., Hill & Lynch, 1983; Quatman & Watson, 2001). Despite research and policy efforts to encourage all students' achievement in sex-typed domains, and evidence that actual achievement gaps between genders are decreasing in areas such as mathematics, gendered stereotypes related to specific academic domains persist (Fredricks & Eccles, 2002).

Many studies have found significant gender differences in competence and expectancy beliefs, and task values. Evidence from studies done in the 1980s and 1990s indicated that compared to girls, adolescent boys had higher ability beliefs and expectancies for success in mathematics and rated math as more important, even when girls in the sample were achieving higher math grades than boys (Eccles, Adler, & Meece, 1984; Marsh et al., 1985). More recently, however, Jacobs et al. (2002) found that adolescent boys' and girls' competence-related beliefs and values for math did not differ. For English, research beginning in the 1980s consistently shows that girls express higher ability beliefs and higher valuing of reading and English than do boys during childhood and adolescence (Eccles et al., 1984; Jacobs et al., 2002).

In a study in which adolescent girls' grade point averages were significantly higher than those of boys, girls should have enjoyed a benefit to their competence beliefs, but no gender difference in self-perceived overall academic competence was found (Quatman & Watson, 2001). Academic competence was found to be a significant predictor of global self-esteem, and because boys consistently outscore girls on measures of global self-esteem, these results paint a troubling picture for adolescent girls (Quatman & Watson, 2001).

The development of competence and motivation in male sex-typed domains may seem a daunting task for adolescent girls; however, subtle changes in classroom envi-
ronment can help. Eccles (1987) reported findings from a study of 89 sixth-grade classrooms, of which 19 classrooms fostered more positive attitudes toward math in girls than in boys, in terms of confidence in math ability, expectations for success, intrinsic interest in math, and plans to take advanced math courses. Students reported that teachers in these "girl-friendly classrooms" treated students more fairly and equally, made math more interesting, and were more likely to explain the importance of math. Students were less likely to compete with each other, including comparing test scores and report cards. In contrast, the classrooms in which boys had the most positive attitudes toward math were characterized by higher levels of social comparison among students. These intriguing results demonstrate that even if girls and boys are not treated differently, they may be affected differently by similar environments. In particular, these young adolescents responded differently to competitive environments, with girls finding them less motivating than did boys. These findings have important implications for researchers and policymakers interested in increasing academic motivation.

The importance of recognizing difficulties faced by both genders is paramount, if positive changes are to be made. Sommers (2000) argued that boys really are the ones at greater risk, reviewing evidence that boys have lower grades in school, are more likely to drop out, are less likely to attend college, and are much more likely to be diagnosed as learning disabled or as having attention deficit disorder, among other things. She concluded that the concern about girls is misplaced, and that schools should be more concerned about the academic lives of boys. Although it is important to recognize the difficulties many boys face, it is unfortunate that this debate is being cast in this way. Rather than arguing either that boys have problems and girls do not, or that girls have problems and boys do not, it seems that members of each gender experience challenges that need attention in school. It therefore does not seem appropriate to focus primarily on either gender, but rather to deal with the separate issues that each gender group faces.

There has been some interesting recent work on how gender and ethnicity interact to influence adolescents' valuing of achievement (see Graham & Taylor, 2002, for review). Graham and her colleagues found that African American and Latino boys in comparison to European American boys tend to devalue academic achievement. Girls from all three ethnic groups valued high achievement. This work illustrates the complexity of the development of achievement values, because the patterns vary across different groups. A further examination of relations between ethnicity and academics is our focus in the next section.

ETHNICITY, IDENTITY, AND ACADEMIC OUTCOMES

In the past few decades, researchers have begun studying ethnic identity development, on the grounds that identity formation may be influenced by the salient and societally important factor of ethnicity. Phinney (1996) defined "ethnic identity" as a fundamental aspect of the self that is related to one's sense of belonging and commitment to an ethnic group, and the part of one's thinking, perceptions, feelings, and behavior that is associated with ethnic group membership. Although research in this area is relatively new, important initial advances have been made in the understanding of ethnic identity development, as well as relations between ethnic identity and different academic outcomes. Indeed, as will be made clear in this section, the relation between ethnicity and academic self-concept, motivation, and competence must be examined with an understanding of the integral role of ethnic identity.

Ethnic Identity Development

Phinney (1989, 1996) developed a three-stage model of ethnic identity formation by modifying and expanding upon Marcia's (1980) model of identity formation. The first stage, *unexamined ethnic identity*, embodies either a lack of ethnic exploration or acceptance of socially ascribed ethnic attitudes (similar to Marcia's diffusion or foreclosure). *Ethnic identity search* (akin to Marcia's moratorium) is characterized by a period of exploration into the meaning of one's ethnicity and can include thinking about the effects of ethnicity on one's life, talking to others about ethnic issues, and learning more about one's ethnicity through books, events, or organizations. The last stage, *ethnic identity achievement* (Marcia's achieved identity), involves a sense of membership in an ethnic group and acceptance of the ethnicity of others. Phinney and her colleagues (e.g., Phinney, 1989; Phinney & Alipuria, 1996) have found strong positive correlations between ethnic identity and self-esteem, and other measures of psychological adjustment, such as sense of mastery, social and peer interactions, and family relations. This model has not been applied to the study of academic outcome variables, however, so future research in this area is warranted.

Ethnic Identity and Academic Achievement

The educational system in the United States has at times been successful, and at times unsuccessful, in providing experiences that foster achievement in members of minority groups (Okagaki, 2001). Many theories have been developed to provide insight into and explanation of the achievement and underachievement of minority students, each of which contributes to a greater understanding of the educative process for minority groups, while leaving some questions unanswered. Theories that focus on conflict between the cultural milieu of education in the United States and the home culture of minority groups that share certain overarching cultural values (e.g., Greenfield & Suzuki, 1998) do not explain fully why some of these groups of minority students thrive in U.S. schools, while others struggle. Theories that emphasize differences among minority groups in the cultural valuing of education (e.g., Okagaki, 2001) do not account for individual variation in academic achievement within ethnic groups. In order to explain achievement differences on an individual as opposed to a generalized group level, it is necessary to examine individual characteristics of members of minority groups (see also Graham, 1994).

In examining specific components of ethnic identity that vary individually, it is possible to obtain an understanding of variation within ethnic groups, while retaining the ability to explore general group trends.

Oyserman and her colleagues (Oyserman, Harrison, & Bybee, 2001; Oyserman et al., 1995) proposed three components of ethnic identity that may be particularly related, either directly or indirectly, to individuals' academic self-concepts: connectedness, awareness of racism, and embedded achievement.

Connectedness has been characterized as positive ingroup identification and pride in one's ethnic group. Ethnic group membership can prescribe group norms, values, and behaviors (Oyserman et al., 2001; Spencer & Markstrom-Adams, 1990). Dependent on the nature of these values and norms in relation to academics, connectedness to an ethnic group may enhance individuals' academic self-concepts and motivation.

Awareness of racism, or negative outgroup perceptions, can have differential effects on academic self-concepts of minority students. Spencer and Markstrom-Adams (1990) noted that identification with one's ethnic group can decrease motivation for academic achievement if one's ethnic group has been negatively labeled by the majority society with respect to academics. In addition, Steele and Aronson (e.g., Steele, 1997; Steele & Aronson, 1995) have researched the detrimental effects of stereotype threat on academic performance. Stereotype threat is experienced as a self-evaluative threat of conforming to a negative stereotype about one's group. Steele and Aronson (1995) found that African American students underperformed on standardized tests relative to European Americans when negative stereotypes were activated.

Embedded achievement refers to the extent to which academic achievement is viewed as an integral part of one's ethnic group (Oyserman et al., 2001). When academic achievement is defined as an ingroup trait or value, tensions between achievement and minority group status may be reduced, and academic motivation increased. In a study done with a high-poverty sample of African American adolescents, Oyserman et al. found that academic efficacy was higher when embedded achievement was high (i.e., when achievement was viewed as part of being African American) than when students indicated low embedded achievement beliefs. This relation between academic efficacy and embedded achievement was found for both girls and boys. However, the interaction of ethnic identity and gender moder-

ated the effect of ethnic identity on academic efficacy. Specifically, high awareness of racism, high connectedness, and low embedded achievement predicted low academic efficacy for girls only. These results indicate that the relation between ethnic identity and academic self-concepts is complex and must be examined for gender-specific effects.

This concept of embedded achievement has important implications for understanding individual differences in academic self-concepts of minority youth. Rather than generalizing the value placed on academics by the culture of an ethnic group as a whole, embedded achievement allows for individual variation. Most parents, regardless of ethnicity, believe education is important and that their children will achieve a high level of schooling (see Galper, Wigfield, Seefeldt, 1997; Stevenson, Chen, & Uttal, 1990). However, a distinction can be made between the abstract value of education and pragmatic beliefs about direct benefits of education (see Mickelson, 1990; Steinberg, Dornbusch, & Brown, 1992). Some theorists argue that institutional- and policy-level treatment of minority groups in the United States limits opportunities for success and may discourage some minority students from exerting effort for academic achievement, because benefits of education are not perceived (e.g., Ogbu, 1981, 1994; Okagaki, 2001). In particular, Ogbu (1994) asserts that minority students from groups not accepted by majority society do not accrue the same benefits from education as majority students, because of a job ceiling and related barriers. In order to improve school success of minority students, he argues, economic resources for minority groups must be increased and improved, such that changes in perceptions of opportunity occur.

There is some evidence supporting ethnic-group differences in the belief that education serves a relevant, pragmatic function. Steinberg et al. (1992) found that African American and Latino adolescents in their socioeconomically diverse sample were more likely to believe they could get the job they wanted without a good education, whereas Asian American and European American students were more likely to report that a good education was necessary for attaining the job they wanted. It has been noted that in Asian cultures, there is an emphasis on educational success that is linked to the importance of bringing honor to one's family (Okagaki, 2001; Oyserman & Sakamoto, 1997). Thus, if bringing honor to one's family is seen as a duty of the child, and academic achievement brings honor to the family, these cultural values may produce motivation to overcome obstacles associated with minority status.

Subjective task-value differences could have important implications for ethnic and socioeconomic group differences in academic motivation and achievement. Academic activity choices are strongly directly predicted by domain-specific value beliefs, and values indirectly predict academic achievement (see Wigfield & Tonks, 2002, for review). The belief that hard work in school will not bring economic and social benefits is associated with low academic motivation (Okagaki, 2001). If pragmatic beliefs about long-term benefits of education are not perceived, subjective values for academic tasks may be low, which would have important implications on academic activity choice and achievement.

In our earlier discussion of the development of competence beliefs and motivation, we discussed how school environments can impact these processes, and often do so in a negative way as adolescents proceed through school. How might schools affect students' identity development? Roeser and Lau's (2002) discussion of this topic, summarized earlier, provides an important beginning, but systematic research is needed to look more carefully at the relations between different school structures, instructional practices, and identity development, including ethnic and gender identity development. We conjecture that practices fostering positive competence and motivation also help students develop a clearer sense of their identity. Practices that tend to undermine students' motivation also may detract from identity development. As discussed earlier, we are beginning to understand which instructional practices enhance adolescents' competence and motivation, and which may undermine them. However, we do not yet know whether the practices that foster competence and motivation work for all students, or whether different practices are needed for different groups of students, such as students from different ethnic groups.

To conclude this section, several considerations must be made in understanding rela-

tions of identity formation to the competence and motivation of adolescents. The process of identity formation is of the utmost importance at this age, and other processes may be seen as subsumed by this task. The development of an academic conception of the self is a part of the process of identity development and is influenced by many factors. Differences related to gendered experiences must be anticipated given existing societal inequalities and differential socialization patterns. In addition, in culturally and ethnically heterogeneous societies, the salience of ethnicity cannot be ignored, and its influences must be examined.

FUTURE RESEARCH DIRECTIONS

We have discussed in this chapter the development of children's beliefs about competence, motivation, and their identities, and how these processes are influenced by psychological factors within the adolescent and contextual factors in the experiences of different adolescents. We have learned much about the development of these processes, but much more remains to be done. With respect to competence-related beliefs and motivation, we think the observed decline in these constructs during the adolescent years continues to be a concern. We now need to look more carefully at patterns of change with different groups of adolescents, in order to understand these changes more fully. There likely are groups of adolescents who maintain positive senses of competence and academic motivation, and others who do not. Understanding these patterns would give us a more complete understanding of the developmental trends in competence and motivation.

Much also remains to be done to understand more clearly the nature of the relations among children's school experiences and the development of their competence beliefs and motivation. An especially important topic is to look to see how schools that have attempted to reform their instructional practices are influencing adolescents' competence beliefs, motivation, and identities. As we understand better the nature of these relations, we can work to develop school structures and environments that facilitate the competence and motivation of adolescents rather than contribute to their decline.

With respect to identity development, there has been much exciting work done on these processes over the last few years, building on the seminal but largely untested work of Erikson (1968). We are particularly excited about the work on gender and ethnic identity development, work that is essential to understanding the increasingly diverse population of adolescents in this country. Theorists have proposed interesting models of gender and ethnic identity development, but (particularly with respect to ethnic identity development) not much research has been done to test these models or to outline the developmental course of ethnic identity in particular. Developing measures of ethnic identity has posed numerous challenges to researchers, particularly measures that can be used with many different ethnic groups (see Phinney, 1992). As discussed earlier in this chapter, we have learned some things about relations of identity development to competence and motivation, but much more remains to be done. Initial research has explored the relations between ethnic identity (particularly, specific components of ethnic identity regarding academics) and variables such as achievement and academic efficacy, but only for certain ethnic groups. More research is needed to examine other variables and other ethnic groups, with particular attention given to interactions with gender.

REFERENCES

Ames, C. (1992). Classrooms: Goals, structures, and student motivation. *Journal of Educational Psychology, 84,* 261–271.

Anderman, E. M., Austin, C. C., & Johnson, D. M. (2002). The development of goal orientation. In A. Wigfield & J. S. Eccles (Eds.), *Development of achievement motivation* (pp. 197–220). San Diego: Academic Press.

Anderman, E. M., & Maehr, M. L. (1994). Motivation and schooling in the middle grades. *Review of Educational Research, 64,* 287–309.

Anderman, E. M., Maehr, M. L., & Midgley, C. (1999). Declining motivation after the transition to middle school: Schools can make a difference. *Journal of Research and Development in Education, 32,* 131–147.

Arnett, J. J. (1999). Adolescent storm and stress, reconsidered. *American Psychologist, 54,* 317–326.

Assor, A., & Connell, J. P. (1992). The validity of students' self-reports as measures of performance affecting self-appraisals. In D. H. Schunk & J. L. Meece (Eds.), *Student self-perceptions in the classroom* (pp. 25–47). Hillsdale, NJ: Erlbaum.

Bandura, A. (1997). *Self-efficacy: The exercise of control.* New York: Freeman.

Bell, L. A. (1989). Something's wrong here and it's not me: Challenging the dilemmas that block girls' success. *Journal for the Education of the Gifted, 12,* 118–130.

Berndt, T. J., & Keefe, K. (1995). Friends' influence on adolescents' adjustment to school. *Child Development, 66,* 1312–1329.

Berzonsky, M. D. (1985). Diffusion within Marcia's identity–status paradigm: Does it foreshadow academic problems? *Journal of Youth and Adolescence, 14,* 527–538.

Blos, P. (1979). *The adolescent passage.* New York: International Universities Press.

Buchanan, C. M. (2002, November). *Views of adolescents and adolescence.* Paper presented at the Festschrift honoring Carol Midgley, University of Michigan, Ann Arbor.

Burke, P. J. (1989). Gender identity, sex, and school performance. *Social Psychology Quarterly, 52,* 159–169.

Byrnes, J. B. (1988). Formal operations: A systematic reformulation. *Developmental Review, 8,* 1–22.

Calsyn, R., & Kenny, D. (1977). Self-concept of ability and perceived evaluations by others: Cause or effect of academic achievement? *Journal of Educational Psychology, 69,* 136–145.

Dornbusch, S. M., Petersen, A. C., & Hetherington, E. M. (1991). Projecting the future of research on adolescence. *Journal of Research on Adolescence, 1,* 7–18.

Dweck, C. S., & Leggett, E. (1988). A social-cognitive approach to motivation and personality. *Psychological Review, 95,* 256–273.

Eccles, J. S. (1987). Gender roles and women's achievement-related decisions. *Psychology of Women Quarterly, 11,* 135–172.

Eccles, J. S. (1994). Understanding women's educational and occupational choices: Applying the Eccles et al. model of achievement-related decisions. *Psychology of Women Quarterly, 18,* 585–609.

Eccles, J. S., Adler, T. F., & Meece, J. L. (1984). Sex differences in achievement: A test of alternate theories. *Journal of Personality and Social Psychology, 46,* 26–43.

Eccles, J. S., & Midgley, C. (1989). Stage/environment fit: Developmentally appropriate classrooms for early adolescents. In R. Ames & C. Ames (Eds.), *Research on motivation in education* (Vol. 3, pp. 139–181). New York: Academic Press.

Eccles, J. S., & Wigfield, A. (1997). Young adolescent development. In J. L. Irvin (Ed.), *What current research says to the middle level practitioner* (pp. 15–29). Columbus, OH: National Middle School Association.

Eccles, J. S., Wigfield, A., Flanagan, C. A., Miller, C., Reuman, D. A., & Yee, D. (1989). Self-concepts, domain values, and self-esteem: Relations and changes at early adolescence. *Journal of Personality, 57,* 283–310.

Eccles, J. S., Wigfield, A., & Schiefele, U. (1998). Motivation to succeed. In N. Eisenberg (Vol. Ed.) & W. Damon (Series Ed.), *Handbook of child psychology* (5th ed., Vol. 3, pp. 1017–1095). New York: Wiley.

Eisenberg, N., Martin, C. L., & Fabes, R. A. (1996). Gender development and gender effects. In D. C. Berliner & R. C. Calfee (Eds.), *Handbook of educational psychology* (pp. 358–396). New York: Macmillan.

Elliot, A. J. (1999). Approach and avoidance motivation and achievement goals. *Educational Psychologist, 34*, 169–189.

Elliot, A. J., & McGregor, H. A. (2001). A 2 × 2 achievement goal framework. *Journal of Personality and Social Psychology, 80*, 501–519.

Epstein, J. L., & Connors, L. J. (1995). School and family partnerships in the middle grades. In B. Rutherford (Ed.), *Creating school/family partnerships* (pp. 37–166). Columbus, OH: National Middle School Association.

Erikson, E. H. (1968). *Identity: Youth and crisis.* New York: Norton.

Fredericks, J. A., & Eccles, J. S. (2002). Children's competence and value beliefs from childhood through adolescence: Growth trajectories in two male-sex-typed domains. *Developmental Psychology, 38*, 519–533.

Galper, A., Wigfield, A., & Seefeldt, C. (1997). Head Start parents' beliefs about their children's abilities, task values, and performances on different activities. *Child Development, 68*, 897–907.

Gilligan, C. (1993). Joining the resistance: Psychology, politics, girls, and women. In L. Weis & M. Fine (Eds.), *Beyond silenced voices* (pp. 143–168). Albany, NY: State University of New York Press.

Gottfried, A. E., Fleming, J. S., & Gottfried, A. I. (2001). Continuity of academic intrinsic motivation from childhood through late adolescence: A longitudinal study. *Journal of Educational Psychology, 93*, 3–13.

Graham, S. (1994). Motivation in African Americans. *Review of Educational Research, 64*, 55–117.

Graham, S., & Taylor, A. Z. (2002). Ethnicity, gender, and the development of achievement values. In A. Wigfield & J. S. Eccles (Eds.), *Development of achievement motivation* (pp. 121–146). San Diego: Academic Press.

Greenfield, P. M., & Suzuki, L. K. (1998). Culture and human development: Implications for parenting, education, pediatrics, and mental health. In W. Damon (Vol. Ed.) & N. Eisenberg (Series Ed.), *Handbook of child psychology* (5th ed., Vol. 4, pp. 1059–1109). New York: Wiley.

Guay, F., Marsh, H. W., & Boivin, M. (2003). Academic self-concept and academic achievement: Developmental perspectives on their causal ordering. *Journal of Educational Psychology, 95*, 124–136.

Hall, G. S. (1904). *Adolescence: Its psychology and its relations to anthropology, sex, crime, religion, and education.* New York: Appleton.

Harter, S. (1981). A new self-report scale of intrinsic versus extrinsic orientation in the classroom: Motivational and informational components. *Developmental Psychology, 17*, 300–312.

Harter, S. (1990). Processes underlying adolescent self-concept formation. In R. Montemayor, G. R. Adams, & T. P. Gullotta (Eds.), *From childhood to adolescence: A transitional period?* (pp. 205–239). Newbury Park, CA: Sage.

Harter, S. (1998). The development of self-representations. In W. Damon (Series Ed.) & N. Eisenberg (Vol. Ed.), *Handbook of educational psychology: Vol. 3. Social, emotional, and personality development* (5th ed., pp. 553–617). New York: Wiley.

Harter, S., & Connell, J. P. (1984). A comparison of alternate models of the relationships between academic achievement and children's perceptions of competence, control, and motivational orientation. In J. G. Nicholls (Ed.), *The development of achievement-related cognitions and behaviors* (pp. 219–250). Greenwich, CT: JAI Press.

Harter, S., Waters, P. L., & Whitesell, N. R. (1997). Lack of voice as a manifestation of false self-behavior: The school setting as a stage upon which the drama of authenticity is enacted. *Educational Psychologist, 32*, 153–174.

Hill, J. P., & Lynch, M. E. (1983). The intensification of gender-related expectations during adolescence. In J. Brooks-Gunn & A. Peterson (Eds.), *Girls at puberty* (pp. 201–228). New York: Plenum Press.

Huston, A. C. (1983). Sex-typing. In P. H. Mussen (Series Ed.) & E. M. Hetherington (Vol. Ed.), *Handbook of child psychology: Vol. 4. Socialization, personality, and social development* (4th ed., pp. 387–467). New York: Wiley.

Jacobs, J. E., & Eccles, J. S. (2000). Parents, task values, and real-life achievement choices. In C. Sansone & J. M. Harackiewicz (Eds.), *Intrinsic and extrinsic motivation: The search for optimal motivation and achievement* (pp. 405–439). San Diego: Academic Press.

Jacobs, J. E., Lanza, S., Osgood, D. W., Eccles, J. S., & Wigfield, A. (2002). Changes in children's self-competence and values: Gender and domain differences across grades one through twelve. *Child Development, 73*, 509–527.

Keating, D. P. (1990). Adolescent thinking. In S. S. Feldman & G. R. Elliott (Eds.), *At the threshold: The developing adolescent* (pp. 54–89). Cambridge, MA: Harvard University Press.

Kindermann, T. A. (1993). Natural peer groups as contexts for individual development: The case of children's motivation in school. *Developmental Psychology, 29*, 970–977.

Kindermann, T. A., McCollam, T. L., & Gibson, E., Jr. (1996). In peer networks and students' classroom engagement during childhood and adolescence. In K. Wentzel & J. Juvonen (Eds.), *Social motivation: Understanding children's school adjustment.* Cambridge, UK: Cambridge University Press.

Mac Iver, D. J., Young, E. M., & Washburn, B. (2002). Instructional practices and motivation during middle school (with special attention to science). In A. Wigfield & J. S. Eccles (Eds.), *The development of achievement motivation* (pp. 333–351) San Diego: Academic Press.

Maehr, M. L., & Midgley, C. (1996). *Transforming school cultures*. Boulder, CO: Westview Press.

Marcia, J. E. (1980). Ego identity development. In J. Adelson (Ed.), *Handbook of adolescent psychology* (pp. 159–187). New York: Wiley.

Markus, H., Cross, S., & Wurf, E. (1990). The role of the self-system in competence. In R. J. Sternberg & J. J. Kolligian (Eds.), *Competence considered* (pp. 205–225). New Haven, CT: Yale University Press.

Marsh, H. W. (1989). Age and sex effects in multiple dimensions of self-concept: Preadolescence to early adulthood. *Journal of Educational Psychology, 81,* 417–430.

Marsh, H. W. (1990a). The causal ordering of academic self-concept and academic achievement: A multiwave, longitudinal path analysis. *Journal of Educational Psychology, 82,* 646–656.

Marsh, H. W. (1990b). The structure of academic self-concept: The Marsh/Shavelson model. *Journal of Educational Psychology, 82,* 623–636.

Marsh, H. W., Byrne, B. M., & Shavelson, R. J. (1988). A multifaceted academic self-concept: Its hierarchical structure and its relation to academic achievement. *Journal of Educational Psychology, 80,* 366–380.

Marsh, H. W., Craven, R., & Debus, R. (1998). Structure, stability, and development of young children's self-concepts: A multicohort-multioccasion study. *Child Development, 69,* 1030–1053.

Marsh, H. W., Smith, I. D., & Barnes, J. (1985). Multidimensional self-concepts: Relations with sex and academic achievement. *Journal of Educational Psychology, 77,* 581–596.

Marsh, H. W., & Yeung, A. S. (1997). Causal effects of academic self-concept on academic achievement: Structural equation models of longitudinal data. *Journal of Educational Psychology, 89,* 41–54.

Mickelson, R. A. (1990). The attitude–achievement paradox among Black adolescents. *Sociology of Education, 63,* 44–61.

Midgley, C., & Edelin, K. C. (1998). Middle school reform and early adolescent well-being: The good news and the bad. *Educational Psychologist, 33,* 195–206.

Moshman, D. (2004). *Adolescent psychological development: Rationality, morality, and identity* (2nd ed.). Mahwah, NJ: Erlbaum.

National Research Council. (2004). *Engaging schools: Fostering high school students' motivation to learn.* Washington, DC: National Academic Press.

Nicholls, J. G. (1984). Achievement motivation: Conceptions of ability, subjective experience, task choice, and performance. *Psychological Review, 91,* 328–346.

Ogbu, J. U. (1981). Origins of human competence: A cultural-ecological perspective. *Child Development, 52,* 413–429.

Ogbu, J. U. (1994). Racial stratification and education in the United States: Why inequality persists. *Teacher's College Record, 96,* 264–299.

Okagaki, L. (2001). Triarchic model of minority children's school achievement. *Educational Psychologist, 36,* 9–20.

Orenstein, P. (1994). *Schoolgirls: Young women, self-esteem, and the confidence gap* (1st ed.). New York: Doubleday.

Oyserman, D., Gant, L., & Ager, J. (1995). A socially contextualized model of African American identity: Possible selves and school persistence. *Journal of Personality and Social Psychology, 69,* 1216–1232.

Oyserman, D., Harrison, K., & Bybee, D. (2001). Can racial identity be promotive of academic efficacy? *International Journal of Behavioral Development, 25,* 379–385.

Oyserman, D., & Markus, H. R. (1990). Possible selves and delinquency. *Journal of Personality and Social Psychology, 59,* 112–125.

Oyserman, D., & Sakamoto, I. (1997). Being Asian American: Identity, cultural constructs, and stereotype perception. *Journal of Applied Behavioral Science, 33,* 435–453.

Pajares, F. (1996). Self-efficacy beliefs in academic settings. *Review of Educational Research, 66,* 543–578.

Parker, J. G., & Asher, S. R. (1987). Peer relations and later personal adjustment: Are low-accepted children at risk? *Psychological Bulletin, 102,* 357–389.

Phinney, J. S. (1989). Stages of ethnic identity development in minority group adolescents. *Journal of Early Adolescence, 9,* 34–49.

Phinney, J. S. (1990). Ethnic identity in adolescents and adults: Review of research. *Psychological Bulletin, 108,* 499–514.

Phinney, J. S. (1992). The multigroup ethnic identity measure: A new scale for use with diverse groups. *Journal of Adolescent Research, 7,* 156–176.

Phinney, J. S. (1996). When we talk about American ethnic groups, what do we mean? *American Psychologist, 51,* 918–927.

Phinney, J. S., & Alipuria, L. L. (1996). At the interface of cultures: Multiethnic/multiracial high school and college students. *Journal of Social Psychology, 136,* 139–158.

Pintrich, P. R. (2000). An achievement goal theory perspective on issues in motivation terminology, theory, and research. *Contemporary Educational Psychology, 25,* 92–104.

Pintrich, P. R. (2003). A motivational science perspective on the role of student motivation in learning and teaching contexts. *Journal of Educational Psychology, 95,* 667–686.

Pintrich, P. R., & Schunk, D. H. (2002). *Motivation in education: Theory, research, and application* (2nd ed.). Upper Saddle River, NJ: Prentice-Hall.

Quatman, T., & Watson, C. M. (2001). Gender differences in adolescent self-esteem: An exploration of domains. *Journal of Genetic Psychology, 162,* 93–117.

Renold, E. (2001a). Learning the "hard" way: Boys, hegemonic masculinity and the negotiation of learner identities in the primary school. *British Educational Research Journal, 22,* 369–385.

Renold, E. (2001b). "Square girls," femininity and the negotiation of academic success in the primary school. *British Educational Research Journal, 27,* 577–588.

Roeser, R. W., & Lau, S. (2002). On academic identity formation in middle school settings during early adolescence. In T. M. Brinthaupt & R. P. Lipka (Eds.), *Understanding early adolescent self and identity: Applications and interventions* (pp. 91–131). Albany: State University of New York Press.

Root, M. P. P. (1998). Experiences and processes affecting racial identity development: Preliminary results from the biracial sibling project. *Cultural Diversity and Mental Health, 4,* 237–247.

Rubin, K. H., Bukowski, W., & Parker, J. G. (1998). Peer interactions, relationships, and groups. In N. Eisenberg (Vol. Ed.) & W. Damon (Series Ed.), *Handbook of child psychology* (5th ed., Vol. 3, pp. 619–700). New York: Wiley.

Ruble, D. N., & Martin, C. L. (1998). Gender development. In N. Eisenberg (Vol. Ed.) & W. Damon (Series Ed.), *Handbook of child psychology* (5th ed., Vol. 3, pp. 933–1016). New York: Wiley.

Ryan, R. M., & Deci, E. L. (2000). Intrinsic and extrinsic motivators: Classic definitions and new directions. *Contemporary Educational Psychology, 25,* 54–67.

Shavelson, R. J., Hubner, J. J., & Stanton, G. C. (1976). Self-concept: Validation of construct interpretations. *Review of Educational Research, 46,* 407–441.

Shell, D. F., Colvin, C., & Bruning, R. H. (1995). Self-efficacy, attribution, and outcome expectancy mechanisms in reading and writing achievement: Grade-level and achievement-level differences. *Journal of Educational Psychology, 87,* 386–398.

Skinner, E. A., Zimmer-Gembeck, M. J., & Connell, J. P. (1998). Individual differences and the development of perceived control. *Monographs of the Society for Research in Child Development, 63*(2–3, Serial No. 254).

Sommers, E. H. (2000). The war against boys. *Atlantic Monthly, 285*(5), 59–62, 64.

Spencer, M. B., & Markstrom-Adams, C. (1990). Identity processes among racial and ethnic minority children in America. *Child Development, 61,* 290–310.

Steele, C. M. (1997). A threat in the air: How stereotypes shape intellectual identity and performance. *American Psychologist, 52,* 613–629.

Steele, C. M., & Aronson, J. (1995). Stereotype threat and the intellectual test performance of African Americans. *Journal of Personality and Social Psychology, 69,* 797–811.

Steinberg, L., Dornbusch, S. M., & Brown, B. B. (1992). Ethnic differences in adolescent achievement:

An ecological perspective. *American Psychologist, 47,* 723–729.

Stevenson, H. W., Chen, C., & Uttal, D. H. (1990). Beliefs and achievement: A study of Black, White, and Hispanic children. *Child Development, 61,* 508–523.

Stipek, D. J., & Mac Iver, D. (1989). Developmental change in children's assessment of intellectual competence. *Child Development, 60,* 521–538.

Weiner, B. (1985). An attributional theory of achievement motivation and emotion. *Psychological Review, 92,* 548–573.

Whitehead, J. M. (1996). Sex stereotypes, gender identity, and subject choice at A-level. *Educational Research, 38,* 147–160.

Wigfield, A. (1994). Expectancy–value theory of achievement motivation: A developmental perspective. *Educational Psychology Review, 6,* 49–78.

Wigfield, A., & Eccles, J. S. (2000). Expectancy–value theory of motivation. *Contemporary Educational Psychology, 25,* 68–81.

Wigfield, A., & Eccles, J. S. (2002). Children's motivation during the middle school years. In J. Aronson (Ed.), *Improving academic achievement: Contributions of social psychology* (pp. 159–184). San Diego: Academic Press.

Wigfield, A., Eccles, J., Mac Iver, D., Reuman, D., & Midgley, C. (1991). Transitions at early adolescence: Changes in children's domain-specific self-perceptions and general self-esteem across the transition to junior high school. *Developmental Psychology, 27,* 552–565.

Wigfield, A., Eccles, J. S., Schiefele, U., Roeser, R., & Davis-Kean, P. (in press). Development of achievement motivation. In W. Damon (Vol. Ed.) & N. Eisenberg (Series Ed.), *Handbook of child psychology* (6th ed.). New York: Wiley.

Wigfield, A., Eccles, J. S., Yoon, K. S., Harold, R. D., Arbreton, A., Freedman-Doan, C., et al. (1997). Changes in children's competence beliefs and subjective task values across the elementary school years: A three-year study. *Journal of Educational Psychology, 89,* 451–469.

Wigfield, A., & Karpathian, M. (1991). Who am I and what can I do?: Children's self-concepts and motivation in achievement situations. *Educational Psychologist, 26,* 233–261.

Wigfield, A., & Tonks, S. (2002). Adolescents' expectancies for success and achievement task values during the middle and high school years. In F. Pajares & T. Urdan (Eds.), *Academic motivation of adolescents* (pp. 53–82). Greenwich, CT: Information Age.

Zimmerman, B. J. (2000). Attaining self-regulation: A social cognitive perspective. In M. Boekaerts, P. R. Pintrich, & M. Zeidner (Eds.), *Handbook of self-regulation* (pp. 13–39). San Diego: Academic Press.

Zimmerman, B. J., & Martinez-Pons, M. (1990). Student differences in self-regulated learning: Relating grade, sex, and giftedness to self-efficacy and strategy use. *Journal of Educational Psychology, 82,* 51–59.

CHAPTER 14

છ

Competence and Motivation in Adulthood and Old Age

Making the Most of Changing Capacities and Resources

JUTTA HECKHAUSEN

This chapter addresses the role of motivation under conditions of radically changing competencies during adulthood and old age. Competence in this context refers to the *potential for effective action* (i.e., primary control) in a given domain of functioning. My aim is to investigate the adaptive strategies that allow individuals to make the most of their waxing and waning competencies during this lifespan period, when many capacities, skills, and expertise rise to their lifespan peak in early or midadulthood, and then in old age plummet back to functional levels attained long before maturity was reached. Making the most of waxing and waning competencies requires sophisticated motivational self-regulation in terms of shepherding oneself through phases of goal engagement, goal adjustment, or goal disengagement. I discuss a theoretical framework for conceptualizing such motivational and self-regulational skills, the lifespan theory of control, and its action-phase model of developmental regulation (Heckhausen, 1999; Heckhausen & Schulz, 1995; Schulz & Heckhausen, 1996). Subsequently, the lifespan theory of control is applied to two distinct yet interrelated areas of competence, namely, intellectual competence and vocational accomplishment.

Note that the approach to motivation used in this chapter does not address interindividual differences in implicit motives of achievement, power, or affiliation (for a discussion of these topics, see Schultheiss & Brunstein, Chapter 3, and Kanfer & Ackerman, Chapter 19, this volume). In this chapter, I focus on the individual's motivational regulation of goal-directed action as it takes up the challenges of change in competence and vocational opportunities during adulthood and old age. Specifically, I examine the goal-*engagement* and -*disengagement* strategies that can optimize the level of motivational investment in different action phases in response to contextual opportunities and constraints at different points in time during the adult life course.

The lifespan theory of control views the striving for control over one's environment, that is, primary control, as the fundamental motivational source of competence striving and development across the lifespan (Heckhausen & Schulz, 1995). Primary control striving is conceptualized as a fundamental motivational orientation underlying other, more thematically specialized strivings (e.g., for achievement or power). Primary control striving thus holds functional primacy in the motivational system not only in humans but also throughout the mammalian strata and most likely well beyond (Heckhausen, 2000a; Heckhausen & Schulz, 1999a).

DEVELOPMENTAL CHANGE IN CONTROL POTENTIAL ACROSS ADULTHOOD AND OLD AGE

The potential for effective action or, in other words, the potential to control the environment, undergoes radical changes across adulthood. These changes are multidimensional and multidirectional (Baltes, Staudinger, & Lindenberger, 1999) in the sense that trajectories of increase, peak, plateau, and decline vary across different domains of functioning. The shape of the age-related trajectory for a given aspect of functioning (e.g., expertise, memory, attention, and social skills) depends on three major factors: the biology of maturation and aging, societal constraints and opportunities to expand competence in the relevant area, and the accumulation of experience and expertise by the individual agent. Throughout this chapter, I discuss each of these three factors—biology, societal scaffolding, and individual agency—for two domains of competence: (1) intellectual and (2) vocational achievements and capacities.

In the first section of this chapter, I focus on the boundary conditions for individual agency, namely, biological maturation and aging, and societal scaffolding. I discuss the role and potential of individual agency in the third section of this chapter, after considering the lifespan theory of control and its model of developmental regulation in more detail (in the second section).

INTELLECTUAL AND VOCATIONAL CAPACITIES AND ACHIEVEMENTS

In this section, the biological boundary conditions for the development of intellectual competence and vocational expertise are discussed first. Research in this area has focused on developmental plasticity as the key to understanding cognitive aging. Experimentally induced and engineered plasticity is a prime strategy in cognitive aging research. Naturally occurring plasticity is, by contrast, very much a product of individual agency directing learning and experience, and is therefore reserved for the later section on individual agency in the regulation of motivational investment. In the last part of this section, I discuss the societal scaffolding of intellectual and vocational capacities in terms of institutional and social–structural constraints and opportunities.

Biological Maturation and Aging

Generally speaking, domains of competence that rely heavily on high-level physical functioning follow change trajectories with steep increases and decreases, and narrow and relatively early peaks. Examples are athletic excellence and world-class performances (Ericsson, 1990; Schulz & Curnow, 1988), which peak at early ages and typically only last for a narrow age window. Differences between various athletic disciplines are based on the extent of challenge of the given sport to physical strength and flexibility relative to the required acquisition time. Thus, individual world-class performance in track-and-field sports peaks earlier than performance in team sports (Schulz & Curnow, 1988).

Age trajectories of extreme competencies reflect early benchmarks for constraints due to biological changes associated with aging. Whereas early declines do not impair performances in most common, everyday activities in work, family, and leisure activities, they do become noticeable in multitask situations, such as when driving and talking, monitoring multiple moving objects (e.g., air traffic controller), or directing groups of diversely acting individuals (e.g., teacher). Research in cognitive aging using dual-task paradigms has uncovered not only drastic declines in multitask performance in early midlife (Li, Lindenberger, Freund, & Baltes, 2001; Lindenberger, Marsiske, & Baltes, 2000) but also specific strategies used by younger and older adults when trying to maintain reasonable performance levels in either task (Kemper, Herman, & Lian, 2003).

With regard to regular cognitive functioning (e.g., as indicated by intelligence tests) decline in performance is typically restricted to fluid intellectual skills (e.g., memorizing nouns, mental rotation) that have fallen out of practice, whereas crystallized abilities (i.e., factual and procedural knowledge) remain stable into old age. Up to very old age, fluid skills can be reactivated by instruction and even minimal practice (Baltes, Dittman-Kohli, & Kliegl, 1986; Baltes, Sowarka, & Kliegl, 1989) and then rise again to levels comparable to those of younger adults. Moreover, older adults can acquire new fluid skills (e.g., memory for nouns, names) and attain levels of performance comparable to those of young adults (Baltes & Kliegl, 1992; Baltes & Lindenberger, 1988; Baltes et al., 1986). For instance, older adults acquired the Method of Loci (i.e., associating memory items with locations on a preset route by forming vivid mental images) to memorize lists of up to 30 nouns and, after some practice, were able to reproduce all nouns, just like their younger adult counterparts. It is only when time constraints (i.e., shortened presentation interval) and cognitive load (i.e., interference from previous lists) are pushed to the limit that older adults fall short of younger adults in their performance (Mayr & Kliegl, 1993; Mayr, Kliegl, & Krampe, 1996) Plasticity of fluid skills fades away only in very advanced old age. For instance, in a sample of adults age 80 years and older, memory training using the Method of Loci produced only modest performance gains immediately after training that were not further enhanced by practice (Singer, Lindenberger, & Baltes, 2003). These decreases in experimentally induced cognitive plasticity mirrored declines found in perceptual speed, memory, and fluency in a population of German older adults, with the old-old segment of this sample showing the steepest decline (Singer, Verhaeghen, Ghisletta, Lindenberger, & Baltes, 2003). Moreover, even recall of factual knowledge, a stable and age-resilient crystallized intellectual ability, showed decline in participants older than 90 years of age.

Thus, for most practical purposes, older adults do not experience a decline in cognitive functioning until very advanced old age. Older adults can use their extensive factual and procedural knowledge effectively in situations that require expertise-relevant and/or overlearned responses (i.e., level 2 cognitive processing, see Kliegl, Krampe, & Mayr, 2003). Basic general cognitive processes (i.e., level 1 cognitive processes) show relatively little aging effects that can be compensated for by increased time investment and focus. However, cognitive aging does show negative effects on competence, when new learning and more complex, coordinated cognitive processing is required (level 3 cognitive processing; Kliegl et al., 2003). An example of the latter is any kind of multiple cognitive demand, such as driving while speaking on the phone or monitoring multiple processes simultaneously. Moreover, individuals in careers requiring highly developed sensory and intellectual abilities may experience constraints in functioning, because their professions push them to the limits of cognitive functioning that is vulnerable to aging-related decline. In the third section on regulating motivational investment as an adaptation to changing capacities, I discuss strategies of motivational regulation that allow the individual to maintain realistic levels of expert functioning into old age, while not despairing at the inevitable loss associated with biological aging.

Societal Opportunities and Constraints

The development and maintenance of high intellectual functioning, expertise, and peak performance is shaped not only by biological changes associated with aging but also by societal factors. On a general level, the greater the sophistication of technology involved in a society's economy, the greater the division of labor and, consequently, the greater the specialization in a society's labor force (Durkheim, 1893/1977). Specialized labor needs to be based on individual aptitude and motivation to build expertise. Rigid class or caste systems that lock individuals into certain positions in society (e.g., serf, vassal, or lord) inevitably imply that there are few or no opportunities for upward mobility. However, any sophisticated system of specialized labor requires a certain degree of social mobility, at least intergenerationally and at best intragenerationally. Thus, modern, highly industrialized societies typically have high degrees of (upward and downward) social mobility that provides substantial "playing fields" for individual agency (Heckhausen & Schulz, 1999b).

Modern, highly industrialized societies, however, differ with regard to intraindividual mobility, especially in adulthood, after academic and vocational education is completed. In the European countries, and in Germany in particular (Blossfeld & Mayer, 1988), social status and vocational careers are typically relatively stable after late adolescence, with little potential for career change in adulthood. Recent trends, however, indicate greater mobility between vocational careers in early adulthood (Heinz, 1999). In the United States, permeability (Hamilton, 1994) between career paths is preserved into midadulthood. Thus, an individual who decides to pursue a midlife career change has much better chances to realize the goal in the United States than in Europe. The downside of this greater permeability is its inevitable companion: less clarity or "transparency" (as Hamilton puts it) of career paths (Sennett, 1998), which turns the entry phase into work life in the United States into a period of floundering (Hamilton, 1990).

What about opportunities for growth in competence beyond early adulthood? For persons in professional careers, growth in challenge and competence often continues well into midlife. However, career development, final promotions, and retirement are constrained by state-regulated and corporate rules about age, timing, and sequencing of promotion. Such institutionalized, age-related constraints for professional development can get in the way of individuals who try to attain long-cherished career goals (Heckhausen, 1999). For example, implicit rules about age limits for moving up the executive ladder in a company can function as deadlines. These implicit, age-normative rules create urgency for corporate executives who get close to the age-related deadline, and futility for those who have already passed the deadline, and obstruct the attainment of long-term career goals when the in-

dividual passes implicit or explicit age deadlines. More generally, social institutional regulations generate patterns of life course and particularly career transitions (Sørensen, 2001). Conditions for competence growth are ideal when the individual's age and position in the career-related sequence of transitions fits with the age and sequence prescribed by the social institution regulating employment. Deviations from such "on-time" patterns require compensatory efforts on the part of the individual to overcome the obstacles associated with "swimming against the stream." For example, returning to school in midlife is possible, but it requires considerable effort, usually is less supported by society (student funding), and implies financial sacrifices that would be less difficult to bear for a younger adult with fewer family obligations (Heckhausen, 1999; Heckhausen & Schulz, 1999b).

Notwithstanding the late-career opportunities in professional vocations, most career tracks do not offer much chance to expand competence after the initial period of establishing oneself. Therefore, most people have limited opportunities to increase competence in their work life after their mid-20s or early 30s. In one such scenario, after attaining an educational degree and completing vocational training on the job, or in a vocational training institution, employees may soon reach the peak and plateau of their occupational career, where they can hope to remain until they retire. This pattern is actually optimistic in view of the development of the labor market in the globalized world economy, which is characterized by less predictability, displacement of skilled by unskilled labor, and a general pattern of temporal jobs replacing stable employment (e.g., Sennett, 1998). Again, differences between countries regarding the permeability of vocational career paths may offer more or less potential to change to a different career that may hold more mastery potential. However, by middle adulthood, such options become extremely costly for the individual who is giving up a career path and starting all over again. This situation of severely constrained potential for growth in competence after early adulthood bears the risk of boredom and loss of meaning for those individuals for whom achievement and growth in competence holds important personal meaning. An example is professions that require college degrees, or even advanced graduate degrees, but become routine after some years of experience, as is the case for some subspecialties of medicine, law, or engineering. In these professions, individuals with an aptitude for intellectual challenge, demonstrated by their successful completion of graduate degrees, end up underchallenged and bored long before it is time to retire.

In order to minimize their discontent, these individuals need to invest effort into motivational adjustments as a central part of their developmental regulation during midlife. I discuss possible strategies for such adjustment in the section on regulating motivational investment.

THE LIFESPAN THEORY OF CONTROL AND ITS IMPLICATIONS FOR MOTIVATION AND DEVELOPMENTAL REGULATION

The lifespan theory of control (Heckhausen, 1999; Heckhausen & Schulz, 1993, 1995; Schulz & Heckhausen, 1996) views individuals as agents in their own development (Brandtstädter & Lerner, 1999), who are actively striving to optimize their potential to control their environments and important outcomes in their lives (i.e., primary control) across the life course. Primary control of one's environment can be conceived in a fundamental sense as competence that is expanded and protected throughout the life course (Brim, 1992). Thus, the lifespan theory of control is about the motivation for competence, and changes and consequences for the individual's active role in lifespan development.

Control Processes Involved in Goal Engagement and Disengagement

The lifespan theory of control proposes two types of control striving: primary and secondary. *Primary control striving* refers to behavior directed at producing effects on the environment (i.e., effects of behavior on tangible outcomes). Examples of this might include trying to construct a Lego house, studying for an exam, applying for a job, or trying to persuade someone to buy one's house. *Secondary control striving* is behav-

ior and cognition directed at one's own motivational resources by either focusing volitional commitment or compensating for a threat to self-esteem. Examples of secondary control striving directed at volition include imagining the benefits of attaining the goal, avoiding tempting distractions, and enhancing one's confidence by being successful with the ongoing primary control striving. Primary and secondary control striving work hand in hand during *goal engagement* to allow the individual to mobilize behavioral (primary control) and motivational (secondary control) resources. Goal engagement involves three kinds of control strategies:

1. *Selective primary control* strategies refer to investing behavioral resources (time, effort, and skills) into goal pursuit (e.g., "I will work hard to have a good career"; from Optimization in Primary and Secondary Control (OPS-Scales); Heckhausen, Schulz, & Wrosch, 1998).
2. *Compensatory primary control* strategies involve getting help or advice from others (e.g., "If I run into obstacles with my career plans, I will ask others for advice") and/or using detours and unusual means toward a desired end (e.g., "I would take a less desirable job now, if it meant I could get the job I wanted in the long run").
3. *Selective secondary control* strategies refer to [volitional] self-regulation that is directed at enhancing one's [volitional] commitment to a chosen goal (e.g., "I often imagine how overjoyed I would be if I found a good job" or "I will be careful that other things do not distract me from getting a good job").

When goal attainment is not feasible (either impossible or too costly), *goal disengagement* is the adaptive response to prevent waste of behavioral and motivational resources that can be more productively applied to other primary control goals. Goal disengagement relies on strategies of *compensatory secondary control* that serve either of two functions: goal disengagement or self-protection. Goal disengagement from unattainable goals is important in order to preserve resources for other, more feasible goal strivings and can be facilitated by devaluing the previously held goal (e.g., "If I am not successful in my career, I will know that it was not the right thing for me anyway"). *Self-protection strategies* help the individual to deflect potential negative effects of failure experiences on self-esteem or action-related optimism. Examples of the self-protective strategies include attributions to external factors, thus avoiding self-blame (e.g., "If I run into problems with my schoolwork, I keep in mind that it is not all my fault") and comparison with others in similar or less favorable circumstances (e.g., "If I'm not successful in my career, I will say to myself that others are in a similar situation").

Action-Phase Model of Developmental Regulation

Throughout life, the individual confronts multiple trajectories of increasing and decreasing opportunities to attain important goals (see Figure 14.1). These rising and falling curves of opportunity have phases of maximum opportunity, when relevant control striving is most effective. Opportunity curves for different developmental goals are stacked across age, resulting in a developmental timetable of goals and transitions. An effective developmental agent would engage in and disengage from developmental

goals in age-graded synchronization, with waxing and waning opportunities across the life course. According to the lifespan theory of control, *optimized goal choice* means making use of favorable opportunities by engaging in "on-time" goals (e.g., "The jobs that I get in the next few years will have a lot of influence on the rest of my life") and avoiding goal engagement when opportunities have diminished or are not yet available. At the same time, long-term consequences of goal engagement need to be taken into account.

The lifespan theory of control and its action-phase model of developmental regulation generates specific predictions about the control processes activated in the sequence-of-action phases comprising a cycle of action around the pursuit of a developmental goal (see Figure 14.2). In the initial phase of goal choice, "metaregulatory" optimization strategies are required (i.e., choosing goals when opportunities are optimal, avoiding negative trade-offs for goals in other domains, and avoiding exclusive reliance on only one goal). Once a decision about a goal (e.g., striving for a promotion, learning a new sport) has been made, the individual should enter the volitional phase of action when goal engagement–related control strategies are activated (i.e., selective primary control,

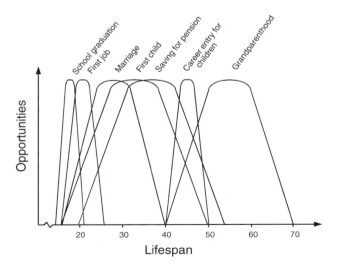

FIGURE 14.1. Age-graded sequencing of opportunity trajectories (hypothetical) for different developmental goals. Adapted from Heckhausen (2000b). Copyright 2000 by Elsevier. Adapted by permission from Elsevier.

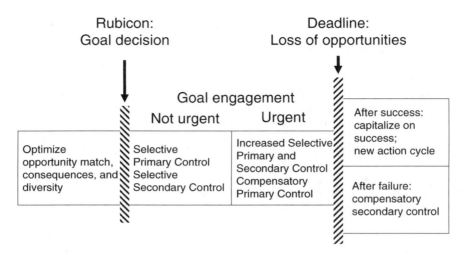

FIGURE 14.2. Action-phase model of developmental regulation. Adapted from Heckhausen (1999). Copyright 1999 by Cambridge University Press. Adapted by permission.

selective secondary control). For goals that are subject to declining opportunities (e.g., training or job opportunities only available in early adulthood), goal engagement becomes more urgent over time, so that goal engagement control strategies need to be employed more completely (i.e., compensatory primary control strategies may provide additional means for goal attainment) and more intensely. In such phases of urgent goal engagement, and particularly when the individual encounters unexpected obstacles, volitional self-regulation is essential to ensure that one's actions stay on track with his or her goals. Thus, under conditions of challenged goal engagement, compensatory primary and selective secondary control strategies may be the hallmark of successful developmental regulation. Finally, when goal attainment opportunities run out, or it becomes clear that the chosen goal is unattainable, the individual should disengage from the now-futile goal and use compensatory secondary control strategies that help him or her to preserve behavioral and motivational resources needed for future goal engagements.

A key proposition of this action-phase model is that transitions between action phases are discrete and organized rather than continuous and disjointed. Thus, when the individual makes a decision about a

goal, the relevant control processes are activated at the moment of crossing the decisional Rubicon and operate in concert. Similarly, when opportunities for goal attainment fade away, the realization of futility and resulting goal disengagement should be discrete in time and orchestrated in means, with multiple compensatory secondary control strategies activated jointly.

Empirical Illustrations of the Lifespan Theory of Control and the Action-Phase Model of Developmental Regulation

The action-phase model of developmental regulation, with its specific predictions about phase-appropriate control strategies, has been employed in several empirical studies (see reviews in Heckhausen & Farruggia, 2003; Schulz, Wrosch, & Heckhausen, 2003). All these studies address shifts in motivation and control processes that are associated with changes in opportunities to attain important goals in life, such as having a child, finding a romantic partner, entering a career, or maintaining one's independence in everyday life. A series of studies investigated the shift from urgent goal engagement to disengagement after having lost opportunities (e.g., to have children), thus passing a developmental deadline for a given life goal. For example, the motivational engagement with the developmental goal of bearing a first child was studied in childless women younger and older than 40 years of age (Heckhausen, Wrosch, & Fleeson, 2001). Moreover, engagement with and disengagement from partnership goals were studied in men and women who had recently separated from or committed to a partnership, and who were either in early adulthood, when remarriage probability is high, or in late middle adulthood, when remarriage probability is low (Wrosch & Heckhausen, 1999). In these studies, before the loss of goal-relevant opportunities (e.g., losing fertility, encountering fewer potential romantic partners), the age groups expressed goal-commitments and control strategies indicative of intense goal engagement, whereas after the loss of opportunities, the age groups endorsed control strategies of goal disengagement and self-protection. For instance, younger, recently separated adults stated that finding a new partner was a high priority goal for them, and that they often imagined how happy they would be when they found a new partner. In contrast, recently separated adults in their 50s endorsed views to the effect that, for them, life could be fulfilled without a partner, and that they did not blame themselves for being single.

Opportunity-congruent goal engagement and disengagement was found not only in explicit self-reports of goals and control strategies but also in selective information processing. Predeadline groups were more likely than postdeadline groups to recall goal-relevant information in an incidental memory task. Most importantly, the degree to which control strategies and information-processing biases were congruent with goal opportunities was positively related to psychological well-being and mental health, both concurrently and across a period of 18 months. Thus, if adults at an age at which the opportunities for goal attainment were favorable reported goal engagement, they were less likely than those who were not goal-engaged at this age to report depressive symptoms. Conversely, among adults at an age in which goal opportunities were unfavorable, those adults who were disengaged reported better mental health than those

who were engaged. To give a specific example, the same statements of goal disengagement ("I can lead a happy life without a partner") were associated with negative affect development in younger adults and positive affect development in late-midlife adults.

This paradigm of investigating developmental regulation during transitions from better to worse was also applied to the study of coping with radical losses in competence associated with disability. It was shown that, depending on the reversibility and, thus, controllability of functional loss associated with the disability, goal engagement (for high controllability) versus goal disengagement (for low controllability) was more adaptive (Wrosch, Heckhausen, & Lachman, 2000; Wrosch, Schulz, & Heckhausen, 2002, 2004). For instance, with acute and more controllable ailments, but not with chronic uncontrollable illnesses, primary control strategies of promoting health and fighting the illness were helpful in reducing depressive symptoms in older adults. Finally, a study of life regrets showed that disengaging from a goal of undoing the regret (e.g., at not having gone to graduate school) and viewing what had been done as out of one's control is adaptive in older adults but maladaptive in younger ones (Wrosch & Heckhausen, 2002). In each of these studies, goal engagement and disengagement that were congruent with available control potential (i.e., engagement with high control potential, disengagement with low control potential) were found to be associated with positive developmental outcomes, whereas incongruent goal engagement was maladaptive.

Currently, studies in several countries are using the lifespan theory of control and its model of action-phases in longitudinal studies. These studies investigate sequential patterns and causal relations between changing opportunities for goal attainment, adaptations of control strategies in terms of goal engagement and disengagement, motivational resources, and physical and mental health. These ongoing longitudinal studies address a wide variety of developmental and self-regulatory challenges, including adaptive and maladaptive pathways in midlife ("Integrative Pathways to Health and Illness—MIDUS II [Midlife in the U.S.]," National Institute on Aging (NIA), PI: Carol Ryff), and old age ("Health and Aging," Canadian Institutes of Health, PI: Judith Chipperfield). Other studies using the lifespan theory of control and its model of developmental regulation focus more on specific challenges, such as the adaptation to caregiving ("Psychiatric and Physical Health Effects of Caregiving," National Institute of Mental Health (NIMH), PI: Richard Schulz), to vision loss (Horowitz, Boerner, Reinhardt, & Brennan, 2002; Wahl Becker, & Burmedi, 2002; "Control Strategies and Mental Health in Impaired Elders," NIMH, PI: Amy Horowitz; "Course and Consequences of Control Regulation in Age-Related Low Vision," German Research Foundation, PI: Hans-Werner Wahl), to cancer treatments (Pinquart & Silbereisen, 2002; "Treatment Decisions and the Revision of Life Plans Among Elderly Cancer Patients," German Cancer Aid, PIs: Martin Pinquart & Rainer Silbereisen), to intergenerational transmission of private business enterprises ("What Facilitates Family Business Transmission?: The Adaptive Roles of Goal Adjustment and Autonomous Motivation," Social Sciences and Humanities Research Council of Canada, PI: Carsten Wrosch), to life regrets (Wrosch & Heckhausen, 2002), and to interpersonal conflict in old age (Rook & Sorkin, 2002; "Impact of Negative Social Exchanges in Later Life," PI: Karen Rook). A number of studies address control strategies employed to manage major transitions in education and career, such as the management of failure and success in the Chinese university entrance exam (Wong, Li, & Shen, 2004), the transition to and persistence in college education ("A Longitudinal Analysis of Career Uncertainty and Technological Uncertainty on Motivation, Achievement, and Attrition of University Students," Social Sciences and Humanities Research Council of Canada, PI: Raymond Perry), the transition from school to vocational training in German adolescents (Heckhausen & Tomasik, 2002; "Developmental Regulation during the Transition from School to Vocational Training: Adaptations in Primary and Secondary Control Striving," German Research Foundation, PIs: Jutta Heckhausen & Olaf Köller), and

the transition from school to college and work in young adults in the United States (Heckhausen, 2003a).

Ascending and Descending Levels of Aspiration for Successful Development

In the most recent development of the lifespan theory of control, the question of how individuals move from one goal-engagement cycle to the next is addressed. More specifically, the issue here is which goal individuals select when they have just succeeded versus failed in a goal pursuit. Does the individual stay within the same domain of control? Which goals can substitute for each other, without challenging the emotional balance and motivational resources of the individual? In their lifespan model of successful aging, Schulz and Heckhausen (1996) distinguished between four levels of control potential: survival, general health, everyday functioning in major domains, and peak performance in select domains of expertise. These levels of successful functioning provide the objectifiable backdrop for identifying successful aging and distinguishing it from suboptimal aging.

After several years of research experience with the action-phase model of developmental regulation, the processes allowing the individual to move between these levels of control potential have become clearer. According to a model of ascending and descending levels of aspiration (Heckhausen, 2003b), individuals disengage from previous goals and engage in new goals in a discrete and organized fashion, akin to the transitions between action phases. For most domains of functioning (i.e., domains of competence), goals can be organized in a staircase manner, with the least difficult, and at the same time most essential, goals at the bottom and the most challenging goals at the top. When experiencing and/or striving for growth in control, individuals move their aspirations from lower to higher level goals in a stepwise fashion. At each time, the individual is engaged with a goal adjusted to his or her currently experienced control capacity, having disengaged from the previous, lower level goal and reengaged with a goal on the next level of control. Conversely, when experiencing loss, individuals withdraw from higher levels of goal challenge to lower levels of difficulty, in accordance with the control potential they experience. This way, at each level of control potential across the life course, individuals can attain or maintain the optimal level of control in their goal pursuits, without wasting resources in futile, overchallenging goal pursuits or missing control opportunities by setting underchallenging goals that fall short of their current control potential. When applied to the area of health psychology and aging, these ascending and descending levels of aspiration can be conceptualized as lines of defense when individuals are fighting disability, and lines of advance when they are striving for rehabilitation (Heckhausen, 2003b). For example, someone with progressive arthritis might give up doing her own grocery shopping, but strive to maintain the capacity to do her own cooking (line of defense). In contrast, someone with the same illness and access to a new physiotherapy might strive to extend his mobility, from being restricted to the house to running errands in the neighborhood.

REGULATING MOTIVATIONAL INVESTMENT AS AN ADAPTATION TO CHANGING CAPACITIES IN INTELLECTUAL COMPETENCE ACROSS ADULTHOOD

In this final section, I discuss how individuals can regulate their motivational investment in response to changing control potential over the life course. For a more detailed discussion of the requirements in executive functioning, see Heckhausen & Mayr (1998). As noted earlier, in this chapter, I do not consider the implications of interindividual differences in achievement and work motivation, but focus on regulatory processes of motivational investment in vocational contexts. A more detailed discussion of work motivation and the role of the achievement motive can be found in Kanfer and Ackerman (Chapter 19, this volume; see also Schultheiss & Brunstein, Chapter 3, this volume for a discussion of the achievement motive).

Given the biological and societal constraints, four scenarios of competence change in adulthood and old age capture the range of challenges to the motivational system: the nonprofessional vocational career, the high-level professional career, the peak performers' developmental course, and the late-life decline and disability in very advanced old age. Here, I discuss the challenges to motivational regulation implied in each of these four scenarios and consider strategies to master these regulatory tasks.

The Nonprofessional Career

As I discussed earlier, most people work in careers (e.g., blue-collar workers, clerks, salesmen) that involve an early phase of training and getting established that does not extend beyond their 20s or early 30s at the most. During this phase of getting established in a career, self-esteem increases after the challenging phase of transition into employment (Dooley, 2003). Also, conceptions about the controllability of outcomes and one's own control potential become more differentiated and integrated, leading to a more stable and realistic world view that integrates both external and internal factors (Hoff, Lempert, & Lappe, 1991).

Once the plateau of vocational achievements is reached by the late 20s or early 30s, the activities the person is involved in during the working day remain pretty invariant, so that further growth in competence is unlikely, if not prevented, at least for those who do not start their own business. These diminished opportunities for growth in competence after the third decade of life should pose a substantial challenge for motivational self-regulation, especially for those individuals who hold strong achievement motives and pursue achievement-related superordinate goals (Heckhausen, 1986). Three alternative paths of motivational self-regulation seem viable in this situation: (1) a disengagement from achievement-related, superordinate goals and/or motives relative to other motives; or (2) a switch of one's investment from work-related pursuits to expanding control and competence outside the work life in leisure activities (e.g., sports); or (3) a switch of career to a field that allows longer term professional growth. All three motivational changes involve goal disengagement that can be expected to be facilitated by the availability of alternative or substitute goals (Aspinwall & Richter, 1999; Wrosch, Scheier, Carver, & Schulz, 2003), and by the employment of compensatory secondary control strategies of disengagement and self-protection. The third path, into a new career, involves high costs, because substantial attainments in the previous career have to be forfeited, and a professionally promising new career typically requires extensive educational investment and a substantial risk of failure. In contrast, the first two paths of self-regulation (the disengagement from superordinate achievement goals and the increased investment in goals outside of work) are facilitated by the predictability in normative career patterns in nonprofessionals. This predictability allows the individual involved in these nonprofessional careers to anticipate the need for motivational adaptation to the fading challenges of the job.

The High-Level Professional Career

Even in late midlife and old age, competence in most professions does not show substantial decline (e.g., Salthouse, 1984; Sparrow & Davies, 1988; Waldman & Avolio, 1986). Moreover, people working in high-level professions typically have to self-regulate their own motivation and, thus, rely on setting their own goals (von Rosenstiehl, Kehr, & Maier, 2000). As a consequence, the degree to which professionals believe the organization (e.g., the company) facilitates goal attainment is crucial to their job satisfaction and organizational commitment. Morever, professional managers experience challenges for professional development and growth well into midlife and, for some, this extends even up to retirement (Kehr, Bles, & von Rosenstiehl, 1999).

One avenue by which professional development is advanced is professional training in midcareer. However, training success is typically constrained by limited transfer of new skills and knowledge to different areas of managerial responsibility. Kehr and colleagues (1999) showed that managers who did not simply adopt the goals proposed by the trainers and supervisors, but carefully evaluated and weighed them in the context of their own needs, experiences, habits, and preferences, were more likely to remember the goals 3 months after completing the training, to experience more positive emo-

tions, and to achieve greater training transfer to their goal realization and criteria fulfillment at work.

In another study, Kehr (2004) investigated the discrepancy among implicit and explicit motives, volitional strength, and their association to subjective well-being in managers of German companies. The results show that across a 5-month period, volitional strength deteriorated with increasing discrepancies between implicit and explicit motives. Moreover, volitional strength mediated the association between implicit–explicit motive discrepancy and subjective well-being over time. Thus, subjective well-being was impacted by implicit–explicit motive discrepancy to the extent that the discrepancy undermined volitional strength.

In summary, in professional, top-level careers, intrinsic motivation plays an even more crucial role than in other career tracks. Having entered their careers with a strong and success-oriented achievement motive, professionals typically cherish these continued challenges and suffer when they are withdrawn or compromised (von Rosenstiehl et al., 2000). The dominant motivational pattern for this group follows a path of contingent success and occasional setbacks, followed by upward or slightly downward adjustments of work and career goals. The overall trajectory is one of continued growth in competence and rise in status. Thus, one can expect that the dominant motivational adjustment is one of habituation to success; when attaining yet another subgoal, enjoyment and pride about the success is relatively moderate and short-lived, and may even reflect a pattern of diminished returns (Lindenberg, 1996). It is essential for these professionals in high-level positions that intrinsic incentives for achievement remain strong. This is not always the case, as power-related activities gain in importance in later stages of professional careers (in business, science, etc.).

Expertise and Peak Performance

Expertise and peak performance careers and their motivational requirements are discussed in more detail, because they represent a testing-the-limits case for management of adjustments in motivational investment.

Peak performances in intellectual competence require the convergence of multiple facilitative factors: biological prime coupled with sufficient training and experience in the domain of expertise, a conducive social context (society, family), and substantial individual investment in the acquisition and perfection of the expertise. Simonton (1994) has investigated achievers of greatness in many domains and across historical time. Based on his extensive data about the life histories of great achievers in the domains of science, art, music, political leadership, business, Simonton developed a normative productivity curve for achieving greatness, displayed in Figure 14.3. According to this curve of greatness across the life course, truly great achievers begin publishing their greatest work sometime in their 20s, ascend to their optimum level near 40 years of age, and show a slow descent in achievements after reaching the optimum. This normative trajectory reflects the life-time it takes to acquire expert levels of knowledge and skill, thus, the relatively late onset (e.g., compared to athletics) in the third decade of life. Moreover, the complexity of knowledge and skills is reflected in the time it takes to develop them to perfection, thus, the optimum level at about 40 years of age. Finally, biological decline and/or other kinds of resource depletion lead to the gradual decline

after age 40, with the gradualness reflecting the individual's efforts to sustain the high level of functioning into old age. Interestingly, Simonton concluded from his analyses that throughout careers of great achievements, the ratio of all works (productivity) to high-quality works (creativity) is stable across age, the "equal-odds rule." Across the life course, the ratio of hits to total output does not appear to change, irrespective of level of expertise.

Research on peak performance in intellectual or artistic domains has revealed the key role of individual motivational investment in acquiring the expertise. Ericsson and his colleagues have shown that for several domains of expertise, most notably for musicians, the highest levels of performance can only be achieved after around 10 years of extensive, daily, deliberate training and practice (Ericsson, Krampe, & Tesch-Römer, 1993). These findings converge with Simonton's analyses of individuals' trajectories of greatness, showing the first top achievements after 20 years of age, if we assume that serious, deliberate practice starts around age 10. According to Ericsson et al. (1993) best achievers in their domains typically accumulated more than 10,000 hours of training and practice until they reach the age of 20 years. Such investment of time and effort requires a highly selective motivational com-

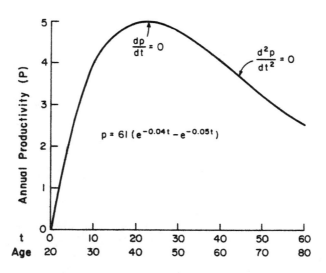

FIGURE 14.3. Annual productivity in all domains of greatness. From Simonton (1994, p. 183). Copyright 1994 by The Guilford Press. Reprinted by permission.

mitment to the domain of expertise, at the expense of other domains of functioning, and with potential high risks should the selected domain of expertise not bear the expected results. Such highly selective investments of time, effort, and motivation early in life can have high costs and bear significant risks, because it narrows the set of viable developmental paths at a very early point in life, when the ultimate fruitfulness of the selected path to peak performance is still highly uncertain (Heckhausen & Schulz, 1999b). The public learns about those who ultimately are successful in this immense investment of life-time and energy; we do not know about the many people who set out on this path and never make it to greatness.

However, those who do achieve peak levels of functioning become highly skilled in optimizing the efficacy of their investments in deliberate training and practice. For example, highly accomplished violin soloists select the times of day when they are most rested for their deliberate practice, practicing in the morning and after a nap in the afternoon (Ericsson et al., 1993).

What happens to the top levels of performance when individuals age? In a study of expert-level (but not world-class level) graphic designers, older designers obtained higher levels in visual imagery than older adults in other professions (Lindenberger, Kliegl, & Baltes, 1992). However, the proficiency in the visual imagery of these older experts fell short of that in any younger participant. Thus, aging-related decline was attenuated but not eliminated by relevant talent, experience, and long-term practice.

A more recent study on solo pianists showed that their fluid intellectual skills undergo similar aging-related decline as nonpianists. However, the older pianists managed to maintain the level of high-speed performance in expertise-related tasks at almost the same level as younger pianists. The findings indicate that the degree to which performance decline was absent in these former concert pianists was associated with the amount of deliberate practice performed in later adulthood. Thus, when these top performers reach midlife and old age, they use deliberate practice to fend off age-related decline in performance that is affecting their basic cognitive skills (Krampe & Ericsson,

1996). Such deliberate practice in advanced age can selectively focus on subcomponents of the skills involved in the expertise, thus resulting in individual-specific patterns of aging effects across subcomponents of the skill. As aging-related decline in sensorimotor and cognitive functioning progresses further, experts have to focus on narrower tasks and allow themselves more time to maintain the selected performance. Goal engagement and its control processes (selective primary, selective secondary, and compensatory primary control) become ever more pronounced and selective, of course, at the expense of other activities (e.g., leisure time and social contacts). This puts considerable strain on the motivational system, because the costs of maintaining the expertise level of functioning will increase ever more with advancing age. Eventually, in more or less advanced old age, most experts and peak performers will have to disengage from their lifelong dedication to top levels of performance in highly selective domain of competence. Such disengagement bears high disruptive potential for self-esteem, life satisfaction, and generally motivational and emotional resources for the primary control projects still feasible in old age. Thus, even and especially for the elderly top expert and previous peak performer, goal disengagement, goal substitution with feasible goals, and self-protective interpretations of the loss in competence are essential. To maintain as much competence as possible given the biological and societal constraints is the key to successful development in adulthood.

Late-Life Decline and Disability

In very advanced old age, chronic illness and disability become a reality for almost everyone who survives into this last phase of human longevity. As for earlier phases of life, successful development in very late life (i.e., after 85 years of age) is a function of the degree to which goal engagement and disengagement strategies match the actual control opportunities. At each level of control compromised by illness and disability, some primary control endeavors are still feasible and adaptive, whereas others have become illusory and are thus wasteful of the precious few control resources. Calibrating one's goal investments to the available control resources is thus ever more important the older an individual is, and the fewer control resources he or she commands. Control investments need to be focused and well orchestrated (i.e., all control strategies of goal engagement should be activated) to be fruitful. Likewise, goal disengagements should be swift and complete, instead of drawn out or hesitant. Thus, the action-phase model of developmental regulation can be applied also to the process of adaptation to constrain control resources that come with old age, disability, and illness.

In a "lines of defense" model, Heckhausen (2003b) has identified five lines of defense as goals for primary control of illness and disability: (1) Avoid disease/disability, (2) protect one's own control (self-reliance) over activities of daily living, (3) use others' help and technical aid to maintain activities of daily living, (4), minimize discomfort, and (5) delay death. With progressing illness and disability, the individual can decide to disengage from a higher level of aspiration (e.g., avoid disease/disability) and instead invest control resources in a lower level (e.g., protect one's own control over activities of daily living). Persisting on a given level in spite of substantially and irreversibly lost primary control potential would be wasteful of control resources and put the individual at risk of sliding uncontrollably further down the cascade of control levels. On the other hand, giving up more control than necessary by dropping down to a lower level than warranted by actual control potential may be maladaptive, too, unless the resources needed for maintaining a given level of disability (e.g., performing activities self-reliantly) prevent the individual from striving for goals (e.g., maintaining a cherished hobby) that are more valued and personally meaningful (Baltes, 1996).

The key proposition of the lines-of-defense model is that goal disengagements and engagements allow for an organized retreat that enables the individual to utilize his or her remaining control potential to defend realistic levels of primary control. The lines-of-defense model can be used for the inverse direction of health-related change of control potential, too, namely, in processes of rehabilitation, during which the individual advances the levels of control for which he or she is striving to higher and higher levels. The greatest regulatory challenges occur when a line of defense is embattled, in the sense that it is not clear from the outset whether the individual will be able to advance or will be forced to retreat from a given level of control. Such situations ensue after a stroke or other serious health event, when rehabilitation may be possible but uncertain. These situations of embattled lines of defense push the individual to the limits of motivational self-regulation, and also confront the advising physician and those close to the individual with unprecedented challenges.

SUMMARY

The biological and societal context brings about changing opportunities and constraints for developing competence during adulthood and old age. Adults in various paths of life need to respond to these changes. Most individuals in the labor force face drastically reduced potential for growth in competence in the forth decade of their lives and, thus, need to accommodate to this change early on in adult life. In contrast, high-level professionals and peak performers may be able to develop their competencies well into midlife, needing to adjust their aspirations much later in life. For the latter group, a strategy of highly focused investment and compensatory efforts may help individuals to maintain high levels of functioning in their domains of expertise until late midlife and, in some domains, even until early old age. However, eventually, everybody needs to disengage from aspirations of maintaining levels of performance attained during one's prime. An action-phase model of developmental regulation identifies transition points in the action cycle that call for discrete and orchestrated engagements and disengagements for most effective, life-course encompassing control striving. In advanced old age, such engagements and disengagements are organized into staircase-structured lines of defense that allow the individual to make the most of his or her remaining control capacities and resources.

REFERENCES

Aspinwall, L. G., & Richter, L. (1999). Optimism and self-mastery predict more rapid disengagement from unsolvable tasks in the presence of alternatives. *Motivation and Emotion, 23,* 221–245.

Baltes, M. M. (1996). *The many faces of dependency in old age.* New York: Cambridge University Press.

Baltes, P. B., Dittman-Kohli, F., & Kliegl, R. (1986). Reserve capacity of the elderly in aging-sensitive tests of fluid intelligence: Replication and extension. *Psychology and Aging, 1,* 172–177.

Baltes, P. B., & Kliegl, R. (1992). Negative age differences in cognitive plasticity of a memory skill during adulthood: Further testing of limits. *Developmental Psychology, 28,* 121–125.

Baltes, P. B., & Lindenberger, U. (1988). On the range of cognitive plasticity in old age as a function of experience: 15 years of intervention research. *Behavior Therapy, 19,* 283–300.

Baltes, P. B., Sowarka, D., & Kliegl, R. (1989). Cognitive training research on fluid intelligence in old age: What can older adults achieve by themselves? *Psychology and Aging, 4,* 217–221.

Baltes, P. B., Staudinger, U. M., & Lindenberger, U. (1999). Lifespan psychology: Theory and application to intellectual functioning. *Annual Review of Psychology, 50,* 471–507.

Blossfeld, H.-P., & Mayer, K. U. (1988). Labor market segmentation in the Federal Republic of Germany: An empirical study of segmentation theories from a life course perspective. *European Sociological Review, 4,* 123–140.

Brandtstädter, J., & Lerner, R. (Eds.). (1999). *Action and self-development: Theory and research through the life-span.* London: Sage.

Brim, O. G., Jr. (1992). *Ambition: How we manage success and failure throughout our lives.* New York: Basic Books.

Dooley, D. (2003). Unemployment, underemployment, and mental health: Conceptualizing employment status as a continuum. *American Journal of Community Psychology, 32,* 9–20.

Durkheim, E. (1977). *De la division du travail social* [Über die Teilung der sozialen Arbeit]. Paris: Übersetzung. (Original work published in 1893)

Ericsson, K. A. (1990). Peak performance and age: An examination of peak performance in sports. In P. B. Baltes & M. M. Baltes (Eds.), *Successful aging: Perspectives from the behavioral sciences* (pp. 164–196). New York: Cambridge University Press.

Ericsson, K. A., Krampe, R. T., & Tesch-Römer, C. (1993). The role of deliberate practice in the acquisition of expert performance. *Psychological Review, 100,* 363–406.

Hamilton, S. F. (1990). *Apprenticeship for adulthood.* New York: Free Press.

Hamilton, S. F. (1994). Employment prospects as motivation for school achievement: Links and gaps between school and work in seven countries. In R. K. Silbereisen & E. Todt (Eds.), *Adolescence in context: The interplay of family, school, peers, and work in adjustment* (pp. 267–303). New York: Springer.

Heckhausen, H. (1986). Achievement and motivation through the life span. In A. B. Sørensen, F. E. Weinert, & L. R. Sherrod (Eds.), *Human development and the life course: Multidisciplinary perspectives* (pp. 445–466). Hillsdale, NJ: Erlbaum.

Heckhausen, J. (1999). *Developmental regulation in adulthood: Age-normative and sociostructural constraints as adaptive challenges.* New York: Cambridge University Press.

Heckhausen, J. (2000a). Evolutionary perspectives on human motivation. In J. Heckhausen & P. Boyer (Eds.), Evolutionary psychology: Potential and limits of a Darwinian framework for the behavioral sciences [Special issue]. *American Behavioral Scientist, 43,* 1015–1029.

Heckhausen, J. (Ed.). (2000b). *Motivational psychology of human development: Developing motivation and motivation development.* Amsterdam: Elsevier.

Heckhausen, J. (2003a). *School-to-work transition in a multi-ethnic sample.* Unpublished research proposal, University of California, Irvine.

Heckhausen, J. (2003b, May). *The life-span theory of control as a paradigm to study illness and disability in old age.* Paper presented at the UC/APA Conference on Health Psychology and Aging, Lake Arrowhead, CA.

Heckhausen, J., & Farruggia, S. P. (2003). Developmental regulation across the life span: A control-theory approach and implications for secondary education. In L. Smith, C. Rogers, & P. Tomlinson (Eds.), *Development and motivation: Joint perspectives* (pp. 85–102). British Journal of Educational Psychology, Monograph Series II: Psychological Aspects of Education—Current Trends. Leicester: British Psychological Society.

Heckhausen, J., & Mayr, U. (1998). Entwicklungsregulation und Kontrolle im Erwachsenenalter und Alter: Lebenslaufpsychologische Perspektiven [Developmental regulation and control in adulthood and old age: Life-span psychological perspectives]. In H. Keller (Ed.), *Lehrbuch für Entwicklungspsychologie* [A developmental psychology textbook]. Bern: Huber.

Heckhausen, J., & Schulz, R. (1993). Optimisation by selection and compensation: Balancing primary and secondary control in life-span development. *International Journal of Behavioral Development, 16,* 287–303.

Heckhausen, J., & Schulz, R. (1995). A life-span theory of control. *Psychological Review, 102,* 284–304.

Heckhausen, J., & Schulz, R. (1999a). The primacy of primary control is a human universal: A reply to Gould's critique of the life-span theory of control. *Psychological Review, 106,* 605–609.

Heckhausen, J., & Schulz, R. (1999b). Biological and societal canalizations and individuals' developmental goals. In J. Brandtstädter & R. Lerner (Eds.), *Action and self-development: Theory and research through the life-span* (pp. 67–103). London: Sage.

Heckhausen, J., Schulz, R., & Wrosch, C. (1998). *Developmental regulation in adulthood: Optimization in Primary and Secondary Control—a multiscale questionnaire (OPS-Scales)* [Technical Report]. Berlin: Max Planck Institute for Human Development.

Heckhausen, J., & Tomasik, M. (2002). Get an apprenticeship before school is out: How German adolescents adjust vocational aspirations when getting close to a developmental deadline. *Journal of Vocational Behavior, 60,* 199–219.

Heckhausen, J., Wrosch, C., & Fleeson, W. (2001). Developmental regulation before and after a developmental deadline: The sample case of "biological clock" for child-bearing. *Psychology and Aging, 16,* 400–413.

Heinz, W. (Ed.). (1999). *From education to work: Cross-national perspectives.* Cambridge, UK: Cambridge University Press.

Hoff, E.-H., Lempert, W., & Lappe, L. (Eds.). (1991). *Persönlichkeitsentwicklung in Facharbeiterbiographien* [Personality development in skilled industrial workers' biographies]. Bern: Hans Huber.

Horowitz, A., Boerner, K., Reinhardt, J., & Brennan, M. (2002, November). *Applying the life-span theory of control to research on adaptation to age-related vision loss.* Paper presented at the 55th Annual Scientific Meetings of the Gerontological Society of America, Boston, MA.

Kehr, H. (2004). Implicit/explicit motive discrepancies and volitional depletion among managers. *Personality and Social Psychology Bulletin, 30,* 315–327.

Kehr, H. M., Bles, P., & von Rosenstiehl, L. (1999). Self-regulation, self-control, and management training transfer. *International Journal of Educational Research, 31,* 487–498.

Kemper, S., Herman, R. E., & Lian, C. H. T. (2003). The costs of doing two things at once for young and older adults: Talking while walking, finger tapping, and ignoring speech or noise. *Psychology and Aging, 18,* 181–192.

Kliegl, R., Krampe, R. T., & Mayr, U. (2003). Formal models of age differences in task-complexity effects. In U. M. Staudinger & U. Lindenberger (Eds.), *Understanding human development: Dialogues with lifespan psychology* (pp. 289–313). Boston: Kluwer Academic.

Krampe, R. T., & Ericsson, K A. (1996). Maintaining excellence: Deliberate practice and elite performance in young and older pianists. *Journal of Experimental Psychology: General, 125,* 331–359.

Li, K. Z. H., Lindenberger, U., Freund, A. M., & Baltes, P. B. (2001). Walking while memorizing: Age-related differences in compensatory behavior. *Psychological Science, 12,* 230–237.

Lindenberg, S. M. (1996). Continuities in the theory of social production functions. In S. M. Lindenberg & H. B. G. Ganzeboom (Eds.), *Verklarende sociologie: Opstellen voor Reinhard Wippler* [Explanatory soci-

ology: Essays for Reinhard Wippler] (pp. 169–184). Amsterdam: Thesis Publishers.

Lindenberger, U., Kliegl, R., & Baltes, P. B. (1992). Professional expertise does not eliminate age differences in imagery-based memory performance during adulthood. *Psychology and Aging, 7,* 585–593.

Lindenberger, U., Marsiske, M., & Baltes, P. B. (2000). Memorizing while walking: Increase in dual-task costs from young adulthood to old age. *Psychology and Aging, 15,* 417–436.

Mayr, U., & Kliegl, R. (1993). Sequential and coordinative complexity: Age-based processing limitations in figural transformations. *Journal of Experimental Psychology: Learning, Memory, and Cognition, 19,* 1297–1320.

Mayr, U., Kliegl, R., & Krampe, R. T. (1996). Sequential and coordinative processing dynamics across the life span. *Cognition, 59,* 61–90.

Pinquart, M., & Silbereisen, R. K. (2002, November). *Cancer patients' control strategies: Associations with age, course of therapy, and subjective well-being.* Paper presented at the 55th Annual Scientific Meetings of the Gerontological Society of America, Boston, MA.

Rook, K. S., & Sorkin, D. H. (2002, July). *Exposure to negative social exchanges in later life: The role of control strivings.* Paper presented at the biennial meeting of the International Association for Relationship Research, Halifax, Nova Scotia.

Salthouse, T. A. (1984). Effects of age and skill in typing. *Journal of Experimental Psychology: General, 113,* 345–371.

Schulz, R., & Curnow, C. (1988). Peak performance and age among superathletes: Track and field, swimming, baseball, tennis, and golf. *Journal of Gerontology: Psychological Sciences, 43,* 113–120.

Schulz, R., & Heckhausen, J. (1996). A life-span model of successful aging. *American Psychologist, 51,* 702–714.

Schulz, R., Wrosch, C., & Heckhausen, J. (2003). The life-span theory of control: Issues and evidence. In S. Zarit, L. Pearlin, & K. W. Schaie (Eds.), *Personal control in social and life course contexts: Societal impact on aging* (pp. 233–262). New York: Springer.

Sennett, R. (1998). *The corrosion of character.* New York: Norton.

Simonton, D. K. (1994). *Greatness: Who makes history and why.* New York: Guilford Press.

Singer, T., Lindenberger, U., & Baltes, P. B. (2003). Plasticity of memory for new learning in very old age: A story of major loss? *Psychology and Aging, 18,* 306–317.

Singer, T., Verhaeghen, P., Ghisletta, P., Lindenberger, U., & Baltes, P. B. (2003). The fate of cognition in very old age: Six-year longitudinal findings in the Berlin Aging Study (BASE). *Psychology and Aging, 18,* 318–331.

Sørensen, A. B. (2001). Careers and employment relations. In I. Berg & A. L. Kalleberg (Eds.), *Sourcebook of labor markets: Evolving structures and pro-

cesses (pp. 295–318). New York: Kluwer Academic/Plenum Press.

Sparrow, P. R., & Davies, D. R. (1988). Effects of age, tenure, training and job complexity on technical performance. *Psychology and Aging, 3,* 307–314.

von Rosenstiehl, L., Kehr, H. M., & Maier, G. W. (2000). Motivation and volition in pursuing personal work goals. In J. Heckhausen (Ed.), *Motivational psychology of human development: Developing motivation and motivating development* (pp. 287–305). Amsterdam: Elsevier.

Wahl, H.-W., Becker, S., & Burmedi, D. (2002, November). *Losing and choosing: Role of control strategies in vision impairment due to age-related macular degeneration.* Paper presented at the 55th Annual Scientific Meeting of the Gerontological Society of America, Boston, MA.

Waldman, D. A., & Avolio, B. J. (1986). A meta-analysis of age differences in job performance. *Journal of Applied Psychology, 71,* 33–38.

Wong, W.-C., Li, Y., & Shen, J. L. (2004). *Chinese students' control processes before and after an academic examination: Evidence for the primacy of primary control.* Paper submitted for publication.

Wrosch, C., & Heckhausen, J. (1999). Control processes before and after passing a developmental deadline: Activation and deactivation of intimate relationship goals. *Journal of Personality and Social Psychology, 77,* 415–427.

Wrosch, C., & Heckhausen, J. (2002). Perceived control of life regrets: Good for young and bad for old adults. *Psychology and Aging, 17,* 340–350.

Wrosch, C., Heckhausen, J., & Lachman, M. E. (2000). Primary and secondary control strategies for managing health and financial stress across adulthood. *Psychology and Aging, 15,* 387–399.

Wrosch, C., Scheier, M. F., Carver, C. S., & Schulz, R. (2003). The importance of goal disengagement in adaptive self-regulation: When giving up is beneficial. *Self and Identity, 2,* 1–20.

Wrosch, C., Schulz, R., & Heckhausen, J. (2002). Health stresses and depressive symptomatology in the elderly: The importance of health engagement control strategies. *Health Psychology, 21,* 340–348.

Wrosch, C., Schulz, R. & Heckhausen, J. (2004). Health stresses and depressive symptomatology in the elderly: A control-process approach. *Current Directions, 13,* 17–20.

PART IV

❦

Contextual Influences

CHAPTER 15

ରୁ

The Role of Parents
in How Children Approach Achievement

A Dynamic Process Perspective

EVA M. POMERANTZ
WENDY S. GROLNICK
CARRIE E. PRICE

Central to children's development is their achievement of a variety of competencies—for example, taking responsibility for themselves, considering the feelings of others, and reading and writing. Indeed, beginning at birth, important issues of achievement arise in almost every area of children's daily life. A key question is how to enable children to approach such issues positively, so that they are successful in navigating the challenges they face over the course of development. Because parents are central figures in most children's lives, they have the potential to shape children's orientation toward achievement. Despite some arguments to the contrary (e.g., Scarr, 1992), much research indicates that parents play a role in children's development along a number of lines (for a review, see Parke & Buriel, 1998). Several diverse strands of this research provide support for the idea that parents contribute to how children tackle issues of achievement that arise as children progress through life (e.g., Frome & Eccles, 1998; Grolnick, 2003; Jacobsen, Wolfgang, & Hofman, 1994).

Our major aim in this chapter is to provide an integrated account of parents' role in children's approach to achievement—that is, what Elliot and Dweck (Chapter 1, this volume) term "competence-relevant motivation," and Eccles, Wigfield, and Schiefele (1998) term the "motivation to succeed." To this end, we highlight how parents and children jointly contribute to children's approach to achievement over the course of development, emphasizing the power of social contextual forces. Achievement is particularly salient in the school context, where children spend a large portion of their day in activities aimed at developing their academic competencies. As a consequence, most of the research on the role of parents in how children approach achievement has been in the academic area. Given this emphasis, our focus in this chapter is on the academic area. However, the issues discussed are likely to be applicable to other areas of children's lives as well (see Elliot & Dweck, Chapter 1, this volume).

A central premise guiding this chapter is that parents enable children to approach achievement positively by aiding them in satisfying their psychological needs. Thus, in the first section, drawing from self-determination theory (Deci & Ryan, 1985, 2000), we discuss the existence of such needs and their importance to children's orientation toward achievement. In the next section, we focus on how parents facilitate children's fulfillment of their psychological needs, thereby shaping the orientation children adopt toward achievement. We delineate three modalities through which parents contribute: behavioral (i.e., parents' practices), cognitive (parents' perceptions and expectancies), and affective (i.e., the sense of relatedness between parents and children). Subsequently, drawing on dynamic process perspectives of socialization (e.g., Bronfenbrenner, 1986; Collins, Maccoby, Steinberg, Hetherington, & Bornstein, 2000), we make the case that parents' contribution to children's approach to achievement is embedded in an ongoing bidirectional socialization process between parents and children, which is influenced by social-contextual forces. In line with this perspective, in the third section, we outline how characteristics of children and the social context moderate parents' influence. In the fourth section, we discuss how characteristics of parents and children shape parents' ability to aid children in meeting their psychological needs. Given the theme of this book, in all the sections, we pay particular attention to matters of competence.

CHILDREN'S PSYCHOLOGICAL NEEDS

Because we view parents' contribution to children's approach to achievement as resting to a large extent on parents' facilitation of children's fulfillment of their psychological needs, we begin by discussing four such needs. Perhaps most centrally, as Elliot

and Dweck highlight in their introduction (Chapter 1, this volume), individuals have an innate need to experience themselves as *competent*—that is, to feel that they are capable of successfully influencing their environment (see Deci & Ryan, 1985, 2000; Elliot, McGregor, & Thrash, 2002; White, 1959). However, a core postulate of Deci and Ryan's (1985, 2000) self-determination theory is that individuals also have an essential need to feel *autonomous*. From birth, individuals need to experience their behavior as emanating from themselves, so that they feel they are acting out of their own choice (see deCharms, 1968). Another fundamental need identified by Deci and Ryan (1985, 2000) is that of feeling *related* to others. Many investigators have emphasized the importance of feeling connected to parents in particular (see Ainsworth, Blehar, Waters, & Wall, 1978; Bowlby, 1988). A fourth need that has not received much attention, but may be important, is that of experiencing the self as *purposeful*. It may be essential for individuals to feel that they are engaged in activities related to meaningful and valuable goals (see Ryff & Singer, 1998).

When these needs are satisfied, children may adopt a positive approach to achievement along three dimensions (see Eccles et al., 1998). First, children's fulfillment of their psychological needs may provide them with regulatory resources that enable them to decide whether they want to achieve and why (Deci & Ryan, 1985, 2000). For example, feelings of competence and autonomy may lead children to be motivated by intrinsic or autonomous reasons (e.g., enjoyment or personal investment) rather than extrinsic or controlled reasons (e.g., punishment or shame). Second, children's fulfillment of their psychological needs may contribute to their beliefs about their capacity for achievement (Deci & Ryan, 1985, 2000), reflected in children's perceptions of competence and efficacy, expectancies for performance, and sense of control. Although children's satisfaction of their competence need is likely to be most relevant, their satisfaction of other needs may also be important (e.g., when children feel connected to their parents, they may feel worthy, which may lead them to feel competent). Third, when children are able to meet their psychological needs, they may develop a variety of learning strategies, such as checking over their work for mistakes, that enhance achievement. Children's experience of themselves as purposeful, for instance, may motivate them to adopt useful learning strategies as they strive to meet goals they view as valuable.

THE ROLE OF PARENTS

We now turn to the question of how parents assist children in satisfying their psychological needs, thereby enhancing the orientation children adopt toward achievement. There are three distinct strands of research investigating parents' role in how children approach achievement; each reflects a different modality by which parents may facilitate children's fulfillment of their needs. First, much attention has been directed toward understanding the influence of parenting practices—that is, parents' actions or *behaviors*, such as involvement in children's schooling. Second, a fairly separate line of research has focused on parents' perceptions of children's competence. We refer to this as parents' *cognition*. Third, a growing body of research has explored the role of the *affective* modality of parenting. This research has focused on relatedness between parents and children along multiple dimensions.

Parental Behavior: Parents' Practices with Children

One of the most critical ways parents help children to approach achievement positively is by being involved in their lives. Parents' involvement is particularly beneficial if it includes structuring children's learning. As we highlight, *how* parents structure children's environment is of utmost important. For structure to be most beneficial, it needs to be autonomy-supportive rather than controlling. Moreover, parents' use of structure is enhanced if it centers on the process of learning rather than on attributes of children, such as their intelligence.

Involvement versus Lack of Involvement

The term "parent involvement" refers to parents' provision of important resources to their children (Grolnick & Slowiaczek, 1994). Such resources may be tangible—for

example, reading with children. However, they may also include supporting children in their endeavors and taking an interest in their lives (Grolnick & Slowiaczek, 1994). Parents' involvement in children's academic lives may manifest itself in a number of ways. Parents may participate in activities at children's school (e.g., take part in conferences with teachers and attend school events), work on schoolwork with children at home, or talk about children's school days with them. In addition, parents may take part in learning experiences, such as talking about current events and going to museums, with children. Parents may also convey their interest in more affective ways, such as showing excitement about children's successes and keeping abreast of what is going on at school.

For several reasons, parents' involvement in children's lives has the potential to enhance how children approach achievement. First, it may assist children in building skills that facilitate their feelings of competence. Second, parents' involvement may also establish a sense of relatedness between parents and children, because it indicates that parents are invested in children, thereby fostering closeness between parents and children (Grolnick & Slowiaczek, 1994). Third, parents' involvement may support children in experiencing themselves as purposeful, because it communicates to children that they are engaged in valuable activities.

Most of the research on parents' involvement in children's schooling has focused on its role in children's academic performance. Using a variety of methods, this research suggests that parents' involvement enhances children's studying, as well as their performance. For example, using teachers' and parents' reports of parental involvement, Epstein (1983) found that elementary school children whose parents are highly involved in their schooling (e.g., attending parent–teacher conferences) have better homework habits and complete more homework than do their counterparts whose parents are not highly involved. Such enhanced effort appears to have positive consequences for children's performance: Stevenson and Baker (1987) showed that during the elementary school and junior high school years, children of parents whom teachers report as highly involved in children's schooling receive high grades. Indeed, much research indicates that parents' interest and participation in school, as reported by children, parents, teachers, and principals, are associated with heightened achievement among elementary and junior high school children (e.g., Grolnick & Ryan, 1989; Grolnick & Slowiaczek, 1994; Herman & Ye, 1983).

It is now clear that parents' involvement is actually a precursor of children's enhanced achievement. Several longitudinal studies using a variety of methods indicate that when parents are involved in children's school lives, children's academic performance benefits over time (e.g., Keith et al., 1993; Pomerantz & Eaton, 2001; Senechal & LeFevre, 2002; Steinberg, Lamborn, Dornbusch, & Darling, 1992). For example, in a three-year study of elementary school children, Izzo, Weissberg, Kasprow, and Fendrich (1999) showed that parents' involvement in children's academic lives both at home and at school (as reported by teachers) predicts enhanced classroom behavior and school performance among children 2 years later, even when children's initial classroom behavior and school performance are taken into account. Such positive effects extend into the adolescent years: When mothers are involved in children's academic lives before children make the transition from elementary school to junior high school, children are less likely to experience a decrease in their reading grades over the transition, adjusting for their grades prior to the transition (Grolnick, Kurowski, Dunlap, & Hevey, 2000).

The positive effects of parents' involvement on children's achievement appear to be due, in part, to children's feelings of competence. Several studies have linked parents' involvement to enhanced perceptions of competence and control among children. For example, involved parents are more likely than their uninvolved counterparts to have elementary school children who perceive themselves as competent in school (Grolnick & Ryan, 1989). Analogous effects have been documented in longitudinal research examining the transition from elementary school to junior high school (Grolnick et al., 2000). In a direct test of whether the feelings of competence fostered by parents' involvement underlie children's enhanced achievement, Grolnick and Slowiaczek (1994) showed that parents'

involvement in their elementary school children's lives is linked to children's school performance through children feeling competent and in control of their school outcomes.

Structure versus Lack of Structure

Once parents are involved in children's schooling, it is important that they create an environment that supports children's competence through information, guidelines, expectations, and feedback. Grolnick and colleagues (e.g., Grolnick, 2003; Grolnick, Deci, & Ryan, 1997) have referred to this dimension of parenting as the degree to which parents provide structure. Parents' use of structure involves providing assistance in a manner that facilitates children's acquisition of skills. This notion of structure is inherent in the idea of scaffolding (see Wood, 1980). Parents' scaffolding involves varying the amount of information they provide about a task according to children's capabilities, and working within the range of difficulty at which children cannot do the task alone, but can do it with support and assistance. When parents' provision of structure is optimally challenging for children, children will naturally use it to increase their skills and to internalize regulations as part of the intrinsically motivated growth process, thereby fulfilling their need to feel competent, autonomous, and related.

In line with this analysis, parents' provision of structure appears to have positive effects on how children approach achievement. For example, Grolnick and Ryan (1989) assessed structure by asking parents of elementary school children about their use of guidelines, limit setting, and rules, as well as their consistency in following through on them. Children of parents who provided high levels of structure reported more knowledge of the sources of control of their performance in school than did their counterparts whose parents were lower on this dimension. Similarly, observational research shows that parents' heightened use of structure in terms of scaffolding and contingent shifting (i.e., decreasing assistance when children are successful, and increasing it when children have difficulty) is associated with heightened engagement and performance among children as young as 3 years of age (Hokoda & Fincham, 1995;

Pratt, Kerig, Cowan, & Cowan, 1988; Winsler, Diaz, McCarty, Atencio, & Chabay, 1999).

Autonomy Support versus Control

The extent to which parents' structuring of children's activities is autonomy-supportive versus controlling plays a key role in how children approach achievement (see Grolnick, 2003). Parental support of autonomy involves allowing children to explore their own environment, initiate their own behavior, and take an active role in solving their own problems. Parents may support children's autonomy by attending to children's work, while allowing them to work on their own; they may also encourage them to generate their own strategies for solving challenges. Controlling behavior, in contrast, involves the exertion of pressure by parents to channel children toward particular outcomes, such as doing well in school. Parents often exert pressure by regulating children's behavior with commands, directives, instructions, orders, love withdrawal, and restrictions, thereby inhibiting children from solving problems on their own.

When parents are autonomy-supportive rather than controlling they enable children to approach achievement positively. The most common explanation given for the beneficial effects of autonomy-supportive rather than controlling parenting is that it supports children's feelings of autonomy by allowing them to take initiative (e.g., Grolnick, Gurland, DeCourcey, & Jacob, 2002; Pomerantz & Ruble, 1998). However, such parenting may also aid children in feeling competent. When parents are autonomy-supportive rather than controlling, they provide children with the experience of solving challenges on their own, which may foster feelings of competence (e.g., Ng, Kenney-Benson, & Pomerantz, 2004; Nolen-Hoeksema, Wolfson, Mumme, & Guskin, 1995; Pomerantz & Ruble, 1998).

The effects of parents' support of autonomy versus controlling behavior begin early in life. Several studies indicate that, prior to the school years, children of parents who are autonomy-supportive rather than controlling are particularly engaged in mastering their environments (e.g., Kelley, Brownell, & Campbell, 2000). For example, using observational methods, Frodi, Bridges, and

Grolnick (1985) showed that 1-year-olds with autonomy-supportive mothers were more mastery-oriented during play 8 months later than were their counterparts with controlling mothers. These initial effects of parents' autonomy support and control are likely to set the stage as children enter school. Indeed, research using a variety of methods suggests that once children enter school, parents' efforts to be autonomy-supportive rather than controlling foster intrinsic motivation and mastery-oriented behavior (e.g., d'Ailly, 2003; Deci, Driver, Hotchkiss, Robbins, & Wilson, 1993; Ginsburg & Bronstein, 1993; Grolnick & Ryan, 1989; Gurland & Grolnick, 2004; Kenney-Benson & Pomerantz, in press; Nolen-Hoeksema et al., 1995).

Parents' autonomy support and control are also important to children's perceptions of competence. A number of studies employing diverse methods show a positive association between parents' autonomy-support and children's perceptions of academic competence during the elementary school years (e.g., Grolnick & Ryan, 1989; Grolnick, Ryan, & Deci, 1991; Wagner & Phillips, 1992). However, such a link is not always evident (e.g., Grolnick & Ryan, 1989; Wagner & Phillips, 1992). It is possible that this may be because children feel competent when their parents are not autonomy-supportive but are involved in their lives and provide them with structure. However, in such circumstances, children's feelings of competence may not be accompanied by feelings of autonomy (i.e., one can feel like a competent pawn). In line with this idea, children's feelings of competence are most positive when parents are high on involvement, structure, and autonomy support. For example, in longitudinal research, adolescents who saw their parents as authoritative (a combination of high involvement, high structure, and high autonomy support) viewed themselves as more competent than did adolescents who saw their parents as authoritarian (a combination of low involvement, high structure, and high control) (e.g., Steinberg, Lamborn, Darling, Mounts, & Dornbusch, 1994).

The enhanced approach to achievement fostered in children by their parents' autonomy-support appears to contribute positively to children's achievement. A number of studies, using a variety of methods, provide evidence for an association between parents' autonomy support and enhanced grades during elementary school (e.g., Grolnick & Ryan, 1989; Ng et al., 2004) and junior high school (e.g., Steinberg, Elmen, & Mounts, 1989). For example, mothers' controlling behavior, particularly appeals to authority, with their 4-year-old children is associated with children not only demonstrating poor school readiness 1 or 2 years later, but also doing poorly in school 8 years later (Hess & McDevitt, 1984). It appears that children's orientation toward achievement underlies the relation between parents' autonomy support versus control and children's achievement. For example, Steinberg and colleagues (1989) showed that adolescents' heightened psychosocial maturity (e.g., positive orientation toward school) mediates the tendency for adolescents' perceptions of their parents as autonomy-supportive to predict an increase in their grades over time (see also Grolnick et al., 1991).

Process versus Person Focus

Another important dimension of parents' practices is whether they are process- versus person-focused. Process-focused practices emphasize the importance of effort and learning (Gottfried, Fleming, & Gottfried, 1994; Kamins & Dweck, 1999; Mueller & Dweck, 1998). Such practices include, but are not limited to, parents responding to children's success by acknowledging their hard work, reacting to children's frustration by emphasizing the learning process, reminding children that what is important is not their actual grades but how hard they are trying, and helping children to develop useful strategies that will enhance their learning. In contrast, person-focused practices emphasize the importance of stable attributes, such as intelligence (Gottfried et al., 1994; Kamins & Dweck, 1999; Mueller & Dweck, 1998). Parents using person-focused practices may respond to children's success by praising their intelligence, highlighting their disappointment when children do not get good grades, linking children's worth to their performance, and pushing children to achieve a good end product, with little attention to the process of doing so.

When parents are process- rather than person-focused, they may foster feelings of competence among children. Because par-

ents' use of process-focused practices emphasizes the importance of effort and learning, children may come to view ability as something malleable, which may be improved by effort, and thus as under their control (see Kamins & Dweck, 1999; Mueller & Dweck, 1998). Such practices may also lead children to attribute their performance to hard work; consequently, failure may signal to them not that they lack competence, but that they need to exert more effort (see Kamins & Dweck, 1999; Mueller & Dweck, 1998). In contrast, when parents are person-focused, they may communicate to children that ability is a stable entity over which children have little control. Moreover, parents' use of person-focused practices may lead children to see their performance as a reflection of their ability; hence, children may attribute their failure to a lack of competence.

Dweck and colleagues have examined process- and person-focused practices by manipulating the type of feedback children are given by a previously unknown adult. For example, Mueller and Dweck (1998) gave elementary school children either process-focused praise (i.e., "You must have worked hard at these problems") or person-focused praise (e.g., "You must be smart at these problems"). Children given process-focused praise were more likely to view ability as malleable, to adopt mastery over performance goals, and to attribute their failure to effort instead of ability than were children given person-focused praise. Children given process-focused praise also persisted to a greater extent, expressed more positive affect, and performed better in the face of failure. Similarly, when preschool children imagined their teachers giving them process-oriented criticism (i.e., "Maybe you could think of another way to do it"), they were less likely than their counterparts imagining person-oriented criticism (e.g., "I am very disappointed in you") to draw negative conclusions about their abilities from their failure, to experience negative affect, and to give up (Kamins & Dweck, 1999).

The effects of parents' use of process- and person-focused practices are quite similar to the effects documented in the laboratory. Using observational methods in the context of a laboratory task with mothers and their elementary school children, Hokoda and Fincham (1995) found that mothers who reacted to children's performance-oriented behavior (e.g., concentrating on how much time is left) with process-focused practices ("That's OK; you did your best") were particularly likely to have mastery-oriented children (see also Gottfried et al., 1994). Other research, in which mothers reported daily on their responses to their elementary school children's academic successes, indicates that when mothers use person-focused rather than process-focused praise, 6 months later, children view ability as a stable entity that cannot be changed and they avoid challenging tasks (Kempner & Pomerantz, 2003). However, Kelley and colleagues (2000) found no evidence of negative effects of mothers' use of person-focused praise in the laboratory on 2-year-olds' mastery motivation. This may be because children at this young age do not yet have a mature understanding of ability and effort (see Dweck, 2002).

Parental Cognition: Parents' Thinking about Children

Although what parents do appears to play a key role in how children approach school, the way parents think also appears to be important. In this section, we focus on two central aspects of parents' thinking. The first is how parents perceive children's competence, which may also be manifest in the expectations parents have for children. Parents may be interpreters of objective information, such as grades and achievement test scores (see Eccles, 1993). As such, parents may help to determine whether children's need to feel competent is satisfied. Second, the value that parents place on children's schooling, particularly on children's academic success, may contribute to how children approach school by facilitating a sense of purposefulness, as well as competence, in children.

Perceptions of Children's Competence and Expectations for Children's Performance

Research beginning as early as the 1950s links parents' heightened expectations and aspirations for children's educational performance with heightened self-esteem, motivation, and achievement among children (e.g., Amato & Ochiltree, 1986; Marjoribanks, 1988; Rosen & D'Andrade, 1959; Winterbottom, 1958). More recently, a wealth of research provides evidence for an association between parents' perceptions of children's competence and children's own perceptions of their competence (e.g., Alexander & Entwisle, 1988; Jodl, Michael, Malanchuk, Eccles, & Sameroff, 2001). Parents' positive perceptions of children's competence, by highlighting children's competence to them, may aid children in satisfying their need to feel competent.

Given that parents' perceptions of children's competence are largely influenced by children's actual achievement, most compelling are studies that take into account children's achievement. For example, Parsons (now Eccles), Adler, and Kaczala (1982) found that children of parents who expect them to do well at math, and view math as easy for them, perceive their competence in math positively, have high expectations for their future performance in math, and see math as easy (see also Jodl et al., 2001). Notably, in this study, parents' perceptions were stronger predictors of children's perceptions than was children's past performance. In fact, in longitudinal research, Frome and Eccles (1998) demonstrated that the associations over time between children's grades in English and math, and their perceptions of competence and difficulty in these areas, are accounted for by parents' perceptions of children's competence in these areas (see also Phillips, 1987). It is noteworthy that children's perceptions of competence are predicted more strongly by parents' perceptions than by teachers' perceptions (Entwisle, 1997; Wigfield, Eccles, Yoon, & Harold, 1997). Parents' perceptions of children's competence also play a role in children's subsequent achievement. For example, one longitudinal study showed that parents' perceptions of children's competence predicted children's achievement over 9 months, even after taking into account children's achievement at the beginning of the study (Halle, Kurtz-Costes, & Mahoney, 1997).

The valence of parents' perceptions of children's competence is clearly significant. However, the accuracy of parents' perceptions appears to be influential as well, particularly as children get older. When parents are accurate in their perceptions of children's competence, they may facilitate the fulfillment of the need to feel competent even among children who do poorly in school, because they are able to provide scaffolding attuned to children's skills. Although parents generally overestimate children's abilities (Pezdek, Berry, & Renno, 2002), the more accurate parents' views of children's academic competence, the better children perform in school (Miller, Manhal, & Mee, 1991). Accuracy becomes a more important factor as children's achievement trajectories become more established: The association between the congruence of parents and teachers' views of children's competence and children's achievement increases over the elementary school years (Peet, Powell, & O'Donnel, 1997).

Research is just beginning to address the mechanisms through which parents' perceptions of children's competence exert their influence on children. There is some indication that such perceptions are associated with parents' practices. For example, parents with high expectations are often very involved in children's schooling (Juang & Silbereisen, 2002). Moreover, parents' perceptions of children's competence may affect the conversations parents and children have about children's achievement (Flannagan, 1997). However, most investigators conclude that there are more subtle and indirect ways that parents' messages find their way into children's belief systems (see Jodl et al., 2001). For example, it is possible that parents' perceptions of children's competence underlie the types of attributions parents make for children's performance. In a laboratory study conducted by Hokoda and Fincham (1995), such attributions were linked to how children respond to failure. These investigators found that when mothers attribute children's failures to lack of ability, children are helpless in coping with failure.

Parents' Values

The extent to which parents value children's schooling also appears to contribute to how children approach school. When parents place importance on children's education, they convey that doing well in school is a valuable endeavor and provide children with a sense of purpose. The few studies examining the extent to which parents value children's schooling suggest that parents who

see children's academic success as important may enhance how children approach school. When parents place heightened importance on their elementary school and junior high school children's schooling, children are more confident about their academic competencies (e.g., Bandura, Barbaranelli, Caprara, & Pastorelli, 1996; Eccles, 1983). However, work by McGrath and Repetti (2000) suggests that these effects may depend on the sex of the parent and child. McGrath and Repetti found that girls, but not boys, felt particularly competent (independent of actual performance) when fathers valued academic success. The value that mothers placed on children's academic success was unrelated to how competent either girls or boys felt. McGrath and Repetti speculate that, given the tendency in our culture to expect less from girls, girls particularly benefit when their fathers stress their academic success. The question of why fathers' value of academic success plays a larger role than that of mothers needs further attention.

Parental Affect: Relatedness between Parents and Children

Because the relationships between parents and children are often the most central ones in children's lives, even in adolescence, when increasing time is spent with peers (see Larson, Richards, Moneta, Holmbeck, & Duckett, 1996; Offer & Offer, 1975), feeling connected to parents is pivotal to children's development (e.g., Allen, Marsh, McFarland, McElhaney, & Land, 2002; Ryan, Stiller, & Lynch, 1994; Sroufe, Fox, & Pancake, 1983). When children feel connected to their parents, they may fulfill their need for not only relatedness but also competence, autonomy, and purposefulness. In this section, we focus on three distinct, albeit related, forms of relatedness between parents and children that appear to influence how children approach achievement: feelings of attachment and closeness between children and their parents, children's sense of obligation to their families, and children's inclusion of their relationships with their parents in their views of themselves (i.e., the extent to which children see their relationships with their parents as an important part of who they are).

Attachment and Closeness

The quality of children's attachment to their parents is a basic form of relatedness that plays a role very early in children's lives in setting the stage for how they approach achievement. Ainsworth et al. (1978) and Bowlby (1988) argue that the quality of children's attachment to parents during infancy contributes to children's constructive exploration of their environment. According to these investigators, children with secure attachments to their parents develop positive internal representations of themselves and others that allow them to explore their environment in a confident, autonomous manner, in part, because they do not have to worry over their relationships with their parents. In essence, fulfilling children's need for relatedness enables children's needs for competence and autonomy to be met. In contrast, children with insecure attachments to their parents develop negative representations of themselves and others that inhibit them from exploring their environment. This may be particularly true for children with insecure attachments, who are anxious about the availability and consistency of their parents.

The role of children's attachment to their parents in their approach to achievement begins early in life. Several studies using observational methods indicate that securely attached infants are more engaged with their environment than are insecurely attached infants, particularly those with preoccupied or disorganized attachment relationships. Children securely attached to their mothers during the second year of life are more enthusiastic, persistent, and competent in the context of problem-solving tasks administered 6–8 months later than are insecurely attached children (Frodi et al., 1985; Matas, Arend, & Sroufe, 1978). In addition, children categorized as securely attached at 18 months are more curious by 4–5 years of age than are their insecurely attached counterparts categorized as preoccupied (Arend, Gove, & Sroufe, 1979).

These effects appear to extend into the elementary school years. Moss and St. Laurent (2001) showed that securely attached young elementary school children were more likely than their insecurely attached counterparts to report taking a mastery-oriented approach to school 2 years later. Moreover, research using a variety of methods indicates that children who are securely attached to their mothers during the early elementary school years are more likely than their insecurely attached counterparts to be engaged in school (e.g., participate in classroom discussions), to have advanced cognitive skills, and to receive high grades not only later in elementary school but also in adolescence (e.g., Jacobsen & Hofman, 1997; Jacobsen et al., 1994). Such effects are accounted for, in part, by securely attached children's heightened feelings of competence (Jacobsen et al., 1994).

As children progress through later life, the quality of their attachment to their parents may be reflected in their feelings of closeness to them. These feelings have effects quite similar to children's earlier attachment. For example, Furrer and Skinner (2003) found that elementary school children's feelings of closeness to their parents predicted heightened engagement in school, as assessed by children's and teachers' reports, over the course of the academic year. During the adolescent years, children who report feeling close to their parents along several dimensions report being both engaged in school and autonomously motivated; they also feel they are in control of their school outcomes and use self-regulated learning strategies (Learner & Kruger, 1997; Ryan et al., 1994). Moreover, in line with the idea that children's preoccupation with their relationships with their parents disrupts how they approach achievement, research using college students' reports of their parents' practices indicates that students' perceptions of their mothers as using love withdrawal is associated with heightened avoidance of failure in school among students (Elliot & Thrash, 2004).

Family Obligation

Other forms of relatedness between parents and children may enhance how children approach achievement by heightening their feelings of purposefulness. Fuligni and colleagues (e.g., Fuligni, 2001; Fuligni, Tseng, & Lam, 1999) have focused on the extent to which children feel obligated to their family. Children's obligation to their family may take three interrelated forms. First, children may feel obligated to provide assistance with household tasks and spend time with their family. Second, children may place importance on respecting and following the wishes of other family members, particularly those of their parents. Third, children may feel obligated to provide support for their families in the future. Although children of Asian and Latino descent are more likely to feel obligated to their family than are children of European descent, even children of European descent report such feelings (Fuligni et al., 1999). When children feel obligated to their family along any of these dimensions, they may feel that it is their duty to achieve the competencies their parents value, giving them a sense of purpose in life (see Fuligni, Alvarez, Bachman, & Ruble, in press). As a consequence, these children may be highly committed to achieving in the academic area—an area on which parents often place much importance.

In line with this idea, adolescents with a heightened sense of obligation to their family report spending much time studying and have very high educational aspirations and expectations (Fuligni et al., 1999). They also place more value on doing well in school than their counterparts who do not feel obligated to their family (Fuligni, 2001). However, although many adolescents with a strong sense of family obligation are more persistent in pursuing higher education than are their counterparts without such a sense of obligation (Fuligni, Yip, & Tseng, 2002), these adolescents do not necessarily earn better grades in school (Fuligni et al., 1999). This may be because, as early as elementary school, children who feel obligated to their family are both intrinsically and extrinsically motivated to do well in school (Fuligni et al., in press); although their intrinsic motivation may enhance their effort and even their emotional well-being, their extrinsic motivation may interfere with their concentration, leading to less productive effort.

Relationships with Parents as Self-Defining

A wealth of theory and research has been concerned with understanding interdependent conceptions of the self, in which the self is viewed as part of an encompassing network of social relationships (for a review, see Markus & Kitayama, 1991). For individuals with interdependent representations of themselves, the self becomes particularly meaningful when it is cast in relation to others. Such individuals define themselves in terms of their relationships with others. Although individuals from Eastern cultures, such as China, are more likely than those from Western cultures, such as the United States, to hold interdependent self-construals, there is considerable variation within cultures in terms of how individuals view themselves (e.g., Cross & Madson, 1997).

Drawing from the theory and research on interdependent self-construals, Wang and Pomerantz (2004) examined the extent to which children define themselves in terms of their relationships with their *parents*. These investigators reasoned that children's inclusion of their relationships with their parents in their views of themselves heightens their motivation to maintain their relationships with their parents, which may increase children's responsiveness to their parents' socialization attempts. Children holding parent-oriented interdependent self-construals may attempt to put themselves in their parents' place, taking on the thoughts and feelings of their parents (see Markus & Kitayama, 1991). As a consequence, such children may be highly invested in meeting the goals set for them by their parents, eventually internalizing them, which may heighten their feelings of autonomy. Because many parents place value on children's achievement in the academic area, children's inclusion of their relationships with their parents in their views of themselves may enhance how they approach achievement in this area, because it allows them to experience themselves as purposeful in the school context.

Consistent with this idea, Wang and Pomerantz (2004) found that children who reported including their relationships with their parents in their views of themselves were particularly likely to report being invested in their schoolwork. Moreover, these children provided autonomous reasons for doing their schoolwork. This heightened investment and autonomous motivation accounted for the tendency of children including their relationships with their parents in their self-construals to be highly engaged in their schoolwork on a daily basis. Interestingly, although this engagement was associated with heightened emotional well-being, it was not associated with better grades in school. This may be because, much like children feeling obligated to their family, children including their relationships with their parents in their views of themselves were motivated by controlled reasons, in addition to autonomous ones, because of a concern with pleasing their parents.

Conclusions

There is substantial evidence that parents influence how children approach achievement. It appears that this takes place through three distinct, albeit related, modalities: behavioral, cognitive, and affective. The effects of each of these modalities have generally been identified in distinct lines of research. Thus, little is known about how they jointly contribute to the approach to achievement that children adopt. There are several possibilities.

The first is an interactive effect, in which the effects of one modality depend on another. In this vein, Darling and Steinberg (1993) argued that parents' general style of interacting with children creates a climate that conveys to children their parents' attitudes toward them. Consistent with this perspective, Steinberg and colleagues (1992) demonstrated that parental involvement is more beneficial for children's achievement when administered by authoritative than by authoritarian parents. In a similar vein, mothers' use of structure on a daily basis is most likely to have positive effects on how children respond to academic failure when mothers accompany it with autonomy support (Pomerantz & Ruble, 1998). Other modalities of parenting may also contribute to such a climate. For example, parents' establishment of feelings of relatedness between children and themselves may be an important aspect of climate.

The second possibility is that different modalities of parenting are important for different children. Along these lines, mothers' use of gentle discipline is particularly likely to enhance temperamentally fearful children's internalization of mothers' standards, presumably because it takes advantage of the optimal level of arousal among these children (e.g., Kochanska, 1991). Although this practice is ineffective with children who are not temperamentally fearful, it is not that mothers are unable to influence these children. Rather, the affective modality is particularly important for children who are not temperamentally fearful: These children internalize their mothers' standards when they have a secure attachment with them, regardless of their mothers' use of gentle discipline. Similar trends may be evident for the role of the different parenting modalities in how children approach achievement.

A third possibility is that the three modalities exert their effects through one another. As we noted earlier, parents' cognition may influence their behavior (see Eccles, 1993). For example, parents who perceive their children as lacking competence may be particularly controlling (see Pomerantz & Eaton, 2001). It is also possible that certain aspects of parents' behavior create a sense of relatedness between parents and children. For example, parents who are involved and autonomy-supportive may establish a secure attachment with children. Once such an attachment is established, it may elicit more positive practices from parents as they engage in a cycle of mutual responsiveness with children (see Kochanska, 1997).

MODERATORS OF THE ROLE OF PARENTS

It is clear that parents contribute to how children approach achievement. However, parents' socialization of children is not a unidirectional process by which parents simply shape children. Indeed, as suggested by dynamic perspectives of socialization (e.g., Bronfenbrenner, 1986; Collins et al., 2000), children's characteristics, as well as social-contextual forces, may influence parents' facilitation of children's fulfillment of their needs. In this section, we focus on the moderators of parents' contribution to how children approach achievement. First, we discuss how children's characteristics influence the effects that parents have on children's approach to achievement. In this context, we focus on the influence of children's need to feel competent. Second, we consider social context as a moderator. Here, attention is directed to the culture in which children and parents reside.

Child Characteristics:
The Need to Feel Competent

Across a number of areas of development, investigators have adopted parent × child models of socialization, in which the effects of parents' practices depend on children's characteristics (e.g., Bates, Pettit, Dodge, & Ridge, 1998; Kochanska, 1993). Research is beginning to suggest that such models are important to understanding parents' role in how children approach achievement. Because parents may contribute to children's orientation toward achievement by aiding children in satisfying their needs to feel competent, autonomous, related, and purposeful, the extent to which children have already fulfilled these needs may moderate parents' contribution. Parents' influence may be strongest among children who do not experience themselves as competent, autonomous, related, or purposeful. In line with the theme of this book, we focus on the moderating role of children's feelings of competence.

As a consequence of a variety of influences (e.g., peer socialization, achievement, and temperament), children come to their interactions with their parents with established perceptions of their competence. Children who experience themselves as incompetent may benefit more than do children who experience themselves as competent when their parents use practices, such as autonomy support, that have the potential to promote feelings of competence. However, children experiencing themselves as lacking competence may be particularly vulnerable when their parents use practices, such as control, that have the potential to detract from feelings of competence. Children with negative perceptions of their competence may be more easily frustrated than are their counterparts with positive perceptions, which may lead them to have more difficulty achieving competence. Parents may be particularly important in providing such children with the skills and opportunities that reduce their frustration, thereby allowing them to experience themselves as competent and, ultimately, to be successful. In essence, because children with negative perceptions of their competence are in greater need than are children with positive perceptions of the competence-related resources that parents can provide, they are more sensitive to their parents' practices bearing on their competence.

The findings of several longitudinal studies using a variety of methods are consistent with this proposal. Low-achieving children are more likely than high-achieving children to benefit when their mothers use autonomy support (Ng et al., 2004). Low-achieving children, for instance, experience greater increments over time in their subsequent performance than do high-achieving children, when their mothers provide support by allowing them to work on their own in the context of a challenging task, and when their mothers respond to their failures with discussion. A similar pattern exists for parents' use of process-focused practices (Pomerantz, Ng, & Wang, 2004b): When mothers are process-oriented in assisting their children with homework, children with negative perceptions of their academic competence are more likely than children with positive perceptions to benefit in terms of their subsequent perceptions of competence, mastery orientation, and positive emotional functioning. Unfortunately, low-achieving children are more likely than high-achieving children to suffer when their mothers use control (Ng et al., 2004; Pomerantz, 2001). For example, when mothers are controlling in the context of assisting children with a challenging task, over time, low-achieving children become less engaged in the task than do high-achieving children. Moreover, when mothers respond to children's failures in a controlling manner, that is, with punishment or reprimands, the performance of low-achieving children suffers more than that of high-achieving children.

Social-Contextual Characteristics:
Cultural Influences

As Bronfrenbrenner (1986) has highlighted, interactions between parents and children take place in a larger social context that not only influences the course these interactions take but also their impact on children. Because of the tendency for children of Asian descent living both inside and outside the United States, to outperform academically their European American counterparts, there has been much attention devoted to understanding how the role of parents in children's academic achievement differs between the two cultures. Although a key focus has been on understanding similarities and differences in the types of practices used by parents' in the two cultures (e.g., C. Chen & Stevenson, 1989), there has been an increasing focus on how the effects on children of parents' use of the *same* practices differ across the two cultures. Children from different cultures may experience the same practices differently, so that the same practices have different functional significance for children from different cultures.

Children of Asian and European cultural heritage may experience their parents' practices differently, in part, because of differences in their views of themselves: Children of Asian descent may include their relationships with others, including their parents, in their views of themselves more than do children of European descent. As a consequence, children from Asian cultures may often take on their parents' goals as their own. This may influence their experience of parents' practices. Children from Asia may not see their parents' practices (e.g., making unilateral decisions for children) as controlling, as they are often seen by children from the United States, which allows them to experience the pursuit of their parents' goals as an autonomous process (see Iyengar & Lepper, 1999). Findings from research manipulating parents' use of control and examining the effects on children's motivation are consistent with this perspective: Iyengar and Lepper (1999) either allowed elementary school children to choose a task on which to work or told them that their mother had chosen one for them. European American children showed more interest in the task that they themselves chose over the one that they were told was chosen for them by their mothers. However, Asian American children preferred the task that they were told was chosen for them by their mothers.

Research comparing the effects of parents' actual use of control in Asia and the United States has generally focused on children's achievement rather than on how they approach achievement. In such research, authoritative parenting tends to have more positive effects than does authoritarian parenting on children of Asian descent (e.g., X. Chen, Dong, & Zhou, 1997), but these effects are often, albeit not always, weaker than they are for children of European descent (e.g., Dornbusch, Ritter, Leiderman, Roberts, & Fraleigh, 1987; Steinberg et al., 1994). Taken together, the findings suggest that the social context in which children reside influences their interpretation of their parents' practices, thereby underscoring the importance of children's understanding of the functional significance of parents' practices.

Conclusions

In accordance with dynamic perspectives of socialization, research suggests that both the characteristics children bring to their interactions with their parents, and the social context in which these interactions take place, influence the role of parents in children's approach to achievement. In terms of children's characteristics, children's experience of themselves as lacking competence heightens the effects of parents' practices that bear on children's competence. It will be key for future research to identify other characteristics of children that moderate the role of parents in how children approach achievement. As suggested earlier, one fruitful line of inquiry may focus on children's experience of themselves as autonomous, related, and purposeful. Also of import is to examine the moderating role of children's gender. Several lines of research suggest that girls are more responsiveness to parents' socialization attempts than are boys (for a review, see Pomerantz, Ng, & Wang, 2004a). As a consequence, parents may play a larger role in how girls approach achievement.

The social context in which children and parents reside also moderates the role of parents in how children approach achievement. We focused on differences in the effects of parenting in Asia and the United States. The evidence to date suggests that parents' practices differentially influence how children approach achievement in the two cultures. Children in these cultures may interpret the same practices differently. As a consequence, parental practices that by American standards might be seen as controlling may not have the same negative effects among Asian children. It will be important for future research to investigate systematically the role of cultural context by examining cultures other than Asia and the United States (e.g., García Coll et al., 2003). It is also critical to examine the moderating role of social-contextual forces within cultures. Research suggesting that the optimal level of parents' structure for children depends on the type of neighborhood in which they live (e.g., Baldwin, Baldwin, & Cole, 1990; Coley & Hoffman, 1996) represents a major stride in this direction.

ANTECEDENTS OF PARENTS' BEHAVIOR, COGNITION, AND AFFECT

Drawing again from dynamic perspectives of socialization, we now turn to the question of what shapes parents' abilities to aid children in satisfying their needs. Although a number of factors have been implicated as influencing parenting (see Belsky, 1984), we focus on those related to competence issues. First, we discuss how characteristics of parents themselves influence their ability to facilitate children's need fulfillment. In this context, we concentrate on the extent to which parents see their worth as hinging on children's achievement. Second, attention is directed to how characteristics of children influence parents' practices. Here, we focus on children's achievement.

Parental Characteristics: Ego Involvement in Children's Achievement

Much research indicates that when parents experience external pressure, such as economic hardship and stressful life events, their parenting suffers (e.g., Dodge, Petit, & Bates, 1994; Grolnick, Weiss, McKenzie, & Wrightman, 1996). However, parents may also experience pressure from within that disrupts their parenting. When individuals are ego-involved in their own performance, their feelings of worth are contingent upon their performance (Crocker & Wolfe, 2001; Nicholls, 1984; Sherif & Cantril, 1947). In other words, they feel good about themselves if they perform well, but bad about themselves if they perform poorly. Al-

though Crocker and Wolfe (2001) have suggested that such ego involvement serves an important regulatory function (see also Pomerantz, Saxon, & Oishi, 2000), it may cause individuals to feel pressured. In line with this idea, work by Ryan (1982) finds that ego involvement is negatively associated with intrinsic motivation. Recent work has expanded the notion of ego involvement in one's own performance to ego involvement in the performance of another. Grolnick and colleagues (2002) reasoned that when parents see children's performance as having ramifications for their own worth, they transfer their experience of pressure onto children, leading them to use controlling rather than autonomy-supportive practices with children.

To test this idea, mothers and their elementary school children worked on homework-like tasks under either an ego-involving, high-pressure condition, in which mothers were led to believe they were responsible for children meeting particular performance standards, or a low-pressure condition deempahsizing children's performance and mothers' responsibility. Mothers under high pressure were more controlling with children than those under low pressure, with mothers who endorsed the use of control being particularly vulnerable to the effects of pressure. Eaton and Pomerantz (2004) examined naturally occurring differences among parents in the extent to which they feel their worth is contingent on children's performance. Similar to the experimental study conducted by Grolnick and colleagues (2002), both mothers and fathers who felt that their worth was contingent on children's performance were more likely to be controlling with children in college, even when children were doing well in school.

Child Characteristics: Achievement

A number of investigators have argued that parenting is determined in part by children's characteristics (e.g., Bell, 1968; Scarr, 1992). In this vein, there is evidence that parents are more likely to become involved in their children's school lives, particularly in terms of assisting them with their homework, when children are having difficulty in school. Several concurrent investigations reveal that parents are more likely to assist children with homework when children are doing poorly in school (e.g., C. Chen & Stevenson, 1989). Although it is possible that this association reflects the negative effects of parents' assistance, research conducted by Pomerantz and Eaton (2001) indicates that this is unlikely. In this research, children's poor performance in school predicted mothers' heightened assistance with homework 6 months later. Mothers apparently increased their assistance with low-achieving children, because they were worried over such children's performance, and they picked up on their children's cues indicating that they felt uncertain about how to do well in school. Indeed, mothers are particularly likely to assist children with homework on the days that they perceive children as helpless in the context of doing their homework (Pomerantz, Wang, & Ng, in press). Importantly, once children's initial achievement is taken into account, mothers' assistance with homework predicts an increase in children's achievement over time (Pomerantz & Eaton, 2001).

Conclusions

The question of what shapes parents' abilities to facilitate children's fulfillment of their needs is important in determining which parents may benefit from help in assisting children to approach achievement positively. However, this question is also critical to understanding the dynamic nature of the process by which parents contribute to children's orientation toward achievement. It is clear that parents play a major role, but it is also clear that children influence this role. The orientation children adopt toward achievement emerges from an ongoing bidirectional socialization process between parents and children. We focused here on how the pressure that parents themselves experience undermines their ability to aid children in satisfying their needs. Other characteristics of parents are also important. For example, parents' personalities (e.g., Clark, Kochanska, & Ready, 2000), feelings of efficacy (e.g., Grolnick, Benjet, Kurowski, & Apostoleris, 1997; Hoover-Dempsey, Bassler, & Brissie, 1992), and educational attainment (Stevenson & Newman, 1986) all appear to influence parenting.

Children are also important. Children's achievement in school appears to influence parents' practices. Other characteristics of children have also been documented as important—for example, children's gender (e.g., Frome & Eccles, 1998; Pomerantz & Ruble, 1998). It is also of note that parents and children interact in a social context that influences what parents do. For example, research indicates that the culture in which parents and children reside determines not only how children respond to their parents' practices but also how parents parent (e.g., C. Chen & Stevenson, 1989). An important direction for future research will be to integrate these multiple influences in understanding the process by which parents contribute to how children approach the achievement of competence.

CONCLUSIONS

Research conducted over the last two decades has established that parents play a central role in how children approach achievement. Critical aspects of parents' behavior, cognition, and affect have been implicated as influential. As a whole, parents have the potential to facilitate children's fulfillment of their psychological needs through multiple modalities, thereby providing children with the resources necessary to approach achievement positively. As investigators continue to study parents' contribution to children's approach to achievement, it will be important to draw on dynamic perspectives of socialization. The initial research conducted from this perspective already reveals that the role of parents is embedded in an ongoing, bidirectional socialization process between parents and children, which is influenced by social-contextual forces.

ACKNOWLEDGMENTS

We are grateful for the constructive feedback on earlier drafts of this chapter provided by Florrie Ng, Qian Wang, and the editors. Writing of this chapter was supported by National Institute of Mental Health and Office of Research on Women's Health (No. R01 MH57505) grants to Eva M. Pomerantz.

REFERENCES

Ainsworth, M. D. S., Blehar, M. C., Waters, E., & Wall, S. (1978). *Patterns of attachment: A psychological study of the strange situation.* Hillsdale, NJ: Erlbaum.

Alexander, K. L., & Entwisle, D. R. (1988). Achievement in the first two years of school: Patterns and processes. *Monographs of the Society for Research on Child Development, 53*(2, Serial No. 218).

Allen, J. P., Marsh, P., McFarland, C., McElhaney, K. B., & Land, D. J. (2002). Attachment and autonomy as predictors of the development of social skills and delinquency during midadolescence. *Journal of Consulting and Clincial Psychology, 70,* 56–66.

Amato, P. R., & Ochiltree, G. (1986). Family resources and the development of child competence. *Journal of Marriage and the Family, 48,* 47–56.

Arend, R., Gove, F., & Sroufe, A. (1979). Continuity of individual adaptation from infancy to kindergarten: A predictive study of ego-resiliency and curiousity in preschoolers. *Child Development, 50,* 950–959.

Baldwin, A. L., Baldwin, C., & Cole, R. E. (1990). Stress-resistant families and stress-resistant children. In J. E. Rolf, A. S. Masten, D. Cicchetti, K. H. Nuechterlein, & S. Weintraub (Eds.), *Risk and protective factors in the development of psychopathology* (pp. 257–280). New York: Cambridge University Press.

Bandura, A., Barbaranelli, C., Caprara, G. V., & Pastorelli, C. (1996). Multi-faceted impact of self-efficacy beliefs on academic functioning. *Child Development, 67,* 1206–1222.

Bates, J. E., Pettit, G. S., Dodge, K. A., & Ridge, B. (1998). Interaction of temperamental resistance to control and restrictive parenting in the development of externalizing behavior. *Developmental Psychology, 34,* 982–995.

Bell, R. Q. (1968). A reinterpretation of the direction of effects in studies of socialization. *Psychological Review, 75,* 81–95.

Belsky, J. (1984). The determinants of parenting: A process model. *Child Development, 55,* 83–96.

Bowlby, J. (1988). *A secure base: Parent–child attachment and healthy human development.* New York: Basic Books.

Bronfenbrenner, U. (1986). Ecology of the family as a context for human development: Research perspectives. *Developmental Psychology, 22,* 723–742.

Chen, C., & Stevenson, H. W. (1989). Homework: A cross-cultural examination. *Child Development, 60,* 551–561.

Chen, X., Dong, Q., & Zhou, H. (1997). Authoritative and authoritarian parenting practices and social and school performance in Chinese children. *International Journal of Behavioral Development, 5,* 81–94.

Clark, L. A., Kochanska, G., & Ready, R. (2000). Mothers' personality and its interaction with child temperament as predictors of parenting behavior.

Journal of Personality and Social Psychology, 79, 274–285.

Coley, R. L., & Hoffman, L. W. (1996). Relations of parental supervision and monitoring to children's functioning in various contexts: Moderating effects of families and neighborhoods. *Journal of Applied Developmental Psychology, 17,* 51–68.

Collins, W. A., Maccoby, E. E., Steinberg, L., Hetherington, E. M., & Bornstein, M. (2000). Contemporary research on parenting: The case for nature and nurture. *American Psychologist, 55,* 218–232.

Crocker, J., & Wolfe, C. T. (2001). Contingencies of self-worth. *Psychological Review, 108,* 593–623.

Cross, S. E., & Madson, L. (1997). Models of the self: Self-construals and gender. *Psychological Bulletin, 122,* 5–37.

d'Ailly, H. (2003). Children's autonomy and perceived control on learning: A model of motivation and achievement in Taiwan. *Journal of Educational Psychology, 95,* 84–96.

Darling, N., & Steinberg, L. (1993). Parenting style as context: An integrative model. *Psychological Bulletin, 113,* 487–496.

deCharms, R. (1968). *Personal causation: The internal affective determinants of behavior.* New York: Academic Press.

Deci, E. L., Driver, R. E., Hotchkiss, L., Robbins, R. J., & Wilson, I. M. (1993). The relation of mothers' controlling vocalizations to children's intrinsic motivation. *Journal of Experimental Child Psychology, 55,* 151–162.

Deci, E. L., & Ryan, R. M. (1985). *Intrinsic motivation and self-determination in human behavior.* New York: Plenum Press.

Deci, E. L., & Ryan, R. M. (2000). The "what" and "why" of goal pursuits: Human needs and the self-determination of behavior. *Psychological Inquiry, 11,* 227–268.

Dodge, K. A., Petit, G. S., & Bates, J. E. (1994). Socialization mediators of the relation between socioeconomic status and child conduct problems. *Child Development, 65,* 649–665.

Dornbusch, S., Ritter, P., Leiderman, P., Roberts, D., & Fraleigh, M. (1987). The relation of parenting style to adolescent school performance. *Child Development, 58,* 1244–1257.

Dweck, C. S. (2002). The development of ability conceptions. In A. Wigfield & J. S. Eccles (Eds.), *Development of achievement motivation* (pp. 57–88). San Diego: Academic Press.

Eaton, M. M., & Pomerantz, E. M. (2004). *When parents feel their self-worth is contingent on their children's performance: Implications for parents' use of control.* Unpublished manuscript.

Eccles, J. S. (1983). Expectancies, values and academic behaviors. In J. T. Spence (Ed.), *Achievement and achievement motives* (pp. 75–146). San Francisco: Freeman.

Eccles, J. S. (1993). School and family effects on the ontogeny of children's interests, self-perceptions, and activity choices. In R. Dienstbier & J. Jacobs (Eds.), *Developmental perspectives on motivation* (Vol. 40, pp. 145–208). Lincoln: University of Nebraska Press.

Eccles, J. S., Wigfield, A., & Schiefele, U. (1998). Motivation to succeed. In N. Eisenberg (Ed.), *Handbook of child psychology: Vol. 3. Social, emotional, and personality development* (5th ed., pp. 1017–1095). New York: Wiley.

Elliot, A. J., McGregor, H. A., & Thrash, T. M. (2002). The need for competence. In E. L. Deci & R. M. Ryan (Eds.), *Handbook of self-determination research*. Rochester, NY: University of Rochester Press.

Elliot, A. J., & Thrash, T. M. (2004). The intergenerational transmission of fear of failure. *Personality and Social Psychology Bulletin, 30,* 957–971.

Entwisle, D. R. (1997). *Children, schools, and inequality*. Boulder, CO: Westview Press.

Epstein, J. L. (1983). Longitudinal effects of family–school–person interactions on student outcomes. In A. Kerckhoff (Ed.), *Research in sociology of education and socialization* (Vol. 4, pp. 101–128). Greenwich, CT: JAI Press.

Flannagan, D. (1997). Associations between the school-related beliefs of Mexican-American and Anglo-American mothers and children. *Journal of Applied Developmental Psychology, 18,* 603–617.

Frodi, A., Bridges, L., & Grolnick, W. S. (1985). Correlates of mastery-related behavior: A short-term longitudinal study of infants in their second year. *Child Development, 56,* 1291–1298.

Frome, P. M., & Eccles, J. S. (1998). Parents' influence on children's achievement-related perceptions. *Journal of Personality and Social Psychology, 74,* 435–452.

Fuligni, A. J. (2001). Family obligation and the academic motivation of adolescents from Asian, Latin, and European American backgrounds. In A. J. Fuligni (Ed.), *Family obligation and assistance during adolescence: Contextual variations and developmental implications* (pp. 61–75). San Francisco: Jossey-Bass.

Fuligni, A. J., Alvarez, J., Bachman, M., & Ruble, D. N. (in press). Family obligation and the academic motivation of young children from immigrant families. In C. R. Cooper, C. Garcia Coll, T. Bartko, H. Davis, & C. Chatman (Eds.), *Hills of gold: Rethinking diversity and contexts as resources for children's developmental pathways*. Mahwah, NJ: Erlbaum.

Fuligni, A. J., Tseng, V., & Lam, M. (1999). Attitudes toward family obligation among American adolescents with Asian, Latin American, and European American backgrounds. *Child Development, 70,* 1030–1044.

Fuligni, A. J., Yip, T., & Tseng, V. (2002). The impact of family obligation on the daily activities and psychological well-being of Chinese American adolescents. *Child Development, 73,* 302–314.

Furrer, C., & Skinner, E. (2003). Sense of relatedness as a factor in children's academic engagement and performance. *Journal of Educational Psychology, 95,* 148–162.

García Coll, C., Akiba, D., Palacios, N., Bailey, B., Silver, R., DiMartino, L., et al. (2003). Parental involvement in children's education: Lessons from three immigrant groups. *Parenting: Science and Practice, 2,* 303–324.

Ginsburg, G. S., & Bronstein, P. (1993). Family factors related to children's intrinsic/extrinsic motivational orientation and academic performance. *Child Development, 64,* 1461–1474.

Gottfried, A. E., Fleming, J. S., & Gottfried, A. W. (1994). Role of parental motivational practices in children's academic intrinsic motivation and achievement. *Journal of Educational Psychology, 86,* 104–113.

Grolnick, W. S. (2003). *The psychology of parental control: How well-meant parenting backfires*. Hillside, NJ: Erlbaum.

Grolnick, W. S., Benjet, C., Kurowski, C. O., & Apostoleris, N. H. (1997). Predictors of parent involvement in children's schooling. *Journal of Educational Psychology, 89,* 538–548.

Grolnick, W. S., Deci, E. L., & Ryan, R. M. (1997). Internalization within the family: The self-determination theory perspective. In J. Grusec & L. Kuczynski (Eds.), *Parenting and children's internalization of values: A handbook of contemporary theory* (pp. 135–161). New York: Wiley.

Grolnick, W. S., Gurland, S. T., DeCourcey, W., & Jacob, K. (2002). Antecedents and consequences of mothers' autonomy support: An experimental investigation. *Developmental Psychology, 38,* 143–154.

Grolnick, W. S., Kurowski, C. O., Dunlap, K. G., & Hevey, C. (2000). Parental resources and the transition to junior high. *Journal of Research on Adolescence, 10,* 465–488.

Grolnick, W. S., & Ryan, R. M. (1989). Parent styles associated with children's self-regulation and competence in school. *Journal of Educational Psychology, 81,* 143–154.

Grolnick, W. S., Ryan, R. M., & Deci, E. L. (1991). Inner resources for school achievement: Motivational mediators of children's perceptions of their parents. *Journal of Educational Psychology, 83,* 508–517.

Grolnick, W. S., & Slowiaczek, M. L. (1994). Parents' involvement in children's schooling: A multidimensional conceptualization and motivational model. *Child Development, 64,* 237–252.

Grolnick, W. S., Weiss, L., McKenzie, L., & Wrightman, J. (1996). Contextual, cognitive, and adolescent factors associated with parenting in adolescence. *Journal of Youth and Adolescence, 25,* 33–54.

Gurland, S. T., & Grolnick, W. S. (2004). *Perceived threat, parental control, and children's achievement orientations*. Manuscript submitted for publication.

Halle, T. G., Kurtz-Costes, B., & Mahoney, J. L. (1997). Family influences on school achievement in low-income African-American children. *Journal of Educational Psychology, 89,* 527–537.

Herman, J. L., & Ye, J. P. (1983). Some effects of parent involvement in schools. *Urban Review, 15,* 11–17.

Hess, R. D., & McDevitt, T. M. (1984). Some cognitive consequences of maternal intervention: A longitudinal study. *Child Development, 55,* 2017–2030.

Hokoda, A., & Fincham, F. D. (1995). Origins of children's helpless and mastery achievement patterns in the family. *Journal of Educational Psychology, 87,* 375–385.

Hoover-Dempsey, K. V., Bassler, O. C., & Brissie, J. S. (1992). Explorations in parent–school relations. *Journal of Educational Research, 85,* 287–294.

Iyengar, S. S., & Lepper, M. R. (1999). Rethinking the value of choice: A cultural perspective on intrinsic motivation. *Journal of Personality and Social Psychology, 76,* 349–366.

Izzo, C. V., Weissberg, R. P., Kasprow, W. J., & Fendrich, M. (1999). A longitudinal assessment of teacher perceptions of parent involvement in children's education and school performance. *American Journal of Community Psychology, 27,* 817–839.

Jacobsen, T., & Hofman, V. (1997). Children's attachment representations: Longitudinal relations to school behavior and academic competency in middle childhood and adolescence. *Developmental Psychology, 33,* 703–710.

Jacobsen, T., Wolfgang, E., & Hofman, V. (1994). A longitudinal study of the relation between representations of attachment in childhood and cognitive functioning in childhood and adolescence. *Developmental Psychology, 30,* 112–124.

Jodl, K. M., Michael, A., Malanchuk, O., Eccles, J. S., & Sameroff, A. (2001). Parents' roles in shaping early adolescents' occupational aspirations. *Child Development, 72,* 1247–1265.

Juang, L. P., & Silbereisen, R. K. (2002). The relationship between adolescent academic capability beliefs, parenting, and school grades. *Journal of Adolescence, 25,* 3–18.

Kamins, M. L., & Dweck, C. S. (1999). Person versus process praise and criticism: Implications for contingent self-worth and coping. *Developmental Psychology, 35,* 835–847.

Keith, T. Z., Keith, P. B., Troutman, G. C., Bickley, P. G., Trivette, P. S., & Singh, K. (1993). Does parent involvement affect eighth-grade students achievement?: Structural analysis of national data. *School Psychology Review, 22,* 474–496.

Kelley, S. A., Brownell, C. A., & Campbell, S. B. (2000). Mastery motivation and self-evaluative affect in toddlers: Longitudinal relations with maternal behavior. *Child Development, 71,* 1061–1071.

Kempner, S., & Pomerantz, E. M. (2003, April). *Mothers' use of praise in their everyday interactions with their children: The moderating role of children's gender.* Paper presented at the Society for Research on Child Development, Tampa, FL.

Kenney-Benson, G. A., & Pomerantz, E. M. (in press). The role of mothers' use of control in children's perfectionism: Implications for the development of children's depressive symptoms. *Journal of Personality.*

Kochanska, G. (1991). Socialization and temperament in the development of guilt and conscience. *Child Development, 62,* 1379–1392.

Kochanska, G. (1993). Toward a synthesis of parental socialization and child temperament in early development of conscience. *Child Development, 64,* 325–347.

Kochanska, G. (1997). Mutually responsive orientation between mothers and their young children: Implications for early socialization. *Child Development, 68,* 94–112.

Larson, R. W., Richards, M. H., Moneta, G., Holmbeck, G., & Duckett, E. (1996). Changes in adolescents' daily interactions with their families from ages 10 to 18: Disengagement and transformation. *Developmental Psychology, 32,* 744–754.

Learner, D. G., & Kruger, L. J. (1997). Attachment, self-concept, and academic motivation in high-school students. *American Journal of Orthopsychiatry, 67,* 485–492.

Marjoribanks, K. (1988). Perceptions of family environments, educational and occupational outcomes: Social-status differences. *Perceptual and Motor Skills, 66,* 3–9.

Markus, H. R., & Kitayama, S. (1991). Culture and the self: Implications for cognition, emotion, and motivation. *Psychological Review, 98,* 224–253.

Matas, L., Arend, R., & Sroufe, A. (1978). Continuity and adaptation in the second year: The relationship between quality of attachment and later competence. *Child Development, 49,* 547–556.

McGrath, E. P., & Repetti, R. L. (2000). Mothers' and fathers' attitudes toward their children's academic performance and children's perceptions of their academic competence. *Journal of Youth and Adolescence, 29,* 713–723.

Miller, S. A., Manhal, M., & Mee, L. L. (1991). Parental beliefs, parental accuracy, and children's cognitive performance: A search for causal relations. *Developmental Psychology, 27,* 267–276.

Moss, E., & St. Laurent, D. (2001). Attachment at school age and academic performance. *Developmental Psychology, 37,* 863–874.

Mueller, C. M., & Dweck, C. S. (1998). Praise for intelligence can undermine children's motivation and performance. *Journal of Personality and Social Psychology, 75,* 33–52.

Ng, F. F., Kenney-Benson, G. A., & Pomerantz, E. M. (2004). Children's achievement moderates the effects of mothers' use of control and autonomy support. *Child Development, 75,* 764–780.

Nicholls, J. G. (1984). Achievement motivation: Conceptions of ability, subjective experience, task choice, and performance. *Psychological Review, 91,* 328–346.

Nolen-Hoeksema, S., Wolfson, A., Mumme, D., & Guskin, K. (1995). Helplessness in children of depressed and nondepressed mothers. *Developmental Psychology, 31,* 377–387.

Offer, D., & Offer, J. B. (1975). *Teenage to young manhood: A psychological study.* New York: Basic Books.

Parke, R. D., & Buriel, R. (1998). Socialization in the family: Ethnic and ecological perspectives. In N. Eisenberg (Ed.), *Handbook of child psychology: Vol. 3. Social, emotional, and personality development* (5th ed., pp. 463–552). New York: Wiley.

Parsons, J., Adler, T., & Kaczala, C. (1982). Socialization of achievement attitudes and perceptions: Parental influences. *Child Development, 53,* 310–321.

Peet, S. H., Powell, D. R., & O'Donnel, B. K. (1997). Mother–teacher congruence in perceptions of the child's competence and school engagement: Links to academic achievement. *Journal of Applied Developmental Psychology, 18,* 373–393.

Pezdek, K., Berry, T., & Renno, P. A. (2002). Children's mathematics achievement: The role of parents' perceptions and their involvement in homework. *Journal of Educational Psychology, 94,* 771–777.

Phillips, D. (1987). Socialization of perceived academic competence among highly competent children. *Child Development, 58,* 1308–1320.

Pomerantz, E. M. (2001). Parent × child socialization: Implications for the development of depressive symptoms. *Journal of Family Psychology, 15,* 510–525.

Pomerantz, E. M., & Eaton, M. M. (2001). Maternal intrusive support in the academic context: Transactional socialization processes. *Developmental Psychology, 37,* 174–186.

Pomerantz, E. M., Ng, F. F., & Wang, Q. (2004a). Gender socialization: A parent × child model. In A. H. Eagly, A. E. Beall, & R. J. Sternberg (Eds.), *The psychology of gender* (2nd ed., pp. 120–144). New York: Guilford Press.

Pomerantz, E. M., Ng, F., & Wang, Q. (2004b). *Mothers' mastery-oriented involvement in children's homework: Implications for the well-being of children with negative perceptions of competence.* Manuscript submitted for publication.

Pomerantz, E. M., & Ruble, D. N. (1998). The role of maternal control in the development of sex differences in child self-evaluative factors. *Child Development, 69,* 458–478.

Pomerantz, E. M., Saxon, J. L., & Oishi, S. (2000). The psychological tradeoffs of goal investment. *Journal of Personality and Social Psychology, 79,* 617–630.

Pomerantz, E. M., Wang, Q., & Ng, F. (in press). Mothers' affect in the homework context: The importance of staying positive. *Developmental Psychology.*

Pratt, M. W., Kerig, P., Cowan, P. A., & Cowan, C. P. (1988). Mothers and fathers teaching 3-year-olds: Authoritative parenting and adult scaffolding of young children's learning. *Developmental Psychology, 24,* 832–839.

Rosen, B. C., & D'Andrade, R. (1959). The psychosocial origins of achievement motivation. *Sociometry, 22,* 185–218.

Ryan, R. M. (1982). Control and information in the intrapersonal sphere: An extension of cognitive evaluation theory. *Journal of Personality and Social Psychology, 43,* 450–461.

Ryan, R. M., Stiller, J. D., & Lynch, J. H. (1994). Representations of relationships to teachers, parents, and friends as predictors of academic motivation and self-esteem. *Journal of Early Adolescence, 14,* 226–249.

Ryff, C. D., & Singer, B. (1998). The contours of positive human health. *Psychological Inquiry, 9,* 1–28.

Scarr, S. (1992). Developmental theories for the 1990s: Development and individual differences. *Child Development, 63,* 1–19.

Senechal, M., & LeFevre, J. (2002). Parental involvment in the development of children's reading skill: A five year longitudinal study. *Child Development, 73,* 445–460.

Sherif, M., & Cantril, H. (1947). *The psychology of ego involvements, social attitudes, and identifications.* New York: Wiley.

Sroufe, L. A., Fox, N. E., & Pancake, V. R. (1983). Attachment and dependency in developmental perspective. *Child Development, 54,* 1615–1627.

Steinberg, L., Elmen, J. D., & Mounts, N. S. (1989). Authoritative parenting, psychosocial maturity, and academic success among adolescents. *Child Development, 60,* 1424–1436.

Steinberg, L., Lamborn, S. D., Darling, N., Mounts, N. S., & Dornbusch, S. (1994). Over-time changes in adjustment and competence among adolescents from authoritative, authoritarian, indulgent, and neglectful homes. *Child Development, 65,* 754–770.

Steinberg, L., Lamborn, S. D., Dornbusch, S. M., & Darling, N. (1992). Impact of parenting practices on adolescent achievement: Authoritative parenting, school involvement, and encouragement to succeed. *Child Development, 63,* 1266–1281.

Stevenson, H. W., & Baker, D. P. (1987). The family-school relations and the child's school performance. *Child Development, 58,* 1348–1357.

Stevenson, H. W., & Newman, R. S. (1986). Long-term prediction of achievement and attitudes in mathematics and reading. *Child Development, 57,* 646–659.

Wagner, B. M., & Phillips, D. A. (1992). Beyond beliefs: Parent and child behaviors and children's perceived academic competence. *Child Development, 63,* 1380–1391.

Wang, Q., & Pomerantz, E. M. (2004). *Children's inclusion of their relationships with their parents in their self-construals: Implications for children's well-being*. Unpublished manuscript.

White, R. H. (1959). Motivation reconsidered: The concept of competence. *Psychological Review, 66*, 297–333.

Wigfield, A., Eccles, J. S., Yoon, K. S., & Harold, R. D. (1997). Change in children's competence beliefs and subjective task values across the elementary school years: A 3-year study. *Journal of Educational Psychology, 89*, 451–469.

Winsler, A., Diaz, R. M., McCarty, M., Atencio, D. J., & Chabay, L. A. (1999). Mother–child interaction, private speech, and task performance in preschool children with behavior problems. *Journal of Child Psychology and Psychiatry and Allied Disciplines, 40*, 891–904.

Winterbottom, M. R. (1958). The relation of need for achievement to learning experiences in independence and mastery. In J. W. Atkinson (Ed.), *Motives in fantasy, action and society* (pp. 453–478). Princeton, NJ: Van Nostrand.

Wood, D. (1980). Teaching the young child: Some relationships between social interaction, language, and thought. In D. Olson (Ed.), *The social foundations of language and thought* (pp. 280–296): New York: Norton.

CHAPTER 16

☙

Peer Relationships, Motivation, and Academic Performance at School

KATHRYN R. WENTZEL

Relationships with peers are of central importance to children throughout childhood and adolescence. They provide a source of companionship and entertainment, help in solving problems, personal validation and emotional support, and especially during adolescence, a foundation for identity development (Brown, Mory, & Kinney, 1994; Parker & Asher, 1993). In turn, children who enjoy positive relationships with peers appear to experience levels of emotional well-being, beliefs about the self, and values for prosocial forms of behavior and social interaction that are stronger and more adaptive than do children without positive peer relationships (Rubin, Bukowski, & Parker, 1998). An additional intriguing finding is that children who enjoy positive relationships with peers also tend to be engaged in and even excel at academic tasks more than those who have peer relationship problems. Children's social competence with peers has been related positively to academic accomplishments throughout the school-age years (Wentzel, 2003).

In light of evidence that links children's adaptive functioning across social and academic domains, a central question that I address in this chapter is how students' social competence with peers might be related to academic motivation and accomplishments. Toward this end, I first provide general criteria for defining social competence that can be applied to students' peer relationships at school. This contextualized focus reflects the fact that children's peer relationships are understood primarily within the context of the school; rarely have researchers looked outside the classroom walls to examine the nature of peer relationships and their correlates. Next, I review the literature on social competence with peers and ways in which social competence might be related to outcomes in the academic domain. Finally, I offer thoughts and provocations for future research.

DEFINING SOCIAL COMPETENCE WITH PEERS

How and why might students' relationships with peers be related to their academic motivation and accomplishments? Is it some aspect of the relationship itself that motivates academic accomplishments or, do social competencies that lead to social approval and acceptance among peers also contribute positively to academic functioning? One approach to answering these questions is to consider first the nature of social competence and how students' relationships with each other reflect a critical component of their social adaptation to school. Toward this end, I begin this section by presenting a definition of "social competence" derived from theoretical perspectives on person–environment fit and personal goal setting. This definition is then applied to the realm of schooling and students' relationships with peers. In this regard, I describe social, as well as academic, correlates of students' competence with peers.

Perspectives on Social Competence

In the social-developmental literature, social competence has been described from a variety of perspectives ranging from the development of individual skills to more general adaptation within a particular setting. In these discussions, social competence frequently is associated with person-level outcomes such as effective behavioral repertoires (Argyle, 1981), social problem-solving skills (Spivack & Shure, 1982), positive beliefs about the self (Bandura, 1986), achievement of social goals (Ford, 1992), and positive interpersonal relationships (Rubin et al., 1998). In addition, central to many definitions of social competence is the notion that contextual affordances and constraints contribute to and mold the development of these individual outcomes in ways that enable them to support the social good (Barker, 1961; Bronfenbrenner, 1989). Social contexts are believed to play an integral role in providing opportunities for healthy social development, as well as in defining the appropriate parameters of social accomplishments. In this chapter, therefore, social competence reflects this balance between the

achievement of positive outcomes for the self and adherence to context-specific expectations for behavior.

Social Competence as Person–Environment Fit

Support for this perspective on social competence can be found in the work of several theorists (e.g., Bronfenbrenner, 1989; Ford, 1992). Bronfenbrenner (1989) argues that competence can only be understood in terms of context-specific effectiveness, being a product of personal attributes such as goals, values, self-regulatory skills, and cognitive abilities, and of ways in which these attributes contribute to meeting situational requirements and demands. Bronfenbrenner further suggests that competence is facilitated by contextual supports that provide opportunities for the growth and development of these personal attributes, as well as for learning what is expected by the social group. Ford (1992) expands on this notion of person–environment fit by specifying four dimensions of competence that reflect personal as well as context-specific criteria: the achievement of personal goals; the achievement of goals that are situationally relevant; the use of appropriate means to achieve these goals; and the accomplishment of goals that result in positive developmental outcomes for the individual.

The application of this perspective on social competence to the realm of schooling results in a multifaceted description of children who are socially competent and well-adjusted. First, socially competent students achieve goals that are personally valued, as well as those that are sanctioned by others. Second, the goals they pursue result in both social integration and positive developmental outcomes for the student. Socially integrative outcomes are those that promote the smooth functioning of social groups at school (e.g., cooperative behavior) and are reflected in levels of social approval and social acceptance; student-related outcomes reflect healthy development of the self (e.g., perceived social competence, feelings of self-determination) and feelings of emotional well-being (Bronfenbrenner, 1989; Ford, 1992). From this description it follows that social competence is achieved to the extent that students accomplish goals that have both personal and social value in a manner that supports continued psychological and emotional well-being. In addition, the ability to be socially competent is contingent on opportunities and affordances of the school context that allow students to pursue multiple social goals.

Social Competence as the Achievement of Social Goals

A goal-based definition of social competence reflects a basic tenet of motivational theories that people set goals for themselves, and that these goals can be powerful motivators of behavior (Austin & Vancouver, 1996; Bandura, 1986; Dweck, 1991). Goal-directed behavior in social domains historically has been viewed as an aspect of competence rather than a type of motivation to achieve mastery of specific outcomes (e.g., Dodge, Asher, & Parkhurst, 1989; Ford, 1985). However, there are similarities between perspectives that describe goal-directed behavior in social and academic domains. First, goal setting is central to theorizing in both social and academic domains (Austin & Vancouver, 1996). In general, theorists define both social and achievement-related goals as cognitive representations of desired future outcomes (e.g., Austin & Vancouver, 1996; Dweck, 1991), although specific definitions of social goals vary to include affiliative needs (McClelland, 1987), reasons for social behavior (Erdley & Asher, 1996), and desires to achieve specific social outcomes (Wentzel, 2002).

In this chapter, I define students' "social goals" with regard to their content, or the social outcomes that students wish to achieve at school. Researchers who focus on the content of students' goals typically examine the frequency of efforts to pursue specific school-related outcomes, and the relation of these efforts to social and academic competencies (e.g., Ford, 1992; Wentzel, 1991a, 1991b, 1993). The content of classroom goals might be task-related, such as mastering subject matter or meeting a specific standard of performance or proficiency, or more cognitive, such as engaging in creative thinking or satisfying intellectual curiosity or challenge. Of concern for this discussion are social goals, such as establishing personal relationships with teachers and peers, gaining approval from others, or behaving cooperatively and responsibly with classmates.

As with task- or academically related outcomes, the achievement of social goals often is evaluated on the basis of standards. However, social standards are rarely discussed in terms of some sort of social excellence. Rather, evaluations of "success" typically are based on a combined judgement of personal satisfaction with and positive social reactions to specific social outcomes. Achieving an acceptable discrepancy between these two sets of evaluations is the hallmark of social competence and is achieved not just by one person's efforts but often as the result of compromise or conflict resolution among two or more individuals.

Finally, social goal pursuit typically is considered within the context of other self-processes that support goal pursuit. Similar to relations identified within the domain of academic motivation, beliefs about ability, personal values, attributions for success and failure, and other social cognitive and affective regulatory processes have been related to positive social outcomes. For instance, beliefs about social competence and efficacy have been related to a range of social outcomes, including helping (Ladd & Oden, 1979), control of aggression (Erdley & Asher, 1996), peer acceptance (Hymel, Bowker, & Woody, 1993), and social assertiveness (Kazdin, 1979). Similarly, attributional styles have been related to a range of social outcomes, including aggression (Hudley & Graham, 1993), peer rejection (Goetz & Dweck, 1980), and help giving (Weiner, 1980). In addition, a specific set of social information-processing and self-regulatory skills have been identified as necessary antecedents of social competence, including the ability to read and process social cues (Crick & Dodge, 1994), social perspective-taking skills (Spivack & Shure, 1982), and interpersonal trust (Rotenberg, 1991).

Summary

"Social competence" is defined in this chapter as the achievement of context-specific social goals that result in positive outcomes not only for the self but also for others. Therefore, a full appreciation of how and why students thrive or fail to thrive at school requires an understanding of a student's social goals, including both those that are personally valued and those that contribute to the stability and smooth functioning of interactions and relationships with others. This definition, however, suggests an additional set of questions: Which goals result in the formation and maintenance of positive relationships with peers at school? How do peers define social competence for each other? Interestingly, much is known about the social standards and expectations that teachers hold for their students (Wentzel, 2003). Indeed, teachers are the primary architects of classroom contexts and of ways in which students can achieve social goals. In contrast, little is known about the goals that students expect each other to achieve, and that lead to social approval among peers. However, it is reasonable to assume that characteristics of students who are well-liked and accepted by their peers also are those that reflect outcomes that are valued by peers and likely to result in peer acceptance and approval. In the following section, student characteristics related to positive relationships with peers are described.

Social Competence with Peers at School

By definition, social competence with peers reflects not only the achievement of personal goals but also those that are valued by the peer group and contribute to positive peer relationships. Therefore, one strategy for understanding the nature of social competence with peers is to identify social characteristics and outcomes related to peer approval and acceptance. Establishing positive relationships with peers can take many forms, ranging from general acceptance or preference by the peer group to involvement in reciprocated friendships. Therefore, identifying the correlates of peer acceptance and approval is not a simple task. However, researchers typically have defined children's involvement in peer relationships in three specific ways: degree of peer acceptance or rejection by the larger peer group, peer group membership, and dyadic friendships. Each of these aspects of peer relationships and their correlates is described in the following sections.

Correlates of Peer Preference and Sociometric Popularity and Rejection

Assessments of peer acceptance and rejection always are based on information obtained from the peer group at large rather than from the individual. In this manner, unilateral assessments of a child's relative standing or reputation within the peer group are used to create a continuum of social preference scores ranging from well-accepted to rejected (e.g., "How much do you like this person?"), or categories of individual students that reflect sociometric status groups (i.e., popular, rejected, neglected, controversial, and average-status children). Although rarely acknowledged as a factor contributing to peer acceptance or rejection, the school and classroom setting has almost always been the context within which peer preference and sociometric status are studied.

Of primary interest for this discussion are sociometrically rejected children, those who are infrequently nominated as someone's best friend and are actively disliked by their peers, and sociometrically popular children, those who are frequently nominated as a best friend and rarely disliked by their peers. A substantial number of studies have yielded consistent findings concerning these groups of children. In general, when compared to average-status peers (i.e., students with scores that do not fall into these statistically defined groups), popular students are more cooperative, helpful, and sociable, demonstrate better leadership skills, and are more self-assertive. In contrast, rejected students tend to be less compliant, less self-assured, less sociable, and more aggressive, disruptive, and withdrawn than their average-status peers (Newcomb, Bukowski, & Pattee, 1993; Rubin et al., 1998; Wentzel & Asher, 1995).

The relevance of the school context for understanding social competence with peers is reflected in consistent findings relating popular status and social acceptance to successful academic performance, and rejected status and low levels of acceptance to academic difficulties (e.g., Austin & Draper, 1984; Buhs & Ladd, 2001; Wentzel, 1991a). Results are most consistent with respect to classroom grades (Buhs & Ladd, 2001; Hatzichristou & Hopf, 1996; Wentzel,

1991a), although peer acceptance has been related positively to standardized test scores (Austin & Draper, 1984), as well as to IQ (Wentzel, 1991a). These findings are robust for elementary-age children, as well as adolescents, and longitudinal studies document the stability of relations between peer acceptance and academic accomplishments over time (e.g., Ladd & Burgess, 2001; Wentzel & Caldwell, 1997).

Correlates of Peer Group Membership

Students also enjoy relationships within peer groups or crowds. In contrast to peer status or preference, group membership is typically assessed by identifying clusters of friends who form a group (see Kindermann, McCollam, & Gibson, 1996), or by asking students to report who actually hangs out in groups with each other (Brown, 1989). Typical adolescent crowds include "Populars," students who engage in positive forms of academic, as well as social behavior, but also in some delinquent activities; "Jocks," students characterized by athletic accomplishments but also relatively frequent alcohol use; more alienated groups (e.g., "Druggies") characterized by poor academic performance and engagement in delinquent and other illicit activities; and "Normals," who tend to be fairly average students who do not engage in delinquent activities. Research on peer group membership has been mostly descriptive, identifying the central norms and values that uniquely characterize various adolescent school-based groups and crowds (e.g., Brown, 1989). Therefore, in contrast to work on sociometric status, there is not a one-to-one correspondence between enjoying high status and being described in a positive light. To illustrate, in contrast to sociometrically popular students, who are typically characterized in positive terms, members of "Popular" crowds are often described by their peers as having undesirable characteristics, such as being dominant and exclusionary, as well as lacking positive prosocial skills (Parkhurst & Hopmeyer, 1998).

As with research on peer acceptance, studies of peer group membership also have focused on academic values and characteristics. For example, ethnographic studies by Brown and his colleagues (Brown, 1989;

Brown, Mounts, Lamborn, & Steinberg, 1993; Stone & Brown, 1999) describe adolescents as characterizing certain crowds in terms of academic standing. "Brains," or students who get high grades, typically enjoy average status in crowd hierarchies, although they are viewed as somewhat disengaged from peer activities. The social status of this crowd also appears to have a developmental trajectory, with Brains' crowd status being highest during middle school and the end of high school, and lowest at the beginning of high school (see Stone & Brown, 1999). Of additional interest, however, is that members of the Popular crowd, who enjoy high status, also are typically characterized as being good students (Brown et al., 1993).

Finally, researchers who identify friendship-based peer groups using statistical procedures also have found relations between group membership and academic performance (Kurdek & Sinclair, 2000; Wentzel & Caldwell, 1997), as well as academic engagement (Kindermann, 1993). Peer group membership in middle school also has been related to changes in the degree to which students perform academically (Ryan, 2001). However, although most of these studies have followed students over time, few have documented long-term relations between group membership and academic performance (e.g., Wentzel & Caldwell, 1997).

Correlates of Friendship

Finally, peer relationships are studied with respect to dyadic friendships. In this case, students are asked to nominate their best friends at school; nominations are then matched to determine reciprocity, or best friendships. An important distinction between friendships and peer group membership is that friendships reflect relatively private, egalitarian relationships, often formed on the basis of idiosyncratic criteria. In contrast, peer groups are characterized by publicly acknowledged and, therefore, fairly consistent characteristics that are valued by the group (Brown, 1989).

Friendships have been described most often with respect to their functions (Furman, 1989) and their qualities (Parker & Asher, 1993). However, simply having a friend at school appears to be related to a range of positive outcomes. Children with friends tend to be more sociable, cooperative, and self-confident compared to their peers without friends (Newcomb & Bagwell, 1995; Wentzel, Barry, & Caldwell, 2004). Children with reciprocated friendships also tend to be more independent, emotionally supportive, altruistic, and less aggressive than those who do not have such friendships (Aboud & Mendelson, 1996; Wentzel et al., 2004). In addition, adolescents report they are satisfied with friends if they are self-disclosing, initiate activities, can manage and resolve conflict, and are emotionally supportive (Aboud & Mendelson, 1996). Research on friendship formation also suggests that personal attributes, such as the ability to engage in responsive communication, to exchange information, to establish common ground, to self-disclose, to extend and elaborate the activities of others, and to resolve conflict (Gottman, 1983), are characteristics that appear to be necessary to develop and maintain positive friendships.

Similar to other types of peer relationships, having friends also has been related positively to grades and test scores in elementary and middle school (Berndt & Keefe, 1995; Wentzel & Caldwell, 1997; Wentzel et al., 2004). Students with friends also tend to be more involved and engaged in school-related activities than those who do not have reciprocated friendships (Berndt & Keefe, 1995; Berndt, Laychak, & Park, 1990; Ladd, 1990; Ladd & Price, 1987).

Summary and Conclusions

The picture of peer-defined social competence that emerges from the literature on sociometric status and friendships is one of frequent displays of prosocial behavior (e.g., helping, sharing, caring), relatively infrequent displays of antisocial and disruptive behavior, and some modicum of academic success. Many of these characteristics also are endorsed by adolescent peer groups, although less predictably. Several issues concerning the nature of social competence with peers, however, remain unresolved.

Perhaps the most glaring omission in the literature on children's competence with peers is definitions of competence obtained directly from students themselves. Indeed,

the correlates of interest to researchers (and therefore, those that are assessed) reflect competencies valued by adults. Limited evidence indicates that students do have common beliefs concerning what they need to be like and how they should behave in order to be accepted by peers. Wentzel and Erdley (1993) found that the vast majority of adolescents in their study believed that showing respect for others, being sociable, and "being yourself" would result in making friends, whereas antisocial behavior, such as physical or verbal aggression, dishonesty, and delinquency, would not. Others have documented characteristics such as physical appearance, athletic abilities, and humor as student-generated correlates of peer acceptance (Rubin et al., 1998). In large part, however, little is yet understood about peer cultures, and what students themselves value and expect of each other in order to gain approval. The complexity of this undertaking is reflected in findings that personal attributes and behavior valued by students also tend to differ as a function of gender, as well as race (Benenson, Apostoleris, & Parnass, 1998; Graham, Taylor, & Hudley, 1998).

Of additional importance is that most researchers who study the correlates of peer interactions and relationships have not considered the role of various qualities and characteristics of peer involvement. For instance, friendships and groups to which students belong differ with respect to stability, status and roles of the individual members of the group or relationship, the degree to which friendships and group membership overlap with other friendships or groups, or overall quality of experiences with the group or friendship (see Newcomb & Bagwell, 1996). In addition, although adolescents are quick to identify school-related groups, they are loath to admit membership in any one group themselves (Matyanowski, 2001). Therefore, much work is still needed to resolve issues concerning how to define and assess various aspects of peer involvement before we can truly understand the role of peers' social demands and expectations in defining socially valued goals for students.

Finally, defining and judging competence from the sole perspective of what the peer environment demands tells us little about what individual students value and the goals they expect to achieve vis-à-vis their peers.

Indeed, the importance of considering the goals that students pursue as an additional component of social competence lies in the fact that pursuit of personal goals can lead to peer acceptance for many reasons. For instance, peer acceptance might be a personally valued outcome in and of itself, and as such, be the primary reason for engaging in peer-valued behavior. In this case, social competence could be assumed if a student's goal to achieve peer acceptance is met. At a more sophisticated level, a student might view demonstrations of specific behaviors and peer acceptance as multiple and interrelated goals, and utilize goal coordination skills to achieve both. If peer values changed, this student would be likely to alter behavior in a way that both sets of goals could still be achieved.

In addition, however, a student might have goals to engage in certain types of behavior irrespective of the fact that they might also be valued by peers. For this student, social competence would reflect a more complex set of outcomes, with peer acceptance being a positive social consequence of goal pursuit but not necessarily an achievement of a personal goal. Over time, peer-related competence might decline if peer values for behavior change. Finally, a student might pursue goals to gain social approval for ulterior motives; acceptance from peers might be pursued in order to enhance feelings of self-worth or to avoid punishment or peer retribution rather than because it holds personal value. In this case, it is possible that peer acceptance could be achieved without personal goals being met. According to the definition adopted for this chapter, this student would not be socially competent if maladaptive outcomes for the self such as social anxieties or fears remain despite social success with peers.

In short, determinations of social competence with peers cannot be made without consideration of students' own personal goals. With respect to peers, students can have goals to gain peer acceptance; they can pursue multiple goals that reflect positive outcomes for themselves, as well as their peers; they might have goals to engage in behaviors that are valued by peers even if peer acceptance is not an important goal to achieve; and they can pursue goals to be socially accepted for ulterior motives. The out-

comes of these various scenarios can have qualitatively different implications for healthy and adaptive functioning. It is clear, however, that peers can play a powerful role in defining socially valued outcomes at school by rewarding specific behaviors and personal characteristics with social acceptance and approval. Moreover, most students want to be accepted by their peers and are likely to behave in ways that will result in positive relationships with their classmates.

What is perhaps least clear in this literature is the role of academic accomplishments in defining social competence with peers. In the case of social preference, and sociometric status especially, there is overwhelming evidence of a positive relation between social acceptance and academic accomplishments. Why this relation exists, however, is not well understood. In the next section, therefore, I discuss models of influence that specify how peer relationships, as well as other social competencies related to peer acceptance and approval, might be related to students' academic pursuits and achievements at school.

RELATING SOCIAL COMPETENCE WITH PEERS TO ACADEMIC MOTIVATION AND ACCOMPLISHMENTS

The literature on peer relationships identifies academic accomplishments as a significant, positive correlate of peer acceptance and approval. Why then, might social competence with peers influence or even be related to academic outcomes? At the simplest level, it is possible that competence with peers and academic accomplishments are correlated but not causally related outcomes. Similarly, peer-related competence might not influence academic accomplishments, but functioning in the two domains might be linked by way of behavioral styles or self-regulatory processes that contribute to positive outcomes in each. Assuming that a causal relation does exist, it is reasonable to speculate that academic achievements can lead to social acceptance if they are valued by the peer group. In contrast, it also is feasible that social competence with peers leads to academic accomplishments, either because interactions with peers facilitate intellectual development (Piaget, 1932/1965, 1983), or because social or cultural norms communicated by peers define the nature of task competence (Vygotsky, 1978). Finally, in line with the definition of "social competence" adopted for this chapter, peer relationships might serve as contextual affordances that support the pursuit of students' personal goals, including those in the academic domain. Each of these possibilities is considered in the following sections.

Correlated but Not Causally Related Domains

Lacking direct evidence of causal influence, it is reasonable to assume that social competence with peers is simply correlated to academic competencies, without any direction of effects. Indeed, positive correlations could reflect reputational biases rather than causal influence. To illustrate, some middle school students attribute positive academic characteristics to sociometrically popular peers but not to other students who also are high achievers but not as well-liked (Wentzel, 1991a; Wentzel & Asher, 1995). This is in contrast to information from teachers, which does not always identify sociometrically popular students as the best students relative to other classmates (Wentzel & Asher, 1995). Therefore, positive correlations between peer acceptance and academic accomplishments might simply reflect a halo effect that leads students to evaluate well-liked classmates positively in both academic and social domains.

Although it is possible that these relations are psychologically meaningless, a more likely explanation is that a third set of factors contributes to competence in both domains. These factors could reflect specific types of social behavior, as well as psychological or emotional processes that support both positive peer relationships and academic excellence. A large body of evidence supports the notion that certain types of social behavior related to peer acceptance also are related to academic accomplishments. Specifically, displays of prosocial behavior, such as helping, sharing, and cooperating, and restraint from disruptive and antisocial forms of behavior in the classroom that have been related consistently and positively to

peer acceptance and approval also are strongly and positively related to intellectual accomplishments, including grades, test scores, and IQ (see Wentzel, 2003, for a review). In further support of this notion, positive forms of classroom participation, such as prosocial and socially responsible behavior, have been found to mediate relations between sociometric status and academic accomplishments in early childhood, as well as during early adolescence (Buhs & Ladd, 2001; Wentzel, 1991a); when these positive forms of behavior are taken into account, significant relations between peer acceptance and academic outcomes become nonsignificant.

A role for positive classroom behavior in mediating relations between peer relationships and academic outcomes is supported by several explanations. Just as prosocial and socially responsible forms of behavior contribute to successful relationships with peers, they also contribute to positive relationships with teachers. Not surprisingly, teachers report social preference and approval for students who cooperate, share, and follow rules (Wentzel, 1991b, 2003). Therefore, it is possible that students are rewarded by teachers for their positive behavior with high grades. It also is likely that displays of positive behavior and a lack of disruptive behavior in the classroom creates an instructional climate conducive to effective teaching and learning of academic material. In this way, social behavior can contribute directly to learning and task mastery, as well as to social approval and acceptance.

Although studied less often, metacognitive and self-regulatory processes also are likely to contribute to adaptive behavior in both social and academic domains. Several theorists have posited goal-setting skills, emotion regulation, self-monitoring, attributions, and means–end thinking and other basic information-processing skills as factors that contribute to the ability to implement strategic and planful behavior in both social and academic domains (Crick & Dodge, 1994). From a motivational perspective, goal networks and hierarchies based on students' beliefs about cause–effect relations also are likely to link performance in both domains. For instance, students might try to demonstrate academic competence to gain social approval, or they might try to behave in socially acceptable ways to get help on academic tasks. Indeed, students who report frequent attempts to behave in socially desirable ways also frequently try to achieve academically (Wentzel, 1989, 1993).

Causally Related Domains

Significant relations between peer relationships and academic accomplishments also might reflect more direct causal relations between the two domains of functioning. One possibility is that, at least for some students, excelling at academic tasks results in peer approval and acceptance. In this case, academic excellence would be one criterion for establishing positive relationships with peers. As noted earlier, this direct relationship between academic accomplishments and positive peer relationships clearly exists for some students, but it is not universal across all peer groups. Another possibility is reflected in models in which positive interactions with peers contribute directly both to competence at academic tasks and to positive forms of social behavior. For example, constructivist models propose that mutual discussion, perspective taking, and conflict resolution with peers can motivate the accommodation of new and more sophisticated approaches to intellectual problem solving (e.g., Piaget, 1932/1965, 1983). Similarly, theorists have argued that peer interactions play a unique role in the development of prosocial tendencies (Youniss & Smollar, 1989b). Children construct an understanding of reciprocity and interpersonal cooperation though discourse, conflict resolution, and social comparison with peers.

An alternative perspective is that all aspects of competence are defined by social and cultural norms (Vygotsky, 1978). In this case, notions of academic excellence and competence would be derived from broader notions of what it means to be competent within the larger culture. Peer relationships would contribute directly to the development of academic skills when competent students teach strategies and standards for performance to peers who are less skilled, or when they scaffold less competent peers to help them learn and perform in culturally prescribed ways (e.g., King, Staffieri, & Adelgais, 1998).

Peer Relationships as Contextual Affordances

A final way to think about the positive relation between peer acceptance and academic accomplishments is to consider the various provisions and opportunities that peer relationships afford to individual students. Recall that definitions of "social competence" are based on notions of social reciprocity: Just as the individual must behave in ways that support and are valued by the social group, so must the social group provide support for the achievement of individual goals. How might peer relationships provide supports for students' pursuit of goals to achieve academically? Models of socialization (e.g., Grusec & Goodnow, 1994) suggest at least two general mechanisms whereby social relationships and experiences might influence goal pursuit. First, ongoing social interactions teach children about themselves and what they need to do to become accepted and competent members of their social worlds. As noted in the previous section, children are likely to develop a set of goals and related standards for behavior that they should strive to achieve within the context of interpersonal interactions with their peers.

In addition, the qualities of children's social relationships are likely to have motivational significance. Ford (1992; see also Wentzel, 2002) suggests that evaluative beliefs about social relationships and settings can play an influential role in decisions to engage in the pursuit of personal goals. Within specific situations, an individual evaluates the correspondence between his or her personal goals and those of others, the degree to which others will provide access to information and resources necessary to achieve one's goals, and the extent to which social relationships will provide an emotionally supportive environment for goal pursuit. Extending this formulation to classroom settings, students who wish to achieve academically should engage in academic activities when they perceive their involvement and relationships with their peers as providing opportunities to achieve academic goals; as being safe and responsive to their academic strivings; as facilitating the achievement of their goals by providing help, advice, and instruction; and as being emotionally supportive and nurturing. In this manner, students' motivation to achieve academic goals should serve to mediate between opportunities afforded by positive relationships with peers and academic accomplishments.

In support of this model is empirical evidence that enjoying positive relationships with peers is related to various aspects of academic motivation. For instance, sociometrically popular students report more satisfaction with school, more frequent pursuit of goals to learn (Wentzel, 1991a, 1994; Wentzel & Asher, 1995), and stronger perceived academic competence (Hymel et al., 1993) than their socially rejected classmates. In contrast, peer rejection has been related to low levels of interest in school (Wentzel & Asher, 1995) and disengaging altogether by dropping out (Parker & Asher, 1987). In addition, Kindermann (1993; Kindermann et al., 1996) reports that elementary-age students tend to self-select into groups of peers that have motivational orientations to school similar to their own. Over the course of the school year, these orientations appear to become stronger and more similar within groups (see also Berndt et al., 1990; Ryan, 2001). During adolescence, dyadic friendships have been found to motivate positive academic behavior such as studying and making plans for college (e.g., Berndt et al., 1990; Epstein, 1983).

In line with Ford's (1992) proposal, ample support also exists for characterizing the opportunities provided by peers along dimensions of instrumental help, clear expectations and opportunities for goal pursuit, safety and responsivity, and emotional support. Therefore, it is reasonable to speculate that these contextual supports provided by peers can explain students' academic accomplishments, because they support the pursuit of academically related goals. In the following sections, I review evidence suggesting that these peer-related supports can promote academic accomplishments by motivating students to engage in positive academic activities.

Providing Expectations and Opportunities

As noted earlier, social contexts can influence goal pursuit if there is correspondence between one's personal goals and those of others. Therefore, a central question concerning students' pursuit of academically related goals is whether students express values and expectations concerning academic accomplishments to each other. Although not well documented, it is reasonable to assume that students communicate to each other values and expectations concerning academic achievement, and provide opportunities for each other that will allow their expression (e.g., Altermatt, Pomerantz, Ruble, Frey, & Greulich, 2002). It is clear, however, that as students advance through their middle school and high school years, the degree to which their goals and values support positive academic accomplishments can become fairly attenuated. In spite of these developmental trends, some adolescent students do report that their classmates expect them to behave appropriately and perform well academically at school. For instance, approximately 70% of adolescents from three predominantly middle-class middle schools reported that their peers expected them to be cooperative and helpful in class either *sometimes* or *always*, and approximately 80% reported similar peer values for academic learning (Wentzel, Looney, & Battle, 2003). Moreover, these perceptions did not appear to differ as a function of grade level. Therefore, it is reasonable to expect that, at least in some schools, peers actively promote the pursuit of positive academic, as well as social, outcomes.

Other evidence suggests that perceived expectations of peers for specific kinds of behavior might play a central role in students' own determination of why it is important to behave in those ways. Specifically, students who perceive relatively high expectations for academic learning and engagement from their peers also report that they pursue goals to learn for internalized reasons (or because its important) rather than because they believe they will get in trouble or lose social approval if they do not (Wentzel & Filisitti, 2003). Peers clearly have the potential to provide the most proximal input concerning whether engaging in a task is important, fun, or interesting. Therefore, peers who model a sense of importance or enjoyment with regard to task engagement are likely to lead others to form similar attitudes toward the task (Bandura, 1986). This is especially likely to occur when students are friends: Students have the opportunity to observe a friend's behavior with greater frequency than a nonfriend's behavior (Crockett, Losoff, & Petersen, 1984), and friendships typically are characterized by strong emotional bonds, thereby increasing the likelihood that friends will imitate each other's behavior (Berndt & Perry, 1986).

Providing Help, Advice, and Instruction

Enjoying positive relationships with peers also can lead directly to resources and information that help students learn. By virtue of the fact that they are socially accepted, it is reasonable to assume that students who get along with their peers will also have access to peer resources that can promote the development of social and academic competencies. These resources can take the form of information and advice, modeled behavior, or specific experiences that facilitate learning. Teachers play the central pedagogical function of transmitting knowledge and training students in academic subject areas. However, students provide each other with valuable resources necessary to accomplish academic tasks (Sieber, 1979). Students frequently clarify and interpret their teacher's instructions concerning what they should be doing and how they should do it, provide mutual assistance in the form of volunteering substantive information and answering questions (Cooper, Ayers-Lopez, & Marquis, 1982), and share various supplies such as pencils and paper.

Classmates also provide each other with important information about themselves by modeling academic competencies (Schunk, 1987), and by comparing work and grades (Butler, 1995; Guay, Boivin, & Hodges, 1999). Such information is likely to influence beliefs concerning their own levels of academic efficacy. Indeed, Altermatt et al. (2002) documented the role of students' evaluative discourse with peers in changing perceptions of academic efficacy over time. Experimental work also has shown that peers serve as powerful models that influence the development of academic self-efficacy (e.g., Schunk, 1987). In turn, students' efficacy beliefs are likely to be a primary motivator of goals to achieve academically (Bandura, 1986).

Providing a Safe and Responsive Environment

Students who are accepted by their peers and who have established friendships with classmates also are more likely to enjoy a relatively safe school environment and less likely to be the targets of peer-directed violence and harassment than their peers who do not have friends (Hodges, Boivin, Vitaro, & Bukowski, 1999; Pelligrini, Bartini & Brooks, 1999; Schwartz et al., 2000). This safety net that friends appear to provide for each other is critical, in that peer-directed violence and harassment is a fairly pervasive problem in American schools and can have an enormous negative impact on students' social and emotional functioning (Elliott, Hamburg, & Williams, 1998; Snyder, Brooker, Patrick, Schreperman, & Stoolmiller, 2003). National surveys indicate that large numbers of students are the target of classmate aggression and take active measures to avoid being harmed physically, as well as psychologically, by peers (National Center for Educational Statistics, 1995).

The general effects of peer harassment on student motivation and school-related competence has not been studied frequently. However, threats to physical safety can have a significant impact on students' emotional functioning at school (Buhs & Ladd, 2001; Elliott et al., 1998). Students who are frequently victimized tend to report higher levels of distress and depression than those who are not routinely victimized (e.g., Boivin & Hymel, 1997; Kochenderfer-Ladd & Waldrop, 2001; Olweus, 1993; Snyder et al., 2003). In turn, other studies have linked psychological distress and depression to interest in school (Wentzel, Weinberger, Ford, & Feldman, 1990) and negative attitudes toward academic achievement (Dubow & Tisak, 1989), as well as academic performance (Wentzel et al., 1990), and ineffective cognitive functioning (Jacobsen, Edelstein, & Hofmann, 1994). Therefore, students' affective functioning appears to mediate the effects of the quality of peer relationships and especially of peer harassment on academic outcomes (Juvonen, Nishina, & Graham, 2000; Wentzel, 1998; Wentzel & Caldwell, 1997; Wentzel & McNamara, 1999).

Providing Emotional Support

In conjunction with providing safe and responsive contexts, peer relationships also have the potential to create a climate of emotional support for students. During adolescence, students report that their peer groups and crowds provide them with a sense of emotional security and a sense of belonging (Brown, Eicher, & Petrie, 1986). In contrast, children without friends, or those who are socially rejected, are often lonely, emotionally distressed and depressed, and suffer from poor self-concepts (Wentzel & Caldwell, 1997; Wentzel et al., 2003). The positive academic effects of emotional support from peers are well documented. Students who perceive that their peers support and care about them also tend to be more engaged in positive aspects of classroom life than are students who do not perceive such support. Perceived support from peers has been associated positively with students' interest in academic pursuits (e.g., Wentzel, 1998; Wentzel et al., 2003). Similarly, young adolescents who do not perceive their relationships with peers as positive and supportive also tend to be at risk for academic problems (e.g., Goodenow, 1993; Wentzel, 1998).

Summary

Why might social competence with peers be related to academic accomplishments? I have argued that multiple models of influence are plausible: Significant relations might be due to additional behavioral styles of self-regulatory processes that contribute to both social and academic outcomes; academic accomplishments might lead to peer acceptance and approval; positive interactions with peers might contribute to the development of intellectual skills; and peer relationships might serve as social contexts that support students' academic goal pursuits and subsequent accomplishments. It is likely that each of these models can partly explain significant relations between positive peer relationships and academic outcomes. In line with the definition of social competence presented in this chapter, the literature also supports the proposal that peers are likely to influence students' adoption and pursuit of academic goals if four basic conditions are met: Clear expectations and opportunities for goal pursuit are communicated by their peers; instrumental help is available from classmates; the peer context is safe and responsive; and emotional support is provided by peers.

Although empirical evidence of the joint contribution of these peer provisions to students' classroom goals has been reported (Wentzel et al., 2003), what it is that develops or is changed on the part of students as a result of these provisions remains unanswered. One area for consideration is the influence of peer provisions on self-regulatory processes that support academic goal pursuit. For example, in a study of middle school and high school students, peer social support, instrumental help, and values explained significant amounts of variance in students' pursuit of academic goals to learn (Wentzel, Battle, & Looney, 2001). Of additional interest is that social support and instrumental help from peers remained significant predictors of efforts to learn when demographic, parenting, and teacher variables were taken into account. However, these peer provisions became nonsignificant predictors when students' academic self-processes (i.e., efficacy for learning, control beliefs, and reasons for learning) were entered into the regression equation. Therefore, although academic motivation in the form of goal pursuit is a likely mediator between peer provisions and students' academic accomplishments, other processes that regulate goal pursuit might be the more proximal targets of peer influence.

In addition to examining further the role of academic self-processes as mediators between provisions of peer relationships and academic goal pursuit, it would be fruitful to focus on other social self-processes that also are likely to influence the degree to which peer contexts orient students toward academic activities. Aspects of social-cognitive processing, such as selective attention, attributions, and social biases and stereotypes, can influence students' interpretations of peer communications, as well as peer reactions to students' behavior (Price & Dodge, 1989). Other individual characteristics, such as attachment security and family functioning (e.g., Fuligni, Eccles, Barber, & Clements, 2001), racial identity (Graham et al., 1998), and the extent that students are oriented toward gaining social approval, are also likely to influence the degree to which they are susceptible to peer influence.

The contribution of different types of peer involvement to academic outcomes also remains a relatively unexplored area of research. On the one hand, friends are believed to play a central role in providing contexts for self-expression, validation, and affirmation (Hartup & Stevens, 1997). Having friends appears to mediate the negative effects of harsh and punitive home environments on children's relations with the broader peer group (Schwartz et al., 2000), and being without friends predicts less than optimal levels of emotional well-being (e.g., Parker & Asher, 1993; Wenz-Gross, Siperstein, Untch, & Widaman, 1997). In addition, friends appear to elicit behavior that would not necessarily be displayed under other circumstances. For example, when children are with friends, they engage in more positive interactions, resolve more conflicts, and accomplish tasks with greater proficiency than when they are with nonfriends (Newcomb & Bagwell, 1995). Children also typically display more affect and emotional intensity with friends than with nonfriends (Parker & Gottman, 1989), and children are more successful at making transitions when friends accompany them (Ladd, 1990; Ladd & Price, 1987). In contrast, friends are believed to play a relatively minor role in socializing each other with respect to larger group norms and expectations (Hartup & Stevens, 1997). If so, the role of friendships in defining and supporting academic competence should be minimal.

On the other hand, adolescent peer groups and crowds are believed to facilitate the formation of identity and self-concept (Brown et al., 1994), and to structure the nature of ongoing social interactions within and across groups (Cairns, Xie, & Leung, 1998). In both of these roles, peer groups and crowds are likely to provide students with values, norms, and interaction styles that are commonly valued and sanctioned; valued behavior is modeled frequently, so that it can be easily learned and adopted by group members (Brown et al., 1994). Ecological perspectives (Bronfenbrenner, 1989; Cairns et al., 1998) also call attention to the roles of peer groups and crowds as interme-

diaries between the individual and broader peer and adult communities. For these reasons, it is likely that peer groups and crowds can play a central role in contributing to students' academic values and accomplishments.

A final question that remains unanswered is whether peers exert a unique influence on students' academic accomplishments when adult socialization processes are considered. The notion that peers can serve as potentially powerful motivators of academic engagement is generally supported in the empirical literature. However, few studies of peer interactions and relationships have taken into account the equally powerful influence of teachers and other adults in defining and promoting students' social and academic competencies. The results of our studies (Wentzel & Filisitti, 2003; Wentzel et al., 2001, 2003) suggest that aspects of students' relationships with peers do predict students' pursuit of academic goals even when certain aspects of teacher and parent influences are taken into account. One explanation for these findings is that peer relationships have a unique influence on students' academic goal pursuit by way of students' emotional well-being. Indeed, in contrast to a growing body of work relating perceived support from peers and students' affective functioning, significant relations between perceived support from teachers and students' levels of emotional distress have not been forthcoming (Wentzel, 1997, 1998; Wentzel & Filisitti, 2003).

An intriguing conclusion based on these findings is that perceptions of social and emotional support from peers are likely to be a critical factor that contributes to students' overall sense of emotional well-being at school, especially during adolescence. Assigning this unique role to peers, however, assumes that all students value peer support, and that peer rejection or lack of friends will automatically lead to emotional distress. In fact, some children are likely to be more adult-oriented than others and thrive despite a lack of close friends. A study of middle school students without friends (Wentzel & Asher, 1995) supports this notion, in that students who had few friends and were neither well-liked or disliked by their peers (sociometrically neglected children), were the most well-liked by their teachers, the most highly motivated students, and were equally self-confident compared to their average-status peers. In a longitudinal study, Wentzel (1998) found that these children remained academically and socially well-adjusted over the course of the middle school years. Whether these findings reflect a disinterest in the peer group and, therefore, a lack of emotional investment in peer relationships, or a dependence on adults for emotional support, remains a question for future research. However, it is likely that peers have little potential to influence some students.

CONCLUSIONS

This chapter began by posing the question of how social competence with peers might be related to academic motivation and accomplishments within the classroom context. I have argued that social competence with peers reflects the degree to which students are able to meet the social expectations of the peer group, as well as pursue their own personal goals; the achievement of these dual sets of goals is reflected in the psychological and emotional well-being of the student, as well as the smooth functioning of peer relationships and interactions. I also have described several pathways whereby students' relationships with peers might be related to academic accomplishments. The bulk of evidence supports a model in which clear expectations and opportunities for academic goal pursuit, instrumental help, safety and responsivity, and emotional support represent provisions of positive peer relationships that support students' pursuit of academic goals and subsequent actual achievements.

Much work, however, remains to be done. At the most general level, we need to address the possible ways in which children, and the various social systems in which they develop, jointly create definitions of social, as well as academic, competence (see Bronfenbrenner, 1989). Similarly, ways in which characteristics of the home, neighborhoods, and schools interact with peer relationships both in and out of school to influence children's functioning must be considered (e.g., Ge, Brody, Conger, Simmons, & Murry, 2002; Pettit, Bates, Dodge, & Meece, 1999).

In this regard, researchers need to identify ways in which students learn to coordinate their own social and academic goals with those prompted by others. Issues concerning cause and effect also necessitate continued focus on underlying psychological processes and skills that promote the development and display of competent outcomes.

Investigations of socially valued goals and expectations also must be conducted within a developmental framework, taking into account the age-related interests and capabilities of the child. From a developmental perspective, the role of peers in motivating academic accomplishments is likely to be especially critical during the middle school and high school years. Although children are interested in and even emotionally attached to their peers at all ages, they exhibit increased interest in their peers, spend more time with them, and exhibit a growing psychological and emotional dependence on them for support and guidance as they make the transition into adolescence (Youniss & Smollar, 1989a). Moreover, whereas friendships are enduring aspects of children's peer relationships at all ages, peer groups and crowds emerge primarily in the middle school years, peak at the beginning of high school, and then diminish in both prevalence and influence by the end of high school (Brown, 1989). Therefore, efforts to understand the influence of peer relationships on academic motivation and outcomes must be sensitive to not only the qualities and types of relationships that students form with each other but also to developmental issues.

In short, the most basic descriptive research has just begun. However, we have gained some initial insights into students' experiences with peers as they relate to academic motivation and achievement. I hope that these insights can serve as a foundation to explore further the social and psychological antecedents and supports of academic motivation and accomplishments of all school-age children.

REFERENCES

Aboud, F. E., & Mendelson, M. J. (1996). Determinants of friendship selection and quality: Developmental perspectives. In W. M. Bukowski, A. F. Newcomb, & W. W. Hartup (Eds.), *The company they* keep: *Friendship during childhood and adolescence* (pp. 87–112). New York: Cambridge University Press.

Altermatt, E. R., Pomerantz, E. M., Ruble, D. N., Frey, K. S., & Greulich, F. K. (2002). Predicting changes in children's self-perceptions of academic competence: A naturalistic examination of evaluative discourse among classmates. *Developmental Psychology, 38,* 903–917.

Argyle, M. (1981). The contribution of social interaction research to social skills training. In J. D. Wine & M. D. Smye (Eds.), *Social competence.* New York: Guilford Press.

Austin, A. B., & Draper, D. C. (1984). The relationship among peer acceptance, social impact, and academic achievement in middle school. *American Educational Research Journal, 21,* 597–604.

Austin, J. T., & Vancouver, J. B. (1996). Goal constructs in psychology: Structure, process, and content. *Psychological Bulletin, 120,* 338–375.

Bandura, A. (1986). *Social foundations of thought and action: A social cognitive theory.* Englewood Cliffs, NJ: Prentice-Hall.

Barker, R. G. (1961). Ecology and motivation. In M. R. Jones (Ed.), *Nebraska Symposium on Motivation* (Vol. 8, pp. 1–50). Lincoln: University of Nebraska Press.

Benenson, J., Apostoleris, N., & Parnass, J. (1998). The organization of children's same-sex peer relationships. *New Directions for Child Development, 80,* 5–23.

Berndt, T. J., & Keefe, K. (1995). Friends' influence on adolescents' adjustment to school. *Child Development, 66,* 1312–1329.

Berndt, T. J., Laychak, A. E., & Park, K. (1990). Friends' influence on adolescents' academic achievement motivation: An experimental study. *Journal of Educational Psychology, 82,* 664–670.

Berndt, T. J., & Perry, T. B. (1986). Children's perceptions of friendships as supportive relationships. *Developmental Psychology, 22,* 640–648.

Boivin, M., & Hymel, S. (1997). Peer expereinces and social self-perceptions: A sequential model. *Developmetnal Psychology, 33,* 135–145.

Bronfenbrenner, U. (1989). Ecological systems theory. In R. Vasta (Ed.), *Annals of child development* (Vol. 6, pp.187–250). Greenwich, CT: JAI Press.

Brown, B. B. (1989). The role of peer groups in adolescents' adjustment to secondary school. In T. J. Berndt & G. W. Ladd (Eds.), *Peer relationships in child development* (pp. 188–215). New York: Wiley.

Brown, B. B., Eicher, S. A., & Petrie, S. (1986). The importance of peer group ("crowd") affiliation in adolescence. *Journal of Adolescence, 9,* 73–96.

Brown, B. B., Mory, M. S., & Kinney, D. (1994) Casting adolescent crowds in a relational perspective: Caricature, channel, and context. In R. Montemayor, G. R. Adams, & T. P. Gullotta (Eds.), *Personal relationships during adolescence* (pp. 123–167). Newbury Park, CA: Sage.

Brown, B. B., Mounts, N., Lamborn, D. D., & Steinberg, L. (1993). Parenting practices and peer group affiliation in adolescence. *Child Development, 64,* 467–482.

Buhs, E. S., & Ladd, G. W. (2001). Peer rejection as an antecedent of young children's school adjustment: An examination of mediating processes. *Developmental Psychology, 37,* 550–560.

Butler, R. (1995). Motivational and informational functions and consequences of children's attention to peers' work. *Journal of Educational Psychology, 87,* 347–360.

Cairns, R., Xie, H., & Leung, M. (1998). The popularity of friendship and the negelct of social networks: Toward a new balance. *New Directions for Child Development, 80,* 25–53.

Cooper, C. R., Ayers-Lopez, S., & Marquis, A. (1982). Children's discourse during peer learning in experimental and naturalistic situations. *Discourse Processes, 5,* 177–191.

Crick, N., & Dodge, K. A. (1994). A review and reformulation of social information-processing mechanisms in children's social adjustment. *Psychological Bulletin, 115,* 74–101.

Crockett, L., Losoff, M., & Petersen, A. C. (1984). Perceptions of the peer group and friendship in early adolescence. *Journal of Early Adolescence, 4,* 155–181.

Dodge, K. A., Asher, S. R., & Parkhurst, J. T. (1989). Social life as a goal coordination task. In C. Ames & R. Ames (Eds.), *Research on motivation in education* (Vol. 3, pp. 107–138). New York: Academic Press.

Dubow, E. F., & Tisak, J. (1989). The relation between stressful life events and adjustment in elementary school children: The role of social support and social problem-solving skills. *Child Development, 60,* 1412–1423.

Dweck, C. S. (1991). Self-theories and goals: Their role in motivation, personality, and development. In R. Dienstbier (Ed.), *Nebraska Symposium on Motivation* (Vol. 38, pp. 199–236). Lincoln: University of Nebraska Press.

Elliott, D. S., Hamburg, B. A., & Williams, K. R. (1998). *Violence in American schools: A new perspective.* New York: Cambridge University Press.

Epstein, J. L. (1983). The influence of friends on achievement and affective outcomes. In J. L. Epstein & N. Karweit (Eds.), *Friends in school* (pp. 177–200). New York: Academic Press.

Erdley, C. A., & Asher, S. R. (1996). Children's social goals and self-efficacy perceptions as influences on their responses to ambiguous provocation. *Child Development, 67,* 1329–1344.

Ford, M. E. (1985). The concept of competence: Themes and variations. In H. A. Marlowe & R. B. Weinberg (Eds.), *Competence development* (pp. 3–49). Springfield, IL: Thomas.

Ford, M. E. (1992). *Motivating humans: Goals, emotions, and personal agency beliefs.* Newbury Park, CA: Sage.

Fuligni, A. J., Eccles, J. S., Barber, B. L., & Clements, P.

(2001). Early adolescent peer orientation and adjustment during high school. *Developmental Psychology*, 37, 28–36.

Furman, W. (1989). The development of children's social networks. In D. Belle (Ed.), *Children's social networks and social supports* (pp. 151–172). New York: Wiley.

Ge, A., Brody, G. H., Conger, R. D., Simons, R. L., & Murry, V. M. (2002). Contextual amplification of pubertal transition effects on deviant peer affiliation and externalizing behavior among African-American children. *Developmental Psychology*, 38, 42–54.

Goetz, T. S., & Dweck, C. S. (1980). Learned helplessness in social situations. *Journal of Personality and Social Psychology*, 39, 246–255.

Goodenow, C. (1993). Classroom belonging among early adolescent students: Relationships to motivation and achievement. *Journal of Early Adolescence*, 13, 21–43.

Gottman, J. M. (1983). How children become friends. *Monographs of the Society for Research in Child Development*, 48(3, Serial No. 201).

Graham, S., Taylor, A., & Hudley, C. (1998). Exploring achievement values among ethnic minority early adolescents. *Journal of Educational Psychology*, 90, 606–620.

Grusec, J. E., & Goodnow, J. J. (1994). Impact of parental discipline methods on the child's internalization of values: A reconceptualization of current points of view. *Developmental Psychology*, 30, 4–19.

Guay, F., Boivin, M., & Hodges, E. V. E. (1999). Predicting change in academic achievement: A model of peer experiences and self-system processes. *Journal of Educational Psychology*, 91, 105–115.

Hartup, W. W., & Stevens, N. (1997). Friendships and adaptation in the life course. *Psychological Bulletin*, 121, 355–370.

Hatzichristou, C., & Hopf, D. (1996). A multiperspective comparison of peer sociometric status groups in childhood and adolescence. *Child Development*, 67, 1085–1102.

Hodges, E. V., Boivin, M., Vitaro, F., & Bukowski, W. M. (1999). The power of friendship: Protection against an escalating cycle of peer victimization. *Developmental Psychology*, 35, 94–101.

Hudley, C., & Graham, S. (1993). An attributional intervention to reduce peer-directed aggression among African-American boys. *Child Development*, 64, 124–138.

Hymel, S., Bowker, A., & Woody, E. (1993). Aggressive versus withdrawn unpopular children: Variations in peer and self-perceptions in multiple domains. *Child Development*, 64, 879–896.

Jacobsen, T., Edelstein, W., & Hofmann, V. (1994). A longitudinal study of the relation between representations of attachment in childhood and cognitive functioning in childhood and adolescence. *Developmental Psychology*, 30, 112–124.

Juvonen, J., Nishina, A., & Graham, S. (2000). Peer harassment, psychological adjustment, and school

functioning in early adolescence. *Journal of Educational Psychology*, 92, 349–359.

Kazdin, A. E. (1979). Nonspecific treatment factors in psychotherapy outcome research. *Journal of Consulting and Clinical Psychology*, 47, 846–851.

Kindermann, T. A. (1993). Natural peer groups as contexts for individual development: The case of children's motivation in school. *Developmental Psychology*, 29, 970–977.

Kindermann, T. A., McCollam, & Gibson, E. (1996). Peer networks and students' classroom engagement during childhood and adolescence. In J. Juvonen & K. R. Wentzel (Eds.), *Social motivation: Understanding children's school adjustment* (pp. 279–312). New York: Cambridge University Press.

King, A., Staffieri, A., & Adelgais, A. (1998). Mutual peer tutoring: Effects of structuring tutorial interaction to scaffold peer learning. *Journal of Educational Psychology*, 90, 134–152.

Kochenderfer-Ladd, B., & Waldrop, J. L. (2001). Chronicity and instability of children's peer victimization experiences as predictors of loneliness and social satisfaction trajectories. *Child Development*, 72, 134–151.

Kurdek, L. A., & Sinclair, R. J. (2000). Psychological, family, and peer predictors of academic outcomes in first- through fifth-grade children. *Journal of Educational Psychology*, 92, 449–457.

Ladd, G. W. (1990). Having friends, keeping friends, making friends, and being liked by peers in the classroom: Predictors of children's early school adjustment. *Child Development*, 61, 1081–1100.

Ladd, G. W., & Burgess, K. B. (2001). Do relational risks and protective factors moderate the linkages between childhood aggression and early psychological and school adjustment? *Child Development*, 72, 1579–1601.

Ladd, G. W., & Oden, S. (1979). The relationships between peer acceptance and children's ideas about helpfulness. *Child Development*, 50, 402–408.

Ladd, G. W., & Price, J. M. (1987). Predicting children's social and school adjustment following the transition from preschool to kindergarten. *Child Development*, 58, 1168–1189.

Matyanowski, M. L. (2001). Adolescent peer group memberships, peer group characteristics, and self-concept. *Dissertation Abstracts International*, 62(1-B), 577.

McClelland, D. C. (1987). *Human motivation*. New York: Cambridge University Press.

National Center for Educational Statistics. (1995). *Student strategies to avoid harm at school* (NCES Publication No. NCES 95–203). Washington, DC: U.S. Government Printing Office.

Newcomb, A. F., & Bagwell, C. L. (1995). Children's friendship relations: A meta-analytic review. *Psychological Bulletin*, 117, 306–347.

Newcomb, A. F., & Bagwell, C. L. (1996). The developmental significanceof children's friendship relations. In W. M. Bukowski, A. F. Newcomb, & W. W.

Hartup (Eds.), *The company they keep: Friendship during childhood and adolescence* (pp. 289–321). New York: Cambridge University Press.

Newcomb, A. F., Bukowski, W. M., & Pattee, L. (1993). Children's peer relations: A metaanalytic review of popular, rejected, neglected, and controversial sociometric status. *Psychological Bulletin, 113*, 99–128.

Olweus, D. (1993). Victimization by peers: Antecedents and long-term outcomes. In K. Rubin & J. B. Asendorf (Eds.), *Social withdrawal, inhibition, and shyness in childhood* (pp. 315–341). Chicago: University of Chicago Press.

Parker, J. G., & Asher, S. R. (1987). Peer relations and later personal adjustment: Are low-accepted children at risk? *Psychological Bulletin, 102*, 357–389.

Parker, J. G., & Asher, S. R. (1993). Friendship and friendship quality in middle childhood: Links with peer group acceptance and feelings of loneliness and social dissatisfaction. *Developmental Psychology, 29*, 611–621.

Parker, J. G., & Gottman, J. M. (1989). Social and emotional developmentin a rleational context: Friendship interaction from early childhood to adoelscence. In T. J. Berndt & G. W. Ladd (Eds.), *Peer relationships in child development* (pp. 95–131). Oxford, UK: Wiley.

Parkhurst, J. T., & Hopmeyer, A. (1998). Sociometric popularity and peer-perceived popularity: Two distinct dimensions of peer status. *Journal of Early Adolescence, 18*, 125–144.

Pellegrini, A. D., Bartini, M., & Brooks, F. (1999). School bullies, victims, and aggressive victims: Factors relating to group affiliation and victimization in early adolescence. *Journal of Educational Psychology, 91*, 216–224.

Pettit, G. S., Bates, J. E., Dodge, K. A., & Meece, D. W. (1999). The impact of after-school peer contact on early adolescent externalizing problems is moderated by parental monitoring, perceived neighborhood safety, and prior adjustment. *Child Development, 70*, 768–778.

Piaget, J. (1965). *The moral judgment of the child.* New York: Free Press (Original published in 1932)

Piaget, J. (1983). Piaget's theory. In P. H. Mussen (Ed.), *Handbook of child psychology* (Vol. 1, pp. 103–128). New York: Wiley.

Price, J. M., & Dodge, K. A. (1989). Peers' contributions to children's social maladjustment: Description and intervention. In T. J. Berndt, & G. W. Ladd (Eds.), *Peer relationships in child development* (pp. 341–370). New York: Wiley.

Rotenberg, K. J. (1991). *Children's interpersonal trust: Sensitivity to lying, deception, and promise violations.* New York: Springer-Verlag.

Rubin, K. H., Bukowski, W., & Parker, J. G. (1998). Peer interactions, relationships, and groups. In W. Damon (Series Ed.) & N. Eisenberg (Vol. Ed.), *Handbook of child psychology: Vol. 3. Social, emo-*

tional, and personality development (5th ed., pp. 619–700). New York: Wiley.

Ryan, A. (2001). The peer group as a context for the development of young adolescent motivation and achievement. *Child Development, 72*, 1135–1150.

Schunk, D. H. (1987). Peer models and children's behavioral change. *Review of Educational Research, 57*, 149–174.

Schwartz, D., Dodge, K. A., Pettit, G. S., Bates, J. E., & the Conduct Problems Prevention Research Group. (2000). Friendship as a moderating factor in the pathway between early harsh home environment and later victimization in the peer group. *Developmental Psychology, 36*, 646–662.

Sieber, R. T. (1979). Classmates as workmates: Informal peer activity in the elementary school. *Anthropology and Education Quarterly, 10*, 207–235.

Snyder, J., Brooker, M., Patrick, M. R., Snyder, A., Schrepferman, & Stoolmiller, M. (2003). Observed peer victimization during early elementary school: Continuity, growth, and relation to risk for child antisocial and depressive behavior. *Child Development, 74*, 1881–1898.

Spivack, G., & Shure, M. B. (1982). The cognition of social adjustment: Interpersonal cognitive problem-solving thinking. In B. B. Lahey & A. E Kazdin (Eds.), *Advances in clinical psychology* (Vol. 5, pp. 323–372). New York: Plenum Press.

Stone, M. R., & Brown, B. B. (1999). Identity claims and projections: Descriptions of self and crowds in secondary school. *New Directions for Child and Adolescent Development, 84*, 7–20.

Vygotsky, L. S. (1978). *Mind in society: The development of higher psychological processes.* Cambridge, MA: Harvard University Press.

Weiner, B. (1980). A cognitive (attribution)–emotion–action model of motivated behavior: An analysis of judgements of help-giving. *Journal of Personality and Social Psychology, 39*, 186–200.

Wentzel, K. R. (1989). Adolescent classroom goals, standards for performance, and academic achievement: An interactionist perspective. *Journal of Educational Psychology, 81*, 131–142.

Wentzel, K. R. (1991a). Relations between social competence and academic achievement in early adolescence. *Child Development, 62*, 1066–1078.

Wentzel, K. R. (1991b). Social competence at school: Relations between social responsibility and academic achievement. *Review of Educational Research, 61*, 1–24.

Wentzel, K. R. (1993). Social and academic goals at school: Motivation and achievement in early adolescence. *Journal of Early Adolescence, 13*, 4–20.

Wentzel, K. R. (1994). Relations of social goal pursuit to social acceptance, classroom behavior, and perceived social support. *Journal of Educational Psychology, 86*, 173–182.

Wentzel, K. R. (1997). Student motivation in middle school: The role of perceived pedagogical caring. *Journal of Educational Psychology, 89*, 411–419.

Wentzel, K. R. (1998). Social support and adjustment in middle school: The role of parents, teachers, and peers. *Journal of Educational Psychology, 90,* 202–209.

Wentzel, K. R. (2002). The contribution of social goal setting to children's school adjustment. In A. Wigfield & J. Eccles (Eds.), *Development of achievement motivation* (pp. 221–246). New York: Academic Press.

Wentzel, K. R. (2003). School adjustment. In W. Reynolds & G. Miller (Eds.), *Handbook of psychology: Vol. 7. Educational psychology* (pp. 235–258). New York: Wiley.

Wentzel, K. R., & Asher, S. R. (1995). Academic lives of neglected, rejected, popular, and controversial children. *Child Development, 66,* 754–763.

Wentzel, K. R., Barry, C., & Caldwell, K. (2004). Friendships in middle school: Influences on motivation and school adjustment. *Journal of Educational Psychology, 96,* 195–203.

Wentzel, K. R., Battle, A., & Looney, L. (2001, April). *Classroom support in middle school: Contributions of teachers and peers.* Paper presented at the biannual meeting of the Society for Research in Child Development, Minneapolis, MN.

Wentzel, K. R., & Caldwell, K. (1997). Friendships, peer acceptance, and group membership: Relations to academic achievement in middle school. *Child Development, 68,* 1198–1209.

Wentzel, K. R., & Erdley, C. A. (1993). Strategies for making friends: Relations to social behavior and peer acceptance in early adolescence. *Developmental Psychology, 29,* 819–826.

Wentzel, K. R., & Filisetti, L. (2003). *Predictors of prosocial behavior in young adolescents: Self-processes and contextual factors.* Manuscript in preparation.

Wentzel, K. R., Looney, L., & Battle, A. (2003). *Social and academic motivation in adolescence.* Manuscript in preparation.

Wentzel, K. R., & McNamara, C. (1999). Interpersonal relationships, emotional distress, and prosocial behavior in middle school. *Journal of Early Adolescence, 19,* 114–125.

Wentzel, K. R., Weinberger, D. A., Ford, M. E., & Feldman, S. S. (1990). Academic achievement in preadolescence: The role of motivational, affective, and self-regulatory processes. *Journal of Applied Developmental Psychology, 11,* 179–193.

Wenz-Gross, M., Siperstein, G. N., Untch, A. S., & Widaman, K. F. (1997). Stress, social support, and adjustment of adolescents in middle school. *Journal of Early Adolescence, 17,* 129–151.

Youniss, J., & Smollar, J. (1989a). Adolescents' interpersonal relationships in social context. In T. J. Berndt & G. Ladd (Eds.), *Peer relationships in child development* (pp. 300–316). New York: Wiley.

Youniss, J., & Smollar, J. (1989b). Self through relationship development. In B. H. Schneider, G. Atilli, J. Nadel, & R. P. Weissberg (Eds.), *Social competence in developmental perspective* (pp. 129–148). Dordrecht: Kluwer.

CHAPTER 17

അ

Competence Motivation in the Classroom

TIM URDAN
JULIANNE C. TURNER

Most prominent approaches to the study of motivation today involve competence in some way, whether it be the desire to become competent, to appear competent to others, to feel competent, or even to avoid feeling or appearing incompetent. In addition, most current conceptualizations of competence motivation were either created by psychologists or derived from earlier theories that were developed by psychologists (e.g., McClelland, Atkinson, White, Lewin). Pintrich (2004) recently argued that motivational science represents "use-inspired basic research" (p. 668). As such, a number of researchers have suggested that each of the various frameworks of motivation has direct implications for classroom practice despite the fact that most of these approaches were developed by psychologists and tested outside of classroom contexts. Our purpose in this chapter is to review the suggested implications for classroom practice of research from various motivational perspectives, to analyze the research evidence supporting these suggested implications, to offer a synthesis across motivational approaches of the best practices for promoting competence

motivation in classrooms, to discuss some cautions that motivation researchers should attend to when trying to apply motivation principles in classrooms, and to suggest future directions for research.

DISTINGUISHING COMPETENCE MOTIVATION FROM OTHER CLASSROOM APPROACHES TO MOTIVATION

Competence motivation is distinct from other motivational theories and perspectives that have been examined and applied in the classroom. By definition, *competence motivation* involves a concern with mastery. The motive, or the impetus for action in a specific direction, is to develop, to attain, or to demonstrate competence. Although the fundamental objective of education is to create competence, a number of efforts to enhance student motivation in classrooms have not focused on competence motivation per se. For example, efforts to enhance students' self-esteem were primarily focused on increasing student motivation, but competence was not the central feature of these efforts. Similarly, token economies and other tangible reward systems are adopted to enhance motivation, but the motivation is often for behaving well, completing classwork, and being punctual rather than for developing competence. There has also been a considerable amount of attention paid to social motivators in schools and classrooms (Coleman, 1961; Ryan, 2001). Research in classrooms has revealed that student engagement and willingness to exert effort on academic tasks can be enhanced by social motives, such as the desire to work with friends and peers (Ryan, 2001), to please parents (Fuligni, 1997), and to please the teacher (Wentzel, 1999). In addition, research has shown that other social factors, such as perceptions of the teachers' social support (Wentzel, 1999), are positively associated with motivation in the classroom. Although none of these social variables and motives represents competence motivation, they may affect competence motivation indirectly by encouraging students to develop and then demonstrate academic competence to parents, peers, or teachers.

Because this volume is devoted to a consideration of competence motivation, we thought it important to define competence motivation in the classroom by distinguishing it from other forms of motivation. In addition, we wanted to foreshadow an argument that we present later in the chapter: A full understanding of the nature of competence motivation *in classrooms* may need to consider additional motivational factors, including the affordances and demands specific to classrooms, and the highly social nature of classroom interactions. We now turn our attention to a consideration of several prominent theories of competence motivation and the suggested implications of each for classroom practice.

OVERVIEW OF MOTIVATIONAL RESEARCH AND SUGGESTED CLASSROOM APPLICATIONS

In this section, we examine the stated implications for classroom practice of several prominent social cognitive conceptualizations of motivation (achievement goals, interest and intrinsic motivation, self-efficacy,

expectancy–value theory, self-determination theory, and attribution theory) as they relate to competence, and review the empirical support for these stated implications. We should note that our attention is limited to research conducted in K–12 settings. Although there has been research conducted in college classrooms (e.g., Harackiewicz, Barron, Tauer, Carter, & Elliot, 2000), it is not clear whether the results of that research generalize to K–12 settings for a variety of reasons. First, college attendance is voluntary whereas most K–12 attendance is coerced. Coercion has serious implications for competence motivation, particularly for theories that include intrinsic motivation. Second, college students, on average, are higher achieving than K–12 students. As such, these students generally fare well in situations involving comparisons of ability and academic competition, which may have implications for the generalizability of results involving the benefits of performance–approach goals (Midgley, Kaplan, & Middleton, 2001). In addition, college students are more likely to be in large classes that involve little personal interaction with the instructor, a fact that may alter the social influences on competence motivation. For these and other reasons (i.e., college students are older, more likely to be enrolled in classes that interest them, etc.), we limit our focus to K–12 settings.

Research on Achievement Goals

Perhaps more than any of the other research programs we discuss, research on achievement goals has been conducted with an eye toward classroom application. This motivational framework posits that individuals have different purposes for engaging (or not engaging) in activities, and these purposes are called *goals or goal orientations* (Dweck, 1992; Elliot, 1997; Maehr & Midgley, 1991). Three types of achievement goals have been most extensively studied: mastery, performance–approach, and performance–avoidance. Whereas performance goals involve a concern with normative performance and appearing able (or avoiding appearing unable), mastery goals represent a concern with developing competence by developing skills and understanding new information. The personal achievement goals that students adopt in a given situation or classroom are believed to be influenced by the goal messages made salient in the achievement context (Ames, 1992). These messages create the *classroom goal structure.* Unlike research on personal goals, the published research on classroom goal structures has generally focused on performance and mastery goal structures, without distinguishing between the approach and avoidance elements (Urdan, 2004).

Stated Implications of Achievement Goal Research

Because mastery goals are more consistently associated with positive motivational and learning outcomes (e.g., increased effort, persistence, positive affect, greater use of elaborative cognitive strategies, attributions of success and failure to controllable factors), goal theorists have often argued that the mastery goal structure should be strengthened in the classroom (Ames, 1992; Maehr & Midgley, 1991; Midgley & Urdan, 1992). Goal researchers have suggested a number of strategies teachers could adopt to create stronger mastery goal structures in their classrooms. Ames (1992) suggested that teachers create academic tasks that are meaningful and personally relevant to students, evaluate students on the basis of improvement and effort rather than relative performance among students, and provide students with a sense of autonomy by giving them choices and a voice in classroom decisions whenever possible. A specific set of suggestions for creating a mastery goal structure in the classroom was offered by Midgley and Urdan (1992), and included recommendations such as making student evaluation and recognition practices as private as possible, emphasizing understanding and challenge, and using cooperative learning.

Empirical Support for the Stated Implications

Research examining classroom goal structures and their effects can be divided into three types: Active manipulations of teacher and classroom practices, survey research, and observational research, or survey-and-observation combinations. The first report of an attempt to manipulate the goals that teachers emphasized in their classrooms was by Ames (1990). In an unpublished study, Ames worked with a group of 66 elementary school teachers, 36 of whom were randomly assigned to a treatment group and 30 others who were assigned to the control group. Teachers in the treatment group implemented a series of mastery-oriented practices in an effort to create mastery goal structures in their classrooms. Students in the treatment classrooms reported no change in their learning strategy use; intrinsic motivation; attitudes toward reading, math, and school; or perceived competence and increases in self-concept of ability; whereas students in the control classrooms reported significant declines in all of these variables except for attitude toward school and self-concept of ability. The second reported goal manipulation effort was from Anderman, Maehr, and Midgley (1999). Analyzing data collected during the Coalition Project described by Maehr and Midgley (1996), they found that when students moved from the last year of elementary school (5th grade) into the treatment middle school (where efforts were under way to create a mastery goal structure), they reported a slight decrease in personal performance–approach goals, whereas students entering the control middle school reported an increase in performance–approach goals. Students moving into control and treatment schools did not differ in their own mastery goal orientations or perceptions of the mastery goal structure in their classrooms.

A number of survey studies have examined the associations between student (and sometimes teacher) reports of the goal structure in the classroom and motivational, affective, and achievement outcomes. The logic of this research has been that if student and teacher reports of the mastery and performance goal structure are related to valued outcomes, such as efficacy or self-regulation, then there is support for teacher attempts to emphasize mastery goal structures and, perhaps, deemphasize performance goal structures (see Urdan, 2004, for a review). Survey measures have typically asked students about their teachers' practices that reflect mastery goals or performance goals. Mastery goal practices include encouraging students to understand the material, viewing mistakes as part of the learning process, and recognizing students for trying hard, whereas performance goal practices include making it obvious which students in the class are doing well and encouraging students to compare their performances with each other (Midgley et al., 2000). Most of this research has revealed that when students perceive a stronger emphasis on mastery goals in the classroom, they are more likely to adopt personal mastery goal orientations (Anderman & Anderman, 1999; Urdan & Midgley, 2003). Across the transition from elementary to middle school, a decline in the perceived classroom mastery goal structure has particularly negative associations with achievement, personal mastery goal pursuit, self-efficacy, and positive affect in school (Urdan & Midgley, 2003). A perceived mastery goal structure is negatively associated with avoidance behaviors, such as avoidance of help seeking, avoidance of novelty, and self-handicapping (Turner et al., 2002). These avoidance behaviors undermine the development of competence and indicate diminished competence motivation.

A limited number of observational studies have also been conducted to identify specific instructional policies and practices that might explain differences among students in their perceptions of classroom goal structures. Meece (1991) found that teachers in classrooms containing students with relatively high personal mastery goal orientations tended to use activities with clearer procedures than did teachers in classrooms containing less mastery-oriented students. Urdan, Kneisel, and Mason (1999) found that the teacher with the most consistent messages of concern for student input and personal relevance of the material had students who perceived the most mastery goal messages in the classroom and most frequently mentioned pursuing mastery goals themselves. Anderman, Patrick, Hruda, and Linnenbrink (2002) found that teachers in classrooms in which students perceived a relatively weak classroom mastery goal structure tended to emphasize the importance of following rules and procedures more than did teachers in classrooms with a stronger perceived mastery goal structure. Turner et al. (2002) discovered that greater motivational, emotional, and social support for learning during instruction was related to students' perceptions of high mastery

classrooms and their reports of low avoidance strategies. Similarly, Stipek, Givvin, Salmon, and MacGyvers (1998) found that teachers who emphasized learning, understanding, and effort, as well as positive affect, had students who reported higher mastery goals, more positive emotions, more enthusiasm, and higher conceptual scores in mathematics than students in other groups.

To summarize, achievement goal research has consistently found that a strong emphasis on mastery goals in the classroom is associated with stronger personal endorsement of mastery goals by students, more positive affect, higher achievement, greater feelings of competence, and less engagement in avoidance behaviors. Active manipulations, survey studies, and observational research have all indicated that when teachers emphasize the relevance of academic work, the importance of effort and personal growth, and are consistent in their mastery goal message, students, on average, are more likely to endorse mastery goals themselves.

Research has also revealed that an emphasis on performance goals in the classroom is related to some detrimental motivational and behavioral variables, such as greater personal performance–avoidance goal pursuit and increased use of self-handicapping (Urdan, Midgley, & Anderman, 1998). Research has often found weaker effects of classroom performance goal structures than of mastery goal structures (Urdan & Midgley, 2003), and goal researchers have more consistently emphasized the importance of strengthening mastery goal structures than of weakening performance goal structures in the classroom (e.g., Ames, 1992). Although important questions remain about how to interpret the research on classroom goal structures (Urdan, 2004), the existing evidence suggests that when teachers emphasize meaning and individual development in the classroom, students' competence motivation is enhanced.

Interest and Intrinsic Motivation

Interest is a potentially important component of competence motivation. Some have argued that human beings have an innate sense of curiosity that leads us, even from infancy, to become interested in novel, moderately challenging, dissonance-creating stimuli (White, 1959). Recent interest research has carefully distinguished between *individual* and *situational* interest (Renninger, 2000). Individual interest refers to the more stable personal disposition toward a specific topic or domain. Situational interest represents a more short-lived, situation-specific attention to a topic (Hidi & Harackiwiewicz, 2000).

Interest may be conceptualized as a component of intrinsic motivation (Hidi, 2000). Intrinsic motivation involves motivation that is free of extrinsic coercion. When intrinsically motivated, individuals engage in activities for the sake of the activity itself (Sansone & Harackiewicz, 2000). Intrinsic motivation may have a variety of sources, including needs for competence (Deci & Ryan, 1985; White, 1959), interest in the material or activity (Renninger, 2000), or perceptions of autonomy (Deci & Ryan, 1985).

Stated Implications of Interest and Intrinsic Motivation Research

Because individual interest is, by definition, idiosyncratic, it would simply be too onerous for classroom teachers to identify the individual interests of all of their students and tailor instruction to the variety of individual interests in a given classroom (Hidi & Harackiewicz, 2000). Rather, teachers should try to "catch" and then "hold" students' situational interest by manipulating the learning environment in a manner that enhances situational interest. A number of suggestions for how to do this include using humor; adding elements of fantasy and variety into the tasks; taking advantage of the social desires of students by having them work together; using puzzles and games; and choosing content that is likely to appeal to most students in the classroom, such as a unit on dinosaurs for a third-grade class (Bergin, 1999; Malone & Lepper, 1987; Pintrich, 2004). Teachers are also encouraged to model their own interest in the material and to provide examples of people who have pursued their interest in a topic. Intrinsic motivation research offers very similar suggestions for practice. Additional suggestions for fostering intrinsic motivation in the classroom include offering moderately challenging tasks to students and contextualizing academic material by linking it to students' personal lives and interests

(Malone & Lepper, 1987). Because intrinsic motivation approaches often include the supposition that individuals are naturally inclined toward developing competence and making sense of their environments, some interest researchers suggest that promoting students' perceptions of autonomy (Ryan & Grolnick, 1986) and emphasizing mastery goals will promote intrinsic motivation in the classroom.

Empirical Support for the Stated Implications

Although a number of studies of interest and intrinsic motivation have been conducted with school-age children, very few have occurred within the natural setting of classrooms. Harter (1982) demonstrated that school-age children distinguish between perceived competence in various domains (cognitive, social, and physical), and that competence is related to intrinsic motivation. Others have also demonstrated an association between intrinsic motivation and perceived competence among children (Boggiano, Main, & Katz, 1988). Research has also demonstrated a link between appropriate challenge and intrinsic motivation (Harter, 1978). What is missing from this research is a direct link to classroom practices (Pintrich, 2004). Although Harter (1978) argued that adult caregivers are important socializing agents of mastery motivation, and Bandura (1986) demonstrated that models and reinforcement influence children's internalization of mastery goals, research conducted in classrooms to determine how teachers affect students' intrinsic motivation is scarce.

Self-Efficacy

Self-efficacy refers to individuals' judgments of their capabilities to perform specific tasks in specific situations (Bandura, 1986; Pajares, 1996). Students are more likely to engage and persist in an activity, and they exert more effort during the activity, when they believe they are able to succeed at the activity. Efficacy beliefs can be as powerful a predictor of achievement as measures of cognitive ability (Pajares & Kranzler, 1995). Of course, because self-efficacy judgments require some consideration of the skills one possesses, ability and efficacy judgments are usually highly correlated.

Bandura (1986) argued that self-efficacy judgments are created from four different sources: (1) experience (i.e., success or failure on similar tasks); (2) vicarious experience, such as observing the success or failure of models, particularly similar models; (3) verbal persuasion, particularly from a respected or otherwise credible source; and (4) physical cues, such as sweating and shortness of breath upon seeing the difficulty of questions on an exam. These four sources of efficacy form the basis for the educational implications of efficacy research.

Stated Implications of Self-Efficacy Research

Teachers can influence their students' self-efficacy by attending to both the definition and sources of efficacy judgments. Because self-efficacy is, by definition, task- or activity-specific, teachers can encourage students to think about the specific skills they have and need to complete a given task rather than to make global judgments about their competence. Even students who think of themselves as poor at math can be encouraged to have high confidence about their ability to succeed at a specific math activity for which they possess the requisite skills. Schunk and Miller (2002) listed several specific strategies that teachers might employ to enhance their students' feelings of self-efficacy. These include helping students set proximal and specific learning goals; specifically teaching students how and when to use various learning strategies; providing students with opportunities to witness models completing the same or similar tasks, particularly models who are similar to students in age or ability; offering students feedback about their performance that focuses on the students' use of specific strategies (e.g., "You did a good job remembering to borrow from the hundreds column on that subtraction problem") rather than general feedback (e.g., "Nice job"); and judiciously using rewards based on performance.

Empirical Support for the Stated Implications

Most of the research examining self-efficacy has not examined educational processes within K–12 classrooms. Therefore, most of the empirical support for the stated implications of self-efficacy research must be inferred from research conducted outside of classrooms. Much of this research was conducted by Schunk and his colleagues in the 1980s (e.g., Schunk, 1984; Schunk, Hanson, & Cox, 1987). All of these studies were experiments rather than classroom-based examinations of students' responses to their teachers' instructional practices. An experimenter typically offered some form of instruction to students individually, and the effects of these instructions on self-efficacy were examined. The research suggests that self-efficacy is enhanced when students observe successful models, develop and pursue proximal goals, and learn how to use (and vocalize the use of) effective self-regulatory strategies.

A number of survey studies have also assessed the associations between self-efficacy and certain motivational and achievement variables among K–12 students in their regular classrooms. Some of these have used authentic tasks (e.g., teacher-designed tests that were counted as part of the students' grades in the class) as the criterion tasks on which self-efficacy judgments were based (Pajares, Miller, & Johnson, 1999; Shell, Colvin, & Bruning, 1995). Although these studies revealed that self-efficacy judgments were strong predictors of achievement in the classroom, they did not examine teacher behaviors or classroom processes that might influence students' self-efficacy judgments. It is difficult to determine whether the stated implications of the experimental and correlational research apply to the question of how competence motivation might be enhanced by increasing self-efficacy in the classroom.

Expectancy–Value Theory

Expectancy–value theory states that both students' expectancy for success and their value for academic activities predict motivational outcomes such as achievement, involvement, and academic choices. It differs from other approaches that emphasize competence as the central motive. Expectancy–value research argues that "even if people are certain they can do a task, they may not *want* to engage in it" (Eccles, Wigfield, & Schiefele, 1998, p. 1028). Expectancy–value research has demonstrated that both expectancy and value make distinct and complementary contributions to students' performance and reports of motivated behaviors, such as effort and persistence (Eccles, 1983; Wigfield & Eccles, 1992), and to the use of self-regulatory strategies (Pintrich & De Groot, 1990). In addition, studies have shown that adolescents' subjective task values predicted taking math and English classes, engaging in sports activities, and choosing a college major (e.g., Eccles, 1983; Meece, Wigfield, & Eccles, 1990).

Although none of this research explicitly examined classroom factors that might contribute to students' expectancy or value beliefs, it was conducted with K–12 students in classroom settings. On the basis of the positive associations found among value, expectancies, motivation, self-regulation, and achievement, expectancy–value theory researchers have argued that their research has important implications for classroom practice.

Stated Implications of Expectancy–Value Theory

To encourage students to develop subjective task value, teachers are encouraged to promote active participation and student control by providing some options, such as when, where, how, and which activities students pursue, and to avoid controlling statements and behaviors. In addition, teachers should select topics and activities that are authentic and meaningful to help their students discover the importance and utility value of the material. To promote a sense of competence and high expectancies for success, teachers are encouraged to provide moderately challenging tasks that help students see improvement. In addition, teachers should emphasize learning by providing specific feedback on progress and strategy use (rather than relative standing), communicating expectations that all students can and will learn, and attributing performance to effort. Teachers are also encouraged to create a supportive and caring classroom community that makes students feel valued and safe to take academic risks.

Empirical Support for the Stated Implications

A series of studies conducted by Eccles, Midgley, and their colleagues examined declines in students' expectancies and values as they made the transition from elementary to middle school. Eccles and Midgley (1989)

hypothesized that these negative changes might be related to a mismatch between students' developmental needs for autonomy, competence, and relatedness, and classroom practices in middle school. Midgley and Feldlaufer (1987) found that after the transition, students desired but had fewer decision-making opportunities than in elementary school. This mismatch predicted a decline in students' value (Mac Iver & Reuman, 1988). After the transition to middle school, practices that may have increased the opportunities for social comparison were related to declines in students' perceptions of competence (Eccles et al., 1989). In addition, students who moved from high- to low-efficacy teachers during the transition had lower expectancies for success in math, lower perceptions of their performance in math, and higher perceptions of the difficulty of math (Midgley, Feldlaufer, & Eccles, 1989). Finally, students who moved from teachers they rated high in supportiveness to teachers rated low in supportiveness during the transition reported a decline in their ratings of intrinsic value, perceived usefulness, and importance of math (Feldlaufer, Midgley, & Eccles, 1988).

In another study (Eccles, 1983), observers attended mathematics classes to determine which teacher behaviors were related to students' motivation. They found that teachers' expectations influenced both achievement expectancies and course taking. For girls, the number of response opportunities and the number of open questions were positively related to value (liking) of math. In summary, data collected in classrooms showed definite relationships between teacher behaviors and students' reports of expectancy and value.

Self-Determination Theory

Self-determination theory (SDT) argues that human beings have three innate needs: competence, autonomy, and relatedness (Deci & Ryan, 1985). It is the satisfaction of these needs that leads to intrinsic motivation. Much classroom-related research has focused on the autonomy component, because SDT contends that only freely chosen, rather than coerced, actions can be experienced as intrinsic. This may provide a theoretical rationale for why some students, even when they learn, feel little joy or pride: learning that is controlled by others is not owned.

SDT theorists acknowledge that not all school learning is intrinsically motivating. Nevertheless, they argue that one can gradually internalize extrinsic reasons for completing necessary, but unappealing, activities and, thus, infuse agency into daily learning activities. As motives for engaging in tasks become more internalized, the potential for self-determination and autonomy increases. If self-determination-promoting teacher behaviors can be shown to promote gradual internalization of extrinsic motivation in the classroom, the SDT model would have important applications in the classroom.

Stated Implications of Self-Determination Theory

Students in K–12 classrooms typically have little control over classroom activities, so much research in this tradition has focused on the negative effects of controlling behaviors. Because some research has revealed that teachers' controlling behaviors are related to decreases in students' intrinsic motivation and achievement, as well as increased feelings of anger and anxiety (Assor, Kaplan, Kanat-Maymon, & Roth, in press), SDT recommends that teachers refrain from overtly controlling student behaviors. Giving students incompetence feedback, imposing strict deadlines, using threats and competition to control behavior, giving frequent directives, interfering with children's natural pace of learning, and not allowing expression of critical or independent opinions are all discouraged by SDT researchers. Instead, teachers are encouraged to provide optimal challenges, informational feedback, interesting and stimulating material and assignments, and opportunities to view effort as a key contributor to performance (Deci & Ryan, 1985). Teachers are also encouraged to show affection, express interest in students' activities, and devote time and resources to students (Assor & Kaplan, 2001).

Empirical Support for the Stated Implications

Most SDT research has used experimental or survey research designs in classrooms. We could find no studies that used observation or interview methods. A few studies used student reports of the autonomy supportiveness of teachers in classrooms, and then linked these reports to measures of student motivation and achievement. Higher perceived support for autonomy in the classroom was related to higher intrinsic motivation, mastery motivation, perceived competence, and self-esteem (Deci, Schwartz, Sheinman, & Ryan, 1981; Ryan & Grolnick, 1986).

Although SDT studies have not taken measures of teachers' actual classroom behaviors, an experimental study of student teachers showed that autonomy-supportive instruction included listening, asking questions about what the student wanted, responding to student-initiated questions, and offering statements that acknowledged the student's perspective (Reeve, Bolt, & Cai, 1999). This study did not examine potential links between these teacher behaviors and student motivation or achievement.

Skinner and Belmont (1993) found that third- to fifth-grade students who perceived the greatest amount of structure, autonomy support, and involvement in the classroom had teachers who were dependable and showed affection for, were attuned to, and dedicated time and energy to, their students. Students of high-involvement teachers also reported the most behavioral engagement, such as effort and persistence, and positive emotion, such as interest and happiness. Assor and Kaplan (2001) investigated the relation between students' perceptions of their teachers' directly controlling and autonomy-supportive behaviors and their motivation while studying. Directly controlling teacher behaviors predicted mostly negative student feelings (i.e., anger, stress, boredom) during learning, whereas autonomy-supportive behaviors predicted positive feelings (i.e., interest and enjoyment). Perceptions of competence were related to enjoyment of learning as well.

Two studies investigated the relation between autonomy-supportive classrooms and dropping out of high school. Each found that teacher autonomy support was related to student perceptions of competence, autonomy, and intention to persist in, or drop out of, school (Hardre & Reeve, 2003; Vallerand, Fortier, & Guay, 1997). Additional research examined predictors of achievement and school adjustment among students with learning disabilities and those with emotional handicaps (Deci, Hodges, Pierson, & Tomassone, 1992). For students with learning disabilities, competence was the best predictor of achievement and adjustment. Interestingly, perceived autonomy best predicted these outcomes for students with emotional handicaps. This study suggests that different needs may be more salient for different students, and that focusing on meeting one need, such as competence, may not serve all students best. In summary, SDT studies have linked autonomy, as well as perceptions of autonomy and competence in the classroom, to achievement and to behavioral, motivational, and emotional outcomes for students. However, studies of how teachers establish autonomy-supportive classrooms have not yet been done.

Attribution Theory and Control Beliefs

The importance of perceived control in the development and support of competence motivation has been a central focus of attribution research and Dweck's (1999) work on theories of intelligence and locus-of-control constructs. The basic premise of this research is that when students believe that their academic achievement depends on controllable factors, they are more motivated and generally achieve at higher levels than when they feel a lack of control over their own learning (Pintrich, 2004; Weiner, 1986). Although it may be more adaptive at the situation-specific level for students to attribute failure to unstable, uncontrollable causes (e.g., bad luck or a particularly difficult exam), at the individual-difference level, greater perceptions of control are associated with increased motivation. As de Charms (1968) argued, it can be difficult to feel competent when one feels like a "pawn" rather than an "origin" of behavior.

Implications of Attribution Theory and Control Beliefs

To help their students develop or maintain a sense of personal control over their learning and achievement, teachers have been encouraged to assess their students' attributions for success and failure, to provide feedback that encourages students to recognize the control they have over their learning,

and to alter attributional styles that diminish their sense of control (i.e., attributional retraining) (Pintrich & Schunk, 2002). Dweck (1999) suggested that when providing students with feedback, teachers should emphasize process factors, such as effort, the use of appropriate strategies, and individual growth, rather than just the end result as a means of encouraging students to adopt an incremental view of ability. Attribution research has highlighted the importance of feedback that is both accurate and, particularly in the case of failure, focused on the unstable, changeable causes for failure (Blumenfeld, Pintrich, Meece, & Wessels, 1982). In some cases, teachers have been encouraged to engage in ongoing attribution retraining with students to help them develop controllable attributions that can replace helpless attribution patterns (Foersterling, 1985).

Empirical Support for the Stated Implications

Although there is substantial evidence from experimental research that attributions for success and failure can be changed from uncontrollable, stable attributions to controllable attributions, there is little research demonstrating a link between teacher behaviors and student attributions in classrooms. Research from the 1980s revealed that teacher feedback about the causes of success and failure can influence students' perceptions of their own ability and effort (Pintrich & Blumenfeld, 1985). But it also revealed that teachers favor effort feedback and rarely offer ability feedback or attributions (Blumenfeld et al., 1982). When teachers do make ability attributions or give ability feedback (e.g., "You must be really smart in math!"), it is likely to be salient, because it is rare. Research on the effects and student interpretations of such unusual feedback is scarce.

Rosenholtz and Simpson (1984) argued that whole-group (rather than cooperative or individualized) instruction, ability grouping, and providing public feedback fostered social comparison and encouraged students to think of ability as stable. Rosenholtz and Wilson (1980) demonstrated this in surveys of fifth- and sixth-grade students. They found that some students were quite able to perceive ability messages that teachers made salient. Such messages may have been particularly damaging to low-ability students, a group most likely to adopt ego-protective strategies (Covington, 1992), reducing effort, persistence, and intrinsic motivation. Experimental studies have also demonstrated that children interpret pity and excessive help as signals to make low-ability attributions and to set lowered expectations for success (Graham, 1984). Also, teachers' use of praise (to preserve the egos of low achievers) and criticism (to express high expectations for high achievers) can influence low-ability students' motivation negatively.

Other Research Related to Competence Beliefs in the Classroom

Motivational Influence of Effective Instruction

Some research on teacher influences on student competence motivation has been conducted outside of the major motivation frameworks described previously. Stipek, Salmon, et al. (1998) argued that "best practices," as advocated in the instructional literature, have positive influences on competence motivation primarily through stressing appropriately challenging and meaningful tasks, emphasizing learning and improvement, and encouraging students' active participation and autonomy. Turner et al. (1998) found that when teachers used appropriately challenging mathematics instruction, students reported the highest intrinsic motivation (and the least boredom).

Teachers' Beliefs and Emotions

Teachers' beliefs regarding ability (malleable vs. fixed), their expectations (Weinstein, 2002) and their own efficacy to teach (Ashton & Webb, 1986; Midgley et al., 1989) should affect the teaching practices used, which, in turn, create a climate that focuses children's attention on either improving or demonstrating competence, or avoiding demonstration of incompetence.

Weinstein (2002) demonstrated that even young children perceive teacher differential treatment and teacher expectations in the classroom. If students perceive low expectations from their teacher, they may develop low perceptions of ability and reduce effort in the classroom. Using interviews with children, Weinstein found that students learned about teacher expectations and perceptions of student ability by attending to the type of work they were assigned, things the teachers said, when and how much they offered help, the type of feedback they give, and even teachers' nonverbal cues, such as facial expressions and tone of voice. Children reported that teachers' feedback was often public and comparative rather than private and focused on individual progress or quality of their work. Children's motivation and liking of the subject matter declined when they perceived low expectations and low-ability cues. Based on classroom observations, Weinstein concluded that certain features were likely to send messages about expectations. They included grouping, materials, evaluation system, motivational strategies, responsibility given to children, and relationships in class (warmth, trust, humor, and concern) with peers, and with teachers.

SUMMARY OF RECOMMENDATIONS FOR ENHANCING COMPETENCE MOTIVATION IN CLASSROOMS

There is quite a bit of overlap across the various motivational approaches previously reviewed regarding the suggestions for promoting competence motivation in the classroom. Synthesizing across research programs, we developed the following list of suggested classroom practices. Table 17.1 summarizes this list, as well as the motivational perspectives that support each recommendation and potential difficulties of implementing them.

1. Develop and assign academic tasks and activities that are personally meaningful and relevant for students.
2. Develop and assign moderately, or appropriately, challenging tasks and material.
3. Promote perceptions of control and autonomy by allowing students to make choices about classroom experience and the work in which they engage. Also, encourage students to view intelligence, learning, and performance as personally controllable by attributing performance to controllable factors such as effort and strategy use. Avoid controlling or coercive language and instructional practices.

4. Encourage students to focus on mastery, skill development, and the process of learning rather than just focusing on outcomes such as test scores or relative performance.
5. Help students develop and pursue proximal, challenging, achievable goals.
6. Infuse the curriculum with fantasy, novelty, variety, and humor.
7. Provide accurate, informational feedback focused on strategy use and competence development rather than social–comparative or simply evaluative feedback.
8. Assess students' confidence, attributional tendencies, and skill levels to help meet their preferences for challenge and to help students approach tasks with realistic expectations and cope with difficulties adaptively.

Despite their appeal, many of these recommendations are not based on classroom research, and the recommendations for the application of these motivational principles have often not been tested in classrooms. In the next section, we raise some questions about the applicability of the empirical support for the stated classroom applications and implications of motivation research.

CAUTIONS ABOUT APPLYING MOTIVATION PRINCIPLES IN CLASSROOMS

With the exception of research on achievement goals and expectancy–value research, there have been few studies examining the association between teacher practices and student motivation in the classroom. There is ample reason to suspect that many of the stated implications of motivation research for classroom practice will not actually work in the classroom as predicted (Blumenfeld, 1992). In fact, some empirical research calls both theoretical claims and recommended practices into question. Although research has explored many of the factors that contribute to individuals' becoming and feeling competent, it is not clear that these conditions can be created regularly in the classroom. In many classrooms, there are greater incentives for students to *be* competent or to *appear* competent than there are for *becoming* competent. Becoming compe-

tent generally involves effort and risking failure. Both of these may be more problematic in classrooms than in experimental research situations. In this section, we consider a nonexhaustive list of several factors that may inhibit the application of motivation principles in the classroom. First, we consider two general questions about the relevance of applying research to practice. Then, we consider how the application of specific motivational principles, simple as they may seem, is complicated by the complex nature of classrooms.

• *Can experimental research be applied to classrooms?* Much of the research on competence motivation has been conducted using experimental methods. In these studies, participants are generally taken out of their regular classrooms and given some sort of individual instruction or training, and the effects of the instruction or training on subsequent motivation are examined (e.g., Schunk's self-efficacy studies in the 1980s, attribution retraining, achievement goal manipulations; Elliot & Harackiewicz, 1996). Although this research has clearly demonstrated that motivation can be influenced by such manipulations, there are a number of reasons to suspect that these experimental conditions cannot be recreated in regular classrooms. First, the sheer number of students in most classrooms makes individualized instruction, such as that used in attribution retraining, difficult. Second, the motivational messages salient in most classrooms tend to be much more mixed than those found in the typical experiment. For example, experimental manipulations of achievement goals typically involve telling participants in different conditions that the purpose of the task is to pursue a single goal (e.g., do better than other students). In classrooms, students are often given mixed goal messages. For example, students may be encouraged to focus on their own improvement but may be evaluated in either normative or absolute grading systems that disregard improvement. Third, the meaning of tasks or instructions may differ in classrooms and experimental conditions. For example, a focus on achieving short-term, proximal goals may enhance efficacy and motivation in experimental settings but may be embarrassing and demotivating in a more

TABLE 17.1. Summary of Recommended Classroom Practices for Enhancing Competence Motivation

Recommended practice	Theoretical proponent	Empirical support	Limitations of empirical support	Barriers to classroom application
1. Develop and assign academic tasks and activities that are personally meaningful and relevant for students.	Achievement goal research, E-V theory, SDT, intrinsic motivation and interest research	Some evidence from E-V research, interest research, intrinsic motivation, and goal theory show an emphasis on meaning related to greater engagement and motivation.	Meaning and relevance of academic work almost never examined in actual classroom settings.	Very difficult to individualize instruction like this; hard to know what is meaningful to all students; more difficult than following prescribed curriculum.
2. Develop and assign moderately or appropriately challenging tasks and material.	Achievement goal research, SDT, intrinsic and interest, E-V, self-efficacy	Experimental research in several motivation programs shows engagement higher on moderately challenging tasks.	As with meaning and relevance, challenge level rarely examined in classrooms. Some evidence that students resist challenge.	Teachers often not good at designing tasks of appropriate challenge; students resist challenge.
3. Promote perceptions of control and autonomy by allowing students to make choices about classroom experience and the work they engage in (e.g., what books to read, how to demonstrate knowledge, etc.). Also encourage students to view intelligence, learning, and performance as personally controllable by attributing performance to controllable factors like effort and strategy use. Avoid controlling or coercive language and instructional practices.	Achievement goal research, attribution theory, Dweck's "theories of intelligence" research, SDT	Attribution research on benefits of controllable attributions; Dweck's research on malleable intelligence theories; E-V research demonstrating declines in value, competence perceptions associated with declines in perceived control; SDT research demonstrates that perceptions of autonomy are related to positive student outcomes including interest, competence perceptions, positive affect, and self-esteem.	Attribution and theory of intelligence research tends to be experimental; little research observing how teachers promote autonomy and control beliefs in the classroom, or how students perceive autonomy-supportive and coercive teacher practices. Mostly survey research in SDT and E-V areas.	Can be difficult for teachers to walk the fine line between promoting autonomy and offering too little scaffolding for learning. Encouraging students to attribute performance to effort can backfire if high effort leads to low performance. Teachers under increasing pressure to follow narrow curriculum; increase in student test scores can cause them to be more coercive with their students.

#	Principle	Related theories/concepts	Research base	Research characteristics	Problems/caveats
4.	Encourage students to focus on mastery, skill development, and the process of learning rather than just focusing on outcomes like test scores or relative performance.	Achievement goal research, attribution theory, self-efficacy, E-V theory, SDT	Student perceptions of mastery goal structures; observational studies of classroom goal structures; Schunk et al. studies of strategy training; attribution retraining studies	Surveys and observations make causal direction difficult to determine, but they were at least looking at genuine classroom processes; variation in perceptions of classroom goal messages; SE, attribution studies were experimental.	Can produce mixed message when grades are based on absolute performance level and test scores are norm-referenced. Social comparison can be motivating for many students; occurs naturally.
5.	Help students develop and pursue proximal, challenging, achievable goals.	Self-efficacy	Series of studies by Schunk and colleagues; Shell and colleagues; Pajares and colleagues	Schunk et al. were experimental—may not replicate in classrooms. Shell, Pajares studies were survey—did not focus on classroom processes.	Requires individualizing instruction which is time-consuming. Difficult for teachers to know level of all students and to design appropriately challenging tasks.
6.	Infuse the curriculum with fantasy, novelty, and humor.	Interest and intrinsic motivation	Summarized by Bergin; Malone & Lepper; Lepper & Henderlong	Based on experiments and computer applications; not examined in classrooms	Can detract from primary concepts to be learned; more difficult than following textbook.
7.	Provide students with competence feedback that is informational, not just evaluative.	Self-efficacy, SDT, E-V, attribution, achievement goal research, teacher expectancies	Schunk experiments; SDT research on controlling practices; Weinstein research on teacher expectancies	Based mostly on experiments in self-efficacy, SDT, and intrinsic motivation research	Summative evaluations are required in school. Grades become most valued feedback for students.
8.	Assess students' knowledge, self-efficacy, and attributional patterns in order to select optimally challenging tasks for them, approach tasks with realistic expectations, and explain failures adaptively.	Self-efficacy, attribution theory, SDT	Alfi, Katz, & Assor; Clifford	There is little or no research reporting teachers' assessments of these student characteristics in real K–12 classrooms.	Difficult to accurately assess skills, attributional tendencies, and self-efficacy for all students in large classes, particularly secondary level. Efficacy attributions may be highly task specific, difficult to assess constantly.

Note. E-V, expectancy–value theory; SDT, self-determination theory.

public setting such as classrooms. Pursuing proximal goals that are much less advanced than one's classmates may be humiliating, whereas focusing on long-range, distal goals, even if they are not achievable, may help some students save face in front of their classroom peers.

• *Do survey and experimental research provide an accurate picture of the classroom?* Students' responses to surveys or behavior in experiments may offer a distorted view of the classroom. As previously mentioned, in experimental situations, students often respond to clear instructions in predictable ways. Similarly, responses to researcher-provided, closed-ended survey questions regularly produce predictable associations between students' perceptions of the classroom motivational climate and their own motivational orientations. But when researchers have actually examined what happens in classrooms, they find that teacher and student behavior does not always conform to theoretical specifications and is often unpredictable. This may be related to the fact that most theory is deductive and based on what is logical rather than empirical (Turner & Meyer, 1999). Urdan and his colleagues (1999) found that teachers rarely discussed goals, and students often did not perceive even the most blatant goal messages, as theory would predict. Miller and Meece (1997) found that even when the teachers they worked with to modify their reading and language arts assignments faithfully implemented the intervention, their third-grade students' achievement and strategy use was not altered. Meece (1991) found that classrooms with higher average levels of student mastery goal orientation did not differ from those with lower average levels of mastery goal orientation in either the cognitive complexity of the tasks assigned or the grouping patterns of students. Patrick, Anderman, Ryan, Edelin, and Midgley (2001) found that classrooms that differed in their perceived levels of mastery and performance goal structures did not differ in the frequency with which students were asked to demonstrate their knowledge publicly or the use of extrinsic rewards. Similarly, Turner and her colleagues (2002) discovered that social comparison in classrooms perceived as having a high performance focus was related less to public evaluation per se and more to nuanced factors, such as teacher af-

fect, and to instructional practices. These observational studies all found that elements of instruction believed to influence the motivational goals of students (e.g., types of tasks, social organization of students, how students were rewarded or recognized, how public demonstration of knowledge was) did not necessarily work in ways predicted by theory or by the results of survey and experimental studies.

Survey and experimental research may also distort the true nature of teacher influence on student motivation in classrooms. Such research typically suggests a unidirectional flow of influence from teachers to students. In reality, the motivational climate in classrooms is produced by a reciprocal exchange of messages that flows constantly between students and teachers, and among students themselves. For example, when students in a classroom report that their teacher uses instructional practices that reflect a mastery goal orientation and create a mastery goal structure in the classroom, it is possible that the teacher has adopted those strategies in response to her perception that the students were motivated by mastery messages. By appropriately responding to students' preferences, the teacher may also reinforce students' mastery goal orientations. It is hard to trace the causal flow of motivational influences in classrooms. Survey studies that reveal an association between teacher practices and students' motivation may not accurately reflect the direction of causal influence.

• *Can teachers really encourage students to seek challenge?* Just as the academic environment provides opportunities to become and feel competent, it offers a wide array of opportunities to be and feel incompetent. Fear of being incompetent can motivate some students to exert additional effort, with an eye toward achieving success, but it can also be demotivating, causing students to adopt an avoidance goal orientation in achievement situations and withdraw effort (Elliot, 1997).

As an example of the double-edged sword of competence motivation, consider the stated implication of a number of motivation approaches that teachers should assign moderately challenging tasks to students. Such tasks are believed to stimulate interest, encourage intrinsic motivation, and spur the adoption of a mastery goal orientation. Although many students find challenging tasks motivating, for a number of students, these types of tasks arouse fear, because challenging tasks carry opportunities for failure. Research has clearly documented a link between fear of failure and the adoption of performance–avoidance goals (Elliot, 1999). When such failure occurs in front of teachers and peers, as it does in classrooms, the fear of appearing and feeling incompetent often causes students to adopt defensive, withdrawing behaviors in class. The same type of activity that can spur competence motivation in an experiment may, for many students, lead to a lack of effort and motivation, and the adoption of self-handicapping strategies (Urdan & Midgley, 2001). Unfortunately, in many classrooms, it may be worse to try and fail than to not try at all.

Even when teachers want to provide challenging tasks for students, there is considerable evidence that their efforts may not be fruitful (Blumenfeld, 1992). Because students understand the inherent dangers of failing at challenging tasks, they often resist this type of work and try to negotiate down the demands of the task with the teacher (Doyle, 1986). In addition, research shows that teachers are not particularly adept at developing or selecting appropriately challenging tasks (Bennett, DesForges, Cockburn, & Wilkinson, 1984). Teachers often select tasks that do not match the skills and abilities of their students well, partly because most classrooms contain students with a wide range of abilities. Finally, teachers do not always understand how to support students when engaged in challenging work, and this may discourage students from persisting (Turner, Meyer, Midgley, & Patrick, 2003). This combination of factors may discourage teachers from assigning creative or challenging work and lead them to settle for lower level facts, algorithms, or even completion as indicators of learning and achievement. To achieve the balance of high cognitive demand and the safety necessary for students to respond positively, challenge needs to be offered in a classroom that stresses mastery goals and the constructive value of error (Clifford, 1984). Most classrooms are not very successful at helping students see error as informational, possibly because many teachers rely on correct answers to know that students are learning.

• *Can teachers provide interesting, meaningful, and relevant tasks*? Many motiva-

tional researchers suggest that teachers create and select interesting and relevant tasks for students. This is very difficult for most teachers to do. Students' interests and values are so varied that it is hard for teachers to find material or tasks that most or all students will find personally meaningful or interesting. Recognizing this difficulty, some researchers have suggested that teachers try to stimulate students' *situational* interest by selecting broadly appealing topics that most children of a certain age would find appealing, or by incorporating elements of fantasy, humor, novelty, and variety into classwork (Bergin, 1999; Hidi, 2000). Although these may be good ideas, in practice, teachers often are confined to following a fairly narrow curriculum that is heavily dependent on textbooks. Research suggests that efforts to enliven the material in textbooks often fail, leading to an obfuscation of the content goals (Brophy & Alleman, 1991). Blumenfeld (1992) argued that trying to make classroom tasks or materials more interesting by adding variety, novelty, and humor can actually "detract from a focus on the real content and problem and probably does not sustain motivation to learn over the long haul" (p. 273). In the end, it may be the teacher's interest in the task that helps students to see its value and relevance, rather than characteristics of the task itself.

• *Can student autonomy and control really be encouraged in classrooms?* Self-determination theory, achievement goal approaches, and attribution theory all emphasize the importance of students' perceiving that they have some control over learning. When students feel that their participation is not voluntary, and that educational outcomes (particularly bad ones) are beyond their control, competence motivation is reduced. Given the compulsory nature of K–12 education, the increasing standardization of the curriculum and emphasis on high-stakes testing, and strong criticism of too much choice offered by "shopping mall" high schools, developing a sense of autonomy in school may be problematic. Can students feel like origins rather than pawns when they are told they must go to school, must read selected textbooks, and must pass certain tests to advance to the next grade or graduate? Even as their choices about which classes to take are being ever reduced? We suspect that students, particularly adolescents, develop an understanding of their lack of autonomy in schools.

Attribution theory suggests that teachers can encourage students to develop a sense of control by encouraging them to view performance, particularly poor performance, as attributable to effort. But when students try hard and fail, as many do, it becomes difficult to avoid attributing failure to a stable, uncontrollable lack of ability. In addition, certain teacher beliefs may clash with the goal of supporting students' perceptions of control. For example, teachers of early adolescents tend to believe that they need to exert more control over students than do teachers of elementary school children, thereby potentially reducing adolescents' sense of autonomy in the classroom (Midgley & Feldlaufer, 1987). Teachers who lack a sense of efficacy to influence the performance of their students, particularly their lower achieving students, have difficulty helping their students view achievement as personally controllable (Tschannen-Moran, Hoy, & Hoy, 1998). In addition, teachers who tend to attribute student achievement to relatively stable factors, such as intelligence, socioeconomic status, or race, may send messages about low expectations and therefore be less inclined to encourage their students to view effort as the cause of academic success and failure (Weinstein, 2002). Finally, as teachers come under increasing pressure to have their students perform well on standardized tests, they may feel the need to exert greater control over their students, thereby reducing students' perceptions of their own agency (Pelletier, Seguin-Levesque, & Legault, 2002).

• *Do teachers understand or value the recommended applications of motivation research?* If principles of motivation research are to be applied in the classroom, teachers will have to endorse them. It is not at all clear that they do, either because they have had little opportunity to learn about research in motivation, or because they do not accept the principles or believe they will work. As previously mentioned, many do not believe that students should have control and voice in the classroom. Although a number of achievement goal researchers have argued that an emphasis on competition in the classroom can produce fears among students that may activate avoidance motivation, research indicates that many teachers believe in the motivational power of competition (Thorkildsen & Nicholls, 1998). Many simply view students as unmotivated and do not endorse the premise that human beings have a natural inclination to understand and master new material. They think that students and families bear responsibility for motivation, not teachers (Urdan, Midgley, & Wood, 1995). Teachers' efficacy and attributions for student achievement influence their beliefs about whether they can influence their students' motivation and, therefore, their willingness to try.

Even if teachers wanted to apply some or all of the motivation principles in their classrooms, a number of practical constraints would inhibit their efforts. One of these is that the jargon of motivation research, usually developed by psychologists, is not readily understood or accessible to teachers (or anyone who has not devoted years to the study of motivation). Another constraint is that the faithful implementation of even one or two of the practices recommended by motivation researchers would require significant changes in teachers' regular practices. Although change is very time-consuming, teachers are afforded little time to change instructional practices. Tollefson (2000) argued that before teachers alter their teaching styles, school structures must be altered to encourage the professional development of teachers. Dividing teachers into separate classrooms teaching large numbers of students in discrete academic disciplines inhibits sharing of information among teachers and leaves little time for meaningful instructional innovation. Simply telling teachers what they should do to enhance the competence motivation of their students is clearly not enough to make it happen. It may take a much larger vision, involving an understanding of how research can contribute to practice (Burkardt & Schoenfeld, 2004). This is a general concern in educational research, not just in motivation.

FUTURE DIRECTIONS

To better understand how competence motivation can flourish in classrooms, we need to expand our focus and our methods, and to develop theories of motivation based on studies of classrooms. Enlarging the focus will entail casting our view beyond the individual to individuals and contexts. It will require generative thinking beyond paradigms that have dominated in psychology. Central to these goals is a way to understand the reciprocal relationships among people and between people and contexts. Such approaches have been used to examine content learning, but they have not been extended to "motivational learning."

Enlarging methods will involve spending time with teachers and students in their own settings, and finding ways to hear their voices, understand their thinking, and interpret their actions. More importantly, researchers and teachers must learn how to communicate their respective knowledge, both research- and practice-based. Enlarging theories might involve one of several possibilities. First, classroom research might help us change, elaborate, or consolidate existing theories of motivation. Second, other theories of learning, such as sociocultural approaches, might be adapted to understand competence motivation in classrooms. Third, new theories might emerge from inductive, grounded studies of motivation in classrooms. The recommendations that follow describe specific approaches that are consistent with our view of future directions in competence motivation research.

Conduct Observational and Ethnographic Studies

We need to identify the types of behaviors that teachers actually engage in during instruction. Descriptions of teacher practices may show that some practices thought to be important are not, or are superceded by others. Similarly, research might help explain under which conditions practices such as social comparison are harmful or neutral. These observations may either reflect the recommendations of motivation research or help construct new theories of motivation. Specifically, how do teachers make material interesting and relevant to students? How do they help students feel efficacious? How do they challenge students without scaring them? How do they encourage students to feel in control of their learning, to attribute their performance to effort, and to think of their ability as malleable? We do not know

enough about what this looks like in classrooms.

Include Students in the Equation

We need to talk to students about specific teacher behaviors and classroom events. Limited qualitative research has already revealed that the presence of motivational cues in the classroom does not ensure that students will attend to them or interpret them as predicted; thus, only certain messages may be relevant to students. Which messages make an impression? Are certain student needs, such as feelings of safety and relatedness in the classroom, prerequisite to satisfying others, such as competence motivation? How much do student characteristics (e.g., age, achievement level, identity) affect their attention to and interpretation of these motivational messages? Assumptions about the transmission process from teachers' practices to students' motivational orientations may not be supported in the classroom and need to be validated through discussions with students.

Conduct Intervention Studies

Teachers often do not apply motivational principles in the classroom spontaneously. For instance, some research indicates that teachers rarely explicitly discuss goals or make a conscious effort to emphasize mastery goals rather than performance goals. Based on findings from observational studies, interventions such as design experiments could be particularly effective in examining how certain motivational principles can be put into practice in specific settings. Once tried and revised in certain settings, the resulting principles could be extended to a larger number of sites in different contexts. This kind of research, although difficult and expensive, would be one way both to discover *what* works and to learn *how* it works.

Expand Our Notion of Competence Motivation

Competence is related not only to beliefs about efficacy but also to other factors, such as value, autonomy, and relatedness. In a classroom, these individual motivations are

likely related and interdependent, so that
satisfying one is positively related to satisfying others. This suggests that there may be
many routes to competence motivation, and
that it is a multidimensional construct. Furthermore, we suggest that satisfying motivational needs is not an individual endeavor,
but is interwoven with the concerns of
teachers, students, and even school and
community cultures. Therefore, ecological
features such as a climate of trust and safety,
built upon serious attention to the social dynamics in the classroom, must exist for approach motivation to succeed over fear and
avoidance motivation. Seeking challenge,
taking responsibility and ownership over
learning, and viewing learning as a developmental process that involves mistakes
(rather than simply a fixed ability) are all
threatening, particularly in large classes
filled with one's peers. For that reason, we
believe that the larger picture, that of the
classroom, should be the focus of our research on competence motivation in the decades ahead.

REFERENCES

Alfi, O., Katz, I., & Assor, A. (2004). Learning to allow
temporary failure: Potential benefits, supportive
practices and teacher concerns. *Journal of Education
for Teaching, 30,* 27–41.
Ames, C. A. (1990, April). *The relationship of achievement goals to student motivation in classroom settings.* Paper presented at the meeting of the American Educational Research Association, Boston, MA.
Ames, C. A. (1992). Classrooms: Goals, structures, and
student motivation. *Journal of Educational Psychology, 84,* 261–271.
Anderman, E. M., Maehr, M. L., & Midgley, C. (1999).
Declining motivation after the transition to middle
school: Schools can make a difference. *Journal of Research and Development in Education, 32,* 131–147.
Anderman, L. H., & Anderman, E. M. (1999). Social
predictors of changes in students' achievement goal
orientations. *Contemporary Educational Psychol-
ogy, 25,* 21–37.
Anderman, L. H., Patrick, H., Hruda, L. Z., &
Linnenbrink, E. A. (2002). Observing goal struc-
tures to clarify and expand goal theory. In C.
Midgley (Ed.), *Goals, goal structures, and patterns
of adaptive learning* (pp. 243–278). Mahwah, NJ:
Erlbaum.
Ashton, P., & Webb, R. (1986). *Making a difference:
Teachers' sense of efficacy and student achievement.*
New York: Longman.

Assor, A., & Kaplan, H. (2001). Mapping the domain
of autonomy support: Five important ways to enhance or undermine student's experience of autonomy in learning. In A. Effklides, J. Kuhl, & R.
Sorrentino (Eds.), *Trends and prospects in motivational research.* Dordrecht: Kluwer Academic.
Assor, A., Kaplan, H., Kanat-Maymon, Y., & Roth, G.
(in press). Directly controlling teacher behaviors as
predictors of poor motivation and engagement in
girls and boys: The role of anger and anxiety.
Learning and Instruction.
Bandura, A. (1986). *Social foundations of thought and
action: A social cognitive theory.* Englewood Cliffs,
NJ: Prentice-Hall.
Bennett, N., DesForges, C., Cockburn, A., &
Wilkinson, B. (1984). *The quality of pupil learning
experiences.* Hillsdale, NJ: Erlbaum.
Bergin, D. A. (1999). Influences on classroom interest.
Educational Psychologist, 34, 87–98.
Blumenfeld, P. C. (1992). Classroom learning and moti-
vation: Clarifying and expanding goal theory. *Jour-
nal of Educational Psychology, 84,* 272–281.
Blumenfeld, P., Pintrich, P. R., Meece, J., & Wessels, K.
(1982). The formation and role of self-perceptions of
ability in the elementary classroom. *Elementary
School Journal, 82,* 401–420.
Boggiano, A. K., Main, D. S., & Katz, P. A. (1988).
Children's preference for challenge: The role of perceived competence and control. *Journal of Personality and Social Psychology, 54,* 134–141.
Brophy, J., & Alleman, J. (1991). Activities as instructional tools: A framework for instructional analysis
and evaluation. *Educational Researcher, 20,* 9–23.
Burkhardt, H., & Schoenfeld, A. H. (2004). Improving
educational research: Toward a more useful, more
influential, and better-funded enterprise. *Educational Researcher, 32,* 3–14.
Clifford, M. M. (1984). Thoughts on a theory of constructive failure. *Educational Psychologist, 19,* 108–
120.
Coleman, J. (1961). *The adolescent society.* Glencoe,
IL: Free Press.
Covington, M. V. (1992). *Making the grade: A self-
worth perspective on motivation and school reform.*
New York: Cambridge University Press.
de Charms, R. (1968). *Personal causation: The internal
affective determinants of behavior.* New York: Academic Press.
Deci, E. L., Hodges, R., Pierson, L., & Tomassone, J.
(1992). Autonomy andcompetence as motivational
factors in students with learning disabilities and
emotional handicaps. *Journal of Learning Disabilities, 25,* 457–471.
Deci, E. L., & Ryan, R. M. (1985). *Intrinsic motivation
and self-determination in human behavior.* New
York: Plenum Press.
Deci, E. L., Schwartz, A. J., Sheinman, L., & Ryan, R.
M. (1981). An instrument to assess adults' orientations toward control versus autonomy with children:
Reflections on intrinsic motivation and perceived

competence. *Journal of Educational Psychology, 73,* 642–650.

Doyle, W. (1986). Classroom organization and management. In M. Wittrock (Ed.), *Handbook of research on teaching* (pp. 392–431). New York: Macmillan.

Dweck, C. S. (1992). The study of goals in human behavior. *Psychological Science, 3,* 165–167.

Dweck, C. S. (1999). *Self-theories: Their role in motivation, personality, and development.* Philadelphia: Taylor & Francis.

Eccles (formerly Parsons), J. (1983). Expectancies, values, and academic behavior. In J. T. Spence (Ed.), *Achievement and achievement motives* (pp. 75–146). San Francisco: Freeman.

Eccles, J. S., & Midgley, C. (1989). Stage–environment fit: Developmentally appropriate classrooms for early adolescents. In R. Ames & C. Ames (Eds.), *Research on motivation in education* (Vol. 3, pp. 139–181). New York: Academic Press.

Eccles, J. S., Wigfield, A., Flanagan, C., Miller, C., Reuman, D., & Yee, D. (1989). Self-concepts, domain values, and self-esteem: Relations and changes at early adolescence. *Journal of Personality, 57,* 283–310.

Eccles, J. S., Wigfield, A., & Schiefele, U. (1998). Motivation to succeed. In W. Damon (Series Ed.) & N. Eisenberg (Vol. Ed.), *Handbook of child psychology: Vol 3. Social, emotional, and personality development* (5th ed., pp. 1017–1095). New York: Wiley.

Elliot, A. J. (1997). Integrating the "classic" and the "contemporary" approaches to achievement motivation: A hierarchical model of approach and avoidance achievement motivation. In M. L. Maehr & P. R. Pintrich (Eds.), *Advances in motivation and achievement* (Vol. 10., pp. 243–279). Greenwich, CT: JAI Press.

Elliot, A. J. (1999). Approach and avoidance motivation and achievement goals. *Educational Psychologist, 34,* 169–189.

Elliot, A. J., & Harackiewicz, J. M. (1996). Approach and avoidance achievement goals and intrinsic motivation: A mediational analysis. *Journal of Personality and Social Psychology, 70,* 968–980.

Feldlaufer, H., Midgley, C., & Eccles, J. S. (1988). Student, teacher, and observer perceptions of the classroom environment before and after the transition to junior high school. *Journal of Early Adolescence, 8,* 133–156.

Foersterling, F. (1985). Attributional retraining: A review. *Psychological Bulletin, 98,* 495–512.

Fuligni, A. J. (1997). The academic achievement of adolescents from immigrant families: The roles of family background, attitudes, and behavior. *Child Development, 68,* 261–273.

Graham, S. (1984). Teacher feelings and students thoughts: An attributional approach to affect in the classroom. *Elementary School Journal, 85,* 91–104.

Harackiewicz, J. M., Barron, K. E., Tauer, J. M., Carter, S. M., & Elliot, A. J. (2000). Short-term and long-term consequences of achievement goals in college: Predicting continued interest and performance over time. *Journal of Educational Psychology, 92,* 316–330.

Hardre, P. L., & Reeve, J. (2003). A motivational model of rural students' intentions to persist in, versus drop out of, high school. *Journal of Educational Psychology, 95,* 347–356.

Harter, S. (1978). Effectance motivation reconsidered: Toward a developmental model. *Human Development, 21,* 34–64.

Harter, S. (1982). The perceived competence scale for children. *Child Development, 53,* 87–97.

Hidi, S. (2000). An interest researcher's perspective: The effects of extrinsic and intrinsic factors on motivation. In C. Sansone & J. Harackiewicz (Eds.), *Intrinsic and extrinsic motivation: The search for optimal motivation and performance* (pp. 309–339). New York: Academic Press.

Hidi, S., & Harackiewicz, J. M. (2000). Motivating the academically unmotivated: A critical issue for the 21st century. *Review of Educational Research, 70,* 151–179.

Lepper, M. R., & Henderlong, J. (2000). Turning "play" into "work" and "work" into "play": 25 years of research on intrinsic versus extrinsic motivation. In C. Sansone & J. M. Harackiewicz (Eds.), *Intrinsic and extrinsic motivation: The search for optimal motivation and performance* (pp. 257–307). New York: Academic Press.

Mac Iver, D. J., & Reuman, D. A. (1988, April). *Decision-making in the classroom and early adolescents' valuing of mathematics.* Paper presented at the annual meeting of the American Educational Research Association, New Orleans, LA.

Maehr, M. L., & Midgley, C. (1991). Enhancing student motivation: A school-wide approach. *Educational Psychologist, 26,* 399–427.

Maehr, M. L., & Midgley, C. (1996). *Transforming school cultures.* Boulder, CO: Westview Press.

Malone, T. W., & Lepper, M. R. (1987). Making learning fun: A taxonomy of intrinsic motivations and learning. In R. E. Snow & M. J. Farr (Eds.), *Aptitude, learning, and instruction: Vol. III. Conative and affective process analyses* (pp. 223–253). Hillsdale, NJ: Erlbaum.

Meece, J. L. (1991). The classroom context and students' motivational goals. In M. L. Maehr & P. R. Pintrich (Eds.), *Advances in motivation and achievement: Vol. 7. Goals and self-regulatory processes* (pp. 261–285). Greenwich, CT: JAI Press.

Meece, J. L., Wigfield, A., & Eccles, J. S. (1990). Predictors of math anxiety and its consequences for young adolescents' course enrollment intentions and performances in mathematics. *Journal of Educational Psychology, 82,* 60–70.

Midgley, C., & Feldlaufer, H. (1987). Students' and teachers' decision making fit before and after the transition to junior high school. *Journal of Early Adolescence, 7,* 225–241.

Midgley, C., Feldlaufer, H., & Eccles, J. S. (1989).

Change in teacher efficacy and student self- and task-related beliefs in mathematics during the transition to junior high school. *Journal of Educational Psychology, 81,* 247–258.

Midgley, C., Kaplan, A., & Middleton, M. (2001). Performance-approach goals: Good for what, for whom, under what circumstances, and at what costs? *Journal of Educational Psychology, 93,* 77–86.

Midgley, C., Maehr, M. L., Hruda, L. Z., Anderman, E., Anderman, L., Freeman, K. E., et al. (2000). *Manual for the Patterns of Adaptive Learning Scales (PALS).* Ann Arbor: University of Michigan Press.

Midgley, C., & Urdan, T. (1992). The transition to middle school: Making it a good experience for all students. *Middle School Journal, 24,* 5–14.

Miller, S. D., & Meece, J. L. (1997). Enhancing elementary students' motivation to read and write: A classroom intervention study. *Journal of Educational Research, 89,* 286–292.

Pajares, F. (1996). Self-efficacy beliefs in achievement settings. *Review of Educational Research, 66,* 543–578.

Pajares, F., & Kranzler, J. (1995). Self-efficacy beliefs and general mental ability in mathematical problem solving. *Contemporary Educational Psychology, 20,* 426–443.

Pajares, F., Miller, M. D., & Johnson, M. J. (1999). Gender differences in writing self-beliefs of elementary school students. *Journal of Educational Psychology, 91,* 50–61.

Patrick, H., Anderman, L. H., Ryan, A. M., Edelin, K. C., & Midgley, C. (2001). Teachers' communication of goal orientations in four fifth-grade classrooms. *Elementary School Journal, 102,* 35–58.

Pelletier, L. G., Seguin-Levesque, C., & Legault, L. (2002). Pressure from above and pressure from below as determinants of teachers' motivation and teaching behaviors. *Journal of Educational Psychology, 94,* 186–196.

Pintrich, P. R. (2004). A motivational science perspective on the role of student motivation in learning and teaching contexts. *Journal of Educational Psychology, 95,* 667–686.

Pintrich, P. R., & Blumenfeld, P. (1985). Classroom experience and children's self-perceptions of ability, effort, and conduct. *Journal of Educational Psychology, 77,* 646–657.

Pintrich, P. R., & DeGroot, E. V. (1990). Motivational and self-regulated learning components of classroom academic performance. *Journal of Educational Psychology, 82,* 33–40.

Pintrich, P. R., & Schunk, D. H. (2002). Motivation in education (2nd ed.) Upper Saddle River, NJ: Merrill/Prentice-Hall.

Reeve, J. M., Bolt, E., & Cai, Y. (1999). Autonomy supportive teachers: How they teach and motivate students. *Journal of Educational Psychology, 91,* 537–548.

Renninger, K. A. (2000). Individual interest and its im-

plications for understanding intrinsic motivation. In C. Sansone & J. M. Harackiewicz (Eds.), *Intrinsic and extrinsic motivation: The search for optimal motivation and performance* (pp. 373–404). New York: Academic Press.

Rosenholtz, S. J., & Simpson, C. (1984). The formation of ability conceptions: Developmental trend or social construction? *Review of Educational Research, 54,* 31–63.

Rosenholtz, S. J., & Wilson, B. (1980). The effect of classroom structure on shared perceptions of ability. *American Educational Research Journal, 17,* 75–82.

Ryan, A. (2001). The peer group as a context for the development of young adolescent motivation and achievement. *Child Development, 72,* 1135–1150.

Ryan, R. M., & Grolnick, W. S. (1986). Origins and pawns in the classroom: Self-report and projective assessments of individual differences in children's perspectives. *Journal of Personality and Social Psychology, 50,* 550–558.

Sansone, C., & Harackiewicz, J. M. (2000). Looking beyond extrinsic rewards: The problem and promise of intrinsic motivation. In C. Sansone & J. M. Harackiewicz (Eds.), *Intrinsic and extrinsic motivation: The search for optimal motivation and performance* (pp. 1–9). New York: Academic Press.

Schunk, D. H. (1984). Enhancing self-efficacy and achievement through rewards and goals: Motivational and informational effects. *Journal of Educational Research, 78,* 29–34.

Schunk, D. H., Hanson, A. R., & Cox, P. D. (1987). Peer-model attributions and children's achievement behaviors. *Journal of Educational Psychology, 79,* 54–61.

Schunk, D. H., & Miller, S. D., (2002). Self-efficacy and adolescents' motivation. In F. Pajares & T. Urdan (Eds.), *Adolescence and education, Vol. 2: Academic motivation of adolescents* (pp. 29–52). Greenwich, CT: Information Age.

Shell, D. F., Colvin, C., & Bruning, R. H. (1995). Self-efficacy, attributions, and outcome expectancy mechanisms in reading and writing achievement: Grade-level and achievement-level differences. *Journal of Educational Psychology, 87,* 386–398.

Skinner, E. A., & Belmont, M. J. (1993). Motivation in the classroom: Reciprocal effects of teacher behavior and student engagement across the school year. *Journal of Educational Psychology, 85,* 571–581.

Stipek, D., Givvin, K., Salmon, J., & MacGyvers, V. (1998). Can a teacher intervention improve classroom practices and student motivation in mathematics? *Journal of Experimental Education, 66,* 319–337.

Stipek, D., Salmon, J., Givvin, K., Kazemi, E., Saxe, G., & MacGyvers, V. (1998). The value (and convergence) of practices suggested by motivation researchers and mathematics education reformers. *Journal for Research in Mathematics Education, 29,* 465–488.

Thorkildsen, T. A., & Nicholls, J. G. (1998). Fifth graders' achievement orientations and beliefs: Individual and classroom differences. *Journal of Educational Psychology, 90,* 179–201.

Tollefson, N. (2000). Classroom applications of cognitive theories of motivation. *Educational Psychology Review, 12,* 63–83.

Tschannen-Moran, M., Hoy, A. W., & Hoy, W. K. (1998). Teacher efficacy: Its meaning and measure. *Review of Educational Research, 68,* 202–248.

Turner, J. C., & Meyer, D. K. (1999). Integrating classroom context into motivation theory and research: Rationales, methods, and implications. In T. Urdan, M. Maehr, & P. R. Pintrich (Eds.), *Advances in motivation* (Vol. 11, pp. 87–121). Greenwich CT: JAI Press.

Turner, J. C., Meyer, D. K., Cox, K. E., Logan, C., DiCintio, M., & Thomas, C. (1998). Creating contexts for involvement in mathematics. *Journal of Educational Psychology, 90,* 730–745.

Turner, J.C., Meyer, D. K., Midgley, C., & Patrick, H. (2003). Teacher discourse and students' affect and achievement-related behaviors in two high mastery/high performance classrooms. *Elementary School Journal, 103,* 357–382.

Turner, J. C., Midgley, C., Meyer, D. K., Gheen, M., Anderman, E. A., Kang, J., et al. (2002). The classroom environment and students' reports of avoidance strategies in mathematics: A multimethod study. *Journal of Educational Psychology, 94,* 88–106.

Urdan, T. (2004). Can achievement goal theory guide school reform? In P. R. Pintrich & M. L. Maehr (Eds.), *Advances in motivation and achievement* (Vol. 13, pp. 361–392). New York: Elsevier.

Urdan, T., Kneisel, L., & Mason, V. (1999). Interpreting messages about motivation in the classroom: Examining the effects of achievement goal structures. In T.

Urdan (Ed.), *Advances in motivation and achievement* (Vol. 11, pp. 123–158). Stamford, CT: JAI Press.

Urdan, T., & Midgley, C. (2001). Academic self-handicapping: What we know, what more there is to learn. *Educational Psychology Review, 13,* 115–138.

Urdan, T., & Midgley, C. (2003). Changes in the perceived classroom goal structure and patterns of adaptive learning during early adolescence. *Contemporary Educational Psychology, 28,* 524–551.

Urdan, T., Midgley, C., & Anderman, E. (1998). The role of classroom goal structure in students' use of self-handicapping strategies. *American Educational Research Journal, 35,* 101–122.

Urdan, T., Midgley, C., & Wood, S. (1995). Special issues in reforming middle level schools. *Journal of Early Adolescence, 15,* 9–37.

Vallerand, R. J., Fortier, M. S., & Guay, F. (1997). Self-determination and persistence in a real-life setting: Toward a motivational model of high school dropout. *Journal of Personality and Social Psychology, 72,* 1161–1176.

Weiner, B. (1986). *An attributional theory of motivation and emotion.* New York: Springer-Verlag.

Weinstein, R. S. (2002). *Reaching higher: The power of expectations in schooling.* Cambridge, MA: Harvard University Press.

Wentzel, K. R. (1999). Social-motivational processes and interpersonal relationships: Implications for understanding students' academic success. *Journal of Educational Psychology, 91,* 76–97.

White, R. (1959). Motivation reconsidered: The concept of competence. *Psychological Review, 66,* 297–333.

Wigfield, A., & Eccles, J. (1992). The development of achievement task values: A theoretical analysis. *Developmental Review, 12,* 265–310.

CHAPTER 18

℘

Motivation in Sport

The Relevance of Competence and Achievement Goals

JOAN L. DUDA

The relevance of competence to performance and participation in the athletic realm is evident to even the most casual observer of or partaker in sport. Anyone who has engaged in a sport contest, watched a sport competition, coached someone learning a new physical skill or aspect of technique, and/or has decided whether to join, stay with, or drop out of sport has clearly witnessed the significance of competence to sport behaviors. Indeed, a perusal of the sport psychology literature readily indicates that ability, in particular, *perceptions* of that ability, is central to task execution (e.g., Weinberg, Gould, Yukelson, & Jackson, 1981) and engagement (e.g., Roberts, Kleiber, & Duda, 1981) or disengagement (e.g., Burton & Martens, 1986) in sport settings. An examination of this literature also reveals that various theoretical models have laid the basis for research on the antecedents and consequences of perceived sport-related competence. A considerable number of studies have been grounded in Bandura's (1977, 1986) social cognitive theory and have centered on judgments regarding task-specific competencies or perceptions of self-efficacy (see Feltz, 1992; Feltz & Lirgg, 2001). Research in youth sport settings (e.g., Babkes & Weiss, 1999; Horn, Glenn, & Wentzel, 1993; Roberts et al., 1981), concerned primarily with developmental and socialization influences on perceived competence, has been based on Harter's competence motivation framework (Harter, 1978, 1981). Eccles's expectancy–value model (Eccles, Jacobs, & Harold, 1990; Eccles & Wigfield, 1995) has been tested in the sport domain as well (e.g., Brustad, 1996; Eccles & Harold, 1991), providing greater awareness of the social factors impacting gender differences in sport competence and interest.

In this chapter, the theoretical emphasis is on contemporary achievement goal frameworks, which have dominated research on achievement motivation in sport since the early 1990s. This line of work has primarily been undergirded by the conceptual contributions of Nicholls (1984, 1989), Dweck (1986, 1999), Ames (1992a, 1992b), and, more recently, Elliot (1997, 1999; Elliot & Harackiewicz, 1996). In particular, the terminology, proposed achievement goal constructs, and theoretical tenets that have stemmed from the writings of Nicholls (1984, 1989) have had a tremendous impact on sport motivation research over the past decade.

It is both interesting and impressive to note that the achievement goal literature specific to the physical domain goes beyond a unitary concern with achievement motivation in organized sport or *athletic* situations. A rather extensive body of research has focused on the motivational processes operating in physical education classes (Biddle, 2001; Duda & Ntoumanis, 2003; Papaioannou, 1995). Studies have also begun to look at exercise motivation from an achievement goal perspective (e.g., Biddle, Soos, & Chatzisarantis, 1999; Kimiecik, Horn, & Shurin, 1996; Lloyd & Fox, 1992).

Delimiting the current discussion specifically to the sport-related literature still leaves a plethora of research directions, study findings, and numerous theoretical and measurement-related issues that are impossible to address with thoroughness in one book chapter (regarding additional reviews in this area, see Duda, 1992, 1993, 2001; Duda & Hall, 2001; Duda & Whitehead, 1998; Roberts, 1992, 2001; Treasure, 2001). Exemplifying the extensiveness of this line of work, a recent systematic review by Biddle, Wang, Kavussanu, and Spray (2003) of published articles (in English) from 1990 to 2000 on the correlates of goal orientations in sport settings involved 98 studies, involving 110 independent samples (total N = 21,076).

With the breadth of this field of inquiry in mind, one aim of this contribution, then, is to provide a synopsis of some of the major questions that *sport* achievement goal researchers have posed and the manner in which they have attempted to answer such questions. Another purpose of this chapter is to encapsulate the prevailing pattern of findings related to these queries. An additional aspiration is to draw attention to the theoretical advancements, and the conceptual and practical issues raised in the existent work on achievement goals in sport.

I begin with a short description of the major constructs embedded in the sport achievement goal literature, namely, the concepts of goal orientations, motivational climate, and goal involvement (Duda, 2001). In each case, I highlight prevailing measurement efforts. The major theoretical tenets, emanating from what are now referred to as dual goal, or dichotomous achievement goal, frameworks, are summarized, and major research trends are described. Recent incorporations of trichotomous and 2 × 2 goal models (Elliot, 1997, 1999; Elliot & Church, 1997; Elliot & McGregor, 2001) in sport research and emergent findings are subsequently reviewed in brief. Such work considers that achievement goals can be both approach- and avoidance-oriented. Throughout the chapter, in the spirit of fostering further work on competence and achievement goals in the sport domain, I propose unresolved issues and potential areas for future inquiry for the reader's consideration.

A fundamental assumption of achievement goal frameworks is that the meaning of achievement activities, such as sport, is what colors ensuing affective responses, cognitions, and behaviors. It is also assumed that this meaning stems from the achievement goals endorsed by individuals (Ames, 1992a; Dweck, 1986; Nicholls, 1984, 1989). In essence, achievement goals are held to be the interpretive lens influencing how we think, feel, and act while engaged in achievement endeavors.

Nicholls (1984, 1989) argued that variation in the construal of competence underlies what achievement goal is adopted in a particular setting. Specifically, in his view, the conception of competence undergirds how success (or subjective goal attainment) is defined. Indicative of the dichotomous goal perspective, two major goals are proposed (i.e., a "task" and an "ego" goal) that reflect two different ways of defining or construing competence. When a task goal is manifested, the concern is with meeting the demands of the task, exerting effort, and developing one's competence. Realizing high competence that is interpreted in a self-referenced manner and inextricably linked to trying one's best is of import when task goals prevail. More specifically, according to Nicholls (1989), people are focused on an "undifferentiated" conception of competence, if striving for task goals. Demonstrating high ability is not distinguished from or dependent on how much effort is given in this case; both are fundamental to subjective success.

When focused on an ego goal, individuals desire to demonstrate superior competence with respect to relevant others and/or normative standards (Nicholls, 1984, 1989). Improving and/or putting forth effort are not sufficient to occasion a sense of success, because there is a fixation with revealing a "differentiated" conception of competence (Nicholls, 1989), in which ability and effort are seen to covary. Thus, if concerned with exhibiting high differentiated competence, one would feel more able and successful if he or she could exhibit outstanding performance with minimal effort. On the other hand, high effort that does *not* result in comparably high performance would be predicted to promote feelings of low competence.

When sport experiences are interpreted through the lens of an ego goal focus, preoccupations with and a greater awareness of the self are likely to be present (Duda & Hall, 2001; Dweck, 1999; Kaplan & Maehr, 1999). When one is centered on ego goals, it is assumed that there is greater apprehension about the adequacy of one's ability (i.e., *proving* oneself rather than *improving* oneself; Dweck, 1999) and a greater likelihood of questioning whether one is good enough in challenging situations. In the demanding and often unpredictable world of competitive sport, it is difficult always to be the best and potentially quite debilitating to be fixated on showing superiority.

ACHIEVEMENT GOALS IN SPORT

Central Constructs

Three central achievement goal constructs that have been examined in the sport domain are dispositional (sport) goal orientations, perceptions of the motivational climate, and goal involvement. With respect to the former, Nicholls (1989) proposed that there are individual differences in the proneness for task and ego goals. More specifically, it is held that, in any achievement activity, individuals vary in their degree of task and ego orientation. Congruent with Nicholls's thinking (1989), these two goal orientations tend to be orthogonal in the sport domain (e.g., Chi & Duda, 1995).

Such independence means that people can be high or low in task and ego orientation, or high in one orientation and low in the other.

In terms of the assessment of sport goal orientations, two measures have dominated the field. Both are bidimensional and capture individual differences in the emphases placed on task- or ego-focused criteria for subjective success (i.e., individuals respond to items following the stem, "I feel successful in sport when . . . "). The Task and Ego Orientation in Sport Questionnaire (TEOSQ; Duda, 1989), developed by Duda and Nicholls, drew from previous instruments designed to tap dispositional goals in classroom settings (Nicholls, 1989). The TEOSQ had been used in 80.6% of the studies considered in the recent systematic review by Biddle and colleagues (2003). The Perceptions of Success Questionnaire (POSQ; Roberts, Treasure, & Balague, 1998) also has been employed in numerous sport-related investigations. Both instruments have been found to be psychometrically sound, have been translated and validated in numerous languages, and have been used to measure achievement goal tendencies among older children through adult participants in a variety of sports at different competitive levels (see Duda & Whitehead, 1998).

A determination of perceived situationally emphasized achievement goals has also been of interest within the sport literature. For the most part, such efforts have pulled from Ames's work on students' perceptions of the motivational climate operating in classrooms (Ames, 1992a, 1992b; Ames & Archer, 1988). This climate is deemed to be composed of various structures (e.g., the system of evaluation, the type of and basis for recognition, the nature of interactions within and between groups, and the source[s] of authority) and is viewed as an overriding psychological environment that impacts the likelihood that individuals will be more or less concerned with exhibiting self- or other-referenced competence.

In the sport domain, the majority of work conducted to date has concentrated on perceptions of the motivational climate created by coaches via either version 1 or 2 of the Perceived Motivational Climate in Sport Questionnaire (PMCSQ-1 or PMCSQ-2; Newton, Duda, & Yin, 2000; Seifriz, Duda,

& Chi, 1992; Walling, Duda, & Chi, 1993). Grounded in a hierarchical measurement model (that assumes the existence of higher order task- and ego-involving dimensions or scales underpinned by more specific situational structures or subscales), the PMCSQ-2 assesses the following task-involving facets of the perceived coach-created motivational climate: the view that the coach emphasizes effort and athletes' personal improvement, contributes to each player feeling that he or she has an important role on the team, and fosters cooperation between team members. In contrast, athletes' appraisals that their coach typically is punitive in response to mistakes, gives the most attention to the most skilled players, and cultivates rivalry among team members constitute the ego-involving subscales of the PMCSQ-2. Contrary to what tends to be the case for the task and ego orientation scales of the TEOSQ or POSQ, the task and ego climate dimensions of the PMCSQ (Vers. 1 or 2) tend to be negatively correlated (i.e., r tends to range from $-.3$ to $-.5$). This suggests that the more a coach is deemed to encourage a focus on self-referenced competence (i.e., a task goal emphasis), the less likely he or she is viewed as promoting a concern with team members demonstrating high sport ability relative to others (i.e., an ego goal emphasis).

As assessed via the PMCSQ (1 or 2), views regarding the coach-emphasized motivational climate operating on particular sport teams have been found to be shared perceptions (Duda, Newton, & Yin, 1999), even though within-team variation among athletes does exist; that is, there is a significant interdependence in the perceptions held by athletes playing on one team when contrasted to the perspectives held by athletes across teams. Such findings suggest that it is important to separate group versus individual effects in analyses of the correlates of the motivational climate in sport.

Measures of the perceived motivational climate created by parents (White, 1996; White, Duda, & Hart, 1992) and, recently, peers (Vazou, Ntoumanis, & Duda, 2004, in press) have also been developed. As athletes' interpretation of and responses to sport are differentially shaped by divergent significant others as they move from childhood into their adult years, a consideration of these sources of the motivational climates surrounding athletes is paramount to a more comprehensive understanding of their socialization experiences. Currently though, there is a daunting challenge facing a researcher who wants to compare the relative significance of the motivational atmospheres created by coaches, parents, peers, and so forth, on athletes' personal goals and achievement patterns; that is, the existent instruments vary with respect to which situational structures are targeted and sometimes include hypothesized correlates of the climate within the measure of the construct itself (see Duda & Whitehead, 1998, for a more extensive discussion of this issue). As a result, if one significant other appeared to be more significant than another in an investigation of social influences on athletes' achievement striving, the researcher could not be sure whether these results are a function of the salience of the particular socializing agent *or* the composition and characteristics of the measures employed.

In general, research has revealed athletes' perceptions of the task-involving features of the climate (regardless of the socializing agent) to be low to moderately correlated with their degree of task orientation. The same holds true with respect to perceptions of an ego-involving climate and ego orientation (Duda, 2001). This literature, though, almost exclusively comprises cross-sectional studies. It is not possible to discern via such a methodology whether dispositional goals influence what athletes "pick up" in their social environments, and/or whether the climate operating has some impact on athletes' tendencies regarding how sport success is defined (Duda, 1993; Ntoumanis & Biddle, 1998). Longitudinal investigations that examine the interplay between goal orientations and perceptions of the motivational climate over time will contribute to the understanding of the independencies between individual differences and situational achievement goals in the athletic setting.

With an eye toward examining perceived situationally emphasized achievement goals in sport, some studies have determined athletes' views of the goal orientations held by significant others, such as parents (e.g., "My dad/mom thinks I am successful in sport when . . . "; e.g., Duda & Hom, 1993; Ebbeck & Becker, 1994). It is important to keep in mind that although perceptions of an important social agent's goal orientations tend to correlate quite strongly with athletes' personal goal orientations, such perceptions are not highly associated with athletes' "take" on the overriding motivational climate created by the significant other in question (Duda, 2001). This is most likely because the perceived motivational climate reflects a composite view of various situational structures and characteristics that inform individuals about how success should be defined and competence construed (Ames, 1992a, 1992b).

Achievement goal frameworks (Dweck, 1999; Nicholls, 1989) hold that individuals, while engaged in achievement activities such as sport, can process those activities in a task- or ego-involved manner. In other words, while actively participating, athletes can be in a state of task or ego involvement (or neither state), perhaps fluctuating from one state to another. Furthermore, it is also assumed that the degree to which an athlete might be task- and/or ego-involved during a particular training or competition would be dependent on his or her dispositional tendencies and the motivational climate manifested (Dweck & Leggett, 1988).

With respect to the assessment of task- and ego-involved states, the achievement goal literature in sport has not progressed to the same degree as has been the case for dispositional goals and perceptions of the prevailing motivational climate. In an attempt to measures sport participants' goal states, some researchers have adopted the TEOSQ or POSQ (e.g., Hall & Kerr, 1997; Williams, 1998) and have tried to discern how athletes are defining success *at that moment*. Others (e.g., Harwood & Swain, 1998) have utilized single-item measures addressing whether the athlete is focused on reaching a high personal standard of performance (regardless of the competitive outcome) *or* on beating others (regardless of how they personally perform) before a competitive event. It has been argued, though, that the former assessment seems to tap "state" goal orientations, or the criteria underlying subjective success at a particular point in time, while the latter is primarily measuring a precompetition emphasis on a process versus outcome goal (Duda, 2001). Drawing from the thinking of Nicholls

(1989), Dweck (1999), and others, it would seem that states of task and ego involvement are more complicated and multidimensional than merely what type of performance standard an athlete is emphasizing or the definition of success he or she is holding at a specific time. In our chapter reviewing advancements in the measurement of achievement goal constructs specific to the sport domain, Whitehead and I (Duda & Whitehead, 1998, p. 42) suggest that the

> assessment of task and ego involvement per se may very well entail the examination of a pattern of variables that represent task and ego processing and preoccupation . . . [and] the measurement of task- and ego-involved goal states would be dynamic and multifaceted. Variations in attentional focus, concerns about what one is doing and how one is doing, the degree of self-/other awareness and task absorption, level of effort exertion, etc., might constitute the constellation of symptoms reflecting task and ego goal states.

Moreover, it is not known at the present time whether task and ego involvement are independent states, or whether it is possible to be (at some level) in both a task- *and* ego-involved state simultaneously (for further discussions of this point, see Harwood, Hardy, & Swain, 2000; Treasure et al., 2001).

Clearly, to determine states of task and ego involvement as suggested earlier, innovative and probably multimethod assessment strategies are necessary. An additional methodological challenge would be for such tools to be suitable for implementation in the real world of sport training and competition, and not be disruptive to athletes' performance. This would be no small feat! As so often seems to be the case, the major question of interest in sport is how a particular performer is going to perform in a given contest (Hardy, 1997; Harwood et al., 2000), and the formulation of conceptually grounded, valid, and reliable measures of task and ego involvement reflects a valued endeavor. This is because achievement goal theory presumes that these goal states, coupled with the athlete's degree of confidence at the time, should be predictive of performance outcomes. However, being able to assess goal involvement effectively would also allow us to test theoretical predictions regarding the hypothesized impact of dispositional and situational goals (and their interaction) on motivational processes and should also provide better insight into the *quality* of the athlete's experiences *while engaged in sport* (Duda, 2001). The latter two benefits, in my mind, are additional important reasons for forging ahead in the pursuit of adequate and appropriate measures of goal states within the athletic milieu.

It should be noted, too, that the achievement goal literature in sport has called for the development of "state" measures of situational factors that could be influencing the perceived motivational climate and athletes' goal involvement during training or competition (Duda & Hall, 2001; Harwood & Swain, 1998). Thus, although there has been impressive advancement in the measurement of key achievement goal constructs in the sport domain (see Duda & Whitehead, 1998, for a review), there is much more work to be done in terms of the refinement of existing measures and the development of new assessment tools.

Theoretical Predictions and Major Findings

Goal Orientations

A plethora of studies have determined the correlates of individual differences in task and ego orientation in the sport domain. Taken in its totality, this work suggests that variations in goal orientations correspond to a multitude of variables reflecting athletes' beliefs about and cognitive, affective, and behavioral responses to sport. This is held to be because achievement goal orientations capture the reasons for engaging in an achievement activity such as sport, and the criteria underpinning judgments of successful performance (Pintrich, 2000).

The foremost achievement-related concomitants of sport goal orientations examined include sport participants' (1) beliefs regarding the causes of success and overall purposes of sport involvement, (2) strategy use in practice and competitive conditions, (3) perceived competence, (4) reported positive and negative affect, and (5) achievement behaviors. Narrative and systematic reviews have described this research in considerable detail. In this chapter, I highlight only the

major findings (and where possible, the strength of those findings).

Numerous studies conducted in various countries, and involving diverse sport participants, such as high school athletes, physically challenged athletes, elite performers, and senior or master's level competitors, have ascertained the interdependencies between goal orientations and beliefs about the causes of success (e.g., Duda, 1989; Newton & Fry, 1998; Roberts & Ommundsen, 1996; Seifriz et al., 1992). In Nicholls's view (1989), dispositional goals and beliefs about success constitute two critical facets of individuals' personal theories of achievement in the context in question. A person's theory about sport, then, would comprise what he or she wants to achieve (i.e., goals or subjective definitions of success) and his or her conceptions of how the situation at hand operates (i.e., views regarding the determinants of success) (Duda & Nicholls, 1992). In Biddle and colleagues' (2003) recent systematic review, a moderate to large effect size (0.47) was found between task orientation and the belief that hard work and training lead to sport success. A similar effect size (0.45) emerged between ego orientation and the belief that the possession of high ability is central to achievement in the athletic setting.

In their review, Biddle and associates (2003) also examined 10 studies (involving over 2,000 participants) that determined the relationship of goal orientations and athletes' beliefs about what the wider purposes of sport involvement should be (e.g., Carpenter & Yates, 1997; Duda, 1989; Treasure & Roberts, 1994). With respect to predominant findings, task orientation tended to correspond to the view that sport participation should promote a work ethic–orientation to mastery (effect size = 0.56), foster social responsibility and citizenship (effect size = 0.32), and encourage an active lifestyle (effect size = 0.37). Ego orientation tended to be coupled with the belief that an important function of sport engagement is to enhance athletes' social status (effect size = 0.53).

Sport studies have looked at the interdependencies between goal orientations and reported learning- and performance-related strategy use. All in all, this line of work suggests that task goal orientation corresponds to more adaptive strategies, while the tactics aligned with ego orientation are more short-term solutions or ways to protect one's sense of adequate ability. For example, Lochbaum and Roberts (1993) found a positive relationship between positive practice and competition strategies (e.g., trying to understand what the coach is conveying within his or her instructions), and task orientation. In research involving French university-level soccer players engaged in a shooting task, Thill and Brunel (1995) found the use of spontaneous and deep-processing strategies to be linked to a task orientation, while the use of more superficial strategies was associated with ego orientation. A series of investigations by Cury and his colleagues (Cury, Famose, & Sarrazin, 1997; Cury & Sarrazin, 1998) indicated that a strong ego orientation (coupled with low task orientation and/or low ability) corresponded to the tendency to reject or disregard objective, task-related feedback. As a performance-related strategy following success, or especially following failure situations, it is difficult to imagine how the latter feedback preference would contribute to the athlete's development!

Achievement goal frameworks (Dweck, 1986, 1999; Nicholls, 1984, 1989) hold that perceptions of ability will be more fragile when individuals are strongly ego-oriented in achievement settings such as sport. With respect to the linkages between task and ego orientation and perceived competence among sport participants, the research to date has examined these relationships in cross-sectional designs (e.g., Duda & Nicholls, 1992). As indicated in the results reported by Biddle and colleagues (2003) in their systematic review, small, positive associations between task and ego orientations and perceived competence tend to be observed (effect sizes = 0.25 and 0.24, respectively). Duda and Nicholls (1992), however, argued that such results are not surprising in the athletic setting. In "slice-in-time" studies of athletes currently involved in sport, one would be unlikely to find many study participants who were strongly ego-oriented and felt their ability to be low. Such individuals would probably have withdrawn from participation. What we do not know at this juncture is what happens to perceptions of competence over time among athletes whose goal orientations vary. Given the predictions of achievement goal theory, it would be particularly intriguing to follow any ensuing changes in perceived sport ability among highly ego-oriented athletes (especially those with a weak task orientation) who are experiencing performance difficulties (Duda, 2001).

A popular research direction in the goal orientation literature has been to determine the interdependencies between dispositional goals and reported positive affect in the athletic domain (e.g., Duda, Fox, Biddle, & Armstrong, 1992). In this research, positive affect is usually operationalized in terms of reported enjoyment, intrinsic interest, satisfaction, or scores on the positive affective responses contained in the Positive and Negative Affect Scale (PANAS). The systematic reviews to date (Ntoumanis & Biddle, 1999a; Biddle et al., 2003) have supported a moderate, positive relationship between task orientation and positive affect (effect size = 0.41 and 0.43, respectively), while no association with ego orientation has emerged.

The correspondence between dispositional goals and negative affect (typically defined with respect to anxiety, boredom, and/or composite negative affect, as assessed with instruments such as the PANAS) among sport populations has also been investigated (e.g., Duda & Nicholls, 1992; Hall & Kerr, 1997). In reviews of this literature (Biddle et al., 2003; Ntoumanis & Biddle, 1999a), a small, negative effect between task orientation and negative affect has been supported. Ego orientation has not been found to relate consistently to negative affect in the sport domain.

Finally, and quite surprisingly, since the prediction of behavior is seminal to the study of motivation, a limited number of investigations have determined the linkages between goal orientations and achievement-related behaviors, such as challenge seeking, performance, and persistence (e.g., Van-Yperen & Duda, 1999). Again, systematic reviews of this work reveal no meaningful associations with ego orientation, although a small, positive effect (effect size = 0.28) has emerged in the case of task orientation.

It seems that when the aim is to predict affective responses (whether positive or negative) and behavioral patterns, a determination of athletes' level of ego orientation alone is not particularly telling. Based on such findings, some researchers have argued (e.g., Hardy, 1997) that there is no evidence to suggest that ego orientation is problematic and/or should be curtailed in the athletic setting. In previous work, I have made three points in regard to such an interpretation of the literature. First, because achievement goal frameworks hold that perceived competence moderates the impact of ego goals on achievement-related responses, it is not surprising that athletes' ego orientation alone would be a significant negative predictor of achievement-related affect, cognitions, and behavior. Work is needed that examines the concomitants of ego goals (again, especially in a longitudinal manner) among athletes who are confident, *as well as* among those who have doubts about their competence. Second, when we look at other correlates of ego orientation (besides achievement-related responses) that provide insight into the meaning of sport and how the athlete is functioning (e.g., moral behavior, indices of well-being), ego orientation (in and of itself) tends to correspond to more negative responses and less adaptive perspectives. Finally, before we make any conclusions about the value or potential negative implications of task and ego goals among sporting populations, it is paramount that we also consider the findings that stem from the research on the correlates of task- and ego-involving sport environments.

In summary, the existent research on the correlates of sport goal orientations supports the premise that dispositional goals act as schemas reflecting the purposes underlying people's behavior and represent an integrated system of interpretations of cognitive and affective responses to achievement experiences (Kaplan & Maehr, 1999). Moreover, as purported by Nicholls (1989, 1992), a determination of athletes' degree of task and ego orientation provides insight into their wider views about the world of sport per se, such as their views regarding what it takes to get ahead in the athletic domain and what should be the consequences of sport participation. It would seem prudent that individual differences in goal orientation need to be considered in any systematic study of human motivation within sport settings.

The Perceived Motivational Climate

In contrast to research on the ramifications of dispositional achievement goals in sport, relatively less work has been conducted on the implications of the motivational climate created by significant others, such as the coach. However, particularly since the development of instruments to tap perceptions regarding the motivational atmosphere manifested in the athletic milieu, this is a growing body of literature (Newton et al., 2000; Seifriz et al., 1992). Moreover, it could be suggested that work on the concomitants of the motivational climate in sport has the most relevance to subsequent intervention efforts in this setting. Although the existing research is primarily correlational and cross-sectional in design, some experimental work on the motivational climate in both laboratory and field settings is evident in previous sport-related investigations (for reviews, see Biddle, 2001; Treasure, 2001).

Overall, the observed findings regarding the motivational climate in sport parallel what has been observed for goal orientations and/or are in accordance with theoretical predictions. For example, a task-involving climate has been found to correspond with greater enjoyment, satisfaction, and positive affect (e.g., Carpenter & Morgan, 1999; Ntoumanis & Biddle, 1999b; Seifriz et al., 1992; Treasure, 1993), the belief that effort is an important contributor to sport success (e.g., Seifriz et al., 1992; Treasure, 1993), subjective and objective performance (e.g., Balaguer, Duda, Atienza, & Mayo, 2002; Pensgaard & Duda, 2004), more adaptive coping strategies (Kim & Duda, 1998), and persistence (e.g., Sarrazin, Vallerand, Guillet, Pelletier, & Cury, 2002). On the other hand, an ego-involving situation has been found to be associated with greater anxiety (Ntoumanis & Biddle, 1998b; Pensgaard & Roberts, 2000), the belief that the possession of ability is central to sport achievement (Seifriz et al., 1992), and dropping out of sport (e.g, Sarrazin et al., 2002). Although such findings are compelling and theoretically consonant, it is important to keep in mind that only the correspondence between perceptions of the motivational climate and positive and negative affect has been tested via meta-analytic techniques (Ntoumanis & Biddle, 1999b).

As the preceding discussion implies, early research on achievement goals in sport primarily focused on either the implications of differences in goal orientations *or* variability in perceptions of the task- and ego-involving features of the environment. More contemporary work tends to incorporate both constructs into the study of achievement outcomes and motivational processes within athletic settings. With respect to this latter line of inquiry, the focal point initially was on identifying which construct (i.e., dispositional or perceived situationally emphasized goals) is the best predictor of the achievement-related cognitions, affect, and/or behavior of interest (e.g., Kavussanu & Roberts, 1996; Seifriz et al., 1992) in a cross-sectional design. In general, and aligned with the proposition of Duda and Nicholls (1992), when the dependent variable in question was more dispositional in nature (e.g., the athlete's level of self-esteem), goal orientations had greater predictive utility. If the aim of the study was to predict a more state-like or situationally specific variable (e.g., how much an athlete enjoys the sport at hand), then perceptions of the motivational climate accounted for more variance.

Aligned with the suggestions of achievement goal theorists (e.g., Dweck & Leggett, 1988), later research (e.g., Newton & Duda, 1999; Treasure & Roberts, 1998) considered the possibility that there may be an interplay between goal orientations and perceptions of the motivational climate. These cross-sectional studies tend to use regression analyses, with the interaction terms entered as predictors following the main effects for task and ego orientation, and task and ego climate variables. Reflecting a better test of the tenets of achievement goal frameworks (Dweck, 1999; Nicholls, 1989), a few of these investigations also included perceived ability as a main effect predictor variable and in interaction with personal and/or situational goals (e.g., Newton & Duda, 1999). All in all, this examination of potential interactions has provided support for the expected interplay between goal orientations and perceptions of the motivational climate (Dweck & Leggett, 1988) but more often than not, significant interaction terms do *not* emerge.

In explicating this lack of significance findings, researchers typically point to insufficient sample sizes and/or limited variability in the predictor variables (Duda, 2001). These type of investigations usually do not have adequate power to detect hypothesized differences. Studies marked by larger and perhaps more heterogeneous samples might help us become more aware of where, when, and how personal and situational achievement goals interact in the sport domain. Longitudinal and experimental protocols would provide even greater insight into the interplay between dispositional goals and the motivational climate(s) operating. Ideographic and qualitative methodologies should also prove informative in terms of this issue (e.g., see Krane, Greenleaf, & Snow, 1997).

MULTIPLE GOAL FRAMEWORKS: THE CASE FOR AVOIDANCE AND APPROACH GOALS

A promising extension of the dichotomous or two-goal models of achievement has been the recent consideration of multiple goals. In particular, Elliot (1997, 1999) and others (Middleton & Midgley, 1997; Skaalvik, 1997) have advocated a revision of the task–ego goal dichotomy by incorporating an approach and avoidance aspect of ego goals. Elliot's (1997, 1999) trichotomous achievement goal framework has had the most impact on contemporary research in sport. This framework holds that three distinct achievement goals are evident in achievement settings, namely, a *mastery or task goal*, in which the emphasis is on the development of competence and mastery; a *performance or ego-approach goal*, which entails a concern about the attainment of favorable judgments of normatively defined competence; and a *performance or ego-avoidance goal*, in which the focus is on avoiding the demonstration of normatively defined competence. The efforts of Elliot and colleagues (Elliot & Church, 1997; Elliot & Harackiewicz, 1996) to assess these three goals in academic contexts have laid the foundation for the formulation of trigoal orientation measures specific to sport (e.g., Cury, 2000; Cury, Laurent, DeTonac, & Sot, 1999).

The trichotomous framework makes a number of assumptions regarding the antecedents to achievement goal adoption (Elliot, 1999). *Personal factors* (i.e., achievement motives, beliefs about ability, competence perceptions) and *environmental factors* (i.e., the degree to which the context at hand is task- and/or ego-involving, and contributes to individual's wanting to demonstrate high competence or avoid demonstrating low competence) are presumed to influence which achievement goal is manifested. The achievement goals, then, are held to be more proximal determinants of ensuing achievement-related processes and outcomes (Elliot, 1999; Elliot & Church, 1997).

One of the important distinctions between the trichotomous model and the existing dichotomous achievement goal framework (Dweck, 1986, 1999; Nicholls, 1984, 1989) revolves around the proposed role of perceived competence. In the latter, perceived competence is assumed to moderate the relationship of ego orientation on achievement responses. With respect to Elliot's (1999) trichotomous framework, perceived competence (typically operationalized as performance expectations in this work) is held to be a precursor of the *valence* of the goal adopted; that is, whether *defined* in terms of task- or ego-related criteria, individuals with perceptions of high competence should be more likely to adopt approach (task and/or ego) goals. On the other hand, when perceived competence is low, individuals are expected to center on avoiding the demonstration of low ability (whether task- or ego-referenced).

Sport research testing assumptions regarding the hypothesized antecedents to goal adoption is in its infancy. However, correlational (Cury, Da Fonseca, Rufo, & Sarrazin, 2002; Cury et al., 1999; Halvari & Kjormo, 1999) and experimental (Cury, Da Fonseca, Rufo, Peres, & Sarrazin, 2003; Da Fonseca, Rufo, & Cury, 2001) studies have provided preliminary support for the assumed relationships. For example, Halvari and Kjormo (1999), in their work involving Olympic-level athletes from Norway, reported a correspondence between fear of failure and performance–ego avoidance goals. Cury and associates (1999) found perceptions of competence to be positively associated with mas-

tery–task and performance–ego approach goals and negatively related to performance–ego avoidance goals in their research on young male French athletes. In the physical education context, perceptions of competence, incremental beliefs about sport ability, and perceptions of a task-involving climate emerged as positive predictors, and a perceived ego-involving climate emerged as a negative correlate of mastery–task goals (Cury, Da Fonseca, et al., 2002). Performance–ego approach goals were positively associated with perceived competence, entity beliefs about sport ability, and perceptions of an ego-involving climate, and negatively linked to incremental beliefs about sport ability. With respect to performance–ego avoidance goals, entity beliefs and a perceived ego-involving climate were positive predictors, while incremental beliefs and perceptions of competence were inversely related.

In an experimental protocol across four testing periods, Da Fonseca et al. (2001) assessed cognitive abilities said to be important to high sport performance among 12 young female athletes. The instructional set for the tests was varied to induce incremental or entity beliefs about the abilities being assessed, and negative versus positive test feedback was provided. Regardless of whether the feedback given was positive or negative, the incremental beliefs manipulation promoted a mastery–task goal focus. Moreover, an interaction between the entity beliefs manipulation and feedback also emerged. Specifically, if the athletes were told that the abilities assessed were fixed and received positive feedback, they were more likely to endorse a performance–ego approach goal. When they were in the entity experimental condition and were provided negative feedback, they tended to emphasize performance–ego avoidance goals.

The trichotomous model (Elliot, 1999) also makes predictions regarding the link between the three goals and motivation-related outcomes. One variable of interest has been intrinsic motivation. Intrinsic motivation is the most self-determined motivational regulation for engagement in an activity (Deci & Ryan, 1985). It has been found to be an important predictor of the quantity and quality of engagement in sport settings (Vallerand, 2001).

Because approach goals reflect a desire to strive for success and view achievement situations as a personal challenge, it is hypothesized that both mastery–task and performance–ego approach goals will correspond to greater intrinsic motivation. When centered on avoidance goals, however, the impetus is to avoid failing. Achievement situations are more likely to be viewed as threatening in this case, and the ensuing threat appraisals and anxiety are assumed to diminish intrinsic interest. Thus, it is predicted that performance–ego avoidance goals would be negatively associated with intrinsic motivation. Research by Cury and associates (1999) on 182 young French athletes and a replication sample of 140 young male athletes supported these hypotheses.

Drawing from the trichotomous model, Cury, Elliot, Sarrazin, Da Fonseca, and Rufo (2002) examined potential mediators of the effect of goals on intrinsic motivation. Young adolescent boys and girls engaged in a basketball dribbling task under one of the three experimental conditions: a mastery–task, a performance–ego, and performance–ego avoidance goal condition. Intrinsic motivation was operationalized with respect to how much time the youngsters spent practicing their dribbling during two free-choice periods. The boys and girls that were assigned to the performance–ego avoidance condition exhibited less intrinsic interest than the other two groups. Competence valuation (i.e., whether one considers the task valuable or important), reported task absorption, and state anxiety were all supported as mediators of the undermining of performance–ego avoidance goals on intrinsic motivation. Similar results were reported by Cury, Da Fonseca, et al. (2003).

In his more recent thinking, Elliot has assimilated the definition (i.e., centered on absolute/intrapersonal [task] or normative [ego] criteria) and valence (i.e., oriented toward the possibility of demonstrating high competence or avoiding the demonstration of low competence) aspects of goals to form a 2 × 2 achievement goal model (Elliot & McGregor, 2001). With respect to goal constructs, the major extension in the 2 × 2 framework is the consideration of what is termed a mastery (or task) avoidance goal perspective. In this case, the individual strives to avoid absolute and/or self-referenced incompetence.

According to Elliot (1999), the 2 × 2 model encapsulates the content universe of competence-based goals assumed to be pertinent in achievement settings. Revising the Achievement Goal Questionnaire of Elliot and McGregor (2001) designed to assess the four goals in academic settings, a 2 × 2 Achievement Goals Questionnaire for Sport has recently been developed (Conroy, Elliot, & Hofer, 2003). This instrument has been found to exhibit adequate factorial validity and temporal stability. Moreover, Conroy and colleagues found all the goals except the task (mastery) approach orientation to be significantly and positively correlated with fear of failure.

Clearly, the trichotomous and 2 × 2 approach–avoidance goal models hold promise for furthering insight into goals and motivational processes in the sport domain. However, several conceptual and measurement-related caveats have been raised in regard to early work on avoidance goals in the athletic domain (Cury, Duda, & Sarrazin, 2003; Smith, Duda, Allen, & Hall, 2002). To begin, questions exist regarding contemporary assessments of multiple goal orientations in sport (e.g., Conroy et al., 2003; Cury et al., 1999). What are the expected interrelationships between the goals? Dichotomous goal orientation measures (that have emanated from the work of Nicholls, 1989, in particular) assume task and ego orientations to be orthogonal. However, that interdependence is not necessarily supported when specifically task- and ego-approach sport goals have been examined (Conroy et al., 2003). Furthermore, the observed associations between the other goals tend to be less specified and potentially problematic. For example, in the work of Conroy and associates on the development of the 2 × 2 sport goal questionnaire, ego approach, task avoidance, and ego avoidance all were correlated low to moderate ($r = .40-.54$), while only the task approach and ego avoidance goals were independent. Does this make conceptual sense?

Another query relates to how avoidance goals, particularly ego avoidance goals, are operationalized in contemporary multiple goal measures (Smith et al., 2002). To date, the questionnaires designed to tap multiple goals in sport have drawn from assessment tools geared to the classroom context (e.g., Conroy et al., 2003; Cury et al., 1999). In their factor analysis of ego avoidance goal items emanating from popular academic scales, Smith and colleagues (2002) found these items to be multidimensional; that is, other constructs, such as impression management, seemed to be embedded in what is considered to be an ego avoidance goal orientation.

One final point that is worthy of further deliberation in sport research, particularly pulling from Elliot's (1999; Elliot & Church, 1997) trichotomous model, revolves around what additional insight is provided by taking into account ego avoidance goals when dichotomous (approach) goals, *along with* perceptions of ability, have already been tapped. Relevant to this issue but specific to the educational setting, we found that ego avoidance goal orientation captured variance above and beyond task and ego (approach) goals, perceived ability, and the ego approach and perceived ability interaction *only* in the case of test anxiety among university students (Duda, Hall, & Reinboth, 2004). The students' motivational regulations, entity–incremental beliefs, and effort regulation were significantly and more effectively predicted by the constructs and tenets rooted in dichotomous achievement goal frameworks (Dweck, 1986, 1999; Nicholls, 1984, 1989).

Moreover, although their valence might differ in terms of a concern with exhibiting or avoiding competence, we should keep in mind that the more traditional ego (approach) goal orientation and its ego avoidance counterpart have a lot in common. For example, in previous sport research, both have been found to correlate significantly with extrinsic motivation, entity beliefs about ability, and fear of failure. Thus, there seems to be a shared belief structure, mutual concerns, and less self-determined–more controlling regulations for engagement underlying these goals. Might it be that a considerable number (if not all?) of the high ego avoidance people in sport were once strongly ego approach-oriented and then came to doubt their competence and/or found themselves in situations that made them more afraid of the consequences of failing (than the joys and sense of accom-

plishment coupled with success)? Recent work by Papaiaonnou, Mylosis, Kosmidou, and Tsiglis (2004) on students engaged in sport-related drills provides preliminary evidence regarding the tenability of this proposition. Specifically, hierarchical multiple regression analyses indicated that the activation of ego approach goals subsequently mobilized ego avoidance goals during the activity. The reverse relationship was *not* supported. In a 12-month longitudinal study of task–ego approach and ego avoidance goal orientations in sport, and with respect to language classes, Papaioannou and associates (2004) also found ego approach goals at Time 1 to significantly predict ego avoidance goals at Time 2, but not vice versa.

IMPLICATION OF ACHIEVEMENT GOALS: BEYOND ACHIEVEMENT

An exciting feature of achievement goal research in the sport domain is that there has been an interest in predicting other responses and perspectives of athletes beyond those that are clearly achievement-related; that is, this literature sheds some light on the role of achievement goals with respect to the *quantity* and *quality* of athletes' motivation (Duda, 2001). The quantity of athletes' motivation is reflected in how they are performing and the degree to which they are invested in sport at a particular point in time. An examination of an athlete's competitive performance at a certain point of time is indicative of the quantity of his or her motivation. A consideration of the quality of motivation entails a broader and more long-term perspective. Is the athlete witnessing personal growth and positive development in terms of his or her psychological, emotional, physical, and moral functioning? Does the athlete want to (and is the athlete able to) persevere in sport and reach his or her potential?

Exemplifying this attention to the quality of athletes' achievement striving, sport studies have found dispositional and/or perceived situationally emphasized achievement goals to predict athletes' moral attitudes and behaviors (e.g., Duda, Olson, & Templin, 1991; Kavussanu & Roberts, 2001). In general, task goals tend to correspond to greater sportspersonship, while ego orientation and/ or a perceived ego-involving motivational climate has been associated with a stronger endorsement of cheating and aggression (Biddle et al., 2003; Duda, 2001). Other studies have found that achievement goals provide insight into health risks among athletic populations (e.g., disordered eating attitudes and behaviors, body image disturbances, and steroid/performance-enhancing substance use; Duda, Benardot, & Kim, 2004). Recent research has also examined the interplay between achievement goals and indicators of athletes' psychological welfare (e.g., Reinboth & Duda, 2004).

One important index of mental and emotional health is an individual's self-esteem (Harter, 1993). With respect to a hypothesized link between achievement goals and self-worth, Kaplan and Maehr (1999) argued that goal orientations may operate as "self-primes." When centered on meeting ego-oriented goals, there is a presumed heightened self-awareness and a concern with validating one's sense of self through the activity; that is, "when an ego goal is endorsed, it focuses attention on who one is, what one can be, or what one can do" (Duda & Hall, 2001, p. 422). In contrast, if geared toward meeting task-oriented criteria for success, the individual is held to be more centered on what he or she is doing.

A number of studies have examined the correspondence between sport goal orientations and athletes' reported self-worth. On the whole, task orientation tends to be positively correlated with level of self-esteem (see Duda, 2001, for a review). It has been argued that understanding the processes underpinning self-worth also entails a consideration of the degree to which an individual's self-esteem varies over time. Individual differences in exhibiting fluctuating self-worth have been termed "labile" (Butler, Hokanson, & Flynn, 1994) or self-esteem stability (Greenier, Kernis, & Waschull, 1995). In our research on a large sample of young British athletes (McArdle, Duda, and Hall, 2004), we attempted to distinguish these participants as a function of their goal orientations and other achievement-related characteristics (i.e., their motivational regulations and perfectionistic tendencies). Relevant to the issue at hand, cluster analysis revealed four groups of athletes. The first

group exhibited moderately high task and ego orientation. The second group was marked by high task orientation and low ego orientation, while the third had high task orientation coupled with moderate ego orientation. A fourth group was characterized by moderately high ego orientation and low task orientation. The athletes who were classified in groups reporting high task orientation had the highest level of self-esteem. The high task-oriented and low ego-oriented athletes revealed the lowest degree of labile self-esteem, while the highly ego-oriented athletes who were not buffered by the possession of high task orientation reported the highest labile self-esteem.

All in all, the findings of McArdle and colleagues (2004) are aligned with the suggestions of Dweck (1999) and Kaplan and Maehr (1999), who argue that an ego goal focus should correspond to an exacerbated awareness of the self and a need to validate oneself through one's performances. With respect to this latter supposition, one possible explanation for why a predominant ego orientation was linked to more unstable self-esteem in the McArdle et al. study (2004) is that these athletes were evaluating themselves as people with respect to how they were doing in sport. In other words, their sense of personal worth was contingent on the demonstration of superior sport ability. Since sport competition makes it a daunting challenge for someone always to be the best, it is understandable why the self-esteem of highly ego-oriented athletes (who are not also highly task-oriented) would be more likely to go up and down.

A recent study by Reinboth and Duda (2004) provides preliminary evidence that is consonant with this argument. In this investigation, we examined the relationship of the perceived motivational climate (in terms of its task- and ego-involving features; Newton et al., 2000) and perceptions of ability to psychological and physical well-being among 265 male adolescent football and cricket players. Level of self-esteem, satisfaction/interest in sport, the physical exhaustion facet of burnout, and physical symptoms were measured as indices of the athletes' mental and physical welfare. However, the degree to which these athletes perceived their self-esteem to be contingent on sport performance was also ascertained.

Contingent self-esteem (as well as physical exhaustion and reported physical symptoms) was found to be positively predicted by perceptions of an ego-involving climate. Moreover, a significant ego-involving climate × perceived ability interaction emerged with respect to level of self-esteem. Aligned with the predictions of achievement goal frameworks (Dweck, 1999; Nicholls, 1989), reported self-worth was lower among the low perceived ability athletes participating in an environment that was perceived to be high in its ego-involving features. Satisfaction/interest in sport was positively related, and physical symptoms were negatively linked to perceived ability and perceptions of a task-involving atmosphere.

As can be seen in this short summary of recent research on aspects of the quality of athletes' sport experience, the work to date has been grounded in dichotomous models of achievement goals. An intriguing direction for subsequent studies would be to examine the implications of both approach and avoidance (task and ego) goals on athletes' moral functioning and well-being within the athletic milieu.

CONCLUSIONS AND FUTURE AREAS OF INQUIRY

Once the work on the implications of achievement goals on achievement-related processes in the academic–cognitive domains caught the attention of sport psychology researchers in the late 1980s, this line of investigation truly burgeoned. Indeed, achievement goal frameworks reflect a (if not *the*) major conceptualization underpinning sport achievement motivation research today. In this chapter, I have attempted to give the reader a feel for the directions this work has taken and the findings to date. In general, results are compatible with what has emerged in educational settings and aligned with theoretical predictions.

Although it is still a source of debate, and certainly not beyond the need for improvement, there have been considerable advancements in the measurement of achievement goal constructs specific to the sport domain. Overall, the measures of sport goal orientations and perceptions of the motivational climate created by coaches and other signifi-

cant others have been repeatedly tested and tend to exhibit acceptable psychometric properties. An interesting and challenging avenue for future work in the sport milieu concerns the assessment of more dynamic states of goal involvement during training and competition.

In terms of the achievement goal literature as a whole, it is fair to say that sport investigations have led the way in terms of looking at the interchange between dispositional and perceived situationally emphasized goals on motivational processes and outcomes. Because both individual differences in sport goal orientations and perceptions of the motivational climate(s) surrounding sport participants play a role in how individuals view and respond to sport, it seems prudent that future work examine their interactive and potentially bidirectional influence in real-life settings over time.

Sport researchers have also extended the general achievement goal literature in other ways. They have taken the existing conceptual frameworks to exciting and relatively uncharted territories, such as contemporary work on athletes' moral functioning and well-being. In research examining the links between achievement goals and intrinsic enjoyment, anxiety, and self-appraisals, they are also moving toward integrations between achievement goal frameworks and other psychological theories of motivation, stress, and self-esteem/self-concept (Duda, 2001).

In closing, it is important for all motivation psychologists to recognize that a great deal of intriguing, insightful, and informative work has been done on achievement goals in the sport domain. The future holds much promise for this trend to continue.

REFERENCES

Ames, C. (1992a). Classrooms, goal structures, and student motivation. *Journal of Educational Psychology*, 84, 261–274.
Ames, C. (1992b). Achievement goals, motivational climate, and motivational processes. In G. C. Roberts (Ed.), *Motivation in sport and exercise* (pp. 161–176). Champaign, IL: Human Kinetics.
Ames, C., & Archer, J. (1988). Achievement goals in the classroom: Students' learning strategies and motivation processes. *Journal of Educational Psychology*, 80, 260–267.

Babkes, M., & Weiss, M. R. (1999). Parental influence on children's cognitive and affective responses to competitive soccer participation. *Pediatric Exercise Science*, 11, 44–62.

Balaguer, I., Duda, J. L., Atienza, F. L., & Mayo, C. (2002). Situational and dispositional goals as predictors of perceptions on individual and team improvement, satisfaction and coach ratings among elite female handball teams. *Psychology of Sport and Exercise*, 3(4), 293–308.

Bandura, A. (1977). Self-efficacy: Toward a unifying theory of behavioral change. *Psychological Review*, 84, 191–215.

Bandura, A. (1986). *Social foundation of thought and action: A social cognitive theory.* Englewood Cliffs, NJ: Prentice-Hall.

Biddle, S. J. H. (2001). Enhancing motivation in physical education. In G. C. Roberts (Ed.), *Advances in sport and exercise motivation* (pp. 101–128). Champaign, IL: Human Kinetics.

Biddle, S. J. H., Soos, I., & Chatzisarantis, N., (1999). Predicting physical activity intentions using goal perspectives and self-determination theory approaches. *European Psychologist*, 4, 83–89.

Biddle, S. J. H., Wang, J., Kavussanu, M., & Spray, C. (2003). Correlates of achievement goal orientations in physical activity: A systematic review of research. *European Journal of Sports Science*, 3(5), 1–19.

Brustad, R. J. (1996). Attraction to physical activity in urban schoolchildren: Parental socialization and gender influences. *Research Quarterly for Exercise and Sport*, 67, 316–323.

Burton, D., & Martens, R. (1986). Pinned by their own goals: An exploratory investigation into why kids drop out of wrestling. *Journal of Sport Psychology*, 8, 183–197.

Butler, A. C., Hokanson, J. E., & Flynn, H. A. (1994). A comparison of self-esteem liability and low trait self-esteem as vulnerability factors for depression. *Journal of Personality and Social Psychology*, 66, 166–177.

Carpenter, P., & Morgan, K. (1999). Motivational climate, personal goal perspectives, and cognitive and affective responses in physical education classes. *European Journal of Physical Education*, 4, 31–44.

Carpenter, P., & Yates, B. (1997). Relationship between achievement goals and the perceived purposes of soccer for semi-professional and amateur players. *Journal of Sport and Exercise Psychology*, 19, 302–312.

Chi, L., & Duda, J. L. (1995). Multi-group confirmatory factor analysis of the Task and Ego Orientation in Sport Questionnaire. *Research Quarterly for Exercise and Sport*, 66, 91–98.

Conroy, D. E., Elliot, A. J., & Hofer, S. M. (2003). A 2 × 2 Achievement Goals Questionnaire for Sport: Evidence for factorial invariance, temporal stability, and external validity. *Journal of Sport and Exercise Psychology*, 25, 1–21.

Cury, F. (2000). Predictive validity of the approach and avoidance achievement in sport model. *Journal of Sport and Exercise Psychology*, 22, S32.

Cury, F., Da Fonseca, D., Rufo, M., Peres, C., & Sarrazin, P. (2003). The trichotomous model and investment in learning to prepare a sport test: A mediational analysis. *British Journal of Educational Psychology*, 73, 529–543.

Cury, F., Da Fonseca, D., Rufo, M., & Sarrazin, P. (2002). Perceptions of competence, implicit theory of ability, perception of the motivational climate, and achievement goals: A test of the trichotomous conceptualization of the endorsement of achievement motivation in the physical education setting. *Perception and Motor Skills*, 95, 233–244.

Cury, F., Duda, J. L., & Sarrazin, P. (2003). *The integration of avoidance motivation in achievement goal theory: Preliminary findings in sport and physical education settings with some caveats and considerations for future work.* Unpublished manuscript.

Cury, F., Elliot, A., Sarrazin, P., Da Fonseca, D., & Rufo, M. (2002). The trichotomous achievement goal model and intrinsic motivation: A sequential mediational analysis. *Journal of Experimental Social Psychology*, 38, 473–481.

Cury, F., Famose, J. P., & Sarrazin, P. (1997). Achievement goal theory and active search for information in a sport task. In R. Lidor & M. Bar-Eli (Eds.), *Innovations in sport psychology: Linking theory and practice. Proceedings of the IX World Congress in Sport Psychology: Part I* (pp. 218–220). Netanya, Israel: Ministry of Education, Culture and Sport.

Cury, F., Laurent, M., De Tonac, A., & Sot, V. (1999). An unexplored aspect of achievement goal theory in sport: Development and predictive validity of the Approach and Avoidance Achievement in Sport Questionnaire (AAASQ). In V. Hosek, P. Tilinger, & L. Bilek (Eds.), *Psychology of sport and exercise: Enhancing quality of life: Proceedings of the 10th European Congress of Sport Psychology—FEPSAC* (pp. 153–155). Prague: Charles University Press.

Cury, F., & Sarrazin, P. (1998). Achievement motivation and learning behaviors in sport tasks. *Journal of Sport and Exercise Psychology*, 20, S11.

Da Fonseca, A., Rufo, M., & Cury, F. (2001). Predictive value of the implicit theories of sport ability in achievement goals. In A. Papaioannou, M. Goudas, & Y. Theodorakis (Eds.), *Tenth World Congress of Sport Psychology proceedings* (Vol. 3, pp. 34–36). Skiathos, Greece, ISSP.

Deci, E. L., & Ryan, R. M. (1985). *Intrinsic motivation and self-determination in human behavior.* New York: Plenum Press.

Duda, J. L. (1989). The relationship between task and ego orientation and the perceived purpose of sport among male and female high school athletes. *Journal of Sport and Exercise Psychology*, 11, 318–335.

Duda, J. L. (1992). Sport and exercise motivation: A goal perspective analysis. In G. Roberts (Ed.), *Motivation in sport and exercise* (pp. 57–91). Champaign, IL: Human Kinetics.

Duda, J. L. (1993). Goals: A social cognitive approach to the study of motivation in sport. In R. N. Singer, M. Murphey, & L. K. Tennant (Eds.), *Handbook on* research in sport psychology (pp. 421–436). New York: Macmillan.

Duda, J. L. (2001). Goal perspectives research in sport: Pushing the boundaries and clarifying some misunderstandings. In G. C. Roberts (Ed.), *Advances in motivation in sport and exercise* (pp. 129–182). Champaign, IL: Human Kinetics.

Duda, J. L., Benardot, D., & Kim, M.-S. (2004). *The relationship of the motivational climate to psychological and energy balance correlates of eating disorders in female gymnasts.* Unpublished manuscript.

Duda, J. L., Fox, K. R., Biddle, S. J. H., & Armstrong, N. (1992). Children's achievement goals and beliefs about success in sport. *British Journal of Educational Psychology, 62,* 313–323.

Duda, J. L., & Hall, H. (2001). Achievement goal theory in sport: Recent extensions and future directions. In R. Singer, H. Hausenblas, & C. Janelle (Eds.), *Handbook of sport psychology* (2nd ed., pp. 417–443). New York: Wiley.

Duda, J. L., Hall, H., & Reinboth, M. (2004). *Predicting motivational regulations, anxiety, and effort regulation in the classroom: Dichotomous versus trichotomous goal predictions.* Unpublished manuscript.

Duda, J. L., & Hom, H. (1993). Interdependencies between the perceived and self-reported goal orientations of young athletes and their parents. *Pediatric Exercise Science, 5,* 234–241.

Duda, J. L., Newton, M. L., & Yin, Z. (1999). Variation in perceptions of the motivational climate and its predictors. *Psychology of sport and exercise: Enhancing the quality of life. Proceedings of the 10th European Congress of Sport Psychology (FEPSAC)* (pp. 167–169). Prague: Charles University Press.

Duda, J. L., & Nicholls, J. G. (1992). Dimensions of achievement motivation in schoolwork and sport. *Journal of Educational Psychology, 84,* 290–299.

Duda, J. L., & Ntoumanis, N. (2003). Correlates of achievement goal orientations in physical education. *International Journal of Educational Research, 39,* 415–436.

Duda, J. L., Olson, L., & Templin, T. (1991). The relationship of task and ego orientation to sportsmanship attitudes and the perceived legitimacy of injurious acts. *Research Quarterly for Exercise and Sport, 62,* 79–87.

Duda, J. L., & Whitehead, J. (1998). Measurement of goal perspectives in the physical domain. In J. Duda (Ed.), *Advances in sport and exercise psychology measurement* (pp. 21–48). Morgantown, WV: Fitness Information Technology.

Dweck, C. S. (1986). Motivational processes affecting learning. *American Psychologist, 41,* 1040–1048.

Dweck, C. S. (1999). *Self-theories: Their role in motivation, personality, and development.* Philadelphia: Psychology Press.

Dweck, C. S., & Leggett, E. L. (1988). A social-cognitive approach to personality and motivation. *Psychological Review, 95,* 256–273.

Ebbeck, V., & Becker, S. L. (1994). Psychosocial predictors of goal orientations in youth soccer. *Research Quarterly for Exercise and Sport, 65,* 355–362.

Eccles, J. S., & Harold, R. (1991). Gender differences in sport involvement: Applying the Eccles expectancy–value model. *Journal of Applied Sport Psychology, 3,* 7–35.

Eccles, J., Jacobs, J., & Harold, R. (1990). Gender role stereotypes, expectancy effects, parents' socialization of gender differences. *Journal of Social Issues, 46*(2), 183–201.

Eccles, J., & Wigfield, A. (1995). In the mind of the actor: The structure of adolescents' achievement task values and expectancy-related beliefs. *Personality and Social Psychology Bulletin, 21*(3), 215–225.

Elliot, A. J. (1997). Integrating the "classic" and "contemporary" approaches to achievement motivation: A hierarchical model of approach and avoidance achievement motivation. In M. L. Maehr & P. R. Pintrich (Eds.), *Advances in motivation and achievement* (Vol. 10, pp. 143–179). Greenwich, CT: JAI Press.

Elliot, A. J. (1999). Approach and avoidance motivation and achievement goals. *Educational Psychologist, 34,* 169–189.

Elliot, A. J., & Church, M. A. (1997). A hierarchical model of approach and avoidance motivation. *Journal of Personality and Social Psychology, 72,* 218–232.

Elliot, A. J., & Harackiewicz, J. M. (1996). Approach and avoidance achievement goals and intrinsic motivation: A mediational analysis. *Journal of Personality and Social Psychology, 70,* 461–475.

Elliot, A. J., & Mc Gregor, H. A. (2001). A 2 × 2 achievement goal framework. *Journal of Personality and Social Psychology, 80,* 501–519.

Feltz, D. L. (1992). Understanding motivation in sport: A self-efficacy perspective. In G. C. Roberts (Ed.), *Motivation in sport and exercise* (pp. 107–128). Champaign, IL: Human Kinetics.

Feltz, D. L., & Lirgg, C. D. (2001). Self efficacy beliefs of athletes, teams and coaches. In R. Singer, H. Hausenblas, & C. Janelle (Eds.), *Handbook of sport psychology* (2nd ed., pp. 340–361). New York: Wiley.

Greenier, K. D., Kernis, M. H., & Waschull, S. B. (1995). Not all high (or low) self-esteem people are the same: Theory and research on stability of self-esteem. In M. H. Kernis (Ed.), *Efficacy, agency, and self-esteem* (pp. 51–71). New York: Plenum Press.

Hall, H. K., & Kerr, A. (1997). Motivational antecedents of precompetitive anxiety in youth sport. *The Sport Psychologist, 11,* 24–42.

Halvari, H., & Kjormo, O. (1999). A structural model of achievement motives, performance approach and avoidance goals and performance among Norwegian Olympic athletes. *Perceptual and Motor Skills, 89,* 997–1022.

Hardy, L. (1997). Three myths about applied consultancy work. *Journal of Applied Sport Psychology, 9,* 277–294.

Harter, S. (1978). Effectance motivation re-considered. *Human Development, 21,* 34–64.

Harter, S. (1981). A model of intrinsic mastery motivation in children: Individual differences and developmental change. In W. A. Collins (Ed.), *Minnesota Symposium on Child Psychology* (Vol. 14, pp. 215–255). Hillsdale, NJ: Erlbaum.

Harwood, C., Hardy, L., & Swain, A. (2000). Achievement goals in sport: A critique of conceptual and measurement issues. *Journal of Sport and Exercise Psychology, 22*, 235–255.

Harwood, C., & Swain, A. (1998). Antecedents of precompetition achievement goals in elite junior tennis players. *Journal of Sport Sciences, 16*, 357–371.

Horn, T. S., Glenn, S. D., & Wentzell, A. B. (1993). Sources of information underlying personal ability judgements in high school athletes. *Pediatric Exercise Science, 5*, 263–274.

Kaplan, A., & Maehr, M. (1999). *Achievement motivation: The emergence, contributions, and prospects of a goal orientation theory perspective.* Unpublished manuscript, Ben Gurion University, Beer Sheva, Israel.

Kavussanu, M., & Roberts, G. C. (1996). Motivation in physical activity contexts: The relationship of perceived motivational climate to intrinsic motivation and self-efficacy. *Journal of Sport and Exercise Psychology, 18*, 254–280.

Kavussanu, M., & Roberts, G. C. (2001). Moral functioning in sport: An achievement goal perspective. *Journal of Sport and Exercise Psychology, 23*, 37–54.

Kim, M.-S., & Duda, J. L. (1998). Achievement goals, motivational climate, and occurrence of and response to psychological difficulties and performance debilitation among Korean athletes. *Journal of Sport and Exercise Psychology, 20*, S124.

Kimiecik, J., Horn, T. S., & Shurin, C. S. (1996). Relationships among children's beliefs, perceptions of their parents' beliefs and their moderate-to-vigorous physical activity. *Research Quarterly for Exercise and Sport, 67*, 324–336.

Krane, V., Greenleaf, C. A., & Snow, J. (1997). Reaching for gold and the price of glory: A motivational case study of an elite gymnast. *The Sport Psychologist, 11*, 53–71.

Lloyd, J., & Fox, K. R. (1992). Achievement goals and motivation to exercise in adolescent girls: A preliminary study. *British Journal of Physical Education Research Supplement, 11*, 12–16.

Lochbaum, M., & Roberts, G. C. (1993). Goal orientations and perceptions of the sport experience. *Journal of Sport and Exercise Psychology, 15*, 160–171.

McArdle, S., Duda, J. L., & Hall, H. K. (2004). *Young athletes striving for perfection: Examining variability in achievement experiences and self perceptions.* Manuscript under review.

Middleton, C., & Midgley, C. (1997). Avoiding the demonstration of lack of ability: An unexplored aspect of goal theory. *Journal of Educational Psychology, 89*, 710–718.

Newton, M. L., & Duda, J. L. (1999). The interaction of motivational climate, dispositional goal orientation and perceived ability in predicting indices of motivation. *International Journal of Sport Psychology, 29*, 1–20.

Newton, M. L., Duda, J. L., & Yin, Z. (2000). Examination of the psychometric properties of the Perceived Motivational Climate in Sport Questionnaire-2 in a sample of female athletes. *Journal of Sport Sciences, 18*(4), 275–290.

Newton, M. L., & Fry, M. (1998). Senior Olympians' achievement goals and motivational responses. *Journal of Aging and Physical Activity, 6*, 256–270.

Nicholls, J. G. (1984). Achievement motivation: Conceptions of ability, subjective experience, task choice, and performance. *Psychological Review, 91*, 328–346.

Nicholls, J. G. (1989). *The competitive ethos and democratic education.* Cambridge, MA: Harvard University Press.

Nicholls, J. G. (1992). The general and the specific in the development and expression of achievement motivation. In G. C. Roberts (Ed.), *Motivation in sport and exercise* (pp. 31–56). Champaign, IL: Human Kinetics.

Ntoumanis, N., & Biddle, S. J. H. (1998). The relationship between competitive anxiety, achievement goals, and motivational climates. *Research Quarterly for Exercise and Sport, 69*, 176–187.

Ntoumanis, N., & Biddle, S. J. H. (1999a). Affect and achievement goals in physical activity: A meta-analysis. *Scandinavian Journal of Medicine and Science in Sport, 9*, 315–332.

Ntoumanis, N., & Biddle, S. J. H. (1999b). A review of motivational climate in physical activity. *Journal of Sport Sciences, 17*, 643–665.

Papaioannou, A. (1995). Motivation and goal perspectives in children's physical education. In S. J. H. Biddle (Ed.), *European perspectives on exercise and sport psychology* (pp. 245–269). Champaign, IL: Human Kinetics.

Papaioannou, A., Mylosis, D., Kosmidou, E., & Tsigilis, N. (2004, June). *A measure of motivational climate and goals at the situational level of generality.* Paper presented at the International Congress of the Moroccan Association of Sports Psychology, Marrakech, Morocco.

Pensgaard, A. M., & Duda, J. L. (2004). *Relationship of situational and dispositional goals to coach ratings, perceived stressors and performance among Olympic athletes.* Manuscript under review.

Pensgaard, A. M., & Roberts, G. C. (2000). The relationship between motivational climate, perceived ability, and sources of distress among elite athletes. *Journal of Sports Sciences, 18*(3), 191–200.

Pintrich, P. R. (2000). An achievement goal theory perspective on issues in motivation terminology, theory, and research. *Contemporary Educational Psychology, 25*, 92–104.

Reinboth, M., & Duda, J. L. (2004). Relationship of the perceived motivational climate and perceptions of ability to psychological and physical well-being in team sports. *The Sport Psychologist, 18,* 237–251.

Roberts, G. C. (1992). Motivation in sport: Conceptual constraints and convergence. In G. C. Roberts (Ed.), *Motivation in sport and exercise* (pp. 3–29). Champaign, IL: Human Kinetics.

Roberts, G. C. (2001). Understanding the dynamics of motivation in physical activity: The influence of achievement goals on motivational processes. In G. C. Roberts (Ed.), *Advances in sport and exercise motivation* (pp. 1–50). Champaign, IL: Human Kinetics.

Roberts, G. C., Kleiber, D. A., & Duda, J. L. (1981). An analysis of motivation in children's sport: The role of perceived competence in participation. *Journal of Sport Psychology, 3*(3), 206–216.

Roberts, G. C., & Ommundsen, Y. (1996). Effects of achievement goal orientations on achievement beliefs, cognitions, and strategies in team sport. *Scandanavian Journal of Medicine and Science in Sport, 6,* 46–56.

Roberts, G. C., Treasure, D. C., & Balague, G. (1998). Achievement goals in sport: The development and validation of the Perception of Success Questionnaire. *Journal of Sports Sciences, 16,* 337–347.

Sarrazin, P., Vallerand, R. J., Guillet, E., Pelletier, L., & Cury, F. (2002). Motivation and dropout in female handballers: A 21-month prospective study. *European Journal of Social Psychology, 32*(3), 395–418.

Seifriz, J., Duda, J. L., & Chi, L. (1992). The relationship of perceived motivational climate to intrinsic motivation and beliefs about success in basketball. *Journal of Sport and Exercise Psychology, 14,* 375–391.

Skaalvik, E. (1997). Self-enhancing and self-defeating ego orientations: Relations with task and avoidance orientation, achievement, self-perceptions, and anxiety. *Journal of Educational Psychology, 89,* 71–81.

Smith, M., Duda, J. L., Allen, J., & Hall, H. (2002). Contemporary measures of approach and avoidance goal orientations: Similarities and differences. *British Journal of Educational Psychology, 2,* 154–189.

Thill, E., & Brunel, P. (1995). Ego involvement and task involvement: Related conceptions of ability, effort, and learning strategies among soccer players. *International Journal of Sport Psychology, 26,* 81–97.

Treasure, D. C. (1993). *A social-cognitive approach to understanding children's achievement behaviour, cognitions, and affect in competitive sport.* Unpublished doctoral dissertation, University of Illinois, Urbana–Champaign.

Treasure, D. C. (2001). Enhancing young people's motivation in youth sport: An achievement goal approach. In G. C. Roberts (Ed.), *Advances in sport*

and exercise motivation (pp. 79–100). Champaign, IL: Human Kinetics.

Treasure, D. C., Duda, J. L., Hall, H. K., Roberts, G. C., Ames, C., & Maehr, M. L. (2001). Clarifying misconceptions and misrepresentations in achievement goal research in sport: A response to Harwood, Hardy, and Swain. *Journal of Sport and Exercise Psychology, 23,* 317–329.

Treasure, D. C., & Roberts, G. C. (1994). Cognitive and affective concomitants of task and ego goal orientations during the middle school years. *Journal of Sport and Exercise Psychology, 16,* 15–28.

Treasure, D., & Roberts, G. C. (1998). Relationship between female adolescents' achievement goal orientations, perceptions of the motivational climate, belief about success, and sources of satisfaction in basketball. *International Journal of Sport Psychology, 28,* 211–230.

Vallerand, R. J. (2001). A hierarchical model of intrinsic and extrinsic motivation in sport and exercise. In G. C. Roberts (Ed.), *Advances in sport and exercise motivation* (pp. 263–320). Champaign, IL: Human Kinetics.

VanYperen, N., & Duda, J. L. (1999). Goal orientations, beliefs about success, and performance improvement among young elite Dutch soccer players. *Scandinavian Journal of Medicine and Science in Sports, 9,* 358–364.

Vazou, S., Ntoumanis, N., & Duda, J. L. (2004, June). *Motivational climate in youth sport: The relative influence of coach and peers.* Paper presented at the annual convention of the North American Society for the Psychology of Sport and Physical Activity, Vancouver, Canada.

Vazou, S., Ntoumanis, N., & Duda, J. L. (in press). Peer motivational climate in youth sport: A qualitative inquiry. *Psychology of Sport and Exercise.*

Walling, M. D., Duda, J. L., & Chi, L. (1993). The Perceived Motivational Climate in Sport Questionnaire: Construct and predictive validity. *Journal of Sport and Exercise Psychology, 15,* 172–183.

Weinberg, R. S., Gould, D., Yukelson, D., & Jackson, A. (1981). The effect of preexisting and manipulated self-efficacy on a competitive muscular task. *Journal of Sport Psychology, 3,* 345–354.

White, S. A. (1996). Goal orientations and perceptions of the motivational climate initiated by parents. *Pediatric Exercise Science, 8,* 122–129.

White, S. A., Duda, J. L., & Hart, S. (1992). An exploratory examination of the Parent-Initiated Motivational Climate Questionnaire. *Perceptual and Motor Skills, 75,* 875–880.

Williams, L. (1998). Contextual influences and goal perspectives among female youth sport participants. *Research Quarterly for Exercise and Sport, 69,* 47–57.

CHAPTER 19

☙

Work Competence

A Person-Oriented Perspective

RUTH KANFER

PHILLIP L. ACKERMAN

In this chapter, we describe the person components and processes involved in the development and expression of competence in the workplace. First, we provide a provisional definition of "work competence" in the context of maximal performance. Next, we outline the major trait and other stable disposition components and processes by which these factors interact to affect work competence. Third, we address the role of situational influences in terms of their effects on both the development and expression of workplace competence, and propose an illustrative model of work competence that takes account of both person and situational influences. Finally, we consider some broad person and contextual issues in the domain of work competence, including the changing nature of work and adult aging.

The process of defining competence in the workplace requires consideration of two issues. First, unlike competence in other life arenas, competence in the workplace typically refers to the potential for, or demonstration of, coordinated actions that accomplish *organizationally valued* tasks, such as installing equipment, planning conferences, resolving customer problems, or creating or selling a product; that is, the definition of competent performance critically depends on the job and work role demands. A restaurant supervisor may be judged competent if food is delivered promptly, even if he or she cannot operate the cash register quickly.

Second, competence is not synonymous with performance. Performance is influenced by a number of factors, including stable trait-like factors internal to the individual (e.g., abilities and skills), external factors (e.g., broken equipment), and transitory factors (e.g., temporary distraction because of an earlier argument with a spouse, or lack of skill with a new computer system). An individual may perform poorly due to incompetence, lack of motivation, and/or environmental factors that impede the effective expression of competence. "Competencies," defined by Landy and Conte (2004; also see Kurz & Bartram, 2002) as "sets of behaviors, usually learned by experience, that are instrumental in the accomplishment of various activities" (p. 116) refer to the integration of individual differences attributes for the purpose of context-specific objectives. In this chapter, we focus on the trait and trait-like factors that contribute to the development of work competencies and competence, and then consider some of the other factors that influence the expression of competence in job performance.

Our explication of competence in the workplace and emphasis on person factors may be further clarified by considering competence in terms of the broader distinction between maximal performance and typical behavior. In the following section, we delineate the differences between these contexts and their implication for defining competence in the workplace.

MAXIMAL PERFORMANCE AND TYPICAL BEHAVIOR

Cronbach (1949) was perhaps the first psychologist to call attention to two different contexts for human behavior. Although Cronbach was most interested in the context of psychological testing and assessment, the distinction is important in academic achievement and work contexts. "Maximal performance" refers to the individual's capabilities. It represents what the individual "can do" when all internal states (amount of sleep, lack of distraction, etc.) are optimal for the individual to focus his or her attention to the task at hand. When psychologists assess aptitudes or abilities, their goal is to elicit the maximal performance of the individual, so that an accurate attribution of the individual's capabilities is made.

In contrast, "typical behavior" refers to what the individual is likely to do, or prefers to do, on a day-to-day basis. When one considers academic aptitude testing, such as is done with the Scholastic Aptitude Test (SAT) or Graduate Record Examination (GRE), examinees are generally willing to expend maximal effort—mainly because the rewards for good performance are obvious and tangible. However, if faced with taking the SAT every day for a year, with no clear rewards for good performance or punishment for poor performance, many individuals would likely reduce their level of effort

during the test administrations. When psychologists assess personality and interest constructs, they usually ask what an individual likes to do, prefers to do, or usually does in various contexts. All of these conditions reflect typical behaviors or, roughly, what the individual is most likely to do (for extensive discussions of these issues, see Ackerman, 1994, 1997).

From this perspective, when we set out to define work competence, we ordinarily refer to the individual's maximal performance rather than his or her typical behavior, since we are, at least initially, most interested in what the individual can do. However, many influences combine to dissociate what the individual can do and what he or she actually will do, and that is the source of additional discussion in this chapter. First, we consider the determinants of maximal performance.

DISTAL DETERMINANTS OF WORK COMPETENCE

Industrial–organizational psychologists often characterize work competence as a complex function of four broad components—knowledge, skills, abilities, and "other" attributes (denoted KSAOs). Our conceptualization takes a similar but not entirely identical categorization. We consider the following components: abilities, knowledge and skills, motivation, personality, and self-concept (which includes self-confidence and self-efficacy). Each of these is treated in turn.

Abilities

Starting about 100 years ago (e.g., Binet & Simon, 1911/1915; Spearman, 1904) and continuing to the present day, differential[1] psychologists and educational psychologists have sought to identify the structure and function of human intellectual abilities. Both historically and pragmatically, there have been two major camps in the debate over the nature of human intelligence. Followers of Spearman (e.g., Jensen, 1998) have emphasized that a single general intellectual ability (denoted g) takes up the major share of individual differences variance across just about any domain of cognitive or intellectual functioning. In contrast, followers of Thorndike (e.g., see Thorndike, Bregman, Cobb, &

Woodyard, 1927), Thurstone (1938), and others have deemphasized the importance of *g* and have focused instead on other lower order factors of intellectual abilities (e.g., spatial, verbal, numerical). Over the past 40 or 50 years, however, the consensus view among researchers in the field is that there is a hierarchy of human abilities, in that lower order abilities exist but are themselves correlated with one another, thus implying that a general factor of intelligence exists and accounts for roughly 50% of the variance in human abilities (e.g., see Carroll, 1993; Vernon, 1950).

However, a developmental perspective, the approach outlined first by Hebb (1942) and later expanded by Cattell (1943), provides an important identification of two major components of human intelligence. The first component, identified as general fluid intelligence (*Gf*) by Cattell, is associated with abstract reasoning, memory, and the cognitive processes associated with solving novel questions. This class of abilities is thought to be most highly associated with biological and genetic factors. Developmentally, *Gf* peaks in late adolescence or early adulthood and declines throughout the rest of adulthood. In contrast, the second major component, called general crystallized intelligence (*Gc*) by Cattell, represents the accumulation of educational and experiential knowledge and skills. Although *Gf* peaks early in an individual's work life, *Gc* often is not only maintained well into middle age but may also continue to develop until relatively old age. Typically, *Gc* is assessed with tests of vocabulary, information, and fluency, but the conceptual representation of *Gc* (e.g., see Ackerman, 1996; Cattell, 1957) is that it encompasses a wide array of academic, vocational, and avocational (e.g., hobbies) knowledge. In most studies of adult intellect, estimates of *Gf* and *Gc* are correlated with one another, but the correlation does not reach levels that would indicate that one general ability is isomorphic to the other (e.g., Horn, 1989; see also Ackerman, 2000, for an empirical example).

Gf and Work Competence

In colloquial terms, individual differences in *Gf* are most important as an indicator of the ability to learn. Measures of *Gf* are often good predictors of learning and academic achievement for adolescents and young adults. When the learning or training environment is novel and challenging, differences in *Gf* can be expected to play an important role in determining the aptitude of individuals for acquiring the knowledge and skills necessary for performing jobs, especially those that are complex, and those that involve substantial continuous investment of attentional resources, such as that of a pilot or an air traffic controller (e.g., see Ackerman & Kanfer, 1993). In this context, *Gf* represents a rough indicator of "potential" for developing competence, and also an indicator for predicting day-to-day competence of individuals in cognitively challenging jobs.

Gc and Work Competence

The role of *Gc* in determining work competence is much more complicated than the role of *Gf*. In the broad context of *Gc* as the entire repertoire of knowledge and skills of the individual, *Gc* is critically important to work competence, because it represents whether the individual has the declarative and procedural knowledge necessary to carry out many job tasks. Indeed, some investigators have suggested that the job knowledge component of *Gc* is a more important determinant of job performance than individual differences in *Gf* (e.g., see Ackerman, 1996; Hunter, 1983). The general sense of this orientation is that, for most individuals, it is both easier and more effective to solve a problem if the solution has been previously learned (i.e., through *Gc*) than to derive the solution from a novel information processing approach (which would be a *Gf*-determined activity).

Investment of Cognitive Resources

Cattell (1971/1987) and, later, Ackerman (1996) have suggested that development of *Gc* is a function of the level of investment of *Gf* resources over extended periods of time; that is, according to Cattell, individual differences in *Gc* arise from differences in the direction and intensity of cognitive effort. For example, whether someone pursues a medical degree, a PhD in psychology, an apprenticeship at carpentry or auto repair, or learns to sell cars for a living is determined by the direction of his or her investment of intellectual effort (i.e., which profession to enter) and the intensity of effort (whether he or she devotes a great deal of effort over an extended period of time or invests little effort, or invests effort over a brief time period). Simonton (1988) and Ericsson, Krampe, and Tesch-Römer (1993) have suggested that in order to become an "expert" in many fields of work, 10 years or so of extended cognitive effort need to be expended. The investment includes pursuit of academic degrees and active engagement in on-the-job performance. The determinants of the direction and intensity of intellectual effort include individual differences in *Gf* but also appear to involve a relatively small set of nonability traits, which we discuss in the next sections.

MOTIVATIONAL TRAITS AND WORK COMPETENCE

Two major aspects of motivational traits are central to the determination of work competence: interests and general motivational tendencies. Interest traits *usually* refer to the direction of investment to which an individual is more or less oriented. As early as the early 1900s, psychologists determined that there is indeed a substantial association between interests in a particular subject matter or profession, measured during adolescence, and the ability or skill for that activity assessed years later. Thorndike (1912) summarized the results of an early study as follows:

> A person's relative interests are an extraordinarily accurate symptom of his [or her] relative capacities. . . . Either because one likes what he [or she] can do well, or because one gives zeal and effort to what he [or she] likes, or because interest and ability are both symptoms of some fundamental feature of the individual's original nature, or because of the combined action of all three of these factors, interest and ability are bound very close together. (cited in Hollingworth, 1929, p. 203)

Assessment of interests has proceeded along two major lines from the 1920s to the present day. In the first approach (exemplified by Strong, 1945), interests are identified through examination of answers to a vast array of questions about individual likes and dislikes. Empirical scoring is used to compare this array of answers to those of job incumbents across many different occupations, in order to find the occupations where job incumbents and the individual examinee have the most similar attitudes and preferences. In contrast, the second approach (e.g., Guilford, Christensen, Bond, & Sutton, 1954; Holland, 1959; Roe, 1956) depends on a theoretically and empirically derived factor structure of interests, which generally is refined to a half-dozen or so different occupational orientations (e.g., in Holland's model, these are realistic, investigative, artistic, social, enterprising, and conventional). Jobs or occupations can also be classified in terms of these factors, so that the end result is a parallel typology of jobs and individual interest profiles. With information from an individual's interest assessments, a vocational psychologist can determine the direction of the individual's orientation (whether toward some domains or away from other domains). These assessments are generally quite effective in identifying the *direction* of interest, they often ignore the *intensity* of interest (though see Holland, 1973, for a theoretical discussion of occupational level, in terms of occupational interests). This brings us to a consideration of motivational intensity for work performance.

Theories and assessment of general motivational traits have generally been developed in parallel to theories and assessment of interests. Perhaps the most well known and most widely investigated motivational trait that refers directly to intensity is the construct of need for achievement (*n* Ach) proposed by Murray and his colleagues (Murray et al., 1938). Murray defined *n* Ach as reflecting the following desires:

> To accomplish something difficult. To master, manipulate or organize physical objects, human being, or ideas. To do this rapidly, and as independently as possible. To overcome obstacles and attain a high standard. To excel one's self. To rival and surpass others. To increase self-regard by the successful exercise of talent (p. 164)

Murray also identified a set of actions associated with high levels of *n* Ach as follows:

> To make intense, prolonged and repeated efforts to accomplish something difficult. To

work with singleness of purpose towards a high and distant goal. To have the determination to win. To try to do everything well. To be stimulated to excel by the presence of others, to enjoy competition. To exert will power; to overcome boredom and fatigue. (p. 164)

Clearly, this definition of *n* Ach is synonymous with an *approach-oriented motivational intensity*, whether through achievement in isolation or achievement by performing better than others (e.g., competitive excellence). Furthermore, the conceptualization of *n* Ach can be represented as an additional component of the structure of intellectual interests discussed earlier (though *n* Ach is not necessarily limited to academic or intellectual achievement orientation). Thus, an individual could have high, moderate, or low *intensity* of interests in any of the half-dozen or so occupational themes described by Holland (1973). For example, the individual could have a dominant direction of interest in artistic activities but have only a low intensity interest to achieve in pursuit of success in the field of art. Conversely, the individual could have a weak orientation to a particular occupational theme, such as investigative interests (which are associated with scientific pursuits), but have a high desire to succeed or compete in attaining success in the field.

Other needs identified by Murray play a role in development and expression of work competence, but the role of these needs in work competence have received less attention. For example, need for affiliation (*n* Aff) may have important consequences for an individual's efforts with respect to work team or group performance, and thus affect how the individual develops competence to be valued by team members.

In the decades of research that followed Murray's seminal work, numerous theoretical investigations (e.g., see Atkinson, 1983) and assessment measures have been designed to assess the broad construct and various hypothetical components of *n* Ach. Most notable among the assessment measures is the Thematic Apperception Test (TAT), which has been subjected to substantial empirical research by McClelland and his colleagues (see Spangler, 1992, for a review). Other measures include the self-report instruments

by Mehrabian (1969) and Helmreich and Spence (1978).

Along the way, it has become clear that *n* Ach is a complex manifestation of three or more related traits (e.g., Elliot & Harackiewicz, 1996). In the organizational domain, for example, Kanfer and Heggestad (1997; see also Heggestad & Kanfer, 2000) identified three major factors underlying the broad construct of achievement motivation. The Motivational Trait Questionnaire (MTQ) provides an assessment of approach-oriented motivation (desire to learn and mastery), and a desire for competitive excellence (competitive excellence and other-referenced goals). The MTQ also provides an assessment of two avoidance-related motivational traits (anxiety in performance contexts and worry in performance contexts), which are distinct from, and relatively uncorrelated with *n* Ach (i.e., the factor defined by the desire to learn and mastery scales; see Heggestad & Kanfer, 2000). Approach-oriented general motivational tendencies represent what has been referred to as a "trait complex", that is, an amalgamation of related but differentiable constructs that together may be important determinants of knowledge and skill acquisition, and also serve as determinants of day-to-day investments of cognitive effort in task performance.

Although Guilford (1959) conceptualized all individual differences (e.g., temperament, attitudes, interests, needs, physiology, morphology, and aptitudes) as aspects of personality, we find that it is useful to consider temperament as a separable domain of individual traits. We next consider the role of temperament or personality traits in the context of work competence.

PERSONALITY TRAITS AND WORK COMPETENCE

Hollingworth (1929) described the importance of personality traits for work performance, as follows:

If aptitude and interest determine what they [employees] do, if competence sets limits to their achievement, there is still to be considered their manner or mode of performance. Two workmen of equal general competence, with identical degree of special skill, will nevertheless differ in temperament and character. One will work calmly, the other more excitedly; one will be steady, the other erratic. (p. 177)

In the past 90 or so years of personality theory and assessment research, there has been a plethora of hypothesized personality traits that may be related to both current work competence and also the development of knowledge and skills over a lifetime. A full review of this domain of research and practice is beyond the scope of this chapter (for details, see Kanfer, Ackerman, Murtha, & Goff, 1995). Here, we review some of the more salient personality traits related to work competence and development.

Early Research

In the early 1900s, two different methods of personality assessment were used to evaluate suitability of individuals for particular jobs. Researchers at the Carnegie Institute of Technology (see Thurstone, 1952, for a review) developed a technique for interviewing job applicants that was used to develop global estimates of suitability. The other method was the use of paper-and-pencil questionnaires to assess a variety of personality traits. This method was exemplified by Woodworth's Personal Data Sheet (see Franz, 1919), which was administered to a large number of conscripts during World War I. The goals of these two methods were somewhat different: The Carnegie group focused on normal personality traits, while the Woodworth approach focused on detecting personality-related psychiatric disorders. The Woodworth approach can be considered an attempt to determine which individuals are unsuitable for a wide range of jobs. Individuals diagnosed as having psychopathological levels of personality traits (such as poor emotional stability) might be considered generally unfit for military service. Later developments with clinical scales (such as the Minnesota Multiphasic Personality Inventory) have been used for similar purposes, such as screening for sensitive jobs (in the military, police, transportation, and security occupations).

In contrast, the Carnegie group's approach was more specific, in that it represented early efforts for matching the personality characteristics of the individual with the specific characteristics of the job. For example, an individual high on extraversion would be considered to be more likely to develop competence in a life insurance sales job but would perhaps be a poor match to a job of book author. In this sense, there was no optimal pattern of personality traits in general, but a greater or lesser match between an individual's traits and the nature of the job to be performed. Later developments of ascendence–submission scales and dominance scales were used for evaluating individual suitability to jobs in sales or management (see Kanfer et al., 1995, for a review).

Five-Factor Model

Through the middle of the 20th century, researchers sought to refine the large corpus of personality traits to a smaller set of five broad factors of normal personality, representing Neuroticism, Extraversion, Openness to Experience, Agreeableness, and Conscientiousness (e.g., Goldberg, 1993; Tupes & Christal, 1961). This approach has been termed the five-factor model (FFM) of personality. Although there is substantial controversy regarding whether or not the FFM is a reasonably complete depiction of the structure of personality (e.g., see Block, 1995), much of the applied research on personality–work competence issues during the past 20 years has focused on the relations between these five factors and job performance. With a few exceptions, this approach can be seen as an extension of the Woodworth approach (which focused on overall suitability for work) to the normal population; that is, most FFM-inspired research has examined broad personality predictors of job performance, in the hope of finding stable predictors across many different job classes.

Over the past two decades, the FFM has been used to reexamine the relationship between personality and job performance. Beginning with the meta-analysis by Barrick and Mount (1991), over a half-dozen meta-analytic studies on personality–performance relations have been conducted (see Kanfer & Kantrowitz, 2002). Results of these studies show several significant relations across a range of criterion measures. Of the five factors, Conscientiousness has been found to exhibit the strongest and most pervasive relation to overall job performance, with estimated criterion-related validity (i.e., the correlation between the predictor variable and a performance criterion) coefficients ranging from .12 to .31, followed by Extraversion (criterion-related validities ranging from .09 to .16) and emotional stability (validities ranging from .08 to .22), though the nature of these relations to performance is generally weaker and inconsistent across job categories and criterion measures. Findings on Openness to Experience have been somewhat mixed, with validities to job performance ranging from −.01 to 27. Overall, the predictive validities for broad personality traits on job competence and job performance are generally lower than validities obtained for general cognitive ability.

Assessment

In many ways, research on the personality determinants of work competence has not made much theoretical progress since the early efforts of Woodworth and others, who focused on suitability for work. The essence of the FFM research in work domains is that, *ceteris paribus*, it is better for a worker to be more conscientious and less neurotic. In contrast to the vocational interest research and theory domains, there has been relatively little work on delineating the best match of personality traits to specific job categories (though for exceptions, see, e.g., Vinchur, Schippmann, Switzer, & Roth, 1998). Although an approach toward matching jobs and personality traits seems to have great intuitive appeal and is supported in the context of overlap between interests and personality traits (e.g., see Holland, 1973), there is much more research needed in this area.

SELF-CONCEPT, SELF-CONFIDENCE, AND SELF-EFFICACY

In addition to abilities, interests, and personality traits, self-concept and self-confidence represent another major source of relatively stable individual differences characteristics related to work competence and job performance. "Self-concept" usually refers to the

individual's evaluation of his or her ability or competence across a wide range of domains, such as academic (e.g., math, spatial, or verbal domains), physical skill (e.g., strength or speed), physical attractiveness, and interpersonal skills. Self-concept can be a normative construct (e.g., "I can read tables and figures better than most others my age"), or it can be an absolute scaled construct (e.g., "I am skilled at getting along in a team work setting"). Where self-concept is generally domain-specific, self-confidence may be a more general construct. Individuals can have high, medium, or low levels of ability to carry out tasks, in a fashion that is functionally independent from self-concept (though, in practice, these are generally substantially positively correlated). However, whereas self-concept is generally stable, self-confidence may fluctuate markedly as a function of environmental conditions or other external variables (e.g., if the individual is sleep-deprived or under stress, he or she may present much lower self-confidence than when the he or she is not sleep-deprived or under stress). Self-efficacy, in this context, is a narrower construct than self-confidence, in that self-efficacy is conceptualized as confidence in performance, specific to a particular time and situation.

In contrast to abilities (where higher levels of ability are associated with higher levels of work competence), however, the relationship between self-concept-type variables and work competence is somewhat more complex. The reason for this complexity has to do with the motivational consequences of high and low self-concept, confidence, or efficacy, and for accurate versus inaccurate self-assessments. At a simple level, self-concept, confidence, and efficacy may be threshold variables that determine whether the individual chooses even to engage a task. On the one hand, if the goal is to run a mile in less than 4 minutes, many individuals with low self-efficacy may not even adopt the goal, and thus not fully devote effort to goal accomplishment. In this sense, having a self-efficacy that is too low for goal accomplishment may lead to disengagement from the task. On the other hand, if self-confidence is high, initial task engagement is a much higher probability outcome.

Current theory and conventional wisdom tell us that self-concept develops in a feedback-feedforward fashion during development, in concert with the individual's experiences. When a child successfully completes math tasks or reading assignments, one can expect that self-concept is incremented in the respective domain. Increments in self-concept also are often thought to yield increases in task-specific interests—mainly because individuals enjoy engaging in tasks in which they usually have success (e.g., Holland, 1973). Increments in self-concept and interests, in turn, raise the probability that the individual will orient toward new tasks in the same domain, creating a positive cycle of task accomplishments (which similarly yield increments in task competence), increasing self-concept and increasing task interest. Conversely, individuals who struggle to complete a task, or who fail at the task, especially repeatedly, will be expected to have a lowered self-concept, leading to a lower level of interest in engaging such tasks in the future. This pattern of experiences and changes can have the pattern of a vicious circle, ultimately resulting in a situation in which the individual has sufficiently low self-efficacy that he or she will refuse to engage in particular kinds of tasks. Ordinarily though, if the individual encounters failures across only some domains but successes in others, interests and self-concept are expected to become increasingly differentiated over the course of child and adolescent development.

SUMMARY OF TRAIT DETERMINANTS OF WORK COMPETENCE AND A DEVELOPMENTAL FRAMEWORK

There are many potential trait determinants of work competence, both from a developmental perspective and from a day-to-day work competence perspective. Developmentally, Gf represents the basic abilities necessary for initial acquisition of Gc knowledge and skills. Through educational and experiential influences, interests and self-concept develop and differentiate, which in turn, lead to differential engagement in the development of specialized Gc domain knowledge and skills. By the time individuals reach adulthood, they tend to have a relatively coherent pattern of Gc, interests and self-concept. In addition, some personality

traits tend to be more or less associated with particular domains of Gc knowledge and skill, and with vocational interests. The communality of various ability and non-ability traits has suggested the existence of a small set of *trait complexes*, that is, groups of traits that are themselves correlated. More specifically, these groups of traits appear to be facilitative or impeding of the acquisition of domain-specific knowledge and skills. To date, we (Ackerman & Heggestad, 1997) have identified at least four broad trait complexes that involve key ability, personality, interest, and self-concept traits. These trait complexes are illustrated in Figure 19.1, and include the following:

1. *Social trait complex*. The social trait complex includes enterprising and social interests, and also extraversion, social potency, and well-being personality constructs, but not any intelligence traits. It is important to note that the social trait complex is essentially orthogonal (uncorrelated) with tradional measures of academic intellectual abilities. There are insufficient data to evaluate whether individuals who score high on this trait complex also have high levels of social or interpersonal intellectual abilities—mainly because there are no validated measures of social or interpersonal intelligence. However, we suggest that such constructs are likely to be related to this constellation of personality and interest constructs.

2. *Clerical/conventional trait complex*. The clerical/conventional trait complex includes conventional interests and similar personality traits, such as conscientiousness, traditionalism, and control. This complex appears to be related to perceptual speed ability—in that individuals who score high on this trait complex tend to prefer high levels of structure in their work environments. This trait complex is also substantially associated with self-concept measures of personal organization and self-reported capabilities to perform well on highly structured and relatively straightforward tasks.

3. *Science/math trait complex*. The science/math trait complex is associated with investigative and realistic interests, and with self-concept in the areas of science, technology, and math. Individuals with high scores on these constituent traits also tend to have substantially higher scores on Gf ability

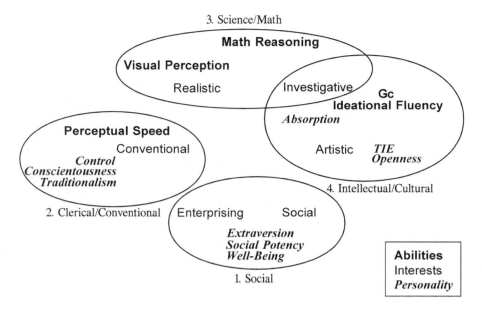

FIGURE 19.1. Trait complexes, including abilities, interests, and personality traits, showing positive commonalities. Shown are (1) social, (2) clerical/conventional, (3) science/math, and (4) intellectual/cultural trait complexes. Ability traits are in **bold**, interests in roman, and personality traits in *italic*. From Ackerman and Heggestad (1997, p. 239). Copyright 1997 by the American Psychological Association. Reprinted by permission.

measures. Interestingly, this trait complex is not associated with any of the traditional measures of personality (see Ackerman & Heggestad, 1997, for a review)

4. *Intellectual/cultural trait complex.* Similar to the science/math trait complex, the intellectual/cultural trait complex is associated with investigative interests. However, the dominant character of the trait complex is that it is highly associated with the educational and experiential aspects of intelligence (*Gc*), artistic interests, and the openness to experience personality construct. In addition, this trait complex is highly associated with a construct called Typical Intellectual Engagement (TIE; see Ackerman, 1994; Goff & Ackerman, 1992). This construct straddles the domains of ability and personality, and reflects a tendency to orient toward intellectual activities (reading for pleasure, attending cultural events, etc.), and away from nonintellectual activities. Self-concept for verbal abilities, general knowledge, and domain-specific knowledge are also substantially positively associated with this trait complex.

PPIK

A theoretical framework that pulls together the previous discussion of determinants of work competence and the notion of trait complexes is shown in Figure 19.2. The framework, called PPIK, for intelligence-as-process, personality, interests, and knowledge, involves a developmental cascade from *Gf*-type abilities (intelligence-as-process) to general knowledge (*Gc*) interacting with personality and interest trait complexes to yield different orientations toward or away from accumulating domain-specific knowledge and skills. The social and clerical/conventional trait complexes represent negative influences on development of academic-type knowledge domains, but positive influences on interpersonal and conventional knowledge and skill domains, respectively. In contrast, the science/math trait complex, along with direct influences of *Gf* and *Gc*, show positive associations with the development of knowledge and skills in scientific, technological, and mathematics domains. The intellectual/cultural trait complex, along with *Gc*, has a positive association with develop-

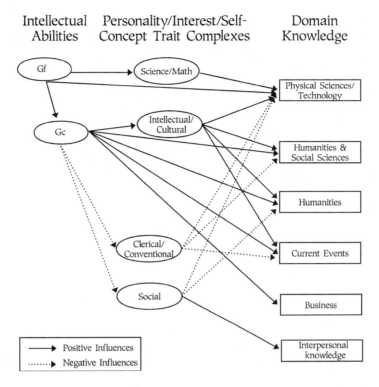

Intellectual   Personality/Interest/Self-   Domain
Abilities   Concept Trait Complexes   Knowledge

FIGURE 19.2. An illustration of PPIK theory. Shown are fluid intelligence (*Gf*) representing intelligence-as-process, crystallized intelligence (*Gc*) representing intelligence-as-knowledge, four trait complexes, composed of personality, interest and self-concept variables, and a set of knowledge domains. Positive influences are indicated by solid arrows; negative influences, by dotted arrows. Adapted from Ackerman, Bowen, Beier, and Kanfer (2001). Copyright 2001 by the American Psychological Association. Adapted by permission.

ment of knowledge and skills across a relatively wide range of domains, such as in the arts, humanities, and social sciences. Support for portions of this framework have been obtained in studies of college students (e.g., Ackerman, Bowen, Beier, & Kanfer, 2001), and of adults from 18 to 70 years of age (e.g., see Ackerman, 2000; Ackerman & Rolfhus, 1999; Beier & Ackerman, 2001, 2003).

SITUATIONAL INFLUENCES ON WORK COMPETENCE

Aside from educational and formal on-the-job training aspects of the work context, other elements of the work situation give rise to differences in work competence. Particularly important are work role demands, work-related goals, and organizational/

work setting culture. We briefly discuss each of these below.

Work Role Demands

On the job, work role demands are imposed by the organization, by members of the work unit, and by the constituencies served. These demands exert specific influences on the development of work-relevant knowledge and skills. In secretarial work, for example, the introduction of computers in the office led to significant changes in work role demands for computer knowledge and word-processing skills, and to the development of organizational training programs to help employees develop competence in these areas. Work role demands can be general (e.g., learning to use Microsoft PowerPoint software) or specific (learning to use a company-specific software program or hardware). These elements of knowledge and skills can be learned to a minimal level, or the individual can attempt to develop a high level of mastery. Although individual differences in motivation control (e.g., see Kanfer & Heggestad, 1997) and mastery orientation (Heggestad & Kanfer, 2000) are likely to be related to the level of skill developed, other situational factors (such as time allocated on the job) will likely set a limit on the opportunity to develop particular skills.

One aspect of work role demands that has received increasing attention during the past two decades pertains to the influence of work structure on the nature of knowledge and skills required for job performance. In the context of teamwork, for example, nontechnical or interpersonal skills may be required to facilitate coordination among team members. Several studies (e.g., Barrick, Stewart, Neubert, & Mount, 1998; Neuman & Wright, 1999; also see Kichuk & Weisner, 1998) indicate that individual job performance in the team context is positively associated with conscientiousness, emotional stability, and agreeableness. From a finding that personality traits have significant criterion-related validities for team process dimensions of job performance, we speculate that the ability and interest variables associated with the social trait complex may prove fruitful for investigating broad person determinants of work team process competence.

Work-Related Task Goals

Task goals represent context-specific objectives for action and the parameters by which to define goal accomplishment. Consistent with goal theories, task goals govern the direction, intensity, and persistence of action. Numerous studies have supported the proposition that task-specific goals, as imposed by the organization, or by a supervisor, can substantially influence learning and performance (see, Locke & Latham, 1990, for a review). More specifically, organizational goal-setting studies indicate a positive relation between goal difficulty and specificity on task performance, particularly among simple tasks and during later phases of skill learning (see Wood, Mento, & Locke, 1987, for a review).

In addition to externally imposed goals, an individual's goal orientation may also in-fluence development and expression of work competence (see Farr, Hofmann, and Ringenbach, 1993). Studies on the effects of "goal orientation," defined in terms of the purpose that individuals hold for goal attainment, suggest a positive relation between learning goal orientation and performance in training and job contexts (Brett & VandeWalle, 1999; Colquitt & Simmering, 1998; Ford, Smith, Weissbein, Gully, & Salas, 1998; Mangos, 2001; Ramakrisha, 2002; Steele-Johnson, Beauregard, Hoover, & Schmidt, 2000; VandeWalle, Brown, Cron, & Slocum, 1999). Consistent with Elliot and Harackiewicz (1996), VandeWalle (1997) proposed that the effects of performance goal orientation on job performance depend upon whether the purpose of the goal is directed toward demonstration of one's ability (i.e., performance prove) or toward avoiding demonstration of one's lack of ability (i.e., performance avoid). Although relatively few studies have used the tripartite distinction in the context of work performance, there have been many studies in academic performance contexts (see, Elliot & McGregor, 2001; Elliot & Moller, in press, for reviews). In the work context, findings obtained by VandeWalle, Cron, and Slocum (2001) indicate a positive relation between performance prove goal orientation and job performance, and a negative relation between performance avoid goal orientation and job performance.

There is also some evidence that personality traits influence task goals in the work setting. In two studies of salespersons, Barrick, Mount, and Strauss (1993) found that the effects of conscientiousness on job performance were mediated by task goals. In a further study of salesperson performance, Barrick, Stewart, and Piotrowski (2002) found that accomplishment and status striving mediated the influence of conscientiousness on job performance. These findings suggest that broad traits may affect job performance through their impact on construal of task-specific goals.

Organizational Culture and Work-Setting Climate

When the work role and goal-setting contexts directly influence the development of competence, other aspects of the organization and the specific work setting will influence the expression of competence. In a supportive organizational culture, workers will be more likely to expend effort toward expressing competence through task performance. However, in too many situations to mention, there are intervening variables that act to prevent a direct relation between work competence and work performance. A few examples illustrate these kinds of situations. First, when there is a climate oriented toward social loafing or a work group that discourages "rate busting" (e.g., Harkins, Latane, & Williams, 1980), workers may be discouraged from expending a maximal degree of effort. In such situations, a bank teller or a grocery store checkout clerk might have the knowledge and skill to accomplish tasks in an efficient and rapid fashion, but does not do so—in order to perform at a level that is typical for the group. Poor interpersonal relations between supervisors and subordinates may also influence withdrawal behaviors (poor effort, excessive off-task behaviors, etc.). An employee who feels that his or her supervisor does not appreciate his or her efforts may find little reason to expend more than a minimal amount of effort on the job, thus creating a dissociation between competence and performance. An organizational lack of procedural fairness (e.g., Greenberg, 1990) may also affect the expression of competent performance. Because a nearly unlimited set of situations result in a breakdown in employee commitment, there are many more reasons for a disassociation between competence and performance to occur than there are reasons for an extremely close association between an employee's competence and performance. However, even if there is otherwise good organizational support, competent job performance is not possible unless the individual has the requisite knowledge and skills for the tasks at hand. Thus, learning opportunities and skill development support and must precede work competence.

A MODEL OF WORK COMPETENCE

The model shown in Figure 19.3 represents an attempt to portray the interplay between the various traits, situational demands, and job performance as they relate to work competence. The broad outline of the PPIK framework provides the distal individual differences determinants of work competence. Work role demands and contextual variables represent the proximal determinants of work competence and job performance. Finally, a path from job performance to work competence provides for the learning mechanism that relates job-related work experiences to increments in work competence. When there is a good match between the individual's trait complexes, his or her acquired work competence, and work role demands, there is a positive effect on both expression and development of work competence. A mismatch among any of these components, however, can result in a breakdown of the individual's future development of work competence.

For example, job performance ratings provide the individual with salient feedback that has consequences for both work motivation and competence. Self-generated and extrinsic performance feedback that are at odds with an individual's percepts of work competence, for example, may create a discrepancy condition that motivates goal choice processes and/or attempts to change work-related knowledge and skill inputs. Poor performance in basic science courses that are requisite for medical school training, for example, may led to alteration of an individual's career goals that shifts the direction of motivation for learning to other knowledge domains. In the job context, outstanding performance in the technical domain may enhance interest and motivation for increasing knowledge and skills in related areas. From a lifespan level of analysis, supervisory and self-generated feedback indicating an age-related decline in technical performance on attention-demanding tasks and slower rates of new skill training may create a motivational paradox in which older workers increase task effort but resist demands for new skill learning. Age-related shifts in the primacy of life goals, from achievement to preservation of competence, may also change the direction of motivation at both broad and specific levels. Midlife employees, for example, may shape work goals in ways that direct effort toward dimensions of performance that may be less valued by the organization (e.g., favoring quality over quantity). In the absence of cor-

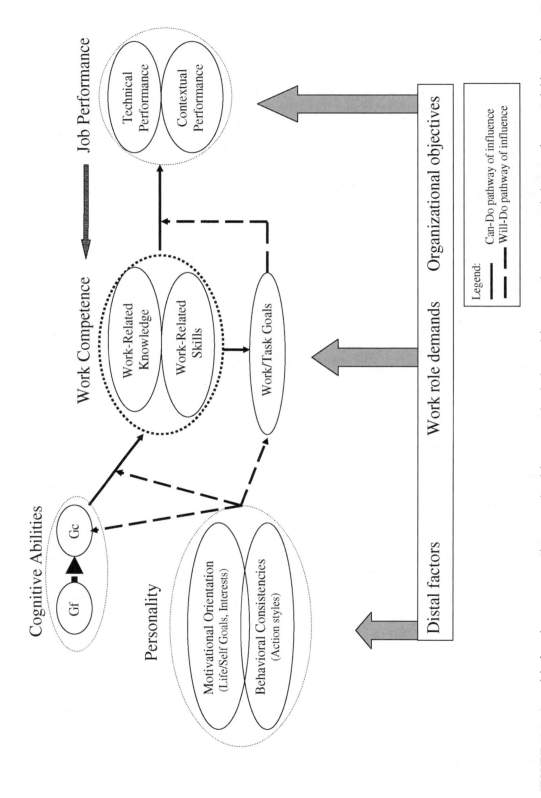

FIGURE 19.3. A model of work competence. Shown are distal factors, work role demand factors, and organizational objective factors. Solid lines indicate "can-do" pathway (maximal performance); dashed lines indicate "will do" pathway (typical behavior).

responding changes in work role demands, within-person changes in motive structure may ultimately reduce job performance and perceptions of work competence.

Individuals usually seek jobs that, among other things, enable them to develop and demonstrate competence. Likewise, organizations seek individuals who will perform well. Effective personnel selection involves careful evaluation of the correspondence between person attributes and job demands. But neither individuals nor organizations are fixed, and work competence may be compromised by changes in the individual and/or changes in the work role. The dynamic nature of both individuals and organizations, and their implications for work competence, is evident in two topics of growing interest to industrial–organizational psychologists: the changing nature of work and the aging workforce.

The Changing Nature of Work

Over the past century, socioeconomic, political, and technological changes in the United States and other developed countries have fundamentally altered the nature of work and the complex of human motivations for skill learning and job engagement. In the United States, fundamental shifts from an agrarian to an industrial to a postindustrial economy have changed the ability, skill, and knowledge requirements for many jobs. Hunt (1995) proposed that job opportunities in the postindustrial economy tend to fall into three broad categories: jobs that place strong demands on higher order problem-solving and reasoning skills (e.g., architect); jobs that place strong demands on interpersonal skills and emotion regulation (e.g., customer service representative); and jobs that place strong demands on behavioral reliability (e.g., cashier).

In addition to changes in job demands, increasing organizational globalization has altered workforce management practices and employee–organization relations. The distribution of organizational operations around the world has increased workforce diversity and increased the use of team structures for work accomplishment. The quickened pace of organizational change in developed countries has also altered psychological assumptions underlying the employment contract.

Large-scale layoffs of long-term employees whose job skills have become obsolete have emphasized the importance of continuous skill learning for sustained employment and the adoption of a protean career model (see Hall & Moss, 1998) that stresses self-managed, successive job changes.

Changes in the workplace have also brought about changes in the mix of motives for demonstrating workplace competence. Economic and achievement motives continue to play a major role. Increasingly, work competence over a career demands that employees demonstrate adaptability and a willingness to update skills and acquire new work competencies. Workers who have high levels of facilitative trait complexes may be expected to continue to invest cognitive resources to maintain competencies and gain new work-related knowledge and skills. Workers who have lower levels of facilitating trait complexes may find their skills increasingly obsolescent, except in low-knowledge jobs, where interpersonal skills may be the major determinant of work competence. However, in knowledge-rich domains, some individuals may nonetheless be sufficiently motivated to learn, when faced with a downward path of earning potential and job status.

The Aging Workforce

From a trait perspective, the transition from early adulthood to middle age and beyond represents a pattern of both stability and change. For abilities, Gf peaks at around the mid-20s, while broad Gc tends to increase well into the 40s and 50s, though to a more modest degree than the declines in Gf. Cross-sectional data (e.g., Ackerman, Beier, & Bowen, 2002) support the notion that the self-concept of middle-age adults tends largely to reflect the changes in abilities associated with aging; that is, middle-age adults have lower self-concept for math and reasoning abilities but preserved self-concept for verbal and other crystallized abilities. Vocational interests tend to be remarkably stable throughout most of the work life (e.g., Strong, 1955). Broad traits of personality tend to be relatively stable as well, though recent findings suggest that personality organization tends to retain a dynamic quality well into middle adulthood (Roberts & DelVecchio, 2000), and that there are mean, age-related changes in trait levels across the lifespan (Jones & Meredith, 1996; Warr, Miles, & Platts, 2001). Motivational traits also tend to be stable, though cross-sectional data suggest that middle-age adults tend to have lower levels of an orientation toward competitive excellence (Kanfer & Ackerman, 2000).

Given these patterns of development and stability for trait determinants of competence, it is important to consider their effects on the development and maintenance of work competence. For well-learned knowledge and skills, just like for broader Gc, it appears that stability across most of the work life is the typical pattern. For tasks that require extensive involvement of Gf-type abilities (e.g., memory, attention, and abstract reasoning) and physical strength, however, day-to-day competence is at risk as individuals age from young to middle adulthood and beyond. An individual might increase his or her effort expended toward task performance (an approach that may compensate for some of the loss in cognitive attentional resources), but jobs such as air traffic controller, neurosurgeon, and fighter pilot are ultimately the province of younger adults. For such jobs, the traditional pattern of promotion to supervisory, administrative, or training roles matches the decline in Gf and compensatory increments in Gc and domain knowledge. This process is described in more detail in the selection, optimization, and compensation model proposed by Baltes and Baltes (1990).

In contrast, knowledge workers often have better prospects for maintenance and development of work competence, without fundamentally changing jobs. Because high levels of domain-specific knowledge facilitate acquisition of new knowledge and skills in the same or similar domains (through near transfer of training), new learning requires less overall investment of effort and time than it does when the domain is novel (new learning, or far transfer of training). The caveat to this assertion is that interruptions in keeping up with new sources of knowledge or new technology may result in more substantial effort and ability demands when the individual finally confronts the need to acquire new knowledge. Failing to continually update knowledge and skills often puts new learning further and further out of reach. At middle-age and beyond, the

investment needed to start learning again may become so high that it results in a poor cost–benefit trade-off (see the analysis by Posner, 1995). In the final analysis, a work environment that is supportive of continuous and lifelong learning is necessary for maximizing the competence of the employees over their work life. When an organization fails to provide this kind of environment, it can be expected that only individuals with high levels of facilitative trait complexes will continue to develop their work competence.

FINAL NOTES

In this chapter, we have provided an outline of the trait and work role determinants of work competence, and a sense of the dynamic interplay of these factors in maintaining competence over the work lifespan. We have described a relatively small set of common factors, called "trait complexes," that appear to be especially facilitative or to impede the development of work competence. We have also provided a conceptual model of work competence, in the context of trait, situation, and performance factors. Implications of these factors were discussed relative to a world in which the nature of work is in flux and individuals also must confront patterns of age-related changes. Individual differences in work competence can be predicted to a significant degree through examination of ability and nonability traits. Expression of work competence can also be predicted though examination of traits, work role demands, and organizational objectives. Individuals who have a favorable pattern of traits and a work situation that encourages knowledge and skill development can be expected, *ceteris paribus*, to maximize competence and performance over the work lifespan. In the final analysis, patterns of growth, stability, or decline in work competence are predicated on all of these components and other factors not considered here (e.g., physical health and work–family conflicts).

NOTE

1. Differential psychology is the study of individual and group differences.

REFERENCES

Ackerman, P. L. (1994). Intelligence, attention, and learning: Maximal and typical performance. In D. K. Detterman (Ed.), *Current topics in human intelligence: Vol. 4. Theories of intelligence* (pp. 1–27). Norwood, NJ: Ablex.

Ackerman, P. L. (1996). A theory of adult intellectual development: Process, personality, interests, and knowledge. *Intelligence, 22,* 229–259.

Ackerman, P. L. (1997). Personality, self-concept, interests, and intelligence: Which construct doesn't fit? *Journal of Personality, 65*(2), 171–204.

Ackerman, P. L. (2000). Domain-specific knowledge as the "dark matter" of adult intelligence: gf/gc, personality and interest correlates. *Journal of Gerontology: Psychological Sciences, 55B*(2), P69–P84.

Ackerman, P. L., Beier, M. B., & Bowen, K. R. (2002). What we really know about our abilities and our knowledge. *Personality and Individual Differences, 34,* 587–605.

Ackerman, P. L., Bowen, K. R., Beier, M. B., & Kanfer, R. (2001). Determinants of individual differences and gender differences in knowledge. *Journal of Educational Psychology, 93,* 797–825.

Ackerman, P. L., & Heggestad, E. D. (1997). Intelligence, personality, and interests: Evidence for overlapping traits. *Psychological Bulletin, 121,* 219–245.

Ackerman, P. L., & Kanfer, R. (1993). Integrating laboratory and field study for improving selection: Development of a battery for predicting air traffic controller success. *Journal of Applied Psychology, 78,* 413–432.

Ackerman, P. L., & Rolfhus, E. L. (1999). The locus of adult intelligence: Knowledge, abilities, and nonability traits. *Psychology and Aging, 14,* 314–330.

Atkinson, J. W. (1983). *Personality, motivation, and action: Selected papers.* New York: Praeger.

Baltes, P. B., & Baltes, M. M. (1990). Psychological perspectives on successful aging: The model of selective optimization with compensation. In P. B. Baltes & M. M. Baltes (Eds.), *Successful aging: Perspectives form the behavioral sciences* (pp. 1–34). Cambridge, UK: Cambridge University Press.

Barrick, M. R., & Mount, M. K. (1991). The Big Five personality dimensions and job performance: A meta-analysis. *Personnel Psychology, 44,* 1–26.

Barrick, M. R., Mount, M. K., & Strauss, J. P. (1993). Conscientiousness and performance of sales representatives: Test of the mediating effects of goal setting. *Journal of Applied Psychology, 78,* 715–722.

Barrick, M. R., Stewart, G. L., Neubert, M. J., & Mount, M. K. (1998). Relating member ability and personality to work-team processes and team effectiveness. *Journal of Applied Psychology, 83,* 377–391.

Barrick, M. R., Stewart, G. L., & Piotrowski, M. (2002). Personality and job performance: Test of the mediating effects of motivation among sales representatives. *Journal of Applied Psychology, 87,* 43–51.

Beier, M. E., & Ackerman, P. L. (2001). Current events knowledge in adults: An investigation of age, intelligence and non-ability determinants. *Psychology and Aging, 16,* 615–628.

Beier, M. E., & Ackerman, P. L. (2003). Determinants of health knowledge: An investigation of age, gender, abilities, personality, and interests. *Journal of Personality and Social Psychology, 84*(2), 439–448.

Binet, A., & Simon, T. (1915). *A method of measuring the development of the intelligence of young children* (C. H. Town, Trans., 3rd ed.). Chicago: Chicago Medical Book Company. (Original published in 1911)

Block, J. (1995). A contrarian view of the five-factor model. *Psychological Bulletin, 117,* 187–215.

Brett, J. F., & VandeWalle, D. (1999). Goal orientation and specific goal content as predictors of performance outcomes in a training program. *Journal of Applied Psychology, 84,* 863–873.

Carroll, J. B. (1993). *Human cognitive abilities: A survey of factor-analytic studies.* New York: Cambridge University Press.

Cattell, R. B. (1943). The measurement of adult intelligence. *Psychological Bulletin, 40,* 153–193.

Cattell, R. B. (1957). *Personality and motivation structure and measurement.* Yonkers, NY: World Book Company.

Cattell, R. B. (1987). *Abilities: Their structure, growth and action* [Revised and reprinted as *Intelligence: Its structure, growth, and action*]. Amsterdam: North Holland. (Original published in 1971)

Colquitt, J. S., & Simmering, M. J. (1998). Conscientiousness, goal orientation, and motivation to learn during the learning process: A longitudinal study. *Journal of Applied Psychology, 83,* 654–665.

Cronbach, L. J. (1949). *Essentials of psychological testing.* New York: Harper.

Elliot, A. J., & Harackiewicz, J. M. (1996). Approach and avoidance achievement goals and intrinsic motivation: A mediational analysis. *Journal of Personality and Social Psychology, 70,* 461–475.

Elliot, A. J., & McGregor, H. A. (2001). A 2 × 2 achievement goal framework. *Journal of Personality and Social Psychology, 80,* 501–519.

Elliot, A. J., & Moller, A. (in press). Performance-approach goals: Good or bad forms of regulation. *International Journal of Educational Research.*

Ericsson, K. A., Krampe, R., & Tesch-Römer, C. (1993). The role of deliberate practice in the acquisition of expert performance. *Psychological Review, 100,* 363–406.

Farr, J. L., Hofmann, D. A., & Ringenbach, K. L. (1993). Goal orientation and action control theory: Implications for industrial and organizational psychology. In C. L. Cooper & I. T. Robertson (Eds.), *International review of industrial and organizational psychology* (Vol. 8, pp. 193–231). New York: Wiley.

Ford, J. K., Smith, E. M., Weissbein, D. A., Gully, S. M., & Salas, E. (1998). Relationships of goal orientation, metacognitive activity, and practice strategies with learning outcomes and transfer. *Journal of Applied Psychology, 83,* 218–233.

Franz, S. I. (1919). *Handbook of mental examination methods* (2nd ed.). New York: Macmillan.

Goff, M., & Ackerman, P. L. (1992). Personality–intelligence relations: Assessing typical intellectual engagement. *Journal of Educational Psychology, 84,* 537–552.

Goldberg, L. R. (1993). The structure of phenotypic personality traits. *American Psychologist, 48,* 26–34.

Greenberg, J. (1990). Employee theft as a reaction to underpayment inequity: The hidden cost of pay cuts. *Journal of Applied Psychology, 75,* 561–568.

Guilford, J. P. (1959). *Personality.* New York: McGraw-Hill.

Guilford, J. P., Christensen, P. R., Bond, N. A., Jr., & Sutton, M. A. (1954). A factor analysis study of human interests. *Psychological Monographs, 68*(4, Whole No. 375), 1–38.

Hall, D. T., & Moss, J. E. (1998). The new protean career contract: Helping organizations and employees adapt. *Organizational Dynamics, 26,* 22–36.

Harkins, S. G., Latane, B., & Williams, K. (1980). Social loafing: Allocating effort or taking it easy? *Journal of Experimental Social Psychology, 16,* 457–465.

Hebb, D. O. (1942). The effect of early and late brain injury upon test scores, and the nature of normal adult intelligence. *Proceedings of the American Philosophical Society, 85,* 275–292.

Heggestad, E., & Kanfer, R. (2000). Individual differences in trait motivation: Development of the Motivational Trait Questionnaire (MTQ). *International Journal of Educational Research, 33,* 751–776.

Helmreich, R. L., & Spence, J. T. (1978). Work and Family Orientation Questionnaire: An objective instrument to assess components of achievement motivation and attitudes toward family and career (Psychological Documents No. 1677). Washington, DC: American Psychological Association.

Holland, J. L. (1959). A theory of vocational choice. *Journal of Counseling Psychology, 6*(1), 35–45.

Holland, J. L. (1973). *Making vocational choices: A theory of careers.* Englewood Cliffs, NJ: Prentice-Hall.

Hollingworth, H. L. (1929). *Vocational Psychology and character analysis.* New York: Appleton.

Horn, J. L. (1989). Cognitive diversity: A framework of learning. In P. L. Ackerman, R. J. Sternberg, & R. Glaser (Eds.), *Learning and individual differences: Advances in theory and research* (pp. 61–116). New York: Freeman.

Hunt, E. (1995). *Will we be smart enough?: A cognitive analysis of the coming workforce.* New York: Russell Sage Foundation.

Hunter, J. E. (1983). A causal analysis of cognitive ability, job knowledge, job performance, and supervisor ratings. In F. Landy, S. Zedeck, & J. Cleveland (Eds.), *Performance measurement and theory* (pp. 257–266). Hillsdale, NJ: Erlbaum.

Jensen, A. R. (1998). *The g factor: The science of mental ability.* Westport, CT: Praeger.

Jones, C. J., & Meredith, W. (1996). Patterns of personality change across the life span. *Psychology and Aging, 11,* 57–65.

Kanfer, R., & Ackerman, P. L. (2000). Individual differences in work motivation: Further explorations of a trait framework. *Applied Psychology: An International Review, 49*(3), 469–481.

Kanfer, R., Ackerman, P. L., Murtha, T., & Goff, M. (1995). Personality and intelligence in industrial and organizational psychology. In D. H. Saklofske & M. Zeidner (Eds.), *International handbook of personality and intelligence* (pp. 577–602). New York: Plenum Press.

Kanfer, R., & Heggestad, E. (1997). Motivational traits and skills: A person-centered approach to work motivation. In L. L. Cummings & B. M. Staw (Eds.), *Research in organizational behavior* (Vol. 19, pp. 1–57). Greenwich, CT: JAI Press.

Kanfer, R., & Kantrowitz, T. M. (2002). Ability and non-ability predictors of job performance. In S. Sonnentag (Ed.), *Psychological management of individual performance* (pp. 27–50). New York: Wiley.

Kichuk, S. L., & Wiesner, W. H. (1998). Work teams: Selecting members for optimal performance. *Canadian Psychology, 39,* 23–32.

Kurz, R., & Bartram, D. (2002). Competency and individual performance: Modeling the world of work. In I. T. Robertson, M. Callinan, & D. Bartram (Eds.), *Organizational effectiveness: The role of psychology* (pp. 227–255). New York: Wiley.

Landy, F. J., & Conte, J. M. (2004). *Work in the 21st century: An introduction to industrial and organizational psychology.* New York: McGraw-Hill.

Locke, E., & Latham, G. (1990). *A theory of goal setting and task performance.* Englewood Cliffs, NJ: Prentice-Hall.

Mangos, P. M. (2001). The role of subjective task complexity in goal orientation, self-efficacy, and performance relations. *Human Performance, 14,* 169–185.

Mehrabian, A. (1969). Measures of achieving tendency. *Educational and Psychological Measurement, 29,* 445–451.

Murray, H. A., Barrett, W. G., Langer, W. C., Morgan, C. D., Homburger, E., MeKeel, H. S., et al. (1938). *Explorations in personality: A clinical and experimental study of fifty men of college age.* New York: Oxford University Press.

Neuman, G. A., & Wright, J. (1999). Team effectiveness: Beyond skills and cognitive ability. *Journal of Applied Psychology, 84,* 376–389.

Posner, R. A. (1995). *Aging and old age.* Chicago: University of Chicago Press.

Ramakrishna, H. V. (2002). The moderating role of updating climate perceptions in the relationship between goal orientation, self-efficacy, and job performance. *Human Performance, 15,* 275–298.

Roberts, B. W., & DelVecchio, W. F. (2000). The rank order consistency of personality traits from childhood to old age: A quantitative review of longitudinal studies. *Psychological Bulletin, 126,* 3–25.

Roe, A. (1956). *The psychology of occupations.* New York: Wiley.

Simonton, D. K. (1988). *Scientific genius: A psychology of science.* New York: Cambridge University Press.

Spangler, W. D. (1992). Validity of questionnaire and TAT measures of need of achievement: Two meta-analyses. *Psychological Bulletin, 112*(1), 140–154.

Spearman, C. (1904). "General intelligence," objectively determined and measured. *American Journal of Psychology, 15,* 201–293.

Steele-Johnson, D., Beauregard, R. S., Hoover, P., & Schmidt, A. M. (2000). Goal orientation and task demand effects on motivation, affect, and performance. *Journal of Applied Psychology, 85,* 724–738.

Strong, E. K., Jr. (1945). *Vocational interests of men and women.* Stanford, CA: Stanford University Press.

Strong, E. K., Jr. (1955). *Vocational interests 18 years after college.* Minneapolis: University of Minnesota Press.

Thorndike, E. L. (1912, November). The permanence of interests and their relation to abilities. *Popular Science Monthly, 81,* 449–456.

Thorndike, E. L., Bregman, E. O., Cobb, M. V., & Woodyard, E. (1927). *The measurement of intelligence.* New York: Teachers College Press.

Thurstone, L. L. (1938). Primary mental abilities. *Psychometric Monographs, 1,* ix–121.

Thurstone, L. L. (Ed.). (1952). *Applications of psychology.* New York: Harper & Brothers.

Tupes, E. C., & Christal, R. E. (1961). *Recurrent personality factors based on trait ratings (ASD-TR-61-97).* Lackland Air Force Base, TX: Aeronautical Systems Division, Personnel Laboratory.

VandeWalle, D. (1997). Development and validation of a work domain goal orientation instrument. *Educational and Psychological Measurement, 57,* 995–1015.

VandeWalle, D., Brown, S. P., Cron, W. L., & Slocum, J. W. (1999). The influence of goal orientation and self-regulation tactics on sales performance: A longitudinal field test. *Journal of Applied Psychology, 84,* 249–259.

VandeWalle, D., Cron, W. L., & Slocum, J. W. (2001). The role of goal orientation following performance feedback. *Journal of Applied Psychology, 86,* 629–640.

Vernon, P. E. (1950). *The structure of human abilities.* New York: Wiley.

Vinchur, A. J., Schippmann, J. S., Switzer, F. S., III, & Roth, P. L. (1998). A meta-analytic review of predictors of job performance for salespeople. *Journal of Applied Psychology, 83,* 586–597.

Warr, P., Miles, A., & Platts, C. (2001). Age and personality in the British population between 16 and 64 years. *Journal of Occupational and Organizational Psychology, 74,* 165–199.

Wood, R., Mento, A. J., & Locke, E. A. (1987). Task complexity as a moderator of goal effects: A meta-analysis. *Journal of Applied Psychology, 72,* 416–425.

CHAPTER 20

୦୫

Legislating Competence

High-Stakes Testing Policies and Their Relations
with Psychological Theories and Research

RICHARD M. RYAN
KIRK W. BROWN

The development of competence in schools is an increasing focus of national concern in countries across the globe. This concern is fueled by the fact that educational outcomes, broadly considered, are linked with the health and economic well-being of nations. Beyond the obvious economic and health value of schooling to the individual person, the general expansion of education within a nation is associated with a host of outcomes, from reduced mortality and fertility to increased economic productivity and positive social change (Sen, 1999).

Because of the importance of the development of competence, governments are also increasingly attempting to legislate ways to enhance educational opportunities and outcomes. Yet much controversy exists about the appropriate ways governments can stimulate improved schools and greater academic achievement, and what kind of improvements in achievement are actually

meaningful for the health and economic well-being of a nation. This issue is international and occupies headlines from Great Britain to South Korea.

In the United States, state and federal government policies aimed at obtaining greater "accountability" and "higher standards" have especially stimulated controversy. These recent policy initiatives attempt to improve school performance through *high-stakes testing* (HST). Specifically, high-stakes policies represent a two-pronged approach to reform. The first prong entails increased testing to gauge how students, teachers, and schools are performing relative to each other, and relative to the *standards* that government agencies determine all students should meet. The second prong carries the motivational component: This testing has teeth. The attainment of standards is motivated or enforced by *high stakes* in the form of rewards and punishments, such as financial incentives and job security for educators, and grade retention versus promotion for students. HST reform has become, in short order, the most dominant pressure in America's public schools and is rapidly reshaping teaching practice and curricular contents across the nation.

What is most interesting about this approach to reform, for the purposes of this volume, is that HST policies reflect particular theories of motivation and achievement. Specifically, high-stakes reform approaches represent a view of competence promotion and teaching that reflects an operant theory of motivation (Kellaghan, Madaus, & Raczek, 1996) and a view of educational outcomes that is more closely aligned with those espousing performance goals rather than mastery or learning goals (Deci & Ryan, 2002); that is, the governmental policy is founded on the idea that making rewards and punishments more salient and contingent on test score outcomes is the most appropriate and effective way of ensuring greater student effort and learning, and more effective teaching. As such, this social policy enacts a behavioristic motivational philosophy and represents a natural experiment in the social psychology of competence. It is a policy that suggests that high-quality educational motivation is a function of external incentives, a view that at least some psychologists support (e.g., Eisenberger, Pierce, & Cameron, 1999; Hidi, 2002).

In contrast, several theories in contemporary motivational psychology predict that attempting to enhance achievement in schools through such external controls will yield some highly negative results, based on the properties of the type of motivation it incites. In particular self-determination theory (Deci & Ryan, 1985; Ryan & Deci, 2000) explicitly predicts important costs of implementing such an approach to motivating competence in public schools. Similarly, some tenets of modern goal theories (e.g., Dweck, 1991; Nicholls, 1984; Elliot, 1999) also suggest potential costs of a focus on demonstrating performance outcomes. Thus, what is scientifically engaging about the social policy debate and implementation is that results of reform should be interpretable, in accord with the varying predictions of these psychological models. What is so-

cially engaging about the debate are the relative costs and benefits to children.

In this chapter, we examine HST reforms in the United States precisely because they illustrate the impact that social policy can have on institutional practice, and the relations (or absence of them) between empirically based research in psychology and education, and governmental policies. We highlight the nature of these test-driven reforms, the legislation surrounding them, and both the theoretically predicted impact and the current empirical data on their effectiveness and consequences. We then discuss the seeming divorce between political reforms and current empirical research in the psychology of competence and education.

To presage some conclusions, our review suggests that, to date, HST has not, in general, produced positive outcomes. Nonetheless, both the positive and negative data that have been obtained can be readily interpreted using the principles outlined in extant theories of motivation. In line with operant theory, and the general recognition of the power of contingent rewards to control behavior, high-stakes policies do indeed change behavior. They lead to increased district, school, and teacher activities intended to raise test scores. In fact, some of the behaviors that these contingencies incite are part of the problem, such as "teaching to the tests," elimination of developmentally enriching activities that are not likely to be tested, manipulation of targeted standards, and "push-outs" of potentially low performers from the pool of test takers. In line with self-determination theory (e.g., Deci & Ryan, 2002; Ryan & LaGuardia, 1999) and some perspectives on performance-focused motivation (e.g., Midgley, Kaplan, & Middleton, 2001), these high-stakes reforms are yielding a variety of collateral or unintended negative consequences, especially in areas involving persistence and quality of learning. Among the concerns is that HST is typically "one size fits all," requiring all students, regardless of their backgrounds, learning differences, and rates of development, to jump the same evaluative hurdles simultaneously. This approach potentially lowers the ability of schools to optimally challenge students of different talents and achievement levels, and it is of special concern regarding students with disabilities. Another concern is the problem of transfer: Rises in high-stakes test scores do not appear to generalize to other indices of improved achievement (e.g., other achievement measures). This poor generalizability is not necessarily due to the invalidity of the tests, but rather to the criterion contamination caused by their high-stakes implementation. The rewards and punishments that prompt an urgency to raise test scores lead to a narrowing of teaching, and therefore learning, and foster classroom dynamics that tend to decrease student motivation and engagement, as well as teacher morale and creativity. Perhaps more importantly, because HST neither provides a good basis for intrinsic motivation nor offers students optimal challenges (because the standards and methods of demonstrating performance are the same for all), reforms based on HST have been associated with increased school dropouts. These dropouts are especially salient among those already at risk, including the urban poor, students with special needs, and those for whom English is a second language—the very children whom many HST advocates have said they do not want to leave behind.

THE HIGH-STAKES
TESTING MOVEMENT

There is little argument that gathering information and providing feedback about performance in educational settings is important for maintaining student and teacher motivation, and for informing educational policy (Linn, 2000; Shepard, 2000). Indeed, feedback regarding outcomes is recognized as a critical feature in improving the function of any organized system (Carver & Scheier, 1998). The function of assessment in gathering information, however, has additional impacts when the outcome data are linked with contingent rewards and punishments, as is the case in HST.

HST has been advocated as a means of motivating students and teachers alike to put in more effort, and thereby raise student achievement (Oakes, 1991; Finn, 1991). Policies instituting HST have taken on varied forms, but the common denominator in such initiatives is that state or federal governments mandate standardized testing of all students and then administer rewards or

sanctions based on the results. Students, teachers, and schools that improve or do well are rewarded, and those that decline or do badly are punished. For students, HST results can be the basis for promotion versus retention, and in some states, failure on a single indicator can result in the denial of a high school diploma. Teachers in schools that perform well may get cash bonuses, while those in other schools are reprimanded or derogated. For the schools, the comparative student performance average can result in increases versus cuts in school budgets, and in some cases, poor student performance may result in administration changes or even school takeovers by the state. When the stakes get high for administrators, local officials can even add to the stakes. For example, schools have offered cash prizes, parties, exemptions from finals, scholarships, candy, and awards to high-scoring students (Keller, 2000). School superintendents have been given personal cash bonuses when scores in their districts improve. However, the principal incentive at the administrative level is the public nature of high-stakes assessments. Schools and districts are publicly compared on their test scores, with the often explicit reasoning that pride or humiliation will be attached to the differences in score attainments. Accordingly, at all levels of educational systems, raising the stakes leads to increased attention to test scores because of the consequences attached to them.

A BRIEF HISTORY
OF HIGH-STAKES TESTING

The modern HST movement has roots dating back to 19th-century England. Utilitarian philosophers such as Jeremy Bentham (1748–1832) and James Mill (1733–1836) formulated principles of motivation based upon hedonic principles and associationism that provided the foundations of what would become modern behaviorism (Rachlin, 1976). In applying these principles, they suggested the systematic use of rewards and punishments to establish good learning habits in schools. The English Parliament was perhaps the first government to put HST into practice, passing numerous laws intensifying examination structures to ensure literacy, including the Revised Code of Regulations (1862), which advocated a "payment by results" scheme that linked the funds awarded to schools to students' performance on the exams. Whereas the Code promoted a wider national school system, it also prompted a rigid narrowing of curricula and an escalation of teacher-centered drill- and repetition-focused instruction. Although the Code was eventually repealed, the ideas of "streaming" or segregation of students according to ability level, evaluation by exams, and the resultant conservative methods instituted by the British system in the 19th century continued into the modern era.

In the United States, the modern instantiation of HST begins with the controversial publication of *A Nation at Risk* in 1983. This document, authored by the National Committee on Excellence in Education, declared that a rising tide of mediocrity was threatening the United States and its ability to compete in the world economy. (Parenthetically, one should note that despite relative stability in achievement standings since 1983, U.S. workers in 2001 were second in the world in global competitiveness according to the World Economic Forum [2002] report). Although one might assume that reform to alleviate "mediocrity" could take any number of directions, the U.S. government's approach under President Reagan was to step up demands for a core curriculum, more homework, more discipline, and more "accountability" (e.g., performance-based pay for teachers and increased testing), not more resources for schools, in part because lawmakers sought reforms that could be easily understood and rapidly implemented. Within several years following the report, virtually all states adopted more stringent graduation requirements, and many added mandatory homework requirements. School days lengthened and extracurricular amenities shrank. Standardized testing and curricula, matched to what those tests could measure, burgeoned.

Echoing the spirit of these reforms, William Bennett, a politician and popular moralist, proclaimed that "accountability is the linchpin, the keystone, the sine qua non of the reform movement" (Toch, 1991, p. 205). The demand for accountability led quickly to a focus on tests and pressure toward better outcomes on them. Policymakers in nearly every state implemented policies to assess educational standards, and in many of these states, high-stakes consequences were attached to these outcomes, presumably as an incentive–punishment system to motivate change. High-performing schools were to be rewarded and underperformers penalized. Thus, the implementation of policy followed a behaviorist paradigm in which contingent rewards were applied to motivate (and control) teachers and students.

Although there were disappointing results from this early round of HST and many well-documented negative effects (see review by Toch, 1991), the late 1990s saw a new infusion of investment in HST policies. Politicians and business groups lobbied for still greater accountability in public schools, and states increasingly developed tests by which to rank and reward schools based on standardized test scores. Some states, such as Texas, aggressively pursued HST policies throughout the 1990s, and in so doing showed increased scores on the specific tests that were the targets of rewards and sanctions (Haney, 2000). By the first year of the new millennium, nearly all states were using HST in an attempt to foster school achievement. Nearly all states now publish school or district report cards on targeted tests, with the explicit purpose of motivating schools through public pressure or ridicule. Nearly half of all states also provide financial rewards to schools that improve on tests, and threats of administrative change or takeover for those that decline. Many states are directly paying school administrators bonus cash awards when schools under their watch improve on test scores.

Finally, states have been increasingly creating high stakes for students, as well as administrators. The most common high stake is that grade passage versus retention, and ultimately graduation, is contingent on passing a state-administered test. The high stakes of grade retention on the basis of a single examination have been applied as early as the fourth grade (e.g., in Florida). It is explicitly assumed by HST advocates that this type of contingency leads students to work harder in school (e.g., Cheney, 1991; Shanker, 1993), a point contested by critics (see Kelleghan et al., 1996). At this point in time, more than half of all states have made graduation from high school contingent on a standardized test performance.

A National Initiative: No Child Left Behind

In 2001, President George W. Bush succeeded in passing, with bipartisan support, landmark legislation entitled No Child Left Behind (NCLB). A stated goal of NCLB is to raise levels of achievement and close the performance gap separating middle-class from poor and underperforming minority students. The plan called for even more testing and more salient stakes for schools and students alike. Specifically, NCLB mandates annual testing in grades 3–8 in math and reading. According to the legislation, scores from such tests are to be used to determine improving and declining achievement, such that penalties and rewards can be attached to them at the level of schools and children. Schools must make steady progress every year toward raising achievement levels on these exams in each of five racial and ethnic subgroups, as well as among low-income students and those with limited English skills or learning disabilities. Failure to demonstrate improvement for *any* of these subgroups for 2 consecutive years results in a school being labeled *low performing*. According to NCLB mandates, schools deemed low performing must facilitate the transfer of students to better schools or provide private tutors for students. Schools that continue to be low performing beyond 2 years can have their administrators and staff replaced. Federal funding is made contingent on compliance with these mandates.

NCLB has many critics. Given the expectable, year-to-year deviations that occur in standardized test results, schools may frequently be categorized as low performing for what amounts to statistical issues rather than reasons of educational quality. However, such logistical concerns are not the ones most pertinent to a critique of HST as a strategy of reform. As noted, HST represents a motivational policy. Yet a number of contemporary motivational theories suggest that a host of unintended negative consequences will stem from the pressure and rewards used to externally control teaching and learning. These include narrowing of curricula, teaching to the test, less creative

teaching, more superficial and nontransferable learning, more controlling behavior at all levels of power, more withdrawal of effort from at-risk students, and increased dropout rates. We turn first to these theoretical predictions, and then to a review of the accumulating empirical findings on the use of HST.

THEORETICAL PERSPECTIVES ON HIGH-STAKES TESTING

High-Stakes Testing as an Operant Approach

HST is based, at least implicitly, on a behaviorist view of student and teacher motivation. By putting contingent reinforcements on outcomes, the policy presumably increases efforts and behaviors associated with improvement; that is, HST advocates reason that whatever behaviors schools adopt to enhance test scores will be reinforced and selected for, whereas those associated with lower scores will be extinguished and, in the case of poor-performing schools, selected out. Not only will the behavior of teachers change, so will that of students. According to Shanker (1993), strong consequences attached to test scores will provide students with "the incentive to work hard and achieve because they know something important . . . is at stake" (p. 7).

The historical link between HST and behaviorism has deep roots. As previously noted, behaviorism emerged from a blend of British associationism and a hedonic view of human motivation, in which learned behaviors were always a function of external controls that punish or reward. It follows from this perspective that educators should utilize these external forces in regulating learning.

This approach to motivation was integral to the work of perhaps the most influential of all behaviorist educators, E. L. Thorndike. The central principle of Thorndike's theory of learning, which he called *connectionism*, was his *law of effect*, which states that if a behavior is followed by a satisfying consequence, it is more likely to occur in the future under similar conditions. Conversely, if a behavior is followed by an unsatisfying consequence, its probability of recurrence will wane. A second principle was that of *frequency*: The more frequently an association is repeated, the more likely it is to recur in similar conditions. Together, these "laws" of learning underwrote educational practices focused on the use of external reinforcements, coupled with practice, drill, and repetition. Although these techniques have characterized conservative approaches to education across history (see Ryan & Lynch, 2003), connectionism gave them a specific theoretical rationale.

Thorndike was also an advocate of testing. As he stated, "Testing the results of teaching and study is . . . the sine qua non of sure progress. It is the chief means to arousing . . . the instinct for achievement" (1962, pp. 65–66). However, interestingly, Thorndike was also cautious about how such tests should be used. As he states: "Great care should be taken in deciding anything about the fate of pupils, the value of methods, the achievement of school systems and the like from scores made in a test" (p. 156).

Thorndike's behaviorism was influential in education for several decades but eventually gave way to the "radical behaviorism" of B. F. Skinner. Skinner similarly advocated the systematic application by teachers of consequences, principally positive reinforcements, to induce learning. Skinner also promoted the idea of "programmed learning," which viewed instruction not as based in relationships or interests, but rather in a well-structured and systematic application of contingent reinforcements.

Today conservative educators continue to advocate the use of rewards to control learning, both at the classroom and school system levels. Behaviorists argue that teaching is most effective when based on control through reinforcements. For example, behaviorists Cameron and Pierce (1994), in the context of reporting a now discredited meta-analysis (see Deci, Koestner, & Ryan, 1999), argued that "teachers have no reason to resist implementing incentive systems in the classroom" (p. 397). At a political level, this theme is echoed loudly. Chester Finn has argued that "the problem is that academic success yields such few rewards [*sic*] and indolence brings few penalties" (1991, p. 120). He, and a broad array of conservative spokespersons, have argued that putting rewards and penalties behind the test scores will effectively alter the behavior of both

teachers and their students. This type of thinking has deeply influenced recent educational reforms in several nations focused on HST. In this view, instruction should be driven by measurement, and the outcomes of measurement should be the basis of rewards and sanctions for both teachers and learners (as discussed in Popham, 1983).

Our interpretation of the HST movement as reflecting an operant strategy has one very important caveat. Operant theory has always been focused on making rewards contingent on target *behaviors*. The twist in the HST movement is that its advocates apply contingent rewards and sanctions to *performance outcomes*; that is, rather than rewarding valued behaviors, such as student effort or work habits, contingencies are instead applied to test outcomes, the control over which is often questionable, especially for at-risk students. Similarly, rather than rewarding excellent teaching activities and approaches, schools are rewarded or sanctioned on their test score results. This practice is not in line with the fundamental tenets of the operant viewpoint. Indeed, we believe that the focus on performance outcomes, rather than on behaviors that students and teachers have direct control over, is one of the features of HST that lead to reinforcement of the wrong behaviors.

This focus on outcomes does find affinity from some theorists who focus on goals as motivating forces in behavior. Among those perspectives that could be aligned with HST-based reforms is the goal theory approach of Locke and Latham (1990), who argue for a high-performance model in which demanding goals are linked with both internal and external rewards to maximize organizational efficiency. Although they developed their model in application to industry, they suggest its generalizability to schooling, arguing that the high-performance model of difficult goals associated with rewards for success "should be made part of our schools as well as our work organizations" (p. 268). Advocating this linkage between measurable outcomes and performance-contingent reinforcements would seem to be fully congruent with the HST approach. A similar advocacy of applying contingent rewards to performance outcomes has also been forwarded by Hidi and Harackiewicz (2000), whose perspective on performance goals we review in discussing theories of mastery and performance goals.

Organismic Perspectives on Learning

A very different view of what motivates learning and competence can be gleaned from what has sometimes been called the "liberal perspective," and sometimes the "organismic perspective," in which learning is seen as an inherent or intrinsic tendency of the person (Ryan & Lynch, 2003). In this tradition, the desire to learn is seen as a natural or basic tendency of humans. Learning is growth. However, like all growth, this inherent initiative or tendency requires support and nutriments. The result is a process (rather than outcome) focus, in which nurturance, mainly in the form of warm relationships, optimal challenges, and supports for autonomy and interest, are the most common elements.

Throughout history, educators embracing this liberal view have argued that students are not optimally motivated by external controls, but rather by support of their inherent tendency to learn. In ancient times, this view was espoused by Quintilian, who recognized that learners of different ages and types have distinct needs and interests, and held that curriculum and methods should be tailored accordingly. He deemphasized the then common use of punishment, instead stressing the importance of making learning interesting and attractive. In the Renaissance, similar views were echoed by Comenius, who focused on the strategic importance of warm student–teacher relationships and enhancing students' interest in learning. Subsequently, Enlightenment philosopher Rousseau laid the groundwork for much modern thinking in the liberal vein, emphasizing children's curiosity and natural inclination to learn under supportive conditions.

Rousseau influenced generations of subsequent educators. Outstanding among them was the Swiss educator, Pestalozzi, who viewed the aims of education not as "imposing on the child fixed doctrines and alien concepts but in helping him to develop his own constructive powers" (Silber, 1973, p. 274). His method of education entailed, first and foremost, an atmosphere of emotional security based in a warm and caring relationship between teacher and child. He advocated that knowledge be gained, when possible, through direct experience rather than through mere words passed from teacher to child. He also downplayed the utility of punishment and fear of evaluation, suggesting that if provided a secure base, the child's nature would lead to discovery and growth. Pestalozzi's philosophy was widely disseminated during the 19th century in Europe and the United States, and became a major influence on a diverse family of practitioners, including Froebel in Germany, and Montessori in Italy.

Finally, in the 20th century, Dewey (1938) emphasized the importance of cultivating interest and inquiry in crafting an education, rather than arbitrarily imposed educational tasks and goals. He stood, in this respect, in stark contrast to his behaviorist contemporary, Thorndike. In the realm of psychology, Rogers (1969) developed an influential perspective on teaching, stemming from his *person-centered approach*. He advocated a classroom experience that grows out of the authentic inquiry of the student. Rogers felt that the external locus of evaluation represented by traditional examinations and normative grading stifled the significant learning that grew out of a student-centered, responsive teaching environment. It was Rogers who faced off with B. F. Skinner in the 1950s and 1960s, debating the value of external control versus self-actualization in the enterprise of learning.

In summary, a long tradition of philosophy and psychology has argued against externally controlling techniques as the *via regia* to student learning. Instead, this tradition focuses on nurturing the natural inclination to learn, the diversity of learning abilities and styles, and the importance of students' developing their powers of self-evaluation. Importantly, the last few decades have seen the emergence of several empirically focused motivation theories that supply some support for this perspective.

Self-determination theory (SDT; Deci & Ryan, 1985; Ryan & Deci, 2000) is one such empirically based organismic perspective that views humans as intrinsically motivated to learn and develop competencies. However, the theory is centrally concerned with the conditions that support versus thwart these intrinsic propensities. SDT is thus particularly interested in the impact of events such as evaluations, praise, and contingent rewards and punishments on behavior and learning.

Specifically, SDT highlights the fact that students' motivation to learn can vary in its relative autonomy, from behaviors motivated by external rewards and punishments (controlled motivations) to those that are energized by interests and values (autonomous motivations). Both evidence and theory based on SDT suggest that, to the extent that one's motivation is based on more autonomous motives, such as intrinsic motivation or well-internalized values, the more quality of learning, persistence, and affective experience are enhanced (Grolnick & Ryan, 1987; Ryan & La Guardia, 1999; Ryan, Stiller, & Lynch, 1994). On the other hand, SDT research has found that motivation based on more controlled motives, such as rewards or punishments (external regulations), or self-esteem-based pressures (e.g., ego involvement) is associated with lower quality learning, lessened persistence, and more negative emotional experience.

Because HST policies are based on the idea that rewards, punishments, and self-esteem-based pressures are effective motivators of learning, the principles of SDT apply (Deci & Ryan, 2002; Ryan & La Guardia, 1999). In what follows, we summarize the theoretical basis for those hypotheses as they relate to teacher and student motivation, and review some of the evidence supporting the validity of these hypotheses.

According to SDT the specific effects of external events such as evaluations or feedback on human motivation depend on the psychological meaning, or *functional significance*, that the events have for the recipient (Deci & Ryan, 1980, 1985, 2000). The theory specifies that the functional significance of an external event, such as a test score, a tangible reward, or praise from a teacher, can be informational, controlling, or amotivating. Events have *informational significance* when they provide effectance-relevant feedback in a noncontrolling way; that is, when an event provides individuals with specific feedback that points the way to being more effective in meeting challenges or becoming more competent, and does so without pressuring or controlling the individuals, it tends to have a positive effect on self-motivation. Events have *controlling sig-*

nificance when they are experienced as pressure toward specified outcomes or as an attempt to control the activity and effort of the individual. According to SDT, when evaluations have controlling significance, they may produce temporary compliance, but they ultimately undermine self-motivation, investment, and commitment in the domain of activity being evaluated. Finally, events have *amotivating significance* when the feedback conveys incompetence to the individuals or supplies no inner or outer rationale for acting. Evaluations or reward structures based on overly challenging standards, or that are perceived to be beyond the reach of the individuals, are thus amotivating: They undermine all motivation and lead to withdrawal of effort. Teaching that does not tap into a student's interests, or that does not supply a basis for the experience of relevance or meaning, can also foster amotivation.

Both experimental and field studies have supported these predictions concerning the impact of events such as feedback and rewards on subsequent motivation. Extensive reviews are available elsewhere, but a few examples are worth detailing. In experiments with rewards, Ryan, Mims, and Koestner (1983) showed that reward structures delivered in an informational manner did not undermine intrinsic motivation, but rewards used to pressure people toward a specified outcome did. In another demonstration, Ryan (1982) showed that students who were pressured to perform by stressing that outcomes reflected ability (an ego-involving induction) were subsequently significantly less likely to engage with the target task than were students who were induced to focus on the task itself rather than task outcomes. In an experiment conducted within an elementary school, Grolnick and Ryan (1987) had students engage in a reading comprehension task under three conditions. In the first, students were told they would not be tested at all. In the second condition, they were told they would be tested, but only to determine what kinds of ideas were learned, so there were no consequences for failure or success. In a third condition, students were told they would be tested and graded, and that the grade would be delivered to their classroom teacher. This third condition represented a controlling use of evaluations. Results showed that the controlling evaluation condition promoted not only short-term, rote memory but also produced a significantly lower level of conceptual learning and knowledge integration than the two noncontrolling conditions. Evidence from these and related studies (e.g., Benware & Deci, 1984) indicates that when tests, evaluations, and rewards are used in controlling ways, they have negative effects on students' interest, motivation, and higher level cognitive outcomes in school. Classrooms studies have added to these findings by showing that when teachers are oriented toward being controlling (e.g., using evaluations and rewards), students are less intrinsically motivated, less desirous of challenge in school, and also less confident in their skills (e.g., Deci, Schwartz, Sheinman, & Ryan, 1981; Ryan & Grolnick, 1986).

How Performance Standards Affect Teachers

The finding that when teachers use controlling strategies and performance pressure to motivate students, the students become less self-motivated and less engaged in school, raises an interesting issue. What factors lead teachers to be controlling? One answer is that they may become controlling when they themselves are pressured to get children to perform. An experiment performed by Deci, Spiegel, Ryan, Koestner, and Kauffman (1982) addressed this issue. Participants simulated teachers with the task of helping students learn a cognitive-perceptual task. The teachers all had the same set of problems to work with and were given the same preparation. However, before entering the teaching session, one group was explicitly told that it was their job to make sure their students performed "up to high standards," whereas another group received no such pressure. The sessions were recorded and rated for differences in teaching strategies. The results showed that the participants who were explicitly pressured to produce high student achievement were more controlling and less supportive of students' autonomy. Specifically, teachers in the performance standards condition engaged in more lecturing, criticizing, praising, and directing—all techniques that have been shown to have a negative impact on students' interest in learning

and their willingness to undertake greater academic challenges. Flink, Boggiano, and Barrett (1990) followed up on this reasoning by examining a newly introduced school-based curriculum for elementary students across several schools. They showed that, as predicted, teachers pressed toward higher standards were more likely to engage in controlling instructional behaviors. In line with SDT, the more they did so, the more their students actually performed more poorly on objective test-score outcomes. This is consistent with a wide body of literature linking evaluative pressure with poorer performance in schools (Kohn, 1996; Ryan & Stiller, 1991), as well as dropout rates (Hardre & Reeve, 2003).

From the SDT perspective, creating a test-driven evaluative focus not only leads teachers to be more controlling but also leads students to be more externally regulated and/or ego involved in their motivational orientation. According to SDT, ego involvement is potentiated whenever a person's esteem is linked with attainment of specific outcomes (deCharms, 1968; Plant & Ryan, 1985; Ryan, 1982). Accordingly, ego involvement can motivate effort, just as rewards can. However, like most performance-contingent rewards, ego involvement is a controlling form of extrinsic motivation, and it runs the risk of undermining internal motivations based in value or interest. Furthermore, unless one is ensured of success when applying effort, ego involvement can have deleterious immediate effects. The more ego involving a context, the more many students, particularly the less confident ones, withdraw effort in order to reduce the diagnosticity of tests and thus protect their self-esteem (Martin, Marsh, & Debus, 2001). Additionally, even for students who try to do well, such evaluation-based motivations tend to foster more superficial and less integrative learning processes, thus debilitating long-term knowledge retention and growth (Golan & Graham, 1990; Grolnick & Ryan, 1987).

Beyond this, the evidence suggests that focusing parents' concerns on performance outcomes will lead them, like teachers, to use pressuring motivational strategies that will backfire, leading to lower achievement over the long term (Ginsburg & Bronstein, 1993; Grolnick, 2003; Grolnick, Gurland, Decourcey, & Jacob, 2002; Grolnick &

Ryan, 1989). In short, pressure (whether it be through rewards or esteem-related threats) to meet externally dictated or controlled standards usually translates into lower quality teaching and less effective motivational practices, unwittingly undermining high-quality performance, as well as the interest and task involvement that facilitate it.

It should also be mentioned that use of uniform evaluative standards for all students regardless of their starting points or resources, which is a invariant feature of HST policies, violates another tenet of SDT's approach to motivation. According to the theory, people are most intrinsically motivated when they are *optimally challenged*—when the tasks set by or for them are within reach. Tasks that are overly challenging have amotivational significance, and thus undermine motivation altogether, leading to lower effort withdrawal, helplessness, and lower confidence and self-esteem (Deci & Ryan, 1985; Ryan & La Guardia, 1999; Vallerand & Reid, 1984). The evidence is clear: If the bar appears to be too high, many students will experience futility and withdraw their effort. People are simply not motivated by the prospect of failure.

Moreover, test-based reforms seem to ignore the diversity of ways in which students both learn and demonstrate learning. As Gardner (1991) has argued, even a well-constructed test may be a nonoptimal challenge for some children, and may present a distorted picture of how well that student has mastered or understood material. Because the hallmark of HST is a single criterion, it favors those who are most apt within its format.

Together, these tenets of SDT would suggest that HST will have a number of negative effects, many of which are undoubtedly unintended (see Ryan & LaGuardia, 1999). The controlling reward structure behind HST should, according to SDT, externally regulate the behavior of teachers. They are thus predicted to engage in those behaviors instrumentally tied to test scores, regardless of their inherent value or worth. One should thus see a narrowing of curricula, more teaching to the test, more controlling motivational techniques used in classrooms, and less positive experience on the part of students and teachers alike. Because of the mo-

tivational dynamics set in motion in the classroom, SDT also predicts greater dropout rates among students, especially those at risk for failure or alienation, since withdrawal of effort is a common fallout of controlling and nonoptimal pressures, and uninspiring classroom practices. Systems such as state and district administrations will, because of the high stakes, be driven to "fuzzy accounting methods" (e.g., wavering standards), pushing out students who might bring down scores, and using other devices to maximize the target outcome, regardless of other costs of such behaviors. Yet, because there is pressure on narrowly defined test-score outcomes, scores on targeted tests should increase, but such increases will not necessarily generalize to other indices of achievement, because these increases were obtained through methods that do not incite more self-motivation, interest, and value for learning.

Achievement Goal Theories: Divided Views on the Value of Performance Goals and High Stakes

Another family of theories that has relevance to HST initiatives is those that concern performance versus mastery goals in the achievement domain, and the conditions that inspire them (e.g., Dweck & Leggett, 1988; Elliot, 1999; Nicholls, 1984; Pintrich, 2000). Although the theories differ in some details, the critically important distinction is between goals that are focused on increasing or *developing* one's competence or knowledge (called mastery or learning goals) and those focused on proving or *demonstrating* one's competence or ability (often called performance goals). HST, by focusing on the demonstration of specific test scores and using rewards to make that demonstration salient, represents an institutional climate that one might expect to catalyze performance goals; that is, by making the demonstration of competence the most salient issue, students, teachers, and administrators alike would be likely to adopt a performance goal orientation.

A large body of evidence suggests that very different behaviors and quality of learning typically follow from performance versus learning and mastery goals. This evidence suggests that the more students are focused on learning or mastery goals, the more extensively they enjoy learning, make greater use of higher level cognitive strategies, experience greater efficacy, and show better integration of what is learned (Ames & Archer, 1987; Elliot, McGregor, & Thrash, 2002; Midgley, Anderman, & Hicks, 1995; Midgley et al., 2001). Performance goals, by contrast, appear to foster a more superficial approach to learning, because the motivation is to demonstrate rather than attain competence. For example, a meta-analysis by Utman (1997) suggests that performance-focused goals can produce enhanced performance at rote or algorithmic tasks but tend to undermine performance at more heuristic or complex tasks. Furthermore, students with learning goals are often more willing to tackle challenges and difficult material, whereas those with performance goals are often more interested in demonstrating competencies already attained (Ames, 1992; Thorkildsen & Nicholls, 1991). Finally, performance goals have been linked to greater self-handicapping (Martin et al., 2001; Urdan, Kneisel, & Mason, 1999) and may leave students more vulnerable to helplessness when failure occurs (Dweck, 2002).

However, despite the numerous advantages of mastery goals in learning contexts, Elliot and his colleagues (see Elliot & Thrash, 2002) introduced an important distinction within goal theories between performance–avoidance and performance–approach goals. *Performance–avoidance* goals concern situations in which the student is primarily motivated to avoid failure or negative outcomes in the demonstration of performance. *Performance–approach* goals refer to a more appetitive desire to positively demonstrate high performance. Much empirical literature supports the view that the adoption of performance–avoidance goals has many negative consequences. By contrast, performance–approach goals seem to show fewer detrimental effects and can inspire some positive consequences (Elliot & Moller, in press).

It is important to realize that current HST systems do not, at least strategically, aim differentially to foster performance–approach rather than performance–avoidance goals. Indeed, the rhetoric of HST suggests that advocates expect that both desire to attain success and fear of failing at these demonstrations are engendered. Indeed, they may activate both to different degrees, both across and within individuals (Elliot & Moller, in press; Midgley et al., 2001).

Nonetheless, among the achievement motivation theorists focused on the performance versus the mastery goal distinction, opinions are divided as to the implications of the findings. Some theorists seem quite positive about having performance goals coupled with rewards be a central focus in classrooms. For example, Harackiewicz, Barron, Carter, Lehto, and Elliot (1997) argued that performance–approach goals are "adaptive" in settings where achievement is competitively defined or based on normative comparisons, because those whose adopted goal is to demonstrate high performance are more likely to do so. Hidi and Harackiewicz (2000) further advocate linking performance goals with extrinsic rewards. They speculated that performance goals linked with reward contingencies may be effective in promoting long-term interest and intrinsic motivation, especially among unmotivated and at-risk students. As Hidi (2002, p. 332) puts it: "Why should we assume that our children will produce high level schoolwork without expecting and receiving rewards?" Such thinking clearly mirrors the philosophy of HST advocates such as Bennett and Finn.

In contrast, other researchers in this domain hold that a focus on promoting performance demonstrations rather than mastery development in real-world classrooms will yield few positive and many negative motivational outcomes. Midgely et al. (2001), for example, highlight the fact that an emphasis on performance goals at best supports and rewards only highly achievement-oriented students who are certain about their abilities, and even for many of them, it leads to an extrinsic and superficial focus, and to vulnerability, if academic setbacks occur. In a context that emphasizes performance goals, they further suggest that many students, especially those with lower or uncertain abilities, will show increased self-protective strategies such as self-handicapping and withdrawal of effort. Thus, performance-focused classrooms may lead some students to be more extrinsically motivated to perform well, but, at the same time, it will lead to lessened intrinsic motivation and withdrawal of effort among those at risk for failure, a prediction in opposition to the view of Hidi and Harackiewicz (2000).

Between these views, Elliot and Moller (in press), even while highlighting the clear benefits of students adopting performance–approach goals, suggest that institutional policies should still be directed toward a mastery focus. For them, performance–approach goals, when they arise, are a natural expression of competence urges (Elliot et al., 2002). However, in their view, policies *aimed* at performance put many students at risk for undermining effects, because many will adopt an avoidance focus under such a circumstance.

Thus, performance–mastery goal theories lack consensus regarding the effects of establishing performance goals as a *modus operandi* in schools and, by implication, on the effects of HST reforms. Some in this tradition suggest a positive influence of performance goals linked with contingent rewards on promoting interest and achievement efforts, whereas others suggest that a performance goal focus backed by high stakes will lead to numerous deleterious results, especially for at-risk students. Still others suggest the need to develop strategies that could foster performance–approach orientations, without simultaneously generating performance–avoidance concerns in the same setting, although ways to do that have not been explicated.

THE RESULTS OF HIGH-STAKES TESTING

Given the clear, yet opposing predictions from theories of motivation on the impact of HST, it is interesting to look at what the accumulating evidence actually shows. It is important to note that full-fledged HST programs are still being phased in within most states; thus, the full impact of HST has not yet been felt. In addition, although anecdotes abound, only a few credible empirical studies are available. Nonetheless, there is a growing body of evidence associated with these initiatives, and we review the most extensive studies to date.

Moon, Callahan, and Tomlinson (2003) surveyed a nationally stratified random sample of teachers on the effects of state HST programs on their classroom practices. Results indicated that classroom practices were strongly affected, especially in schools serving students in the lowest socioeconomic strata. Teacher reports suggested that HST was indeed salient, and that increases in test scores are not necessarily a result of student academic attainment, but are more due to test preparation. Test preparation associated with HST was reported to drive out other instructional activities, because much time was taken in the classroom to review and practice for state testing. Test preparation was especially intense in poorer districts. The authors speculated that one result of HST is a narrowing of the curriculum and the implementation of practices that may actually run counter to effective instruction, student self-direction and autonomy, and opportunities for interaction between students. Indeed, the authors suggested that the very salience of HST in the minds of teachers may be restricting educational opportunities, particularly among those from the most impoverished areas. Moon et al. further suggested that when teachers specifically teach to the test, the scores may no longer represent the broader domain of knowledge for which they are supposed to be an indicator, especially in schools serving disadvantaged students, where the test preparation was reported to be more intensive.

A study by McNeil and Valenzuela (2000) of Texas teachers arrived at similar conclusions. They found that teachers were encouraged or required to reallocate time away from core subjects not tested on the state examinations, and to eliminate or curtail special projects, experiments, library research, extensive writing, or oral assignments. This was especially true in schools that might be lower in absolute performance levels (i.e., those serving less affluent students). Much time was also reported being spent specifically on test-taking strategies rather than substantive issues.

Evidence that HST leads to "teaching to the test," which in turn crowds out the teaching of skills not on the tests and the provision of enriched experiences that might better engage students' interest in additional knowledge seeking, may underlie the concern with the generalizability of score gains. This issue can be partly addressed by examining *transfer*, or the extent to which gains on HST are reflected in evidence of improved achievement on other, nontargeted measures. Little research exists on the validity of test-score increases on HST, despite the fact that it is a crucial bone of contention between HST advocates and their opponents.

Perhaps the most comprehensive look at this issue was an 18-state study by Amrein and Berliner (2002). To test the transfer of score increases on high-stakes examinations, they obtained scores on non-HST that overlap with HST in their assessment of achievement domains. These were the ACT (established by the American College Testing Program), Scholastic Aptitude Test (SAT), National Assessment of Educational Progress (NAEP), and Advanced Placement (AP) tests. Their evidence suggested, contrary to that of HST advocates, that when transfer is considered, level of learning in those states with salient HST policies remains level or falls below previous levels once HST is implemented. In contrast, states without high-stakes graduation tests were more likely than states that had imposed them to show improvements on these outside tests. Indeed more than two-thirds of states posted decreases on ACT performance after high-stakes graduation exams were implemented.

Neil and Gaylor (2001), using the NAEP as a metric, similarly showed that states without HST were more likely to show score improvements than states with them; that is, NAEP scores were not improved by HST initiatives, and they also had many other potentially negative consequences. They specifically suggested that HST may widen educational outcome inequities between the rich and the poor rather than ameliorate them.

With so much attention paid to test scores, an equally important gauge of school performance is high school dropout rate. Although dropouts are hard to track and are often systematically misreported (Orfield, Iosen, Wald, & Swanson, 2004), available data show that both dropouts and students leaving high schools for equivalency diplomas are on the rise, with notable escalation in the past few years as HST policies have intensified. Indeed, Reardon and Galindo (2002), for example, studying students between 8th- and 10th-grade in districts with and without HST policies, estimated that the imposition of HST increased the odds of dropout by 39%.

Although accounts differ, one possibility is that as states required students to pass tests for promotion, more pupils were held back. In turn, convincing data suggests that the mere fact of retention dramatically increases the probability of dropout (Natriello, 1998). In addition, if one assumes that HST imposes even modestly more difficult standards, that, too, could lead to a motivation and discouragement among students already at risk for failure.

A related issue is the concern that HST may lead many students to seek a general equivalency diplomas (GED). Studies comparing high school graduates to young people who received equivalency diplomas show that even among those with similar academic scores, those who complete high school have higher earnings, secure better employment, and commit fewer crimes. One reasonable account of this is that the confidence, self-esteem, and work habits of young adults is greater if they graduate from high school than if they drop out to earn a GED, and that confidence translates into better adult outcomes. In other words, if HST drives students out of school, this has costs, most of which will be borne by children from lower income families.

Jacob (2001) examined the effects of high-stakes high school examinations on student retention, especially among low achievers, who, some have argued, would most benefit from a performance-based focus (e.g., Hidi & Harackiewicz, 2000). His findings, based on analysis of data from 15 states, showed that students in the bottom 20th percentile of achievement who faced such requirements were 25% more likely to drop out in states with tests. He also found, however, that use of the tests had no significant effect on subsequent academic achievement for the population considered as a whole.

Another way to examine the impact of HST policies is to examine the results in Texas, where the most widely cited and lauded HST program has been in place since the early 1990s. HST policies in Texas have been described in the press as the "Texas Miracle," and have become a model for other reform efforts, including the federal NCLB program. This enthusiasm was partially based on the fact that scores on the

Texas State Achievement Tests (the TAAS) had shown large gains under the high-stakes regimen; TAAS scores provided evidence of a decreasing gap between minority and white students. An independent report by Grissmer, Flanagan, Kawata, and Williamson (2000) of the RAND Corporation initially suggested that the high-stakes policies themselves might have facilitated this positive trend. However a subsequent report by RAND investigators (Klein, Hamilton, McCaffrey, & Stecher, 2000) found that such gains in TAAS scores did not match trends on other measures, raising serious questions about the meaning of these achievement gains, or their transfer, and about the validity of the score gains. With regard to the achievement gap, results from other tests besides the TAAS also suggested that the gap might have slightly widened in Texas, over the same period that TAAS scores suggested it was closing.

At the same time, evidence of higher grade retention and dropout rates in Texas has accumulated (Haney, 2000), and outright cheating on results has been documented (Hoff, 2000; Johnston, 1999). Haney (2000) found that increased dropout rates in Texas were especially high among Latino and African American students. Haney linked these dropouts with aggregate score gains, arguing that Texas students' gains in NAEP scores were directly related to exclusion rates. Haney concluded that the apparent rise in scores was illusory. Tracking these dropouts, Haney found that approximately one-third of students leave school before graduation, often as a direct result of being retained in grade 9 by schools focused on obtaining good HST scores.

Moreover, evidence from Texas points to considerable teaching to the test, again, especially intensively in low-performing schools serving pockets of poverty and minority students. Such teaching to the test can give the appearance of "closing the gap" when that is not occurring, because of the criterion contamination this behavior causes (Carnoy, Loeb, & Smith, 2000; McNeil & Valenzuela, 2000). For such reasons, Popham (1999) concludes that judgments about school quality based on changes in HST scores are not likely to be valid.

Despite the limitations of the empirical studies thus far conducted, it is not unrea-

sonable to suggest that the evidence points to the very kinds of changes predicted by some of the motivational theories we reviewed. Under HST, outcome-focused behavior change does indeed occur, no doubt due to the power of rewards and sanctions. Yet these changes are often a "monkey's paw," representing deleterious classroom and institutional processes that hurt especially the most vulnerable populations. This in turn suggests that the HST policies may be exacerbating the problem they are designed to correct. Nonetheless, these negative results should not be taken as a definitive summary or as the final chapter. We reiterate that the results of HST policies are still unfolding. At the same time, there are clearly problems with the impact of HST, which predictably motivates counterproductive processes in both classroom and school administration arenas. It is ultimately the economically disadvantaged students, as well as the frontline teachers who serve them, that appear to suffer the most serious costs.

MOTIVATION THEORIES AND EDUCATIONAL REFORM

One conclusion we reach from reviewing this material concerns the relevance of debates between theories of motivation to policies attempting to legislate competence in schools. We have underscored how policymakers have, at both state and federal levels, enacted policies driven by a naive behaviorism in their attempts to motivate improvements in school performance. Unlike behaviorists, however, they have applied rewards and sanctions contingently upon performance outcomes (test scores) rather than desired behaviors, and they have also not appreciated the well-documented deleterious effects that even a well-structured contingency management approach can yield in domains such as learning and education. At the same time, results bespeak the power of such contingencies to change behavior, if not necessarily for the better.

The specific deleterious effects of such high-stakes policies have been predictable, and sometimes explicitly predicted by some motivational perspectives, whereas others have not addressed these "collateral" consequences. Most notably, self-determination theory has specifically argued that these reforms would foster teaching to the test, narrowing of the learning experience, relatively poor transfer of knowledge, and increased dropouts among those most disadvantaged (Ryan & LaGuardia, 1999; Ryan & Stiller, 1991). All of these predictions have come home to roost in states that have used HST. Similar deleterious effects may have been predictable from some goal theories as well, particularly the perspectives of Dweck (2002) and Midgeley et al. (2001). These views stand in contrast to the views of those who have advocated greater emphasis on performance goals in classrooms linked with high stakes. Rather than facilitating achievement in at-risk students, such motivational interventions seem especially harmful to vulnerable groups. If nothing else, one lesson we should learn from this is that our theoretical and empirical differences are far from merely "academic."

SOME POLICY IMPLICATIONS

Empirical research is critical to informed policy in education, yet the gulf between the types of reforms suggested by educational research and those being implemented by policymakers appears vast. In part, this stems from the fact that policymakers want clear-cut actions, an urge that the implementation of high-stakes and standardized tests appears to satisfy. At the same time, as the effects of this "natural experiment" unfold, we should make sense of the results and outcomes, learning from the implementation (Hamilton, Stecher, & Klien, 2002). To do so we use the lens of SDT, which has specifically predicted many of these effects.

The SDT perspective suggests that tests can have both informational and controlling effects, and the high-stakes approach has largely undermined the informational value of standardized testing. Policymakers might first remember the purpose of testing: To gain information that can be used to advocate for those assessed. The informational use of tests would be represented by using tests to help identify students who may be most disadvantaged and in need of resources, and perhaps to identify curricular issues or problems with teaching methods.

Informational use of tests would also require that they be useful to teachers—that they would not simply be a scorecard at the end of a year, but a useful indicator of gaps in knowledge, while there is still time to redress the situation. The current practice in most HST states is year-end testing, with individual score reports often not going to the teacher who taught the subject matter until the following year, which is of little educational benefit to the participating students.

More importantly, the positive effects that can come from the informational function of tests are undermined when policymakers place high stakes behind test outcomes. The implementation of high-stakes contingencies based upon test performance, which are intended as "motivators," actually do have a strong impact. They lead to practices that distort the validity of the outcomes, and that instigate deleterious institutional behaviors. They narrow curricula, decrease individualized approaches, and make even more vulnerable those students who are at risk for retention and dropout. Taking the stakes out of the heart of testing policies would make the testing more informationally valuable. Whereas high stakes contaminate the criterion, removing the stakes might make standardized testing all the more useful, and less engendering of damaging processes.

A further important issue concerns the fact that any standardized paper-and-pencil measure may be a poor fit with the learning and performance styles of some learners, making it inappropriate as a sole criterion for attaining credentials. "One size fits all" as a model of outcomes is a regressive step in schools, where for years educators have been developing approaches to address more effectively diversity in learning styles, interests, and skills. Moreover, basing high-stakes decisions on a single indicator is unfair to students, and even unethical, given the lack of validity of most of the tests for this purpose (American Educational Research Association, 2000). Accountability does not need to be actualized by only a single, uniform test. Instead, schools that use alternative approaches and curricula could develop and justify alternative assessments. This would in fact lead toward greater innovation rather than drying up choice and diversity, which has been the trend under HST.

In a context where testing was used for informational rather than controlling purposes, educational experiments might actually permit better judgement on their effectiveness, and indeed catalyze more innovation and progress. For instance, there appears to be growing evidence that high schools organized into small schools or learning communities, where personalized attention is available, are effective in promoting achievement (e.g., Howley & Bickel, 2000; Meier, 1998; National Research Council, 2004). Effective non-high-stakes testing could both verify and extend such data, and be a basis for justifying such structural reforms to policymakers and taxpayers. Similarly, an innovative and highly successful experiment in redesigning urban high schools was the creation of the New York Performance Standards Consortium (NYPSC) schools. These schools had served as models and were recognized for their high educational standards, high attendance, and low dropout and college success rates (Darling-Hammond, Ancess, & Ort, 2002). However, NYPSC schools were built around a portfolio-based assessment system that was deemed integral to the form of instruction, which itself was highly individualized rather than standardized. These successful schools are being forced under New York's rigidly enacted high-stakes regimen to change their practices and teach to the tests. In a non-high-stakes atmosphere, standardized tests might have been one among several useful indices affirming their efficacy, but in a high-stakes atmosphere, the curriculum will be bent to the shape of tests, and a successful innovation stifled.

An important take-home point is that the introduction of high stakes behind test scores distorts the validity of tests as an indicator of true excellence in the classroom, or of school quality. Amrein and Berliner (2002) described this distortion effect by evoking the *Heisenberg Uncertainty Principle*. According to the principle, the more important any quantitative indicator becomes in decision making, the more likely it will distort and corrupt the process it is intended to monitor. Because high-stakes policies attach reward and punishment contingent on test scores, they especially have such distorting and corrupting consequences. They make the meaning of test score changes questionable, and they make inferences from

score changes problematic. Combined with the fact that most states use percentage-passing rates on tests that are not equivalent from year to year, many of the inferences concerning the outcomes of reform are without a sound scientific basis.

While the massive educational experiment called HST is still in progress, it is clear that what is driving national and state education policy is not sound educational theory or research, but a blend of political expediency and naive faith in the efficacy of rewards and punishments. Research that has accumulated points to complex, and often negative, effects that may not be willingly received by politicians who, in many instances, may "have already decided" that HST is an effective approach (Hamilton et al., 2002). On a more positive note, we suggest that current work in the field of motivational psychology is highly relevant to, and capable of, meaningfully informing the process of education reform. The question is, who might be listening?

REFERENCES

American Educational Research Association. (2000). Position statement of the American Educational Research Association concerning high stakes testing in pre K–12 education. *Educational Researcher, 29,* 24–25.

Ames, C. (1992). Classrooms: Goals, structures, and student motivation. *Journal of Educational Psychology, 84,* 261–271.

Ames, C., & Archer, J. (1987). Mothers' beliefs about the role of ability and effort in school learning. *Journal of Educational Psychology, 79,* 409–446.

Amrein, A. L., & Berliner, D. C. (2002, March 28). High-stakes testing, uncertainty, and student learning. *Education Policy Analysis Archives, 10*(18). Retrieved January 14, 2003, from *http://epaa.asu.edu/epaa/v10n18/*.

Benware, C., & Deci, E. L. (1984). Quality of learning with an active versus passive motivational set. *American Educational Research Journal, 21,* 755–765.

Cameron, J., & Pierce, W. D. (1994). Reinforcement, reward, and intrinsic motivation: A meta-analysis. *Review of Educational Research, 64,* 363–423.

Carnoy, M., Loeb, S., & Smith, T. L. (2000, April). *Do higher state test scores in Texas make for better high school outcomes?* Paper presented at the Annual Meeting of the American Educational Research Association, New Orleans, LA.

Carver, C. S., & Scheier, M. F. (1998). *On the self-regulation of behavior.* Cambridge, UK: Press Syndicate of Cambridge University.

Cheney, L. (1991). Proponents of national tests of student achievement argue that such tests, if required by college officials or employers, would motivate students to work harder in school: Do you agree?: Response of Lynne Cheney. *Association for Supervision and Curriculum Development Update, 33,* 7.

Darling-Hammond, L., Ancess, J., & Ort, S. (2002). Reinventing high school: Outcomes of the coalition campus schools project. *American Educational Research Journal, 39,* 639–673.

deCharms, R. (1968). *Personal causation: The internal affective determinants of behavior.* New York: Academic Press.

Deci, E. L., Koestner, R., & Ryan, R. M. (1999). A meta-analytic review of experiments examining the effects of extrinsic rewards on intrinsic motivation. *Psychological Bulletin, 125,* 627–668.

Deci, E. L., & Ryan, R. M. (1980). Self-determination theory: When mind mediates behavior. *Journal of Mind and Behavior, 1,* 33–43.

Deci, E. L., & Ryan, R. M. (1985). *Intrinsic motivation and self-determination in human behavior.* New York: Plenum Press.

Deci, E. L., & Ryan, R. M. (2000). The "what" and the "why" of goal pursuits: Human needs and the self-determination of behavior. *Psychological Inquiry, 11,* 227–268.

Deci, E. L., & Ryan, R. M. (2002). The paradox of achievement: The harder you push, the worse it gets. In D. I. Cordova & J. Aronson (Eds.), *Improving academic achievement: Contributions of social psychology* (pp. 61–87). New York: Academic Press.

Deci, E. L., Schwartz, A. J., Sheinman, L., & Ryan, R. M. (1981). An instrument to assess adults' orientations toward control versus autonomy with children: Reflections on intrinsic motivation and perceived competence. *Journal of Educational Psychology, 73,* 642–650.

Deci, E. L., Spiegel, N. H., Ryan, R. M., Koestner, R., & Kauffman, M. (1982). The effects of performance standards on teaching styles: The behavior of controlling teachers. *Journal of Educational Psychology, 74,* 852–859.

Dewey, J. (1938). *Experience and education.* New York: Collier.

Dweck, C. (1991). Self theories and goals: Their role in motivation, personality, and development. In R. Dienstbier (Ed.), *Nebraska Symposium on Motivation* (Vol. 38, pp. 199–235). Lincoln: University of Nebraska Press.

Dweck, C. S. (2002). Messages that motivate: How praise molds students' beliefs, motivation, and performance (in surprising ways). In J. Aronson (Ed.), *Improving academic achievement: Impact of psychological factors on education* (pp. 38–61). San Diego: Academic Press.

Dweck, C. S., & Leggett, E. L. (1988). A social-cognitive approach to personality and motivation. *Psychological Review, 95,* 256–273.

Eisenberger, R., Pierce, W. D., & Cameron, J. (1999). Effects of reward on intrinsic motivation—negative, neural, and positive: Comment on Deci, Koestner, and Ryan (1999). *Psychological Bulletin, 125,* 677–691.

Elliot, A. J. (1999). Approach and avoidance motivation and achievement goals. *Educational Psychologist, 34,* 169–189.

Elliot, A. J., McGregor, H. A., & Thrash, T. M. (2002). The need for competence. In E. L. Deci & R. M. Ryan (Eds.), *Handbook of self-determination research* (pp. 361–387). Rochester, NY: University of Rochester Press.

Elliot, A. J., & Moller, A. C. (in press). Performance–approach goals: Good or bad forms of regulation? *International Journal of Educational Research.*

Elliot, A. J., & Thrash, T. M. (2002). Approach–avoidance motivation in personality: Approach and avoidance temperaments and goals. *Journal of Personality and Social Psychology, 83,* 804–818.

Finn, C. E. J. (1991). *We must take charge: Our schools and our future.* New York: Free Press.

Flink, C., Boggiano, A. K., & Barrett, M. (1990). Controlling teaching strategies: Undermining children's self-determination and performance. *Journal of Personality and Social Psychology, 59,* 916–924.

Gardner, H. (1991). *The unschooled mind: How children think and how schools should teach.* New York: Basic Books.

Ginsburg, G. S., & Bronstein, P. (1993). Family factors related to children's intrinsic/extrinsic motivational orientation and academic performance. *Child Development, 64,* 1461–1474.

Golan, S., & Graham, S. (1990, April). *The impact of ego and task-involvement on levels of processing.* Paper presented at the annual meeting of the American Educational Research Association, Boston, MA.

Grissmer, D., Flanagan, A., Kawata, J., & Williamson, S. (2000). *Improving student achievement: What state NAEP test scores tell us* [MR-924-EDU]. Santa Monica, CA: RAND.

Grolnick, W. S. (2003). *The psychology of parental control: How well-meant parenting backfires.* Mahwah, NJ: Erlbaum.

Grolnick, W. S., Gurland, S. T., DeCourcey, W., & Jacob, K. (2002). Antecedents and consequences of mother's autonomy support: An experimental investigation. *Developmental Psychology, 38,* 143–155.

Grolnick, W. S., & Ryan, R. M. (1987). Autonomy in children's learning: An experimental and individual difference investigation. *Journal of Personality and Social Psychology, 52,* 890–898.

Grolnick, W. S., & Ryan, R. M. (1989). Parent styles associated with children's self-regulation and competence in school. *Journal of Educational Psychology, 81,* 143–154.

Hamilton, L. S., Stecher, B. M., & Klein, S. P. (2002). *Making sense of test-based accountability in education.* Santa Monica, CA: RAND Corporation.

Haney, W. (2000). The myth of the Texas miracle in education. *Education Policy Analysis Archives, 8*(41).

Retrieved December 16, 2003, from *http:// epaa.asu.edu/epaa/v8n41*

Harackiewicz, J. M., Barron, K. E., Carter, S. M., Lehto, A. T., & Elliot, A. J. (1997). Predictors and consequences of achievement goals in the college classroom: Maintaining interest and making the grade. *Journal of Personality and Social Psychology, 73,* 1284–1295.

Hardre, P. L., & Reeve, J. (2003). A motivational model of rural students' intentions to persist in, versus drop out of, high school. *Journal of Educational Psychology, 95,* 347–356.

Hidi, S. (2002). An interest researcher's perspective: The effects of extrinsic and intrinsic factors on motivation. In C. Sansone & J. M. Harackiewicz (Eds.), *Intrinsic and extrinsic motivation: The search for optimal motivation and performance* (pp. 311–342). San Diego: Academic Press.

Hidi, S., & Harackiewicz, J. M. (2000). Motivating the academically unmotivated: A critical issue for the 21st century. *Review of Educational Research, 70,* 151–179.

Hoff, D. J. (2000). As stakes rise, definition of cheating blurs. *Education Week, 19,* 1–4.

Howley, C., & Bickel, R. (2000). *Results of four-state study: Smaller schools reduce harmful impact of poverty on student achievement.* Washington, DC: Rural School and Community Trust.

Jacob, B. (2001). Getting tough?: The impact of high school graduation exams. *Educational Evaluation and Policy Analysis, 23,* 99–121.

Johnston, R. C. (1999). Texas presses districts in alleged test-tampering cases. *Education Week, 18,* 22, 28.

Kellaghan, T., Madaus, G. F., & Raczek, A. (1996). *The use of external examinations to improve student motivation.* Washington, DC: American Educational Research Association.

Keller, B. (2000). Incentives for test-takers run the gamut. *Education Week, 19,* 1–3.

Klein, S. P., Hamilton, L. S., McCaffrey, D. F., & Stecher, B. M. (2000). What do test scores in Texas tell us? *Education Policy Analysis Archives, 8*(49). Retrieved April 24, 2003, from *http://epaa.asu.edu/ epaa/v8n49/*

Kohn, A. (1996). By all available means: Cameron and Pierce's defense of extrinsic motivators. *Review of Educational Research, 66,* 1–4.

Linn, R. L. (2000). Assessments and accountability. *Educational Researcher, 29*(2), 4–16.

Locke, E. A., & Latham, G. P. (1990). *A theory of goal setting and task performance.* Englewood Cliffs, NJ: Prentice-Hall.

Martin, A. J., Marsh, H. W., & Debus, R. L. (2001). Self-handicapping and defensive pessimism: Exploring a model of predictors and outcomes from a self-protection perspective. *Journal of Educational Psychology, 93,* 87–102.

McNeil, L., & Valenzuela, A. (2000). *The harmful impact of the TAAS system of testing in Texas: Beneath the accountability rhetoric.* Cambridge, MA: Harvard University Civil Rights Project.

Meier, D. (1998). Changing the odds. In E. Clinchy (Ed.), *Creating new schools: How small schools are changing American education.* New York: Teachers College Press.

Midgley, C., Anderman, E., & Hicks, L. (1995). Differences between elementary and middle school teachers and students: A goal theory approach. *Journal of Early Adolescence, 15,* 90–113.

Midgley, C., Kaplan, A., & Middleton, M. (2001). Performance–approach goals: Good for what, for whom, under what circumstances, and at what cost? *Journal of Educational Psychology, 93,* 77–86.

Moon, T. R., Callahan, C. M., & Tomlinson, C. A. (2003, April 28). Effects of state testing programs on elementary schools with high concentrations of student poverty-good news or bad news? *Current Issues in Education, 6*(8). Retrieved May 14, 2003, from *http://cie.ed.asu.edu/volume6/number8/*

National Commission on Excellence in Education. (1983). *A nation at risk: The imperative for educational reform.* Washington, DC: U.S. Government Printing Office.

National Research Council and Institute of Medicine of the National Academies. (2004). *Engaging schools: Fostering high school students' motivation to learn.* Washington, DC: National Academies Press.

Natriello, G. (1998). Failing grades for retention. *School Administrator, 55,* 14–17.

Neil, M., & Gaylor, K. (2001). Do high-stakes graduation tests improve learning outcomes?: Using state-level NAEP data to evaluate the effects of mandatory graduation tests. In G. Orfield & M. L. Kornhaber (Eds.), *Raising standards or raising barriers?: Inequality and high-stakes testing in public education.* New York: Century Foundation Press.

Nicholls, J. G. (1984). Achievement motivation: Conceptions of ability, subjective experience, task choice, and performance. *Psychological Review, 91,* 328–346.

Oakes, J. (1991). The many-sided dilemmas of testing. In *Voices from the field: 30 expert opinions on America 2000: The Bush administration strategy to "reinvent" America's schools* (pp. 17–18). New York: William T. Grant Foundation Commission on Work, Family and Citizenship Institute for Educational Leadership.

Orfield, G., Iosen, D., Wald, J., & Swanson, C. B. (2004, February 25). *Losing our future: How minority youth are being left behind by the graduation crisis.* Boston: Harvard Civil Rights Project. Retrieved April 4, 2004, from *http://www.civilrightsproject. harvard.edu/research/dropouts*

Pintrich, P. R. (2000). Multiple goals, multiple pathways: The role of goal orientation in learning and achievement. *Journal of Educational Psychology, 92,* 544–555.

Plant, R., & Ryan, R. M. (1985). Intrinsic motivation and the effects of self-consciousness, self-awareness, and ego-involvement: An investigation of internally controlling styles. *Journal of Personality*, *53*, 435–449.

Popham, W. J. (1983). Measurement as an instructional catalyst. *New Directions for Testing and Measurement*, *17*, 19–30.

Popham, W. J. (1999). Educators' indifference to the misuse of standardized tests is having calamitous consequences. *Education Week*, *18*, 48–32.

Rachlin, H. (1976). *Introduction to modern behaviorism* (2nd ed). San Francisco: Freeman.

Reardon, S. F., & Galindo, C. (2002, April). *Do high stakes tests affect students' decisions to drop out of schools?* [Evidence from NELS]. Paper presented at the American Educational Research Association, New Orleans, LA.

Rogers, C. (1969). *Freedom to learn*. Columbus, OH: Merrill.

Ryan, R. M. (1982). Control and information in the intrapersonal sphere: An extension of cognitive evaluation theory. *Journal of Personality and Social Psychology*, *43*, 450–461.

Ryan, R. M., & Deci, E. L. (2000) Self-determination theory and the facilitation of intrinsic motivation, social development and well-being. *American Psychologist*, *55*, 68–78.

Ryan, R. M., & Grolnick, W. S. (1986). Origins and pawns in the classroom: Self-report and projective assessments of individual differences in children's perceptions. *Journal of Personality and Social Psychology*, *50*, 550–558.

Ryan, R. M., & La Guardia, J. G. (1999). Achievement motivation within a pressured society: Intrinsic and extrinsic motivations to learn and the politics of school reform. In T. Urdan (Ed.), *Advances in motivation and achievement* (Vol. 11, pp. 45–85). Greenwich, CT: JAI Press.

Ryan, R. M., & Lynch, M. (2003). Motivation and classroom management. In R. Curren (Ed.), *A companion to the philosophy of education* (pp. 260–271). Malden, MA: Blackwell.

Ryan, R. M., Mims, V., & Koestner, R. (1983). Relation of reward contingency and interpersonal context to intrinsic motivation: A review and test using cognitive evaluation theory. *Journal of Personality and Social Psychology*, *45*, 736–750.

Ryan, R. M., & Stiller, J. (1991). The social contexts of internalization: Parent and teacher influences on autonomy, motivation and learning. In P. R. Pintrich & M. L. Maehr (Eds.), *Advances in motivation and achievement: Vol. 7. Goals and self-regulatory processes* (pp. 115–149). Greenwich, CT: JAI Press.

Ryan, R. M., Stiller, J., & Lynch, J. H. (1994). Representations of relationships to teachers, parents, and friends as predictors of academic motivation and self-esteem. *Journal of Early Adolescence*, *14*, 226–249.

Sen, A. (1999). *Development as freedom*. New York: Knopf.

Shanker, A. (1993, May 23). Where we stand: Goals 2000. *New York Times*, p. A7.

Shepard, L. (2000). The role of assessment in a learning culture. *Educational Researcher*, *29*, 4–14.

Silber, K. (1973). *Pestalozzi: The man and his work*. New York: Schocken.

Thorkildsen, T. A., & Nicholls, J. G. (1991). Students' critiques as motivation. *Educational Psychologist*, *26*, 347–368.

Thorndike, E. L. (1962). *Psychology and the science of education*. New York: Teachers College, Columbia University.

Toch, T. (1991). *In the name of excellence: The struggle to reform the nation's schools, why it's failing, and what should be done*. New York: Oxford University Press.

Urdan, T. C., Kneisel, L., & Mason, V. (1999). Interpreting messages about motivation in the classroom: Examining the effects of achievement goal structures. In M. L. Maehr & P. R. Pintrich (Series Eds.) & T. C. Urdan (Vol. Ed.), *Advances in motivation and achievement: Vol. 11. The role of context* (pp. 123–158). Greenwich, CT: JAI Press.

Utman, C. H. (1997). Performance effects of motivational state: A meta-analysis. *Personality and Social Psychology Review*, *1*, 170–182.

Vallerand, R. J., & Reid, G. (1984). On the causal effects of perceived competence on intrinsic motivation: A test of cognitive evaluation theory. *Journal of Sport Psychology*, *6*, 94–102.

World Economic Forum. (2002). *The Global Competitiveness Report, 2001–2002*. Geneva, Switzerland: WEF Publications.

PART V

❦

Demographics and Culture

CHAPTER 21

ભ

Gender, Competence, and Motivation

JANET SHIBLEY HYDE
AMANDA M. DURIK

The second half of the 20th century witnessed remarkable changes in women's achievements in the realms of education and occupations. For example, in 1970, 8% of MD degrees went to women, compared with 41% in 1996 (Costello & Stone, 2001; Rix, 1988). In 1975, 31% of all college and university professors were women, compared with 42% in 1998 (Costello & Stone, 2001). Yet many occupations have not seen these dramatic shifts and remain highly gender-segregated. For example, women were 0.5% of auto mechanics in 1975 and 0.8% of auto mechanics in 1998 (Costello & Stone, 2001).

Both theory and research in psychology place strong emphasis on the role of motivation and personal competence beliefs in determining achievements and, in particular, in determining gendered patterns of achievement behaviors. In this chapter, we focus first on gender and competence beliefs, reviewing Eccles's expectancy–value theory, Bussey and Bandura's social cognitive theory, empirical data on and developmental approaches to understanding gender and competence beliefs, and the role of stereotype threat in creating gender differences in competence beliefs. We then turn to research and theory on gender and achievement motivation, first considering McClelland's classic theory and research, and critiques of it, followed by motive to avoid success, and most recently, achievement goal theory. Finally, we consider the role of ethnicity and culture in determining patterns of gender differences in competence beliefs. First, however, we highlight three overarching issues: the importance of a balanced consideration of gender differences and gender similarities, the importance of adopting a developmental approach, and the distinction between gender as a person variable and gender as a stimulus variable.

GENDER DIFFERENCES AND GENDER SIMILARITIES

Scholars approaching topics in gender and psychology tend to be drawn to findings of gender differences, as the moth is to the flame. Nonetheless, numerous meta-analyses have found evidence of psychological gender similarities in areas as diverse as mathematical performance (Hyde, Fennema, & Lamon, 1990), verbal ability (Hyde & Linn, 1988), and self-esteem (Kling, Hyde, Showers, & Buswell, 1999; see Hyde & Plant, 1995, for a review). At the same time, moderate to large gender differences have been found in areas such as aggression (Eagly & Steffen, 1986; Hyde, 1984) and sexuality (Oliver & Hyde, 1993). Consideration of questions of gender, competence, and motivation should provide a balanced acknowledgment of both gender differences and gender similarities. Both are interesting and important.

A DEVELOPMENTAL APPROACH

Gendered patterns of motivation and competence are not present at birth (or if they are, no one has yet presented the evidence). Rather, they emerge in the course of development, as a result of the cumulation of experiences with parents, peers, teachers, sports, and so on. If we are to understand gender differences in motivation and competence, we must understand their developmental origins. Therefore, we present developmental evidence whenever possible in this review.

GENDER AS A PERSON VARIABLE VERSUS GENDER AS A STIMULUS VARIABLE

Gender may be conceptualized as either a person variable or a stimulus variable (e.g., Deaux & Major, 1987; Grady, 1979); that is, gender can, on the one hand, be thought of as a characteristic of the person, an individual differences variable. Research on psychological gender differences implicitly assumes this approach. On the other hand, gender can be conceptualized as a stimulus variable. A person's gender serves as a cue to others interacting with and responding to that person, and people respond differently depending on whether they are interacting with a man or a woman, or a boy or a girl. The classic research assessing sex bias in the evaluation of work using the John McKay/Joan McKay paradigm (reviewed by Swim, Borgida, Maruyama, & Myers, 1989) used

this approach of considering gender to be a stimulus variable. As we consider gender, competence, and motivation, we should be alert to findings of gender differences; at the same time, we should be mindful of the fact that gender is a stimulus variable. The individual's gender affects the responses he or she receives from others, which in turn may influence his or her motivation or self-efficacy.

GENDER AND COMPETENCE BELIEFS

Theory

Major theorizing on gender and competence beliefs comes from Eccles's expectancy–value theory (e.g., Eccles, 1987a; Fredricks & Eccles, 2002; Meece, Eccles-Parsons, Kaczala, Goff, & Futterman, 1982) and Bussey and Bandura's (1999) cognitive social-learning theory. Each is reviewed in turn.

Eccles: Expectancy–Value Theory

Eccles' expectancy–value theory of achievement-related choices is a general model that, at the same time, is particularly dedicated to understanding gender differences in these choices (Eccles, 1987a, 1987b, 1994). According to the model, a person will undertake a challenging achievement task—such as taking calculus in high school or applying to medical school—only if he or she expects to succeed at it and values the task. Here, we focus on the path to expectations for success; the question of values is discussed by Eccles in Chapter 7, this volume.

A major force shaping expectations for success at a particular achievement task is one's self-concept of one's abilities (Eccles, 1994), or competence beliefs. Gender differences in competence beliefs, then, will have a profound influence on the achievement tasks that males and females undertake. Competence beliefs themselves, according to the model, are shaped by not only people's past achievement experiences but also a variety of social and cultural factors, including (1) the behaviors and beliefs of important socializers, such as parents and teachers; and (2) cultural gender roles that prescribe certain qualities, such as aggressiveness, as appropriate or inappropriate for males or females, and gender stereotypes about particular activities (e.g., professional football is played only by men).

Numerous empirical studies by Eccles and others have provided support for links in this model, including the gender-related links. This research is reviewed later in the chapter.

Bussey and Bandura: Social Cognitive Theory

Bussey and Bandura (1999) extended Bandura's (1986) social cognitive theory to address the issue of gender learning and development. Their model of triadic reciprocal causation, which is intrinsically developmental, specifies that person factors, behavior, and environment all exert reciprocal influences on each other. The individual's perceived self-efficacy in a given domain, such as mathematics, is one kind of person factor. (We take Bussey and Bandura's construct of self-efficacy to be roughly equivalent to Eccles's concept of competence beliefs.) According to the model, self-efficacy has a profound impact on behavior; as Bussey and Bandura put it, "Perceived efficacy is, therefore, the foundation of human agency" (1999, p. 691). It influences the challenges that people undertake, and how long they persevere in pursuing a goal.

Self-efficacy comes into play in a particularly powerful way in the area of occupational choice. Most adolescents and young adults eliminate vast numbers of jobs from personal consideration, because their sense of self-efficacy tells them that they cannot do the job or master the knowledge necessary for the job. Gender enters the picture, because occupations are highly gender-segregated (Costello & Stone, 2001). Many adult women and men, then, are making gendered occupational choices. A number of influences are involved, including hostile environments for women in some occupations, but one powerful factor is self-efficacy beliefs that have developed over time. Male college students feel about as efficacious in traditionally female-dominated careers as they do in traditionally male-dominated careers; female undergraduates, however, have a weaker sense of efficacy in traditional male occupations compared with traditional female occupations (Betz & Hackett, 1981).

Gender differences disappear, though, when students judge their efficacy at a task presented in a stereotypically feminine context (Betz & Hackett, 1983), suggesting that women's sense of self-efficacy is not chronically low, but rather responds to situational factors related to gender, as the research on stereotype threat, reviewed below, demonstrates.

Mathematics skill and self-efficacy are a major factor in occupational choice, because they are essential for scientific and technical careers. Mathematics self-efficacy encourages choice of mathematics courses in high school and college, which further bolsters mathematics self-efficacy. Research shows that the effect of gender on mathematics performance is mediated by perceived self-efficacy (Pajares & Miller, 1994). Moreover, mastery experiences eliminate gender differences in mathematics self-efficacy (Schunck & Lilly, 1984).

Self-efficacy, according to social cognitive theory, develops in four ways (Bussey & Bandura, 1999): (1) through graded mastery experiences; (2) through social modeling, such as seeing people like oneself succeed because of effort; (3) through social persuasion, in which another person expresses confidence in one's ability to succeed; and (4) by reducing stress and depression, building physical strength, and changing misinterpretations of bodily states. The second factor, social modeling, is particularly relevant to gender and occupational choice. In everyday life and in the media, children observe the gender segregation of occupations—that almost all nurses and elementary school teachers are women, and that almost all professional basketball players and all presidents of the United States are men. Girls therefore see people like themselves—women—succeeding as nurses and teachers, and boys see people like themselves—men—succeeding as basketball players and presidents. The result is that girls develop a greater sense of self-efficacy at being a nurse or teacher, making them likelier to pursue that career choice. Boys develop a greater sense of self-efficacy in athletics and leadership roles, encouraging a choice of careers in those areas.

Numerous empirical studies by Bussey, Bandura, and others support various aspects of social cognitive theory as it applies to gender differentiation in self-efficacy and achievements (reviewed by Bussey & Bandura, 1999). For example, concerning social persuasion as one of the factors influencing self-efficacy, research shows that as early as kindergarten, mothers have higher expectations for their daughters in reading, and higher expectations for their sons in math (Lummis & Stevenson, 1990). When boys and girls are matched for math performance, parents rate daughters' mathematical ability as less than sons' (Yee & Eccles, 1988). In a daily checklist study, when praising children for an achievement, mothers of sons were more likely than mothers of daughters to connect the praise to the child's ability (Pomerantz & Ruble, 1998).

A Comparison of the Two Theories

Both Eccles and colleagues' expectancy–value theory and Bussey and Bandura's social cognitive theory contribute to a fuller understanding of how achievement expectations, beliefs, and behaviors become gendered over time. At this point, it is worthwhile to highlight some of the similarities and differences we see in these two approaches in order to understand how they might best be used to inform future research.

These models are similar in that both place importance on the influence of socializers such as parents and peers, the impact of expectations for success, and the pivotal role of individual choice in shaping beliefs about gender and achievement. However, there are also subtle differences in these models in their specific focus on how these variables combine to predict and explain the intersection of gender and achievement. For example, Bussey and Bandura elaborate on specific processes of social learning that might unfold to explain how parents' beliefs and behavior about achievement are learned by children. Because parents serve as models in this framework, the extent to which children learn gendered beliefs from parents should vary in response to specific parameters, such as the attention children focus on the model at a given time, the similarities between the child and the model, and whether there are inconsistencies between the model's behavior and what the model explicitly teaches. Processes such as these help specify when and how socializers affect children's beliefs about achievement. Adding processes such as these to the expectancy–

value framework should be helpful. Second, the Eccles and colleagues and the Bussey and Bandura models also differ slightly in how they treat the relationship between competence beliefs and task value. Specifically, Eccles's model, as an explicit expectancy–value model, predicts that achievement choices are impacted both by expectancies for success and task values. In this way, believing that one is skilled at a task and that the task is worthwhile can operate independently. In this model, task value is determined by factors in addition to competence beliefs, such as short- and long-term goals, and these values can contribute to expectancy beliefs, as well as combine with them to predict achievement behavior. In contrast, Bussey and Bandura's model implies that efficacy beliefs affect achievement choices, and the role of values is given little attention.

These theories provide frameworks within which to describe and predict achievement behaviors, and how these behaviors might differ by gender. Although similar in some ways, they each offer specificity in different areas. It is important to draw from each theory in order for us, as researchers, to reach a more thorough understanding of gender, competence, and achievement.

Gender Socialization and the Gender Segregation Effect

In this section, we shift the focus to empirical findings on the role of parents, teachers, and peers in the development of gender differences in competence beliefs. A thorough review of all studies on gender socialization relevant to motivation and competence is beyond the scope of this chapter. Bussey and Bandura (1999) reviewed many of the relevant studies. Here, we focus on some key ones and others that are exemplars of various categories of evidence.

Lytton and Romney (1991) conducted a meta-analysis of 172 studies of parents' differential rearing of boys compared with girls. The studies used a variety of methods, including reports by the child, interviews and questionnaires for parents, and direct observations. The studies also covered a wide array of domains that included encouraging achievement, warmth, encouraging dependency, restrictiveness, discipline, and encouraging sex-typed activities. The most relevant domain for this discussion of gender and the development of competence is encouragement of achievement. For North American studies, the effect size was $d = 0.05$; that is, there was essentially no difference in the extent to which parents encouraged achievement in girls compared with boys. Does that imply that parental socialization is not a force? Not in the least. A more substantial effect size was found for encouragement of sex-typed activities ($d = 0.34$). Measures in these studies assessed practices such as encouraging boys to play with trucks or to shovel the sidewalk, and girls to play with dolls and help with vacuuming. To the extent that parents encourage boys to play with trucks, they are building a sense of competence in a particular domain in their sons more than in their daughters. The same is true for encouragement of girls in activities such as playing with dolls. This meta-analysis is helpful insofar as a general impression exists that parents treat boys and girls entirely differently; the results, in contrast, show that, on the whole, parents treat their sons and daughters quite similarly. Encouragement of sex-typed activities, however, is a major exception, and this tendency can easily lay the foundation for different senses of competence in girls compared with boys; that is, these results indicate that girls and boys will become differentiated not in their global sense of competence, but rather in their sense of competence in specific domains.

Teachers, too, are socializers. Research based on classroom observations in preschools and elementary schools indicates that teachers treat boys and girls differently. Teachers, on average, pay more attention to boys than to girls (DeZolt & Hull, 2001; Golombok & Fivush, 1994). When teachers praise students, the compliments go to girls for decorous conduct and to boys for good academic performance (Dweck, Goetz, & Strauss, 1980; Golombok & Fivush, 1994). Teachers, then, are socializing a sense of academic competence for boys more than girls.

Maccoby (1990, 1998) has argued that one of the most potent forces encouraging gender differentiation is the largely self-imposed gender segregation that occurs in childhood. By 3 years of age, children have a tendency to seek out and play with other children of their own gender and to avoid playing with children of the other gender. The tendency grows stronger by the time

children are in elementary school. It occurs regardless of the gender socialization principles in their families, and in villages in developing nations as much as in the United States. Importantly, all-girl and all-boy groups differ in terms of their activities. Boys' play is rougher and involves more risk, confrontation, and striving for dominance. All-girl groups are more likely to use conflict-reducing strategies in negotiating with each other and to engage in more self-disclosure. All-girl groups also tend to maintain communication with adults, whereas boys separate themselves from adults, test the limits, and seek autonomy. Later, in adolescence, heterosexual attraction brings the sexes back together again, but that cannot undo the effects of the years of segregation.

The net effect of gender segregation in childhood, and the differentiation of activities intertwined with it, is that girls and boys have success experiences and build their sense of competence in different domains. Boys develop a sense of competence in rough, active pursuits that will contribute to competence beliefs in athletics and other competitive domains. Girls' practice at communication and maintaining harmonious relationships within the group will build their sense of competence in the domain of relationships. And these are precisely the domains in which the culture at large expects competence from girls and women compared with boys and men.

Development of Competence Beliefs in Girls and Boys

As reviewed earlier, several processes might contribute to gender differences in competence beliefs. Therefore, a crucial initial question surrounding gender and motivation within achievement settings concerns whether there are indeed gender differences in competence beliefs. If gender differences in competence beliefs exist, the next pressing issues are when and how these differences emerge. At first blush, evidence concerning the presence versus absence of gender differences in competence beliefs is mixed. In general, there is little empirical evidence to suggest that gender differences in competence beliefs exist at a global level. For example, most studies investigating academic competence beliefs in general indicate no or very small gender differences (e.g., Cole et al.,

2001; Jambunathan & Hurlbut, 2000). Although these studies report data from U.S. samples, this pattern of gender similarity appears to characterize non-U.S. samples as well. A study of elementary school students' achievement-related beliefs in several cities around the world (East and West Berlin, Berne, Los Angeles, Moscow, Prague, and Tokyo) revealed that girls and boys hold similar beliefs about their general academic competence (Stetsenko, Little, Gordeeva, Granshof, & Oettingen, 2000).

Research addressing competence beliefs within specific domains reveals a pattern that is more gender-differentiated. For example, several studies have found that boys report more competence in math, science, and athletics, and girls report less competence in these domains (Crain, 1996; Debacker & Nelson, 2000; Eccles, Wigfield, Harold, & Blumenfeld, 1993; Fredricks & Eccles, 2002; Jacobs, Finken, Griffin, & Wright, 1998; Lummis & Stevenson, 1990; Marsh & Young, 1998; Malpass, O'Neil, & Hocevar, 1999; Wigfield et al., 1997). A meta-analysis of studies of gender differences in attitudes toward math indicated that boys had somewhat higher competence beliefs in math than girls, and that this difference was widest during high school (Hyde, Fennema, Ryan, Frost, & Hopp, 1990). In contrast, girls report feeling more competent than do boys in language arts (Crain, 1996; Eccles, Wigfield, et al., 1993; Lummis & Stevenson, 1990; Marsh & Young, 1998; Wigfield et al., 1997). It is noteworthy that these domain-specific gender differences have emerged among samples from Taiwan and Japan, as well as the United States (Lummis & Stevenson, 1990).

Consistent with theorizing by Eccles and her colleagues, girls and boys come to develop nuanced beliefs about gender, and these beliefs are intimately tied to specific achievement domains. The developmental patterns of gender differences in competence beliefs within different domains are less clear. Although there is evidence to suggest that there are larger gender differences in competence beliefs among older children than younger children (Eccles, 1987a; Eccles, Adler, & Meece, 1984; Hyde, Fennema, Ryan, et al., 1990), most work has not examined the competence beliefs of the same group of individuals over a long enough span of time to determine the trajectory of gender differences across different ages.

However, a recent study provided a comprehensive analysis of gender differences in three different domains from childhood through adolescence (Jacobs, Lanza, Osgood, Eccles, & Wigfield, 2002). In this longitudinal study, participants reported their competence beliefs in math, language arts, and sports from first through 12th grades. The results indicated that the patterns of gender variations were specific to domain. In the domain of math, although in first grade boys' beliefs in their math competence was higher than those of girls, the difference disappeared in high school. The nature of this pattern, however, is revealing about competence beliefs in math more generally. Both girls' and boys' feelings of competence in math decreased through childhood and adolescence. However, because boys' competence beliefs decreased at a faster rate than those of girls, by late high school, girls' and boys' competence beliefs concerning math were the same. These results suggest that there might be more global social or contextual processes operating within schools and beyond that cause both genders' math competence beliefs to decrease (Eccles & Midgley, 1989; Eccles, Midgley, et al., 1993) and thereby converge over time. These effects are different from those reported in earlier work that revealed a larger gender difference in math competence in high school than in middle school (Eccles, 1994). Because the data collected from the cohort reported by Jacobs et al. (2002) were more recent than those reported by Eccles (1994), this narrowing gender difference from childhood through adolescence could be taken as a promising sign of social changes that promote greater gender equality. Consistent with this, meta-analyses of gender differences in math performance revealed larger gender differences among older studies than among more recent studies (Hyde, Fennema, & Lamon, 1990). Although this is promising, it is still worrisome that both boys' and girls' beliefs in their mathematics competence plummet through elementary and secondary school.

The pattern of results found by Jacobs et al. (2002) concerning competence in language arts tells a different story. Girls believe they are more competent in language arts than do boys, and this difference actually becomes more pronounced over time. In this domain, the widening gender gap occurred as a consequence of boys' accelerated decline in competence beliefs concerning language arts. As in the math domain, both genders evidenced a decline in competence beliefs in language arts, but boys' decline was more steep .

These results lend themselves to a discussion of the effects that varying levels of competence might have on later academic, extracurricular, and career choices. In the Jacobs et al. (2002) study, the researchers also assessed students' valuation of math and language arts, and found that beliefs about competence predicted the extent to which children valued the given domain. As a consequence, children's feelings of competence are likely to affect their interests and the activities that they pursue (Eccles, 1994; Eccles & Midgley, 1989; Eccles et al., 1984). This becomes increasingly important as children grow older, because course taking in high school and college becomes increasingly more driven by interests.

Before continuing, it is worth noting that the gender differences in *beliefs* about competence exceed any differences in actual achievement. For example, meta-analyses indicate that there is only a small gender difference in math performance favoring males, and that this becomes apparent only in late high school and college ($d = 0.32$; Hyde, Fennema, & Lamon, 1990). Similarly, a meta-analysis of studies on gender and verbal abilities revealed essentially no difference ($d = -0.11$; Hyde & Linn, 1988). The presence of gender differences in competence beliefs, especially given that there are virtually no differences in actual achievement, inspires curiosity concerning environmental influences that affect children's beliefs about competence. For a review of how parents affect children's beliefs about competence and their achievement behaviors, see Chapter 15, this volume.

Competence Beliefs and Stereotype Threat

Steele introduced the concept of stereotype threat to capture the ways in which stereotypes can have a deleterious impact on performance (Steele, 1997; Steele & Aronson,

1995). His original research dealt with ethnic stereotypes—specifically, the stereotype that African Americans are less intellectually competent than their white peers. When the researchers activated stereotype threat by telling participants that a test was diagnostic of intelligence, highly talented black students at Stanford performed worse than a control group that was told the test was not diagnostic of intelligence. White students' performance was unaffected by instructions about the test.

Later researchers tested whether stereotype threat applies to gender stereotypes, in particular, the stereotype that women are bad at math (Brown & Josephs, 1999; Quinn & Spencer, 2001; Spencer, Steele, & Quinn, 1999; Walsh, Hickey, & Duffy, 1999). In an experiment by Spencer et al. (1999, Study 2), male and female college students with equivalent mathematics backgrounds were tested. Half were told that the math test had shown gender differences in the past, and half were told that the test had been shown to be gender-fair, and that men and women had performed equally on it. Under stereotype threat conditions, women underperformed compared with men, whereas when gender fairness was assured, there were no gender differences in performance. This effect has been replicated a number of times (Brown & Josephs, 1999; Davies, Spencer, Quinn, & Gerhardstein, 2002; Spencer et al., 1999).

What mediates the effect of stereotype threat conditions on performance? Several possible mediators have been proposed, including self-evaluative anxiety (Spencer et al., 1999; Steele, 1997), dejected mood (Keller & Dauenheimer, 2003), and feelings of competence or self-efficacy (Spencer et al., 1999; Steele, 1997). Here, we focus on sense of competence. Spencer et al. (1999, Study 3) specifically tested whether sense of self-efficacy, measured by items such as "I am uncertain whether I have enough mathematical knowledge to do well on this test," mediated the experimental effects of stereotype threat on performance on a mathematics test. The results indicated that self-efficacy was not a significant mediator. However, this experiment (Spencer et al., 1999, Study 3) did not include a condition of explicit stereotype threat activation; it simply gave no information about the math test or instructed participants that there were no gender differences on the test. Therefore, the failure to find mediation effects for self-efficacy may have been a result of the absence of an experimental condition involving explicit stereotype threat activation. Clearly these questions should be pursued with additional research.

A developmental approach is useful in understanding the origins of these effects. Ambady, Shih, Kim, and Pittinsky (2001) found that gender stereotype threat effects on mathematics performance occurred among middle school girls, as they expected. Surprisingly, the same effect was found for lower elementary girls, but not for upper elementary girls. This particular study involved Asian American girls and also activated their ethnic identity in some conditions, which improved their performance. These results seem to derive from a complex interplay of gender and ethnic stereotype awareness. Perhaps most importantly, they indicate that the effects of gender stereotype threat appear early. Unfortunately, sense of competence in mathematics was not measured in this study.

The research on stereotype threat demonstrates that although mathematics performance, competence, and gender differences in competence are generally thought of as trait-like, one's sense of competence at a particular task can also be quite sensitive to situational cues or context. Thus, gender differences in feelings of competence may appear or disappear, depending on the task and contextual cues.

Expectations and Performance Feedback

The research on stereotype threat indicates that performance can be undermined when group status is salient and one's group is believed to be disadvantaged in that particular domain. This raises the possibility that, by undermining performance, stereotype threat can undermine feelings of competence. With this in mind, it is worth examining how individuals respond *after* they receive feedback about their performance within gender-stereotyped domains.

Limited research exists on the effects of performance feedback (either positive or negative) on females' and males' motivation within gender-typed domains. One notable study examined third graders' and junior high school students' achievement-related beliefs just before and a few days after taking a math exam (Stipek & Gralinski, 1991). Consistent with the work reviewed earlier, prior to the test, boys expected to do better on the exam than girls did. However, the focus of the study was students' reactions after they received their scores. Girls and boys attributed their success and failure to different sources. Girls who performed well on the test were less likely to attribute their success to high ability than were boys who performed similarly well. These girls did not reap the confidence-building benefits of success. Moreover, girls who performed poorly were more likely to attribute their failure to low ability and to want to hide their exam papers from others, compared with boys who performed similarly. These girls made more harsh attributions about their performance. Finally, the researchers found that girls' attributional patterns could ultimately lead them to avoid math activities. This study nicely illustrates the insidious nature of stereotypes within achievement domains. Performing in the domain is only the beginning of the process, and research attention should also focus on what happens after individuals find out how they performed. Receiving feedback and either altering or affirming one's personal beliefs about competence in a given domain are all part of the continuing process whereby individuals develop beliefs about their abilities.

The previous study involved a situation in which individuals received fairly objective feedback about their performance (i.e., scoring math tests relies very little on subjective judgments). However, interpreting feedback is more difficult when the criteria for evaluation are less clear, as might be the case in occupational and interpersonal contexts. Crocker and Major (1989) have examined the difficulty that individuals in stigmatized groups can have when interpreting evaluations from others who are aware of their group membership. Specifically, these researchers pointed out that when stigmatized individuals interpret feedback from others, there is ambiguity, because the feedback could be based on actual performance, or be tainted by information about group membership. For example, imagine a woman who works for a male supervisor in a primarily male engineering firm. Upon receiving her end-of-the-year evaluation, she might be cautious about how to interpret it. Specifically, if the evaluation is positive, she might wonder whether her evaluation is based on her true merit or influenced by the fact that she is a woman. For example, she might wonder whether her boss judged her by lower standards than those used for her male peers or was afraid of giving negative feedback because he was concerned that she might think he was sexist. Although attributional ambiguity can buffer the effects of negative feedback on self-esteem (Crocker & Major, 1989), this example illustrates how it can prevent stigmatized individuals from fully enjoying positive feedback (Crocker, Voelkl, Testa, & Major, 1991).

The research described earlier identifies some of the difficulties women encounter when performing in domains in which men are believed to perform better than women. There is surprisingly little research investigating how men behave when they perform in domains in which women are believed to perform better than men. For example, it is very possible that boys make different attributions for success and failure than girls on reading-related tasks. Perhaps boys in these situations are less likely to attribute success to high ability and more likely to attribute failure to low ability. Advancing research within domains believed to be both female- and male-typed will help us better understand the system that is set in motion when an individual performs in a domain where his or her group is believed to be disadvantaged.

GENDER AND ACHIEVEMENT MOTIVATION

History of Research on Gender and Achievement Motivation

McClelland's traditional method of measuring achievement motivation, developed in the 1950s, uses a projective technique in which people's stories in response to an ambiguous picture cue are scored for achievement imagery (McClelland, Atkinson, Clark, & Lowell, 1953). Most of the classic literature reviews concluded that there were gender differences in achievement motivation, with females showing a lower level of moti-

vation than males (Hoffman, 1972; Tyler, 1965). In the late 1960s and 1970s, these differences were thought to be important in explaining why women had not achieved as much as men in the realm of adult occupations. Theories were constructed to explain the developmental forces, such as socialization, that might lead girls to display less achievement motivation (Hoffman, 1972). It was also believed that females were motivated more by a need for affiliation than by a need for achievement (Hoffman, 1972).

In their watershed review, however, Maccoby and Jacklin (1974) challenged these views, concluding that there was little evidence for lower achievement motivation in females. Their conclusions are complicated by the variety of ways in which achievement motivation can be measured. In the neutral or relaxed condition for the McClelland et al. (1953) measure, females actually show higher achievement motivation than males. Under achievement arousal conditions, however, males' achievement motivation increases sharply, whereas females' does not.

A number of scholars criticized McClelland and Atkinson's classic theory of achievement motivation as applied to questions of gender (e.g., Spence & Helmreich, 1983). Stewart and Chester (1982) noted substantial flaws in the experimental methods used by McClelland and Atkinson to arouse achievement motivation. McClelland and Atkinson's theory specified that achievement motivation should increase under achievement arousal conditions—for example, when participants were told that the test measured capacity to act as a leader. Males' behavior was consistent with this prediction, whereas females' behavior was not, so McClelland and Atkinson excluded females from later empirical studies. Indeed, McClelland went so far as to say: "Clearly we need a differential psychology of motivation for men and women" (1966, p. 481), never questioning the adequacy of his own theory, but instead concluding that someone else would have to develop a theory to account for women's behavior.

In an effort to create new theory and methods, Spence and Helmreich (1983) developed a nonprojective, self-report measure of motivation that, additionally, expanded on the classic unidimensional view of achievement motivation to recognize multiple domains of achievement motivation. Their research uncovered three dimensions of achievement motivation: work, mastery, and competitiveness.

Also following on the research from the 1950s and 1960s indicating that females had a lower level of achievement motivation than did males, evidence suggests that women's achievement motivation has increased over time. Veroff, Depner, Kukla, and Douvan (1980) found that achievement motivation increased among American women from 1957 to 1976, and Jenkins (1987) found similar increases from 1967 to 1981. The most recent studies show no gender differences in achievement motivation (Mednick & Thomas, 1993).

What can account for these changes over time? It seems likely that the opening of educational opportunities and career options for women over the last three decades has increased achievement motivation for women as they gain experience in careers, and for girls as they anticipate jobs with exciting possibilities for achievement. Jenkins (1987) found that achievement motivation in female students who were college seniors in 1967 predicted their employment in achievement-oriented occupations 14 years later. Even more intriguing is the finding that women employed as college professors or as business entrepreneurs showed significant increases in their achievement motivation compared with their scores in college, whereas those in other occupations showed no change in achievement motivation (Jenkins, 1987).

Motive to Avoid Success

Seeking alternatives to traditional models of achievement motivation, Horner (1969) formulated the construct of a motive to avoid success, or fear of success, among bright, high-achieving women. In attempting to understand the gender differences in achievement that were present in the 1960s, Horner observed that achievement situations were more anxiety provoking for females than for males. To measure this phenomenon, Horner devised a projective test in which respondents completed a story that began "After first-term finals, Anne (John) finds herself (himself) at the top of her (his) medical school class." Women wrote about Anne and men, about John.

Men's stories in response to this cue generally indicated happiness and feelings of satisfaction over achievement. Women's responses, in contrast, were far more negative, indicating fears of social rejection, worries about maintaining womanhood, and denial of the reality of success. In Horner's sample from the University of Michigan, 65% of the women showed such negative responses, compared with 10% of the men.

Horner collected her original data in 1965 for her doctoral dissertation. The publication of the findings in 1969 attracted widespread attention from the popular media, and the *Psychology Today* article was required reading for students in many courses. The research was appealing, because it appeared at the time of the emergence of the women's movement and concern over women's equal opportunity. The research seemed to offer a believable explanation for why more women had not succeeded in high-status occupations—they simply feared success.

More than 30 years later, the research does not seem nearly as appealing. It has been criticized on a number of grounds (Mednick, 1989; Shaver, 1976; Tresemer, 1977; Zuckerman & Wheeler, 1975):

1. Other studies using Horner's techniques often found men displaying as much motive to avoid success as women. Therefore, there is no reason to believe that it is found only in women, or even that it is more frequent in women. If that is the case, it cannot be used to explain women's lesser occupational achievements.
2. Anne's success was in a field that, at the time, was stereotyped as male-oriented, namely, medical school. Therefore, the research might not indicate a generalized fear of success so much as a fear of being successful in a way that violates gender stereotypes. Indeed, when Anne was presented as successful in nursing school, women did not show anxiety about her success (Cherry & Deaux, 1978).
3. The research method confounded gender of stimulus person with gender of respondent; that is, women wrote about Anne, and men wrote about John. Perhaps

women are not anxious about their own success, but rather Anne's success stimulates anxiety, whether a woman or man writes about her and, in fact, one study showed exactly that (Monahan, Kuhn, & Shaver, 1974).

Today, research on motive to avoid success has virtually disappeared. Nonetheless, it provides an important object lesson on the popular appeal of attributing women's lesser achievements to internalized, intrapsychic factors and how, ultimately, such factors were unsuccessful in accounting for the striking gender differences in occupational achievement that characterized the 1950s and 1960s. As we search for productive research approaches for the future, models that assume widespread intrapsychic deficits in women are unlikely to be productive. The models reviewed next show far more promise.

Gender and Achievement Goal Theory

Achievement goals are cognitive representations that define individuals' desired outcomes concerning competence (Ames, 1992; Dweck, 1986; Nicholls, 1989; see other chapters in this volume for discussions of achievement goal theory). As such, achievement goals orient individuals toward competence and help organize behavior in order to attain competence. Although very little research has been done to examine relationships between gender and achievement goals (Pintrich & Schunk, 2002), two primary questions are of interest. The first concerns whether there are gender differences in the extent to which women and men adopt achievement goals for themselves. The second question concerns whether the processes initiated by the adoption of achievement goals differ depending on gender. Overall, the answers to these questions appear to be somewhat mixed, although most studies do not find large gender differences of either kind.

Several authors have noted the paucity of research on gender and achievement goals (e.g., Pintrich & Schunk, 2002). To begin to remedy this situation, we undertook a brief review of studies in which gender was included in analyses of mastery and performance–approach achievement goals, al-

though gender was rarely the focus of these studies. Our review indicated that many studies reveal no gender differences in self-set mastery and performance–approach achievement goals (e.g., Barron & Harackiewicz, 2001; Fukada, Fukada, & Hicks, 1993; Gernigon & Le Bars, 2000; Pajares, Britner, & Valiante, 2000; Sachs, 2001). However, some studies do report gender differences; in these studies, the general pattern was that females reported adopting higher levels of goals than males, and often higher levels of mastery goals in particular (e.g., Bouffard, Boisvert, Vezeau, & Larouche, 1995; Elliot & Church, 1997; Harackiewicz, Barron, Carter, Lehto, & Elliot, 1997; Nolen, 1988; Pajares et al., 2000; Wentzel, 1993). In order to try to make sense of this mixed set of results, we reexamined these studies to determine whether there was a pattern in the types of studies that revealed differences versus similarities across gender. Specifically, given the data reported earlier suggesting that task domain is a crucial determinant of competence beliefs for females and males, we examined whether the presence or absence of observed gender differences in achievement goals systematically differed by domain.

Overall, this analysis revealed some general patterns. Of the studies indicating that women adopted higher levels of mastery goals than men, two were in psychology (Elliot & Church, 1997; Harackiewicz et al., 1997), one was in language arts (Pajares et al., 2000), one was in science (Nolen, 1988), and two were in academics in general (Bouffard et al., 1995; Wentzel, 1993). In contrast, the domains in which women and men did not show differences in adopted mastery goals seemed to be more stereotypically masculine: one in math (Barron & Harackiewicz, 2001), one in science (Pajares et al., 2000), one in educational research (Sachs, 2001), and two in athletics (Fukada et al., 1993; Gernigon & Le Bars, 2000).

Only four studies revealed gender differences in performance goals. The studies reporting that women adopted higher levels of performance goals than men were in academics generally (Bouffard et al., 1995; Wentzel, 1993), and in psychology (Harackiewicz et al., 1997). Only one of the studies indicated that men adopted higher levels of performance goals than women, and this was a study of math (Middleton & Midgley, 1997).

Given the apparent domain specificity, suggesting that individuals are more likely to set approach achievement goals in domains where their gender is favored, a fascinating question is whether an inverse pattern would be observed for the adoption of avoidance goals. Performance–avoidance goals are focused on *not* performing poorly relative to others. Specifically, individuals might be more likely to adopt avoidance achievement goals in domains in which their gender is believed to be disadvantaged. Imagine two high school calculus students, Jennifer and Sam. Most likely, both Sam and Jennifer will focus on performing well and achieving success on an upcoming examination. However, if Jennifer is concerned about confirming the stereotype that girls do not perform as well as boys in calculus, then she might also adopt a performance–avoidance goal not to do poorly relative to the boys in the class. This possibility is bolstered by data suggesting that competence beliefs are inversely related to the adoption of avoidance goals (Elliot & Church, 1997). If girls believe they are not as good at math as boys, then girls will be more likely to adopt performance–avoidance goals. Moreover, performance–avoidance goals are associated with a host of negative outcomes, including lower interest and lower performance (Elliot & Church, 1997). This is especially interesting in light of the earlier discussion on the undermining effects of stereotype threat on performance. As more research on avoidance goals accumulates, it will be interesting to determine whether members of the gender that is believed to be disadvantaged in a given domain are more likely to adopt performance–avoidance goals in those contexts.

Finally, few gender differences are evident when considering whether gender moderates the effects of goals on other outcomes. For example, in laboratory studies in which goals are experimentally manipulated, the effects of these goals are typically not found to differ by gender (e.g., Barron & Harackiewicz, 2001; Elliot & Harackiewicz, 1994). However, there is some evidence to suggest that the motivational benefits of adopting performance–approach goals are stronger for males than for females (e.g., Bouffard et al., 1995; Linnenbrink, Ryan, &

Pintrich, 2000). In general, there is little consensus on what processes related to achievement goals differ by gender. There is much to be gained from research in the area—both identifying consistent patterns (either patterns of gender similarity or difference) and understanding why those patterns emerge.

Overall, there is much more work to be done in this area to synthesize results across studies, identify meaningful patterns, and gain a better understanding of when gender differences do and do not emerge, but the trends indicate that gender differences in achievement goals depend on domain and are generally consistent with gender stereotypes about competence in domains such as mathematics, athletics, and psychology.

CULTURE AND ETHNICITY

A thorough understanding of gender, competence, and motivation should involve a consideration of the cultural contexts in which gendered beliefs develop and change over time. This includes a consideration of how variations across ethnicity and cultures affect gender roles and beliefs about gender and competence, and how achievement is demonstrated by and expected from each gender. The issues surrounding culture and ethnicity, as they relate to competence and motivation, are addressed in other chapters of this volume (see Chapters 22–26), and as research accumulates, it will be possible to understand better how gender intersects with various social and cultural factors. Here, we review two empirical examples of how gender and cultural norms can affect competence behaviors and beliefs.

One facet of culture concerns the extent to which social roles are divided by gender. As a consequence, we might expect larger gender differences in motivation and achievement among groups that adhere to more rigid gender roles. However, layered on top of traditional roles is a more dynamic process, in which some cultures are becoming more egalitarian in terms of gender. Cialdini, Wosinska, Dabul, Whetstone-Dion, and Heszen (1998) proposed a process by which individuals from cultures that have seen social movements toward gender equality might reject their traditional roles and respond in nontraditional ways. The cultural norm examined in this study involved the traditional expectation that women be modest about their achievements and successes. Cialdini et al. argued that American women, compared with Polish women, would respond in a way counter to the traditional female role (less modestly) when gender roles were made salient, because the women's movement in the United States would cause American women to want to reject their traditional role. Consistent with hypotheses, American women evidenced more reduced modesty about their achievements when traditional gender roles were salient than when they were not salient. In contrast, gender role salience did not affect the reports of modesty made by American men, or Polish men and women.

These results are intriguing not only because American women were likely to display less modesty in their achievements but also because this process might predict that individuals would reject traditional gender roles in other ways as well. For example, some women might come to care about doing well in math in order to reject rather than conform to traditional gender roles. Moreover, although these data on role rejection might seem contradictory to the research on stereotype threat reviewed earlier, they might actually be parts of the same process. Accordingly, wanting very much to reject the stereotype about one's group might exacerbate performance problems.

A few studies have examined the intersection of race and gender within the context of stereotype threat. For example, Asian American women are in a particularly interesting situation when it comes to the domain of mathematics: They are stereotyped to be skilled at math because they are Asian, and unskilled at math because they are female. Pursuing this phenomenon, Shih, Pittinsky, and Ambady (1999) found that the aspect of identity that was activated (either Asian or female) predicted whether Asian American women evidenced performance decrements or enhancements under stereotype threat conditions. When their ethnic identity was primed, they evidenced performance enhancements. In contrast, they showed performance decrements when their gender was salient.

Similarly, because women are stereotyped to be less competent in math than men, and Latinos are stereotyped to be less competent at math than whites, Latina women are double-stereotyped to be unskilled at math. One study has examined whether performance decrements due to stereotype threat are additive in this sense (Gonzales, Blanton, & Williams, 2002). In this study, white and Latino men and women were randomly assigned to perform a math task either under stereotype threat conditions or not. Whereas white men evidenced performance enhancement under stereotype threat conditions, white women and Latino men evidenced some performance decrements, and Latina women evidenced the greatest performance decrements. Importantly, all participants scored similarly when the task was not performed under stereotype threat conditions. These data suggest that the effects of both gender and ethnic stereotype threat can accumulate and have an additive effect on performance.

SUMMARY AND CONCLUSIONS

Rapid advances over the past 30 years in women's educational and occupational achievements have been paralleled by advances in theory and research on gender, competence beliefs, and motivation. Eccles's expectancy–value theory and Bussey and Bandura's (1999) social cognitive theory provide similar—although not identical—accounts of how gender differences in competence beliefs might be created. Both theories allow for the conceptualization of self-efficacy as domain-specific rather than general. Both highlight the importance of input from significant socializers, such as parents, teachers, and peers, and from the culture more broadly (in the form of gender stereotypes and gender segregation of adult occupations) in shaping competence beliefs.

We view competence beliefs as the result of developmental processes. In both mathematics and language arts, patterns of gender differences in self-efficacy shift from early elementary school through high school. Maccoby (1998) highlighted the importance of gender segregation in childhood in creating gender differences in behavior and competence beliefs. Stereotype threat may affect competence beliefs both acutely, in a particular situation, and chronically, as many experiences of stereotype threat accumulate for the developing child. These effects may be particularly relevant to issues of girls and mathematics achievement.

In the realm of achievement motivation, research and theory have shifted rapidly from the 1950s, when girls and women were believed to be low in achievement motivation and were excluded from much research, to the 1980s, when gender similarities seemed to be the rule for achievement motivation. The construct of motive to avoid success emerged in 1969 as a complement to the classic research on achievement motivation, but researchers uncovered many problems with the construct, and it has largely faded from contemporary research. Achievement goal theory is now the dominant approach; research based on this model often fails to detect gender differences in achievement goals. When gender differences are detected, they tend to fall along stereotypical lines, for example, with women adopting higher mastery achievement goals than men in areas such as psychology and language arts.

We have noted the importance of considering the intersection of gender and ethnicity when studying competence, achievement motivation, and stereotype threat. Gender and ethnicity may in some cases create a double-dose of stereotype threat that attacks competence beliefs, as in the case of Latinas and mathematics. In other cases, gender and ethnic effects may act in opposite directions, as in the case of Asian American women and mathematics. Only by studying gender and ethnicity simultaneously will we be able to understand the complexity of these influences.

For the most part, gender differences in self-efficacy and in achievement goals are small and domain-specific. Gender similarities may prove to be the rule. Our belief is that, rather than studying main effects of gender, researchers should consider gender interactions. For example, are performance goals more beneficial for men than for women? Do some categories of women and other categories of men respond to achievement challenges with enhanced competence beliefs? These more complex approaches will be necessary for research to advance.

REFERENCES

Ambady, N., Shih, M., Kim, A., & Pittinsky, T. L. (2001). Stereotype susceptibility in children: Effects of identity activation on quantitative performance. *Psychological Science, 12,* 385–390.

Ames, C. (1992). Classrooms: Goals, structures, and student motivation. *Journal of Educational Psychology, 84,* 261–271.

Bandura, A. (1986). *Social foundations of thought and action: A social cognitive theory.* Englewood Cliffs, NJ: Prentice-Hall.

Barron, K. E., & Harackiewicz, J. M. (2001). Achievement goals and optimal motivation: Testing multiple goal models. *Journal of Personality and Social Psychology, 80,* 706–722.

Betz, N. E., & Hackett, G. (1981). The relationship of career-related self-efficacy expectations to perceived career options in college women and men. *Journal of Counseling Psychology, 28,* 399–410.

Betz, N. E., & Hackett, G. (1983). The relationship of mathematics self-efficacy expectations to the selection of science-based college majors. *Journal of Vocational Behavior, 23,* 329–345.

Bouffard, T., Boisvert, J., Vezeau, C., & Larouche, C. (1995). The impact of goal orientation on self-regulation and performance among college students. *British Journal of Educational Psychology, 65,* 317–329.

Brown, R. P., & Josephs, R. A. (1999). A burden of proof: Stereotype relevance and gender differences in math performance. *Journal of Personality and Social Psychology, 76,* 246–257.

Bussey, K., & Bandura, A. (1999). Social cognitive theory of gender development and differentiation. *Psychological Review, 106,* 676–713.

Cherry, F., & Deaux, K. (1978). Fear of success versus fear of gender-inappropriate behavior. *Sex Roles, 4,* 97–102.

Cialdini, R. B., Wosinska, W., Dabul, A. J., Whetstone-Dion, R., & Heszen, I. (1998). When social role salience leads to social role rejection: Modest self-presentation among women and men in two cultures. *Personality and Social Psychology Bulletin, 24,* 473–481.

Cole, D. A., Maxwell, S. E., Martin, J. M., Peeke, L. G., Serocynski, A. D. Tram, J. M., et al. (2001). The development of multiple domains of child and adolescent self-concept: A cohort sequential longitudinal design. *Child Development, 72,* 1723–1746.

Costello, C. B., & Stone, A. J. (Eds.). (2001). *The American woman 2001–2002: Getting to the top.* New York: Norton.

Crain, R. M. (1996). The influence of age, race, and gender on child and adolescent multidimensional self-concept. In B. A. Bracken (Ed.), *Handbook of self-concept: Developmental, social, and clinical considerations* (pp. 240–280). New York: Oxford University Press.

Crocker, J., & Major, B. (1989). Social stigma and self-esteem: The self-protective properties of stigma. *Psychological Review, 96*, 608–630.

Crocker, J., Voelkl, K., Testa, M., & Major, B. (1991). Social stigma: The affective consequences of attributional ambiguity. *Journal of Personality and Social Psychology, 60*, 218–228.

Davies, P. G., Spencer, S. J., Quinn, D. M., & Gerhardstein, R. (2002). Consuming images: How television commercials that elicit stereotype threat can restrain women academically and professionally. *Personality and Social Psychology Bulletin, 28*, 1615–1628.

Deaux, K., & Major, B. (1987). Putting gender into context: An interactive model of gender-related behavior. *Psychological Review, 94*, 369–389.

Debacker, T. K., & Nelson, R. M. (2000). Motivation to learn science: Differences related to gender, class type, and ability. *Journal of Educational Research, 93*, 245–254.

DeZolt, D., & Hull, S. (2001). Classroom and school climate. In J. Worell (Ed.), *Encyclopedia of gender* (pp. 246–264). San Diego: Academic Press.

Dweck, C. S. (1986). Motivational processes affecting learning. *American Psychologist, 41*, 1040–1048.

Dweck, C. S., Goetz, T., & Strauss, N. L. (1980). Sex differences in learned helplessness: IV. An experimental and naturalistic study of failure generalization and its mediators. *Journal of Personality and Social Psychology, 38*, 441–452.

Eagly, A. H., & Steffen, V. J. (1986). Gender and aggressive behavior: A meta-analytic review. *Psychological Bulletin, 100*, 309–330.

Eccles, J. S. (1987a). Gender roles and women's achievement-related decisions. *Psychology of Women Quarterly, 11*, 135–172.

Eccles, J. S. (1987b). Gender roles and achievement patterns: An expectancy value perspective. In J. M. Reinisch, L. A. Rosenblum, & S. A. Sanders (Eds.), *Masculinity/femininity: Basic perspectives* (pp. 240–280). New York: Oxford University Press.

Eccles, J. S. (1994). Understanding women's educational and occupational choices: Applying the Eccles et al. model of achievement-related choices. *Psychology of Women Quarterly, 18*, 585–610.

Eccles (formerly Parsons), J. S., Adler, T., & Meece, J. L. (1984). Sex differences in achievement: A test of alternate theories. *Journal of Personality and Social Psychology, 46*, 26–43.

Eccles, J., & Midgley, C. (1989). Stage/environment fit: Developmentally appropriate classrooms for young adolescents. In R. E. Ames & C. Ames (Eds.), *Research on motivation and education* (Vol. 3, pp. 139–186). New York: Academic Press.

Eccles, J. S., Midgley, C., Wigfield, A., Buchanan, C. M., Reuman, D., Flannagan, C., et al. (1993). Development during adolescence: The impact of stage–environment fit on young adolescents' experiences in schools and families. *American Psychologist, 48*, 90–101.

Eccles, J. S., Wigfield, A., Harold, R. D., & Blumenfeld, P. (1993). Ontogeny of children's self-perceptions and subjective task values across activity domains during the early elementary school years. *Child Development, 64*, 830–847.

Elliot, A. J., & Church, M. A. (1997). A hierarchical model of approach and avoidance achievement motivation. *Journal of Personality and Social Psychology, 72*, 218–232.

Elliot, A. J., & Harackiewicz, J. M. (1994). Goal setting, achievement orientation, and intrinsic motivation: A mediational analysis. *Journal of Personality and Social Psychology, 66*, 968–980.

Fredricks, J. A., & Eccles, J. S. (2002). Children's competence and value beliefs from childhood through adolescence: Growth trajectories in two male-sex-typed domains. *Developmental Psychology, 38*, 519–533.

Fukada, H., Fukada, S., & Hicks, J. (1993). Stereotypical attitudes toward gender-based grade-level assignment of Japanese elementary school teachers. *Journal of Psychology, 127*, 345–351.

Gernigon, C., & Le Bars, H. (2000). Achievement goals in aikido and judo: A study among beginner and experienced practitioners. *Journal of Applied Sport Psychology, 12*, 168–179.

Golombok, S., & Fivush, R. (1994). *Gender development.* New York: Cambridge University Press.

Gonzalez, P. M., Blanton, H., & Williams, K. (2002). The effects of stereotype threat and double-minority status on the test performance of Latino women. *Personality and Social Psychology Bulletin, 28*, 659–670.

Grady, K. E. (1979). Androgyny reconsidered. In J. H. Williams (Ed.), *Psychology of women: Selected readings* (pp. 172–177). New York: Norton.

Harackiewicz, J. M., Barron, K. E., Carter, S. M., Lehto, A. T., & Elliot, A. J. (1997). Predictors and consequences of achievement goals in the college classroom: Maintaining interest and making the grade. *Journal of Personality and Social Psychology, 73*, 1284–1295.

Hoffman, L. W. (1972). Early childhood experiences and women's achievement motives. *Journal of Social Issues, 28*(2), 129–155.

Horner, M. S. (1969). Fail: Bright women. *Psychology Today, 3*(6), 36.

Hyde, J. S. (1984). How large are gender differences in aggression?: A developmental meta-analysis. *Developmental Psychology, 20*, 697–706.

Hyde, J. S., Fennema, E., & Lamon, S. J. (1990). Gender differences in mathematics performance: A meta-analysis. *Psychological Bulletin, 107*, 139–155.

Hyde, J. S., Fennema, E., Ryan, M., Frost, L. A., & Hopp, C. (1990). Gender comparisons of mathematics attitudes and affect: A meta-analysis. *Psychology of Women Quarterly, 14*, 299–324.

Hyde, J. S., & Linn, M. C. (1988). Gender differences in verbal ability: A meta-analysis. *Psychological Bulletin, 104*, 53–69.

Hyde, J. S., & Plant, E. A. (1995). Magnitude of psychological gender differences: Another side to the story. *American Psychologist, 50,* 159–161.

Jacobs, J. E., Finken, L. L., Griffin, N. L., & Wright, J. D. (1998). The career plans of science-talented rural adolescent girls. *American Educational Research Journal, 35,* 681–704.

Jacobs, J. E., Lanza, S., Osgood, D. W., Eccles, J. S., & Wigfield, A. (2002). Changes in children's self-competence and values: Gender and domain differences across grades one through twelve. *Child Development, 73,* 509–527.

Jambunathan, S., & Hurlbut, N. L. (2000). Gender comparisons in the perception of self-competence among four-year-old children. *Journal of Genetic Psychology, 161,* 469–477.

Jenkins, S. R. (1987). Need for achievement and women's careers over 14 years: Evidence for occupational structure effects. *Journal of Personality and Social Psychology, 53,* 922–932.

Keller, J., & Dauenheimer, D. (2003). Stereotype threat in the classroom: Dejection mediates the disrupting threat effect on women's math performance. *Personality and Social Psychology Bulletin, 29,* 371–381.

Kling, K. C., Hyde, J. S., Showers, C. J., & Buswell, B. N. (1999). Gender differences in self-esteem: A meta-analysis. *Psychological Bulletin, 125,* 470–500.

Linnenbrink, E., Ryan, A., & Pintrich, P. R. (2000). The role of goals and affect in working memory functioning. *Learning and Individual Differences, 11,* 213–230.

Lummis, M., & Stevenson, H. W. (1990). Gender differences in beliefs and achievement: A cross-cultural study. *Developmental Psychology, 26,* 254–263.

Lytton, H., & Romney, D. M. (1991). Parents' differential socialization of boys and girls: A meta-analysis. *Psychological Bulletin, 109,* 267–296.

Maccoby, E. E. (1990). Gender and relationships: A developmental account. *American Psychologist, 45,* 513–520.

Maccoby, E. E. (1998). *The two sexes: Growing up apart, coming together.* Cambridge, MA: Harvard University Press.

Maccoby, E. E., & Jacklin, C. N. (1974). *The psychology of sex differences.* Stanford, CA: Stanford University Press.

Malpass, J. R., O'Neil, H. F., Jr., & Hocevar, D. (1999). Self-regulation, goal orientation, self-efficacy, worry and high stakes math achievement for mathematically gifted high school students. *Roeper Review, 21,* 281–288.

Marsh, H. W., & Young, A. S. (1998). Longitudinal structural equation models of academic self-concept and achievement: Gender differences in the development of math and English constructs. *American Educational Research Journal, 35,* 705–738.

McClelland, D. C. (1966). Longitudinal trends in the relation of thought to action. *Journal of Consulting Psychology, 30,* 479–483.

McClelland, D. C., Atkinson, J. W., Clark, R. A., & Lowell, F. L. (1953). *The achievement motive.* New York: Appleton–Century–Crofts.

Mednick, M. T. (1989). On the politics of psychological constructs: Stop the bandwagon, I want to get off. *American Psychologist, 44,* 1118–1123.

Mednick, M. T., & Thomas, V. G. (1993). Women and the psychology of achievement: A view from the eighties. In F. L. Denmark & M. A. Paludi (Eds.), *Psychology of women: A handbook of issues and theories* (pp. 585–626). Westport, CT: Greenwood.

Meece, J. L., Eccles-Parsons, J., Kaczala, C. M., Goff, S. B., & Futterman, R. (1982). Sex differences in math achievement: Toward a model of academic choice. *Psychological Bulletin, 91,* 324–348.

Middleton, M. J., & Midgley, C. (1997). Avoiding the demonstration of lack of ability: An underexplored aspect of goal theory. *Journal of Educational Psychology, 89,* 710–718.

Monahan, L., Kuhn, D., & Shaver, P. (1974). Intrapsychic versus cultural explanations of the "fear of success" motive. *Journal of Personality and Social Psychology, 29,* 60–64.

Nicholls, J. G. (1989). *The competitive ethos and democratic education.* Cambridge, MA: Harvard University Press.

Nolen, S. B. (1988). Reasons for studying: Motivation orientations and study strategies. *Cognition and Instruction, 5,* 269–287.

Oliver, M. B., & Hyde, J. S. (1993). Gender differences in sexuality: A meta-analysis. *Psychological Bulletin, 114,* 29–51.

Pajares, F., Britner, S. L., & Valiante, G. (2000). Relation between achievement goals and self-beliefs of middle school students in writing and science. *Contemporary Educational Psychology, 25,* 406–422.

Pajares, F., & Miller, M. D. (1994). Role of self-efficacy and self-concept beliefs in mathematical problem solving: A path analysis. *Journal of Educational Psychology, 86,* 193–203.

Pintrich, P. R., & Schunk, D. H. (2002). *Motivation in education: Theory, research and applications.* Englewood Cliffs, NJ: Merrill/Prentice-Hall.

Pomerantz, E. M., & Ruble, D. N. (1998). The role of maternal control in the development of sex differences in child self-evaluative factors. *Child Development, 69,* 458–478.

Quinn, D. M., & Spencer, S. J. (2001). The interference of stereotype threat with women's generation of mathematical problem-solving strategies. *Journal of Social Issues, 57,* 55–72.

Rix, S. E. (Ed.). (1988). *The American woman 1988–89.* New York: Norton.

Sachs, J. (2001). A path model for adult learner feedback. *Educational Psychology, 21,* 267–275.

Schunk, D. H., & Lilly, M. W. (1984). Sex differences in self-efficacy and attributions: Influence of performance feedback. *Journal of Early Adolescence, 4,* 203–213.

Shaver, P. (1976). Questions concerning fear of success and its conceptual relatives. *Sex Roles*, 2, 305–320.

Shih, M., Pittinsky, T. L., & Ambady, N. (1999). Stereotype susceptibility: Identity salience and shifts in quantitative performance. *Psychological Science*, 10, 80–83.

Spence, J. T., & Helmreich, R. L. (1983). Achievement-related motives and behaviors. In J. T. Spence (Ed.), *Achievement and achievement motives: Psychological and sociological approaches* (pp. 7–74). San Francisco: Freeman.

Spencer, S. J., Steele, C. M., & Quinn, D. M. (1999). Stereotype threat and women's math performance. *Journal of Experimental Social Psychology*, 35, 4–28.

Steele, C. C. M. (1997). A threat in the air: How stereotypes shape intellectual identity and performance. *American Psychologist*, 52, 613–629.

Steele, C. M., & Aronson, J. (1995). Stereotype threat and the intellectual test performance of African Americans. *Journal of Personality and Social Psychology*, 69, 797–811.

Stetsenko, A., Little, T. D., Gordeeva, T., Granshof, M., & Oettingen, G. (2000). Gender effects in children's beliefs about school performance: A cross-cultural study. *Child Development*, 71, 517–527.

Stewart, A. J., & Chester, N. L. (1982). The exploration of sex differences in human social motives: Achievement, affiliation, and power. In A. J. Stewart (Ed.), *Motivation and society* (pp. 172–218). San Francisco: Jossey-Bass.

Stipek, D. J., & Gralinski, J. H. (1991). Gender differences in children's achievement-related beliefs and emotional responses to success and failure in mathematics. *Journal of Educational Psychology*, 83, 361–371.

Swim, J., Borgida, E., Maruyama, G., & Myers, D. G. (1989). Joan McKay versus John McKay: Do gender stereotypes bias evaluations? *Psychological Bulletin*, 105, 409–429.

Tresemer, D. (1977). *Fear of success*. New York: Plenum Press.

Tyler, L. E. (1965). *The psychology of human differences*. New York: Appleton–Century–Crofts.

Veroff, J., Depner, C., Kukla, R., & Douvan, E. (1980). Comparison of American motives: 1957 versus 1976. *Journal of Personality and Social Psychology*, 39, 1004–1013.

Walsh, M., Hickey, C., & Duffy, J. (1999). Influence of item content and stereotype situation on gender differences in mathematical problem solving. *Sex Roles*, 41, 219–240.

Wentzel, K. R. (1993). Motivation and achievement in early adolescence: The role of multiple classroom goals. *Journal of Early Adolescence*, 13, 4–20.

Wigfield, A., Eccles, J. S., Yoon, K. S., Harold, R. D., Arbreton, A. J. A., Freedman-Doan, C., et al. (1997). Change in children's competence beliefs and subjective task values across the elementary school years: A 3-year study. *Journal of Educational Psychology*, 89, 451–469.

Yee, D. K., & Eccles, J. S. (1988). Parent perceptions and attributions for children's math achievement. *Sex Roles*, 19, 317–333.

Zuckerman, M., & Wheeler, L. (1975). To dispel fantasies about the fantasy-based measure of fear of success. *Psychological Bulletin*, 82, 932–946.

CHAPTER 22

ℭ℞

Race and Ethnicity in the Study of Motivation and Competence

SANDRA GRAHAM
CYNTHIA HUDLEY

About 10 years ago, one of us wrote a review on motivational processes in African Americans (Graham, 1994). That article summarized what was known at the time about five motivational constructs that had been studied in African American participants. Because those constructs are pertinent to the theme of this volume on motivation and competence, one strategy for organizing our chapter on race and ethnicity might be to take the Graham review as a starting point. For example, we could update what has been documented since 1994 on attributions, expectancies, and self-perceived competence in African Americans and other ethnic groups. We could expand our analysis by synthesizing current research on other contemporary motivation constructs represented in this *Handbook*—such as achievement goals, values, and efficacy beliefs—that were not well studied in ethnic minority groups at the time of the Graham review.

We have chosen not to take this approach to writing our chapter for two reasons. The first reason is a fairly practical one. There simply is not enough of a contemporary empirical literature with ethnic populations on any of the motivation constructs that now dominate the field. It is not that researchers have failed to consider the thoughts and feelings that energize or impede achievement strivings among ethnic groups in this country; but that work has not been situated within the literatures on motivation and competence.

Our second reason is more conceptual. The Graham review was guided by an intrapersonal view of motivation (individual needs, self-directed thoughts and feelings), with little attention to the larger context in which achievement strivings unfold. The review started with person-oriented theories of motivation about, for example, causal attributions or personal control, and then examined whether or not hypotheses derived from those theories were supported in African Americans. We now recognize the limitations of that approach. The significance of race and ethnicity for understanding motivation and competence requires that we cast a broader net and begin with factors that are unique to the everyday lives of people of color. Some of those factors are historical and structural in nature. Many racial and ethnic minority groups in contemporary America are positioned at the bottom of a status hierarchy wherein barriers to opportunity often override personal strivings for achievement. In an influential conceptual analysis, Garcia-Coll and colleagues (1996) identified experiences with racism and discrimination as meaningful macro-system variables that compromise the outcomes of children of color. Following their lead, we therefore begin our chapter with a discussion of perceived discrimination and coping with racial and ethnic stereotypes as structural variables that influence achievement strivings and the quest for competence among persons of color.

Members of racial and ethnic groups have proven to be remarkably resilient in the face of structural barriers such as those to be considered in the first two parts of this chapter. One important psychological variable that may contribute to that resilience is racial or ethnic identity, defined as one's attitudes and feelings about membership in his or her group (see Phinney, 1996). In the third part of this chapter, we examine research on racial/ethnic identity, with a particular focus on how that literature sheds light on motivation and competence in minority group members. The psychological meaning of race and ethnicity in the United States has been reshaped by the driving forces of immigration, and in the fourth section of our chapter, we consider how achievement strivings might be influenced by immigrant history and generational status. The four main topics reviewed—reactions to discrimination, coping with stereotypes, racial and ethnic identity, and the immigration experience—encompass vast literatures that have been just as much the intellectual terrain of sociologists and anthropologists as of psychologists. Therefore, we cannot do them justice in the context of this chapter. Rather, our goal is to use our knowledge of the topics as a framework for discussing the unique challenges of racial and ethnic groups as they strive for mastery and competence.

We use the terms "race" and "ethnicity" throughout the chapter, so we want to be clear about how we define those terms. In theory, "race" is an ascribed category, with a race being a group of persons with shared genetic, biological, and physical features. Using that definition, we think of blacks, whites, and Asians as different races, and we refer to them as such in this chapter. However, we also realize that race is more socially constructed than biologically determined, in that the meaning of racial group membership changes across time and context, and that the variability within racial groups far exceeds that between groups (Yee, Fairchild, Weizmann, & Wyatt, 1993). "Ethnicity," on the other hand, has been defined as a category, either ascribed or voluntary, that reflects a group's common history, nationality or geography, language, and culture. For example, Black Haitian immigrants and African Americans are different in many significant ways despite sharing a common racial designation, and the construct of ethnicity allows us to capture many of those differences. Some advocate consolidating the two terms into a single identifier for the sake of clarity (Phinney, 1996). Others argue that such an approach obscures important differences between theoretically distinct constructs (Helms & Talleyrand, 1997). We take the position that the two constructs are distinct but not mutually exclusive, consistent with what sociologists refer to as the *new ethnicity* approach (Cornell & Hartmann, 1998). Thus we frequently use the two terms in tandem in this chapter. However, when describing distinct research literatures (e.g., racial identity development vs. ethnic identity development) we use the specific term most appropriate to that literature.

REACTIONS TO DISCRIMINATION

One of the major challenges faced by racial and ethnic minority groups in the United States is the experience of discrimination. By "discrimination," we mean negative or harmful behavior toward persons because of their membership in a particular group (see

Jones, 1997). We also focus on personal experiences or the *perception* of harmful treatment because of one's racial or ethnic group membership rather than actual (documented) group discrimination in the legal sense.

Despite the economic, political, and social gains of the second half of the last century among people of color, experiences with racial discrimination continue to be quite prevalent in contemporary America. Survey data reveal that at least two-thirds of African Americans report that they have been discriminated against in the last year (e.g., Broman, Mavaddat, & Hsu, 2000; Kessler, Mickelson, & Williams, 1999). Even children as young as age 10 have reported race-based mistreatment, especially in schools and public places (Simons et al., 2002), and middle-class samples are just as likely to be targets of racial discrimination as their economically disadvantaged counterparts (Cose, 1993; Feagin, 1991).

Perceived discrimination can occur in almost any arena. It can be blatant, intended, and obvious; or subtle, unintended, and not easy to detect. Some researchers have used the term "microaggressions" to capture a particularly subtle but pernicious kind of degradation that many people of color encounter on an almost daily basis (Pierce, 1995). Examples of microaggressions include being ignored or overlooked while waiting in line, being suspected of cheating because one received a good grade on a test, being followed or observed while in public places, or being mistaken for someone who serves others (Harrell, 2000; Solorzano, 2000). One of us (S. G.) is reminded of a particularly painful example of microaggression that her husband (an African American) encountered during his first year of medical school. Beginning his first clinical rotation, the aspiring young physician entered the university hospital, dressed in a white medical coat, shirt and tie, and with a stethoscope around his neck. As he rushed down the corridor on the way to Grand Rounds, a patient raised her hand, caught his attention, and signaled him to come to her room, by calling, "Oh, waiter, I'm ready for my tray." On the face of it, one such experience may seem fairly benign. But cumulative microaggressions can surely take their toll on mental health.

Consequences of Discrimination for Motivation and Competence

Many of the negative consequences of discrimination have implications for motivation and competence. People who perceive themselves to be chronic targets of others' mistreatment often lose confidence in themselves and in their ability to be self-efficacious. Because coping with discrimination is recognized as a major stressor for ethnic minorities, it also has been linked to a number of physical health problems associated with stress, including hypertension, decreased immune functioning, and heart disease (Clark, Anderson, Clark, & Williams, 1999). And because discrimination often takes the form of social exclusion, it can threaten one of the most fundamental human motives—the need to belong (Baumeister & Leary, 1995). Many studies have documented that even mild forms of laboratory-induced social exclusion can lead to both distressed affect and depletion of the cognitive resources needed to function productively (e.g., Baumeister, Twenge, & Nuss, 2002; Eisenberger, Lieberman, & Williams, 2003).

Most of the research on the mental and physical health consequences of discrimination has been conducted with adults, but there is a growing literature on the correlates of perceived race-based maltreatment among adolescents. Among the most prevalent kinds of unfair treatment reported by ethnic minority youth is that which takes place in school settings. Receiving a lower grade than deserved or being the recipient of unusually harsh discipline are common experiences of mistreatment in school reported by youth of color (Fisher, Wallace, & Fenton, 2000). Such experiences have been linked to more depression among early adolescents of color (Simons et al., 2002), drug use (Gibbons, Gerrard, Cleveland, Wills, & Brody, 2004), decreased perceptions of mastery (Phinney, Madden, & Santos, 1998) and increased negative attitudes about school (Brand, Felner, Shim, Seitsinger, & Dumas, 2003). Perceived discrimination can lead to mistrust of teachers and to the general belief that the school rules and policies are unfair. A number of studies now document that personal experiences with discrimination, in combination with racial mistrust, can contribute to academic disengagement and other problem behaviors at school (e.g., Taylor, Casten, Flickinger, Roberts, & Fulmore, 1994).

Attributions to Discrimination: Risk or Protective Factor?

If discrimination is so ubiquitous, then how do ethnic minority targets manage to cope with it? One explanation pertinent to motivation and perceived competence focuses on the attributions of stigmatized groups (including racial and ethnic minorities) for their negative outcomes. Imagine for example, an African American student who receives a low grade on a test despite the fact that she thought she had answered all of the questions correctly. Because the failure was unexpected, she is likely, implicitly or explicitly, to ask, "Why?" Although attributional reasoning is complex, involving multiple causes, a basic distinction has been made in attribution research between causes that are internal (e.g., "It is something about *me*— my ability or effort") versus external (e.g., "It is something about my teacher; he's prejudiced") (Weiner, 1985; Chapter 5, this volume). External attributions for failure protect personal esteem by shifting blame away from the self. In an influential theoretical review, Crocker and Major (1989) drew on attribution research to argue that attributions to prejudice were an important self-protective mechanism that members of stigmatized groups use to maintain their self-esteem in spite of disparaging treatment by others.

Empirical support for the adaptiveness of external attributions for discrimination has been found in experimental research (see Major, Quinton, & McCoy, 2002, for a review), correlational studies (e.g., Moghaddam, Taylor, Lambert, & Schmidt, 1995), and longitudinal analyses (LaVeist, Sellers, & Neighbors, 2001). For example, LaVeist et al. (2001) found that African American adults who attributed discrimination to external factors (what the authors labeled as *system blame*) were more likely to be alive 13 years later than were their counterparts who attributed the same outcome to their own characteristics (self-blame). Lower mortality among the external attribution group was upheld even after controlling for the known correlates of survival, such as age, health status, and income.

The idea that external attributions can be self-protective for stigmatized groups provides a compelling theoretical account for why low-status groups have positive self-views *in spite of* their disadvantaged position. In recent years, however, empirical support for the esteem-protecting function of attributions to prejudice has been questioned (see Major et al., 2002). It has been argued, for example, that stigmatized groups only make external attributions when evaluator prejudice is very salient (Ruggiero & Taylor, 1995). In causally ambiguous contexts, targets are more likely to blame themselves in order to maintain personal control. There also appear to be social costs to making attributions to prejudice that may result in the dampening rather than maintenance of high self-esteem. Kaiser and Miller (2001) found that an African American target person who attributed a negative job evaluation to racial discrimination was perceived as irritating and troublesome, even when it was clear that the evaluator had reacted in a biased manner. Ethnic minorities may also be less likely to endorse attributions to prejudice when those causes need to be stated in the presence of a high-status evaluator (Stangor, Swim, Van Allen, & Sechrist, 2002). These studies suggest that people may be motivated to minimize attributions to prejudice to avoid devaluation, exclusion, or retaliation by others.

Some of the inconsistent findings in the attributional literature on discrimination may be due to an overly simplistic conception of an attribution to prejudice. Because perceived discrimination implicates personal characteristics (one's race or ethnicity), as well as the characteristics of external agents, it may be perceived as both internal and external on the locus dimension of causality (for related discussions, see Major et al., 2002; Schmitt & Branscombe, 2002). Moreover, internal and external causes differ along two other causal dimensions identified in attribution theory (i.e., stability and controllability) that also have motivational consequences. We suspect that the key attributional dimension for predicting how individuals cope with discrimination may be stability rather than locus. Stable causes for an outcome, whether internal or external, lead to the expectation that the same outcome will occur again, and that expectation, in turn, predicts cognitions, affect, and behavior associated with one's future prospects (Weiner, 1985). Cumulative experiences with discrimination and the perception that the causes of discrimination are stable will lead to depressed affect (e.g., feelings of hopelessness) and giving up in the face of challenge. Those stability–expectancy linkages, which mirror research findings on the negative consequences of discrimination reviewed earlier, bear little relation to self-esteem and the locus of attributions to discrimination.

Summary

Experiences with discrimination are a significant risk factor for undermining motivation and competence in children, adolescents, and adults of color. Causal attributions for discrimination appear to be an important mechanism for understanding the effects of unfair treatment on subsequent adjustment. However, the properties of that causal explanation and their relation to adjustment have not been fully explored. We believe that the stability of attributions for discrimination, rather than locus, may be especially meaningful for understanding the relations between coping with discrimination and competence motivation.

RACIAL STEREOTYPES

Stereotypes are culturally shared beliefs, both positive and negative, about the characteristics and behaviors of particular groups. For example, the notion that blondes have more fun or that adolescents are victims of "raging hormones" is part of our culturally endorsed beliefs about the attributes of those social groups. An important distinction has been made in the stereotype literature between one's own privately held beliefs about members of social groups (personal stereotypes) and the consensual or shared understanding of those groups (cultural stereotypes), for the latter are primarily of interest in this chapter.

Most of the racial stereotype literature in the United States has focused on African Americans, and there is much evidence that the cultural stereotypes of that group remain largely negative. Even though privately held beliefs have become more positive over the last 50 years (e.g., Schuman, Steeh, Bobo, & Krysan, 1997), studies of cultural stereotypes continue to show that respondents associate being black (and male) with low intelligence, hostility, aggressiveness, and violence (e.g., Devine & Elliot, 1995; Krueger, 1996). The much smaller stereotype literature on other ethnic groups in the United States also portrays the more marginalized groups in a negative light. For example, cultural stereotypes of Latinos represent them as illegal immigrants who prefer menial jobs, thus driving down wages, while driving up the costs of social services (e.g., Kao, 2000). Similar to African Americans, adolescent Latino males are perceived as unintelligent, antisocial, and with little personal ambition (Cowan, Martinez, & Mendiola, 1997; Neimann, Pollack, Rogers, & O'Connor, 1998). So pervasive are these linkages that they are sometimes endorsed even by members of the target ethnic groups. In our own research, for example, we found that African American and Latino adolescents were just as likely as their white classmates to associate being male and black or Latino with academic disengagement and socially deviant behavior (Graham, Taylor, & Hudley, 1998; Hudley & Graham, 2001).

Racial Stereotypes about Intelligence

African Americans and Stereotype Threat

Because the notion of race differences in intelligence has such a long history in the United States, it is not surprising that people continue to believe that African Americans are innately less intelligent than whites. Recall the enormous media attention to *The Bell Curve* but a decade ago (Herrnstein & Murray, 1994). For many, the book was derided as scientific racism; but for others, it was heralded as reviving a scientific truth.

Long before and after publication of *The Bell Curve*, social scientists have been writing about the negative consequences of stereotypes that associate being black with low intelligence. One particularly provocative program of research relevant to motivation and competence has between carried out by Claude Steele, Joshua Aronson, and their colleagues on a phenomenon that they label *stereotype threat* (Steele, 1997; Steele &

Aronson, 1995). Because that phenomenon is the subject of an entire chapter in this *Handbook*, we only briefly describe it here.

"Stereotype threat" is the awareness that individuals have about negative stereotypes associated with their group. Although considered to be a general psychological state applicable to any negative group stereotype, the construct originated in the achievement domain, and it has been applied to African American students' awareness of the cultural stereotype associating their race with intellectual inferiority. That awareness can be quite debilitating, especially for those African American students who are invested in doing well in school. For example, in a series of studies with black and white students attending Stanford University, Steele and Aronson (1995) found that black students performed more poorly than whites on test items taken from the Graduate Record Examination (GRE) when they were told that the test was diagnostic of their abilities. When told that the test was a problem-solving activity unrelated to ability, there was no difference in the performance of the two racial groups. In ability-related contexts, therefore, what became threatening for African American students was the fear that they might confirm the stereotype or be treated and judged by others based on that stereotype. Steele and Aronson suggested that stereotype-threatened students often are dividing their attention between the task itself (e.g., taking a GRE) and ruminating about the meaning of their performance (e.g., "What does this say about *me* or about members of my racial group?").

Stereotype threat researchers have documented two motivational consequences of the anxiety associated with thinking about race and intelligence in highly evaluative achievement contexts (Steele, 1997). Some African American students may choose to work especially hard as a way of disconfirming the stereotype. Of course, high effort in the face of increasing academic challenge may be difficult to sustain and may even lead one to question his or her abilities. Stereotype threat can also have the opposite effect, causing students to minimize effort and downplay the importance of doing well in school. Steele coined the term academic "disidentification" to describe students who no longer view academic achieve-

ment as a domain that is either important to them or their self-definition. Disidentification has been operationalized as the absence of a relationship between academic performance and self-esteem, and it has been associated with declining achievement from middle school to high school, particularly among African American boys (Osborne, 1997). A similar process, labeled academic "disengagement," occurs when students begin to discount the feedback they receive about their performance or to devalue achievement altogether (e.g., Major, Spencer, Schmader, Wolfe, & Crocker, 1998; Major & Schmader, 2001). Thus, while disidentification and disengagement may be self-protecting mechanisms for coping with negative racial stereotypes, in the long run, their detrimental effects on achievement strivings may outweigh any short-term self-enhancing effects.

Asian Americans and the Model Minority Stereotype

Unlike African Americans, the cultural stereotype about Asians is that they are hardworking and intellectually gifted high achievers who are especially competent in math and science (Kao, 1995). The term "model minority" was coined in the 1960s by social scientists and journalists to capture those characteristics and to account for the seemingly unprecedented successful entry of East Asian immigrants into mainstream American society (Sue & Okazaki, 1990). Many studies have now documented that Asians and non-Asians alike are aware of the culturally shared association between high academic achievement strivings and being an Asian American (e.g., Kao, 1995, 2000; Lee, 1994). Asked to describe the stereotypes about their group, over 80% of Asian American college students in one study listed terms such as "smart," "nerdy," and "overachiever" (Oyserman & Sakamoto, 1997).

While it may be more tolerable to know that one's ethnic group is viewed as smart and hardworking rather than as lazy and dumb, that stereotype also has its own unique set of challenges. Ethnographic, survey, and experimental research all point to psychological and emotional costs associated with living up to the model minority stereotype. Ethnographic studies, for example, detail the anxiety that many Asian American students feel when forced to cope with the perception of their group as academic superstars (see Lee, 1994). Many report feeling frustrated and pressured to attain or maintain high academic achievement because of the expectations placed upon them. As one Asian American student poignantly disclosed:

> They [whites] will have stereotypes, like we're smart. . . . They are so wrong, not everyone is smart. They expect you to be this and sometimes you tend to be what they expect you to be and you just lose your identity. . . . When you get bad grades, people look at you really strangely because you are sort of distorting the way they see an Asian. It makes you feel really awkward if you don't fit the stereotype. (in Lee, 1994, p. 419)

Consequences of those pressures have also been confirmed in laboratory experimental studies. Cheryan and Bodenhausen (2000) had Asian American women college students complete a set of math problems under conditions that manipulated whether their ethnicity was salient at the time of testing. Women in whom ethnic group membership had been primed performed more poorly and reported greater difficulty concentrating than those in a neutral condition. The authors suggested that positive stereotypes about academic ability can lead to "choking" under pressure if there is concern about failure to live up to high expectations about one's group. It also has been documented that Asian students were punished more for poor performance on a math tests than non-Asians who achieved the same outcome (Ho, Driscoll, & Loosbrock, 1998), implying that their evaluators perceived them as not trying hard. From an attributional perspective, failure attributed by others to lack of effort, given high ability, is maximally punished (Weiner, 1995).

Teacher Expectancies (Stereotypes?) as Self-Fulfilling Prophecies

Thus far, we have argued that intelligence-related stereotypes about African American and Asian American students are prevalent, and that these stereotypes influence students' motivation and perceptions of competence. It is reasonable also to ask whether teachers hold stereotypes linking race to intelligence and, if so, whether such stereotypes have an impact on student motivation and competence. Rosenthal and Jacobson's (1968) classic study, *Pygmalion in the Classroom*, was the first to document how teachers' inaccurate expectancies about students' intelligence actually produced changes in students' IQ scores that were consistent with their expectancies. Teacher expectancies became self-fulfilling prophesies (Merton, 1957), because an initially false definition of a situation evoked behaviors that subsequently made the false belief true. Stereotypes are often conceptualized as inaccurate expectations about individuals based on group membership, and a number of experimental studies have now documented the behavior-confirming (i.e., self-fulfilling) potential of social stereotypes (for recent examples, see Bargh, Chen, & Burrows, 1996; Chen & Bargh, 1997).

There is not a lot of concrete evidence that teacher expectations function as self-fulfilling prophesies (see review in Jussim, Eccles, & Madon, 1996). When found, however, those effects are often stronger when the expectations are low rather than high, and when they are held for African American compared to white students (see Rubovits & Maehr, 1973, for an early example and Jussim et al., 1996, for a more contemporary example). In the Jussim et al. study of sixth-grade math teachers and their students, teacher perceptions of low math ability in the fall predicted actual (low) achievement in the spring, over and above that explained by students' measured abilities. That effect was especially powerful for African American students, suggesting that these children are particularly vulnerable to confirming the beliefs of teachers who have low expectations about their academic potential.

How are negative teacher expectations communicated to students in self-fulfilling ways? One possible mechanism is the use of instructional practices that indirectly communicate low ability messages. For example, one of us (Graham, 1991) has found that undifferentiated praise for success at easy tasks, unsolicited offers of help, and too much sympathy following failure can lead students to attribute their academic setbacks to low ability (see also Mueller & Dweck,

1998 on the praise–low ability relation). Furthermore, altering pedagogical practices to be more effort- rather than ability-oriented can have immediate impact on students' motivation, even among those who are highly identified with the achievement domain. Cohen, Steele, and Ross (1999) found that African American college students displayed more subsequent task motivation when poor performance feedback was accompanied by criticism and communicated high expectations than when the same criticism was accompanied by general praise as a buffer. Such feedback, labeled "wise" by Cohen et al. (1999), can shift the attribution for failure away from low ability and toward those factors, such as lack of effort, that are under volitional control.

Racial Stereotypes about Antisocial Behavior

Arguably, *the* most pernicious racial stereotype affecting motivation and competence is the culturally shared belief that African Americans are violent, dangerous, aggressive, and antisocial. As we stated earlier, there is a great deal of evidence that this stereotype remains a part of the contemporary American psyche (e.g., Devine & Elliott, 1995).

Racial stereotypes about antisocial behavior have been linked to the disproportionately harsh treatment of African American youth in both the juvenile justice system and in the area of school discipline. For example, African American youth ages 10–17 are three to five times more likely than whites to be confined in the juvenile system (Poe-Yamagata & Jones, 2000). Some of that racial disparity is due to bias, inasmuch as African American offenders often receive harsher sentences than do whites, even after controlling for legal variables such as crime severity and prior offense history (Bridges & Steen, 1998; Leonard, Pope, & Feyerherm, 1995). In the school domain, Zero Tolerance and related "get tough" policies have produced racial disparities in the use of disciplinary practices. In a recent study of school suspension across 10 large school districts in the United States, the suspension rate for African American students was from two to five times greater than their representation in the school population (Applied Research Center, 2000). As in the justice system, racial disparities are evident, because many studies document that black students are punished more harshly than white students for the same school offense, and they appear to be disciplined for less severe and more subjectively perceived transgressions, such as behaving in a threatening or disrespectful manner (Skiba, 2001).

While many social scientists have argued that disproportionately harsh treatment of African American students and young offenders can be attributed to the presence of racial stereotypes, at present, there is little empirical research that directly tests those linkages. We believe that the stereotypes do exist, and that they influence decision making about African American youth largely at an unconscious level (e.g., Graham & Lowery, 2004). That belief is consistent with a growing literature in social psychology documenting that stereotypes can be activated and used outside of conscious awareness (e.g., Greenwald & Banaji, 1995). Unconscious stereotypes are *unintentional*, because they are not planned responses; *involuntary*, since they occur automatically in the presence of an environmental cue; and *effortless*, in that they do not deplete an individual's limited information-processing resources (Bargh & Chartrand, 1999). By automatically and effortlessly categorizing people according to the stereotypes that they hold about them, perceivers can manage information overload and make social decisions more efficiently. Particularly among perceivers at the front end of a system, such as police officers in the justice system or teachers dealing with classroom disorder, decisions often must be made quickly, under conditions of cognitive and emotional overload (e.g., perceived threat), and where much ambiguity exists. These are the very conditions that are known to activate unconscious beliefs (Fiske, 1998).

Situating the study of racial stereotypes in basic social cognitive processes provides new opportunities to think about intervention at the individual level. Even if stereotypes are largely automatic, they are still amenable to change (Blair, 2002). For example, perceivers can unlearn negative stereotypes with enough practice ("Just say no"), and they can be taught to focus on counterstereotypical associations with mental imagery (Kawakami, Dovidio, Moll, Hermsen, & Russin, 2000). Thus, decision makers in our courts, schools, and other social arenas can be educated to be more aware of the nature of their biases and how to change them.

Summary

Stereotypes that associate being African American with low intelligence, or those that associate being Asian American with high intelligence, can undermine the motivation and perceived competence of the targets of those stereotypes. The stereotype threat literature suggests that some African American students fear that their performance will confirm a negative stereotype; the model minority literature proposes that some Asian American students fear that their performance will disconfirm a positive stereotype. We suspect that coping with ability-related stereotypes in the academic domain, either negative or positive, can lead to performance–avoidance goals (i.e., being oriented toward a negative possibility), which have known negative consequences for motivation and performance (see Elliot, 1999; Chapter 4, this volume). Thus, students of color may often define their achievement goals according to the stereotypical images of their group. Racial stereotypes about antisocial behavior have been linked to punitive outcomes that cut off opportunities to be competent. Linking stereotypes to faulty information processing provides new directions for cognitive intervention at the individual level that can complement activism to combat racism at the institutional level.

RACIAL AND ETHNIC IDENTITY

Research on stereotypes and discrimination provides a natural bridge to racial identity because social psychologists have become very interested in the ways in which ethnic identity might moderate the relationship between perceived discrimination and adjustment. For example, it has been suggested that a strong racial identity can buffer the negative effect of discrimination on mental health (Sellers & Shelton, 2003). That finding is consistent with a growing literature on racial and ethnic identity, and the role that

they play in healthy adjustment. In this section, we turn to that literature in the context of academic achievement.

We define racial (ethnic) identity as a person's sense of belonging to his or her group and the meaning attached to that group membership (e.g., Phinney, 1990). Sense of belonging has many dimensions, including self-labeling (e.g., Do I describe myself as *Mexican American?*); level of knowledge about one's group, including its history and culture; and participation in activities and practices of the group. Psychological meaning includes the importance of ethnic membership, one's feelings of pride associated with membership in the group, and one's attitudes about his or her group, particularly the way it is perceived in the eyes of others (Sellers, Smith, Shelton, Rowley, & Chavous, 1998).

In a multiethnic society, members of minority groups are constantly called upon to negotiate their identity. They must weigh the relative value of maintaining a distinct group identity versus taking on some, if not all, of the perceived characteristics of the dominant group. Ethnic identity negotiation can be challenging. Some of the challenge relates to forging an ethnic identity when one's group historically has been devalued by the larger society, as in the case of African Americans. Other difficulties concern reconciling bicultural identities with both country of origin and country of residence, as is true for many Latino and Asian youth with recent immigrant histories. For children and adolescents, the school context is one of the primary environments in which identity negotiation is enacted, and the consequences of that negotiation may significantly influence a child's motivation for and commitment to school learning. While a strong identification with one's ethnic group may facilitate achievement motivation, an alternative perspective suggests that a strong ethnic identity may pose a significant barrier to achievement strivings.

Ethnic Identity as Educational Risk Factor

Conceptualizing ethnic identity as an educational risk factor is perhaps most clearly represented by John Ogbu's cultural ecological theory (Ogbu, 1978, 2003). That theory examines achievement striving in the context of a minority group's historical, social, cultural, and linguistic relationship to the dominant culture. Two interlocking influences are seen as central to the achievement strivings of ethnic minority youth. One is what Ogbu refers to as "the system," or the manner in which the larger society and its institutions have incorporated and treated the minority group. The other is "the community," or the collective adaptation of the group to the dominant society and to its minority status.

Cultural ecological theory argues that each ethnic or cultural group in a pluralistic society tends to perceive its identity according to how it has historically been incorporated into the social system. Involuntary minorities are those that have been incorporated into the dominant society without their consent, through slavery, conquest, or colonization. Members of these groups understand the racism and discrimination that they experience as an expression of their forced subordinate status and see the dominant cultural forms taught in "the system's" public schools as tools used against them for the purpose of oppression. In response to repeated experiences of discrimination and subordination by the dominant group, involuntary minority groups may develop a system of secondary cultural differences that are formed by a process known as "cultural inversion."

Oppositional Identity

Through the process of cultural inversion, certain behaviors and symbols are assigned exclusively to the dominant group, and the minority group adopts behaviors and symbols in direct contradiction to those of the dominant group. This process of cultural inversion creates among members of involuntary minority groups what cultural ecological theory refers to as an "oppositional identity." In an effort to maintain cultural boundaries, anything labeled as a characteristic of the dominant group (e.g., academic motivation, school engagement, and success) is, by definition, not appropriate for members of their own ethnic group. Rather, the involuntary minority group must be defined by characteristics (e.g., school disengagement) that are the direct opposite (i.e., an in-

version) of the dominant group. In school, student members of involuntary minority groups may reject achievement striving and displays of effort to preserve their ethnic or cultural identity.

Consistent with oppositional identity, several ethnographies have concluded that African American adolescents believe that working hard for school success may be viewed by their black peers as "acting white," or supplanting one's own ethnic identity with that of the dominant culture (Fordham, 1996; Fordham & Ogbu, 1986; Tatum, 1997). It has been proposed that highly academically motivated African American students must adopt a "raceless" identity (Fordham, 1996) and often endure the rejection and outright ridicule of peers who espouse an oppositional identity. Furthermore, even among middle-class African American families and students, suspicion of racial inequity often creates an oppositional frame of interaction between schools and families and an oppositional identity among students, who reject achievement striving in favor of aspirations for sports or entertainment careers (Ogbu, 2003). A few ethnographic studies of oppositional identity have also been carried out with other marginalized (involuntary) ethnic groups and report similar findings. For example, a study of Mexican-descent high school students revealed that youth with a particular type of ethnic identification (e.g., *cholo*) endorsed beliefs about barriers to opportunity, experienced identity conflict, and displayed the same kinds of oppositional behaviors that Fordham and Ogbu (1986) have attributed to African Americans (Matute-Bianchi, 1991). In addition, Lee (1994) reported that some Asian-identified students, labeled as *New Wavers*, showed similar disdain for academic achievement, not only as a reaction to the model minority stereotype, but also because they associated being popular with academic disengagement.

The discourse surrounding oppositional identity during adolescence has become very lively among public intellectuals, as well as researchers, at least partly because it provides a motivational explanation for the achievement gap between black and white students. One would be hard pressed to find an article on academic motivation in African American adolescents in the last 10 years that does not explicitly or implicitly make reference to oppositional identity. That construct also has been linked to other motivational phenomena discussed earlier in this chapter, such as stereotype threat and disidentification, as a way to fully capture the academic challenges that African American students face (Steele, 1992).

Aside from the ethnographic studies, however, there is not much empirical support for the phenomenon of oppositional identity. For example, two studies (Ainsworth-Darnell & Downey, 1998; Cook & Ludwig, 1997) tested hypotheses about oppositional identity using data from the National Education Longitudinal Study (NELS), a nationally representative panel study of 25,000 ethnically diverse students, their parents, and their teachers, who were assessed when students were in 8th, 10th, and 12th grade. Examining 10th-grade data, but using different analytic strategies, neither Ainsworth-Darnell and Downey (1998) nor Cook and Ludwig (1997) found clear evidence for attitudes resembling oppositional identity in African American high school students. Black students reported *more* proschool attitudes than their white counterparts, had equally high expectations for their future, and felt that high-achieving black peers were indeed among the most popular in school. To be sure, African American students in NELS analyses had lower school achievement than whites on virtually every indicator. But to the degree that antiachievement peer norms were present, they were the same for the two racial groups.

Some scholars have countered that large-scale surveys such as NELS are not sensitive enough to capture the more nuanced cultural and school contexts that do indeed promote oppositional identity among involuntary minorities (e.g., Farkas, Lleras, & Maczuga, 2002). Yet other qualitative studies do not find that African American adolescents believe either that doing well in school threatens their racial identity or that high achievers are rejected by the peer group (Bergin & Cooks, 2002; Datnow & Cooper, 1997). Rather than being oppositional, a strong racial identity was promotive of achievement strivings. In the next section, we turn to other research that argues for positive associations between ethnic identity and motivation.

Ethnic Identity as a Protective Factor

Although lacking a provocative conceptual framework like that of Fordham and Ogbu, a growing empirical literature has documented the motivational benefits of strongly identifying with one's ethnic group. Rather than cultural anthropology, this literature is grounded in more psychological approaches that measure ethnic identity with established scales and then relate strength of measured identity to a number of outcomes. For African Americans in particular, supportive results have been found with samples from childhood to young adulthood. Among elementary school students, for example, self and teacher ratings of school interest and school adjustment relate significantly to measures of racial identity (Thomas, Townsend, & Belgrave, 2003). Furthermore, a racial identity that includes the attitude that academic achievement is a part of being black has been shown to predict subsequent motivation and achievement (Oyserman, Harrison, & Bybee, 2001) as well as self-perceptions of ability and career aspirations in African American middle school students (Smith, Walker, Fields, Brookins, & Seay, 1999). Similarly, recent data indicate that African American middle school students with a positive racial identity are more likely to have high academic self-concepts and to be academically more successful than their counterparts who endorse a Eurocentric identity (Spencer, Noll, Stoltzfus, & Harpalani, 2001). Spencer et al. have been particularly vocal in criticizing the "acting white" phenomenon.

Consistent with findings from younger students, positive attitudes toward racial identity are also predictive of high academic self-concept and achievement among African American high school students (O'Connor, 1999; Witherspoon, Speight, & Thomas, 1997). In one of few studies to examine racial identity in a longitudinal design, Chavous et al. (2003) documented that 12th graders who perceived their racial identity to be central to their self-concept attended school more regularly, achieved higher grades, and were more likely to graduate from high school and go on to college. As might be expected from the foregoing results, positive racial identification is also predictive of achievement motivation and academic success in African American college undergraduates (Cokley, 2001; Sellers, Chavous, & Cooke, 1998).

The effects of a strong ethnic identity seem to generalize to other racial and ethnic groups as well. Research on Native American college students has consistently linked a positive psychosocial connection to Native culture with academic motivation, persistence, and achievement (Montgomery, Miville, Winterowd, Jeffries, & Baysden, 2000). This literature suggests that the most motivated students construct a unique academic identity that explicitly incorporates Indian ways of knowing, including the value of guides, the wisdom of elders, and the reciprocally supportive relationship between the Native community and the student. Among Latino students across grade levels, strong ethnic identity has been associated with school engagement, intrinsic motivation, and a belief in the value of schooling, although these findings appear to be more robust for Latino females than for males (e.g., Okagaki, Frensch, & Dodson, 1996; Lasley-Barajas & Pierce, 2001)

What are the origins of strong ethnic identity in youth of color? One important factor appears to be the way parents socialize their children about race and ethnicity. Two types of attitude about race that parents transmit to their offspring have been identified: (1) the communicated messages that instill racial and ethnic pride, including learning about one's history, heritage and culture; and (2) preparation for experiences with racial bias and discrimination (Bowman & Howard, 1985; Hughes & Chen, 1997). An underlying theme in this socialization research is that ethnic minority parents begin to teach their children about their ethnic history, heritage, and culture as early as the preschool years, and that preparation for coping with discrimination increases as children get older, especially in African American families. These communicated messages are related not only stronger to ethnic identity but also to higher academic achievement, more perceived mastery, and better problem-solving skills.

Summary

There are two competing hypotheses in the literature about the relationship between ethnic identity and achievement strivings.

Using qualitative methods, cultural ecological theorists argue that positive achievement attitudes and behaviors can threaten the identity of involuntary minority groups. On the other hand, contemporary programs of research using survey methods and self-report measures of identity find that strong ethnic identity is related to successful academic outcomes. It also is evident that parental socialization about race contributes to the positive relation between identity and achievement. What is missing from this literature is an understanding of process, or the mechanisms by which identity promotes motivation and competence. For example, the process may be primarily affective (e.g., ethnic pride enhances the subjective feeling of being competent), cognitive (e.g., strong identity enables one to filter out negative, ability-related messages of others), or some combination of feeling and thinking sequences. These are issues for future research.

THE IMMIGRANT EXPERIENCE

Census 2000 completely redefined the racial and ethnic landscape in the United States. Although whites are still the majority group in the nation as a whole, Asians and Latinos are now the fastest growing ethnic groups. In some states, such as California, that growth has been so dramatic that it is no longer meaningful to talk about majority and minority groups, inasmuch as no single ethnic group holds the numerical balance of power. The increased presence of immigrant children of color in the schools has led to an interest in the psychosocial impact of acculturation on academic motivation and adjustment, and we concentrate our review on that literature. As schools become more multicultural, immigrant students cope simultaneously with increased cross-ethnic contact and pressures to adjust to the dominant culture. These acculturation pressures are presumed to impact a number of areas, including mental health, coping with discrimination, ethnic identity, and orientation toward school.

Segmented Assimilation

Traditional theories about immigration were guided by the experiences of European immigrants in the early 20th century (e.g., Gordon, 1964). Those "melting pot" theories proposed that social and economic mobility should increase across successive generations of residence as the descendants of early immigrants are steadily assimilated into the American fabric. Thus, second- and third-generation residents should achieve better outcomes than their first-generation forbears to the extent that they adopt the language, culture, and values of the host society and become more similar to (indistinguishable from) mainstream Americans.

The outcomes for immigrants since the 1960s, who are largely of African, Latino, and Asian rather than European descent, have not supported the assimilationists' theory of upward mobility across successive generations. A growing literature on the psychosocial adjustment of youth as a function of immigrant history documents poorer adjustment across successive generations of residence in the United States (see review in Zhou, 1997). For example, in some studies, first- and second-generation adolescents of Latino, Asian, or black (Caribbean) descent did better in school and maintained more positive attitudes about achievement than did same-ethnicity youth whose families had resided in this country for three or more generations (Fuligni, 1997; Kao & Tienda, 1995; Matute-Bianchi, 1991; Rong & Brown, 2001). Lower self-esteem also has been associated with longer residence among adolescent children of immigrants (Rumbaut, 1994). Such findings have led immigration researchers to propose that there might be multiple pathways to immigrant success, not all of which involved rapid assimilation (Portes & Zhou, 1993). The theory of segmented assimilation suggests that adopting the characteristics of the host culture, while relinquishing one's culture of origin, can lead either to upward mobility and absorption into the middle class, or to downward mobility and absorption into the urban underclass. Yet a third pathway involves upward mobility, while holding on to the values embedded in one's culture and maintaining close ties with one's immigrant community. In the following sections, we consider research on family socialization and on ethnic identity across generations to illustrate these divergent pathways.

Family Socialization and Motivation

Communicated parental values about hard work and the importance of a good education appear to be among the most important factors accounting for higher achievement among immigrants and children of immigrants (second generation) compared to their counterparts of third generation and beyond. For example, Fuligni (1997) found that the higher academic performance of Asian and Latino first- and second-generation adolescents could be traced to higher parental expectations that they do well in school and higher parental aspirations for their educational attainment. Much of the parental socialization around achievement involves encouragement of children to overcome setbacks, because their educational opportunities are perceived to be much greater in the United States than those available in their home countries.

Parental socialization about obligation to the family has been similarly linked to higher achievement strivings among relative newcomers to this country. "Family obligation" refers to how much family members feel a sense of duty to help one another and to take into account family needs when making personal decisions (Fuligni, Tseng, & Lam, 1999). It has been shown that Latino and Asian immigrant youth are more likely than their American-born counterparts to report a belief in family duty, although both groups display more family loyalty than European American peers (Fuligni et al., 1999; Suarez-Orozco & Suarez-Orozco, 1995). Family obligation also is correlated with achievement values, inasmuch as many of the youth feel that doing well in school is something that they owe their parents.

Identity Development

Picture two second-generation adolescents, one whose parents were born in Mexico, and the other whose parents were born in Haiti. If we were to ask these youth the perennial "Who am I?" question by selecting an ethnic label, what would each choose? Will the youth of Mexican origin self-identify as *Mexican, Mexican American, or Latino*? Will the youth of Haitian origin self-identify as *Haitian, African American,* or *black*? More generally, are immigrant youth more likely to adopt pan-ethnic labels, such as *Mexican American* or *African American*, that link them to American-born peers with similar (albeit distant) ethnic heritages, or are they more likely to self-identify in ways that tie them more closely to the immigrant experience and their country of origin? While complex and not easy to answer, this question is very relevant to our chapter. How children with recent immigration histories negotiate their ethnic identity has important implications for motivation and competence.

A number of studies that have addressed this question with diverse immigrant groups reached similar conclusions. For example, in a study of adolescent children of Vietnamese immigrants in New Orleans, Bankston and Zhou (1997) found that adolescents who remained highly integrated within their ethnic communities (e.g., had Vietnamese friends, preferred Vietnamese food and music, maintained close family ties) were doing better in school and were better socially adjusted than those who had come to identify with local American youth. Waters (1994) studied second-generation Haitian and West Indian adolescents in New York City. The middle-class youth in that study, and those who were doing well in school, preferred to be identified with their country of origin. Such youth consciously rejected being viewed as African American because of the negative stereotypes associated with that group. In contrast, lower socioeconomic scale and lower achieving blacks were more likely to identify with African Americans, to be particularly sensitive to discrimination, and to adopt many of the negative attitudes about school that have been associated with oppositional identity. In research on Mexican-descent high school students in central California, Matute-Bianchi (1991) distinguished between second-generation students, who identified with traditional Mexican culture, values, and language (Mexican-oriented), and their native-born counterparts, who were least likely to self-identify as such (*Chicanos* and *Cholos*). Mexican-oriented students were more liked and respected by their teachers, reported being more engaged in school, and experienced higher academic achievement than *Chicanos* and *Cholos*. These latter groups, in fact,

were among the most troubled in the school, suggesting that their identities had been transformed in way that alienated them from both their school context and traditional Mexican culture. Thus, a common theme in all of these studies is that adolescents with recent immigration histories fare better when they strongly identify with their country of origin rather than distancing themselves from it.

The notion of segmented assimilation, its relationship to identity negotiation, and multiple pathways to upward or downward mobility is complementary to Ogbu's cultural ecological theory introduced earlier. While some students may adopt attitudes and display behaviors characteristic of an involuntary minority, those children who experience a more modified acculturation process and retain their traditional ethnic identity are consistent with Ogbu's definition of "voluntary minorities." Members of this group have chosen minority status in the dominant American culture, with the expectation of a better life, rather than having that status forced upon them, as is the case with involuntary minorities. As such, voluntary minorities believe in the value of schooling as a means to get ahead, they retain their original cultural values and language rather than developing a unique secondary culture in opposition to the dominant culture, and they tend to experience school success at much higher rates than involuntary minorities. Thus, Ogbu's typology of voluntary–involuntary minorities and the theory of segmented assimilation lead to similar conclusions about the impact of acculturation on motivation and competence. The key to success appears to be the development of a strong bicultural competence (LaFromboise, Coleman, & Gerton, 1993), or the ability to function effectively in the dominant culture, while retaining a primary ethnic identity.

GENERAL SUMMARY

The study of race and ethnicity in motivation and competence needs to begin with the unique experiences of people of color in this society. We have focused on a set of interrelated factors that draw on the historical circumstances and cultural forces that have shaped those experiences and that have motivational significance. Coping with discrimination and cultural stereotypes is meaningful because it sheds light on what Weiner (Chapter 5, this volume) has labeled the "social psychology of competence." The way other people perceive the abilities of ethnic minority members, and how those perceptions are communicated and enacted, partly determine what ethnic group members think and feel about themselves. Perceptions of others also affect the goals toward which people of color strive (e.g., to disconfirm negative stereotypes about competence), their causal explanations for discrimination (e.g., Is it *me* or is it *them*?), and the perceived costs and benefits of sustained achievement strivings.

Discrimination and racial stereotypes are structural variables that impact motivation and perceived competence of people of color, an impact that is filtered by how individuals think about their membership in a particular racial or ethnic group. We therefore have focused on ethnic identity as the lens through which people of color interpret the reactions of dominant group members. Our interpretation of the literature is that ethnic identity is a protective factor, particularly during adolescence. When adolescents of color are strongly identified with their ethnic group, they are more motivated to achieve and have a greater repertoire of skills to ward off threats to their competence. A task for the future is to better understand process, or the psychological mechanisms by which ethnic identity serves this buffering role.

Finally, we have incorporated the immigration experience as a way of acknowledging the changing racial and ethnic landscape in this country. There was a time when the discourse about race and psychological variables was limited to African Americans and the ways in which they were similar to or different from whites. The large influx of ethnic immigrants from Latin America, the Caribbean, and Southeast Asia has fundamentally altered that discourse. The serious researcher who wants to study how ethnicity shapes achievement strivings and the pursuit of competence will have to address immigrant and generational status. For some ethnic groups, motivation and competence can be impaired over time and across generations.

TOWARD THE FUTURE

We conclude with a set of guidelines for research on motivation and competence in racial and ethnic groups that evolves from our focus in this chapter. None of the guidelines is discussed in detail, and they surely reflect our biases. We offer them as food for thought, and in some cases, as cautionary notes.

The Intersection of Social Class and Gender

Some scholars, critical of how race has been studied in psychological research, have argued that most of what the field attributes to racial or ethnic differences is really a function of social and economic disparities, and that the latter is where our emphasis should be placed. We agree in part with this position, because we are well aware that ethnic minority groups are overrepresented among those who endure social and economic marginality. However, many of the phenomena examined in this chapter transcend social class differences. Coping with discrimination and stereotypes and identity negotiation are challenges faced by ethnic group members across all socioeconomic strata (e.g., Feagin, 1991). Those challenges might inform debate on the achievement gap (e.g., Jencks & Phillips, 1998) and on physical health disparities (e.g., Adler & Snibbe, 2003), two contexts wherein differences between African Americans and whites remain even when social class is taken into account. After reviewing the literature on relations between socioeconomic status and physical health, Adler and Snibbe (2003) concluded that "although a substantial portion of the racial–ethnic differences in health is due to social disadvantages associated with low SES, unique effects specific to race–ethnicity also exist, reflecting experiences of discrimination, residential segregation, negative stereotypes, and other circumstances" (p. 122). We agree with this conclusion. There is something unique about being an ethnic minority, over and above poverty or affluence, and that uniqueness should not be ignored in the study of motivation and competence.

There also are particular circumstances

associated with being *male* and a member of an ethnic minority that have not adequately been recognized in motivation research. In most gender research on motivation, a dominant theme is the heightened vulnerability of girls to motivational deficits. Some argue that gender role socialization and cultural stereotypes about women and achievement lead many girls to question their academic competence more, particularly in math; to display more maladaptive reactions to failure, including low-ability attributions; to perceive more barriers to success; and to experience more conflict between individual achievement strivings and social conformity (see reviews in Eccles, Wigfield, & Schiefele, 1998; Ruble & Martin, 1998). Even research on stereotype threat in young adults underscores that developmental gender literature because it draws many parallels between the academic plight of African Americans and that of women in math and science (Steele, 1997).

We believe that gender analyses in motivation research may need to be reframed. In research on motivation and achievement that examines both ethnic and gender differences, it is evident that ethnic minority males (i.e., African American and Latino) are faring more poorly than females (e.g., Graham et al., 1998; Matute-Bianchi, 1991; Osborne, 1997; Taylor et al., 1994). The ethnicity-by-gender differences increase across the school years and are particularly apparent when the measures are so-called "markers" of adolescent success (i.e., high school graduation) and young adult mobility (i.e., enrollment in and completion of college; see review in Sidanius & Pratto, 1999). The outcomes of racial stereotypes about antisocial behavior, such as school suspension and confinement in the justice system, also fall disproportionately on African American males. We believe that ethnic minority males, more so than other groups, must cope with the dual stressors of academic challenge and negative stereotypes about their group. Such stressors create particular needs that can be addressed with appropriate pedagogical intervention (Hudley, 1995, 1997). Therefore, research on motivation and competence must be particularly sensitive to gender-by-ethnicity interactions in order to uncover other kinds of challenges that are unique to ethnic minority boys.

Beyond Self-Esteem

If we were to base our appraisal of racial differences in motivation and competence on what research participants *say*, we would find a perplexing, some might say, counterintuitive pattern of findings. African American children and adolescents' perceptions of their competence, whether measured by general or academic-specific measures of self-esteem, are equal to or more positive than those of their white counterparts, even when achievement data indicate that they are doing more poorly in school. This robust finding is documented in several reviews (Crocker & Major, 1989; Graham, 1994; Gray-Little & Hafdahl, 2000). Important theoretical contributions have emerged from scholars' attempts to understand how African Americans can continue to report feeling good about themselves when achievement outcomes indicate otherwise. In the literature on external attributions for discrimination, reviewed in this chapter, a good example is Crocker and Major's (1989) influential analysis of the self-protective (esteem-enhancing) strategies employed by stigmatized groups. As important as that work has been (it certainly dispelled the myth of black self-hatred), we believe that the study of motivation and competence in racial and ethnic groups should move beyond personal esteem and related self-appraisal constructs. Among African Americans at least, self-perceived competence is not a reliable predictor of actual competence. We suspect that there is more to be learned by focusing on constructs that tap perceived barriers to opportunity or the payoff of persistence in spite of those barriers. These are expectancy- rather than esteem-related constructs.

Importance of Multiple Methods

Motivation research on racial and ethnic groups needs to employ multiple methods. At least one phenomenon that we have considered in this chapter—oppositional identity—so captured the interest of motivation researchers that it had an impact on our field even in the absence of a strong empirical base. Not until the ethnographic studies were complemented with survey methods did the literature begin to question whether, how, and when African American (involuntary minority) youth actually displayed the attitudes and behavior associated with oppositional identity. Other phenomena examined in this chapter also have been linked to a single empirical approach. For example, stereotype threat and teacher expectancies as self-fulfilling prophesies have mainly been documented in laboratory experimental studies; vulnerability to the model minority stereotype has been best illustrated in the qualitative approach of ethnography; and contemporary ethnic identity research mainly draws on correlational studies that measure individual differences in the strength of one's allegiance to his or her group. We believe that experimental, ethnographic, and correlational approaches are all necessary to capture fully the dynamics of motivation and striving for competence in ethnic minority groups. Also needed are longitudinal analyses that track growth and change in these phenomena over time. We do not know of any longitudinal studies in which the primary focus is the development of motivation in ethnic minority youth.

Revitalizing the Socialization (Child-Rearing) Antecedents of Achievement Strivings

In the history of motivation research with racial and ethnic groups, parental socialization once played a pivotal role. Early research from the 1950s on the achievement syndrome by Bernard Rosen and colleagues attempted to examine how child-rearing practices, such as early training in mastery and independence, were related to achievement aspirations and values (e.g., Rosen & d'Andrade, 1959). Yet it was never clearly documented that any components of the achievement syndrome were related to racial and ethnic differences in child-rearing practices, and by 1980, that genre of socialization research had faded from view.

As motivation researchers, we do not lament the early demise of socialization research in ethnic minority youth. Even in general motivation research, it is not clear that particular child-rearing practices are systematically related to specific motivational characteristics in children. That weak empirical literature also frequently portrayed black families in a negative light (see Graham, 1994). More promising, we believe, is a re-

newed interest in socialization influences, within the context of research on parental socialization about race and ethnicity among American ethnic groups and the socialization of achievement attitudes and values among children of immigrants. We are especially encouraged by this newer literature, because it focuses on normative rather than deviant child-rearing and on adaptive rather than pathological functioning in families of color.

Ethnicity in Context

Throughout this chapter, we have emphasized the importance of situating the study of motivation and competence in the broader social context. We certainly are not unique in this claim. All of the contributors to this *Handbook* acknowledge that personal motivation is responsive to contextual influences. Less clear, however, is *how* to study context when one's primary focus is race and ethnicity. We think of context in the Bronfenbrenner (1979) framework as nested levels of influence with varying degrees of proximity to the individual. Thus, students are nested within peer groups, which in turn are nested within classrooms that are within schools, and so forth. Using this framework, one promising approach to studying ethnicity within context might be to examine how individual motivation and competence develop in classrooms and schools that vary in ethnic composition. For example, do children of color develop stronger ethnic identity (and presumed higher motivation) when their ethnic group is the numerical majority in their school and they have many same-ethnicity peers with whom to affiliate? Or does ethnic identification intensify when one's group is the minority and there are distinct boundaries between groups (e.g., "us" vs. "them")? Is perceived discrimination more psychologically harmful when the target is a numerical ethnic minority? In our research (Bellmore, Witkow, Graham, & Juvonen, 2004; Graham & Juvonen, 2002), we found that targets of mistreatment by peers tend to feel worse when they are members of the *majority* ethnic group in their classroom or school, and that those targets are particularly vulnerable to self-blaming attributions (it may be hard to make an external attribution to the prejudice of same-race others). One might also ask how these same processes are influenced by a changing ethnic context, such as transitioning from a small and relatively homogeneous elementary school to a large and ethnically heterogeneous middle school. School transitions are important turning points in which students lose social status when they go from being the oldest to the youngest in their school, and that loss may be exacerbated by the shift from ethnic majority to minority status.

These kinds of questions are guided by our belief that it is not so much ethnicity per se, but rather ethnicity within a particular social context (e.g., numerical majority vs. minority) that will inform future motivation research. We have to look back to the aftermath of *Brown v. Board of Education* and the desegregation studies of the 1960s and 1970s to find any substantive empirical literature on the psychological impact of racially homogeneous versus heterogeneous school contexts. Regrettably, that literature had all but disappeared by 1980 (see Schofield, 1991), and its only real legacy was that black children had higher self-esteem when they attended racially segregated rather than integrated schools. On the 50th anniversary of *Brown v. Board of Education*, the time seems right to revisit that legacy. Studying ethnicity in context may shed new light on how racial and ethnic diversity can foster achievement strivings and greater competence in people of color.

REFERENCES

Adler, N., & Snibbe, A. (2003). The role of psychosocial processes in explaining the gradient between socioeconomic status and health. *Current Directions in Psychological Science, 12,* 119–123.

Ainsworth-Darnell, J., & Downey, D. (1998). Assessing the oppositional culture explanation for racial/ethnic differences in school performance. *American Sociological Review, 63,* 536–553.

Applied Research Center. (2000). *Facing the consequences: An examination of racial discrimination in U.S. public schools.* Oakland, CA: Author.

Bankston, C., & Zhou, M. (1997). Valedictorians and delinquents: The bifurcation of Vietnamese American youth. *Deviant Behavior, 18,* 343–364.

Bargh, J., & Chartrand, T. (1999). The unbearable automaticity of being. *American Psychologist, 54,* 462–479.

Bargh, J., Chen, M., & Burrows, L. (1996). Automaticity of social behavior: Direct effects of trait construct and stereotype activation on action. *Journal of Personality and Social Psychology, 71,* 230–244.

Baumeister, R., & Leary, M. (1995). The need to belong: Desire for interpersonal attachment as a fundamental human motivation. *Psychological Bulletin, 117,* 497–529.

Baumeister, R., Twenge, J., & Nuss, C. (2002). Effects of social exclusion on cognitive processes: Anticipated aloneness reduces intelligent thought. *Journal of Personality and Social Psychology, 83,* 817–827.

Bellmore, A., Witkow, M., Graham, S., & Juvonen, J. (2004). Beyond the individual: The impact of ethnic context and classroom behavioral norms on victims' adjustment. *Developmental Psychology, 40,* 1159–1172.

Bergin, D., & Cooks, H. (2002). High school students of color talk about accusations of "acting white." *Urban Review, 34,* 113–134.

Blair, I. (2002). The malleability of automatic stereotypes and prejudice. *Personality and Social Psychology Review, 6,* 242–261.

Bowman, P., & Howard, C. (1985). Race-related socialization, motivation, and academic achievement: A study of black youths in three-generation families. *Journal of the American Academy of Child Psychiatry, 24,* 134–141.

Brand, S., Felner, R., Shim, M., Seitsinger, A., & Dumas, T. (2003). Middle school improvement and reform: Development and validation of a school-level assessment of climate, cultural pluralism, and school safety. *Journal of Educational Psychology, 95,* 570–588.

Bridges, G. S., & Steen, S. (1998). Racial disparities in official assessments of juvenile offenders: Attributional stereotypes as mediating mechanisms of juvenile offenders. *American Sociological Review, 63,* 554–571.

Broman, C., Mavaddat, R., & Hsu, S. (2000). The experience and consequences of perceived racial discrimination: A study of African Americans. *Journal of Black Psychology, 26,* 165–180.

Bronfenbrenner, U. (1979). *The ecology of human development: Experiments by nature and design.* Cambridge, MA: Harvard University Press.

Chavous, T., Bernat, D., Schmeelk-Cone, K., Caldwell, C., Kohn-Wood, L., & Zimmerman, M. (2003). Racial identity and academic attainment among African American adolescents. *Child Development, 74,* 1076–1090.

Chen, M., & Bargh, J. (1997). On the automaticity of self-fulfilling prophesies: The nonconscious effects of stereotype activation on social interaction. *Journal of Experimental Social Psychology, 33,* 541–560.

Cheryan, S., & Bodenhausen, G. (2000). When positive stereotypes threaten intellectual performance: The psychological hazards of "model minority" status. *Psychological Science, 11,* 399–402.

Clark, R., Anderson, N., Clark, V., & Williams, D. (1999). Racism as a stressor for African Americans:

A biopsychosocial model. *American Psychologist*, *54*, 805–816.

Cohen, G., Steele, C., & Ross, L. (1999). The mentor's dilemma: Providing critical feedback across the racial divide. *Personality and Social Psychology Bulletin*, *25*, 1302–1318.

Cokley, K. (2001). Gender differences among African American students in the impact of racial identity on academic psychosocial development. *Journal of College Student Development*, *42*, 480–487.

Cook, P., & Ludwig, J. (1997). Weighing the "burden of 'acting white' ": Are there race differences in attitudes toward education? *Journal of Policy Analysis and Management*, *16*, 256–278.

Cornell, S., & Hartmann, D. (1998). *Ethnicity and race: Making identities in a changing world.* Thousand Oaks, CA: Pine Forge Press.

Cose, E. (1993). *The rage of the privileged class.* New York: HarperCollins.

Cowan, G., Martinez, L., & Mendiola, S. (1997). Predictors of attitudes toward illegal Latino immigrants. *Hispanic Journal of Behavioral Sciences*, *19*, 403–415.

Crocker, J., & Major, B. (1989). Social stigma and self-esteem: The self-protective properties of stigma. *Psychological Review*, *96*, 608–630.

Datnow, A., & Cooper, R. (1997). Peer networks of African American students in independent schools: Affirming academic success and racial identity. *Journal of Negro Education*, *66*, 56–72.

Devine, P. G., & Elliot, A. J. (1995). Are racial stereotypes really fading?: The Princeton trilogy revisited. *Personality and Social Psychology Bulletin*, *21*, 1139–1150.

Eccles, J., Wigfield, A., & Schiefele, U. (1998). Motivation to succeed. In N. Eisenberg (Ed.), *Handbook of child psychology* (5th ed., Vol. 3, pp. 1017–1095). New York: Wiley.

Eisenberger, N., Lieberman, M., & Williams, K. (2003). Does rejection hurt?: An fMRI study of social exclusion. *Science*, *302*, 290–292.

Elliot, A. (1999). Approach and avoidance motivation and achievement goals. *Educational Psychologist*, *34*, 169–189.

Farkas, G., Lleras, C., & Maczuga, S. (2002). Does oppositional culture exist in minority and poverty peer groups? *American Sociological Review*, *67*, 148–155.

Feagin, J. (1991). The continuing significance of race: Anti-black discrimination in public places. *American Sociological Review*, *56*, 101–116.

Fisher, C., Wallace, S., & Fenton, R. (2000). Discrimination distress during adolescence. *Journal of Youth and Adolescence*, *29*, 679–694.

Fiske, S. (1998). Stereotyping, prejudice, and discrimination. In D. Gilbert, S. Fiske, & G. Lindzey (Eds.), *Handbook of social psychology* (Vol. 2, 4th ed., pp. 357–411). Boston: McGraw-Hill.

Fordham, S. (1996). *Blacked out.* Chicago: University of Chicago Press.

Fordham, S., & Ogbu, J. (1986). Black students' school success: Coping with the "burden of 'acting White.' " *Urban Review*, *18*, 176–206.

Fuligni, A. (1997). The academic achievement of adolescents from immigrant families: The roles of family background, attitudes, and behavior. *Child Development*, *68*, 351–363.

Fuligni, A., Tseng, V., & Lam, M. (1999). Attitudes toward family obligations among American adolescents with Asian, Latin American, and European backgrounds. *Child Development*, *70*, 1030–1044.

Garcia-Coll, C., Lamberty, G., Jenkins, R., McAdoo, H., Crnic, K., Wasik, B., et al. (1996). An integrative model of developmental competencies in minority children. *Child Development*, *67*, 1891–1914.

Gibbons, F., Gerrard, M., Cleveland, M., Wills, T., & Brody, G. (2004). Perceived discrimination and substance use in African American parents and their children: A panel study. *Journal of Personality and Social Psychology*, *77*, 826–838.

Gordon, M. (1964). *Assimilation in American life: The role of race, religion, and national origins.* New York: Oxford University Press.

Graham, S. (1991). Communicating low ability in the classroom: Bad things good teachers sometimes do. In S. Graham & V. Folkes (Eds.), *Attribution theory: Applications to achievement, mental health, and interpersonal conflict* (pp. 17–36). Hillsdale, NJ: Erlbaum.

Graham, S. (1994). Motivation in African Americans. *Review of Educational Research*, *64*, 55–117.

Graham, S., & Juvonen, J. (2002). Ethnicity, peer harassment, and adjustment in middle school: An exploratory study. *Journal of Early Adolescence*, *22*, 173–199.

Graham, S., & Lowery, B. (2004). Priming unconscious racial stereotypes in the juvenile justice system. *Law and Human Behavior*, *28*, 483–504.

Graham, S., Taylor, A., & Hudley, C. (1998). Exploring achievement values among ethnic minority early adolescents. *Journal of Educational Psychology*, *91*, 606–620.

Gray-Little, B., & Hafdahl, A. (2000). Factors influencing racial comparisons of self-esteem: A quantitative review. *Psychological Bulletin*, *126*, 26–54.

Greenwald, A. G., & Banaji, M. R. (1995). Implicit social cognition: Attitudes, self-esteem, and stereotypes. *Psychological Review*, *102*, 4–27.

Harrell, S. (2000). A multidimensional conceptualization of racism-related stress: Implications for the well-being of people of color. *American Journal of Orthopsychiatry*, *70*, 42–57.

Helms, J., & Talleyrand, R. (1997). Race is not ethnicity. *American Psychologist*, *52*, 1246–1247.

Herrnstein, R., & Murray, C. (1994). *The bell curve: Intelligence and class structure in American life.* New York: Free Press.

Ho, C., Driscoll, D., & Loosbrock, D. (1998). Great expectations: The negative consequences of falling short. *Journal of Applied Social Psychology*, *28*, 1743–1759.

Hudley, C. (1995). Assessing the impact of separate schooling for African-American male adolescents. *Journal of Early Adolescence, 15*, 38–57.

Hudley, C. (1997). Issues of race and gender in the educational achievement of African-American children. In B. Bank & P. Hall (Eds.), *Gender, equity, and schooling* (pp. 113–133). New York: Garland Press.

Hudley, C., & Graham, S. (2001). Stereotypes of achievement strivings among early adolescents. *Social Psychology of Education, 5*, 201–224.

Hughes, D., & Chen, L. (1997). When and what parents tell children about race: An examination of race-related socialization among African American families. *Applied Developmental Science, 1*, 200–214.

Jencks, C., & Phillips, M. (1998). The black–white test score gap: An introduction. In C. Jencks & M. Phillips (Eds.), *The black–white test score gap* (pp. 1–51). Washington, DC: Brookings Institution Press.

Jones, J. (1997). *Prejudice and racism* (2nd ed). New York: McGraw-Hill.

Jussim, L., Eccles, J., & Madon, S. (1996). Social perception, social stereotypes, and teacher expectations: Accuracy and the quest for the powerful self-fulfilling prophesy. *Advances in Experimental Social Psychology, 29*, 281–388.

Kaiser, C., & Miller, C. (2001). Stop complaining!: The social costs of making attributions to discrimination. *Personality and Social Psychology Bulletin, 27*, 254–263.

Kao, G. (1995). Asian Americans as model minorities?: A look at their academic performance. *American Journal of Education, 103*, 121–159.

Kao, G. (2000). Group images and possible selves among adolescents: Linking stereotypes to expectations by race and ethnicity. *Sociological Forum, 15*, 407–431.

Kao, G., & Tienda, M. (1995). Optimism and achievement: The educational performance of immigrant youth. *Social Science Quarterly, 76*, 1–19.

Kawakami, K., Dovidio, J. F., Moll, J., Hermsen, S., & Russin, A. (2000). Just say no (to stereotyping): Effects of training in the negation of stereotypic associations on stereotype activation. *Journal of Personality and Social Psychology, 78*, 871–888.

Kessler, R., Mickelson, K., & Williams, D. (1999). The prevalence, distributions, and mental health correlates of perceived discrimination in the United States. *Journal of Health and Social Behavior, 40*, 208–230.

Krueger, J. (1996). Personal beliefs and cultural stereotypes about racial characteristics. *Journal of Personality and Social Psychology, 71*, 536–548.

LaFromboise, T., Coleman, H., & Gerton, J. (1993). Psychological impact of biculturalism: Evidence and theory. *Psychological Bulletin, 114*, 395–412.

Lasley-Barajas, H., & Pierce, J. (2001). The significance of race and gender in school success among Latinas and Latinos in college. *Gender and Society, 15*, 859–878.

LaVeist, T., Sellers, R., & Neighbors, H. (2001). Perceived racism and self and system blame attribution: Consequences for longevity. *Ethnicity and Disease, 11*, 711–721.

Lee, S. (1994). Behind the model-minority stereotype: Voices of high- and low-achieving Asian American students. *Anthropology and Education Quarterly, 25*, 413–429.

Leonard, K., Pope, C., & Feyerherm, W. (Eds.). (1995). *Minorities in juvenile justice.* Thousand Oaks, CA: Sage.

Major, B., Quinton, W., & McCoy, S. (2002). Antecedents and consequences of attributions to discrimination: Theoretical and empirical advances. In M. Zanna (Ed.), *Advances in experimental social psychology* (Vol. 34, pp. 252–330). New York: Academic Press.

Major, B., & Schmader, T. (2001). Coping with stigma through psychological disengagement. In J. Swim & C. Sangor (Eds.), *Prejudice: The target's perspective* (pp. 219–241). San Diego, CA: Academic Press.

Major, B., Spencer, S., Schmader, T., Wolfe, C., & Crocker, J. (1998). Coping with negative stereotypes about intellectual performance: The role of psychological disengagement. *Personality and Social Psychology Bulletin, 24*, 34–50.

Matute-Bianchi, M. (1991). Situational ethnicity and patterns of school performance among immigrant and nonimmigrant Mexican-descent students. In M. Gibson & J. Ogbu (Eds.), *Minority status and schooling: A comparative study of immigrant and involuntary minorities* (pp. 205–247). New York: Garland Press.

Merton, R. (1957). *Social theory and social structure.* New York: Free Press.

Moghaddam, F., Taylor, D., Lambert, W., & Schmidt, A. (1995). Attributions and discrimination: A study of attributions to the self, the group, and external factors among Whites, Blacks, and Cubans in Miami. *Journal of Cross Cultural Psychology, 26*, 209–220.

Montgomery, D., Miville, M., Winterowd, C., Jeffries, B., & Baysden, M. (2000). American Indian college students: An exploration into resiliency factors revealed through personal stories. *Cultural Diversity and Ethnic Minority Psychology, 6*, 387–398.

Mueller, C., & Dweck, C. (1998). Praise for intelligence can undermine children's motivation and performance. *Journal of Personality and Social Psychology, 75*, 33–52.

Niemann, Y., Pollack, K., Rogers, S., & O'Connor, E. (1998). Effects of physical context in stereotyping of Mexican-American males. *Hispanic Journal of Behavioral Sciences, 20*, 349–362.

O'Connor, C. (1999). Race, class, and gender in America: Narratives of opportunity among low-income African American youths. *Sociology of Education, 72*, 137–157.

Ogbu, J. (1978). *Minority education and caste: The American system in cross-cultural perspective.* New York: Academic Press.

Ogbu, J. (2003). *Black students in an affluent suburb: A study of academic disengagement.* Mahwah, NJ: Erlbaum.

Okagaki, L., Frensch, P., & Dodson, N. (1996). Mexican American children's perceptions of self and school achievement. *Hispanic Journal of Behavioral Sciences, 18,* 469–484.

Osborne, J. (1997). Race and academic disengagement. *Journal of Educational Psychology, 89,* 728–735.

Oyserman, D., Harrison, K., & Bybee, D. (2001). Can racial identity be promotive of academic efficacy? *International Journal of Behavioral Development, 25,* 379–385.

Oyserman, D., & Sakamoto, I. (1997). Being Asian American: Identity, cultural constructs, and stereotype perception. *Journal of Applied Behavioral Science, 33,* 435–453.

Phinney, J. (1990). Ethnic identity in adolescents and adults: Review of research. *Psychological Bulletin, 108,* 499–514.

Phinney, J. (1996). When we talk about American ethnic groups, what do we mean? *American Psychologist, 51,* 918–927.

Phinney, J., Madden, T., & Santos, L. (1998). Psychological variables as predictors of perceived ethnic discrimination among minority and immigrant adolescents. *Journal of Applied Social Psychology, 28,* 937–953.

Pierce, C. (1995). Stress analogs of racism and sexism: Terrorism, torture, and disaster. In C. Willie, P. Reiker, & B. Brown (Eds.), *Mental health, racism, and sexism* (pp. 277–293). Pittsburgh: University of Pittsburgh Press.

Poe-Yamagata, E., & Jones, M. (2000). *And justice for some: Differential treatment of minority youth in the justice system.* Washington, DC: Building Blocks for Youth.

Portes, A., & Zhou, M. (1993). The new second generation: Segmented assimilation and its variants among post-1965 immigrant youth. *Annals of the American Academy of Political and Social Science, 530,* 74–96.

Rong, X., & Brown, F. (2001). The effects of immigrant generation and ethnicity on educational attainment among young African and Caribbean Blacks in the United States. *Harvard Educational Review, 71,* 536–565.

Rosen, B., & d'Andrade, R. (1959). The social origins of achievement motivation. *Sociometry, 22,* 185–217.

Rosenthal, R., & Jacobson, L. (1968). *Pygmalion in the classroom: Teacher expectations and student intellectual development.* New York: Holt, Rinehart & Winston.

Ruble, D., & Martin, C. (1998). Gender development. In N. Eisenberg (Ed.), *Handbook of child psychology* (5th ed., Vol. 3, pp. 993–1016). New York: Wiley.

Rubovits, P., & Maehr, M. (1973). Pygmalion black and white. *Journal of Personality and Social Psychology, 25,* 210–218.

Ruggierro, K., & Taylor, D. (1995). Coping with discrimination: How disadvantaged group members perceive the disadvantage that confronts them. *Journal of Personality and Social Psychology, 68,* 826–838.

Rumbaut, R. (1994). The crucible within: Ethnic identity, self-esteem, and segmented assimilation among children of immigrants. *International Migration Review, 28*(4), 748–794.

Schmitt, M., & Branscombe, N. (2002). The internal and external causal loci of attributions to prejudice. *Personality and Social Psychology Bulletin, 28,* 620–628.

Schofield, J. (1991). School desegregation and intergroup relations: A review of the literature. *Review of Research in Education, 17,* 335–409.

Schuman, H., Steeh, C., Bobo, L., & Krysan, M. (1997). *Racial attitudes in America: Trends and interpretations.* Cambridge, MA: Harvard University Press.

Sellers, R., Chavous, T., & Cooke, D. (1998). Racial ideology and racial centrality as predictors of African American college students' academic performance. *Journal of Black Psychology, 24,* 8–27.

Sellers, R., & Shelton, J. (2003). The role of racial identity in perceived racial discrimination. *Journal of Personality and Social Psychology, 84,* 1079–1092.

Sellers, R., Smith, M., Shelton, J., Rowley, S., & Chavous, T. (1998). Multidimensional model of racial identity: A reconceptualization of African American identity. *Personality and Social Psychology Review, 2,* 18–39.

Sidanius, J., & Pratto, F. (1999). *Social dominance.* New York: Cambridge University Press.

Simons, R., Murry, V., McLoyd, V., Lin, K., Cutrona, C., & Conger, R. (2002). Discrimination, crime, ethnic identity, and parenting as correlates of depressive symptoms among African American children: A multilevel analysis. *Development and Psychopathology, 14,* 371–393.

Skiba, R. J. (2001). When is disproportionality discrimination?: The overrepresentation of black students in school suspension. In W. Ayers, B. Dohrn, & R. Ayers (Eds.), *Zero tolerance: Resisting the drive for punishment in our schools* (pp. 176–187). New York: New Press.

Smith, E., Walker, K., Fields, L., Brookins, C., & Seay, R. (1999). Ethnic identity and its relationship to self-esteem, perceived efficacy and prosocial attitudes in early adolescence. *Journal of Adolescence, 22,* 867–880.

Solorzano, D. (2000). Critical race theory, racial microaggressions, and campus racial climate: The experiences of African American college students. *Journal of Negro Education, 69,* 60–73.

Spencer, M., Noll, E., Stoltzfus, J., & Harpalani, V. (2001). Identity and school adjustment: Revisiting the "acting White" assumption. *Educational Psychologist, 36,* 21–30.

Stangor, C., Swim, J., Van Allen, K., & Sechrist, G.

(2002). Reporting discrimination in public and private contexts. *Journal of Personality and Social Psychology, 82,* 69–74.

Steele, C. (1992, April). Race and the schooling of Black Americans. *Atlantic Monthly,* pp. 68–78.

Steele, C. (1997). A threat in the air: How stereotypes shape the intellectual identities of women and African Americans. *American Psychologist, 52,* 613–629.

Steele, C., & Aronson, J. (1995). Stereotype threat and the intellectual performance of African Americans. *Journal of Personality and Social Psychology, 69,* 797–811.

Suarez-Orozco, C., & Suarez-Orozco, M. (1995). *Transformations: Migration, family life, and achievement motivation among Latino adolescents.* Stanford, CA: Stanford University Press.

Sue, S., & Okazaki, S. (1990). Asian American educational achievements: A phenomenon in search of an explanation. *American Psychologist, 45,* 913–920.

Tatum, B. (1997). *Why are all the Black kids sitting together in the cafeteria?* New York: Basic Books.

Taylor, R., Casten, R., Flickinger, S., Roberts, D., & Fulmore, C. (1994). Explaining the school performance of African-American adolescents. *Journal of Research on Adolescence, 4,* 21–44.

Thomas, D., Townsend, T., & Belgrave, F. (2003). The influence of cultural and racial identification on the psychosocial adjustment of inner-city African American children in school. *American Journal of Community Psychology, 32,* 217–228.

Waters, M. (1994). Ethnic and racial identities of second-generation Black immigrants in New York City. *International Migration Review, 28,* 795–820.

Weiner, B. (1985). An attributional theory of achievement motivation and emotion. *Psychological Review, 92,* 548–573.

Weiner, B. (1995). *Judgments of responsibility: A foundation for a theory of social conduct.* New York: Guilford Press.

Witherspoon, K., Speight, S., & Thomas, A. (1997). Racial identity attitudes, school achievement, and academic self-efficacy among African American high school students. *Journal of Black Psychology, 23,* 344–357.

Yee, A., Fairchild, H., Weizmann, F., & Wyatt, G. (1993). Addressing psychology's problems with race. *American Psychologist, 48,* 1132–1140.

Zhou, M. (1997). Growing up American: The challenge confronting immigrant children and children of immigrants. *Annual Review of Sociology, 23,* 63–95.

CHAPTER 23

CR

Children's Competence and Socioeconomic Status in the Family and Neighborhood

JEANNE BROOKS-GUNN
MIRIAM R. LINVER
REBECCA C. FAUTH

In 2001, 16% of children in the United States lived in poverty. Although this figure has dropped in the last decade, the poverty rates in the United States surpass those of other industrialized nations (Federal Interagency on Child and Family Statistics, 2003). Rates for children residing in female-headed households and for minority children are even higher (i.e., 54% and 30%, respectively). Growing up in poverty has detrimental impacts on young children's well-being across multiple domains, including children's school readiness and educational outcomes, as well as their physical and mental health (see Brooks-Gunn & Duncan, 1997; Leventhal & Brooks-Gunn, 2002). Other outcomes, including children's competence, while important to children's future well-being and adjustment (Dweck, 2002; Elliot & Thrash, 2001; Harackiewicz, Barron, Tauer, & Elliot, 2002), have been studied less often as correlates of childhood poverty.

Although family income and poverty status are the most frequently studied indicators of family socioeconomic status (SES), empirical work has identified other correlates of child well-being, the most important of these is parental education (see e.g., Duncan, Brooks-Gunn, & Klebanov, 1994; Magnuson, 2003; Smith, Brooks-Gunn, & Klebanov, 1997). Family structure (typically measured as living in a two-parent vs. single-parent family, or living with both biological parents vs. living with one biological parent and a stepparent), parental occupation, and especially in the case of mothers, parental employment are also important (Bornstein & Bradley, 2003; Brooks-Gunn, Duncan, & Rebello, 1999; Hoffman & Youngblade, 1999; Leventhal & Brooks-Gunn, 2000; McLanahan & Sandefur, 1994; Smith, Brooks-Gunn, & Jackson, 1997). Neighborhood SES may also be associated with child well-being, independent of (or over and above) family SES, although the evidence for these links is less clear than the evidence for family SES (Jencks & Mayer, 1990; Leventhal & Brooks-Gunn, 2000).

In this chapter, we define SES broadly for several reasons. First, there are multiple indicators of SES (i.e., income, wealth, parental education, family structure, and occupation), all of which theoretically may have independent associations with child well-being. Second, these SES conditions usually co-occur, such that even when studies present results for individual conditions (via regression analyses), they cannot always be neatly unpacked. Analyses based on regressions represent an "ideal" child rather than a "real" child (Zhao, Brooks-Gunn, McLanahan, & Singer, 1999). More person-oriented approaches to the links between SES and child well-being are not reviewed in this chapter, due to the paucity of relevant research. However, we wish to highlight this limitation of the extant regression-based work. Third, SES conditions vary over time.

This chapter explores in detail the topic of links between SES and children's well-being. In the first section, we discuss common ways of measuring income poverty and SES, and potential limitations of the current measures. Second, we review research documenting direct associations between family and neighborhood SES measures and child well-being; we focus on children, because not all relevant studies include adolescent samples. Associations between SES and children's well-being are likely indirect, operating through a variety of pathways involving family (parental mental health, parenting practices) and neighborhood (environmental toxins, neighborhood resources, and community norms).

MEASUREMENT OF SOCIOECONOMIC STATUS

Family Socioeconomic Status

In this chapter, we review four family-level SES conditions: measures of economic conditions (e.g., earned income, wealth/assets, income-to-needs ratios), human capital variables (e.g., parental education, cognitive skills), parental employment, and family structure–turbulence (e.g., marital dissolution, residential mobility).

Economic Conditions

Family-level economic conditions are frequently measured via money, wealth/assets, government cash transfers and tax benefits, and, for low-income families, poverty thresholds. Earned income is the most common indicator of family economic well-being. Because population income distributions are often positively skewed (i.e., many families cluster at the low end of the distribution), the logged form of income is often used in regression models (Conley, 1999; Duncan, Yeung, Brooks-Gunn, & Smith, 1998; Mayer, 1997b). Other scholars use hourly earnings as an assessment of family economic conditions, especially in lower income samples, where employees often earn an hourly wage versus a salary (Petersen, 1989). Larger families presumably need more resources than smaller families to live comfortably, so the number of household members is often included in analytic models in order to place the proper weight on income (Phillips, Brooks-Gunn, Duncan, Klebanov, & Crane, 1998). Furthermore, due to increased measurement stability, a sum of several years of income data compared with a single-year measure is the preferred measure in most economic and sociological studies (Duncan et al., 1994; Mayer, 1997b).

Some scholars suggest that assets, including savings accounts, stocks, and homes, are more stable indicators of SES than yearly earned income measures given the variability of the latter (Mayer, 1997a). An obvious problem with using asset measures is that low-income individuals may not have any assets. Another issue involves cash transfers, such as Temporary Assistance for Needy Families (TANF), child support, and the Earned Income Tax Credit (EITC). These transfers supplement family income and thus should be considered in assessments of families' economic conditions, especially in low-income samples. Assessments of families' disposable income should include both money income from all sources and the value of in-kind benefits, such as food stamps and housing vouchers (Citro & Michael, 1995).

In the United States, income poverty is defined via an absolute rather than a relative threshold. The current measure, developed in 1959, is based on expected food expenditures for families of varying sizes and adjusted annually for the cost of living. As seen in Figure 23.1, the child poverty rate exceeded 25% in 1959, the first year official poverty rates were available, declined in the 1960s, and then began rising in the 1970s and 1980s. In 2003, the poverty threshold for a single mother raising two children was $14,824, and for a two-parent, two-child family, it was $18,660 (U.S. Bureau of the Census, 2003).

Studies of basic family budgets suggest that the current U.S. poverty threshold may be too low, because even families above the poverty level (especially in metropolitan versus rural areas), are not able to "make ends meet" (Edin & Jencks, 1992; Edin & Lein, 1997; Mayer & Jencks, 1988). Researchers have also noted that the current poverty measure has never been revised. Thus, the cutoff, based on food expenditures as approximately one-third of families' expenses, overestimates the proportion of families' income allotted to food. Today, food spending has decreased to approximately one-fifth of the family budget (Citro & Michael, 1995),

due in part to large increases in the proportion of income needed to maintain housing. Other critiques of the absolute poverty threshold measure currently used in the United States include its lack of attention to regional differences in the cost of living (Betson & Michael, 1997), its exclusion of cash transfers (e.g., TANF, child support) and housing subsidies in calculations of families' income, and that the threshold measure does not take into account expenses associated with employment (e.g., transportation, child care) or benefits such as food stamps or health insurance.

Because the United States poverty threshold is so low, poverty is often defined up to 150% of the threshold (or, in a single-parent family, $22,236, and in a two-parent, two-child family, $27,990). Indeed, some federal programs use 185% of the poverty threshold as the eligibility cutoff including the Women, Infants, and Children (WIC) program, the federal nutrition program, and Medicaid (Currie, 1997; Devaney, Ellwood, & Love, 1997). The income-to-needs ratio, a frequently used extension of the standard

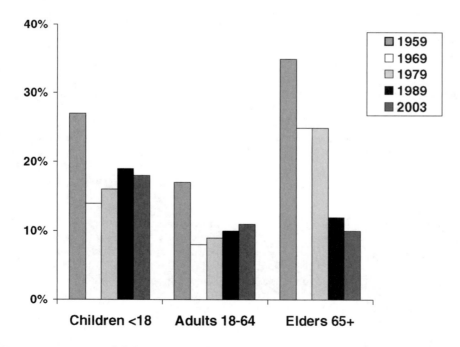

FIGURE 23.1. Percentage of children and adults who were poor from 1959 to 2003. From U.S. Bureau of the Census (2003).

poverty measure, is calculated to adjust income for household size. For example, an income-to-needs ratio of 1.0 indicates that the family is living at the poverty threshold, a ratio of 0.5 is indicative of living at half of the poverty threshold (i.e., deep poverty), and a ratio of 2.0 is defined as living at twice the poverty threshold (Duncan & Brooks-Gunn, 1997).

Human Capital

Human capital, another facet of families' SES, captures personal attributes that are productive in an economic market (Becker & Tomes, 1986). Parental cognitive skills are an example of human capital, because they represent an endowment that may benefit children. These skills are assessed using a variety of instruments, including short-word definition tests (e.g., the General Social Survey asked adults to provide definitions for 10 words over the telephone), receptive verbal ability (e.g., pointing to one of four pictures when given a word, as in the Peabody Picture Vocabulary Test), cognitive test batteries (e.g., the Armed Forces Qualification Test includes arithmetic reasoning, math knowledge, paragraph comprehension, and word knowledge), achievement tests (e.g., Peabody Individual Achievement Test, Woodcock–Johnson Tests of Achievement), and full-scale intelligence tests (e.g., Weschler Adult Intelligence Scale, Stanford–Binet Intelligence Scale).

Parents' formal education is another indicator of human capital, because education is an investment with likely returns in the form of wage earnings. Education is usually operationally defined as the number of years of completed schooling.[1] Completed schooling is influenced by both cognitive and noncognitive competencies, including both personality and motivational constructs (e.g., planfulness, orderliness, and efficiency, as recent work has shown; Dunifon, Duncan, & Brooks-Gunn, 2001, 2004).[2]

Low education may impair adults' ability to complete basic tasks, such as counting change during a purchase, reading labels on food/grocery items, understanding medication directions, comprehending public transportation maps and timetables, and understanding government forms and applications (e.g., for housing, social services, TANF, EITC). Measures that have been developed to assess these basic skills have been shown to be predictive of adult success over and above education levels (Baydar, Brooks-Gunn, & Furstenberg, 1993).

Employment

Employment, as it relates to families' SES, is often assessed via occupational complexity and/or status measures and is associated with educational attainment and income (Menaghan & Parcel, 1995; Smith et al., 1997). Measurement is sometimes limited to the head of household, which in two-parent families is the father (regardless of which parent earns more or is more highly educated), and for single-parent families is considered the residential parent (in the vast majority of cases, the mother). Other, less frequently used measures of occupation include percentage of females in a particular occupation, work hazards, and part- versus full-time employment. Parental time allocation is also a consideration, especially for low-income families, because it creates a conflict between availability of parents to engage in child-rearing versus time spent earning money.

Other Measures

Other commonly used measures of families' SES include family structure and turbulence. Single mothers and unwed parents tend to be more disadvantaged than married parents, because these families cannot pool their monetary resources in the same manner as cohabiting and married couples (Jackson, Tienda, & Huang, 2001; McLanahan & Sandefur, 1994; Wilson & Brooks-Gunn, 2001). Turbulence includes marital dissolution (McLanahan & Sandefur, 1994), the birth of another child (Menaghan & Parcel, 1995), and residential moves (Astone & McLanahan, 1994; Haveman, Wolfe, & Spaulding, 1991; Simpson & Fowler, 1994; Tucker, Marx, & Long, 1998). It may also affect families' SES in either direction; that is, whereas divorce, the birth of another child, and moving to a neighborhood with few economic or child care opportunities may deplete families economically, remarriage and/or moving to a resource-rich neighborhood may boost families' SES.

Neighborhood Socioeconomic Status

Each decade, the U.S. Bureau of the Census canvasses the country to provide extensive geographical and socioeconomic information on census tracts and blocks, two commonly used indicators of neighborhood boundaries. Census tracts are small, relatively permanent county (or equivalent) subdivisions containing between 1,000 and 8,000 individuals; tracts are frequently marked via visible, permanent features, such as railroad stations (U.S. Bureau of the Census, 2002). Each tract can be broken down into one to four blocks or block groups in order to gauge more nuanced descriptors of a particular area; tracts cannot be broken down further because of confidentiality concerns. Many census measures parallel those discussed earlier in relation to family SES. Various indicators of structural neighborhood SES are often averaged together to create a single construct (e.g., neighborhood affluence or neighborhood poverty; Leventhal & Brooks-Gunn, 2000).

Economic Conditions

Neighborhood affluence or poverty is generally measured via median or per capita income for a particular tract. Additionally, the fraction of residents living within various income ranges (e.g., less than $10,000 per year, $10,000–$14,999 per year, $15,000–$24,999 per year, and $25,000 or more per year) is also available. The percentage of residents living below the poverty line and the percentage receiving public assistance are other commonly used economic variables.

Human Capital

Human capital can be measured using educational attainment data from the census. For example, the percentage of residents over the age of 25 years with a high school degree is a commonly used indicator. For wealthier tracts, similar variables delineating the percentage of residents with college and/or graduate degrees are also available.

Employment

Labor force status aggregated across individuals in a tract is a community-level indicator of employment. The percentage of residents in management or professional occupations can be used as an assessment of occupational status. Similarly, data regarding the fraction of residents in service, sales, farming, or production industries are also available. Length of travel time to work may be used to gauge access to convenient employment opportunities.

Other Measures

Other commonly used indicators of neighborhood SES include the percentage of residents residing in female-headed households, the percentage of residents who have resided in a tract for less than 5 years, the percentage of minority or foreign-born residents, and the percentage of owner-occupied (vs. rental) housing.

BEHAVIORAL AND SOCIAL ASPECTS OF SOCIOECONOMIC STATUS

Research groups led by Conger (Conger, Rueter, & Conger, 2000; Conger & Elder, 1994), Elder (Elder & Caspi, 1988), and McLoyd (McLoyd, Jayaratne, Ceballo, & Borquez, 1994) have included behavioral aspects in their conceptualization of family economic pressure or hardship, such as families' perceived inability to make ends meet, their sense of not having money for bills and other necessities, and economic adjustments as a result of insufficient resources. Inclusion of these behavioral constructs often accounts for additional variance above and beyond family income, suggesting that although these constructs overlap with income (i.e., they are correlated), they are distinct, to some extent.[3]

FAMILY SOCIOECONOMIC STATUS AND CHILD WELL-BEING

Indicators of child well-being reviewed here include cognitive and academic competence, and behavior problems. These terms are first defined, followed by a discussion of how each is linked with SES.

Cognitive and Academic Competence

Typically, children's cognitive competence is examined by verbal or mathematics ability and is assessed via standardized tests that measure basic skills related to the subject and may serve as predictors of future school performance. The Peabody Picture Vocabulary Test (PPVT) is one example of a receptive verbal ability assessment that measures children's skills related to reading, language, and vocabulary. Academic competence and achievement are related constructs that may be defined by the level a child has reached in a particular subject area (Stipek & Ryan, 1997). For example, the Woodcock–Johnson Tests of Achievement measures achievement and learning in various domains, including letter–word identification and applied problems.

Links between family poverty and lower cognitive test scores are found, starting at 2 to 3 years of age and continuing through childhood (Klebanov, Brooks-Gunn, McCarton, & McCormick, 1998; McLoyd, 1998). These associations are lowered, but do no disappear, when maternal cognitive skills and education are controlled (Crane, 1996; Duncan et al., 1998; Fish & Pinkerman, 2003; Huston, McLoyd, & Garcia Coll, 1994; Korenman, Miller, & Sjaastad, 1995; Liaw & Brooks-Gunn, 1994; McLoyd, 1998). In general, differences between poor and nonpoor children's IQ scores, assessed at 2–5 years of age range from 2 to 4 points (Duncan et al., 1994; Klebanov et al., 1998; Smith, Brooks-Gunn, & Klebanov, 1997). Moreover, test score differences are sustained as children begin formal schooling and may lead to lower achievement, grade retention, and possibly school drop-out over time for poor children (Axinn, Duncan, & Thornton, 1997). Researchers have examined aspects of family SES in addition to income, such as maternal education and single parenthood (Blau, 1999; Smith, Brooks-Gunn, & Klebanov, 1997; Dearing, McCartney, & Taylor, 2001). It is not clear whether income or human capital is more predictive of children's cognitive outcomes (Blau, 1999; Dearing et al., 2001).

When considering the effects of poverty on cognitive and academic competence, it is essential first to consider nuances of poverty, including the timing, depth, and duration of poverty in the child's life. Children fare the worst when the family lives in deep poverty, when family poverty is experienced early in the child's life, and when the child's family lives in poverty for a long time (Brooks-Gunn & Duncan, 1997). Effect sizes are small to moderate; children ages 3–8 years old living in deep poverty scored between 6 and 13 points lower on standardized tests of achievement, IQ, and verbal ability than more affluent children living in families with incomes 1.5–2 times the poverty threshold (Brooks-Gunn & Duncan, 1997; Brooks-Gunn et al., 1994; Korenman et al., 1995; Smith et al., 1997). Smaller test differences are found for children in families who live closer to (but still below) the poverty threshold compared to more affluent children (Smith et al., 1997). Second, family income over an individual's childhood is often unstable (Duncan, 1988). With respect to timing, early childhood poverty is more predictive of high school completion than is middle childhood or early adolescent family poverty (Duncan et al., 1998). For example, a $10,000 increase in family income during the first 5 years of life for children in the bottom half of the income distribution was associated with a 1-year increase in completed schooling. Third, children age 5 living in persistent poverty (in this study, defined as being poor over a 4-year span) scored 6–9 points lower on test scores than children who were never poor (Smith et al., 1997). Long-term poverty (measured over a 13-year time span) had a greater impact on children than short-term poverty (family poverty in the year before cognitive scores measured), even after controlling for a number of demographic characteristics (Korenman et al., 1995).

Behavior Problems

Behavior problems are discussed with respect to more global mental health, including attention and self-regulation. Children's self-regulation is usually captured via a number of constructs, including motor control, cognitive control, delay of gratification, and sustained attention (see McCabe, Hernandez, Lara, & Brooks-Gunn, 2000; McCabe, Hernandez, Rebello-Britto, & Brooks-Gunn, 2004). Early self-regulation is associated with fewer behavior problems later in childhood (Rothbart & Bates, 1998). One study reported that sustained attention and inhibitory control tasks moderated the association between family SES (measured via maternal education) and children's level of hyperactivity, with high self-regulators (compared with low self-regulators) being more sensitive to declines in SES (Miech, Essex, & Goldsmith, 2001). Children's motor control abilities and attention have been studied as correlates of early health risk factors such as low birth weight, lead exposure, and poor nutrition, which are more common among low-income children (Hack, Klein, & Taylor, 1995; McMichael et al., 1988; Starfield et al., 1991; Taylor, Klein, Minich, & Hack, 2000).

Parents of poor children are more likely than parents of nonpoor children to report that their child has ever had an emotional or behavioral problem and been treated for such problems (Korenman et al., 1995; McLeod & Shanahan, 1993). Family income and poverty status, over and above maternal education and family structure, have small-to-moderate effects on young children's externalizing and internalizing behaviors (Brooks-Gunn, Duncan, Klebanov, & Sealand, 1993; Duncan et al., 1994; Klebanov, Brooks-Gunn, & McCormick, 1994; Smith et al., 1997). Associations between family SES and children's mental health are generally smaller than those found between family SES and children's cognitive outcomes. Lower parental education and living in a single-parent home are associated with behavior problems; family structure has a greater effect on behavior problems than achievement, while parental education has more influence on achievement compared to behavior problems (Amato, 2000; Linver, Brooks-Gunn, & Kohen, 2002).

The timing, depth, and duration of childhood poverty may differentially affect children's mental health outcomes. Early childhood poverty has been associated with depression that persists until late childhood and may also impact adolescent's antisocial behavior, anxiety, and hyperactivity (McLeod & Shanahan, 1996; Pagani, Boulerice, & Tremblay, 1997). Compared with nonpoor peers, young children living in persistent poverty have higher internalizing problem scores (Duncan et al., 1994). Some researchers have found that persistent poverty is associated with externalizing problems (e.g., Hanson, McLanahan, & Thomson, 1997). A recent study of American Indian children revealed that the higher levels of psychiatric symptoms exhibited by poor children were attenuated 4 years later among children who were no longer living in poverty, particularly for externalizing symptoms (Costello, Compton, Keeler, & Angold, 2003). Elevated psychiatric symptoms were only seen among the persistently poor children. Finally, deep poverty is more strongly associated with children's behavior problems than less poor children living at the poverty threshold (Smith, Bastiani, & Brooks-Gunn, 1998).

NEIGHBORHOOD SOCIOECONOMIC STATUS AND CHILD WELL-BEING

In the following sections, we review associations between neighborhood SES and children's well-being. Poor children and families are more likely than their nonpoor counterparts to grow up in disadvantaged neighborhoods characterized by unemployment and crime. Neighborhood residence may be more important for adolescents than for children, due to their increased independence from parents and their peer group interaction (Aber, Gephart, Brooks-Gunn, & Connell, 1997; Graber & Brooks-Gunn, 1996). Studies have examined associations between various neighborhood SES dimensions and children's outcomes. This review summarizes only studies that simultaneously controlled for family-level SES indicators to avoid attributing neighborhood effects to family effects. Whenever possible, results are presented by the type of neighborhood SES condition indicator utilized, including neighborhood poverty or affluence (median income, percentage of poor, percentage on public assistance), employment rates, racial/ethnic diversity, and residential stability.

Cognitive and Academic Competence

Research using data from large longitudinal studies (e.g., Infant Health and Development Program [IHDP], Children of the National

Longitudinal Survey of Youth [NLSY-CS]) has documented positive associations between neighborhood affluence (e.g., proportion of residents earning $30,000 or more per year, proportion of adult residents with 13 or more years of schooling, proportion of professional workers) and children's school readiness and achievement outcomes. Neighborhood-level effects, though significant, are much smaller than family-level effects. Although neighborhood SES was not a significant predictor of very young children's (i.e., 2 years or younger) IQ scores (Klebanov et al., 1998), neighborhood affluence was positively associated with preschool-age children's IQ and vocabulary scores, especially for boys and white children (Brooks-Gunn, Duncan, et al., 1993; Chase-Lansdale, Gordon, Brooks-Gunn, & Klebanov, 1997). These associations persisted once children entered kindergarten or first grade (Chase-Lansdale & Gordon, 1996; Chase-Lansdale et al., 1997; Duncan et al., 1994) and among a slightly older sample of fifth graders for various outcomes, including IQ scores and reading achievement (Shumow, Vandell, & Posner, 1999). Experimental evidence from the Moving to Opportunity (MTO) for Fair Housing Demonstration, in which low-income, minority children were randomly selected to move out of housing projects in high-poverty areas to private housing in low-poverty neighborhoods, revealed minimal achievement differences between children who moved to low-poverty neighborhoods and children in the original, high-poverty neighborhoods approximately 6 years following moves (Orr et al., 2003). However, in this experiment, children did not move to higher quality schools (Leventhal & Brooks-Gunn, 2004).

Although less common, associations between neighborhood poverty (e.g., percentage of poor, percentage on public assistance, percentage of unemployed, and percentage of female-headed households) and measures of children's cognitive ability and achievement outcomes have been found. Most studies have documented negative links between neighborhood disadvantage and children's cognitive outcomes (Halpern-Felsher et al., 1997; Kohen, Brooks-Gunn, Leventhal, & Hertzman, 2002; McCulloch & Joshi, 2001). The degree of racial/ethnic diversity

in a neighborhood was negatively associated with outcomes in a few studies, especially for white children (Brooks-Gunn, Duncan et al., 1993; Chase-Lansdale et al., 1997).

Neighborhood effects on children's outcomes may be moderated by family SES. For example, one study using a nationally representative sample of eighth graders found the negative association between neighborhood disadvantage and children's math scores was moderated by family SES, with the largest associations found for high-SES children (Catsambis & Beveridge, 2001). Another study, with a slightly older sample, reported strong positive associations between neighborhood income and children's PPVT scores, when family income was low (Gordon et al., 2003). In the same study, a mismatch between family and neighborhood income was associated with elevated attention-deficit/hyperactivity disorder symptoms.

Behavior Problems

Most frequently, associations between neighborhood low-SES (vs. high-SES) and behavior problems have been documented. A British study documented associations between residence in poor neighborhoods and more behavior problems among 2-year-olds (Caspi, Taylor, Moffitt, & Plomin, 2000). High adult male unemployment and low percentages of professional workers have been associated with more problems for 3- to 4-year-olds (Brooks-Gunn, Duncan et al., 1993; Chase-Lansdale et al., 1997). Several international studies reported similar links between neighborhood SES and 4- to 7-year-old children's behavior problems (Boyle & Lipman, 2002; Kalff et al., 2001; Kohen et al., 2002). Results for 5- to 6-year-olds' externalizing problems are similar (Chase-Lansdale et al., 1997). However, residence in affluent neighborhoods was also associated with higher levels of internalizing problems (Chase-Lansdale & Gordon, 1996). Are neighborhood effects conditional on family SES? High-SES in one domain (i.e., family or neighborhood) attenuated negative associations between disadvantage in the other domain on children's behavior problems and self-esteem (Boyle & Lipman, 2002; Turley, 2002).

PATHWAYS BETWEEN SOCIOECONOMIC STATUS AND CHILD WELL-BEING

Child development occurs within several distinct but interrelated ecological systems, including the family, the school, the neighborhood, and the wider network of community and government institutions (Bronfenbrenner, 1979). Here, we consider poverty's influences on child well-being, through family- and neighborhood-level characteristics and resources. Risk factors within and between ecological levels frequently co-occur; children who experience poverty are also likely to experience additional risk factors, such as attending a lower quality school or living in an impoverished neighborhood (Brooks-Gunn & Duncan, 1997). In fact, cumulative effects of multiple risk factors are greater than the additive combination of the effects of individual risks (Liaw & Brooks-Gunn, 1994; Sameroff, Seifer, Baldwin, & Baldwin, 1993; Sameroff, Seifer, Baroas, Zax, & Greenspan, 1987).

Family Mechanisms

As reviewed previously, associations between income and SES on young children's well-being are consistently found. The family stress model and the investment model have hypothesized pathways through which low income operates.

The Family Stress Model

The family stress model (and related models) hypothesizes that low income, unemployment, and income loss lead to family financial strain, which in turn influences parental mental health and parenting behavior (Conger, Conger, & Elder, 1997; Elder, 1999; McLoyd, 1989, 1990). The proposed pathways differ somewhat from scholar to scholar: Some believe that parenting behavior may be directly influenced by financial strain, while others believe that such associations are usually mediated through parental mental health.

Parental mental health, notably, emotional health (e.g., depression, anxiety), may link family SES with children's outcomes. Maternal depression has been shown to predict decreased cognitive and academic competence among children (Downey & Coyne, 1990; Murray, Fiori-Cowley, Hooper, & Cooper, 1996), as well as increased behavior problems (Alpern & Lyons-Ruth, 1993; Cicchetti, Rogosch, & Toth, 1998; Downey & Coyne, 1990; Hubbs-Tait et al., 1996; Leadbeater, Bishop, & Raver, 1996; Marchand & Hock, 1998; Shaw & Vondra, 1995). Additionally, parental psychopathologies, including substance abuse, antisocial behavior, and depression, are related to conduct disorder and hyperactivity in children (McGee, Williams, & Silva, 1984; Webster-Stratton, 1998).

Parenting practices are another pathway that link family SES with children's well-being. Warm, nonharsh, and responsive parenting is favorably associated with children's cognitive and mental health outcomes (Bornstein, 1995; Collins, Maccoby, Steinberg, Hetherington, & Bornstein, 2000; McLoyd & Smith, 2002). Moreover, empirical work has demonstrated that economic hardship diminishes parental abilities to provide warm, responsive parenting and contributes to an increase in the use of harsh punishment (McLoyd et al., 1994; Sampson & Laub, 1993; Smith & Brooks-Gunn, 1997).

Warm parenting mediates the relation between economic hardship and academic school performance (Conger et al., 1992, 1993), and harsh parenting mediates the relation between economic hardship and externalizing behavior problems (Conger, Ge, Elder, Lorenz, & Simons, 1994; Conger, Patterson, & Ge, 1995). A recent study reported that 6% of the differences in poor and nonpoor children's behavior problems was explained by maternal depressive affect and parenting practices, yet only 2% of the differences in children's IQ scores was explained by the same factors, indicating that family stress processes are likely more predictive of children's emotional health compared to cognitive outcomes (Linver et al., 2002).

Parental Investments

Income enables families to purchase materials, experiences, and services (including schools, child care, food, housing, stimulating learning materials and activities, and extracurricular activities) to invest in human capital of their children. Children in low-income families tend to have less favorable developmental outcomes due to limited access to resources. This view has been termed the "human capital," "financial resources," or "investment model" (Becker & Tomes, 1986; Haveman & Wolfe, 1994; Mayer, 1997b).

Provision of learning experiences in the home has been associated strongly with child cognitive outcomes (Bradley, 1995; Bradley et al., 1989; Gottfried, Fleming, & Gottfried, 1998; Mayer, 1997b). Many studies use the Home Observation for Measurement of the Environment (HOME) Inventory, to assess the home environment. The HOME is based on observation and interview during a home visit (i.e., types of play materials in the home are observed, and mothers are asked about reading materials and amount of time spent reading to the child). The ways in which parents read to their children are associated with their preschooler's language skills, over and above the amount of reading that occurs in the home (Snow, 1986; Whitehurst et al., 1994; Whitehurst & Lonigan, 1998). In a related vein, help and support provided by mothers during a problem-solving assessment have been associated with young children's enthusiasm and persistence toward the task (Bornstein, 1989; Spiker, Ferguson, & Brooks-Gunn, 1993). Our group has found that providing a stimulating environment in the home (including book reading) mediates the association between income, and children's behavioral and cognitive outcomes (Linver et al., 2002; Yeung, Linver, & Brooks-Gunn, 2002). This follows directly from the investment model, wherein parents with diminished economic conditions have less access to resources (e.g., books, quality child care, and extracurricular lessons) that lead to a more stimulating home environment (Becker & Tomes, 1986; Haveman & Wolfe, 1994).

Involvement in extracurricular activities is another example of a human capital investment in children. The New Hope experiment in Milwaukee, which offered low-income working families job search assistance, earnings supplements, and affordable health and child care, provided some evidence for the importance of extracurricular activities on children's well-being. Elementary school boys whose families received the New Hope supplements were rated by teachers as doing better in school than boys who did not receive additional benefits (Morris, 2002). Additional analyses revealed that boys in the experimental group were more likely to be enrolled in extracurricular activities than boys in the control group, who did not receive services.

Other work using data from the Panel Study of Income Dynamics (PSID) has examined conscientiousness or organization as correlates of earnings (Dunifon et al., 2001; 2004). Specifically, during annual home visits between 1968 and 1972, interviewer assessment of clean house was collected and linked to respondents' earnings in the mid-1990s. Controlling for a rich array of background characteristics and housework, the clean house assessment was modestly predictive of higher earnings. Stronger support for the benefits of a clean house was found for children of the original respondents (also assessed in the mid-1990s). Even after controlling for potentially confounding parent characteristics, including housework, years of schooling, test scores, and measures of psychological-oriented constructs (i.e., efficacy and fear of failure), parents' clean house was positively associated with children's earnings nearly 25 years later.

The clean home measure might be tapping efficiency, as well as organization, both of which might be related to personality or motivational factors. In fact, conscientiousness, which encompasses orderliness, effort, constraint, dependability, and will, is one of the five personality domains identified in many studies of adults (Goldberg, 1990; Wiggins & Pincus, 1992). A long-term study of Harvard College students revealed that conscientiousness during college was associated with income and lower rates of smoking, alcohol abuse, and psychiatric treatment 45 years later (Soldz & Vaillant, 1998). Other work has also reported links between conscientiousness and employment success (Schmidt & Hunter, 1998).

This research review leads to the question of whether parents in cleaner homes relative to parents in less clean homes are more organized and efficient in general, such that they are providing more structure in the home, more family routines, and perhaps more cognitive simulation. The HOME Inventory has a clean home item (Bradley & Caldwell, 1984; Caldwell & Bradley, 1984). Although it does not contain an assessment of clean home per se, the CHAOS (Confusion, Hubbub, and Order) scale was negatively associated with responsive parenting (Corapci & Wachs, 2002; Matheny, Wachs, Ludwig, & Phillips, 1995); for example, lack of order within the home may be associated with low scores on measures of children's task persistence (Evans, Saltzman, & Cooperman, 2001). Whether this is due to internal conditions, such as physical crowding in the home, and/or external environmental conditions, such as traffic and noise, or more generally, the orderliness of the internal environment (independent of crowding and outside traffic), is not known.[4]

Comparing Pathways

Much of the research examining family effects on children's well-being focuses on one or two spheres in isolation. For example, the focus is on how parenting practices affect children's emotional or cognitive well-being or on how family income is correlated with school success. Few researchers have combined multiple domains in order to understand how these contexts may work together to influence children's development. In contrast, some recent work has examined family processes that may serve as links between family economic and human capital indicators and young children's well-being, combining the family stress model with the investment perspective.

For example, in a study of low-wage-earning single black mothers in New York City, we found approximately one-third to one-half of the effects of income on achievement and cognition operated through maternal mental health and parenting behavior (Jackson, Brooks-Gunn, Huang, & Glassman, 2000). Specifically, maternal education and earnings were directly related to financial strain, which in turn was associated with maternal depressive symptoms. Depressive affect was associated with mothers' provision of cognitive stimulation and emotional support to their 3- to 5-year-old children. Completing the link, preschoolers' scores on a school readiness measure directly related to these parenting practices; however, an indirect pathway from financial strain to de-

pression, to parenting, and then to school readiness was not found (Jackson et al., 2000).

When our research group conducted similar models with a large, nationally representative sample, we found evidence of these indirect pathways (Yeung et al., 2002). Family stress model mediators included economic pressure, maternal depressive affect, warm parenting, and parents' use of physical discipline. The physical environment of the home, child care costs, provision of stimulating materials, and parents' activities with the child were included to assess the investment model. Child well-being outcomes included math and reading achievement, and externalizing behaviors. Our results revealed that different mediating mechanisms were at work for different child outcomes. Much of the association between income and children's cognitive test scores was mediated by the family's investment in providing an environment beneficial to children's learning. In contrast, results for children's behavior problems demonstrated that maternal emotional distress was the primary mediator of income associations with children's behavior (Yeung et al., 2002).

Neighborhood Mechanisms

Neighborhood processes that may serve as an important link between neighborhood-level SES and children's competence include environmental toxins, neighborhood resources (child care and schools), and families' sense of community within their neighborhoods, represented by neighborhood collective efficacy (Sampson, Morenoff, & Earls, 1999; Sampson, Raudenbush, & Earls, 1997).

Environmental Toxins

Experimental and nonexperimental studies have documented associations between neighborhood SES and children's health outcomes (e.g., injuries, asthma), which may be due in part to environmental quality (Durkin, Davidson, Kuhn, & O'Connor, 1994; Katz, Kling, & Liebman, 2001; Spengler et al., 2002). There seems to be an asthma epidemic among low-income minority children, particularly those who live in poor urban neighborhoods. Children's breathing problems are associated with exposure to high levels of diesel exhaust (via major roadways), the presence of incinerators, and factories (Carr, Zeitel, & Weiss, 1992; Northridge et al., 1999). One study reported negative associations between children's prenatal exposure to industrial compounds, and their scores on memory and visual discrimination tasks measured at 4 years of age, but not their sustained attention (Jacobson, Jacobson, Padgett, Brumitt, & Billings, 1992). Postnatal exposure via breast-feeding was not associated with children's outcomes, indicating the elevated importance of protecting unborn children from toxins. Children's cognitive well-being may also be affected indirectly by the presence of environmental toxins, because of school absences due to persistent health problems such as asthma (Potasova, 1998).

Resources

Although little empirical evidence is available, the presence or absence of neighborhood resources is a likely conduit between neighborhood SES and children's well-being. Public schools often service children residing in a particular locale. Research has shown that neighborhood SES is a correlate school quality, with lower quality schools clustered in low-income neighborhoods (Jencks & Mayer, 1990). Thus, a child residing in a more affluent neighborhood is likely to receive a higher quality education than a child living in a poor neighborhood. Child care may operate differently for low-income families, because publicly funded child care (e.g., universal prekindergarten programs, Head Start) may be clustered within very low-income areas, and the center-based care accessible to low-income families in these locales is likely to be of higher quality than other arrangements including kith and kin care or unregulated center care (National Institute of Child Health and Development Early Child Care Research Network, 1997; Zigler & Styfco, 2004). Work on family-level economic status indicates that the association between income and child care quality is curvilinear, with families in the middle quintiles receiving lower quality care than families on the top and bottom quintiles (National Institute of Child Health and Human Development Early Child Care Research Network, 1997; Phillips, Voran, Kisker, Howes, & Whitebook, 1994). This trend may extend to neighborhood SES.

What is it about child care and school environments specifically that affect children's well-being? Aspects of the school environment, including school expenditures (Greenwald, Hedges, & Laine, 1996; Hanushek, 1986; Hedges, Laine, & Greenwald, 1994), class size (Finn, 1998; Finn & Achilles, 1990; Glass, Cahen, Smith, & Filby, 1982; Mosteller, 1995; Robinson & Whittebols, 1986; U.S. Department of Education, 1998), teacher qualifications (Darling-Hammond, 2000; Henke, Choy, Chen, Geis, & Alt, 1997; U.S. Department of Education, 1999, 2001), and teacher involvement (Howes & Hamilton, 1992; Skinner & Belmont, 1993; Tucker et al., 2002), may affect children's well-being, although links are often not found. Important aspects of child care quality include health and safety provisions, caregiver quality, developmentally appropriate curriculum, provision of learning activities, small staff-to-child ratios, and staff development, among others (Brooks-Gunn, Fuligni, & Berlin, 2003; Scarr, Eisenberg, & Deater-Deckard, 1994).

Other neighborhood resources, including health clinics, libraries, parks, and recreational programs, may also affect children's well-being. Neighborhood disadvantage may be associated with the type of medical care available (Brooks-Gunn, McCormick, Klebanov, & McCarton, 1998), as well as the prevalence of recreation programs and museums (Catsambis & Beveridge, 2001). Use of recreation programs was higher among families in high-poverty neighborhoods compared with those in moderately poor neighborhoods (Rankin & Quane, 2000), indicating that, if present, families residing in impoverished environments make use of such resources.

Collective Efficacy

Collective efficacy captures shared values among residents and their willingness to intervene on behalf of the community. Collective efficacy is linked with favorable outcomes for children and youth, including achievement (Ainsworth, 2002), school involvement and affiliation with academically oriented peers (Fletcher & Shaw, 2000;

Rankin & Quane, 2002), and avoidance of problematic behavior (Elliott et al., 1996; Gorman-Smith, Tolan, & Henry, 2000; Greenberger, Chen, Beam, Whang, & Dong, 2000; O'Neil, Parke, & McDowell, 2001). Neighborhood disadvantage, residential instability, immigrant concentration, observed neighborhood disorder, and crime are negatively associated with collective efficacy (Raudenbush & Sampson, 1999; Sampson, 1997; Sampson et al., 1997, 1999).[5]

The absence of community-level institutions is associated with exposure to risks including danger, violence, crime, and access to illegal or harmful substances. One study found strong negative associations between neighborhood disorder (e.g., persons arguing, shouting, or fighting in a hostile or threatening manner, as observed by interviewers) and preschool-age children's verbal ability, after controlling for family and neighborhood structural dimensions, as well as maternal mental health (Kohen et al., 2002).

Children and youth reared in poor neighborhoods are likely to be exposed to violence, whether by witnessing or personal victimization (Buka, Stichick, Birdthistle, & Earls, 2001; Martinez & Richters, 1993; Richters & Martinez, 1993). Exposure to violence and disadvantage may lead to hostile attribution bias, wherein children view positive or neutral events through a negative lens (see Bennett & Fraser, 2000). Violent environments may also leave children feeling helpless and with diminished expectations for the future (see Garbarino, 1999). A large body of work has documented the deleterious effects of violence exposure on children's outcomes, ranging from mental health problems to poor academic functioning, attentional difficulties, and low perceived competence (Aneshensel & Sucoff, 1996; Buka et al., 2001; Gorman-Smith & Tolan, 1998; Margolin & Gordis, 2000; Osofsky, 1999; Schwab-Stone et al., 1995, 1999).

Each of the potential neighborhood-level pathways reviewed is directly impacted by neighborhood SES, and in turn, affects children's well-being. Thus, changes in neighborhood SES may not alter children's well-being if they are not coupled with changes in some or all of the potential pathways. Moreover, it is likely that family and neighborhood SES additively influence children, such that low-income children residing in affluent neighborhoods may experience different outcomes than higher income children residing in the same neighborhoods.

SUMMARY, POLICY IMPLICATIONS, AND FUTURE DIRECTIONS

In this chapter, we have focused our review on outcomes for young children; SES in early childhood has lasting impacts on children's well-being. The National Academy of Science's groundbreaking *Neurons to Neighborhoods* concluded that early development "matters a lot, not because this period of development provides an indelible blueprint for adult well-being, but because it sets either a sturdy or fragile stage for what follows" (Shonkoff & Phillips, 2000, p. 5). Children's well-being can have a significant impact on future competencies and successes in adolescence and adulthood, including high school graduation, delayed childbearing, and future earnings; these are all associated with family SES (Brooks-Gunn, Guo, & Furstenberg, 1993; Furstenberg & Hughes, 1995; Trusty, 2000; White & Glick, 2000; Willie, 2001).

Low family and neighborhood SES is problematic for children's well-being. Although economic disadvantage has both harmful and widespread effects on child development, it may be difficult to disentangle the effects of SES from the effects of other risk factors, including, for example, ethnicity, immigrant status, and gender. As detailed in this chapter, SES is directly and indirectly linked with child well-being. The family SES–child outcome link is mediated by familial factors such as parenting, parent mental health, and parental investments, while neighborhood SES is related to child outcomes via environmental toxins, neighborhood resources, and collective efficacy. Researchers are cautioned to examine the effects of SES on child well-being carefully; statistical and methodological techniques are available to consider complex models that can take into account diverse contexts and extensive covariates. More importantly, it is essential to design studies and devise research questions that address the complex relations and contexts linking SES to children's well-being.

Our research findings comparing pathways of SES–child outcome links underscore the importance of trying to understand the process of how family—and wider—contexts are associated with children's well-being. In particular, parenting stands out in our statistical models as a strong mediator, often explaining much of the association between income and child developmental outcomes. However, the connection between parenting and children's well-being is not straightforward. Indeed, other factors, such as the home environment (e.g., single- vs. two-parent family, parental employment, parental mental health), individual characteristics (e.g., race/ethnicity, cognitive functioning), neighborhood characteristics (e.g., access to resources, exposure to violence), and even societal factors (e.g., current policy climate must be taken into account when examining parenting and child well-being).

Children's race/ethnicity is usually controlled for in analyses examining SES and child outcomes. The use of race/ethnicity as a statistical control, however, does not specifically address how race/ethnicity matters for children's well-being. Our group has participated in a line of research parceling out racial test score gaps. White and black children in the United States have vastly different experiences in school and the broader society. Test score gaps are found as early as 3 years of age and persist. Parent education and verbal ability differences account for a large portion of the gap. In addition, we found that the black–white test score gap was influenced by quality of maternal high school, over and above maternal education, maternal verbal ability, and a host of demographic characteristics (including grandparent characteristics) (Phillips et al., 1998). When such characteristics were controlled, the test score gap decreased by 40–85%. This work indicates that parents' schooling influences have lasting impacts on their ability to provide a stimulating environment for their children.

A large body of work has shown negative associations between disadvantage—both at the family and neighborhood levels—and children's well-being, but few researchers have attempted to address how and why this connection is so strong and persists throughout childhood and into adolescence (Jencks & Phillips, 1998). Exploring the processes

that link SES with child well-being is especially critical when thinking about how to improve the school readiness of poor children. Programs geared toward improving young children's cognitive skills may work best if they focus on providing children with cognitively stimulating materials, increasing family literacy, or encouraging parents to engage in reading activities and/or stimulating outings, as well facilitating positive parenting skills (Brooks-Gunn, Berlin, & Fuligni, 2000; Fuligni & Brooks-Gunn, 2000). If a program's goal is to promote healthy development of children across multiple domains, a multipronged approach may be most appropriate. For example, a package of services could be offered to families that includes cash benefits, as well as services that target family literacy, stress relief, parenting practices, and provision of high-quality child care.

ACKNOWLEDGMENTS

We would like to thank the National Institute of Child Health and Human Development Research Network on Child and Family Well-Being, the National Institute of Mental Health Consortium on Child and Adolescent Research, as well as the Family and Work Network of the MacArthur Foundation.

NOTES

1. It is important to note that this definition does not capture differences in quality of education. For example, one study found a negative association between the number of white students at mothers' high schools and the test score gap between black and white children, indicating that attending schools with large proportions of white students (a proxy for school quality) led to smaller race differentials in children's vocabulary scores than attending schools with large minority student bodies, even controlling for mothers' years of school and cognitive ability (Phillips et al., 1998). Virtually all of the current national longitudinal studies collect some data on cognitive skills, as well as education.
2. Cognitive skills and education are highly, but not perfectly, correlated (i.e., correlation coefficients of .40 to .60, in most studies).
3. Whether or not a family lives above the poverty line is not necessarily indicative of the difficulty of making ends meet (Jackson et al.,

2000). Some families living below the poverty line have their basic needs met through, for example, subsidized housing, publicly funded health insurance, TANF payments, child support, and/or food stamps. A working poor family, in contrast, will likely have higher reported income but may lack eligibility for any or all of the benefits just listed, and thus, the family may report high financial strain. A recent study documented this phenomenon with welfare recipients who entered the workforce compared with those who did not; the former reported higher strain than the latter (Gyamfi, Brooks-Gunn, & Jackson, 2001).

4. Although in the analyses using PSID data, the number of individuals in the home and the presence of an individual with health limitations in the home were controlled for in analyses (Dunifon et al., 2001).

5. Although this chapter is most concerned with children, much of the extant research on collective efficacy focuses on adult and youth samples.

REFERENCES

Aber, J. L., Gephart, M. A., Brooks-Gunn, J., & Connell, J. P. (1997). Development in context: Implications for studying neighborhood effects. In J. Brooks-Gunn, G. J. Duncan, & J. L. Aber (Eds.), *Neighborhood poverty: Vol. 1. Context and consequences for children* (pp. 44–61). New York: Russell Sage Foundation.

Ainsworth, J. W. (2002). Why does it take a village?: The mediation of neighborhood effects on educational achievement. *Social Forces, 81*(1), 117–152.

Alpern, L., & Lyons-Ruth, K. (1993). Preschool children at social risk: Chronicity and timing of maternal depressive symptoms and child behavior problems at school and at home. *Development and Psychopathology, 5*, 371–387.

Amato, P. R. (2000). The consequences of divorce for adults and children. *Journal of Marriage and the Family, 62*(4), 1269–1287.

Aneshensel, C. S., & Sucoff, C. A. (1996). The neighborhood context of adolescent mental health. *Journal of Health and Social Behavior, 37*, 293–310.

Astone, N. M., & McLanahan, S. S. (1994). Family structure, residential mobility, and school drop out: A research note. *Demography, 31*, 575–584.

Axinn, W., Duncan, G. J., & Thornton, A. (1997). The effects of parents' income, wealth and attitudes on children's completed schooling and self-esteem. In G. J. Duncan & J. Brooks-Gunn (Eds.), *Consequences of growing up poor* (pp. 518–540). New York: Russell Sage Foundation.

Baydar, N., Brooks-Gunn, J., & Furstenberg, F. F., Jr. (1993). Early warning signs of functional illiteracy:

Predictors in childhood and adolescence. *Child Development, 64*, 815–829.

Becker, G. S., & Tomes, N. (1986). Human capital and the rise and fall of families. *Journal of Labor Economics, 4*, S1–S139.

Bennett, M. D. J., & Fraser, M. W. (2000). Urban violence among African American males: Integrating family, neighborhoods, and peer perspectives. *Journal of Sociology and Social Welfare, 27*(3), 93–117.

Betson, D. M., & Michael, R. T. (1997). Why so many children are poor. *Future of Children, 7*(2), 25–39.

Blau, D. M. (1999). The effect of income on child development. *Review of Economics and Statistics, 81*, 261–276.

Bornstein, M. H. (1989). Between caretakers and their young: Two models of interaction and their consequences for cognitive growth. In M. H. Bornstein & J. S. Bruner (Eds.), *Interactions in human development* (pp. 197–214). Hillsdale, NJ: Erlbaum.

Bornstein, M. H. (Ed.). (1995). *Handbook of parenting*. Mahwah, NJ: Erlbaum.

Bornstein, M. H., & Bradley, R. H. (Eds.). (2003). *Socioeconomic status, parenting, and child development*. Mahwah, NJ: Erlbaum.

Boyle, M. H., & Lipman, E. L. (2002). Do places matter?: Socioeconomic disadvantage and behavioral problems of children in Canada. *Journal of Consulting and Clinical Psychology, 70*(2), 378–389.

Bradley, R. H. (1995). Environment and parenting. In M. H. Bornstein (Ed.), *Handbook of parenting, Vol. 2: Biology and ecology of parenting* (pp. 235–261). Mahwah, NJ: Erlbaum.

Bradley, R. H., & Caldwell, B. M. (1984). The HOME Inventory and family demographics. *Developmental Psychology, 20*(2), 315–320.

Bradley, R. H., Caldwell, B. M., Rock, S. L., Ramey, C. T., Barnard, K. E., Gray, C., et al. (1989). Home environment and cognitive development in the first three years of life: A collaborative study involving six sites and three ethnic groups in North America. *Developmental Psychology, 25*(2), 217–235.

Bronfenbrenner, U. (1979). *The ecology of human development*. Cambridge, MA: Harvard University Press.

Brooks-Gunn, J., Berlin, L. J., & Fuligni, A. S. (2000). Early childhood intervention programs: What about the family? In J. P. Shonkoff & S. J. Meisels (Eds.), *Handbook of early childhood intervention* (2nd ed., pp. 549–588). New York: Cambridge University Press.

Brooks-Gunn, J., & Duncan, G. J. (1997). The effects of poverty on children. *Future of Children, 7*, 55–71.

Brooks-Gunn, J., Duncan, G. J., Klebanov, P. K., & Sealand, N. (1993). Do neighborhoods influence child and adolescent development? *American Journal of Sociology, 99*, 353–395.

Brooks-Gunn, J., Duncan, G. J., & Rebello, P. (1999). Are socioeconomic gradients for children similar to those for adults?: Achievement and health in the United States. In D. Keating & C. Hertzman (Eds.),

Developmental health and the wealth of nations: Social, biological and educational dynamics (pp. 94–124). New York: Guilford Press.

Brooks-Gunn, J., Fuligni, A. S., & Berlin, L. J. (2003). *Early child development in the 21st century: Profiles of current research initiatives.* New York: Teachers College Press, Columbia University.

Brooks-Gunn, J., Guo, G., & Furstenberg, F. F. (1993). Who drops out of and who continues beyond high school?: A 20-year follow-up of Black urban youth. *Journal of Research on Adolescence, 3*(3), 271–294.

Brooks-Gunn, J., McCarton, C., Casey, P., McCormick, M., Bauer, C., Berenbaum, J., et al. (1994). Early intervention in low birth weight, premature infants: Results through age 5 years from the Infant Health and Development Program. *Journal of the American Medical Association, 272,* 1257–1262.

Brooks-Gunn, J., McCormick, M. C., Klebanov, P., & McCarton, C. (1998). Health care use of 3 year-old low birthweight premature children: Effects of family and neighborhood poverty. *Journal of Pediatrics, 132,* 971–975.

Buka, S. L., Stichick, T. L., Birdthistle, I., & Earls, F. J. (2001). Youth exposure to violence: Prevalence, risks, and consequences. *American Journal of Orthopsychiatry, 71*(3), 298–310.

Caldwell, B. M., & Bradley, R. H. (1984). *Home Observation for Measurement of the Environment.* Little Rock: University of Arkansas Press.

Carr, W., Zeitel, L., & Weiss, K. (1992). Variations in asthma hospitalizations and deaths in New York City. *American Journal of Public Health, 82*(1), 59–65.

Caspi, A., Taylor, A., Moffitt, T. E., & Plomin, R. (2000). Neighborhood deprivation affects children's mental health: Environmental risks identified in a genetic design. *Psychological Science, 11,* 338–342.

Catsambis, S., & Beveridge, A. A. (2001). Does neighborhood matter?: Family, neighborhood, and school influences on eight-grade mathematics achievement. *Sociological Focus, 34*(4), 435–457.

Chase-Lansdale, P. L., & Gordon, R. A. (1996). Economic hardship and the development of five- and six-year-olds: Neighborhood and regional perspectives. *Child Development, 67,* 3338–3367.

Chase-Lansdale, P. L., Gordon, R. A., Brooks-Gunn, J., & Klebanov, P. (1997). Neighborhood and family influences on the intellectual and behavioral competence of preschool and early school-age children. In J. Brooks-Gunn, G. J. Duncan, & J. L. Aber (Eds.), *Neighborhood poverty: Vol. 1. Context and consequences for children* (pp. 79–118). New York: Russell Sage Foundation.

Cicchetti, D., Rogosch, F. A., & Toth, S. L. (1998). Maternal depressive disorder and contextual risk: Contributions to the development of attachment insecurity and behavior problems in toddlerhood. *Development and Psychopathology, 10,* 283–300.

Citro, C. F., & Michael, R. T. (Eds.). (1995). *Measuring poverty: A new approach.* Washington, DC: National Academy Press.

Collins, W. A., Maccoby, E. E., Steinberg, L., Hetherington, E. M., & Bornstein, M. H. (2000). Contemporary research on parenting: The case of nature and nurture. *American Psychologist, 55,* 218–232.

Conger, K. J., Rueter, M. A., & Conger, R. D. (2000). The role of economic pressure in the lives of parents and their adolescents: The family stress model. In L. J. Crockett & R. K. Silbereisen (Eds.), *Negotiating adolescence in times of social change* (pp. 201–223). New York: Cambridge University Press.

Conger, R. D., Conger, K. J., & Elder, G. H., Jr. (1997). Family economic hardship and adolescent adjustment: Mediating and moderating processes. In G. J. Duncan & J. Brooks-Gunn (Eds.), *Consequences of growing up poor* (pp. 288–310). New York: Russell Sage Foundation.

Conger, R. D., Conger, K. J., Elder, G. H., Lorenz, F. O., Simons, R. L., & Whitbeck, L. B. (1992). A family process model of economic hardship and adjustment of early adolescent boys. *Child Development, 63,* 526–541.

Conger, R. D., Conger, K. J., Elder, G. H., Lorenz, F. O., Simons, R. L., & Whitbeck, L. B. (1993). Family economic stress and adjustment of early adolescent girls. *Developmental Psychology, 29,* 206–219.

Conger, R. D., & Elder, G. H. (1994). *Families in troubled times: Adapting to change in rural America.* New York: Aldine de Gruyter.

Conger, R. D., Ge, X., Elder, G. H., Lorenz, F. O., & Simons, R. L. (1994). Economic stress, coercive family process, and development problems of adolescents. *Child Development, 65,* 541–561.

Conger, R. D., Patterson, G. R., & Ge, X. (1995). It takes two to replicate: A mediational model for the impact of parents' stress on adolescent adjustment. *Child Development, 66,* 80–97.

Conley, D. (1999). *Being Black, living in the red: Race, wealth, and social policy in America.* Los Angeles: University of California Press.

Corapci, F., & Wachs, T. D. (2002). Does parental mood or efficacy mediate the influence of environmental chaos upon parenting behavior? *Merrill–Palmer Quarterly, 48,* 182–201.

Costello, E. J., Compton, S. N., Keeler, G., & Angold, A. (2003). Relationships between poverty and psychopathology: A natural experiment. *Journal of the American Medical Association, 290*(15), 2023–2029.

Crane, J. (1996). Effects of home environment, SES, and maternal test scores on mathematics achievement. *Journal of Educational Research, 89*(5), 305–314.

Currie, J. M. (1997). Choosing among alternative programs for poor children. *Future of Children, 7,* 113–131.

Darling-Hammond, L. (2000). Teacher quality and student achievement: A review of state policy evidence. *Education Policy Analysis Archives, 8.* Retrieved September 4, 2003, from *http://epaa.asu.edu/epaa/v8n1/.*

Dearing, E., McCartney, K., & Taylor, B. A. (2001). Change in family income-to-needs matters more for children with less. *Child Development, 72,* 1779–1793.

Devaney, B. L., Ellwood, M. R., & Love, J. M. (1997). Programs that mitigate the effects of poverty on children. *Future of Children, 7,* 88–112.

Downey, G., & Coyne, J. C. (1990). Children of depressed parents: An integrative review. *Psychological Bulletin, 108,* 50–76.

Duncan, G. J. (1988). Volatility of family income over the life course. In P. B. Baltes, D. L. Featherman, & R. M. Lerner (Eds.), *Life-span development and behavior* (pp. 317–358). Hillsdale, NJ: Erlbaum.

Duncan, G. J., & Brooks-Gunn, J. (Eds.). (1997). *Consequences of growing up poor.* New York: Russell Sage Foundation.

Duncan, G. J., Brooks-Gunn, J., & Klebanov, P. (1994). Economic deprivation and early-childhood development. *Child Development, 65,* 296–318.

Duncan, G. J., Yeung, W. J., Brooks-Gunn, J., & Smith, J. R. (1998). How much does childhood poverty affect the life chances of children? *American Sociological Review, 63,* 406–423.

Dunifon, R., Duncan, G. J., & Brooks-Gunn, J. (2001). As ye sweep, so shall ye reap. *American Economic Review, 91*(2), 150–154.

Dunifon, R., Duncan, G. J., & Brooks-Gunn, J. (2004). The long-term impact of parental organization and efficiency. In A. Kalil & T. DeLeire (Eds.), *Family investments in children: Resources and behaviors that promote success* (pp. 85–118). Mahwah, NJ: Erlbaum.

Durkin, M. S., Davidson, L. L., Kuhn, L., & O'Connor, P. (1994). Low-income neighborhoods and the risk of severe pediatric injury: A small-area analysis in northern Manhattan. *American Journal of Public Health, 84*(4), 587–592.

Dweck, C. S. (2002). The development of ability conceptions. In A. Wigfield & J. S. Eccles (Eds.), *Development of achievement motivation: A volume in the educational psychology series* (pp. 57–88). San Diego: Academic Press.

Edin, K., & Jencks, C. (1992). Welfare. In C. Jencks (Ed.), *Rethinking social policy* (pp. 204–235). Cambridge, MA: Harvard University Press.

Edin, K., & Lein, L. (1997). *Making ends meet: How single mothers survive welfare and low-wage work.* New York: Russell Sage Foundation.

Elder, G. H. (1999). *Children of the great depression: Social change in life experience.* Boulder, CO: Westview Press.

Elder, G. H., & Caspi, A. (1988). Economic stress in lives: Developmental perspectives. *Journal of Social Issues, 44*(4), 25–45.

Elliot, A. J., & Thrash, T. M. (2001). Achievement goals and the hierarchial model of achievement motivation. *Educational Psychology Review, 13*(2), 139–156.

Elliott, D. S., Wilson, W. J., Huizinga, D., Sampson, R. J., Elliott, A., & Rankin, B. (1996). The effects of neighborhood disadvantage on adolescent development. *Journal of Research in Crime and Delinquency, 33,* 389–426.

Evans, G. W., Saltzman, H., & Cooperman, J. L. (2001). Housing quality and children's socioemotional health. *Environment and Behavior, 33*(3), 389–399.

Federal Interagency on Child and Family Statistics. (2003). *America's children: Key national indicators of well-being 2003.* Washington, DC: U.S. Government Printing Office.

Finn, J. (1998). *Class size and students at risk: What is known? What is next?* Washington, DC: U.S. Department of Education, Office of Educational Research and Improvement, National Institute on the Education of At-Risk Students.

Finn, J., & Achilles, C. (1990). Answers and questions about class size: A statewide experiment. *American Educational Research Journal, 27,* 557–577.

Fish, M., & Pinkerman, B. (2003). Language skills in low-SES rural Appalachian children: Normative development and individual differences, infancy to preschool. *Applied Developmental Psychology, 23,* 539–565.

Fletcher, A. C., & Shaw, R. A. (2000). Sex differences in associations between parental behaviors and characteristics and adolescent social integration. *Social Development, 9*(2), 133–148.

Fuligni, A. S., & Brooks-Gunn, J. (2000). The healthy development of young children: SES disparities, prevention strategies, and policy opportunities. In B. D. Smedley & S. L. Syme (Eds.), *Promoting health: Intervention strategies from social and behavioral research* (pp. 170–216). Washington, DC: National Academy of Sciences.

Furstenberg, F. F., Jr., & Hughes, M. E. (1995). Social capital and successful development among at-risk youth. *Journal of Marriage and the Family, 57,* 580–592.

Garbarino, J. (1999). The effects of community violence on children. In L. Balter & C. S. Tamis-LeMonda (Eds.), *Child psychology: A handbook of contemporary issues* (pp. 412–425). Philadelphia: Taylor & Francis.

Glass, G., Cahen, L., Smith, M., & Filby, N. (1982). *School class size.* Beverly Hills, CA: Sage.

Goldberg, L. R. (1990). An alternative "description of personality": The Big-Five factor structure. *Journal of Personality and Social Psychology, 59,* 1216–1222.

Gordon, R. A., Savage, C., Lahey, B. B., Goodman, S. H., Jensen, P. S., Rubio-Stipec, M., et al. (2003). Family and neighborhood income: Additive and multiplicative associations with youths' well-being. *Social Science Research, 32,* 191–219.

Gorman-Smith, D., & Tolan, P. (1998). The role of exposure to community violence and developmental problems among inner-city youth. *Developmental Psychopathology, 10,* 101–116.

Gorman-Smith, D., Tolan, P., & Henry, D. B. (2000). A developmental–ecological model of the relation of family functioning to patterns of delinquency. *Journal of Quantitative Criminology, 16*(2), 169–198.

Gottfried, A. E., Fleming, J. S., & Gottfried, A. W. (1998). Role of cognitively stimulating home environment in children's academic intrinsic motivation: A longitudinal study. *Child Development, 69*, 1448–1460.

Graber, J. A., & Brooks-Gunn, J. (1996). Transitions and turning points: Navigating the passage from childhood through adolescence. *Developmental Psychology, 32*(4), 768–776.

Greenberger, E., Chen, C., Beam, M., Whang, S.-M., & Dong, Q. (2000). The perceived social contexts of adolescents' misconduct: A comparative study of youths in three cultures. *Journal of Research on Adolescence, 10*(3), 365–388.

Greenwald, R., Hedges, L. V., & Laine, R. D. (1996). The effect of school resources on student achievement. *Review of Educational Research, 66*, 361–396.

Gyamfi, P., Brooks-Gunn, J., & Jackson, A. P. (2001). Associations between employment and financial and parenting stress in low-income single black mothers. *Women and Health, 32*(1), 119–135.

Hack, M., Klein, N. K., & Taylor, H. G. (1995). Long-term developmental outcomes of low birth weight infants. *Future of Children, 5*, 176–196.

Halpern-Felsher, B., Connell, J. P., Spencer, M. B., Aber, J. L., Duncan, G. J., Clifford, E., et al. (1997). Neighborhood and family factors predicting educational risk and attainment in African American and white children and adolescents. In J. Brooks-Gunn, G. J. Duncan, & J. L. Aber (Eds.), *Neighborhood poverty: Vol. 1. Context and consequences for children* (pp. 146–173). New York: Russell Sage Foundation.

Hanson, T. L., McLanahan, S., & Thomson, E. (1997). Economic resources, parental practices, and children's well-being. In G. J. Duncan & J. Brooks-Gunn (Eds.), *Consequences of growing up poor* (pp. 190–238). New York: Russell Sage Foundation.

Hanushek, E. A. (1986). The economics of schooling: Production and efficiency in public schools. *Journal of Economic Literature, 24*, 1141–1177.

Harackiewicz, J. M., Barron, K. E., Tauer, J. M., & Elliot, A. J. (2002). Predicting success in college: A longitudinal study of achievement goals and ability measures as predictors of interest and performance from freshman year through graduation. *Journal of Educational Psychology, 94*(3), 562–575.

Haveman, R., & Wolfe, B. (1994). *Succeeding generations: On the effects of investments in children.* New York: Russell Sage Foundation.

Haveman, R., Wolfe, B., & Spaulding, J. (1991). Child events and circumstances influencing high school completion. *Demography, 28*(1), 133–158.

Hedges, L. V., Laine, R. D., & Greenwald, R. (1994). Does money matter?: A meta-analysis of studies of the effects of differential school inputs on student outcomes. *Educational Researcher, 23*, 5–14.

Henke, R. R., Choy, S. P., Chen, X., Geis, S., & Alt, M. N. (1997). *America's teachers: Profile of a profession, 1993–94* (No. NCES 97–460). Washington, DC: National Center for Education Statistics.

Hoffman, L. W., & Youngblade, L. M. (1999). *Mothers at work: Effects on children's well-being.* New York: Cambridge University Press.

Howes, C., & Hamilton, C. E. (1992). Children's relationships with caregivers: Mothers and child care teachers. *Child Development, 63*(4), 859–866.

Hubbs-Tait, L., Hughes, K. P., Culp, A. M., Osofsky, J. D., Hann, D. M., Eberhart-Wright, A., et al. (1996). Children of adolescent mothers: Attachment representation, maternal depression, and later behavior problems. *American Journal of Orthopsychiatry, 66*, 416–426.

Huston, A. C., McLoyd, V. C., & Garcia Coll, C. T. (1994). Children and poverty: Issues in contemporary research. *Child Development, 65*, 275–282.

Jackson, A. P., Brooks-Gunn, J., Huang, C.-C., & Glassman, M. (2000). Single mothers in low-wage jobs: Financial strain, parenting, and preschoolers' outcomes. *Child Development, 71*(5), 1409–1423.

Jackson, A. P., Tienda, M., & Huang, C.-C. (2001). Capabilities and employability of unwed mothers. *Children and Youth Services Review, 23*(4/5), 327–351.

Jacobson, J. L., Jacobson, S. W., Padgett, R. J., Brumitt, G. A., & Billings, R. L. (1992). Effects of prenatal PCB exposure on cognitive processing efficiency and sustained attention. *Developmental Psychology, 28*(2), 297–306.

Jencks, C., & Mayer, S. (1990). The social consequences of growing up in a poor neighborhood. In L. Lynn & M. McGeary (Eds.), *Inner-city poverty in the United States* (pp. 111–186). Washington, DC: National Academy Press.

Jencks, C., & Phillips, M. (Eds.). (1998). *The Black–White test score gap.* Washington, DC: Brookings Institution Press.

Kalff, A. C., Kroes, M., Vles, J. S. H., Hendriksen, J. G. M., Feron, F. J. M., Steyaert, J., et al. (2001). Neighborhood level and individual level SES effects on child problem behaviour: A multilevel analysis. *Journal of Epidemiology and Community Health, 55*, 246–250.

Katz, L. F., Kling, J. R., & Liebman, J. B. (2001). Moving to Opportunity in Boston: Early results of a randomized mobility experiment. *Quarterly Journal of Economics, 116*, 607–654.

Klebanov, P. K., Brooks-Gunn, J., McCarton, C., & McCormick, M. C. (1998). The contribution of neighborhood and family income to developmental test scores over the first three years of life. *Child Development, 69*, 1420–1436.

Klebanov, P. K., Brooks-Gunn, J., & McCormick, M. C. (1994). Classroom behavior of very low birth weight elementary school children. *Pediatrics, 94*, 700–708.

Kohen, D., Brooks-Gunn, J., Leventhal, T., & Hertzman, C. (2002). Neighborhood income and physical and social disorder in Canada: Associations with young children's competencies. *Child Development*, 73(6), 1844–1860.

Korenman, S., Miller, J. E., & Sjaastad, J. E. (1995). Long-term poverty and child development in the United States: Results from the NLSY. *Children and Youth Services Review*, 17, 127–155.

Leadbeater, B. J., Bishop, S. J., & Raver, C. C. (1996). Quality of mother–toddler interactions, maternal depressive symptoms, and behavior problems in preschoolers of adolescent mothers. *Developmental Psychology*, 32, 280–288.

Leventhal, T., & Brooks-Gunn, J. (2000). The neighborhoods they live in: Effects of neighborhood residence upon child and adolescent outcomes. *Psychological Bulletin*, 126, 309–337.

Leventhal, T., & Brooks-Gunn, J. (2002). Poverty and child development. *International Encyclopedia of the Social and Behavioral Sciences*, 3(14, Article 78), 11889–11893.

Leventhal, T., & Brooks-Gunn, J. (2004). A randomized study of neighborhood effects on low-income children's educational outcomes. *Developmental Psychology*, 40(4), 488–507.

Liaw, F. R., & Brooks-Gunn, J. (1994). Cumulative familial risks and low birth weight children's cognitive and behavioral development. *Journal of Clinical Child Psychology*, 23, 360–372.

Linver, M. R., Brooks-Gunn, J., & Kohen, D. E. (2002). Family processes as pathways from income to young children's development. *Developmental Psychology*, 38(5), 719–734.

Magnuson, K. (2003). *The effect of increases in welfare mothers' education on their young children's academic and behavioral outcomes: Evidence from the National Evaluation of Welfare-to-Work Strategies Child Outcomes Study* (No. 1274–03). Madison, WI: University of Wisconsin, Institute for Poverty Research.

Marchand, J. F., & Hock, E. (1998). The relation of problem behaviors in preschool children to depressive symptoms in mothers and fathers. *Journal of Genetic Psychology*, 159, 353–366.

Margolin, G., & Gordis, E. B. (2000). The effects of family and community violence on children. *Annual Review of Psychology*, 51, 445–479.

Martinez, P., & Richters, J. E. (1993). The NIMH Community Violence Project: II. Children's distress symptoms associated with violence exposure. *Psychiatry*, 56, 22–35.

Matheny, A. P., Wachs, T. D., Ludwig, J. L., & Phillips, K. (1995). Bringing order out of chaos: Psychometric characteristics of the Confusion, Hubbub, and Order Scale. *Journal of Applied Developmental Psychology*, 16(3), 429–444.

Mayer, S. E. (1997a). Trends in the economic well-being and life chances of America's children. In G. J. Duncan & J. Brooks-Gunn (Eds.), *Consequences of growing up poor* (pp. 49–69). New York: Russell Sage Foundation.

Mayer, S. E. (1997b). *What money can't buy: Family income and children's life chances*. Cambridge, MA: Harvard University Press.

Mayer, S. E., & Jencks, C. (1988). Poverty and the distribution of material hardship. *Journal of Human Resources*, 24, 88–113.

McCabe, L. A., Hernandez, M., Lara, S. L., & Brooks-Gunn, J. (2000). Assessing preschoolers' self-regulation in homes and classrooms: Lessons from the field. *Behavioral Disorders*, 26(1), 53–69.

McCabe, L. A., Hernandez, M., Rebello-Britto, P., & Brooks-Gunn, J. (2004). Games children play: Observing young children's self-regulation across laboratory, home, and school settings. In R. DelCarmen-Wiggins & A. Carter (Eds.), *Handbook of infant–toddler mental health assessment* (pp. 491–521). New York: Oxford University Press.

McCulloch, A., & Joshi, H. E. (2001). Neighborhourhood and family influences on the cognitive ability of children in the British National Child Development Study. *Social Science and Medicine*, 53, 579–591.

McGee, R., Williams, S., & Silva, P. A. (1984). Background characteristics of aggressive, hyperactive, and aggressive–hyperactive boys. *Journal of the American Academy of Child Psychiatry*, 23, 280–284.

McLanahan, S., & Sandefur, G. (1994). *Growing up with a single parent: What hurts and what helps*. Cambridge, MA: Harvard University Press.

McLeod, J. D., & Shanahan, M. J. (1993). Poverty, parenting, and children's mental health. *American Sociological Review*, 58, 351–366.

McLeod, J. D., & Shanahan, M. J. (1996). Trajectories of poverty and children's mental health. *Journal of Health and Social Behavior*, 37, 207–220.

McLoyd, V. C. (1989). Socialization and development in a changing economy: The effects of paternal job and income loss on children. *American Psychologist*, 44, 293–302.

McLoyd, V. C. (1990). The impact of economic hardship on black families and children: Psychological distress, parenting, and socioemotional development. *Child Development*, 61, 311–346.

McLoyd, V. C. (1998). Socioeconomic disadvantage and child development. *American Psychologist*, 53, 185–204.

McLoyd, V. C., Jayaratne, T. E., Ceballo, R., & Borquez, J. (1994). Unemployment and work interruption among African American single mothers: Effects on parenting and adolescent socioemotional functioning. *Child Development*, 65(2), 562–589.

McLoyd, V. C., & Smith, J. (2002). Physical discipline and behavior problems in African American, European American, and Hispanic children: Emotional support as a moderator. *Journal of Marriage and the Family*, 64(1), 40–53.

McMichael, A. J., Baghurst, P. A., Wigg, N. R.,

Vimpani, G. V., Robertson, E. F., & Roberts, R. J. (1988). Port Pirie cohort study: Environmental exposure to lead and children's abilities at the age of four years. *New England Journal of Medicine, 319,* 468–475.

Menaghan, E. G., & Parcel, T. L. (1995). Social sources of change in children's home environments: The effects of parental occupational experiences and family conditions. *Journal of Marriage and the Family, 57*(1), 69–84.

Miech, R., Essex, M. J., & Goldsmith, H. H. (2001). Socioeconomic status and the adjustment to school: The role of self-regulation during early childhood. *Sociology of Education, 74,* 102–120.

Morris, P. A. (2002). The effects of welfare reform policies on children. *Social Policy Report: Society for Research in Child Development, 16.*

Mosteller, F. (1995). The Tennessee study of class size in the early grades. *Future of Children, 5,* 113–127.

Murray, L., Fiori-Cowley, A., Hooper, R., & Cooper, P. (1996). The impact of postnatal depression and associated adversity on early mother–infant interactions and later infant outcomes. *Child Development, 67,* 2512–2526.

National Institute of Child Health and Human Development Early Child Care Research Network. (1997). Child care in the first year of life. *Merrill–Palmer Quarterly, 43*(3), 340–360.

Northridge, M. E., Yankura, J., Kinney, P. L., Santella, R. M., Shepard, P., Riojas, Y., et al. (1999). Diesel exhaust exposure among adolescents in Harlem: A community-driven study. *American Journal of Public Health, 89*(7), 998–1002.

O'Neil, R., Parke, R. D., & McDowell, D. J. (2001). Objective and subjective features of children's neighborhoods: Relations to parental regulatory strategies and children's social competence. *Applied Developmental Psychology, 22,* 135–155.

Orr, L., Feins, J. D., Jacob, R., Beecroft, E., Sanbonmatsu, L., Katz, L. F., et al. (2003, September). *Moving to Opportunity for Fair Housing Demonstration interim impacts evaluation.* Retrieved, September 4, 2003 from *http://www.huduser.org/publications/fairhsg/mtofinal.html*

Osofsky, J. D. (1999). The impact of violence on children. *Future of Children, 9*(3), 33–49.

Pagani, L., Boulerice, B., & Tremblay, R. E. (1997). The influence of poverty on children's classroom placement and behavior problems. In G. J. Duncan & J. Brooks-Gunn (Eds.), *Consequences of growing up poor* (pp. 311–339). New York: Russell Sage Foundation.

Petersen, T. (1989). The earnings function in sociological studies of earnings inequality: Functional form and hours worked. *Research in Social Stratification and Mobility, 8,* 221–250.

Phillips, D. A., Voran, M., Kisker, E., Howes, C., & Whitebook, M. (1994). Child care for children in poverty: Opportunity or inequity? *Child Development, 65*(2), 472–492.

Phillips, M., Brooks-Gunn, J., Duncan, G. J., Klebanov, P., & Crane, J. (1998). Family background, parenting practices, and the Black–White test score gap. In C. Jencks & M. Phillips (Eds.), *The Black–White test score gap* (pp. 103–145). Washington, DC: Brookings Institution Press.

Potasova, A. (1998). Cognitive functions of preschool children affected by environmental toxins. *Studia Psychologica, 40*(4), 335–338.

Rankin, B. H., & Quane, J. M. (2000). Neighborhood poverty and the social isolation of inner-city African American families. *Social Forces, 79,* 139–164.

Rankin, B. H., & Quane, J. M. (2002). Social contexts and urban adolescent outcomes: The interrelated effects of neighborhoods, families, and peers on African-American youth. *Social Problems, 49*(1), 79–100.

Raudenbush, S. W., & Sampson, R. J. (1999). Assessing direct and indirect effects in multilevel designs with latent variables. *Sociological Methods and Research, 28,* 123–153.

Richters, J. E., & Martinez, P. (1993). The NIMH Community Violence Project: I. Children as victims of and witnesses to violence. *Psychiatry, 56,* 7–21.

Robinson, G., & Whittebols, J. H. (1986). *Class size research: A related cluster analysis for decision making.* Arlington, VA: Educational Research Service.

Rothbart, M. K., & Bates, J. E. (1998). Temperament. In W. Damon & N. Eisenberg (Eds.), *Handbook of child psychology* (Vol. 3, pp. 105–176). New York: Wiley.

Sameroff, A. J., Seifer, R., Baldwin, A., & Baldwin, C. (1993). Stability of intelligence from preschool to adolescence: The influence of social and family risk factors. *Child Development, 64,* 80–97.

Sameroff, A. J., Seifer, R., Baroas, R., Zax, M., & Greenspan, S. (1987). Intelligence quotient scores of 4-year old children: Social–environmental risk factors. *Pediatrics, 79,* 343–350.

Sampson, R. J. (1997). Collective regulation of adolescent misbehavior: Validation results from eighty Chicago neighborhoods. *Journal of Adolescent Research, 12,* 227–244.

Sampson, R. J., & Laub, J. H. (1993). *Crime in the making: Pathways and turning points through life.* Cambridge, MA: Harvard University Press.

Sampson, R. J., Morenoff, J., & Earls, F. (1999). Beyond social capital: Spatial dynamics of collective efficacy for children. *American Sociological Review, 64,* 633–660.

Sampson, R. J., Raudenbush, S. W., & Earls, F. (1997). Neighborhoods and violent crime: A multilevel study of collective efficacy. *Science, 277,* 918–924.

Scarr, S., Eisenberg, M., & Deater-Deckard, K. (1994). Measurement of quality in child care centers. *Early Childhood Research Quarterly, 9,* 131–151.

Schmidt, F. L., & Hunter, J. E. (1998). The validity and utility of selection methods in personnel psychology: Practical and theoretical implications of 85 years of research findings. *Psychological Bulletin, 124*(2), 262–274.

Schwab-Stone, M. E., Ayers, T. S., Kasprow, W., Voyce, C., Barone, C., Shriver, T., et al. (1995). No safe haven: A study of violence exposure in an urban community. *Journal of the American Academy of Child and Adolescent Psychiatry, 34,* 1343–1352.

Schwab-Stone, M. E., Chen, C., Greenberger, E., Silver, D., Lichtman, J., & Voyce, C. (1999). No safe haven II: The effects of violence exposure on urban youth. *Journal of the American Academy of Child and Adolescent Psychiatry, 38,* 359–367.

Shaw, D. S., & Vondra, J. I. (1995). Infant attachment security and maternal predictors of early behavior problems: A longitudinal study of low-income families. *Journal of Abnormal Child Psychology, 23,* 335–357.

Shonkoff, J. P., & Phillips, D. A. (Eds.). (2000). *From neurons to neighborhoods: The science of early child development.* Washington, DC: National Academy of Sciences.

Shumow, L., Vandell, D. L., & Posner, J. (1999). Risk and resilience in the urban neighborhood: Predictors of academic performance among low-income elementary school children. *Merrill–Palmer Quarterly, 45*(2), 309–331.

Simpson, G. A., & Fowler, M. G. (1994). Geographic mobility and children's emotional/behavioral adjustment and school functioning. *American Academy of Pediatrics, 93,* 303–309.

Skinner, E. A., & Belmont, M. J. (1993). Motivation in the classroom: Reciprocal effects of teacher behavior and student engagement across the school year. *Journal of Educational Psychology, 85*(4), 571–581.

Smith, J. R., Bastiani, A., & Brooks-Gunn, J. (1998). Poverty and mental health. In H. Friedman (Ed.), *Encyclopedia of mental health* (Vol. 3, pp. 219–228). San Diego: Academic Press.

Smith, J. R., & Brooks-Gunn, J. (1997). Correlates and consequences of harsh discipline for young children. *Archives of Pediatric and Adolescent Medicine, 151,* 777–786.

Smith, J. R., Brooks-Gunn, J., & Jackson, A. (1997). Parental employment and children. In R. Hauser, B. Brown & W. Prosser (Eds.), *Indicators of children's well-being* (pp. 279–308). New York: Russell Sage Foundation.

Smith, J. R., Brooks-Gunn, J., & Klebanov, P. K. (1997). Consequences of living in poverty for young children's cognitive and verbal ability and early school achievement. In G. J. Duncan & J. Brooks-Gunn (Eds.), *Consequences of growing up poor* (pp. 132–189). New York: Russell Sage Foundation.

Snow, C. E. (1986). Conversations with children. In P. Fletcher & M. Garman (Eds.), *Language acquisition: Studies in first language development* (pp. 69–89). Cambridge, UK: Cambridge University Press.

Soldz, S., & Vaillant, G. E. (1998). A 50-year longitudinal study of defense use among inner city men: A validation of the DSM-IV defense axis. *Journal of Nervous and Mental Disease, 186*(2), 104–111.

Spengler, J. D., Jaakkola, J., Parise, H., Kislitsin, V., & Kuzmin, S., & Kosheleva, A., et al. (2002, July). *Housing characteristics and children's respiratory health.* Paper presented at the Indoor Air Conference, Monterey, CA.

Spiker, D., Ferguson, J., & Brooks-Gunn, J. (1993). Enhancing maternal interactive behavior and child social competence in low birth weight, premature infants. *Child Development, 64,* 754–768.

Starfield, B., Shapiro, S., Weiss, J., Liang, K. Y., Ra, K., Paige, D., et al. (1991). Race, family income, and low birth weight. *American Journal of Epidemiology, 134,* 1167–1174.

Stipek, D. J., & Ryan, R. H. (1997). Economically disadvantaged preschoolers: Ready to learn but further to go. *Developmental Psychology, 33,* 711–723.

Taylor, H. G., Klein, N., Minich, N. M., & Hack, M. (2000). Verbal memory deficits in children with less than 750 g birth weight. *Child Neuropsychology, 6,* 49–63.

Trusty, J. (2000). High education expectations and low achievement: Stability of educational goals across adolescence. *Journal of Educational Research, 93,* 356–365.

Tucker, C. J., Marx, J., & Long, L. (1998). "Moving on": Residential mobility and children's school lives. *Sociology of Education, 71,* 111–129.

Tucker, C. M., Zayco, R. A., Herman, K. C., Reinke, W. M., Trujillo, M., Carraway, K., et al. (2002). Teacher and child variables as predictors of academic engagement among low-income African American children. *Psychology in the Schools, 39*(4), 477–488.

Turley, R. N. L. (2002). Is relative deprivation beneficial?: The effects of richer and poorer neighbors on children's outcomes. *Journal of Community Psychology, 30*(6), 671–686.

U.S. Bureau of the Census. (2002). *Census 2000 basics.* Washington, DC: U.S. Government Printing Office.

U.S. Bureau of the Census. (2003). *Poverty thresholds for 2003 by size of family and number of related children under 18 years.* Retrieved April 26, 2004, from *http://www.census.gov/hhes/poverty/threshld/thresh03.html*

U.S. Department of Education. (1998). *Reducing class size: What do we know?* Retrieved September 4, 2003, from *http://www.ed.gov/pubs/reducingclass/index.html*

U.S. Department of Education. (1999). *The initial report of the secretary on the quality of teacher preparation.* Available online at *http://www.ed.gov/about/reports/annual/teachprep/initialreport4.pdf*

U.S. Department of Education. (2001). *Monitoring school quality: An indicators report.* Retrieved September 4, 2003, from *http://nces.ed.gov/pubs2001/2001030.pdf*

Webster-Stratton, C. (1998). Preventing conduct problems in Head Start children: Strengthening parenting competencies. *Journal of Consulting and Clinical Psychology, 66,* 715–730.

White, M. J., & Glick, J. E. (2000). Generation status,

social capital, and the routes out of high school. *Sociological Forum, 15*, 671–691.

Whitehurst, G. J., Arnold, D. S., Epstein, J. N., Angell, A. L., Smith, M., & Fischel, J. E. (1994). A picture book reading intervention in day care and home for children from low-income families. *Developmental Psychology, 30*, 679–689.

Whitehurst, G. J., & Lonigan, C. J. (1998). Child development and emergent literacy. *Child Development, 69*, 848–872.

Wiggins, J. S., & Pincus, A. L. (1992). Personality: Structure and assessment. *Annual Review of Psychology, 43*, 473–504.

Willie, C. V. (2001). The contextual effects of socioeconomic status on student achievement test scores by race. *Urban Education, 36*, 461–478.

Wilson, M., & Brooks-Gunn, J. (2001). Health status and behaviors of unwed fathers. *Children and Youth Services Review, 23*(4/5), 377–401.

Yeung, W. J., Linver, M. R., & Brooks-Gunn, J. (2002). How money matters for young children's development: Parental investment and family processes. *Child Development, 73*(6), 1861–1879.

Zhao, H., Brooks-Gunn, J., McLanahan, S., & Singer, B. (1999). Studying the real child rather than the ideal child: Bringing the person into developmental studies. In L. R. Bergman & R. B. Cairns (Eds.), *Developmental science and the holistic approach* (pp. 393–419). Mahwah, NJ: Erlbaum.

Zigler, E., & Styfco, S. J. (2004). Moving Head Start to the states: One experiment too many. *Applied Developmental Science, 8*(1), 51–55.

CHAPTER 24

☙

Stereotypes and the Fragility of Academic Competence, Motivation, and Self-Concept

JOSHUA ARONSON
CLAUDE M. STEELE

Human intelligence is among the most fragile things in nature. It doesn't take much to distract it, suppress it, or even annihilate it.

—NEIL POSTMAN (1988)

Despite occasional statements like this from education researchers and commentators, most people think of intellectual competence as a stable thing. We expect children who do well in grammar school to perform well in junior high and high school; we expect those who score well on tests this week to score well next week, and so on. But we are often wrong about this. Although clearly not the most fragile thing in nature, competence is much more fragile—and malleable—than we tend to think. Consider a few examples:

In a recent study by Baumeister, Twenge, and Nuss (2002), college students were given bogus feedback from a personality test; for some, the test was said to indicate that others would one day reject them. This bad news dramatically interfered with their performance on a standard IQ test they took shortly afterward; they solved about six fewer items than equally smart students in control groups, who got either a different kind of negative feedback or no feedback at all.

Mueller and Dweck (1998) gave students a problem-solving task (engineered to guarantee high performance) and then praised students for their success. The feedback varied by condition, so that some students were praised for their intelligence ("You must be really smart at these"), while others received effort praise ("You must have worked hard"), and members of a third group were told simply that their score was very high. Later, on a subsequent set of harder problems, those praised for being smart performed significantly worse than the other groups.

College freshmen signed up for a study conducted by Wilson and Linville (1982) because they were struggling academically: They were performing less well than they wanted to, felt intellectually inferior to their classmates, and were generally anxious about doing well in college. By the flip of a coin, some of these students were assigned to receive an intervention— lasting all of a few minutes—wherein they learned that their struggles were not unique, and that many struggling students improve over time in college. Compared to the control group, these students solved significantly more items on a standardized test taken a short while later and dramatically improved their grade point averages (GPAs) in the following year.

Such examples not only show how competence is both fragile and responsive to intervention but also point to why. Specifically, in many contexts, intellectual competence is not just something inside a person's head (Sternberg, 2002). Rather, it is quite literally the product of real or imagined interactions with others. How a student construes the way he or she is viewed and treated by others matters a lot: how welcomed or excluded, how respected, how tuned in to others' difficulties and triumphs—these perceptions can exert a profound influence on intellectual competence, on motivation, and ultimately upon a student's academic self-concept. Competence is fragile, then, because it is transacted within a web of social relations. The social psychology and education literatures are full of examples of how things that influence social relations also influence motivation, learning, and performance (e.g., National Research Council, 2003), but too often we fail to appreciate these social forces.

To be sure, we do sometimes acknowledge impediments to competence—especially our own competence—as when we experience *stage fright, writer's block,* or some other temporary hindrance. Yet particularly when judging others, we have what amounts to an "innate ability bias" (Aronson, 2002a; Aronson & Jones, 1992); we are apt to assume that people's intellectual accomplishments are products of internal forces like giftedness, rather than situational ones, like an encouraging social climate (e.g., Dweck, 1999; Jones, 1989). Thus, unless we have prior knowledge to the contrary, students who score poorly on tests or get bad grades in school will probably just seem untalented or lazy. These impressions may be correct some of the time, but in many cases, as in the earlier examples, there is more to the story; social forces are at play that may be hard to see or appreciate, but that nonetheless undermine people's academic achievement in important ways.

In this chapter, we focus on one set of forces, the influence of stereotypes on academic performance, engagement, and self-concept, which together comprise what we see as fundamental to *competence.* There is much evidence, beginning with research in the 1960s, to suggest that teachers' expectations about their students can play a significant role in the nurture (or neglect) of student competence (see Rosenthal, 2002). We briefly review similar, more recent, research that applies a similar logic to stereotypes, which are expectations based on category membership. Our own research in this area began several years ago with a search for new answers to the decades-old question about why African American and other minority students' test performance and achievement lags behind that of white students, even when comparing students who attend the same schools, whose parents are comparably well off and well educated, who come from comparable neighborhoods, and so on (e.g., Herrnstein & Murray, 1994; Jencks & Phillips, 1998; Ogbu & Davis, 2003). The fact that equating students on such background factors reduces yet fails to eliminate the gap in achievement frustrated the standard arguments about genetic or cultural influences on test and school performance, because these arguments rest upon the notion that ability, skills, and preparation account for nearly all the variance in achievement. But because black students with equal ability and preparation so frequently underperformed in college relative to identically scoring whites (Jensen, 1980), there seemed to be an unaccounted factor at play, something beyond the things to which we customarily attribute achievement. Our research, and that of many others, suggests that part of the problem is rooted in the psychology of stereotyping and stigma, namely, the way people are influenced by stereotypes of intellectual inferiority that surround certain groups in American society.

STEREOTYPES SHAPE SOCIAL INTERACTIONS

One way stereotypes influence competence is that they cause stereotype targets to be perceived and treated differently than nontargets. Stereotypes were nicely described long ago by Walter Lippman (1922/1997) as "the pictures in our heads" that simplify the world by saving us the trouble of thinking when we come into contact with people. These pictures function as expectations of what people in particular categories (boys, girls, blacks, Latinos, etc.) will be like and what they can and cannot do, thus allowing us to fill in the blanks when information is ambiguous or incomplete. The problem, of course, is that stereotypes are overgeneralizations; they encourage simplistic thinking that ignores individual differences between people who belong to certain categories.

There is no shortage of stereotypes about the reputed abilities of social groups, and by a surprisingly young age, Americans become familiar with their content (Aboud, 1988; Huston, 1983). Thus, by middle childhood, most American children have learned that blacks and Latinos are less intelligent than whites, that Asians are good at math, while girls are not, that blacks are better athletes than whites, and so on (e.g., McKown & Weinstein, 2003; Smith, 1990). Not everyone believes the stereotypes, but most people in the culture are aware of them, targets as well as nontargets. Regardless of whether we come to hold these stereotypes as strong convictions or merely as familiar-but-distrusted images, knowledge of their content alone can bias perceptions of stereotype targets (Devine, 1989).

Teachers

This can pose a measurable problem for students who happen to belong to groups alleged to lack academic competence. For example, in a recent study, Arnold and Cross (2003) had teachers rank-order the children in their Head Start classes with respect to their interest in math activities. The teachers rated the Asian children as far more interested than African American or Anglo children, quite in line with the stereotypical image of Asians as math-oriented. But the picture in the teachers' heads was misleading: Expert objective observers found nothing to confirm the teachers' rankings of math orientation—neither the children's self-reports nor objective recordings of children's observed interest in playing math games revealed any differences. The black and Latino kids liked math just as much as the Asian kids, but the teachers missed it.

The problem, as we know from years of research, is that these distorted perceptions are not inert; people act upon them, treating the targets as if the stereotypes are true. Beginning with Rosenthal's Pygmalion studies (Rosenthal & Jacobson, 1968; Rosenthal, 2002), research shows that stereotyped expectations shape social interactions and over time can result in the stereotype's fulfillment, a process known as a "self-fulfilling prophecy." Specifically, if a student's social identity suggests high ability, interest, or potential, he or she may be treated accordingly by a teacher—receiving more warmth, more challenging material, more patience, and so on—and over time, develop into the bright student the teacher imagined initially. By the same token, negative expectancies based on group reputation can have the opposite effect, leading a teacher to create a colder, less challenging environment for students from these groups. For example, teachers in a study by Brophy and Good (e.g., 1974), treated differently students they had labeled as strong or weak. When a "strong" student faltered, say, during a reading task, teachers were more likely to give subtle clues until the student came upon the solution. When a "weak" student faltered, teachers were more likely to simply supply the correct answer, thus depriving the student of the opportunity to build skill and a sense of accomplishment. The process can be subtle and nonverbal, and it can occur without intention among individuals who consciously (and even adamantly) reject the stereotyped notions (Darley & Gross, 1983; Word, Zanna, & Cooper, 1974; Fazio, Jackson, Dunton, & Williams, 1995).

Sometimes the differential treatment is not so unconscious or unwitting. Evidence from various studies shows that teachers sometimes use stereotypes in not-so-subtle ways, attaching social identity to negative behavior or poor performance, such as when the poorest, least liked, children are seated at the back of the room (Rist, 1970), or when incompetence or unruly behavior is openly attributed to race (Tyson, 2003). Whether blatant or subtly expressed, teacher expectations can shape student performance, leading some scholars to cite low expectations—based on stereotypes—as a significant factor in the achievement gap between blacks and whites (e.g., Ferguson, 1998; Weinstein, 2002), and the gap between students of high and low socioeconomic status (e.g., Croizet & Dutrévis, in press).

Parents

Parents, surprisingly, are not immune to the influence of stereotypes. For example, there is research to suggest that the "girls-can't-do-math" stereotype distorts the way parents evaluate their children's interests and abilities. Parents in various studies have been found to see their daughters as less interested and adept than their sons at math and science, to see their girls succeeding through effort, but their boys succeeding by dint of natural ability. These attributions shape the messages that parents send their kids, a process very similar to the self-fulfilling prophecy described earlier for teachers. For example, recent research conducted by Tenenbaum and Leaper (2003) found that parents asked more cognitively challenging questions of boys when working through a science problem than when discussing a less male-associated topic, such as interpersonal relations. Remarkably, other research further showed that parents' beliefs predicted their child's self-efficacy (confidence) better than actual performance (e.g., Frome & Eccles, 1998). This means that parental ex-

pectations—which are influenced by gender stereotypes—can matter more than a child's actual ability, interests, and performance in shaping their child's academic self-concept.

There are, of course, a variety of ways that a child's orientation to achievement can be shaped by parent beliefs, such as the way they respond to a child's successes, or with criticism or praise (see Dweck, 1999, for a review), or withdrawal of affection (Elliot & Thrash, 2004; Jones & Berglas, 1978), or the schools, media, or playmates they choose for their children (Harris, 1998). What is clear is that stereotyped notions about intellectual ability can influence the way parents respond to their children, and that these responses, in turn, have effects on various aspects of competence.

Peers

Needless to say, fellow students play a tremendous role in a child's developing competence and achievement-related self-conceptions. There seems to be validity to the claim that adolescents in American schools care about belonging—fitting in socially with their peers—more than they care about nearly anything else (e.g., Arroyo & Zigler, 1995; Coleman, 1961). Indeed, peer influence is so important that some scholars have been compelled to conclude that teacher or parental influence is secondary to that of other children (e.g., Harris, 1998). Statistics suggest that this is particularly true during the middle school and high school years, when social concerns reach their apex. One sees clues that stereotypes create academic problems at this stage in the fact that this is precisely when many bright and high-achieving students begin to falter academically (e.g., Aronson & Good, 2002; Wigfield & Eccles, 2002), and when most children attain an awareness that certain groups are broadly stereotyped in society (McKown & Weinstein, 2003). Minority students are at increased risk for social exclusion by peers, which, as suggested by the Baumeister et al. (2002) study described earlier, can have direct effects on academic performance. School-based studies confirm that peer rejection imperils school performance and engagement (e.g., the likelihood of dropping out), particularly if those excluded are seen as hostile, or when teachers are thought to dislike the excluded student (see Harrist & Bradley, 2002, for a review). Children get excluded for a number of reasons—being unattractive, aggressive, or just different (see Killen, Lee-Kim, McGlothin, & Stangor, 2002, for a review). Racial and ethnic minorities appear to experience more than their fair share of peer rejection (Kistner, Metzler, Gatlin, & Risi, 1993); thus, by itself, minority status appears to lead to differential treatment by classmates and can thereby put students at risk for academic problems. This appears most likely in classrooms where competition is stressed (Aronson & Patnoe, 1997; Sherif & Sherif, 1969).

Social pressures come from within minority groups as well. For example, there is some evidence to suggest that minority students, more than their nonminority classmates, must choose between academic and social success within their ethnic group, because engaging academically invites charges of "acting white" and abandoning one's social group (Fordham & Ogbu, 1986). Although any student is likely to pay a social price for being too "nerdy," some peer nomination studies—which ask students to list who is cool, admirable, and influential in their school—suggest that black and Latino males pay the highest social penalties for engaging academically (e.g., Graham, Taylor, & Hudley, 1998). If this is so, then it may partly explain why, as a group, African American males appear to be the least academically identified students in America (Osborne, 1997). In many middle and high schools, there is a trade-off for students between social or academic success that varies in intensity depending on race and gender.

It is important to note that the evidence for peer sanctions against achievement is mixed. For example, studies using national samples of data suggest that adolescents do not generally devalue education (e.g., Spencer, Iserman, Davies, & Quinn, 2001), and that the "acting white" or "oppositional culture" hypothesis may be an overgeneralization from ethnographic case studies (Cook & Ludwig, 1998). Yet these large survey studies have their own limitations as well. There appears to be enough evidence to suggest that, at least under some circumstances and in some schools and classrooms,

social success and academic engagement have inverse relationships, and this may interfere with the development of competence among some minority students.

In sum, stereotypes about academic abilities can inhibit the expression and development of competence by prompting differential treatment by teachers, parents, and peers. For the remainder of the chapter we focus in considerably more detail on different route by which negative stereotypes influence competence.

STUDENTS REACT TO STEREOTYPES

Stereotype Threat

Our research over the last decade shows that a student need never encounter actual prejudice or differential treatment of the sort described earlier to be meaningfully affected by stereotypes. Just as mere knowledge of a stereotype can influence the thinking and behavior of a teacher, parent, or peer, it can also, in a variety of ways, impact the student more directly. Our initial hypothesis (Steele 1992; Steele & Aronson, 1995) was that students targeted by negative stereotypes are bothered by the implications of the intellectual inferiority stereotype—the possibility that they will be viewed through its negative lens, and that the stereotype could accurately characterize them or their group. Confirming a stereotype through low performance poses a threat to at least three important human motives: the need for competence (e.g., White, 1959), the need to appear competent to others (e.g., Jones, 1989), and the need to belong socially in a domain that one values (Baumeister & Leary, 1995).

Thus, our argument goes, compared to people not targeted by stereotypes, in situations where academic competence is relevant—taking a test, speaking up in class, working on a project with peers, or even doing one's homework, stereotype targets will feel extra pressure not to fail. This extra burden, therefore, could induce black students, Latino students, or women working in male-dominated arenas (i.e., math and science) to perform less well, thereby confirming the stereotype that they want to disprove. Ten years later, we have ample confirmation that this phenomenon—which we named "stereotype threat"—is real, and that it contributes to the gap in performance between minorities and whites. Over a hundred studies conducted since we coined that term have revealed much about the conditions under which stereotype threat undermines performance, the groups susceptible to it, individual risk factors that amplify its effects, the processes by which it interferes with achievement, and some useful techniques for reducing its impact on achievement (e.g., Aronson, 2002b; Steele, Spencer, & Aronson, 2002). We begin with research demonstrating its effects on standardized test performance.

Stereotype Threat and Test Performance

In our early studies, we started with a simple hypothesis: If concerns about confirming a negative stereotype undermine standardized test performance, then arranging situations to minimize those concerns should boost performance of individuals stereotyped as intellectually inferior. To those not stereotyped as inferior, the change of situation should have little or no effect on performance. To test this reasoning, we had African American and Caucasian college students take a difficult standardized verbal test, which we constructed by culling some of the more difficult items from an old Graduate Record Examination (GRE). The students took this test under one of two conditions. In the "stereotype threat" condition we presented the test the way such tests are typically presented: as a diagnostic tool we were using to measure their verbal ability. This explicit scrutiny of ability, we thought, should bring to the fore concerns about confirming the stereotype. In the "no stereotype threat" condition, we presented the same test as a nonevaluative exercise aimed at teaching us about the psychology of verbal problem solving. In other words, we made it clear to the students that although we wanted them to try hard to get the problems right, we were not the least bit interested in how smart they were. We thought that, framed in this way, the students should be less worried about confirming the stereotype.

The results suggested we were right. As shown in Figure 24.1, after we statistically controlled for individual differences in preparation and verbal aptitude (we covaried out students' verbal Scholastic Aptitude Test [SAT] scores), we found that black students performed dramatically better in the no ste-

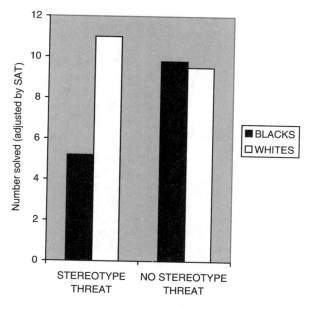

FIGURE 24.1. Test performance under stereotype threat versus no stereotype threat conditions. Adapted from Steele and Aronson (1995). Copyright 1995 by the American Psychological Association. Adapted by permission.

reotype threat condition than they did in the stereotype threat condition. Caucasian test takers were not meaningfully affected by the framing of the test.

Follow-up studies using the same diagnostic–nondiagnostic manipulation provided some clues about the experience of stereotype threat—and to some extent validated our conception of the phenomenon. For example, Steele and Aronson (1995, experiment 3) found that black students who thought that we were interested in measuring their intelligence (on an upcoming test) had more stereotypes on their mind. Specifically, we used an implicit memory measure, which supplies a long list of partial words and asks people to quickly fill in the blanks to make an English word. Cognitive psychologists have found that people completing such tasks will tend to construct words that fit with recently activated (thought about) ideas. Thus, given the word stem (_ _ C E), one might come up with a number of different completions (MICE, RICE, FACE, PACE, etc.), depending upon recently encountered stimuli or thoughts. What we found is that black students in our diagnostic condition were significantly more likely to come up with the word RACE—as well as other words associated with black stereotypes on other word stems. They seemed, in other words, to have racial stereotypes on their mind as a result of having their intelligence evaluated. This we took as evidence that stereotypes are indeed linked to the experience of evaluative scrutiny in a domain where competence is relevant. When the evaluative stakes are raised, so too are thoughts about racial stereotypes, suggesting that the two contexts are cognitively associated for African Americans but not for whites.

Moreover, our data suggest the desire on the part of stereotype-threatened black test takers to disprove the negative stereotype. Immediately after the word stem task, our students were given a survey. The survey asked about the kinds of activities they enjoyed—the kinds of sports they played, the kind of music they enjoyed, and so on. Some of these preferences were clearly stereotypical of African Americans (liking rap music, playing basketball, being lazy, and so on). There was a very telling difference in the way that black students filled out the survey.

Those who thought we would be diagnosing their intelligence later on distanced themselves from the stereotypical portrayals of themselves. They reported liking basketball, rap music, being lazy, and so on, significantly less than their counterparts, who thought the upcoming exam was not going to diagnose their abilities. And most (75%) of these students chose the option of not indicating their race at the end of this survey, whereas all the black students in the no-stereotype-threat condition (and all the white students in both conditions) indicated their race. It seemed clear, therefore, that the evaluative nature of the situation made them think about stereotypes and be wary of confirming them.

A subsequent experiment nailed down the role of this wariness in the impairment of test performance among African American students. In this study (Steele & Aronson, 1995, experiment 4), all test takers were put in the nondiagnostic condition of the previous experiment; they were told we would not be evaluating their abilities. But for half, we made their racial identity salient; we asked them just prior to beginning the test to indicate their race on a demographic questionnaire (this time it was not optional). Whereas this mere mention of race had no effect on white test takers, it rather dramatically impaired the black test takers, cutting in half the number of items they correctly solved. This is clear evidence that our attention to race spurred evaluative concerns—and a nice illustration of Postman's claim that it does not take much to suppress human intelligence.

Generality of Stereotype Threat Effects

But this raises a critical question: To what extent do such effects generalize to other groups of humans? Is the experience of stereotype threat limited to African Americans? While stereotype threat may be most likely and most keenly felt among historically stigmatized groups such as African Americans, it is a predicament that can trouble the member of any group, because it is largely a product of circumstances that threaten basic human motives—being competent, appearing competent, and being accepted by others (e.g., Aronson, Quinn, & Spencer, 1998). Thus, anyone who conceivably could be targeted by a stereotype alleging inferiority could experience pressure to disprove the stereotype. This would be important, because to remove barriers to all students' demonstrating and developing their competence, it is critical to know the extent to which these barriers originate from something unique to their social group, or something more general operating in the situations most students confront. Research conducted over the past decade has mostly supported the generality hypothesis.

For example, similarly dramatic affects using a different manipulation have been found by Spencer, Steele, and Quinn (1999) among women taking mathematics tests. In their study, highly math-proficient male and female college students (they were in the upper 15% of the university population in terms of SAT scores) took a very challenging math test. In the control group, the women performed significantly less well than the men. In the experimental condition, stereotype threat was nullified with a simple statement: "This test has never produced gender differences in the past." In this condition, women's performance rose markedly, equaling that of the men. Other research finds similar effects with Latino students, importantly, with variations on the manipulation of stereotype threat (Aronson & Salinas, 2001), and in another case (Gonzales, Blanton, & Williams, 2002), examining the role of "double-minority status." The former study found impaired performance when the issue of bias in standardized testing was raised; the latter suggested that conditions that make Latina women aware of their ethnicity make them especially likely to underperform on a math test.

Similarly, research has found that the stereotype suggesting that old people's memories are faulty and deteriorating can be similarly disruptive to its targets. When the elderly participants in one experiment were subtly reminded of the stereotype regarding old age and senility, they performed worse on a test of short-term memory than when they were reminded of the more positive "old-people-are-wise" stereotype instead (Levy, 1996). In a subsequent study by Hess, Auman, Colcombe, and Rahhal (2003), older adults read mock newspaper articles on research about aging and memory. Half of the articles presented negative findings

that suggested mental declines were inevitable. The other half presented more positive findings, which implied that some mental skills lasted into old age, and that cognitive declines could be slowed. After reading the articles, the subjects were given a memory test in which they had to recall a list of words. Those who read the positive article performed about 30% better on the test than those who read the negative article.

Jean Claude Croizet and his colleagues have found that stereotype threat effects extend to students of low socioeconomic status (Croizet & Claire, 1998; Croizet & Dutrévis, in press). This suggests that the stereotype of poor people as less intelligent may contribute to the oft-cited correlation between socioeconomic status and test performance.

Perhaps the most persuasive findings regarding the generality of these effects is that stereotype threat can impair the performance of even those groups who are neither minority nor broadly stereotyped as intellectually inferior—for example, white males at top tier universities. In a simple experiment (Aronson, et al., 1999), we asked highly competent white males to take a difficult math test. Both groups were told that the test was aimed at determining their math abilities. For one group we added a stereotype threat: We told them that one of our reasons for doing the research was to understand why Asians seemed to perform better on these tests. In this condition, these highly competent and confident males—most of whom were mathematics or engineering majors—lost a significant number of items on the test. These were students with extremely high skills—most had earned near perfect scores on the math portion of the SAT. Thus, if they can experience stereotype threat, anyone who plausibly can be targeted by a stereotype can feel it (for similar findings with white males see Leyens, Désert, Croizet, & Darcis, 2000; Smith & White, 2002). The rather exotic situation that we imposed upon them—a direct comparison with a supposedly superior group—is, in form, similar to the predicament of blacks and Latinos, who contend daily with such settings in any integrated academic setting. For us, these findings make it easier to accept a situational account of their relatively low academic outcomes; it proves that lower competence or motivation need not be involved in their underperformance.

Studies aimed at discovering the developmental onset of stereotype threat effect show that children, as well as adults, can be impaired by making their stereotyped social identity relevant to an ability test (Aronson & Good, 2002; McKown & Weinstein, 2003). In the Aronson and Good studies, stereotype threat effects did not emerge in children in the fifth grade but showed up reliably among sixth graders—girls on math tests, and Latinos on verbal tests. The McKown and Weinstein studies suggested that children at this stage become stereotype-vulnerable because they are able to grasp the fact that their group is broadly stereotyped in society. Whatever the exact mechanism, it is clear that by middle childhood, children, like adults, can become unnerved by the negative stereotypes about their group's intellectual abilities.

Stereotype threat effects also generalize to other performance domains. In a particularly notable example, Stone, Lynch, Sjomeling, and Darley (1999) found that when a game of miniature golf was framed as a measure of "sport strategic intelligence," black athletes performed worse at it than whites. Interestingly, by framing this same golf game as a measure of "natural athletic ability," the pattern reversed, and the black athletes outperformed the whites. Similarly, Garcia, Helms, and Garcia (2003) report results of a study suggesting that white athletes jumped less high when observed by an African American coach than when observed by a white coach, suggesting a stereotype threat—and therefore partly situational—explanation involving the stereotype that "white men can't jump." Such studies show not only the group-by-situation variability of stereotype threat but also suggest its generalizability in real life across groups, settings, and types of behavior. Studies that we discuss shortly further reinforce the breadth of stereotype threat effects.

Mediation of Test Performance

What mediates the effects of stereotype threat on test performance? That is, how does stereotype threat turn into lower performance? Various researchers have asked this question and, as it turns out, have found almost as many mediators as they have looked for.

Anxiety

Our original hypothesis (Steele & Aronson, 1995) was this: trying extra hard to disprove the negative stereotype arouses anxiety, which in turn interferes with performance. Although our original studies tested for this—we used standard self-report measures of test anxiety, evidence was spotty at best; we would find it in one study but not in another. Other researchers using self-reports (typically administered retrospectively after the exam) have found similarly inconclusive mediation data. Two research studies used more direct measures and confirmed that anxiety plays at least a partial role. Blascovich, Spencer, Quinn, and Steele (2001) had black and white college students take a difficult verbal test under "stereotype threat" or "no stereotype threat" conditions (the diagnostic test was described as "racially fair" in the no stereotype threat condition). The test takers' blood pressure was monitored throughout the test in all conditions. The study yielded a typical pattern of stereotype threat effects on performance: Blacks performed worst when the test was represented as diagnostic of verbal ability, best when represented as racially fair. But for blacks in the stereotype threat condition, blood pressure rose sharply and significantly above baseline levels, whereas for all other test takers, it dropped. Interestingly, on questionnaires probing for anxiety, there were no differences, suggesting that self-reports may be inaccurate indicators of internal states in stereotype threat situations.

Another way of assessing the role of anxiety is to compare the effects of testing conditions on complex versus simple tasks. Anxiety has long been known to boost performance on simple tasks but interfere with performance on complex tasks. Thus, if stereotype threat did the same, this would be more evidence that anxiety is involved in stereotype threat. In a recent experiment, O'Brien and Crandall (2003) showed just this. Women under stereotype threat performed better on an easy math test than women under no stereotype threat but, replicating earlier stereotype threat studies (e.g., Spencer et al., 1999), stereotype threat impaired their performance on the difficult math test.

That stereotype threat arouses anxiety squares nicely with important work on achievement goals. Specifically, Elliot and colleagues find that people experience more anxiety and perform worse when they pursue performance avoidance goals—when they try to avoid comparing poorly to others, as opposed to just doing their best (Elliot & Church, 1997; Elliot, McGregor, & Gable, 1999). Such a mind-set appears to be the least productive and enjoyable way to approach achievement, and it aptly describes the hypothesized goal—and the observed achievement outcomes—of people subjected to stereotype threat. Research is currently under way that directly examines the mediational role of performance avoidance goals in stereotype threat–related underperformance.

Expectations

The previous studies do not, however, force the conclusion that anxiety is the sole mediator of stereotype threat; other processes may be involved. One possible comediator is performance expectations. Some researchers have found that activating stereotypes lowers performance expectations (Stangor, Carr, & Kiang, 1998), but in this study, performance was not assessed, so it is unclear whether these lowered expectations would have translated into lower performance. Other studies (e.g., Spencer et al., 1999; Stone et al., 1999) found no such direct effect of stereotype threat on expectations, despite the fact that stereotype threat impaired performance. Still other studies find that raising performance expectations fails to "wipe out" the effects of stereotype threat on performance. The role of expectations in stereotype threat is therefore likely to be a complex one; because, for one thing, initial expectations based on situational cues that arouse or nullify stereotype threat can change as soon as one encounters success or difficulties while progressing from item to item on a test.

Effort

One would think that a likely response to stereotype threat might be simply to give up or withdraw effort and, thereby, perform worse. Yet studies that have measured effort—how long people work on the test, how many problems they attempt, how much effort they report putting in, and so on—have revealed no evidence that this happens. In one study, Aronson and Salinas (2001) had participants complete a difficult math test with electrodes on their wrists that purportedly monitored the effort they expended during the test. Participants also understood that they would have to retake the test until an acceptable amount of effort was detected. Despite this elaborate effort-assuring ruse, stereotype threat effects still emerged, suggesting that reduced effort is not a necessary mediator of stereotype threat effects. This hardly forces the conclusion that effort withdrawal *never* mediates these effects. After all, most studies have involved strong students, people who are highly invested in academics, who take a test that is portrayed as an important indicator of their ability. And they work on the test for a relatively short time (usually 20–30 minutes). These are the conditions likely to produce maximal effort. It does not seem unreasonable to assume that less invested students involved in more drawn out tasks might respond to stereotype threat with lower effort. Future research will sort out the conditions under which this strategy is most likely to occur. What can be said with confidence is that lower performance due to stereotype threat can occur without the withdrawal of effort, and this is important to know.

Cognitive Load

Earlier, we noted evidence that black test takers in stereotype threat situations seem to have more stereotypes on their mind, which suggests that stereotype threat imposes an extra cognitive burden. Various studies have examined this situation and found that being stereotype threatened eats up valuable cognitive resources. Schmader and Johns (2003), for example, found that stereotype threat reduces working memory capacity. Croizet, Desprès, Gauzins, Huguet, and Leyens (2003) found that it increases heart rate variability, an index of cognitive load. Steven Spencer and his colleagues (2001) have found evidence that people under stereotype threat actively try to suppress the negative stereotypes and attendant unpleasant thoughts, a mentally taxing—and largely futile—exercise that consumes resources needed for test performance. Inzlicht, McKay, and Aronson (2004) found that stereotype threat taxes self-regulation capacity, mental energies needed for important executive functions, such as self-control, memory, and organizational skills. In one study, they showed that, under stereotype threat, people were less able to maintain a tight squeeze on an exercise handgrip, a common, nonreactive measure of self-regulation energy. In sum, just about every study that has examined a cognitive-load or divided-attention explanation for stereotype threat effects has found supportive evidence. The exceptions are those studies that employed self-report measures (e.g., Steele & Aronson, 1995; Aronson et al., 1999).

Ideomotor Effects?

One of the most intriguing findings to have emerged in the past several years is that when a stereotype is mentally activated without conscious awareness, people display a remarkable tendency to behave in line with it. Subtly expose college students to words suggesting old age and they will walk more slowly away from an experiment. Do the same with words suggesting rudeness, and they will be more likely to interrupt a conversation a few moments later (Bargh, Chen, & Burrows, 1996). These are called "ideomotor" effects, because they occur automatically, with no apparent mediator between thought and action. Research like this suggests that test performance could likewise be impaired—or lifted—by "priming" social stereotypes associated with high or low ability. In a particularly striking example of such effects, Shih, Pittinsky, and Ambady (1999), found that when primed with their Asian identity, women performed better on a math test. But if they were primed to think of their female identity, they performed worse. These effects do not appear to require any sense of threat or anxiety; people need only know the stereotype's content. Accordingly, even young students, who are familiar with the stereotypes but are not yet aware of how broadly they are applied, can nonetheless be susceptible to their influence (Ambady, Shih, Kim, & Pittinsky, 2001). The extent to which these direct effects of stereotypes are involved in underperformance in the real world (where many stereotypes are activated simultaneously) is unclear. It is important to recognize that even in the sterile confines of a laboratory experiment, the effect of such subtle primes on performance is often quite modest: In most studies, they produce no meaningful difference in the number of items solved, but instead impair performance accuracy (the number of items solved divided by the number attempted). Still, more research needs to be conducted to sort out the degree to which this process mediates underperformance of stereotyped groups (Wheeler & Petty, 2001; Steele et al., 2002).

All of these mediation findings suggest that negative stereotypes, in one way or another, impair performance by depleting cognitive resources away from the performance task, by arousing anxiety, or by simply prompting people to unconsciously behave as the stereotype prescribes—or by some combination of these. That researchers have found evidence for several mediators does not, we think, indicate empirical murkiness. Rather, it reflects the complexity and fragility of human performance: there are many ways to fail. Indeed, the fact that one can find several different pathways between the presence of stereotypes and impaired performance should, if anything, strengthen our confidence in the relationship between negative stereotypes and performance difficulties. All the pathways seem to lead to the same result.

Situational Risk Factors for Stereotype Threat

Implicit in the findings of much of the research discussed earlier is that certain situations are likely to give rise to stereotype threat. For example, in the Steele and Aronson (1995) studies, both ability evaluation and the salience or implied relevance of racial identity induced the underperformance among black students. Likewise, cues about the biased or fair nature of this tests were sufficient to turn on or off stereotype threat in other studies, such as the Aronson and Salinas (2001), Blascovich et al. (2001), and Spencer et al. (1999) studies. Thus, one can see the inherent difficulty in arranging situations to reduce stereotype threat, given that the evaluation of abilities is endemic to most testing situations, and that in diverse classrooms in America, the salience of race and gender are difficult to reduce.

This latter point is underscored by recent experiments conducted by Michael Inzlicht and colleagues, which show how group composition can matter. In one study (e.g., Inzlicht & Ben-Zeev, 2000), highly competent female undergraduates took a difficult math exam in small groups. Depending on the condition of the experiment, the researchers added one or more men to this testing session. The mere presence of one male test taker was enough to significantly impair the performance of the female test takers in the group. Moreover, adding another male into the testing session, such that women were outnumbered, produced an increase in stereotype threat and a corresponding drop in the women's performance, a linear effect of gender integration on underperformance. Inzlicht, Aronson, Good, and McKay (2003) reported effects that suggest African Americans are sometimes susceptible to such effects as well. The critical variable in these studies seems to be the salience of one's negatively stereotyped social identity, which minority status activates and apparently amplifies. Studies also show that the variety of cues regarding social identity—the gender or race of the test administrator, or a recently viewed TV spot in which women are depicted stereotypically—can have disruptive effects on performance (e.g., Marx & Roman, 2002; Davies, Spencer, Quinn, & Gerhardstein, 2002). In sum, there are two primary triggers that can turn the performance of challenging cognitive tasks into a stereotype-threatening situation—ability evaluation, and the salience of a social identity that is stereotyped as inferior in the ability domain.

Stereotype Vulnerability: Individual Risk Factors for Underperformance

Such triggers are not equally unnerving to all individuals. Important individual differences make some individuals more vulnerable than others to the kind of underperformance we have been discussing. The sum of these risk factors can be thought of as "stereotype vulnerability." The following factors appear to contribute to an individual's level of stereotype vulnerability.

Domain Identification

In his remarkable book, *A Hope in the Unseen*, Ron Suskind (1999) tells the true story of a high school student, Cedric Jennings, who beats the odds: Poor, black, and schooled in the worst high school in Washington, DC, he succeeds through grit, determination, and intelligence to make it into the Ivy League. When Cedric gets his score on the SAT, he is disappointed but remains determined. He buckles down hard and studies his SAT prep virtually night and day, hoping to lift his score when he takes it again several months later. He goes at his studies with the devotion and drive that we hope to find and cultivate in our students. In the language of educational psychology, Cedric is a highly *engaged* or *identified* student. He cares. When he gets his scores back, we see the ironic fruits of his labor—his score has *dropped* significantly.

This is a perfect illustration of a commonplace finding in our research: Stereotype threat it is most keenly felt by the individuals who care most about doing well. In a number of studies, we have measured the degree to which people care about a particular domain—how much they value doing well in math, science, or any particular domain of academic achievement, and how much doing poorly in the domain threatens their self-esteem. What we find is that underperformance under stereotype threat is more pronounced for those who really want to do well (Aronson et al., 1999; Aronson & Good, 2001a). This is quite logical, of course. We would not expect to be unnerved by a stereotype alleging a lack of ability if that ability was trivial. The irony is that we increasingly see high-stakes testing used to evaluate our students' progress or suitability for admissions to institutions of higher learning, or to advance from one grade level to the next. It is unfortunate that, in a sense, we punish those minority students—like Jennings—who care the most about doing well, and who will go through hell and high water to succeed.

Group Identification

The best available research suggests further that people who feel a deep sense of attachment to their ethnic or gender group are also more at risk for feeling stereotype threat. Some individuals are less invested than others in their gender or racial identity, and initial research into this area of research, while not yet definitive, suggests that the less attached to or identified with one's group, the less one will be bothered by stereotypes impugning that group's abilities (e.g., Schmader, 2002). Apparently, in some cases, there can be an unfortunate trade-off for feelings of group pride and solidarity; deep identification with one's own group can create difficulty navigating integrated situations in which stereotypes may be relevant. Group identification may in part explain the fact that black immigrants, such as West Indians, have been found to be less vulnerable to stereotype threat despite the fact that they are seen and often treated as African Americans—and are quite aware of the negative stereotypes. They simply have less identification with African American identity and can easily draw positive benefits from their West Indian identity. This is particularly true among first-generation West Indians; those from the second generation, who identify more with an African American identity, appear to be more vulnerable to underperformance than their first-generation counterparts (Deaux et al., 2003).

Stigma Consciousness and Rejection Sensitivity

One reason group pride may heighten stereotype threat is that it often comes along with higher expectations for discrimination. Studies of "racial socialization" find that African Americans who have experienced discrimination in their lives often attempt to prepare and shield their children from such discrimination by teaching them to expect it—and to counter it with pride in their group (e.g., Hughes & Chen, 1999). Thus, along with a sense of group pride, some children also develop a heightened sense of what Pinel (1999) calls "stigma consciousness" and what Mendoza-Denton, Purdie, Downey, and Davis (2002) call "race-based rejection-sensitivity." Both measure the tendency to expect and to be bothered by prejudice, and people who score high on these measures perform worse in evaluative testing situations (e.g., Brown & Pinel, 2003; Aronson & Inzlicht, 2004).

Acceptance of the Stereotype

One need not believe a stereotype in order to feel threatened by its implications. Even if one rejects the premise of a stereotype, one nevertheless must contend with others and what they think. One can still feel uneasy or alienated in academic settings if there is a suspicion of inferiority—and these feelings, we have shown, are sufficient to undermine performance (Aronson, et al., 1999). But it seems reasonable to assume that some people may suspect that a stereotype may have some validity, a "kernel of truth," and such individuals would presumably be more threatened by the stereotype. Using subtle measures of people's implicit acceptance of stereotypes, recent research shows that the more people accept the stereotypes as true, the more vulnerable they are to stereotype threat (Spicer & Monteith, 2001; Schmader, 2002).

Self-Monitoring?

Because stereotype threat, as suggested earlier, stems partly from concern regarding other's impressions, people who are particularly good at managing impressions may be less susceptible to stereotype threat. Some recent research led by Michael Inzlicht (Inzlicht et al., 2003) suggests that this is indeed the case. In this research, black students took standardized tests either in the presence of other black students or one or more white students. The results showed that self-monitoring mattered. Only those black students who were "low self-monitors" were impaired in the presence of whites. Low self-monitors are typically less concerned with creating positive impressions; they just want to be themselves. As a result, they may be less practiced at the art of contending with situations where they are at risk of looking bad. More research is under way to examine these results, but they are also mirrored in studies involving women and mathematics, which suggest a robust relationship between self-monitoring and reactions to stereotype threat.

Beyond Test Performance

Stereotype threat effects such as we have described have been observed for many different populations and by numerous researchers. They have also been found on a variety of different tests, such as the GRE (Steele & Aronson, 1995), the Texas Assessment of Academic Skills (Aronson & Good, 2001b), Raven's Progressive Matrices (Croizet & Dutrévis, in press), and the Advanced Placement (AP) Calculus exam (Stricker & Ward, 1998), among others. If the influence of stereotype threat were limited to performance on standardized tests, this would be bad enough; performance on these tests is associated with important life outcomes, such as admission to college, advanced placement in college, and eventual earnings (e.g., Jencks & Phillips, 1998). But recent research suggests the role in other important indices of competence, such as the avoidance of challenge, identification with academics, and academic self-image.

Avoidance of Challenge

It is axiomatic in educational psychology that intellectual growth requires intellectual challenge. Yet when stereotypes are salient, challenge can signal the potential for racial or gender devaluation—in others' eyes and in one's own eyes as well. Aronson and Good (2001b) wanted to see whether, in addition to performance differences, children would respond to an evaluative setting by shying away from challenging problems in favor of easy, success-ensuring ones. They found that at the 6th grade (but not before), children did just this: They selected easier problems on an evaluative test but selected problems appropriate for their grade level when the test was framed as nondiagnostic of their abilities. This was true of both Latinos on a reading test and girls on a math test, a finding that mirrored precisely the performance differences we found for 6th graders. Jeff Stone (2002) has found nearly identical results: Under stereotype threat, athletes were more likely to avoid practice. Similarly, Pinel (1999) showed that women most prone to stereotype threat avoided tests in domains in which women are stereotypically alleged to be inferior to men. Such avoidance tactics are quite related to self-handicapping, in which individuals interfere with their own performance in order to have a plausible excuse for failure. One can well imagine that when given the choice

of curriculum that is challenging or not, the potential for encountering stereotype-threatening circumstances may steer people toward lower threat alternatives, and as a result, missed opportunities for developing competence.

Grades

In an important study, Massey, Charles, Lundy, and Fischer (2003) conducted a longitudinal survey of over 4,000 freshmen from different ethnic backgrounds attending over 28 U.S. colleges. These students were surveyed each year, and their performance in college was monitored throughout their undergraduate careers. Unsurprisingly, Massey et al. found the common achievement gaps observed between groups; Asians and whites outperformed blacks and Latinos, even when controlling for SAT scores, family income, and other important background factors. But when students' responses to questions probing their degree of stereotype vulnerability were controlled, the grade gaps disappeared; the degree of stereotype threat they felt as freshmen was associated with lower grades. This not only tells us that stereotype threat influences GPA, it tells us that it is a phenomenon that operates in the real world, outside the psychology laboratory.

Disidentification

After blunders or failures, people tend to rationalize. When people fail a math test and then claim the test was biased against them or that they do not really care about math anyway, we refer to this response as devaluing—and nearly everyone engages in some form of it (Major, Quinton, & McCoy, 2002). But when the response becomes so chronic that people adjust their self-concepts, divesting their self-esteem from the domain, this response can thwart achievement. We call this chronic adaptation "disidentification." We noted earlier that stereotype threat is strongest among students who are most invested in doing well, those who are highly identified with an intellectual domain. Disidentification helps by reducing sensitivity to failure. Although failure in and of itself is enough to prompt disidentification, stereotype threat appears to make it a more common response among blacks and Latinos, because the stereotype suggests not only a lack of ability but also limited belongingness in the domain (Cohen & Steele, 2002). But disidentification in the long run will hurt achievement because some degree of psychological investment is necessary; caring about doing well underlies the motivation for achievement (Osborne, 1997; Steele, 1992, 1997).

Rejection of Feedback

Targets of stereotypes suspect that others hold negative views about their group. Whether or not it is justified by actual prejudice, this can create an atmosphere of mistrust in any situation where those stereotypes are relevant (e.g., Cohen & Steele, 2002; Major et al., 2002). Thus, when a black student receives feedback from a white evaluator, it may be rejected as prejudiced. As Crocker and Major (1989) have shown, this "discounting" of feedback preserves self-esteem. But as Cohen and Steele's (2002) research suggests, it also impairs motivation. It is as if the student asks, "Why try hard to do a good job when whatever I do will be devalued?" Indeed, even positive feedback is often discounted. In a recent study by Lawrence and Crocker (2002), we see just how tricky the business of giving feedback can be in the context of a negative stereotype. White evaluators gave both blacks and whites a test that was engineered to produce high performance. For half the participants, she simply wrote the score on the exam. For the other half, she added the words "great job." The white students reacted quite differently to this detail: The black students thought the evaluator had lower expectations of them when they received the praise, as though surprised by a black student's high performance.

Thus, although there are clear benefits in terms of self-esteem maintenance, discounting feedback has serious drawbacks; one loses motivation and, presumably, important information about how to improve one's performance whenever one rejects feedback. Moreover, Aronson and Inzlicht (2004) have found that those most vulnerable to stereotype threat (as measured by questionnaire responses) have unclear academic self-concepts; that is, they are less aware of their strengths and weaknesses than individuals who are not stereotype-vulnerable. Because this sort of awareness is a key component of competence—one needs to know one's weaknesses to improve on them or compensate for them—lacking clarity can be a risk factor (e.g., Sternberg, 1996). Thus, all of these self-image protective strategies—avoiding challenge, avoiding practice, avoiding evaluation, and discounting feedback—reveal another irony about stereotype threat: Often, *feeling* competent matters more than becoming competent.

BOOSTING THE PERFORMANCE OF STEREOTYPE-VULNERABLE STUDENTS

One advantage to explaining underperformance in terms of situational variables is that this both implies and points the way to situational solutions to boosting performance. At the same time, given the nature of the triggers to stereotype threat—evaluative situations and social identity salience—changing situations to reduce the threat may be more difficult in the real world. Although schoolteachers can work to create a nonevaluative atmosphere in class, doing so on tests is another matter. Likewise, since the mere mixing of students can arouse stereotype threat even in the absence of evaluation, the diverse classroom or testing center is likely to be rife with apprehension for minority students who are invested in doing well.

Yet there is mounting evidence from both laboratory and field studies that the gaps in performance can be narrowed with careful attention to how situations are created and to what students can be taught.

Situational Approaches

Cooperation

Stereotyping and intergroup tensions tend to thrive in the competitive settings, as in traditional American classrooms. A number of interventions have yielded impressive gains in the academic achievement of minority youth by structuring classroom or study environments to minimize the performance-undermining processes akin to those have discussed here. E. Aronson's "Jigsaw Classroom" (Aronson & Patnoe, 1997) and Uri Treisman's (1992) work with African American math students are outstanding examples in this regard. In the Jigsaw Classroom, lessons are broken up into several pieces, with one piece distributed to each member of the group, who must learn the material and teach it to the others. To perform well, therefore, students must cooperate, because the piece of the puzzle held by each student is vital to everyone's successful learning and performance. Studies of the Jigsaw Classroom show that the technique typically raises the minority students' grades (by about a letter grade), raises their self-esteem, increases friendships between ethnic group members, and leads to greater enjoyment among students of all backgrounds. (In some cases, the nonminority students also benefit academically, but in no case do they ever do worse than in the traditional classroom.) In Treisman's calculus workshops, there is also cooperative group study outside of class in special homework sessions, but the cooperation is not rigidly divided as in the Jigsaw Classroom. Moreover, the work is very challenging, going beyond what is covered in class. Treisman's program lifted the African Americans' calculus achievement to surprising levels; they earned grades as high as the Asian students in the class. Getting children or adult students to work cooperatively not only reduces prejudice (and thus stereotype threat), but it also ensures that all students feel a sense of belongingness. These studies are touchstones; they prove that group differences are tractable, that achievement gaps narrow under the proper social conditions.

Drawing on the Treisman work, Steele, Spencer, Davies, Harber, and Nisbett (2001) designed a comprehensive program for first-year students at the University of Michigan. This program sought to reduce stereotype threat through a number of tactics. First, students were recruited to the program in a way that emphasized that they had already met the tough admission standards at the University of Michigan. During the program, students participated in weekly seminars throughout the first semester that allowed them to get to know one another and to learn some of the common problems they shared. They also participated in subject mastery workshops in one of their courses that exposed them to advanced material that went beyond material in the class. These tactics were designed to convey three vital messages: that instructors and peers believed in their potential to excel academically, that they would not stereotype them, and that they believed they belonged at the university. Several years of the program demonstrate that such practices can lead to a substantial increase in African American's performance in school. On average, African Americans randomly assigned to the program do .4 of a grade point better than African Americans randomly assigned to a control group. This increase in performance, despite diminishing somewhat over time, led to higher retention rates. What makes the program work? Analysis of survey data collected from the program participants and the control group suggests that the program decreases stereotype threat, which in turn promotes identification with school, which leads to better grades and retention.

Individual Approaches

Forewarning

Can awareness of one's susceptibility to processes such as stereotype threat release one from its effects? In other words, is forewarned forearmed? Apparently so, according to two recent studies. In one (Aronson & Williams, 2004), prior to being tested in the Steele and Aronson paradigm described earlier, black college students were sent and instructed to read a pamphlet describing either the stereotype threat effect, the phenomenon of test anxiety, or a completely unrelated topic. Those in the first two conditions performed just as well as those who took the test under no stereotype threat conditions; those in the control group performed significantly less well, as low as those students under stereotype threat but not forewarned. A very similar study (Johns & Schmader, 2004) found precisely the same effect with women taking a difficult math test. These studies are important for those of us who are interested in interventions to boost student achievement, but they also provide relief for those of us who worry that teaching their psychology students about the research might create rather than reduce a vulnerability to stereotypes.

Reframing Ability

Based on research by Carol Dweck (e.g., 1999), Aronson (1999) predicted that stereotype threat would be least problematic for students who conceived of their abilities as malleable. After all, if the stereotype gains power by implying a lack of ability, stereotype threat should be less threatening if one sees ability as expandable. To test this reasoning, students took a difficult GRE verbal test presented as a test of an ability that was either malleable or fixed. As predicted, the African Americans—and to a lesser degree the whites—performed much better and reported lower performance anxiety when the test was said to diagnose an ability that could be expanded with practice. The utility of seeing ability as malleable is further underscored in a similar study (Aronson, 1997). In this study, undergraduates were led to believe they had either performed well or poorly on a test measuring their speed-reading ability. Prior to receiving the feedback, the test takers had been led to believe either that speed-reading was a highly improvable skill, or that it was an endowed ability that could not be improved much with practice. At issue was how the feedback and the conception of the ability would interact to influence how much the students devalued the importance of speed-reading. The results were clear. When speed-reading was presented as a trait that could not be improved, test takers who received positive feedback gave it high ratings ("Speed-reading is an extremely valuable skill"). In contrast, test takers who received negative feedback did not believe that speed-reading was an important skill. This devaluing did not occur when the test takers were led to believe that they could get better at speed-reading. Students in both groups in this condition—those who got positive feedback and those who got negative feedback—said that speed-reading was an important skill. Thus thinking of a skill as malleable appears to reduce the tendency to disidentify in the face of failure.

A pair of field interventions built upon these findings. One program involving African American and European American college students (Aronson, Fried, & Good, 2002) employed numerous tactics of attitude change to get them to adopt the malleable intelligence mind-set. Attitudes toward academic achievement and actual performance were assessed 4 months later and at the end of the school year. The results were highly encouraging. On average, African American students improved their grades (overall GPA) by .4 grade point. In a second program (Good, Aronson, & Inzlicht, 2003), college students mentored Latino and European American junior high students. The mentors conveyed to their students different attitudes that we hypothesized would help the students navigate the difficult transition year from elementary school to junior high school. For one group of students, the mentors focused on the idea that intelligence is expandable; for another group of students, the mentors discussed the perils of drug use. At year's end, students mentored in the malleability of intelligence received higher scores on the statewide standardized test of reading ability than students who received the antidrug message. Similar results were found for girls' math performance on the mathematics test. When the malleability message was not incorporated into the mentoring, girls underperformed relative to boys. When they were taught about the expandability of intelligence, their performance increased substantially. Similarly positive results were found in an additional condition, in which the students were taught to attribute any difficulties or anxieties they were experiencing to the normal difficulties of junior high rather than any lack of ability. This is a replication of the intervention by Wilson and Linville (1982), described at the beginning of this chapter. This research shows that although stereotype threat is a real phenomenon, it is certainly not insurmountable; there are many ways to overcome its effects. What remains to be studied is the extent to which elements in each of these studies can be combined to produce additive effects on performance.

In considering the effect of stereotypes on achievement, we think it is vital to realize that competence is both fragile and malleable. Social relations—how people think about and treat one another—can make a big difference for achievement. The good news is that understanding this can help us reduce some of the achievement inequities that continue to perplex researchers, educators, and policymakers. But we hasten to underscore that arguing that stereotypes can undermine student performance, motivation and self-concept should not be taken to mean that these are the *primary* sources of the achievement gap. There are bigger factors at play, most notably, inequities in socioeconomic background, schools, and teacher quality that put many minorities at a distinct disadvantage. But we do think that stereotypes account for a meaningful portion of the gap that remains when these factors are equivalent. The fact that the minority–white achievement gap persists—and continues to puzzle those who study it—lies partly in the difficulty of recognizing the forces that can make human competence more fragile than we customarily think.

REFERENCES

Aboud, F. E. (1988). *Children and prejudice*. New York: Blackwell.

Ambady, N., Shih, M., Kim, A., & Pittinsky T. L. (2001). Stereotype susceptibility in children: Effects of identity activation on quantitative performance. *Psychological Science, 12*, 385–390.

Arnold, D. H., & Cross, B. D. (2003). *The relationship of student ethnicity and gender to teacher perceptions of math interest in Head Start preschoolers*. Unpublished manuscript, University of Massachusetts, Amherst.

Aronson, E., & Patnoe, S. (1997). *The jigsaw classroom*. New York: Longman.

Aronson, J. (1997). *The effects of conceptions of ability on task valuation*. Unpublished manuscript, New York University, New York.

Aronson, J. (1999). *The effects of conceiving ability as fixed or improvable on responses to stereotype threat*. Unpublished manuscript, New York University, New York.

Aronson, J. (2002a, August). *Narrowing the minority–white achievement gap: Lessons from psychology*. G. Stanley Hall Lecture, American Psychological Association, Chicago, IL.

Aronson, J. (2002b). Stereotype threat: Contending and coping with unnerving expectations. In J. Aronson (Ed.), *Improving academic achievement: Impact of psychological factors on education*. San Diego: Academic Press.

Aronson, J., Fried, C., & Good, C. (2002). Reducing the effects of stereotype threat on African American college students by shaping theories of intelligence. *Journal of Experimental Social Psychology, 38*, 113–125.

Aronson, J., & Good, C. (2001a). *Personal versus situational stakes and stereotype threat: A test of the vanguard hypothesis*. Manuscript in preparation.

Aronson, J., & Good, C. (2001b). *Stereotype threat and the avoidance of challenging work*. Manuscript in preparation.

Aronson, J., & Good, C. (2002). The development and consequences of stereotype vulnerability in adolescents. In F. Pajares & T. Urdan (Eds.), *Adolescence and education*. New York: Information Age.

Aronson, J., Inzlicht, M. (2004). The ups and downs of attributional ambiguity: Stereotype vulnerability and the academic self-knowledge of African American college students. *Psychological Science, 15*, 829–836.

Aronson J., & Jones, E. E. (1992). Inferring abilities after influencing performance. *Journal of Experimental Social Psychology, 28*, 277–299.

Aronson, J., Lustina, M., Good, C., Keough, K., Steele, C., & Brown, J. (1999). When white men can't do math: Necessary and sufficient factors in stereotype threat. *Journal of Experimental Social Psychology, 35*, 29–46.

Aronson, J., Quinn, D., & Spencer, S. J. (1998). Stereotype threat and the academic performance of minorities and women. In J. Swim & C. Stangor (Eds.), *Prejudice: The target's perspective*. San Diego: Academic Press.

Aronson, J., & Salinas, M. F. (2001). *Stereotype threat, attributional ambiguity, and Latino underperformance*. Unpublished manuscript, New York University, New York.

Aronson, J., & Williams, J. (2004). *Stereotype threat: Forewarned is forearmed*. Manuscript in preparation.

Arroyo, C. G., & Zigler, E. (1995). Racial identity, academic achievement, and the psychological well-being of economically disadvantaged adolescents. *Journal of Personality and Social Psychology, 69*, 903–914.

Bargh, J. A., Chen, M., & Burrows, L. (1996). Automaticity of social behavior: Direct effects of trait construct and stereotype priming on action. *Journal of Personality and Social Psychology, 71*, 230–244.

Baumeister, R. F., & Leary, M. R. (1995). The need to belong: Desire for interpersonal attachments as a fundamental human motivation. *Psychological Bulletin, 117*, 497–529.

Baumeister, R. F., Twenge, J. W., & Nuss, C. K. (2002). Effects of social exclusion on cognitive processes: Anticipated aloneness reduces intelligent thought. *Journal of Personality and Social Psychology, 83*, 817–827.

Blascovich, J., Spencer, S. J., Quinn, D. M., & Steele, C. M. (2001). Stereotype threat and the cardiovascular reactivity of African-Americans. *Psychological Science, 12*, 225–229.

Brophy, J. E., & Good, T. (1974). *Teacher–child dyadic relationships: Causes and consequences*. New York: Holt, Rhinehart & Winston.

Brown, R. P., & Pinel, E. C. (2003). Stigma on my mind: Individual differences in the experience of stereotype threat. *Journal of Experimental Social Psychology, 39*, 626–633.

Cohen, G. L., & Steele, C. M. (2002). A barrier of mistrust: How stereotypes affect cross-race mentoring. In J. Aronson (Ed.), *Improving academic achievement: Impact of psychological factors on education.* San Diego: Academic Press.

Coleman, J. S. (1961). *The adolescent society.* New York: Free Press.

Cook, P., & Ludwig, J. (1998). The burden of "acting white": Do black adolescents disparage academic achievement? In C. Jencks & M. Phillips (Eds.), *The black–white test score gap.* Washington, DC: Brookings Institution Press.

Crocker, J., & Major, B. (1989). Social stigma and self-esteem: The self-protective properties of stigma. *Psychological Review, 96,* 608–630.

Croizet, J. C., & Claire, T. (1998). Extending the concept of stereotype threat to social class: The intellectual underperformance of students from low socioeconomic backgrounds. *Personality and Social Psychology Bulletin, 24,* 588–594.

Croizet, J. C., Després, G., Gauzins, M., Huguet, P., & Leyens, J. (2003). *Stereotype threat undermines intellectual performance by triggering a disruptive mental load.* Unpublished manuscript, Université Blaise Pascal, Clermont-Ferrand, France.

Croizet J. C., & Dutrévis, M. (in press). Socioeconomic status and intelligence: Why test scores do not equal merit. *Journal of Poverty.*

Darley, J. M., & Gross, P. (1983). A hypothesis-confirming bias in labeling effects. *Journal of Personality and Social Psychology, 44,* 20–33.

Davies, P. G., Spencer, S. J., Quinn, D. M., & Gerhardstein, R. (2002). All consuming images: How demeaning commercials that elicit stereotype threat can restrain women academically and professionally. *Personality and Social Psychology Bulletin, 28,* 1615–1628.

Deaux, K., Steele, C. M., Gilkes, A., Blikmen, N., Ventumeac, A., Joseph, Y., et al. (2003). *Becoming American: Stereotype threat effects in black immigrant groups.* Unpublished manuscript, Graduate Center, City University of New York.

Devine, P. (1989). Stereotypes and prejudice: Their automatic and controlled components. *Journal of Personality and Social Psychology, 56,* 5–18.

Dweck, C. S. (1999). *Self-theories: Their role in motivation, personality, and development.* Philadelphia: Taylor & Francis.

Elliot, A. J., & Church, M. A. (1997). A hierarchical model of approach and avoidance achievement motivation. *Journal of Personality and Social Psychology, 72,* 218–232.

Elliot, A. J., McGregor, H., & Gable, S. (1999). Achievement goals, study strategies, and exam performance: A mediational analysis. *Journal of Educational Psychology, 91,* 549–563.

Elliot, A. J., & Thrash, T. M. (2004). The intergenerational transmission of fear of failure. *Personality and Social Psychology Bulletin, 30,* 957–971.

Fazio, R. H., Jackson, J. R., Dunton, B. C., & Williams, C. J. (1995). Variability in automatic activation as an unobtrusive measure of racial attitudes: A bona fide pipeline? *Journal of Personality and Social Psychology, 69,* 1013–1027.

Ferguson, R. F. (1998). Teacher's perceptions and expectations and the black–white test score gap. In C. Jencks & M. Phillips (Eds.), *The black–white test score gap.* Washington, DC: Brookings Institution Press.

Fordham, S., & Ogbu, J. (1986). Black students' school success: Coping with the "burden of acting white." *Urban Review, 18,* 176–206.

Frome, P. M., & Eccles, J. S. (1998). Parents' influence on children's achievement-related perceptions. *Journal of Personality and Social Psychology, 74,* 435–452.

Garcia, J., Helms, W., & Garcia, L. (2003). *White men can't jump?: Stereotype threat and triggering cues.* Unpublished manuscript, Tufts University, Cambridge, MA.

Gonzales, P. M., Blanton, H., & Williams, K. J. (2002). The effects of stereotype threat and double-minority status on the test performance of Latino women. *Personality and Social Psychology Bulletin, 28,* 659–670.

Good, C., Aronson, J., & Inzlicht, M. (2003). Improving adolescents' standardized test performance: An intervention to reduce the effects of stereotype threat. *Journal of Applied Developmental Psychology, 24,* 645–662.

Graham, S., Taylor, A., & Hudley, C. (1998). Exploring achievement values among ethnic minority early adolescents. *Journal of Educational Psychology, 90*(4), 606–620.

Harris, J. R. (1998). *The nurture assumption.* New York: Touchstone.

Harrist, A. W., & Bradley, D. (2002). Teachers and students as agents of change. In J. Aronson (Ed.), *Improving academic achievement: Impact of psychological factors on education.* San Diego: Academic Press.

Herrnstein, R. J., & Murray, C. (1994). *The bell curve.* New York: Free Press.

Hess, T. M., Auman, C., Colcombe, S. J., & Rahhal, T. (2003). The impact of stereotype threat on age differences in memory performance. *Journal of Gerontology, 58,* 3–11.

Hughes, D., & Chen, L. (1999). Parents' race-related messages to children: A developmental perspective. In C. Tamis-Lemonda & L. Balter (Eds.), *Child psychology: A handbook of contemporary issues.* New York: New York University Press.

Huston, A. C. (1983). Sex typing. In E. M. Hetherington (Ed.), *Handbook of child psychology* (Vol. 4). New York: Wiley.

Inzlicht, M., Aronson, J., Good, C., & McKay, L. (2003). *Monitoring's moderating muscle: Why being outnumbered does not always threaten stigmatized groups.* Unpublished manuscript, New York University, New York.

Inzlicht, M., & Ben-Zeev, T. (2000). A threatening intellectual environment: Why females are susceptible to experiencing problem-solving deficits in the presence of males. *Psychological Science, 11,* 365–371.

Inzlicht, M., McKay, L., & Aronson, J. (2004). *Losing control: How being the target of stigmatization depletes the ego.* Unpublished manuscript, New York University, New York.

Jencks, C., & Phillips, M. (1998). *The black–white test score gap.* Washington, DC: Brookings Institution Press.

Jensen, A. R. (1980). *Bias in mental testing.* New York: Free Press.

Johns, M., & Schmader, T. (2004, January). *Knowing is half the battle.* Paper presented at the annual meeting of the Society for Personality and Social Psychology, Austin, TX.

Jones, E. E. (1989). The framing of competence. *Personality and Social Psychology Bulletin, 15,* 477–492.

Jones, E. E., & Berglas, S. (1978). Control of attributions of the self through self-handicapping strategies: The appeal of alcohol and the role of underachievement. *Personality and Social Psychology Bulletin, 4,* 200–206.

Killen, M., Lee-Kim, J., McGlothin, H., & Stangor, C. (2002). How children and adolescents evaluate gender and racial exclusion. *Monographs of the Society for Research in Child Development, 67,* 45–83.

Kistner, J., Metzler, A., Gatlin, D., & Risi, S. (1993). Classroom racial proportions and children's peer relations: Race and gender effects. *Journal of Educational Psychology, 85,* 446–452.

Lawrence, J. S., & Crocker, J. (2002, August). *Does academic praise communicate stereotypic expectations to Black students?* Paper presented at the American Psychological Association Annual Convention, Chicago, IL.

Levy, B. (1996) Improving memory in old age through implicit self-stereotyping. *Journal of Personality and Social Psychology, 71,* 1092–1107.

Leyens, J. P., Désert, M., Croizet, J. C., & Darcis, C. (2000). Stereotype threat: Are lower status and history of stigmatization preconditions of stereotype threat? *Personality and Social Psychology Bulletin, 26,* 1189–1199.

Lippmann, W. (1997). *Public opinion.* New York: Macmillan. (Original work published 1922)

Major, B., Quinton, W. J., & McCoy, S. K. (2002). Antecedents and consequences of attributions to discrimination: Theoretical and empirical advances. In M. Zanna (Ed.), *Advances in experimental social psychology* (Vol. 34). San Diego: Academic Press.

Marx, D. M., & Roman, J. S. (2002). Female role models: Protecting women's math test performance. *Personality and Social Psychology Bulletin, 28,* 1183–1193.

Massey, D. S., Charles, C. Z., Lundy, G. F., & Fischer, M. J. (2003). *The source of the river: The social origins of freshmen at America's selective colleges and universities.* Princeton, NJ: Princeton University Press.

McKown, C., & Weinstein, R. S. (2003). The development and consequences of stereotype-consciousness in middle childhood. *Child Development, 74*(2), 498–515.

Mendoza-Denton, R., Purdie, V., Downey, G., & Davis, A. (2002). Sensitivity to status-based rejection: Implications for African American students' college experience. *Journal of Personality and Social Psychology, 83,* 896–918.

Mueller, C. M., & Dweck, C. S. (1998). Praise for intelligence can undermine children's motivation and performance. *Journal of Personality and Social Psychology, 75,* 33–52.

National Research Council. (2003). *Engaging schools: Fostering high school students' motivation to learn.* Washington, DC: National Academy Press.

O'Brien, L., & Crandall, C. (2003). Stereotype threat and arousal: Effects on women's math performance. *Personality and Social Psychology Bulletin, 29,* 782–789.

Ogbu, J., & Davis, A. (2003). *Black American students in an affluent suburb.* Mahwah, NJ: Erlbaum.

Osborne, J. W. (1997). Race and academic disidentification. *Journal of Educational Psychology, 89,* 728–735.

Pinel, E. C. (1999). Stigma consciousness: The psychological legacy of social stereotypes. *Journal of Personality and Social Psychology, 76,* 114–128.

Postman, N. (1988). *Conscientious objections.* New York: Knopf.

Rist, R. (1970). Student social class and teacher expectations: The self-fulfilling prophecy in ghetto education. *Harvard Educational Review, 40*(3), 411–451.

Rosenthal, R. (2002). The Pygmalion effect and its mediating mechanisms. In J. Aronson (Ed.), *Improving academic achievement: Impact of psychological factors on education.* San Diego: Academic Press.

Rosenthal, R., & Jacobson, L. (1968). *Pygmalion in the classroom.* New York: Holt, Rinehart & Winston.

Schmader, T. (2002). Gender identification moderates the effects of stereotype threat on women's math performance. *Journal of Experimental Social Psychology, 38,* 194–201.

Schmader, T., & Johns, M. (2003). Converging evidence that stereotype threat reduces working memory capacity. *Journal of Personality and Social Psychology, 85,* 440–452.

Sherif, M., & Sherif, C. W. (1969). *Social psychology.* New York: Harper & Row.

Shih, M., Pittinsky, T. L., & Ambady, N. (1999). Stereotype susceptibility: Identity salience and shifts in quantitative performance. *Psychological Science, 10,* 80–83.

Smith, J. L., & White, P. H. (2002). An examination of implicitly activated, explicitly activated and nullified stereotypes on mathematical performance: It's not just a women's issue. *Sex Roles, 47,* 179–191.

Smith, T. W. (1990). *Ethnic images* [GSS Topical Report

No. 19]. National Opinion Research Center, Chicago.

Spencer, S. J., Iserman, E., Davies, P. G., & Quinn, D. M. (2001). *Suppression of doubts, anxiety, and stereotypes as a mediator of the effect of stereotype threat on women's math performance.* Unpublished manuscript, University of Waterloo, Ontario, Canada.

Spencer, S. J., Steele, C. M., & Quinn, D. M. (1999). Stereotype threat and women's math performance. *Journal of Experimental Social Psychology, 35,* 4–28.

Spicer, C. V., & Monteith, M. J. (2001). *Implicit outgroup favoritism among African Americans and vulnerability to stereotype threat.* Unpublished manuscript, College of Charleston, SC.

Stangor, C., Carr, C., & Kiang, L. (1998). Activating stereotypes undermines task performance expectations. *Journal of Personality and Social Psychology, 75,* 1191–1197.

Steele, C. M. (1992, April). Race and the schooling of black Americans. *The Atlantic Monthly,* pp. 44–54.

Steele, C. M. (1997). A threat in the air: How stereotypes shape the intellectual identity and performance. *American Psychologist, 52,* 613–629.

Steele, C. M., & Aronson, J. (1995). Stereotype threat and the intellectual test performance of African Americans. *Journal of Personality and Social Psychology, 69,* 797–811.

Steele, C. M., Spencer, S. J., & Aronson, J. (2002). Contending with group image: The psychology of stereotype and social identity threat. In M. P. Zanna (Ed.), *Advances in experimental social psychology* (Vol. 34, pp. 379–440). San Diego: Academic Press.

Steele, C. M., Spencer, S. J., Davies, P. G., Harber, K., & Nisbett, R. E. (2001). *African American college achievement: A "wise" intervention.* Unpublished manuscript, Stanford University, Stanford, CA.

Sternberg, R. J. (1996). *Successful intelligence.* New York: Simon & Schuster.

Sternberg, R. J. (2002). Intelligence is not just inside the head. In J. Aronson (Ed.), *Improving academic achievement: Impact of psychological factors on education.* San Diego: Academic Press.

Stone, J. (2002). Battling doubt by avoiding practice: The effects of stereotype threat on self-handicapping in White athletes. *Personality and Social Psychology Bulletin, 28,* 1667–1678.

Stone, J., Lynch, C. I., Sjomeling, M., & Darley, J. M. (1999). Stereotype threat effects on Black and White athletic performance. *Journal of Personality and Social Psychology, 77,* 1213–1227.

Stricker, L. J., & Ward, W. (1998). Inquiring about examinee's ethnicity and sex: Effects on AP calculus AB examination performance (College Board Report 98-1; l Educational Testing Service Research Report No. 98-5). New York: College Entrance Examination Board.

Suskind, R. (1999). *A hope in the unseen.* New York: Broadway Books.

Tenenbaum, H., & Leaper, C. (2003). Parent–child conversations about science: The socialization of gender inequities? *Developmental Psychology, 1,* 34–47.

Treisman, U. (1992). Studying students studying calculus: A look at the lives of minority mathematics students in college. *College Mathematics Journal, 23*(5), 362–372.

Tyson, K. (2003). Notes from the back of the room: Problems and paradoxes in the schooling of young black students. *Sociology of Education, 76,* 326–343.

Weinstein, R. S. (2002). *Reaching higher: The power of expectations in schooling.* Cambridge, MA: Harvard University Press.

Wheeler, S. C., & Petty, R. E. (2001). The effects of stereotype activation on behavior: A review of possible mechanisms. *Psychological Bulletin, 127,* 797–826.

White, R. W. (1959). Motivation reconsidered: The concept of competence. *Psychological Review, 66,* 297–333.

Wigfield, A., & Eccles, J. S. (2002). Students' motivation during the middle school years. In J. Aronson (Ed.), *Improving academic achievement: Impact of psychological factors on education.* San Diego: Academic Press.

Wilson, T. D., & Linville, P. W. (1982). Improving the academic performance of college freshmen: Attribution therapy revisited. *Journal of Personality and Social Psychology, 42,* 367–376.

Word, C. O., Zanna, M. P., & Cooper, J. (1974). The nonverbal mediation of self-fulfilling prophecies in interracial interaction. *Journal of Experimental Social Psychology, 10,* 109–120.

CHAPTER 25

ॐ

The "Inside" Story

A Cultural–Historical Analysis of Being Smart and Motivated, American Style

VICTORIA C. PLAUT
HAZEL ROSE MARKUS

A popular video used in social science and education courses, *Preschool in Three Cultures*, presents highlights of a study comparing preschool practices in the United States, Japan, and China. In the video (Tobin, Wu, & Davidson, 1989), teachers from each of the three cultural contexts comment on each other's teaching and classroom practices. In the Japanese segment, a boy called Hiroki is obviously disrupting his class. He stands on the table, tosses around cards from a sorting game, tells jokes, sings, and engages other kids in noisy conversation while the teacher is giving a lesson. The teacher ignores him. The American teachers are alarmed by Hiroki's behavior, but are even more concerned by the teacher's inaction. They wonder aloud why the teacher does not intervene to stop Hiroki. They suggest that because he is very intelligent, perhaps gifted, and obviously bored by classroom routine, he should be given some individualized or special instruction. The Japanese teachers are taken back by this characterization. While agreeing that Hiroki disrupts the class, they question how he could possibly be "very intelligent" if he does not even know how to control his behavior and fit in with his fellow students.

The example of Hiroki is instructive about competence and motivation, American[1] style. The American preschool teachers assume, as do many American teachers, supervisors, and employers, that intelligence displays itself in verbal output and through behavioral expressions that are in some ways distinctive. Their comments further reveal their belief that competent behavior requires that the student be personally interested and engaged. The surprise of the Japanese teachers at the American reflections highlights different understandings of competence and motivation. From their perspective, it is impossible to see Hiroki as a competent or gifted student. Competence and intelligence, Japanese style, requires knowing how to behave properly. A sensitivity to others and their expectations is the signature of motivation.

The mutual bewilderment of the two sets of teachers at what is regarded as smart or motivated by teachers in the other cultural context points to the influence of invisible networks of culture-specific assumptions about the social world. These assumptions include solutions to questions: What is a person? What are the sources of behavior? and What is the good and right way "to be" within this social world? We call these culture-specific sets of meanings and practices "cultural models." These typically tacit models render the actions in the Japanese classroom meaningful and coherent to the Japanese observers, and, simultaneously, peculiar to the American observers who are using different models to make sense of the classroom.

In this chapter, we examine the importance of cultural models to both scientific and lay understandings of competence and motivation. We (1) provide some examples of sociocultural diversity in models of competence and motivation, (2) describe the origins and nature of the common European American model that underlies most psychological theorizing and research, and (3) review recent comparative empirical research that illuminates the sociocultural specificity of many findings in the competence and motivation literature.

In examining cultural models, we draw on the cultural psychological literature. "Cultural psychology" is the interdisciplinary study of how cultural practices and meanings, and psychological processes and structures depend on each other (Fiske, Kitayama, Markus, & Nisbett, 1998; Miller, 1994; Shweder, 1991). A cultural psychology approach focuses on the interpretive structures of the world within which the person is a participant. We analyze cultural models of competence and motivation as significant features of cultural contexts that fashion individual experience (Bruner, 1990; Holland, Lachicotte, Skinner, & Cain, 1998). Being competent and motivated, as well as identifying competence and motivation in others, entails engagement with cultural models.

Although a variety of models of competence and motivation are possible and indeed exist in various contexts, the most prevalent and well-elaborated lay and scientific models within American contexts represent these phenomena as innate individual properties and locate them firmly "inside" the individual. As these models are taken for granted and absorbed in the everyday practices of teaching and testing, their organizing force is made transparent, so that the search for the sources of competence and motivation focuses on the internal properties of brains, minds, and people. There are, of course, and have always been other theories and perspectives suggesting that competence and motivation—in fact, all of human behavior—is best understood by focusing on the outside: the external, the contextual, the social, the cultural, and the historical (e.g., Lewin, 1935; Vygotsky, 1978). Likewise, there have always been theories proposing that the self is socially constructed (Cooley, 1902; Mead, 1934). Why the "inside" story tenaciously persists as the most prevalent interpretation of differences in competence and motivation is the story of this chapter.

The view that competence and motivation are primarily individual and internal forces is not the result of the unfettered observations of the way humans "actually are"; instead, this view reflects the incorporation of historically derived, widely dispersed systems of meanings and ideas about humans, the self, the role of others in action, and the consequences of action. This vast interpretive matrix is essential for human behavior; it affords individual experience. Yet a comparative approach reveals that the "inside" cultural model of competence and motivation is in many ways discretionary. It could have been, and perhaps could still be, otherwise.

SOCIOCULTURAL HISTORICAL MODELS: THE INVISIBLE FOUNDATION OF COMPETENCE AND MOTIVATION

What does it mean to be competent? In many American workplaces and schools, the answer is obvious. Competence, unless it is qualified (e.g., athletic or social competence), refers to intellectual competence. The focus is on the nature of the mind, thinking, and knowledge. The competent person is quick, sharp, able to express him- or herself, has a lot of knowledge, and is able to use it successfully to make connections and solve problems or intellectual puzzles. The social context, social skills, relationships, and other people and their expectations are largely irrelevant and external to the domain of intellectual competence.

Most psychological concepts of "competence" (defined in this volume as ability or success, including phenomena such as aptitude, intelligence, proficiency, skill, etc.) are rooted in deeply entrenched but rarely articulated cultural models of intelligence (e.g., Carugati, 1990; Polanyi, 1957). These models include tacit assumptions, images, and metaphors that carry a far ranging set of commitments. For example, they define what competence is, what it does, where it comes from, and where to look for it.

A Machine or a Root?: Divergent Metaphors of Mind

Metaphors provide the initial blueprints for understanding competence and the source of competence (Sternberg, 1990; Weiner, 1991). For example, according to Lakoff and Johnson (1999), the mind is often conceptualized as

> a container image defining a space that is inside the body and separate from it. Via metaphor, the mind is given an inside and an outside. Ideas and concepts are internal, existing somewhere in the inner space of our minds, while what they refer to are things in the external, physical world. This metaphor is so deeply ingrained that it is hard to think about the mind in any other way. (p. 266)

In Western philosophy and in the science that is built on its philosophical assumptions, the mind is also often metaphorized as a mechanical device, a switchboard, a machine, a set of gears that "works" (Lakoff & Johnson, 1999). As people think, they can feel that the "wheels are turning" and have a sense that they are "cranking out a solution." Sometimes the mind is a calculator that counts and sums (e.g., "To what does it all add up?" or "What is the bottom line?" or "Give me 'an account' of what happened"). Problems are solved with "power" from the "engine" of the brain. In recent theorizing, the machine that is the mind is a computer: The mind is the software; the brain is hardware (Minsky, 1986). When the mind machine is experiencing difficulties, it

is said to be a little rusty or to be experiencing a mental breakdown. In an extreme statement, but one that aptly characterizes empirical work in psychology, Shweder (1990) argues that psychology

> assumes that its subject matter is a central (abstract and transcendent = deep or interior or hidden) processing mechanism inherent (fixed and universal) in human beings, which enables them to think (classify, infer, remember, imagine) . . . and that "all the other stuff—stimuli, contexts, resources, values, meanings, knowledge, religion, rituals, language, technologies, institutions—is conceived to be external to or outside of the central processing mechanism. (pp. 45–46)

Machine metaphors are central to Western conceptions of mind and thinking, and they simultaneously define what is involved in being a competent person. In many European American cultural contexts, the person is represented and realized as a separate, bounded, autonomous entity—an individual (Markus & Kitayama, 1991; Shweder & Bourne, 1984). Individual actions result from the attributes or the properties of the person that are activated and then cause behavior. Competence is one such individual property. Accordingly, competence is located *in* the individual, *in* the mind, *in* the brain. European American competence is active; it cranks, works, churns, turns, hums, percolates, crackles, and illuminates, and out come solutions and products. Typically, it involves technical intelligence that is distinctly separate from socioemotional expertise or skills (Goleman, 1995; Rogoff & Chavajay, 1995). People are understood to be powered by what is inside. Whether the right stuff is DNA, genes, neurons, hormones, traits, abilities, motivation, drive, or talent, it is what is inside that counts. The inside view sets up the powerful inside–outside dichotomy that pervades lay thinking and scientific theorizing alike. If the inside is good, the outside (the world, others and their expectations) is irrelevant, or maybe even corrosive to the inside.

Minds and intellectual competence take a different form in many non-Western contexts (Greenfield, 1997; Harkness, Super, & Keefer, 1992). In East Asian cultural contexts, minds are not containers with fixed boundaries marking inside and outside. Instead, they are entities more likely to be of the natural world, like wind or water, or organisms, like plants or roots, which are interdependent with the environment and require the sun and nutrients of the soil (Markus, Kitayama, & Heiman, 1996). In some East Asian contexts, the "good" mind is not cranking and churning but is instead clear or blank or still, and is often described through metaphors of water. It is "a mind as clear and reflective as water is central . . for it is accurate information, whether it is in the detection of an opponent's next move in judo, or the anticipation of a subtle shift in consumer taste in automobiles that forms the basis for creative action" (Kraft, as quoted in Goleman, Kaufman, & Ray, 1992, p. 42).

In Korean cultural contexts, the mind and self are sometimes metaphorized as a white root. When a white root is planted within red soil, it becomes red; when planted within green soil, it becomes green. Similarly, in Japan, the mind becomes a willow and the self is a rice plant (Ohnuki-Tierney, 1995). Willows and rice plants are appropriate metaphors, because they grow and mature; they are flexible and bend, as should good minds, according to the requirements of social conditions and the press of one's responsibilities and obligations. Through these metaphors, the mind, competence, and motivation become inherently relational in nature and take form as a transaction between inside and outside. People and their actions are understood to be dependent on time, place, and circumstance. From a Western point of view, imagining the mind as a plant may seem like a demotion for such a critical and powerful entity. Yet once the mind is likened to a plant rather than to a machine, it is evident that the soil, the culture—what is often from a Western point of view, construed as the "outside"—is critical for development and growth of the mind.

A number of research groups within Western cultural contexts have sought alternative metaphors for the mind. Extending Mead's idea of thought as conversation with a generalized other, they have converged on notions of thinking as shared, collaborative, communicative, or intersubjective (Ickes, Stinson, Bissonnette, & Garcia, 1990; Zajonc, 1992). Other researchers have challenged the long-standing distinction between the cognitive and the social (Greeno, 1988), and have described cognitive systems as social systems (Minsky, 1986). Others have described becoming competent as joining a conversation (Bruner, 1990), and learning as a process of becoming a member of a sustained community of practice (Lave & Wenger, 1991; Rogoff, Baker-Sennett, Lacasa, & Goldsmith, 1995). These evocative ideas, however, have not been widely accepted in research on competence and motivation.

WHAT IS GOOD THINKING?

Gaining Knowledge

Metaphors of mind and intelligence carry with them assumptions about the nature and purpose of thinking, which are in turn tied to understandings about good thinking and desirable modes of being. In most Western conceptions, competence involves gaining knowledge, figuring things out, good reasoning, and problem solving. According to Aristotle, "All men by nature desire to know." The powerful underlying belief is that the world is systematic, and that it is possible to gain knowledge of it (Lakoff & Johnson, 1999). Gaining this knowledge is an effortful, individual pursuit and involves the application of reason to discover the truth. The preference for self-generated knowledge reflects the Socratic tradition, which is skeptical of the beliefs of others and prizes only truth that is "neither prescribed by authority figures nor socially negotiated. Rather it is found by the self" (Tweed & Lehman, 2002, p. 91). Rodin's sculpture, *The Thinker*, captures the essence of good thinking, Western style. Prototypical good thinking is a highly effortful, private, and internal activity. It is done with eyes closed, the body hunched over, while the world is held at bay.

To assume that the goal of using the mind is to know or to gain information also fits well with a Cartesian world view, in which the pursuit of knowledge, truth, or reason is valued more than activities of doing, being, or feeling (Misra & Gergen, 1993). Given that knowledge is the goal, the more knowledge the thinker can gain, the better. Hence, rapid thinking or mental processing that quickly produces a general understanding is most highly valued. The analysis of information processing from this perspective has led to discoveries of tendencies to "go beyond the information given" (Bruner, 1957), to find meaningful patterns, to take salient examples that are prototypical of the relevant general phenomenon, and to draw probabilistic, rather than determinate, conclusions (Fiske & Taylor, 1994). These tendencies, however, may reflect not basic human tendencies but instead Western mentalities that derive in part from Western assumptions about the purpose and meaning of thinking and intellectual competence (Goodnow, 1990).

In an analysis of American implicit theories of intelligence, Sternberg, Conway, Ketron, and Bernstein (1981) asked laypeople and experts to list characteristics of intelligence. The most important factor was problem-solving ability, which included behaviors such as "reasons logically and well," "identifies connections among ideas," and "sees all aspects of a problem." A second factor was verbal ability, which included "speaks clearly and articulately" and "converses well." Finally, a third but less important factor was social competence, which included "admits mistakes" and "displays interest in the world at large." These implicit theories reveal the pervading influence of a metaphor that conceptualizes intelligence as something internal to and contained within the person (Sternberg, 1990).

Dweck and her colleagues have also examined theories of intelligence and found two general types of implicit theories or meaning systems (Dweck, Chui, & Hong, 1995; Dweck & Leggett, 1988). Some people believe that intelligence is relatively fixed (an entity view), while others hold that intelligence is relatively malleable (an incremental view). The view that intelligence is an entity locates competence somewhere inside the person, away from influence. The view that intelligence is malleable and grows and changes focuses attention on the importance of effort and persistence in competence, and can signal a more social and relational view of competence. Such an incremental construction of intelligence can draw attention to the learner trying to meet the expectations and standards of others, and to the role of others in encouraging such persistence (Hong, 2001). Still, many descriptions of intelligence as incremental or malleable are relatively intrapersonal and foster an inside view of competence (Ames & Archer, 1988; Maehr & Yamaguchi, 2001). From the incremental, inside perspective, others serve primarily to evaluate performance, while the potential for mastery comes as a consequence of individual differences in internal qualities such as effort or intrinsic motivation.

Responding to Others

In many contexts other than European American ones, competence, thinking, and intelligence are associated with very different meanings and practices. These differences are linked to alternative ideas of what it means to be a person. The person is an interdependent being, a part that becomes whole only in relation to others (Markus et al., 1996). Consequently, the intelligence or competence of this interdependent being is naturally and decidedly more social and relational. The goal of good thinking is to maintain relations with others. Competence is not developed *within* individuals but is fostered *through* relations, particularly attending to the expectations of others. Using a methodology similar to that of Sternberg et al. (1981), Azuma and Kashiwagi (1987) found that when characterizing intelligence, Japanese respondents gave much greater emphasis to interpersonal qualities than to problem-solving and verbal ability (Shapiro & Azuma, 2004). The first interpersonal factor was characterized by sociability, humor, and leadership, and the second, by characteristics such as sympathy, social modesty, and the ability to take another's perspective. Notably, another important aspect of competence, Japanese style, was the ability to regulate or to achieve control over one's inner state.

Competence in many East Asian contexts is imagined not so much in terms of internal properties of the head, but instead in terms of relationships among hearts. And social competence is the litmus test for general competence. Lewis (1995) reported that Japanese educators emphasize "the relationship of hearts, the nurturing of bonding between the teacher's and children's hearts" (p. 56). Thus, Hiroki's problem in the opening example is that he was not properly responsive to others and to his socializing milieu (White & LeVine, 1986). A smart child is one who is intelligent enough to know how to listen to others. According to the Japanese Ministry of Education, the goal of preschool is not academic preparation but instead to build the proper relationships and good habits that will become the bedrock of later competence (Peak, 1991; Shapiro & Azuma, 2004). In many Western schools and educated contexts, relating to others in the academic context is fraught with potentially negative associations; for example, a reliance on others to solve a problem is classified as cheating. In the everyday situations of many other cultural settings, however, not using a companion's assistance is regarded as folly or egoism (Rogoff & Chavajay, 1995).

Living in the Right Way

According to many diverse and richly elaborated Indian philosophical works (Das, 1994; Srivastava & Misra, 1999), competent persons are those who are reflective and sensitive to context, and who select the appropriate behavior for the situation. An emphasis is placed on "waking up, noticing, recognizing, understanding, and comprehending" (Srivastava & Misra, p. 160). Knowledge acquisition, while important, appears as a way station on the path to understanding. Knowing is not for its own sake; instead, thinking is for the purpose of living in the right way. Intelligence is not neutral. Instead, intelligence and morality are interwoven, and good intelligence is constructive and associated with happiness, pleasure, and prosperity, while bad intelligence is destructive and leads to unhappiness. Competence, then, both reflects and fosters karma, the doctrine by which one's deeds are related to the quality of one's life both currently and in the future incarnations.

Examining what it means to be intelligent in India, Srivastava and Misra (1999) identified hundreds of Sanskrit Suktis and proverbs spoken in Hindi that had some relevance to intelligence as it is commonly understood. These sukti and proverbs were coded for their meaning and were then grouped into a few broad categories. Across both sets of texts, intelligence and competence involved being good or smart at life.

The notion of being privately smart in a way that is not useful for life was relatively infrequent. A key aspect of social competence was situational sensitivity and knowing how to behave appropriately according to time, place, and person. Showing respect to parents, elders, and guests was another feature of intelligent behavior.

In Chinese cultural contexts, thinking also has a very important relational function, in particular, a hierarchy-maintaining function. When thinking in the presence of an elder, for example, tradition requires acknowledging one's relative incompetence. In such situations, one should wait to be addressed or questioned before beginning conversation. The lower status person should not direct the conversation, introduce topics, or begin a reply until the teacher or superior is finished, or answer a question if there is someone else for whom it is more appropriate to do so (Legge, 1967, as described in Scollon & Scollon, 1994, pp. 144–155). Learning is less likely to be associated with evaluating, questioning, and generating knowledge, which is referred to as "critical" thinking in the West; it is instead tuning into the insights and wisdom of those in the collective who have been recognized as exemplars (Tweed & Lehman, 2002). Within cultural contexts influenced by Confucianism, it may follow then that intelligence, competence, or good thinking, at least in the social domain, may not require snap judgments, rapid distinctions, quick inferences, or going beyond the information given to impose meaning, but instead requires listening, receiving, accepting, applying multiple frames, reflecting, letting meanings arise or reveal themselves, hesitating, or making a judgment only after an extended period.

An emphasis on social competence as the defining feature of competence is not confined to East Asia or to India. In fact, in virtually all contexts other than middle-class American ones, competence is in large part explicitly social. For example, in a comparison between Puerto Rican families in Puerto Rico's metropolitan areas and Anglo families in New Haven, Connecticut, Harwood, Miller, and Irizarry (1995) found striking differences in what parents valued and hoped to foster in competent children. Anglo mothers valued autonomy (children exploring settings on their own), self-control (rather than control by others), initiative, and self-maximization. Puerto Rican mothers, like many mothers outside of middle-class American settings, valued displaying proper social demeanor and maintaining harmony within the group. The proper child in Puerto Rican settings would be "calm, obedient, and respectfully attentive to the teachings of his or her elders, in order to become skilled in the interpersonal and rhetorical competencies that will someday be expected of the well-socialized adult" (p. 98). Indeed in some settings, beyond an emphasis on harmonious and stable intergroup relations, there is a distinct prescription for intelligent people to conform. Harkness et al. (1992), report, for example, that in Kenya, parents defined intelligence as the "ability to do what is needed to be done around the homestead without being asked" (p. 105).

In studies conducted in Uganda, Wober (1974) asked samples of villagers, teachers, and medical students that differed in their level of education and contact with Western ideas to rate various concepts related to intelligence on 9-point semantic differential scales (consisting of pairs of adjectives with opposite meanings). Although there were important differences among the samples of Ugandans, there was also considerable overlap. Most notably, intelligence was not associated with haste or mental speed. Many respondents thought of intelligence as slow, careful, straightforward, and sane. The villagers were also likely to associate intelligence with terms such as "friendly" and "public," suggesting that a productive use of the mind is to be found in a reaching out to others and in a prosocial or public-spirited orientation. Wober's study reveals, however, that with exposure to Western ideas, intelligence becomes less social, and becomes instead a more individual and private entity. In contrast to the villagers, students were more likely to associate intelligence with rapid response, and not with pause or delay.

The literature on competence is replete with compelling theoretical statements (e.g., Berry, 1996; Luria, 1981) urging those who are interested in the nature of the mind, intelligence, or competence to attend carefully to the environment that the mind has been shaped to meet. These views, as well as a variety of recent ones (Shapiro & Azuma, 2004; Sternberg & Grigorenko, 2004), find

that different ecologies and situations recruit and create different ideas of competence and intelligence; thus, competence will necessarily assume a variety of forms. Moreover, recent theories of competence and motivation, for example, Gardner's (1993) multiple intelligences, Sternberg's (1997) triarchic theory of intelligence, Cantor's social intelligence (Cantor & Kihlstrom, 1985), Goleman's (1995) emotional intelligence and Mischel and Shoda's (1995) cognitive–affective theory, increasingly reflect within a Western context some of the understandings of Hiroki's preschool teachers, and explicitly delineate the importance of the interpersonal context and the requirements and expectations of others in developing competence. Yet given the dominance of the "inside" story of competence in both lay and scientific imaginations, the theories of competence and motivation that challenge the inside–outside dichotomy and that instead conceptualize them as context-dependent and fundamentally interpersonal social phenoman (for a review, see Salili, Chiu, & Hong, 2001) have tremendous difficulty taking hold (Farr, 1996).

IMAGINING AGENCY: CONCEPTIONS OF TRYING AND DOING

The Force Within

Because competence and related concepts such as ability and intelligence often fail to adequately account for variation in achievement, other explanatory constructs have become necessary. The concept of motivation, like the concept of competence, is tied to a set of culture-specific understandings and practices that describe what motivation is and why it is necessary. Motivation is generally understood as the reason for behaving in some way, or the explanation for stopping one action and beginning another (Mook, 1986). The concept of motivation serves to justify and explain the direction and purposefulness that seem to characterize human action, at least in European American contexts (Stewart & Bennett, 1991).

Although the source of individual behavior could theoretically be social, relational, or located outside the person, in the most popular lay accounts of motivation, is an inside entity, a feeling of interest or enthusiasm, or a personal or individual force. Motivation is one of the set of internal attributes that defines the person and that causes behavior. Why is Hiroki misbehaving? Because he is not excited and interested by the lesson. He is bored; he is not intrinsically motivated. According to this account, people perform well or successfully because they are motivated, or they fail because they have insufficient motivation. Motivation is extremely important in European American contexts; a growing motivation industry produces speakers, seminars, books, tapes, and CDs exhorting people to feel the power of the force "within them" and to understand that what lies behind, or what lies ahead, is nothing compared to what lies "within." Lance Armstrong, six-time winner of the Tour de France bicycle race is described in an advertisement for Subaru cars to be "driven by what's inside." Similarly, in analyzing the outcome of a game, sports commentators often make statements such as "The losing team didn't have enough drive," or "The winning team was hungrier." Americans, in fact, are quick to make internal attributions for behavior relative to situational attributions (Ross, 1977), more so than people in other cultural contexts such as China and India (Miller, 1984; Morris & Peng, 1994).

In analyzing metaphors of motivation, Weiner (1991) finds two dominant ones: the person as a machine and as a god. He argues that the machine metaphor has been attractive to Western theorists, because it incorporates concepts from the natural sciences related to energy, force fields, and associative connections, and seems to account parsimoniously for the initiation, maintenance, and termination of behavior. Freud construed the person as a steam engine that was allotted a fixed amount of energy to realize desired end states. Hull (1943), in what was characterized as drive theory, saw the behaving organism as "a completely self-maintaining robot" (p. 27).

The second metaphor for motivation, according to Weiner, is the person as a god. This metaphor was invoked as theorists grappled with how to explain individual choices and decisions. The idea is that people are perfectly rational and all-knowing. Such a metaphor provides the basis for theories of the person as a rational decision

maker and as a scientist. More recently, Weiner (2001) suggested that people are also judges, and when an individual acts, a field of others considers the action, and then judges the person—good or bad, responsible or not, moral or immoral, deserving sympathy or anger. The judge metaphor helps highlight the particular cultural models that guide our observations and attributions. People are assumed to "have" high or low ability. Those with high ability who do not work or try are judged harshly. Potential is an innate attribute, and not realizing it is regarded very negatively. Those with less ability but who nonetheless succeed through effort are regarded somewhat more positively. Despite the importance of effort, however, in many settings, those who succeed without much effort, working "smart" rather than hard, are often admired. The nature of these evaluations reveals the operation of a dense network of assumptions about the nature of competence and motivation, and how they work together to generate performance. As we explore later, these assumptions are not natural or human but are instead rooted in the Protestant ethic, which values overcoming obstacles through hard work, and in other assumptions about natural virtues (Spence, 1985; Weiner, 2001).

Agency in the World

The most common metaphors of agency are alike in their location of the driving force of behavior as inside the individual. Metaphors of agency in other contexts conceptualize the person as a more porous, fractional, and interdependent entity. In holistic world views, in which there is no clear division between the human and the natural or supernatural, agency is projected outward and located in the world at large (Misra & Gergen, 1993). Agency can be located in spirits, in the Evil Eye, in hexes or curses, in the imbalance of various forces, or more simply in social practices—the routine scripted social activities that structure life and require participation (Landrine & Klonoff, 1994). Drawing on his fieldwork among the Miamin in Papua, New Guinea, Gardner (1987) observes, "The concept of agency employed by the Miamin is embedded in social practices; far from there being any abstractions from these practices, in the form of a model of human nature, the characteristics of specifically human agency are projected upon the world at large" (p. 174). Stewart and Bennett (1991) quote a Ghanaian government employee as saying, "We do not concern ourselves with motivation as the Americans do. We know what our job is and we do it" (p. 78). From this perspective, problems with individual performance are not located inside the individual but instead stem from role confusion, or from some difficulty in the social context, such as antagonism among groups.

Miller (1984, 1988) was among the first to draw attention to the social and interpersonal nature of motivation. For example, in American contexts, doing one's duty or sacrificing one's self for others is tantamount to giving up one's own agency or to being extrinsically motivated (Markus & Kitayama, 1994). In Hindu Indian contexts, on the other hand, performing interpersonal responsibilities–doing what relevant others oblige one to do—is more frequently experienced as agentic and intrinsically motivated.

In Western contexts, the individualist assumption that people are separate from others is the cornerstone assumption in the most prevalent models of agency. To explain the actions of isolated individuals requires the postulation of a force to propel them, something to move them to work or achieve and to define them. One such force is the "achievement motive" (McClelland, 1961), variously defined as the desire to overcome obstacles, to exert power, or to do something as well as possible, or to master or manipulate it. Markus and Kitayama (2004) suggest, however, that if the individual is not described as an independent, autonomous self who seeks to express itself through action, but instead is characterized as an interdependent self who requires a relationship or a social setting in order to "be," then the characterization of motivation will take new forms. Motivation will involve other people and social situations, and independent actions or achievements will be less relevant or significant. Of greater importance will be behaving according to obligations, duties, rules, and privileges. Such motivations have often been regarded in European American settings as "outside," and therefore less legitimate, authentic, or powerful than internal factors.

Although the recognition of individuality and of purposeful agency appears to be universal, Markus and Kitayama (2004) contend that this recognition does not require a commitment to the European and American ideology of individualism and its particular normative models of human nature. In describing the various ways in which actions can be constructed, these authors use the word "agency" to refer to the "self in action." They propose that how actions are understood is tied to conceptions of the self. They find that European American contexts reflect an implicit cultural model of agency, in which normatively good actions originate in an independent autonomous self, and the actions of this self are *disjoint*, that is, in some ways separate or distinct from the actions of others. By contrast, East Asian contexts often reveal another implicit cultural model of agency, in which normatively good actions originate in an interdependent self, and the actions of this self are *conjoint*, that is, in some ways impelled by interactions or relationships with others.

This distributed view of agency is not restricted to New Guinea, Africa, India, or East Asia. Wherever there are contexts that encourage strong notions of relationality among people or between people and nature, agency and motivation are less likely to be viewed as abstractions detached from the world and as properties of people, and instead are assumed to be social in origin and conceptualized as shared. Lamont (2000), for example, notes that in both French and American working-class contexts, respondents in in-depth interviews signal an awareness that their actions and their fate are interdependent with others, and that their actions are responsive to the need to be responsible to others and uphold the moral order. Similarly, Markus, Ryff, Curhan, & Palmerscheim (2004) find that those engaged in working-class settings are more likely to be attuned to the requirements of others and to the demands of the situation. Given their occupations and living arrangements, they are more likely to understand themselves as maintaining their integrity and controlling themselves in uncertain material and social worlds, and may therefore be less likely to view themselves as freely choosing their own actions (Snibbe & Markus, in press).

In recent writings, achievement motivation theorists appear to be shifting the focus away from the inside, blurring the dichotomy between person and environment. Weiner (2001) underscores that success and failure do not occur in a vacuum, but "in a social context which affects and is affected by achievement performance" (p. 19). He also emphasizes that motivation has a strong interpersonal component. Other theorists are examining how the environment or the context influences the nature of an individual's goals (Steele & Sherman, 1999). Thus, task goals, or similar constructs such as mastery or learning goals (e.g., Dweck, 1986), draw somewhat more attention to the social nature of motivation, because they implicate others, and the expectations of others, more than performance goals, or similar constructs such as relative ability goals or ego goals (e.g, Maehr, 1984). When learning goals are present, for example, students are more willing to seek out others for academic help. And whether or not learning goals are present depends on the goal structure of the classroom (Urdan, 2001). Research explaining the performance gap between middle- and working-class students (Croizet & Claire, 1998), or between white and black students (Steele, 1997), is also explicitly training theoretical and empirical attention on more external, contextual factors in motivation. Thus, Graham (2001) argues that motivation is interpersonal, and that the broader context of cultural and social influences may provide a set of untapped clues for understanding minority achievement. Whether the "it's what's inside that counts" story of motivation, with its focus on internal and intrinsic factors, will be challenged by the accounts that illuminate interpersonal contexts will depend on how well theorists can create metaphors, narratives, and models that can effectively communicate and represent their more social perspectives on motivation.

HISTORICAL AND IDEOLOGICAL FOUNDATIONS OF THE INSIDE STORY

Why is the inside story of competence and motivation so powerful in many European American contexts? Why is it difficult for a more contextual, social, or relational account to take hold? The historical and ideological foundation of the inside story has been forged out of a set of powerful and sometimes conflicting collective beliefs, including beliefs in inherited traits, in the power of the environment, and in the need for the self to feel autonomy and control to develop to its full potential.

Innate Faculties

The notion of innate faculties takes root in the ancient Greek concept of essentialism—that objects have inherent qualities. For example, Socrates spoke of God creating people of gold, silver, or brass and iron, which defined their place in society (e.g., as a commander vs. a craftsman) and that of their offspring. This concept of inborn competencies that are naturally occurring properties of a person has survived in some form throughout American history. The belief that people have innate faculties figured prominently in the discourse of the Founding Fathers during and after the formation of the American republic (Wiley, 1994). They believed, for example, that a natural aristocracy existed among men (Lemann, 1999) and that some (e.g., free white persons) were fit for self-government, whereas others (e.g., Indians and slaves) were not (Jacobson, 1998).

The notion that certain desirable qualities were heritable gained prominence in the latter part of the 19th century with the rise of Social Darwinism. This movement promoted the application of quasi-evolutionary principles, such as "survival of the fittest," to human behavior and social and psychological attributes. The popularity of Social Darwinism was made possible by the growing knowledge of the work of three British scientists: Darwin's evolutionary theory, Mendel's genetics, and Galton's behavioral genetics. In particular, in *Hereditary Genius*, Galton (1869/1978) explored the importance of genetics for the transmission of intelligence by analyzing families of "eminent" men. Galton also promoted the use of selective breeding techniques to improve the intelligence of the human race—a concept that he dubbed "eugenics." Influenced by Galton, psychologists such as McDougall, who conducted studies on inherited characteristics and believed that individuals are motivated by inherited instincts, helped to introduce the study of eugenics and heredity to the United States. From roughly the 1890s to the 1920s, the eugenics movement spread through American academic and political institutions. The movement, which heralded the biological engineering of the body politic, was motivated in large part by recent waves of immigration to the United States from Southern and Eastern Europe, and the concomitant fear that these immigrants would pollute the American genetic pool.

The significant immigration during this time period, together with the establishment of compulsory education and American involvement in World War I, also produced a perceived need for identifying and classifying large numbers of people (Chapman, 1988)—a need soon satisfied by the development and widespread use of mental tests. American psychologist J. Cattell (1890), who had briefly worked with Galton, originated the term "mental test." At the turn of the century, Thorndike, one of his students, was developing a variety of intelligence measures. The American initiative to develop mental tests was also advanced by similar work in Europe. In 1904, the French government asked Binet and Simon to develop a test to identify slow learners, so that they could be given special help. The resulting Binet–Simon Intelligence Scale (1905, 1911) was meant as a measure of current performance, not innate intelligence. In 1916, Terman, a Stanford professor known to have eugenicist proclivities, adapted the Binet–Simon for Americans. At this point, the test lost its basis in performance and shifted to innate intelligence. The test measured IQ and was renamed the Stanford–Binet Intelligence Scale. Mass testing of intelligence received a further boost during World War I, when the military needed a way to assess quickly and classify large numbers of new recruits. The first large-scale mental test was an IQ test administered to nearly 2 million recruits.

With the use of large-scale group testing, the American public began to accept the inside account of intelligence and the idea that people could be sorted into different levels of mental abilities. Testing became more widespread in schools and industry. A variation of the IQ test—the Scholastic Aptitude Test (SAT)—was first administered in 1926. Broad-scale SAT testing emerged soon afterwards, aided by World War II, the GI Bill, the Cold War, the founding of the Educational Testing Service, and the vision of Harvard administrators of an elite democratically chosen on the basis of mental test scores (Lemann, 1999).

Testing has not been confined to the United States. In China, for example, civil service tests have long been used to assess knowledge of geography, law, military, and agriculture. In France, Germany, and Great Britain, students must pass the Baccalaureat, Abitur, and A-levels, respectively, to gain placement in university. In contrast to American tests, however, these tests are primarily knowledge-based. In the United States, the culture of testing has focused more on assessing how "smart" a person is rather than how much knowledge he or she has accumulated, or how much he or she has learned. This concern with native intelligence has manifested itself in the development and widespread administration of intelligence tests throughout the 20th century, and both IQ tests and the SAT are still in use today. For many, intelligence testing had appeal, because it presented a way to assess and sort students according to their capabilities. According to Lemann (1999), "Testing touched upon the deepest mythic themes: the ability to see the invisible (what was inside people's heads), the oracular ability to predict the future (what someone's grades would be in courses he hadn't even chosen yet)" (p. 18). These themes were made real when they were incorporated into practice. Once people were given an intelligence score, by definition, they were seen as "having intelligence and potential within them," or not.

Other countries have overtly rejected American-style mental testing, often because of its social implications. In the Soviet Union, for example, mental testing was abandoned, because it was believed to reinforce class structure. In the United States, the relationship of mental testing with race—rather than social class—has generally been a primary area of concern, although it has seldom been used as the basis for eliminating this form of testing. Instead, eugenicist ideas linking race and intelligence frequently reappear, perhaps owing to the widespread acceptance of the innate model of competence.

For example, in a 1969 article, "How Much Can We Boost IQ and Scholastic Achievement?," Jensen argued that racial differences in intelligence are due to heredity rather than to social factors such as poverty and discrimination. In 1994, Herrnstein and Murray published *The Bell Curve*, in which they discussed the relationship of intelligence (genetically determined) to social structure and argued that whites are genetically superior to blacks with respect to IQ.

Although some controversy exists within the field about the conceptualization of intelligence, the vast majority of theories still posit that intelligence is internal—confined to what is inside the head. At the height of the testing movement, one of the most influential theories, British psychologist Spearman's (1927) *g* factor, catapulted the notion of general intellectual ability into academic and public discourse. Other theorists, although still working with the model of intelligence as inside the head, subsequently presented more multifaceted views of intelligence (e.g., Gardner's multiple intelligences [1993], Sternberg's triarchic theory [1985]). Nonetheless, the idea of *g* and IQ still resonate strongly, not just in the field of psychometrics but also in education, the military, and corporate America (see, e.g., Gladwell, 2002).

The Power of the Environment

Despite its predominance, the "inside" story has been paralleled by an "outside" story. Many scholars have voiced the opinion that what is "outside" (e.g., the environment, culture) has a significant influence on individuals' behavior and development. For example, in the 17th century, the idea of the mind as a "blank slate," written on by experience, was introduced by Locke (1690/ 1979), who wrote:

> Let us then suppose the mind to be, as we say, white paper, void of all characters, without any ideas; How comes it to be furnished? Whence comes it by that vast store, which the busy and boundless fancy of man has painted on it, with an almost endless variety? Whence has it all the materials of reason and knowledge? To this I answer, in one word, from experience. (p. 104)

Locke believed education, not natural genius, to be the prime determinant of success: "I think I may say, that of all the Men we meet with, Nine Parts of Ten are what they are, Good or Evil, useful or not, by their Education. 'Tis that which makes the great Difference in Mankind" (1693/1989, p. 83). Locke's influence in academic psychology came in part from his empiricism, the idea that knowledge must be based on observable things and events. He proposed that people do not possess innate ideas but experience the world through their senses, that a person's ideas are mental models of experienced reality, and that mind is a receptacle of input meanings. Locke believed that unequal faculties were the effect unequal environments (Wiley, 1994).

This idea lay somewhat dormant during the 19th century, and the influence of environmental circumstance on the individual resurfaced with the rise of behaviorism. For many behaviorists, the mind was, in a sense, the ultimate blank slate, while for others, there was no slate to be written on, because what was inside the mind did not affect the stimulus–response sequence. In either case, from the behaviorist perspective, intelligence testing and the innate faculties approach in general were an erroneous way of understanding human behavior. In staunch opposition to the notion of innate faculties, Watson (1924) famously said,

> Give me a dozen healthy infants . . . and my own specified world to bring them up in and I'll guarantee to take any one at random and train him to become any type of specialist I might select—doctor, lawyer, artist, merchant . . . regardless of his talents, penchants, tendencies, abilities, vocations, and race of his ancestors. (p. 82)

From this perspective, environmental conditions were seen as much more powerful predictors of human potential than how an individual scored on an IQ test.

During this same period, in anthropology, Boas and his students proposed that culture casts a shadow on biology as the prime determinant of social behavior. The Boasian vision of environmentalism, culture, and human changeability, unlike Social Darwinism, explained human variation in a way that was compatible with an egalitarian form of government (Wiley, 1994). The concept of culture thus gained popularity in part as a reaction to the events in Nazi Germany. In the 1950s, M. Mead, a student of Boas, helped increase the popularity and prevalence of the concept of culture in the social sciences. However, with the discovery of the double helix in the mid-1950s, the pendulum began to swing back in the direction of the inside, natural story. By the 1980s, the computer metaphor had taken hold in psychology, and sociocultural approaches that attempted to see how psychological processes are grounded were met with resistance, in favor of the notion of basic, universal psychological processes.

The Rise of the Self

While the study of environmental and cultural influence, which shifted focus away from the self and articulated a more external and social view, did penetrate the American public and academic discourse, other ideologies and psychological theorizing sustained a powerful American belief that the key to being successful lay within the self. In the 19th century, in an address on the elements of success, R. Cushman stated: "The things which are really essential for a successful life are not circumstances, but qualities, not the things which surround a man, but the things which are in him; not the adjuncts of his position, but the attributes of his character" (1848, as quoted by Wyllie, 1954, p. 21). And in the 20th century, although it was acknowledged that intelligence and aptitude tests could shed light on the inner contours of the mind, success was still seen as emanating from a person's willpower, perseverance, ambition, and industry. Through a combination of American ideology and psychological theorizing, the self became seen as the key to being competent and motivated. In particular, ideas about the self's independence and self-reliance, personal responsibility and control, and psychological theories of optimal self-development were fueled and invigorated by the foundational ideologies of independence, the Protestant ethic, and the American Dream.

Independence and Self-Reliance

American institutions, practices, and psychological tendencies reflect an ethos of independence and individualism (Baumeister, 1987; Plaut, Markus, & Lachman, 2002). Locke's "liberal individualism"—the idea that societies are made up of autonomous individuals who form governments in order to protect their natural rights—forms the philosophical foundation of the U.S. Declaration of Independence. Lockean philosophy reflects an ontological individualism whereby the individual is seen as prior to society; moreover, this philosophy is atomistic, in that it views society as an aggregation of independent entities. This model of the person as independent and free from others has survived throughout American history (Bellah, Madsen, Sullivan, Swidler, & Tipton, 1985; Fiske et al., 1998). Freedom is, according to Bellah et al., "perhaps the most resonant, deeply held American value" (1985, p. 23). American notions of freedom and autonomy include wanting to be left alone by others and not to be imposed upon by other people's values, beliefs, or lifestyles. Whereas some cultural contexts may stress the importance of tradition and meeting social standards, U.S. culture emphasizes a "socially unsituated self" that thrives on "separating oneself from the values imposed by one's past or by conformity to one's social milieu, so that one can discover what one really wants" (p. 24). In American contexts, this emphasis on independence leads to respect for the individual and fosters initiative and creativity (Bellah et al., 1985).

Independence and self-reliance became key to the American understanding of success in the 19th century. Transcendentalists such as Emerson and Thoreau articulated and helped popularize these concepts. For example, Emerson (1950) wrote in his 1841 essay "Self-Reliance" that one should "trust thyself" (p. 146), that "[s]ociety everywhere is in conspiracy against the manhood of every one of its members," and that to be a man, one need "be a nonconformist" (p. 148). Moreover, Emerson espoused the belief that the key to success lay within the person, evidenced, for example, in the following statement: "The reason why this man or that man is fortunate is not to be told. It lies in the man" (p. 367). In his 1840 commentary on democracy in America, de Tocqueville (1840/2000) made the following observation about Americans: "They are in the habit of always considering themselves in isolation, and they willingly fancy that their whole destiny is in their hands" (p. 484). Indeed, the independent, self-reliant, self-made man, who rose out of obscurity on his own personal merit without external help, soon became a powerful image in American society (Wyllie, 1954).

Personal Responsibility and Control

Notions of personal responsibility and control have contributed significantly to American models of competence and motivation. Two ideologies in particular, the Protestant ethic and the American Dream, have contributed to the individualistic focus of current conceptions of success and achievement in American culture (Spence, 1985).

The Protestant Ethic. Success in America has long been associated with moral superiority. Success and morality are linked under the Protestant ethic, which emphasizes the duty to pursue one's calling and the moral superiority of industriousness and hard work. According to Weber (1904/1958), under the Protestant ethic, the individual's highest moral obligation is to fulfill his duty in worldly affairs. This idea is derived from the Calvinist doctrine of predestination, which holds that God predetermines who will be saved from damnation. People cannot work toward becoming one of the few "elect"; however, they should regard themselves as chosen, as an act of faith, and should demonstrate that faith by pursuing success in a calling. Attaining that success came to be regarded as a sign that a person was in a state of grace. Calvinism, according to Weber, supplies the moral energy and drive of the capitalist entrepreneur. This is in contrast to a religion such as Confucianism, for example, which set as the ideal the harmonious adjustment of the individual to the established order of things (Munro, 1969).

The link between religion, hard work, and success has a long history in American discourse, reflected in, for example, the lessons of Benjamin Franklin. Franklin, a product of Puritan Boston, was highly influenced by Cotton Mather, who wrote that God approved of business callings and rewarded virtue with wealth (Wyllie, 1954). Franklin's adages, such as "Early to bed and early to rise, makes a man healthy, wealthy, and

wise" and "Remember that time is money," reflected a can-do ideology—the idea that one can get ahead on one's own initiative. They also implied that virtues (e.g., industry, frugality, honesty, and integrity) both lead to and reflect success. This ideology, also called utilitarian individualism (Bellah et al., 1985; Spence, 1985), is considered to be a secular version of the Protestant ethic.

Whereas Weber (1904/1958) claimed that by Franklin's time, the religious basis of capitalism had "died away" (p. 180), others have demonstrated a strong link between the church and economic practices. Many Congregational clergy wrote on success, and both clergy and secular writers continued to stress the importance of the secular calling, the pursuit of wealth as a religious duty, the importance of frugality, and the moral superiority of the rich (Wyllie, 1954). De Tocqueville (1840/2000) remarked that, in America, the spirit of religion and the spirit of freedom "united intimately with one another: they reigned together on the same soil" (p. 282). More recently, psychologists have commented that religion in U.S. contexts is tied to ideas of personal control and independence (Cohen, Hall, Koenig, & Meador, 2003; Snibbe & Markus, 2002).

Regardless of whether the Protestant ethic endures in a religious or secular form, the ideology continues to influence ideas about the person. Well into the 20th century, "[p]uritanism lingered on, not so much as a search for individual salvation or as a celebration of the virtues of thrift and industry but as a recognition of the dignity of the individual and of his duty to achieve both spiritual and material prosperity" (Commager, 1950, p. 410), so that the Protestant ethic remains one of America's core values (Hsu, 1972). Lamont's (1992) cultural sociological study comparing American and French workers in the 1980s reveals that in the United States, ambition and hard work are seen as central to moral character, that dynamism and energy signal competence, and that hard work and competence are seen as signs of moral purity (at least in upper-middle-class male culture). The Protestant ethic ideology continues to be reflected in American patterns of psychological well-being and attitudes toward work (Plaut et al., 2002; Quinn & Crocker, 1999).

The American Dream. American notions of competence and motivation have also been shaped by the American Dream ideology. The American Dream is a central ideology in American culture and is the cornerstone of American individualism, combining success and self-interest, and promoting the idea that the greatest good is to be as individually successful as possible (Bellah et al., 1985; Hochschild, 1995). This ideology has promoted a perspective of optimism in one's capacity for success and of personal control and determination in achieving success.

The American Dream took root in the promise of "a new world where anything can happen and good things might" (Hochschild, 1995, p. 15). From the colonial period to the present, the United States has been perceived as a land of opportunity and plenty (Potter, 1954), and many immigrants have come with hopes of improving their economic status (Takaki, 1993). The United States has long promoted the idea that it is not where one came from or what one did before that matters, but what one does now: One can shed the past and invent a better future. This emphasis on opportunity, imagining the future, and starting over has been embodied in many American institutions (e.g., western land grants of the 19th century, the Civil Rights Acts), in common practices (e.g., political campaigns run on "change," change management), in cultural artifacts (e.g., Horatio Alger's rags-to-riches stories), and in popular ideas (e.g., the frontier, Manifest Destiny) (McElroy, 1999; Turner, 1920).

A central assumption of the American Dream is that people can remodel themselves if they possess determination; thus, seeking success is under their control. Nineteenth-century guides for success touted maxims such as "*Will* it and it is thine" and "To the man of vigorous will there are few impossibilities" (quoted in Wyllie, 1954, p. 40). More recently, in a 1993 speech, President Clinton remarked: "The American Dream that we were all raised on is a simple but powerful one—if you work hard and play by the rules you should be given a chance to go as far as your God-given ability will take you" (quoted in Hochschild, 1995, p. 18). The American Dream promises that everyone, regardless of ascribed traits, family background, or personal history, may

reasonably seek success through actions and traits under their own control (Hochschild, 1995), and implies that it is important to possess such a mind-set.

In addition, the American Dream ideology's focus on optimism, control, and determination fosters an expectation of success and an association between success and individual satisfaction. Success is central to Americans' self-image, and Americans not only expect or hope to achieve but are also not gracious about failure (Hochschild, 1995; Spindler & Spindler, 1990). De Tocqueville (1840/2000) famously wrote that every American is "devoured by the desire to rise" (p. 599). In a 19th-century business self-help book, Marden wrote, "The Creator made man a success-machine, and failure is as abnormal to him as discord is to harmony" (quoted in Wyllie, 1954, p. 37). Although the American Dream's emphasis on material rewards may seem to suggest that the focus is solely on external contingencies, it is a thoroughly "inside" story. The American Dream involves doing better and getting ahead not just for the sake of material wealth but also out of a sense of personal investment in and commitment to one's work and to personal advancement. Feeling personally satisfied and fulfilled, and that one has "made it," are integral to this ideology.

The American Dream is not just a relic of the past; it is still alive and well. For example, a recent television commercial for the financial services company American Century states, "American determination, American enlightenment, American optimism," while showing a graduate running across a college campus; NBC has entitled a new prime-time drama, *American Dreams*; and multimillionaire Latina singer–actress Jennifer Lopez has recently been called the perfect Horatio Alger story.

Psychological Theorizing

Pragmatism. In psychology, many scholars have channeled independence, the Protestant ethic, and/or the American Dream in their theorizing. For example, Pragmatism, introduced in the early 20th century by James (1978), who built on the work of Pierce, was a highly individualistic philosophy. Pragmatism attempted to make philosophy more practical, stressing that the meaning of a belief depends on the practical difference it makes in one's life. Thus, Pragmatism emphasized personal experience, the effect of one's thoughts or actions, and changing existing realities. Pragmatism therefore reflected qualities in the American character: "It assigned to each individual, as it were, a leading role in the drama of salvation, gave him a share and a responsibility in making what he held good come true . . . and decreed that he succeeded or failed through his own efforts . . . [and] emphasized his uniqueness rather than his conformity" (Commager, 1950, p. 95). Pragmatism suggested that people held the future in their own hands and encouraged optimism.

Drives and Needs. Many theories of motivation developed in the United States have conceived of motivation as the internal processes that cause individuals to move toward a goal. For example, Hull (1943), arguably the most influential drive theorist, believed that human behavior could be reduced to the drive—the major underlying instigator of behavior. Also depending on a view of motivation as emanating from within the individual, McClelland and colleagues (McClelland, Atkinson, Clark, and Lovell, 1953) developed a theory of motivation based on intrinsic motivational needs. Building on the work of Murray (1938), who developed the concept of achievement motivation and the Thematic Apperception Test, McClelland et al. (1953) distinguished between people high in need for achievement (*n* Ach) and those low in *n* Ach. This theory of achievement motivation captured the spirit of the traditional work ethic (Spence, 1985), and is reminiscent of de Tocqueville's observation that Americans are eaten up with longing to rise.

Self and Psychological Development

Self-Actualization. Although it opposed drive theories and incentive–goal theories, the humanist perspective on motivation also focused on processes within the autonomous individual. According to humanism (e.g., Maslow, 1970; Rogers, 1977), people's actions are influenced by a need for personal growth and fulfillment, and people have free will to determine their destiny. People create their own perceptions of the world and actively choose their own life experiences. A key concept in humanism is self-actualization, which is thought to be a fundamental need that motivates people to fulfill their potential and is seen as the ultimate level of psychological development. Self-actualization theory has been influential in business, psychotherapy, and education. Perhaps its popularity outside of academic psychology stems in part from its focus on the independent, self-determined, satisfaction-seeking individual, consistent with the American Dream ideology. After all, self-actualization theory regards the individual as capable of overcoming repressive social constraints in order to achieve the highest level of psychological development (Hewitt, 1989). And, although it was influenced in part by Buddhism and Hinduism (Wilson, 1997) and stimulated by a rejection of materialist goals, self-actualization has been referred to as "another facet of unbridled individualism" (Spence, 1985, p. 1290).

Competence, Self-Efficacy, and Control. Theories of competence (White, 1959) and self-efficacy (Bandura, 1977, 1997) also hinge on a model of the person as autonomous and in control of his or her environment and actions. White introduced to the study of motivation the notion of "competence," defined as the capacity to interact effectively with the environment. According to White, the motivation needed to attain competence could not come from drives alone and required effectance motivation to produce a feeling of efficacy. The need for efficacy was considered to be a fundamental motive that was highly important in the growth of personality. "Self-efficacy" is defined by Bandura (1997) as "beliefs in one's capabilities to organize and execute the courses of action required to produce given attainments" (p. 3). It is perceived as necessary for success. A strong relationship has been established between self-efficacy beliefs and cognitive engagement, academic performance, and persistence (Pintrich & Schrauben, 1992; for a meta-analysis, see Multon, Brown, & Lent, 1991).

A vast literature on control has also emerged in psychology. Rotter's (1966) work on locus of control and Weiner's (1985) model of attribution, for example, center on notions of personal responsibility and beliefs about the individual's ability to control events (Miller, 1996). Research on illusions of control emphasizes the positive consequences of believing that one has control over one's outcomes (Taylor & Brown, 1988). Other work has introduced a distinction between primary and secondary control, the former involving behaviors aimed at changing the world to fit the needs of the individual, and the latter involving behaviors aimed at fitting in with the world (Rothbaum, Weisz, & Snyder, 1982). Heckhausen and Schultz (1995) have claimed that across cultures and history, primary control has functional primacy over secondary control in development, while secondary control takes on a support role.

In response to notions of control as individual and primary, cross-cultural research has suggested some important cultural variation. Some have suggested that that people in East Asian contexts emphasize secondary control more than do people in Western contexts (Gould 1999; Weisz, Rothbaum, & Blackburn, 1984). Others believe that the important distinction is between indirect and direct primary control, and argue that the Japanese evince more indirect primary control, which involves the modification of existing reality not through direct confrontations but by deliberately using tactics that are expected eventually to modify behavior in appropriate directions (Kojima, 1984). Others have suggested that the Japanese meaning of success is control over one's inner state as opposed to achieving control over external circumstances, which is more common in U.S. contexts (Shapiro & Azuma, 2004). Markus and Kitayama (2004) have distinguished between disjoint and conjoint models of agency, with disjoint agency permeating U.S. contexts and conjoint agency occurring more frequently in East Asian contexts. Researchers have also looked at variation within the United States by comparing the models of agency that are prevalent in working-class or high school-educated versus middle-class or college-educated contexts (Snibbe & Markus, in press).

Self-Determination and Intrinsic Motivation. A class of theories of motivation has rested on the assumption that human beings have an inborn need to exert mastery, or control, over their external environment (deCharms, 1968; Deci, 1975). It is generally assumed that these innate intrinsic motives serve as the milieu out of which springs intrinsic motivation (Spence, 1985). According to Spence, the belief in the intrinsic value of work is a permutation of the Protestant work ethic. This view encourages the notion that work should be engaged in primarily because it is inherently satisfying, and it assigns greater value to intrinsic than to extrinsic motivation.

Researchers have constructed a dichotomy between motivation that comes from internal as opposed to external sources and have repeatedly demonstrated that external sources can undermine intrinsic motivation (e.g., Deci, 1971; Lepper, Greene, & Nisbett, 1973). According to cognitive evaluation theory (Deci & Ryan, 1980), events that negatively affect a person's experience of autonomy or competence diminish intrinsic motivation, whereas events that support perceived autonomy and competence enhance intrinsic motivation. To the degree that the controlling aspect of an external reward is salient, the reward will undermine intrinsic motivation because of the perceived external locus of causality (deCharms, 1968), which is the sense that the behavior stems from a source outside the self. Furthermore, according to self-determination theory (Deci & Ryan, 1985), external goals and rewards (e.g., social recognition and money) can provide only indirect satisfaction of basic psychological needs for autonomy, relatedness, and competence. And focusing on external cues and contingencies as the basis for regulating behavior instead of on internal needs and feelings can have significant personal and interpersonal costs (Ryan & Connell, 1989). Decades of research indeed have revealed that people (at least in U.S. contexts) are most motivated when able to initiate and direct their own behavior (Condry, 1977; Rotter, 1966). Choice and control have been found to affect intrinsic motivation positively (Cordova & Lepper, 1996; Deci & Ryan, 1985). In contrast, removing choice (Brehm, 1966; Wicklund, 1974) or imposing someone else's choice (Iyengar & Lepper, 1999) has been shown to affect intrinsic motivation negatively.

COMPETING STORIES: COMPARATIVE EMPIRICAL EXAMPLES

Models of competence and motivation are not merely cultural construals used to interpret behavior after it has occurred. Rather, they are lived; that is, they are institutionalized and given a material form, thereby structuring behavior. For example, in the American novels of the must-read humanities canon, the heroes are most often those who show competence and motivation, American style. Their competence and motivation spring from private, internal stores, and they are capable of standing out from the group and going their own way. Many educational practices, such as testing and ability tracking, also reflect the commitments of these models, and play a role in identifying and fostering competence and motivation as personal, internal entities. People live their lives in terms of the blueprints provided by these models, thereby making them reality (Adams & Markus, 2004). If people's worlds are set up in such a way as to foster a particular model of competence and motivation, then, on average, the behavioral tendencies of many people engaged with these contexts will reflect that model. Through people's actions, which reproduce the model, the inside story becomes the real story and the true story.

Yet the inside story is a particular one, a historically and socioculturally specific one. In other contexts, there are other models of competence and motivation. A growing number of empirical studies carried out in contexts other than European and American ones reveal patterns of behavior that reflect these different models. Major dimensions of cultural variation include whether achievement is considered to be individual or social; how self-efficacy relates to performance; perceptions of the roles of effort and ability in success; the relationship between choice, control, and intrinsic motivation; and styles of competence and acknowledgment of different styles.

Achievement: An Individual or Social Construct?

Empirical evidence suggests that cultural contexts differ in the extent to which people seek more affiliative, or social, as opposed to individual goals. This line of inquiry arose, in part, in response to the need for achievement literature that was prevalent in the 1960s and deemed to reflect individualistic achievement values (Salili, 1996). In the subsequent three decades, researchers have explored cross-cultural differences in the achievement construct, arguing that this construct takes on different meanings in different cultures, and that it is important to understand these sociocultural variations (Fryans, Salili, Maehr, & Desai, 1983; Maehr, 1974; Niles, 1998).

Divergent Goals: Individual versus Social

Research in this area has generally revealed more individual-oriented achievement motivation in U.S. and other Western contexts than in Asian and Latin American contexts, where a socially oriented motivation is more prevalent. For example, Japanese and Native Hawaiians have been found to associate achievement with goals of affiliation and social belonging more than with individual goals (De Vos, 1973; Gallimore, Boggs, & Jordan, 1974). Research in India also has revealed more emphasis on group-related goals than on individual ones (Agrawal & Misra, 1987; Singhal & Misra, 1989). Similarly, Niles (1998) found Sri Lankan adults to be more family- and group-oriented in their achievement goals than Australians, although Sri Lankans were also found to have important individual goals. In a study comparing Chinese and Australian gymnasts, the Chinese rated affiliation motivations as more important than did the Australians (Kirkby, Kolt, & Liu, 1999). In a review of learning style and achievement orientation in Asian contexts, Salili (1996) argued that socially oriented achievement motivation is more common in Asian than in Western cultures because of cultural differences in attitudes toward learning and education; for Asian students, success is defined in terms of recognition and smooth social relationships. In Japanese contexts, "success only for oneself has been considered a sign of excessive, immoral egoism" (De Vos, 1973, p. 181).

Some research suggests that individual and social motivation may be more entangled in Asian than in U.S. contexts, where affiliative and individualistic achievements are seen as mutually exclusive. In a study of university students in the Philippines and in the United States, Church and Katigbak (1992) found a closer relationship between intrinsic task motives and affiliative motives in the Filipino than in the American sample. They suggested that school is a more interpersonal experience for Filipinos, and that need for achievement and for affiliation are more intertwined in Filipino contexts. Similarly, Salili (1994) found that for Chinese adult students, affiliative and individualistic achievement were closely related.

These types of differences have also been examined within the United States. Results of one study revealed that Mexican American and black subjects scored higher on family achievement than did Anglo subjects (Ramirez & Price-Williams, 1976). "Family achievement" was defined as goals from which the family would benefit or that would gain recognition from family members. Notably, Mexican American and black subjects emphasized both family and individual achievement, indicating that, in some cultural contexts, the achievement for purposes of self and family are not considered contradictory. In some U.S. minority contexts, achievement may be pursued for the purpose of family and peer-group solidarity and identification, rather than, or in addition to, individual and independent attainment (Gallimore et al., 1974; Ramirez & Price-Williams, 1976). According to Fryberg and Markus (2004), learning in American Indian settings reflects a concern with family and with community relationality.

Pleasing Parents and Family Pressure

Research in this area has also revealed that pleasing parents, parental pressure, and responsibility felt toward one's family are strong motivations for achievement in Asian and Latino contexts. Azuma (1994) observed that pleasing the mother was one of top three reasons Japanese fifth graders gave for doing well on tests. Similarly, Salili and Ching (1992, cited in Salili, 1996) found that when they asked Chinese students to rate their reasons for working hard, both low and high achievers rated pleasing parents as the most important reason. In an investigation of Asian American students' success in high school, Reglin and Adams (1990) found Asian American high school

students to be more influenced by their parents' desire for success than were their non-Asian counterparts. The authors argued that, for Asian American students, perceived parental desire for success creates pressure to achieve, motivating them to spend more time on homework. In examining Asian children's adaptation to U.S. schools, Hirayama (1985) argued that parents emphasize the welfare of the family as a whole, and children assume the moral burden of succeeding for the whole family.

Similar observations have been made about the role of the family in Latin American and Latino contexts. For example, Mexican children feel responsible for the honor of the entire family, and Central American refugee students whose families have experienced misfortune in coming to the United States feel both guilt and responsibility (Suarez-Orozco, 1987). Trueba and Delgado-Gaitan (1985) have argued that education-relevant motivations change as immigrant children learn different motivations in U.S. schools, such as competition and individualism.

Predicting Achievement

Cultural variation has also surfaced in predicting achievement. In one study, need for affiliation, rather than need for achievement, predicted reading achievement for Native Hawaiians (Gallimore, 1974). Another study revealed that qualities found to be predictive of achievement in U.S. samples, such as high mastery, high work orientation, and low competitiveness, did not predict academic achievement in Fijians (Basow, 1984). Fryberg and Markus (2004) found that self-ratings of interdependence predicted grades for American Indian high school students but not for European American high school students.

Feelings of Competence and Self-Efficacy: Tied to Performance and Persistence?

Relationship between Performance and Self-Efficacy, Competence, and Fear of Failure

The link between self-efficacy and performance that is strong in North American contexts, and that reflects and promotes the incorporation of the inside story, does not obtain in Asian and Asian American contexts. One study revealed that although Taiwanese children rated themselves significantly lower on perceived competence than American children, they outperformed the Americans academically (Stigler, Smith, & Mao, 1985). In a similar study, Kwok (1995) found that Chinese children downgraded their competence, as compared with Canadian children. Eaton and Dembo (1997) examined differences in motivational beliefs and performance on a word unscrambling task among Asian American and non-Asian (mostly Anglo) ninth graders. While Asian American students reported lower levels of self-efficacy beliefs, they outperformed their non-Asian counterparts. Similarly, Whang and Hancock (1994) found that Asian American students scored higher than non-Asian students on standardized math tests but reported lower self-concepts for mathematical ability relative to non-Asian students. According to Eaton and Dembo (1997), Asian Americans focus less on self-efficacy, or perceptions of capability to complete a task, and more on the importance of excelling at a task. In contrast, non-Asian children in U.S. contexts may overestimate their abilities. Children in these contexts are encouraged to maintain self-esteem regardless of their academic performance, which may contribute to self-protective illusions, or overestimating one's competencies relative to actual performance (Oettingen, Little, Lindenberger, & Baltes, 1994; Taylor & Brown, 1988).

Whereas self-efficacy concerns individuals in non-Asian U.S. contexts, failure seems to weigh on the minds of individuals in Asian contexts. In a study by Steinberg, Dornbusch, and Brown (1992), Asian American students showed simultaneously the highest academic achievement and the highest fear of failure. Eaton and Dembo (1997), in the same study described earlier, discovered that fear of the consequence of academic failure best explained the performance of Asian American participants but least explained results for non-Asian students. Their main explanation for these findings relates to the previous discussion of parental pressure: Fear of academic failure stems from Asian American parental stress on academic success for their children (Siu, 1992).

Self-Enhancing versus Self-Improving Motivations

Whether self-efficacy is tied to motivation may depend on whether motivation centers on enhancing the self, reflective of an internal, individualistic model of motivation, or on improving the self and meeting expected standards, reflective of a more relational model. In a study of Filipino and American university students, for example, Church and Katigbak (1992) found that approval and self-improvement motives ranked higher for Filipino college students than for American students. Similarly, Heine et al. (2001) tested the hypothesis that Japanese students focus more on self-improving motivations, while North American students focus more on self-enhancing motivations. Results confirmed their hypothesis: North Americans persisted more on a creativity task after success than after failure, whereas Japanese persisted more after failure than after success. Moreover, North Americans, but not Japanese, were more likely to view creativity as important for life success if they had done well, while Japanese were more likely to view creativity as important for life success if they had done poorly. Finally, North Americans felt better after success than did Japanese. The authors concluded that although individuals in both cultures want to do their best, North Americans pursue this goal by focusing on their strengths, while Japanese pursue this goal by focusing on their shortcomings. Oishi and Diener (2003) likewise found that European Americans' choice of a second task was based on how well they thought they had done on an earlier task, but this did not hold for Asian Americans. Furthermore, choice was related to more enjoyment of the second task for the European Americans, but not for the Asian Americans.

If one is interested in self-advancement, one will work harder to stick out, which is more common in American cultural contexts. In contrast, if self-improvement is the goal, one will work harder to avoid sticking out, which is more prevalent in Asian cultural contexts. In these contexts, fulfilling role obligations may be a more salient goal, requiring more attention to meet a minimum standard than to surpass the standard (Su et al., 1999).

Perceived Determinants of Success: Ability or Effort?

If an individual assumes that motivation is linked to actualizing one's potential and displaying one's ability, as is more common in American contexts, then he or she most likely will view ability as relatively fixed and most predictive of success (Heine et al., 2001). However, if one believes that motivation is linked to discovering shortcomings and correcting them, as is more prevalent in Japanese contexts, one most likely will view ability as malleable and may believe that effort plays a larger role in determining success than does innate ability. Heine et al. tested the hypothesis that cultures differ in their emphasis on entity versus incremental theories and found cultural variation on the Beliefs in Incremental Abilities Scale. This scale asked participants to respond to concrete behavioral scenarios (e.g., "Imagine that Michelle, a sophomore, scored the highest grade in her history class. Only knowing this about Michelle, please do your best to estimate what percentage of her performance in the class was due to her natural-born ability and how much was due to her effort and studying"). The Japanese believed that abilities were more incremental (i.e., more effort-based) than did European Americans. Moreover, on an item that asked what percentage of intelligence is due to natural ability versus effort, European Americans reported on average that 36% was due to effort, Japanese reported 55%, and Asian Americans reported 45%.

Although implicit theories of intelligence are conceptualized primarily as an individual difference construct (e.g., see Dweck & Leggett, 1988), it seems likely that they will also vary by cultural context, insofar as models of competence and motivation also vary. Moreover, if an incremental view predominates, tasks will likely be understood as reflecting process (e.g., effort), and performance will not likely be linked with underlying traits and self-worth. If an entity view prevails, however, tasks will likely be understood as measuring permanent intelligence (e.g., intelligence tests in the United States) and achievement. Empirical observations indicate that Japanese and Chinese respondents' beliefs about achievement outcomes center primarily on effort, while American respondents assign more importance to ability (Lewis, 1995; Stevenson & Stigler, 1992; White, 1987). Thus, one reason for Hiroki's teachers' surprise at the Americans' insistence that he was gifted, as described earlier, is that in Japanese contexts, "the notion that children's success and failure and their potential to become successful versus failed adults has more to do with effort and character and thus with what can be learned and taught in school than with raw inborn ability" (Tobin et al., 1989, p. 24).

Research on attributions for academic achievement also has suggested cultural variation in perceptions of the importance of ability and effort, with individuals in U.S. contexts generally seeing ability as the primary determinant of success, and individuals in Asian contexts attributing academic success and failure to effort (Holloway, 1988; Stevenson & Stigler, 1992). In one study, American undergraduate and graduate students attributed academic achievement significantly more often to ability than did Asian (Japanese, Korean, Chinese, and Southeast Asian) students (Yan & Gaier, 1994). American students also believed that effort was more important for success than lack of effort was for failure, whereas Asian students believed effort to be equally important for success and failure. Hess, Chang, and McDevitt (1987) compared the attributions of Chinese mothers living in China, Chinese American mothers, and Caucasian American mothers. Whereas Chinese mothers in China viewed lack of effort as the major cause of their children's low performance, Caucasian American mothers attributed least to effort and distributed responsibility more evenly across the options. Chinese American mothers also viewed lack of effort as important but assigned considerable responsibility to other sources. Holloway, Kashiwagi, Hess, and Azuma (1986) examined attributions for math performance by Japanese and American mothers and children. Whereas American mothers and children emphasized ability, Japanese respondents emphasized effort, particularly when assessing low performance.

Studies also show that Americans support rewarding people for their accomplishments rather than for their efforts

(Hochschild, 1995). In Japanese cultural contexts, on the other hand, the process is just as important as the outcome and must involve *gambaru*, which means working hard and persisting (White, 1987). In work by Mashima, Shapiro, and Azuma (1998), 70% of Americans described success or failure in terms of achieving some effortful goal, in contrast with only 29% of Japanese. Instead, Japanese described the internal process of exerting effort, without mentioning whether the final outcome had been achieved.

Research indicates that although individuals in American and Asian contexts use the categories of effort and ability to understand achievement, the meaning and relationship of these categories differs (Miller, 1996). For example, whereas in U.S. contexts, ability and effort are perceived as having a compensatory relationship, in Chinese contexts, they are often seen as being positively related, implying that ability can be increased through effort (Hong, 2001; Salili, 1996). Under Chinese models of competence and motivation, "people working hard have higher ability and those who have high ability must have worked hard" (Salili & Hau, 1994, p. 233).

Intrinsic Motivation: Personal Choice and Control Required?

Theories of achievement motivation developed in U.S. and other Western contexts generally have been based on individualism, emphasizing personal choice and responsibility (Miller, 1996; Spence, 1985). In so doing, these theories have also contributed to the development and perpetuation of the inside story. Under the predominant model of motivation, controlling one's environment, self-determination, and freedom of choice are associated with higher intrinsic motivation, whereas feelings of being controlled can decrease intrinsic motivation (Deci & Ryan, 1985). The relationship between intrinsic motivation and control may assume a different form in cultural contexts in which alternative models of motivation prevail—ones that stress indirect or secondary modes of control, relational sources of control, tolerance, and flexibility (e.g., see Weisz et al., 1984).

Internal and External Sources of Control

Iyengar and Lepper (1999) questioned the assumption that intrinsic motivation and the provision of individual choice and self-determination go hand in hand by examining the relationship between choice and motivation across cultures. In one study, Anglo American and Asian American grade-school children were asked to work on an anagrams task. Anglo American children performed best and spent more time working on the anagrams when they chose which anagrams they would work on for themselves, while Asian American children performed best and spent more time working on the anagrams when they thought that their mothers had chosen the anagrams for them. Iyengar and Lepper obtained similar results when children were told that an outgroup (children at another school) or ingroup (their own classmates) had made the selections.

Asian American children may perform best and appear to enjoy tasks most when valued ingroup members choose for them, because of the different models of motivation that permeate their cultural contexts. It is not surprising that children are more motivated by "what Mom thinks" in a cultural context that stresses the relational nature of motivation than in one that stresses the independent, internal sources of motivation. Moreover, boundaries between intrinsic and extrinsic motivation are culturally defined (Iyengar & Brockner, 2001; Iyengar & Lepper, 1999). Iyengar and Lepper note that in American society, if someone behaves in order to please someone else or conform to their ideals, then that behavior is viewed as extrinsically motivated (deCharms, 1968; Deci, 1975). In East Asian settings, external sources of motivation may not inherently contradict or interfere with internal motives. For example, Church and Katigbak (1992) found a closer relationship between intrinsic task motives and affiliative motives among Filipino than among American university students. Salili, Chiu, and Lai (2001) observed that in Chinese cultural contexts, extrinsic and intrinsic motivation may work side by side. According to Tweed and Lehman (2002), in Chinese contexts, external goals, such as social recognition, are positively associated with mastery goals, suggesting that the Confucian emphasis on pragmatic learning does not preclude learning-related goals.

Practices of Choice and Control

Different cultural contexts also provide varying degrees of opportunity for exercising choice and control. For example, whereas in American contexts, choice may figure prominently in daily life, having and making choices is not part of a students' normal daily routine in Japanese contexts (Lewis, 1995). Instead, conforming to the preferences of a social group or adjusting to others is more prevalent. Furthermore, according to Tweed and Lehman (2002), the Socratic approach to learning common in Western cultures is associated with a desire for self-directed tasks, but cultures that stress Confucian approaches to learning may not foster self-determination to the same extent. A recent study by Morling, Kitayama, and Miyamoto (2002) examined cultural variation in the affordance of direct control. They asked Americans and Japanese to describe actual social situations in which "you have influenced or changed the surrounding people, events, or objects according to your own wishes" or in which "you have adjusted yourself to surrounding people, objects and events." Respondents also indicated when the events had occurred. Americans recounted more recent influencing events than adjusting events, but Japanese recounted more recent adjusting than influencing events.

The inside story, although common in American cultural contexts, is not uniformly distributed across social settings. For example, studies find that people in working-class contexts are less likely to be acting upon the world by expressing their own preferences through choice, and are perhaps more likely to be adjusting to the world by conforming to relational norms and meeting obligations (Kusserow, 1999; Lamont, 2000). As a result, working-class participants may respond differently to choice than do middle-class participants. For example, Snibbe and Markus (in press) examined social class differences in personal choice within the United States. Results indicated that college-educated participants, but not high school-educated participants, like an object better if they have chosen it themselves.

Competence: Competing Perspectives?

Different Styles of Competence

Models of competence and motivation can also be linked to the styles of thinking that pervade a cultural context (Cole & Scribner, 1974; Nisbett, Peng, Choi, & Norenzayan, 2001). Consistent with the more relational models in Eastern cultures, holistic or relational–contextual thought predominates in these cultures. In holistic thought, there is greater attention to the field in which objects are embedded. In contrast, and consistent with the inside story, an analytic approach to the world is more characteristic of Western cultures. Analytic thought emphasizes paying attention primarily to the object and to the categories to which it belongs. For example, Ji and Nisbett (2001) examined Chinese and American participants' use of relationships versus categories as bases for grouping objects together. They found that Chinese participants were more likely to group objects on the basis of relationship (e.g., "Because the sun is in the sky"), while Americans were more likely to group objects on the basis of category or shared object features ("Because the sun and the sky are both in the heavens"). In a study by Masuda and Nisbett (2001), which also examined cultural variation in thinking styles, Japanese and American students saw animated vignettes of underwater scenes. Subsequently, they were shown figures that had either been previously seen or not seen, and that were either in their original setting or in some other setting. Japanese students recognized previously presented figures more accurately when seen with the original background than with the new background, whereas the latter manipulation had no effect on American subjects.

Awareness of Difference

Within American contexts, some researchers who focus on explaining differences between ethnic and racial groups in academic performance achievement motivation have drawn attention to the role of the context in performance (Jones, 1999; Markus, Steele, & Steele, 2001; Steele, 1997). Mainstream contexts typically inscribe the ideas and practices of the majority. Thus, those who examine these contexts from the perspective of the minority are often in a good position to see the context, which is often invisible to the majority. The mainstream context can facilitate performance for some and impair it for others. Without acknowledging that the context of learning and motivation may differ for those in the majority and those in the minority, explaining the gap among students and employees from different backgrounds in terms of internal factors can seem reasonable. And historically, researchers have pursued this exact explanatory path, thereby continually reinforcing the inside story. Even social psychologists have leaned toward explanations that focus on internal basic processes. As Steele and Sherman (1999) argue, despite the initial impact of Lewin's theoretical formulations, researchers have paid relatively little attention to "the 'life–space' contexts of people's lives—their socioeconomic position in society, their position in a family, their group identities, the cultures they are immersed in, the status they enjoy, the stigmas they endure, and the opportunities and resources they possess" (pp. 393–394).

Charting the particulars of the relevant contexts reveals, for example, that those in the majority, compared to those in the minority (e.g., white students compared to black students in a predominantly white school), are not in the same context. They are often assumed by teachers, principals, and other students to be able to succeed, and they are expected to succeed. Furthermore, whites are likely to have benefited from contexts with relatively better schools and more prepared teachers, to have better educated parents, and to live in homes and neighborhoods with more school-relevant resources (Lamont & Lareau, 1988; Ogbu, 1991). Whites also are relatively free from a whole concert of negative stereotypes and limiting evaluations that are often associated with minority groups in academic contexts (Crocker & Major, 1989). Steele and colleagues (Steele, 1997; Steele & Aronson, 1995) found that if negative stereotypes of academic ability of black students are present in a context, then even well-qualified black students can experience a threat to

their identity and perform less well than they do in a context free of these stereotypes. Seen from the point of view of the minority, many elements of the context and its potential impact on competence and motivation are in relatively high relief.

Given the prevalence of the inside story in mainstream American cultural contexts, majority members are less likely to notice how the context may be more supportive and less toxic for them than it is for those in the minority. Since the scaffolding provided by the supportive social context is rarely delineated, especially when the context is supportive and affirming, the inside story gains credibility. Competence and motivation are seen to stem from their internal traits and properties. The ways in which the assumptions, expectations, representations, and practices of the context afford the inside view are hidden. For majority learners or observers in a majority context, it is as if they were "born on third base" (with all of its relative advantages), yet believe, thanks to the automatic engagement of the inside cultural model, that they have "hit a triple."

Most American mainstream educational contexts, while seemingly fostering a "general" or "basic" model of education, promote mainstream or European American ideas and practices of education (Bruner, 1996). Students who have been socialized according to this model may have an important, yet largely unseen, advantage over those with very different frameworks of understandings relevant to education and competence. For example, Fryberg and Markus (2004) found that education in American Indian contexts involves fostering a trusting relationship between student and teacher. Yet schooling, as practiced in mainstream settings, focuses on the autonomous, independent individual and may be experienced as threatening to valued relationships. Oyserman, Gant, and Ager (1995) found that, whereas for white students, achievement is related to individualism and the Protestant work ethic, for blacks, it is related to collectivism and ethnic identity. A reasonable congruence between the models that the student invokes and the models that are predominant in the student's school setting is likely to facilitate academic success, while a lack of congruence may decrease the likelihood of such success.

CONCLUDING REMARKS

As with all psychological phenomena, competence and motivation are multiply afforded and maintained. Surely, both individual differences in capacities identified as internal, as well as differences in individual engagements with the social context, will prove to be significant in the analysis of competence and motivation. The main point of the chapter, however, is that the story of being smart and motivated in America has been, and continues to be, primarily an inside story. It is an inside story, not because the weight of the evidence overwhelmingly supports this perspective, but because the inside understanding of competence and motivation fits like Cinderella's slipper to the predominant cultural model of behavior. When parents, teachers, and employees seek to explain variation in competence and motivation, they most commonly look to what is believed to be inside the person—to an entity or a set of entities, or to a force or energy that powers and controls behavior. Whether these entities or forces are presumed to be innately given faculties or the result of effort and persistent engagement with the relevant tasks, they are believed to reside inside the person and to be subject to individual, willful control.

Given the historical and ideological foundations of the American and European contexts in which these theories have developed, peering inward is natural and obvious. In individualistic cultures that prize, above all, freedom (both freedom from the constraint of others and the freedom to express one's self through choice and control), it is unthinkable to locate the sources of positive, desirable behavioral tendencies (those associated with achievement and success) anywhere but inside the person. Many analyses of competence and motivation then quite reasonably seek and find these phenomena or processes within the person. Given the ideological landscape and the extensive system of practices and institutions that accord these ideas a real and objective status, the relative underdevelopment of a social or relational understanding of competence and motivation is hardly surprising. A collective preference for a view of the actor as independently mastering the environment obscures the potential role of the social context.

Our argument is that the inside model is prominent and powerful, not that it is the only model of competence and motivation that has been theorized in American and European contexts. Certainly, the role of the social context, particularly the expectations of others, has been explored. However, these views are swimming upstream against a dense and forceful flow of meanings and practices, both in science and in the everyday world, and these more social views of competence and motivation have not caught on and have not stuck. Our review of the literature reveals that in contexts in which the person is regarded as an interdependent part of an encompassing social network, the social nature of competence and motivation is decidedly more obvious and natural. Our review of these studies serves primarily to underscore that the prevalent, implicit cultural models in a given context shape the scientific search, analysis, and interpretation strategies in ways that are important to identify and delineate. As a science, have we searched for the sources of competence and motivation and found them "inside" because they are there, or have we searched where the cultural spotlight is brightest?

Is it a problem that an "it's what's inside that counts" cultural context has "it's what's inside that counts" theories and practices of competence and motivation? Our view is that it is a problem if the scientific goal is to develop a comprehensive human psychology, not a particular or a partial one. Socially and practically, within European and American contexts, it matters because, as a growing number of empirical studies suggest, the social context is important for competence and motivation, but this may be the case particularly for those outside mainstream contexts—those who engage or have engaged in cultural contexts different from the middle-class European American one—and for those who have been historically marginalized and excluded from full participation in mainstream contexts. For these individuals, failures to manifest competence or motivation may result from different understandings and approaches to motivation, but they are often immediately explained with inside accounts (e.g., these people are stupid or lazy). The role of the context, as well as the potential mismatch between the prevalent models in a context and those that students or employees bring with them, may be relatively invisible and unidentified. To be competent and motivated in a given context requires behaving in a culturally appropriate manner. Those who are motivated by friends and family more than by their own interests may be judged as followers; those who are very receptive to others, and to relations with others, may be seen as dependent and uncreative; those who criticize rather than enhance themselves may be judged as unmotivated or may not be noticed at all. Moreover, those who expect that a positive and effective context is an interdependent, relational one may not respond well in contexts requiring separation, independence, and relative autonomy from others. Finally, failures to manifest competence and motivation that arise because people are required to contend with the pressure of being stereotyped, devalued, and otherwise limited may go completely undetected. Under the influence of the inside model, those in this predicament may be readily labeled as incompetent or unmotivated.

The situation of Hiroki, whom Americans judged as gifted and Japanese judged as unintelligent, is a powerful reminder of the importance of explicitly examining the prevailing implicit cultural models of competence and motivation. What does it mean to be competent or motivated in this situation? What is the source of this understanding? Does the arrangement of classrooms and workplaces foster one model of competence and motivation at the expense of others? Who is privileged by this arrangement of the context, and who is disadvantaged? What is missing in many European American contexts is the idea that competence and motivation arise from complex, dynamic relations between people and their social environment. Enriching the inside story with a more social view will serve to generate more competence and motivation. The inside story, while a best-seller, is not the full story, and it leaves a lot of competence and motivation on the shelf.

NOTE

1. When we refer to "American" or "American style," we mean pertaining to "mainstream" U.S. cultural contexts and to those who have engaged with dominant, middle-class U.S. ideas and practices and participated in U.S. institutions. Depending on the literature being reviewed or the studies being portrayed, in some places, we use the term "European American" to denote Americans of European descent, and "Anglo" to mean Americans of British descent. By "Western," we mean from countries that are culturally Western, most of which are located in Europe and North America, and have been strongly influenced by Greek and Roman culture and Christianity.

REFERENCES

Adams, G., & Markus, H. R. (2004). Toward a conception of culture suitable for a social psychology of culture. In M. Schaller & C. S. Crandall (Eds.), *The psychological foundations of culture* (pp. 335–360). Mahwah, NJ: Erlbaum.

Agarwal, R., & Misra, G. (1987). Towards conceptualizing achievement in Indian context. *Psychologia*, *30*(4), 228–234.

Ames, C. A., & Archer, J. (1988). Achievement goals in the classroom: Students' learning strategies and motivation processes. *Journal of Educational Psychology*, *80*(3), 260–267.

Azuma, H. (1994). Two modes of cognitive socialization in Japan and the United States. In P. M. Greenfield & R. R. Cocking (Eds.), *Cross-cultural roots of minority child development* (pp. 275–284). Hillsdale, NJ: Erlbaum.

Azuma, H., & Kashiwagi, K. (1987). Descriptors for an intelligent person: A Japanese study. *Japanese Psychological Research*, *29*(1), 17–26.

Bandura, A. (1977). Self-efficacy: Toward a unifying theory of behavioral change. *Psychological Review*, *84*, 191–215.

Bandura, A. (1997). *Self-efficacy: The exercise of control*. New York: Freeman.

Basow, S. A. (1984). Ethnic group differences in educational achievement in Fiji. *Journal of Cross-Cultural Psychology*, *15*, 435–451.

Baumeister, R. F. (1987). How the self became a problem: A psychological review of historical research. *Journal of Personality and Social Psychology*, *52*, 163–176.

Bellah, R. N., Madsen, R., Sullivan, W. M., Swidler, A., & Tipton, S. M. (1985). *Habits of the heart: Individualism and commitment in American life*. New York: Harper & Row.

Berry, J. W. (1996). A cultural ecology of cognition. In I. Dennis & P. Taspfield. (Eds.), *Human abilities: Their nature and measurement* (pp. 19–37). Hillsdale, NJ: Erlbaum.

Binet, A., & Simon, T. (1905). Méthodes nouvelles pour le diagnostic du niveau intellectuel des anormaux [New methods for the diagnosis of the intellectual level of abnormals]. *L'Année Psychologique, 11*, 191–244.

Binet, A., & Simon, T. (1911). *A method of measuring the development of the intelligence of young children*. Lincoln, IL: Courier.

Brehm, J. W. (1966). *A theory of psychological reactance*. New York: Academic Press.

Bruner, J. S. (1957). Going beyond the information given. In J. S. Bruner, E. Brunswik, L. Festinger, F. Heider, K. F. Muenzinger, C. E. Osgood, & D. Rapaport (Eds.), *Contemporary approaches to cognition* (pp. 41–69). Cambridge, MA: Harvard University Press.

Bruner, J. S. (1990). *Acts of meaning*. Cambridge, MA: Harvard University Press.

Bruner, J. S. (1996). *The culture of education*. Cambridge, MA: Harvard University Press.

Cantor, N., & Kihlstrom, J. F. (1985). *Social intelligence: The cognitive basis of personality*. Ann Arbor: University of Michigan Press.

Carugati, F. F. (1990). Everyday ideas, theoretical models and social representations: The case of intelligence and its development. In G. R. Semin & K. J. Gergen (Eds.), *Everyday understanding: Social and scientific implications* (pp. 130–150). Thousand Oaks, CA: Sage.

Cattell, J. M. (1890). Mental tests and measurements. *Mind, 15*, 373–381.

Chapman, P. D. (1988). *Schools as sorters: Lewis M. Terman, applied psychology, and the intelligence testing movement, 1890–1930*. New York: New York University Press.

Church, A. T., & Katigbak, M. S. (1992). The cultural context of academic motives: A comparison of Filipino and American college students. *Journal of Cross-Cultural Psychology, 23*(1), 40–58.

Cohen, A. B., Hall, D. E., Koenig, H. G., & Meador, K. G. (2003). *Social versus individual motivation: Implications for normative definitions of religious orientation*. Unpublished manuscript, Duke University, Durham, NC.

Cole, M., & Scribner, S. (1974). *Culture and thought: A psychological introduction*. New York: Wiley.

Commager, H. S. (1950). *The American mind: An interpretation of American thought and character since the 1880's*. New Haven, CT: Yale University Press.

Condry, J. (1977). Enemies of exploration: Self-initiated versus other-initiated learning. *Journal of Personality and Social Psychology, 35*, 459–477.

Cooley, D. H. (1902). *Human nature and the social order*. New York: Scribners.

Cordova, D. I., & Lepper, M. R. (1996). Intrinsic motivation and the process of learning: Beneficial effects of contextualization, personalization, and choice. *Journal of Educational Psychology, 88*, 715–730.

Crocker, J., & Major, B. (1989). The self-protective properties of stigma. *Psychological Review, 96*, 608–630.

Croizet, J. C., & Claire, T. (1998). Extending the concept of stereotype and threat to social class: The in-

tellectual underperformance of students from low socioeconomic backgrounds. *Personality and Social Psychology Bulletin, 24*, 588–594.

Das, J. P. (1994). Eastern views of intelligence. In R. J. Sternberg (Ed.), *Encyclopedia of human intelligence* (Vol. 1, pp. 387–391). New York: Macmillan.

deCharms, R. (1968). *Personal causation: The internal affective determinants of behavior*. New York: Academic Press.

Deci, E. L. (1971). Effects of externally mediated rewards on intrinsic motivation. *Journal of Personality and Social Psychology, 18*, 105–115.

Deci, E. L. (1975). *Intrinsic motivation*. New York: Plenum Press.

Deci, E. L., & Ryan, R. M. (1980). Self-determination theory: When mind mediates behavior. *Journal of Mind and Behavior, 1*, 33–43.

Deci, E. L., & Ryan, R. M. (1985). *Intrinsic motivation and self-determination in human behavior*. New York: Plenum Press.

de Tocqueville, A. (2000). *Democracy in America* (H. C. Mansfield & D. Winthrop, Trans.). Chicago: University of Chicago Press. (Original work published in 1840)

De Vos, G. A. (1973). *Socialization for achievement: Essays on the cultural psychology of the Japanese*. Berkeley: University of California Press.

Dweck, C. S. (1986). Motivational processes affecting learning [Special issue: Psychological science and education]. *American Psychologist, 41*(10), 1040–1048.

Dweck, C. S., Chiu, C., & Hong, Y. (1995). Implicit theories and their role in judgments and reactions: A world from two perspectives. *Psychological Inquiry, 6*(4), 267–285.

Dweck, C. S., & Leggett, E. L. (1988). A social-cognitive approach to motivation and personality. *Psychological Review, 95*, 256–273.

Eaton, M. J., & Dembo, M. H. (1997). Differences in the motivational beliefs of Asian American and non-Asian students. *Journal of Educational Psychology, 89*(3), 433–440.

Emerson, R. W. (1950). *The complete essays and other writings*. New York: Modern Library.

Farr, R. M. (1996). *The roots of modern social psychology*. Oxford, UK: Blackwell.

Fiske, A. P., Kitayama, S., Markus, H. R., & Nisbett, R. E. (1998). The cultural matrix of social psychology. In D. T. Gilbert, S. T. Fiske, & G. Lindzey (Eds.), *Handbook of social psychology* (4th ed., pp. 915–981). New York: McGraw-Hill.

Fiske, S. T., & Taylor, S. E. (1994). *Social cognition* (2nd ed.). Reading, MA: Addison-Wesley.

Fryans, L. J., Salili, F., Maehr, M. L., & Desai, K. A. (1983). A cross-cultural exploration into the meaning of achievement. *Journal of Personality and Social Psychology, 44*(5), 1000–1013.

Fryberg, S., & Markus, H. R. (2004). *Models of education in American Indian, Asian American, and European American cultural contexts*. Unpublished manuscript, University of Arizona.

Gallimore, R. (1974). Affiliation motivation and Hawaiian-American achievement. *Journal of Cross-Cultural Psychology, 5*, 481–491.

Gallimore, R., Boggs, J. W., & Jordan, C. (1974). *Culture, behavior, and education: A study of Hawaiian-Americans.* Beverly Hills, CA: Sage.

Galton, F. (1978). *Hereditary genius: An inquiry into its laws and consequences.* London: Julian Friedmann. (Original work published 1869)

Gardner, D. S. (1987). Spirits and conceptions of agency among the Miamin of Papau New Guinea. *Oceania, 57*, 161–177.

Gardner, H. (1993). *Frames of mind: the theory of multiple intelligences.* New York: Basic Books.

Gladwell, M. (2002, July 22). The talent myth. *The New Yorker*, pp. 28–33.

Goleman, D. (1995). *Emotional intelligence.* New York: Bantam.

Goleman, D., Kaufman, P., & Ray, M. (1992). *The creative spirit.* New York: Dutton.

Goodnow, J. J. (1990). The socialization of cognition: What's involved? In J. Stigler, R. Shweder, & G. Herdt (Eds.), *Cultural psychology: Essays on comparative human development* (pp. 259–286). New York: Cambridge University Press.

Gould, S. J. (1999). A critique of Heckhausen and Schulz's (1995) life-span theory of control from a cross-cultural perspective. *Psychological Review, 106*(3), 597–604.

Graham, S. (2001). Inferences about responsibility and values: Implication for academic motivation. In F. Salili, F. Chiu & Y. Hong (Eds.), *Student motivation: The culture and context of learning* (pp. 31–59). Dordrecht: Kluwer Academic.

Greenfield, P. M. (1997). You can't take it with you: Why ability assessments don't cross cultures. *American Psychologist, 52*(10), 1115–1124.

Greeno, J. G. (1988). *Situations, mental models, and generative knowledge* (Report No. IRL88-0055). Palo Alto, CA: Institute for Research on Learning.

Harkness, S., Super, C. M., & Keefer, C. H. (1992). Learning to be an American parent: How cultural models gain directive force. In R. G. D'Andrade & C. Strauss (Ed.), *Human motives and cultural models* (pp. 163–178). New York: Cambridge University Press.

Harwood, R. L., Miller, J. G., & Irizarry, N. L. (1995). *Culture and attachment: Perceptions of the child in context.* New York: Guilford Press.

Heckhausen, J., & Schulz, R. (1995). A life-span theory of control. *Psychological Review, 102*, 284–304.

Heine, S. J., Lehman, D. R., Ide, E., Leung, C., Kitayama, S., Takata, T., et al. (2001). Divergent consequences of success and failure in Japan and North America: An investigation of self-improving motivations and malleable selves. *Journal of Personality and Social Psychology, 81*(4), 599–615.

Herrnstein, R. J., & Murray, C. (1994). *The bell curve: Intelligence and class structure in American life.* New York: Free Press.

Hess, R. D., Chang, C. M., & McDevitt, T. M. (1987). Cultural variables in family beliefs about children's performance in mathematics: Comparisons among People's Republic of China, Chinese-American, and Caucasian-American families. *Journal of Educational Psychology, 79*, 179–188.

Hewitt, J. (1989). *Dilemmas of the American self.* Philadelphia: Temple University Press.

Hirayama, K. K. (1985). Asian children's adaptation to public schools. *Social Work in Education, 7*(4), 213–230.

Hochschild, J. L. (1995). *Facing up to the American Dream: Race, class, and the soul of the nation.* Princeton, NJ: Princeton University Press.

Holland, D., Lachicotte, W., Jr., Skinner, D., & Cain, C. (1998). *Identity and agency in cultural worlds.* Cambridge, MA: Harvard University Press.

Holloway, S. D. (1988). Concepts of ability and effort in Japan and the United States. *Review of Educational Research, 58*(3), 327–345.

Holloway, S. D., Kashiwagi, K., Hess, R. D., & Azuma, H. (1986). Causal attribution by Japanese and American mothers about performance in mathematics. *International Journal of Psychology, 21*, 269–286.

Hong, Y. (2001). Chinese students' and teachers' inferences of effort and ability. In F. Salili, F. Chiu, & Y. Hong (Eds.), *Student motivation: The culture and context of learning* (pp. 105–120). Dordrecht: Kluwer Academic.

Hsu, F. L. K. (1972). American core values and national character. In F. L. K. Hsu (Ed.), *Psychological anthropology* (pp. 241–262). Cambridge, MA: Schenkman.

Hull, C. L. (1943). *Principles of behavior.* New York: Appleton–Century–Crofts.

Ickes, W., Stinson, L., Bissonnette, V., & Garcia, S. (1990). Naturalistic social cognition: Empathic accuracy in mixed-sex dyads. *Journal of Personality and Social Psychology, 59*, 730–742.

Iyengar, S. S., & Brockner, J. (2001). Cultural differences in self and the impact of personal and social influences. In W. Wosinska, R. B. Cialdini, D. W. Barrett, & J. Reykowski (Eds.), *The practice of social influence in multiple cultures* (Vol. 18, pp. 13–32). Mahwah, NJ: Erlbaum.

Iyengar, S. S., & Lepper, M. R. (1999). Rethinking the value of choice: A cultural perspective on intrinsic motivation. *Journal of Personality and Social Psychology, 76*, 349–366.

Jacobson, M. F. (1998). *Whiteness of a different color: European immigrants and the alchemy of race.* Cambridge, MA: Harvard University Press.

James, W. (1978). *Pragmatism and the meaning of truth.* Cambridge, MA: Harvard University Press.

Jensen, A. R. (1969). How much can we boost IQ and scholastic achievement? *Harvard Educational Review, 39*, 1–123.

Ji, L., & Nisbett, R. E. (2001). *Culture, language and categories.* Unpublished manuscript, University of Michigan, Ann Arbor.

Jones, J. M. (1999). Cultural racism: The intersection

of race and culture in intergroup conflict. In D. A. Prentice & D. T. Miller (Eds.), *Cultural divides: Understanding and overcoming group conflict* (pp. 465–490). New York: Russell Sage Foundation.

Kirkby, R. J., Kolt, G. S., & Liu, J. (1999). Participation motives of young Australian and Chinese gymnasts. *Perceptual and Motor Skills, 88,* 363–373.

Kojima, H. (1984). A significant stride toward the comparative student of control. *American Psychologist, 39*(9), 972–973.

Kusserow, A. (1999). De-homogenizing American individualism: Socializing hard and soft individualism in Manhattan and Queens. *Ethos, 27,* 210–234.

Kwok, D. C. (1995). The self-perception of competence by Canadian and Chinese children. *Psychologia, 38*(1), 9–16.

Lakoff, G., & Johnson, M. (1999). *Philosophy in the flesh: The embodied mind and its challenge to Western thought.* New York: Basic Books.

Lamont, M. (1992). *Money, morals and manners: The culture of the French and American upper-middle class.* Chicago: University of Chicago Press.

Lamont, M. (2000). *The dignity of working men.* New York: Russell Sage Foundation.

Lamont, M., & Lareau, A. (1988). Cultural capital. *Sociological Theory, 6,* 153–168.

Landrine, H., & Klonoff, E. A. (1994). Cultural diversity in causal attributions for illness: The role of the supernatural. *Journal of Behavioral Medicine, 17,* 181–193.

Lave, J., & Wenger, E. (1991). *Situated learning: Legitimate peripheral participation.* Cambridge, UK: Cambridge University Press.

Lemann, N. (1999). *The big test: The secret history of the American meritocracy.* New York: Farrar, Straus & Giroux.

Lepper, M. R., Greene, D., & Nisbett, R. E. (1973). Undermining children's intrinsic interest with extrinsic rewards: A test of the "overjustification" hypothesis. *Journal of Personality and Social Psychology, 28,* 129–137.

Lewin, K. (1935). *A dynamic theory of personality.* New York: McGraw-Hill.

Lewis, C. C. (1995). *Educating hearts and minds.* New York: Cambridge University Press.

Locke, J. (1979). *An essay concerning human understanding.* (P. H. Nidditch, Ed.). Oxford, UK: Clarendon. (Original work published 1690)

Locke, J. (1989). *Some thoughts concerning education.* Oxford, UK: Clarendon. (Original work published 1693)

Luria, A. R. (1981). *Language and cognition* (J. V. Wertsch, Trans.). New York: Wiley.

Maehr, M. (1974). Culture and achievement motivation. *American Psychologist, 29,* 887–896.

Maehr, M. L. (1984). Meaning and motivation: Toward a theory of personal investment. In E. Ames & C. Ames (Eds.), *Research on motivation in education* (Vol. 1, pp. 115–144). New York: Academic Press.

Maehr, M. L., & Yamaguchi, R. (2001). Cultural diversity, student motivation and achievement. In F. Salili,

F. Chiu, & Y. Hong (Eds.), *Student motivation: The culture and context of learning* (pp. 123–148). Dordrecht: Kluwer Academic.

Markus, H. R., & Kitayama, S. (1991). Culture and the self: Implications for cognition, emotion, and motivation. *Psychological Review, 98,* 224–253.

Markus, H. R., & Kitayama, S. (1994). A collective fear of the collective: Implications for selves and theories of selves. *Personality and Social Psychology Bulletin, 20,* 568–579.

Markus, H. R., & Kitayama, S. (2004). Models of agency: Sociocultural diversity in the construction of action. In V. Murphy-Berman & J. Berman (Eds.), *The 49th Annual Nebraska Symposium on Motivation: Cross-cultural differences in perspectives on self* (pp. 1–57). Lincoln: University of Nebraska Press.

Markus, H. R., Kitayama, S., & Heiman, R. (1996). Culture and "basic" psychological principles. In E. T. Higgins & A. W. Kruglanski (Eds.), *Social psychology: Handbook of basic principles* (pp. 857–913). New York: Guilford Press.

Markus, H. R., Ryff, C. D., Curhan, K. B., & Palmerscheim, K. (2004). In their own words: Well-being at midlife among high school and college educated adults. In O. G. Brim, C. D. Ryff, & R. C. Kessler (Eds.), *How healthy are we?: A national study of well-being at midlife* (pp. 273–319). Chicago: University of Chicago Press.

Markus, H. R., Steele, C. M., & Steele, D. M. (2000). Colorblindness as a barrier to inclusion: Assimilation and nonimmigrant minorities. *Daedalus, 129*(4), 233–259.

Mashima, M., Shapiro, L., & Azuma, H. (1998). Sakubun kadai ni yoru mokuhyou kouzou to shourai tenbou ni kansuru kenkyu: "Mokuteki wo motte doryoku shita koto: no nichibei hikaku" (chuukan houkoku) [Research on goal structure and future time perspective in an essay task: A U.S.–Japan comparison of "conscious goal-directed efforts" (an interim report)]. *Human Development Research, Journal of the Center of Developmental Education and Research, 13,* 106–118.

Maslow, A. H. (1970). *Motivation and personality* (Rev. ed.). New York: Harper & Row.

Masuda, T., & Nisbett, R. E. (2001). Attending holistically versus analytically: Comparing the context sensitivity of Japanese and Americans. *Journal of Personality and Social Psychology, 81,* 922–934.

McClelland, D. C. (1961). *The achieving society.* Oxford, UK: Van Nostrand.

McClelland, D. C., Atkinson, J. W., Clark, R. A., & Lowell, E. L. (1953). *The achievement motive.* New York: Appleton–Century–Crofts.

McElroy, J. H. (1999). *American beliefs: What keeps a big country and a diverse people united.* Chicago: Ivan R. Dee.

Mead, G. H. (1934). *Mind, self, and society.* Chicago: University of Chicago Press.

Miller, J. G. (1984). Culture and the development of everyday social explanation. *Journal of Personality and Social Psychology, 46,* 961–978.

Miller, J. G. (1988). Bridging the content structure di-chotomy: Culture and the self. In M. Bond (Ed.), *The cross-cultural challenge to social psychology* (pp. 266–281). Beverly Hills, CA: Sage.

Miller, J. G. (1994). Cultural psychology: Bridging dis-ciplinary boundaries in understanding the cultural grounding of self. In P. K. Bock (Ed.), *Handbook of psychological anthropology* (pp. 139–170). West-port, CT: Greenwood.

Miller, J. G. (1996). Culture as a source of order in so-cial motivation. *Psychological Inquiry, 7*(3), 240–243.

Minsky, M. L. (1986). *The society of mind.* New York: Simon & Schuster.

Mischel, W., & Shoda, Y. (1995). A cognitive-affective system theory of personality: Reconceptualizing the invariances in personality and the role of situations. *Psychological Review, 102*(2), 246–268.

Misra, G., & Gergen, K. J. (1993). On the place of cul-ture in psychological science. *International Journal of Psychology, 28*(2), 225–243.

Mook, D. G. (1986). *Motivation: The organization of action.* New York: Norton.

Morling, B., Kitayama, S., & Miyamoto, Y. (2002). Cultural practices emphasize influence in the United States and adjustment in Japan. *Personality and Social Psychology Bulletin, 28*(3), 311–323.

Morris, M. W., & Peng, K. (1994). Culture and cause: American and Chinese attributions for social and physical events. *Journal of Personality and Social Psychology, 67,* 949–971.

Multon, D. K., Brown, S. D., & Lent, R. W. (1991). Re-lation of self-efficacy beliefs to academic outcomes: A meta-analytic investigation. *Journal of Counseling Psychology, 38,* 30–38.

Munro, D. (1969). *The concept of man in early China.* Stanford, CA: Stanford University Press.

Murray, H. A. (1938). *Explorations in personality.* New York: Oxford University Press.

Niles, S. (1998). Achievement goals and means: A cul-tural comparison. *Journal of Cross-Cultural Psy-chology, 29*(5), 656–667.

Nisbett, R. E., Peng, K., Choi, I., & Norenzayan, A. (2001). Culture and systems of thought: Holistic ver-sus analytic cognition. *Psychological Review, 108,* 291–310.

Oettingen, G., Little, T. D., Lindenberger, U., & Baltes, P. B. (1994). Causality, agency and control beliefs in East versus West Berlin children: A natural experi-ment on the role of context. *Journal of Personality and Social Psychology, 66,* 579–595.

Ogbu, J. U. (1991). Minority coping responses and school experience. *Journal of Psychohistory, 18,* 433–456.

Ohnuki-Tierney, E. (1995). *Rice as self: Japanese identi-ties through time.* Princeton, NJ: Princeton Univer-sity Press.

Oishi, S., & Diener, E. (2003). Culture and well-being: The cycle of action, evaluation, and decision. *Per-sonality and Social Psychology Bulletin, 29,* 1–11.

Oyserman, D., Gant, L., & Ager, J. (1995). A socially contextualized model of African American identity: Possible selves and school persistence. *Journal of Personality and Social Psychology, 69*(6), 1216–1222.

Peak, L. (1991). *Learning to go to school in Japan: The transition from home to preschool life.* Berkeley: University of California Press.

Pintrich, P. R., & Schrauben, B. (1992). Students' moti-vational beliefs and their cognitive engagement in ac-ademic tasks. In D. Schunk & J. Meece (Eds.), *Stu-dent perceptions in the classroom* (pp. 149–183). Hillsdale, NJ: Erlbaum.

Plaut, V. C., Markus, H. R., & Lachman, M. E. (2002). Place matters: Consensual features and regional vari-ation in American well-being and self. *Journal of Personality and Social Psychology, 83,* 160–184.

Polanyi, K. (1957). *The great transformation.* Boston: Beacon Press.

Potter, D. (1954). *People of plenty: Economic abun-dance and the American character.* Chicago: Univer-sity of Chicago Press.

Quinn, D. M., & Crocker, J. (1999). When ideology hurts: Effects of belief in the Protestant ethic and feeling overweight on the psychological well-being of women. *Journal of Personality and Social Psychol-ogy, 77,* 402–414.

Ramirez, M., & Price-Williams, D. R. (1976). Achieve-ment and motivation in children of three ethnic groups in the United States. *Journal of Cross-Cultu-ral Psychology, 7,* 49–60.

Reglin, G. L., & Adams, D. R. (1990). Why Asian-Amer-ican high school students have higher grade point av-erages and SAT scores than other high school stu-dents. *High School Journal, 73*(3), 143–149.

Rogers, C. R. (1977). *On personal power: Inner strength and its revolutionary impact.* New York: Delacorte.

Rogoff, B., Baker-Sennett, J., Lacasa, P., & Goldsmith, D. (1995). Development through participation in sociocultural activity. In J. J. Goodnow, P. Miller, & F. Kessel (Eds.), *Cultural practices as contexts for de-velopment* (pp. 45–65). San Francisco: Jossey-Bass.

Rogoff, B., & Chavajay, P. (1995). What's become of research on the cultural basis of cognitive develop-ment. *American Psychologist, 50*(10), 859–877.

Ross, L. (1977). The intuitive psychologist and his shortcomings. In L. Berkowitz (Ed.), *Advances in ex-perimental social psychology* (Vol. 10, pp. 174–220). New York: Academic Press.

Rothbaum, F., Weisz, J. R., & Snyder, S. S. (1982). Changing the world and changing the self: A two-process model of perceived control. *Journal of Per-sonality and Social Psychology, 42,* 5–37.

Rotter, J. B. (1966). Generalized expectancies for inter-nal vs. external control of reinforcement. *Psycholog-ical Monographs: General and Applied, 80,* 1–28.

Ryan, R. M., & Connell, J. P. (1989). Perceived locus of causality and internalization. *Journal of Personality and Social Psychology, 5,* 749–761.

Salili, F. (1994). Age, sex, and cultural differences in the meaning and dimensions of achievement. *Personality and Social Psychology Bulletin, 20*, 635–648.

Salili, F. (1996). Learning and motivation: An Asian perspective. *Psychology and Developing Societies, 8*(1), 55–81.

Salili, F., Chiu, C., & Hong, Y. (2001). *Student motivation: The culture and context of learning.* Dordrecht: Kluwer Academic.

Salili, F., Chiu, C., & Lai, S. (2001). The influence of culture and context on students' achievement orientations. In F. Salili, F. Chiu, & Y. Hong (Eds.), *Student motivation: The culture and context of learning* (pp. 221–247). Dordrecht: Kluwer Academic.

Salili, F., & Hau, K. T. (1994). The effect of teachers' evaluative feedback on Chinese students' perceptions of ability: A cultural and situational analysis. *Educational Studies, 20*, 223–236.

Scollon, R., & Scollon, S. (1994). Face parameters in East–West discourse. In S. Ting-Toomey (Ed.), *The challenge of facework* (pp. 133–157). Albany: State University of New York Press.

Shapiro, L. J., & Azuma, H. (2004). Intellectual, attitudinal, and interpersonal aspects of competence in the United States and Japan. In R. J. Sternberg & E. L. Grigorenko (Eds.), *Culture and competence: Contexts of life success* (pp. 187–205). Washington, DC: American Psychological Association.

Shweder, R. A. (1990). Cultural psychology: What is it? In J. W. Stigler, R. A. Shweder, & G. Herdt (Eds.), *Cultural psychology: Essays on comparative human development* (pp. 1–46). Cambridge, UK: Cambridge University Press.

Shweder, R. A. (1991). *Thinking through cultures: Expeditions in cultural psychology.* Cambridge, MA: Harvard University Press.

Shweder, R. A., & Bourne, L. (1984). Does the concept of the person vary cross-culturally? In R. A. Shweder & R. A. LeVine (Eds.), *Culture theory: Essays on mind, self, and emotion* (pp. 158–199). New York: Cambridge University Press.

Singhal, R., & Misra, G. (1989). Variations in achievement cognitions: The role of ecology, age, and gender. *International Journal of Intercultural Relations, 13*(1), 93–107.

Siu, S. F. (1992). *Toward an understanding of Chinese American educational achievement* (Report No. 2). Washington DC: U.S. Department of Health and Human Services, Center on Families, Communities, Schools and Children's Learning.

Snibbe, A. C., & Markus, H. R. (2002). The psychology of religion and the religion of psychology. *Psychological Inquiry, 13*, 229–234.

Snibbe, A. C., & Markus, H. R. (in press). You can't always get what you want: Educational attainment, agency, and choice. *Journal of Personality and Social Psychology.*

Spearman, C. (1927). *The abilities of man.* London: Macmillan.

Spence, J. T. (1985). Achievement American style: The rewards and costs of individualism. *American Psychologist, 40*(12), 1285–1295.

Spindler, G., & Spindler, L. (1990). *The American cultural dialogue and its transmission.* London: Falmer Press.

Srivastava, A. K., & Misra, G. (1999). An Indian perspective on understanding intelligence. In W. J. Lonner, D. L. Dinnel, D. K. Forgays, & S. A. Hayes (Eds.), *Merging past, present, and future in cross-cultural psychology: Selected papers from the 14th International Congress of the International Association for Cross-Cultural Psychology* (pp. 159–172). Lisse: Swets & Zeitlinger.

Steele, C. M. (1997). A threat in the air: How stereotypes shape intellectual identity and performance. *American Psychologist, 52*(6), 613–629.

Steele, C. M., & Aronson, J. (1995). Stereotype threat and the intellectual test performance of African Americans. *Journal of Personality and Social Psychology, 69*(5), 797–811.

Steele, C. M., & Sherman, D.A. (1999). The psychological predicament of women on welfare. In D. A. Prentice & D. T. Miller (Eds.), *Cultural divides: understanding and overcoming group conflict.* New York: Russell Sage Foundation.

Steinberg, L., Dornbusch, S. M., & Brown, B. B. (1992). Ethnic differences in adolescent achievement: An ecological perspective. *American Psychologist, 47*, 723–729.

Sternberg, R. J. (1985). *Beyond IQ: A triarchic theory of intelligence.* New York: Cambridge University Press.

Sternberg, R. J. (1990). *Metaphors of mind: Conceptions of the nature of intelligence.* New York: Cambridge University Press.

Sternberg, R. J. (1997). The triarchic theory of intelligence. In D. P. Flanagan, J. L. Genshaft, & P. L. Harrison (Eds.), *Contemporary intellectual assessment: Theories, tests, and issues* (2nd ed., pp. 92–104). New York: Guilford Press.

Sternberg, R. J., Conway, B. E., Ketron, J. L., & Bernstein, M. (1981). People's conceptions of intelligence. *Journal of Personality and Social Psychology, 41*(1), 37–55.

Sternberg, R. J., & Grigorenko, E.L. (Eds.). (2004). *Culture and competence: Contexts of life success.* Washington, DC: American Psychological Association.

Stevenson, H. W., & Stigler, J. W. (1992). *The learning gap: Why our schools are failing and what we can learn from Japanese and Chinese education.* New York: Summit Books.

Stewart, E. C., & Bennett, M. J. (1991). *American cultural patterns: A cross-cultural perspective* (Rev. ed.). Yarmouth, ME: Intercultural Press.

Stigler, J. W., Smith, S., & Mao, L. (1985). The self-perception of competence by Chinese children. *Child Development, 56*, 1259–1270.

Su, S. K., Chiu, C.-Y., Hong, Y.-Y., Leung, K., Peng, K.,

& Morris, M. W. (1999). Self organization and social organization: American and Chinese constructions. In T. R. Tyler, R. Kramer, & O. John (Eds.), *The psychology of the social self* (pp. 193–222). Mahwah, NJ: Erlbaum.

Suarez-Orozco, M. M. (1987). Becoming somebody: Central American immigrants in U.S inner-city schools. *Anthropology and Education Quarterly, 18,* 287–298.

Takaki, R. (1993). *A different mirror: A history of multicultural America.* Boston: Little, Brown.

Taylor, S. E., & Brown, J. D. (1988). Illusion and well-being: A social psychological perspective on mental health. *Psychology Bulletin, 103,* 193–210.

Tobin, J. J., Wu, D. Y. H., & Davidson, D. H. (1989). *Preschool in three cultures: Japan, China, and the United States.* New Haven, CT: Yale University Press.

Trueba, H. T., & Delgado-Gaitan, C. (1985). Socialization of Mexican children for cooperation and competition: Sharing and copying. *Journal of Educational Equity and Leadership, 5,* 189–204.

Turner, F. J. (1920). *The frontier in American history.* New York: Holt.

Tweed, R. G., & Lehman, D. R. (2002). Learning considered within a cultural context: Confucian and Socratic approaches. *American Psychologist, 57*(2), 89–99.

Urdan, T. (2001). Contextual influences on motivation and performance: An examination of achievement goal structures. In F. Salili, F. Chiu, & Y. Hong (Eds.), *Student motivation: The culture and context of learning* (pp. 171–201). Dordrecht: Kluwer Academic.

Vygotsky, L. S. (1978). *Mind in society: The development of higher psychological processes.* In M. Cole, V. John-Steiner, S. Scribner, & E. Souberman (Eds.), Cambridge, MA: Harvard University Press.

Watson, J. B. (1924). *Behaviorism.* New York: Norton.

Weber, M. (1958). *The Protestant ethic and the spirit of capitalism* (T. Parsons, Trans.). New York: Scribner. (Original work published 1904)

Weiner, B. (1985). An attributional theory of achievement motivation and emotion. *Psychological Review, 92*(4), 548–573.

Weiner, B. (1991). Metaphors in motivation and attribution. *American Psychologist, 46,* 921–930.

Weiner, B. (2001). Intrapersonal and interpersonal theories of motivation from an attribution perspective. In F. Salili, C. Chiu, & Y. Hong (Eds.), *Student motivation: The culture and context of learning* (pp. 17–30). Dordrecht: Kluwer Academic.

Weisz, J. R., Rothbaum, F. M., & Blackburn, T. C. (1984). Standing out and standing in: The psychology of control in America and Japan. *American Psychologist, 39,* 955–969.

Whang, P. A., & Hancock, G. R. (1994). Motivation and mathematics achievement: Comparison between Asian-American and non-Asian students. *Contemporary Educational Psychology, 19,* 302–322.

White, M. (1987). *The Japanese educational challenge: A commitment to children.* New York: Free Press.

White, M. I., & LeVine, R. A. (1986). What is an *li ko* (good child)? In H. Stevenson, H. Azuma, & K. Hakuta (Eds.), *Child development and education in Japan* (pp. 55–62). New York: Freeman.

White, R. W. (1959). Motivation reconsidered: The concept of competence. *Psychological Review, 66,* 297–333.

Wicklund, R. A. (1974). *Freedom and reactance.* Potomac, MD: Erlbaum.

Wiley, N. (1994). *The semiotic self.* Chicago: University of Chicago Press.

Wilson, S. R. (1997). Self-actualization and culture. In D. Munro, J. F. Schumaker, & S. C. Carr (Eds.), *Motivation and culture* (pp. 85–96). New York: Routledge.

Wober, M. (1974). Towards an understanding of the Kiganda concept of intelligence. In J. W. Berry & P. R. Dasen (Ed.), *Culture and cognition: Readings in cross-cultural psychology.* London: Methuen.

Wyllie, I. G. (1954). *The self-made man in America: The myth of rags to riches.* New York: Free Press.

Yan, W. F., & Gaier, E. L. (1994). Causal attributions for college success and failure: An Asian-American comparison. *Journal of Cross-Cultural Psychology, 25*(1), 146–158.

Zajonc, R. B. (1992). *Cognition, communication, consciousness: A social psychological perspective.* Unpublished manuscript, University of Michigan, Ann Arbor.

CHAPTER 26

∝

Cultural Competence

Dynamic Processes

CHI-YUE CHIU
YING-YI HONG

The rapid increase in global interconnectedness has created a pressing demand for a model of cultural competence in many areas, including management, medical professions, counseling, social services, and education (e.g., Bernal & Castro, 1994; Sue, 1998). Experts in the field have different opinions on what "cultural competence" is, despite the strong agreement on its importance (Cunningham, Foster, & Henggeler, 2002). Most practitioners believe that cultural competence involves self-understanding, knowledge of others whose cultural origins and values are different from one's own, and adapting one's own behaviors to the needs of culturally diverse groups (e.g., Hansen, Pepitone-Arreola-Rockwell, & Greene, 2000). However, little is known about the roles of awareness, knowledge, and skills in enabling people to function effectively in a variety of cultures.

In this chapter, drawing on recent research in cultural and cross-cultural psychology, we offer a framework for conceptualizing the nature of cultural competence, and for identifying its major components. We also dis-

cuss the relationships between multicultural experiences and cultural competence, and the implications of our conceptual framework for studying the psychology of culture.

THE NATURE OF CULTURAL COMPETENCE

There is a lesson that cultural competence researchers can learn from the social competence literature. In his seminal paper, Edward Thorndike (1920) defined "social competence" as a kind of intelligence analogous to abstract academic intelligence. Whereas abstract academic intelligence is "the ability to understand and manage ideas and symbols," social intelligence is "the ability to understand and manage men and women, boys and girls—to act wisely in human relations" (p. 228). Inspired by Thorndike's idea, numerous attempts have been made by researchers to identify the specific expertise and skills (e.g., expertise in decoding communicative behaviors, expertise in judging people, tacit knowledge about managing other people) that define social competence (e.g., Sternberg & Smith, 1985). Many such attempts have failed (e.g., Brown & Anthony, 1990; Ford & Tisak, 1983). Then some investigators realized that although expertise and specific skills are necessary for competent social behavior, they are not sufficient for attaining personal goals and promoting interpersonal relationships. Two crucial components of social competence have been overlooked: sensitivity to subtle cues about the psychological meanings of *changing* situations, and *discriminative* use of social knowledge and skills across situations (Cheng, Chiu, Hong, & Cheung, 2001; Chiu, Hong, Mischel, & Shoda, 1995). In this chapter, learning from the experience of studying social competence, we highlight four major components of cultural competence, namely, sensitivity to both inter- and intracultural variations in cultural meanings, use of context-appropriate cultural knowledge in intercultural interaction, flexibility in switching cultural frames for sense making, and use of cultural knowledge to foster creativity.

In psychological research, "culture" is often defined in terms of relatively static qualities (traits, essence, values, beliefs) shared by individuals in a delineated population (see Lehman, Chiu, & Schaller, 2004). According to this entity view of culture, a person who enters a new culture must accept as a fixed reality the qualities that make up the new culture. To behave competently in an unfamiliar culture, people need to acquire knowledge of the culture's essences, and adapt their responses to the seemingly unalterable reality. Indeed, much psychological research has focused on the shock experiences and psychological stress that people need to overcome when they adapt to a new culture (Ward, Bochner, & Furnham, 2001). Not surprisingly, many cultural competence training programs emphasize learning the characteristic patterns of thoughts and actions in other cultures, reflecting on one's own thoughts and actions, and adapting one's thoughts and actions to the expectations in other cultures (e.g., Dogra, 2001).

A different view of culture, which emphasizes the dynamic and agentic aspects of culture and behavior, is assumed in our conceptualization of cultural competence. In this view, culture consists of a network of knowledge and practices that is produced, distributed, and reproduced among a collection of interconnected people. In addition, by taking an agentic perspective to culture and psychology, we assume that people may use culture as a resource to attain their goals. Accordingly, people are not passive carriers of culture. Instead, they express and exercise agency via culture, and apply cultural knowledge flexibly and discriminatively across situations. Because this conception of culture, which is crucial to understanding cultural competence in a multicultural environment, is relatively novel in the psychological literature (Hong & Chiu, 2001), we elaborate on the major assumptions of this conceptual approach to culture.

Culture as Distributed Knowledge

As mentioned, we use culture to designate a coalescence of loosely organized knowledge (or learned routines) that is produced, distributed, and reproduced among a collection of interconnected individuals. The idea that culture consists of a network of distributed knowledge has gained considerable support in anthropology (e.g., Shore, 1996; Sperber, 1996) and in psychology (Chiu & Chen, 2004; Hong & Chiu, 2001; Kashima, Woolcock, & Kashima, 2000). Two important aspects of this conception of culture should be highlighted. First, our usage of knowledge is most similar to the one proposed by Barth (2002), which refers to "all the ways of understanding that we use to make up our experienced, grasped reality" (p. 1), and includes all learned routines of thinking, feeling, and interacting with other people. In this usage, knowledge is a necessary accompaniment to action, and vice versa. As Barth (p. 1) put it, while "knowledge provides people with materials for reflection and premises for action, . . . actions become knowledge to others" after the fact. Thus, knowledge and practice form a circular causal chain. Second, these learned routines are not just personal knowledge in the heads of individuals. Instead, they are shared, albeit incompletely, among individuals in a delineated population. Because cultural knowledge in a delineated population is not perfectly shared, cultures are not homogeneous monoliths. Although many researchers (e.g., Appadurai, 1996; Friedman,

1994) have commented on the danger of treating cultures as static monoliths, one commonly held view is that people will act competently in a new culture if they possess knowledge about the average proclivities of members of the new culture. If cultures are not static monoliths, such knowledge is more likely to be overgeneralization than to be veridical knowledge. To act competently across cultures, individuals need to be sensitive to *both* intercultural and intracultural variations in knowledge.

Culture and Psychology: An Agentic Perspective

Culture can be compared to a toolkit that can be put to manifold uses (DiMaggio, 1997). People in a cultural group can sample knowledge tools from their cultural toolkit to construct their experiences. In addition, people are not passive carriers of cultural meanings; they express their agency via culture and participate actively in culture (Chiu & Chen, 2004). In other words, culture should be understood in terms of how cultural agents use cultural knowledge in particular social contexts to fulfill their goals.

Consistent with the idea that culture is a collection of consensually validated interpretive tools (DiMaggio, 1997), research has shown that people are likely to apply cultural knowledge in problem solving when the situation calls for a consensually validated, conventionalized solution (Briley, Morris, & Simonson, 2000), or when the problem solver lacks the capability, motivation, or resources to consider alternative solutions (Chiu, Morris, Hong, & Menon, 2000; Knowles, Morris, Chiu, & Hong, 2001; Morris & Fu, 2001).

People may also use culture to fulfill their identity needs (Chiu & Chen, 2004). Culture and identity are related. When a cultural identity is made salient, its attendant cultural knowledge becomes cognitively accessible (Hong, Ip, Chiu, Morris, & Menon, 2001; Rhee, Uleman, Lee, & Roman, 1995). In addition, people might use cultural knowledge to express or defend their social identity (Jetten, Postmes, & Mcauliffe, 2002) and threat against mortality (Greenberg, Solomon, & Pyszczynski, 1997; Solomon, Greenberg, & Pyszczynski, 1991). In short, what is interesting in an agentic analysis of

culture and identity is the possibility that people may use culture to fulfill some identity needs.

Finally, in intercultural interactions, individuals can use their knowledge about another culture to guide their interaction with people from that culture.

COMPONENTS OF CULTURAL COMPETENCE

Cultural Sensitivity

As mentioned, sensitivity to intercultural and intracultural variations in behavior contributes to culturally competent behavior. However, to what kind of inter- and intracultural variations would a culturally competent person attend? Before we can answer this question, we need to identify the major sources of inter- and intracultural variations.

Intercultural Variations

Cultural Differences in Meanings. Culture legislates what kinds of behaviors are deemed to be acceptable or desirable expressions of the same basic psychological process. When psychological differences between two cultural groups are observed, it is important to determine whether the differences reflect different psychological processes in the two groups, or whether they are different expressions of the same psychological process in two different populations. We illustrate this point with a recent debate in the psychology of human agency, a construct that is at the heart of any definition of human competence.

Both social cognitive theory of personality (Bandura, 2001) and self-determination theory (Ryan & Deci, 2000) take an agentic perspective to human motivation. In social cognitive theory, agentic individuals are efficacious persons, who believe that they can intentionally influence their functioning and life circumstances. In self-determination theory, an agentic self is also an autonomous self, whose actions are driven by personal choice or intrinsic aspirations. In both theories, a subjective sense of agency energizes agentic actions and enables people to devise ways of adapting flexibly to remarkably diverse environments.

Some recent findings in culture and motivation research seem to question the universality of human agency as a primary source of human motivation. First, compared to Westerners,[1] East Asians have lower self-esteem (Heine, Lehman, Markus, & Kitayama, 1999; Hetts, Sakuma, & Pelham, 1999), and are less likely to reduce postdecision dissonance by justifying their personal choices (Heine & Lehman, 1997). East Asians also use more negative descriptions and fewer positive descriptions than do Westerners to describe themselves, particularly when they do so in front of an authority figure (Kanagawa, Cross, & Markus, 2001). In some studies, East Asians even exhibited a significant bias toward self-criticism (Hetts et al., 1999). Also, they do not view criticism or negative feedback as a threat to self-esteem. In response to failure feedback, they do not defend their self-esteem by derogating high performers, as Westerners often do (Brockner & Chen, 1996).

Second, compared to Westerners, Asians are less motivated by success, and more motivated by avoidance of failure. For example, among Westerners, success-foregone events are perceived to be more important than failure-avoidance events (Lee, Aaker, & Gardner, 2000), success situations have more influence on self-esteem than do failure situations (Kitayama, Markus, Matsumoto, & Norasakkunkit, 1997), and success feedback is more motivating than failure feedback (Heine et al., 2001). By contrast, Asians pursue more avoidance goals than do Westerners (Eaton & Dembo, 2001; Elliot, Chirkov, Kim, & Seldon, 2001). Asians also perceive failure-avoidance events to be more important than success-foregone events (Lee et al., 2000), and think that failures would decrease their self-esteem more than success would increase their self-esteem (Kitayama et al., 1997).

Third, Iyengar and Lepper (1999) reported that whereas European American children show more intrinsic motivation when they make their own task choices than when choices are made for them by others, Asian American children are most intrinsically motivated when choices are made for them by trusted figures or peers. These findings seem to question whether personal choice generally enhances motivation for people in different cultural contexts.

In summary, compared to the Western self, the East Asian self seems to be a less efficacious agent. However, Asians do not appear to have more motivation deficiencies than do Westerners. On the contrary, compared to Westerners, Asians are oftentimes more persistent and mastery-oriented in the face of setbacks, work more diligently toward their goals, and have higher performance (Blinco, 1992; Chen & Stevenson, 1995; Eaton & Dembo, 2001; Heine et al., 2001). On the surface of it, these findings seem to cast doubt on the centrality of agency in East Asian cultures.

In response, Bandura (2002) argued that cultural psychologists have misrepresented the construct of agency. According to Bandura, people can exercise their agency through the self (direct personal agency), other people who act on the self's behest (proxy agency), or group action (collective agency). Successful functioning requires an agentic blend of these three modes of agency. When this expanded conception of agency is adopted, agency is central to personal development, adaptation, and change in diverse cultural milieus. By contrast, confining agency to direct personal agency would inevitably result in a distorted view of agency, in which collective efficacy is disembodied from personal efficacy.

Similarly, Ryan and Deci (2000) argued that in some East Asian societies, people often identify with choices made for them by significant others, and experience autonomy through pursuing a self-identified collective choice. Consistent with this contention, research has shown that in East Asian societies, successful pursuit of self-identified collective choices (vs. externally imposed goals) contributes to psychological well-being (Chirkov, Kim, Ryan, & Kaplan, 2003).

It is important to distinguish between the generic and specific senses of agency. The "generic" sense of agency refers either to the universal capability to participate in or to the state of engaging in generative and proactive (or goal-directed) actions. The "specific" sense of agency refers to concrete, culturally constructed models for exercising agency. These agency models differ in the pathway(s) they prescribe for exercising agency. However, all agency models function to orient people to pursue and to develop the capability to pursue their valued goals.

From this perspective, the East–West differences that appear to challenge the universality of agency should be construed as differences arising from societies' choices between different models of agency. Every society has its unique collection of agency models, and societies differ systematically in how they weigh the relative importance of different agency models. For example, Chinese societies emphasize group agency more than they do direct personal agency. In contrast, in North America, direct personal agency is emphasized over group agency (Chiu et al., 2000; Menon, Morris, Chiu, & Hong, 1999; Su et al., 1999). Whereas European American students tend to define "individual competence" as success in projects that are important to the self, Chinese students tend to define it as success in socially recognized projects (Chang, Wong, & Teo, 2000; Tao & Hong, 2000; Yu & Yang, 1994). Furthermore, in North America, people are encouraged to construct their self-worth based on generalized self-competence. In many East Asian contexts, people are encouraged to construct their self-worth on the basis of how successfully they adhere to socially approved standards (Tafarodi, Lang, & Smith, 1999).

Moreover, people may choose to use the most widely accepted agency model in their society as a tool to attain important goals in life. Consistent with the idea, research has shown that people in different societies may adopt different strategies to achieve the same valued goals. For example, positive self-image and favorable public image are valued among individuals in most societies. People may seek to enhance their self-image by rating themselves on attributes that are highly valued in their cultural context. Compared to East Asians, European Americans are more inclined to self-enhance by rating the self as being above average on personal attributes (Heine & Lehman, 1997; Heine & Renshaw, 2002). East Asians also self-enhance, but they are more inclined than European Americans to do so by holding positive—sometimes unrealistically positive—views of the self when they appraise themselves on communal traits and collectivistic attributes (Kurman, 2001; Sedikides, Gaertner, & Toguchi, 2003).

In a recent study, we (Ip, Chen, & Chiu, 2003) found a similar pattern in management of public self-image. In this study, Chinese and European American undergraduates responded to Paulhus's (1984) measure of social desirability, which assesses two components of socially desirable responding: impression management and self-deception. Compared to their European American counterparts, Chinese undergraduates have a greater tendency to manage impression by attributing to the self socially approved behavior with low occurrence probabilities (e.g., "I have never dropped litter on the street"). By contrast, European American undergraduates have a greater tendency to self-deceive by attributing to the self extremely positive personal attributes ("I am fully in control of my own fate").

Finally, people feel happy when they succeed in meeting the standards of an agentic self in their society (Suh, Diener, Oishi, & Triandis, 1998). For example, in countries where personal goals are valued, factors relating to direct personal agency (self-esteem, identity consistency, personal freedom, pursuit and attainment of individual goals) and personal affect predict life satisfaction, whereas factors relating to feelings of connectedness (pursuit and attainment of interdependent goals, quality of interpersonal relationship) do not. In countries where collective goals are also emphasized, both factors relating to personal agency and personal affect, and those relating to feelings of connectedness predict life satisfaction (e.g., Kwan, Bond, & Singelis, 1997; Oishi & Diener, 2001; Oishi, Diener, Lucas, & Suh, 1999; Schimmack, Radhakrishnan, Oishi, & Dzokoto, 2002; Suh, 2002).

In short, when marked behavioral differences between individuals from different cultures are observed, it is tempting to conclude that culture influences some basic psychological processes, although such behavioral differences could be different manifestations of the same psychological process. To understand the behavior of a person from a different culture, one must go beyond mere descriptions of cultural differences in behavior. It is not enough just to identify the behavior that "they" do and "we" do not (e.g., "Unlike Japanese, we don't self-efface"), and the behavior that "we" do and "they" do not (e.g., "Unlike us, Japanese do not desire self-esteem, and do not need to self-enhance"). It is a common tendency to use one's own experiences with a psychological process as the anchor to evaluate cultural similarities and differences. Cultural sensitivity requires suspension of this tendency and calls for attention to the nuances in the meanings of behavioral differences in cultures.

Differences in Prevalence and Chronic Accessibility of Cultural Knowledge. A body of knowledge may be more prevalent or widely distributed in one culture than in another. To be able to interact competently with a person from another cultural group, one also needs to be sensitive to the distribution of knowledge in the target's cultural group. For example, in one study, Li and Hong (2001) found that mainland Chinese students studying in Hong Kong differed among themselves in how much they knew the distribution of values in Hong Kong society. Those who were more knowledgeable had more competent social interactions with Hong Kong students.

A body of knowledge that is widely distributed in a culture often has high chronic accessibility. Chronic accessibility of a body of cultural knowledge is a product of frequent use of that body of knowledge (Higgins, 1996). A body of cultural knowledge that is frequently used in a group is usually widely shared (Lau, Chiu, & Lee, 2001; Lau, Lee, & Chiu, 2004; Sechrist & Stangor, 2001), more frequently reproduced in communication (Lyons & Kashima, 2001), widely represented in external or public carriers of culture (Menon & Morris, 2001), and cognitively accessible to members of the group (Hong, Morris, Chiu, & Benet-Martinez, 2000).

For example, in Asian contexts, group agency and aspects of the interdependent self are relatively well represented in commercial advertisements (Han & Shavitt, 1994; Kim & Markus, 1999), newspaper articles (Menon et al., 1999) and the languages (Kashima & Kashima, 1998). By contrast, in Western contexts, direct personal agency and aspects of the independent self are relatively well represented in these media. In addition, when asked to describe themselves, Asians spontaneously mention more interdependent or group-related self-statements, and fewer independent self-statements than do Westerners, indicating that the interdependent or group-related self is more

cognitively accessible to Asians than to Westerners (Rhee et al., 1995; Wang, 2001).

Sensitivity to the distribution of knowledge in a foreign culture may develop from frequent intercultural contacts. There is some preliminary evidence for this idea. Although both Hong Kong and New York City are cosmopolitan cities, Hong Kong people have more exposure to New York culture than do New Yorkers to Hong Kong culture. Given such asymmetry in the direction of cultural contacts, Lee (2002) found that Hong Kong undergraduates are more accurate in estimating the distribution of knowledge (e.g., general knowledge about flowers and landmarks) among New York undergraduates than are New York undergraduates in estimating the distribution of knowledge among Hong Kong undergraduates.

In a recently completed study, we (Ip et al., 2003) asked American undergraduates, Hong Kong Chinese undergraduates, and Beijing Chinese undergraduates to estimate how American undergraduates would respond to the Regulatory Focus Questionnaire (Higgins et al., 2001), which measures one's personal history of fulfilling personal aspirations (promotion pride) and meeting parental expectations (prevention pride). The American students also indicated how they themselves would respond to this measure. On their self-report, American students scored slightly higher on promotion pride than on prevention pride. American students' estimations of their own group's difference in promotion and prevention pride were highly accurate. Beijing Chinese undergraduates had relatively limited exposure to American culture, and they overestimated by a factor of three the difference between promotion pride and prevention pride among American students. Hong Kong students, who had more exposure to American culture than did Beijing students, were more accurate than Beijing students and less accurate than American students in estimating American students' difference in promotion and prevention pride.

Intracultural Variations

Interdomain and Situational Variations. In psychology, a common practice is to use global, stable cultural dimensions or culture-prototypical self-construals to explain broad East–West differences in psychological processes. Writing against this practice, Bandura (2002) maintained that "cultures are diverse and dynamic social systems not static monoliths" (p. 275). A recent review of the extant literature on country differences in individualism and collectivism adds ammunitions to Bandura's criticism. In this review, Oyserman, Coon, and Kemmelmeier (2002) found that, contrary to popular assumptions in cross-cultural and cultural psychology, "European Americans were not more individualistic than African Americans, or Latinos, and not less collectivistic than Japanese or Koreans" (p. 3). In addition, there are remarkable interdomain variations in country differences in individualism and collectivism. For example, in the case of U.S.–Japan differences, Americans are more collectivistic than Japanese in most domains, which include accepting hierarchy, striving to maintain group harmony, defining oneself contextually, as well as sense of belonging to groups. Japanese are more collectivistic than Americans only in the domain of preference for working in a group. Comparisons of European Americans with other countries all point to the same conclusion: The nature of the country difference depends on which domain of individualism or collectivism is being assessed.

Cultural differences are also situation-dependent (see Lehman et al., 2004). For example, well-documented East–West differences in perception disappear when the research participants have control over the test procedures (Ji, Peng, & Nisbett, 2000). Seemingly robust East–West differences in the preference for holistic versus analytical thinking style vanish when the contradictions between the two thinking styles are not salient (Norenzayan, Smith, Kim, & Nisbett, 2002).

The intracultural variations reviewed earlier have created a crisis in cultural analysis of psychological processes. Is it useful to employ broadly and diffusely defined psychological constructs to explain group differences in cognition, motivation, and behavior? Is it legitimate to accept any country difference as evidence of cultural influence (Oyserman et al., 2002)?

In response to this challenge, Kitayama (2002) argued that attitude and value measures have failed to capture the coherence of culture, because culture resides in external, public representations, not in people's mind. According to Kitayama, "Within-cultural variation usually draws on individual difference, which is a source of variance that is entirely separate from the sources of variance relevant for between-cultural variation" (p. 91). Culture cannot be reduced to knowledge represented in the minds of individual members of a cultural group. Instead, culture is "out there," in the form of external realities and collective patterns of behavior, which include verbal and nonverbal symbols (e.g., language and media), daily practices and routines (e.g., gossips, behavioral scripts), tools (e.g., mobile phones and the Internet), and social institutions and structures (e.g., reward allocation and legal systems).

By externalizing culture to artifacts and collective behavioral patterns, Kitayama (2002) attributed a special status to these artifacts and behavioral patterns: They represent the "authentic" aspects of people's shared life. These artifacts and behavioral patterns are also granted the final authority in interpreting cultural meanings. This conceptualization of culture draws researchers' attention to the importance of analyzing cultural affordances, but at the expense of objectifying culture. It is inconceivable how meanings of cultural materials could exist independent of the subjective interpretation of the researcher and the people who participate in the culture (Shweder & Sullivan, 1990).

Externalizing culture will not save the project of identifying discrete, homogeneous cultures, unless one also assumes homogeneity in the public meanings that are represented in the social institutions and practices in a cultural group. This assumption flies in the face of the fact that diversity in social institutions and practices in most contemporary societies has pluralized cultural meaning in these societies. In some societies, such as the United States, representation of pluralistic heritage cultures is encouraged, and cultural diversity is celebrated. In Japan, one also finds representations of different philosophical–religious traditions, including Confucianism, Buddhism, Shintoism, and Christianity. Some commentators (Gjerde & Onishi, 2000) have referred to the representation of Japanese culture as a homogeneous monolith as "the psychological imagination of the Japanese in the era of globalization" (p. 216).

In addition, inconsistent and contrastive cultural ideas are represented in the same external carrier of cultural meanings. For example, popular sayings and idioms carry widely shared evaluative, prescriptive, or proscriptive beliefs, and are embedded in many conversation scripts. Thus, popular sayings and idioms are important carriers of cultural meanings. Ho and Chiu (1994, Study 1) analyzed the contents of 2,056 Chinese popular sayings. Of these sayings, 70 are related to autonomy or conformity, and 98 are related to independence or interdependence. Of the 70 sayings relating to autonomy or conformity, 51 (72.9%) express either affirmation of conformity or negation of autonomy; the remaining sayings (27.1%) express either affirmation of autonomy or negation of conformity. Of the 98 sayings relating to independence or interdependence, 64 (65.3%) express either affirmation of independence or negation of interdependence, and 34 (34.7%) express either affirmation of interdependence or negation of independence. In another study (Ho & Chiu, 1994, Study 2), Hong Kong Chinese undergraduates indicated their extent of agreement with the Chinese popular sayings related to independence and interdependence. They agreed strongly both with sayings expressing interdependence (e.g., "A single hand can hardly make a sound," "If two persons are united with a single purpose, soil turns into gold"), and with sayings expressing independence ("Rather than to ask for help, better rely on oneself," "One accepts the consequences for what one does").

Some culture travelers may enter a new culture with the expectation that behaviors in the new culture are coherently organized around a few broad themes (e.g., Japanese are collectivistic and value interpersonal interdependence). Given the huge amount of intracultural variability, when these cultural travelers get around in the culture, they may find that such knowledge can at best serve as a crude guide after having made many jumbled moves. However, as we argue presently, such intracultural variations should not be treated as random or unpredictable variability. Instead, sensitivity to the psychological

factors that give rise to meaningful patterns amid seemingly uncharted variability underlies cultural competence.

Factors That Underlie Meaningful Patterns. To discern meaningful cultural patterns, it is important to discern the range of applicability of broad cultural themes, and to identify the domain-specific beliefs that mediate behaviors across different life domains, as well as the distribution of these beliefs in the culture.

Some cultural dimensions, such as individualism and collectivism, have a broad range of applicability; they are applicable in situations that involve interests of the self and/or those of the collective. However, cultural differences in individualism and collectivism are target-specific (Hui, 1988): A cultural group (e.g., Japanese) may encourage collectivism in interactions with coworkers, and individualism in interactions with strangers (see Oyserman et al., 2002), while another cultural group (e.g., Chinese) may value collectivism in family interactions, and individualism in interactions with strangers (Ho & Chiu, 1994). Thus, target specificity in the application of broad cultural dimensions can account for a portion of the interdomain variability within a culture.

Differences between cultural groups are also mediated by knowledge with a relatively narrow range of applicability. For example, East Asians believe more strongly than do European Americans in the malleability of intelligence (Heine et al., 2001) and personality (Norenzayan, Choi, & Nisbett, 2002), but European Americans believe more strongly than do East Asians in the malleability of social institutions (Chiu, Dweck, Tong, & Fu, 1997). Beliefs about the malleability of intelligence, personality, and social institutions are only slightly correlated at the individual level (Dweck, Chiu, & Hong, 1995) and at the cultural level (Su et al., 1999). In addition, malleability beliefs in a given domain predict behaviors in the same domain but not in other domains (Chiu, Dweck, et al., 1997). For example, (1) East–West differences in perceived malleability of intelligence predict East–West differences in the likelihood of displaying persistent and mastery-oriented responses in the face of setbacks in an ability task (Heine et al., 2001); (2) East–West differences in perceived malleability of personality predict East–West differences in reliance on broad personality traits to understand social behavior (Norenzayan, Choi, et al., 2002); and (3) East–West differences in perceived malleability of social institutions predict East–West differences in the way people respond to injustices (Chiu, Dweck, et al., 1997).

Because culturally constructed knowledge is not perfectly shared in a cultural group, there is substantial heterogeneity among individuals within the group. For instance, although Easterners as a collectivity believe more strongly in the malleability of intelligence and personality than do Westerners as a collectivity, a sizeable proportion of East Asians subscribe to a fixed theory of intelligence (Hong, Chiu, Dweck, Lin, & Wan, 1999) or personality (Chiu, Hong, & Dweck, 1997; Tong & Chiu, 2002). Similarly, a substantial percentage of European Americans subscribe to a malleable view of intelligence (Dweck, 1999; Dweck et al., 1995) and personality (Dweck, Hong, & Chiu, 1993; Dweck et al., 1995; Gervey, Chiu, Hong, & Dweck, 1999).

Evidence from experimental studies also supports the idea that seemingly contrastive ideas about the self are available to both East Asians and Westerners. Contextual cues may increase the temporary accessibility of a body of knowledge and momentarily raise the probability that this body of knowledge will be applied (Higgins, 1996). Although the independent self has high chronic accessibility among American undergraduates, American undergraduates mention more group attributes and fewer personal attributes when their collective self is primed than when their private self is primed. This finding reveals that both personal and collective self-construals are available to some American undergraduates, and contextual priming calls out one or the other kind of self-construal (Gardner, Gabriel, & Lee, 1999; Trafimow, Triandis, & Goto, 1991). Similar findings have been obtained among Chinese students (Gardner et al., 1999; Trafimow, Silverman, Fan, & Law, 1997).

In short, cultural knowledge is domain-specific, imperfectly shared, and not entirely internally consistent. These properties of cultural knowledge give rise to intracultural variability. Sensitivity to the range of applicability, target specificity, and prevalence of specific cultural knowledge will enhance people's cultural sensitivity and cultural competence.

Contextual Shift in Cultural Meanings. Another factor that contributes to intracultural variability in behavior is shift of cultural meanings in different situational contexts. Sometimes, cultural meanings are assumed to be invariant across situational contexts. This assumption may be valid in most experimental situations, in which contextual features are carefully sampled to ensure comparability of responses in different experimental conditions. In real-life situations, the motivational context of behavior is usually much richer, and cultural meanings may shift as the motivational context changes. For example, effort is emphasized in East Asian achievement contexts (Hong, 2001). However, as illustrated in the following two studies, the meaning of effort may change as the motivational context changes.

Attributing achievement setbacks to lack of effort (vs. abilities) is usually accompanied by more task enjoyment, greater task persistence, and better performance after failure (Dweck, 1999). Grant and Dweck (2001) found that this relationship changes when students feel a sense of responsibility to their group for their own performance, as students in some East Asian contexts often do. When individual performance becomes a social responsibility, the emphasis on effort may give rise to the perception one has not tried hard enough to meet group expectations, which in turn produces feelings of anxiousness, embarrassment, guilt, and humiliation following failures.

In another study, Salili, Chiu, and Lai (2001) compared the achievement motivation of Hong Kong Chinese high school students with Canadian Chinese and European Canadian high school students. Compared to the European Canadian group, Hong Kong Chinese students and Canadian Chinese students placed heavier emphasis on teacher-, family-, and peer-oriented goals, but the two Chinese groups did not differ from each other in perceived importance of these socially oriented goals, suggesting that the two groups of Chinese students shared the strong socially oriented achievement motivation that is highly encouraged in Chinese culture. However, there were salient differences in the motivational contexts in Hong Kong and Canada. In Hong Kong, students with poorer grades were made to work harder; there was a negative correlation between time spent on studying and academic performance. In Canada, students who worked harder had better grades; the correlations between effort and academic performance in both Chinese Canadian and European Canadian student groups were positive. Expectedly, Hong Kong Chinese students and Canadian Chinese students attributed different meanings to effort. Among Hong Kong Chinese students, time spent on studying was unrelated to self-efficacy but positively related to test anxiety (cf. Hong, 2001). Among Canadian Chinese students, time spent on studying was positively related to self-efficacy and unrelated to test anxiety.

In summary, intracultural variations across individuals, contexts, and domains are not random or unwanted residual variances (Hong & Mallorie, 2004). To behave competently in a culture, instead of ignoring such variations, a person would need to decode the subtle meanings of such variations.

Use of Cultural Knowledge in Social Interaction

Cultural knowledge empowers people by providing them with tools for sense making and adaptive, flexible problem solving. Culturally competent individuals make use of these tools in intercultural interactions, and there is evidence that multicultural experiences foster the ability to use cultural knowledge flexibly in intercultural contacts. As noted, in Lee's (2002) studies, Hong Kong undergraduates are more accurate in estimating the distribution of knowledge among New York undergraduates than are New York undergraduates in estimating the distribution of knowledge among Hong Kong undergraduates. In addition, Hong Kong undergraduates are capable of applying their knowledge about New York undergraduates when they formulate communicative messages for New York undergraduates. New York undergraduates, by comparison, have less accurate knowledge about Hong Kong undergraduates and tend not to use such knowledge when they formulate messages for Hong Kong undergraduates.

Within the United States, Chinese American bicultural individuals are familiar with both Chinese and American cultures, whereas most European Americans are familiar with mainstream American cultures only. In a recently completed study, we (Leung, Chiu, & Hong, 2004) found that, compared to European Americans, Chinese American bicultural individuals were more accurate in their knowledge about Chinese American differences in promotion versus prevention pride. In addition, when asked to persuade a Chinese or American target to purchase an insurance policy, Chinese American bicultural individuals were more likely to tailor arguments according to the ethnicity of the target based on their knowledge (i.e., they chose more promotion-focused arguments for an American target than for a Chinese target). By contrast, the target's ethnic identity did not affect European Americans' choice of persuasive messages.

Flexible Deployment of Cultural Knowledge

Flexible switching of cultural frames is an experience familiar to people with multicultural background. In our research, we (Hong, Benet-Martinez, Chiu, & Morris, 2003; Hong, Chiu, & Kung, 1997) primed bicultural individuals (Hong Kong Chinese, Chinese Americans) with either Chinese cultural icons (e.g., the Chinese dragon) or American cultural icons (e.g., Mickey Mouse). When primed with Chinese (vs. American) cultural icons, these bicultural individuals were more inclined to use a group agency model to interpret an ambiguous event; they made more group attributions and fewer individual attributions. Analogous culture priming effects have been found on spontaneous self-construal (Ross, Xun, & Wilson, 2002) and cooperative behaviors (Wong & Hong, in press). In addition, the culture priming effect has also been replicated in studies that used different bicultural samples (Chinese Canadians, Dutch Greek bicultural children), and a variety of cultural primes (e.g., language, experimenter's cultural identity; Ross et al., 2002; Verkuyten & Pouliasi, 2002).

Cultural frame switching (Hong et al., 2000) is a good example of flexible and discriminative use of cultural knowledge to grasp experiences in a changing sociocultural milieu. The reflectivity, sensitivity, and flexibility that define the conceptual core of cultural competence are epitomized in the following reflection from Susanna Harrington, a multicultural informant of South American origin in Sparrow's (2000) study.

> I think of myself not as a unified cultural being but as a communion of different cultural beings. Due to the fact that I have spent time in different cultural environments I have developed several cultural identities that diverge and converge according to the need of the moment. (p. 190)

When bicultural individuals switch between cultural frames, they attend to cultural frames' applicability in the immediate context. In a recent series of culture priming experiments, we (Hong et al., 2003) found that among Chinese American bicultural individuals, culture priming affected the likelihood of applying a group agency model or an individual agency model only when we highlighted the tension between group agency and individual agency in the stimulus event, making the two agency models applicable in the judgment context.

In another study, Wong and Hong (in press) asked Chinese American bicultural participants to engage in Prisoner's Dilemma games with friends or strangers after the participants were primed with Chinese, American, or neutral cultural icons. The cultural primes only affected the participants' cooperative behaviors in the predicted direction (i.e., more cooperative in the Chinese than in the American priming condition) toward friends but had no effect toward strangers. These findings again show that the context limits the applicability of cultural models.

Every society has a collection of knowledge tools. Individuals use these tools to pursue important goals. The availability of multiple tools in every society leaves room for choices, and people often switch their tools as the context changes. Choosing between different tools also presupposes a reflective and agentic self (Sokefeld, 1999), which is at the heart of human competence.

Creativity and Reduction of Culturocentrism

The self is an active cultural agent that proactively engages in transactions with culture. However, the self is always embedded in a cultural context, and always sees the world through a cultural lens. If a cultural lens is used frequently enough to make sense of the environment, it becomes a learned routine and a part of "routinized" culture (Ng & Bradac, 1993). For this reason, although culture provides conventional tools for sense making and problem solving, it also impedes creativity. For example, most creative activities involve instances of conceptual expansion, in which people extend the boundaries of a conceptual domain by creating novel instances of the concept. When people engage in creative conceptual expansion, it is difficult to avoid the influence of exemplars high in chronic accessibility (Ward, Patterson, Sifonis, Dodds, & Saunders, 2002). Such exemplars are also the normative anchors of the concept in the culture. Thus, there might be a limit to the generativity of cultural agency.

However, at least in the domain of conceptual expansion, it is possible to overcome this limit when people are exposed to dissimilar graded category structures of the same concept. Such structures are likely to come from cultures with very different intellectual traditions. For example, in the United States, the most accessible instance of the self is a bounded, distinctive, autonomous, and self-contained entity. When American psychologists learned that the most accessible instance of the self in Japan is socially embedded and defined in relation to a person's position in a relational network, they became aware of the culturocentric nature of their conceptualization of the self. In addition, creative ideas emerge when two seemingly incompatible cultural traditions are combined (Hampton, 1997; Wan & Chiu, 2002). Instead of keeping contrastive cultural construals in juxtaposition, attempts to integrate contrastive ideas from diverse cultures into a coherent conceptual framework should facilitate creative synthesis.

By the same argument, laypeople may also become aware of the culturocentric nature of their own cultural beliefs as they expose themselves to ideas from foreign cultures. Gradually, they may attempt to weave seemingly inconsistent strands of ideas from diverse cultures into their cultural life, and in the process of doing so become a creative and generative agent in a rich and dynamic culture (Nemeth & Kwan, 1985). Consistent with this idea, there is evidence that exposure to diverse cultural experiences weakens the constraints of conventionalized socialization on creative thinking (Simonton, 2000). For example, the experience of growing up when a nation breaks up into several peacefully coexisting independent states is conducive to development of creativity (Simonton, 1975). In addition, the level of creativity in a country tends to increase when it opens itself to foreign influences (Simonton, 1997). Finally, although children in some Eastern countries (e.g., China, Indonesia) tend to do more poorly than their European counterparts on standardized tests of creativity (Jellen & Urban, 1989), Asian children with rich multicultural experiences (e.g., Hong Kong Chinese children) and Chinese American children outperformed European American children in standardized creativity tests (Niu & Sternberg, 2002; Rudowicz, Lok, & Kitto, 1995). In short, cultural diversity may facilitate creativity (Simonton, 2000).

BOUNDARY CONDITIONS OF MULTICULTURAL EXPERIENCES

Thus far, we have introduced four components of cultural competence. From the literature we have reviewed, it seems that cultural competence develops from cultural contacts. However, under some circumstances, cultural contacts may also promote culturocentrism and intercultural animosity. The Israelis and Palestinians are not deprived of opportunities for intercultural contact. Despite this, when this chapter was written, the two groups were still inflicting harm to each other. Openness to alternative cultural constructions is a necessary condition for intercultural contacts to produce productive intercultural interactions. However, when people are cognitively busy, under time pressure, or accountable to their cultural group, intercultural contacts may increase culturocentrism, or the tendency to

rely on culturally received knowledge in their cultural group to guide perceptions and behaviors (Richter & Kruglanski, 2004). As we mentioned at the beginning of this chapter, other potential boundary conditions for the beneficial effects of intercultural contacts include identity threat and mortality salience. Together, these contextual factors create the boundary conditions for the beneficial effects of intercultural contacts.

PSYCHIC UNITY: THE BASIS OF INTERCULTURAL UNDERSTANDING AND CULTURAL COMPETENCE

David Hume (1784/1894, p. 358) had written in favor of psychic unity: "It is universally acknowledged that there is a great uniformity among the actions of men [sic], in all nations and ages, and that human nature still remains the same, in its principles and operations." According to this view, despite phenotypical variations in behaviors across cultures, there is a universal psychological infraculture that enables communication of minds across the globe. In this sense, psychic unity is the universal foundation for intercultural communication and cultural competence. In the past 15 years, cultural psychological research has uncovered striking group differences in cognition, motivation, emotion, and behavior. On the surface, these findings seem to challenge the notion of psychic unity. In our view, psychic unity and cultural differences are not antithetical to each other.

To resolve the apparent contradiction between psychic unity and cultural differences, cultural psychologists can borrow a lesson from Kelly's personal construct theory. As Kelly (1955) pointed out, when two persons use similar constructs to construe their experience, they go through similar psychological processes. However, people do not need to employ similar constructs or go through similar psychological processes in order to understand each other. As long as one person can cognitively represent the construction processes of another person, social understanding can be achieved. Invariably, people look through a cultural lens when they construe the reality. However, they are also capable of acquiring and momentarily wearing another cultural lens. In cosmopolitan societies, frequent intercultural contacts have resulted in extensive global interconnectedness. Many cultural lenses are available to a cultural group, and people can and do see the world through different cultural lenses. The ability to construct reality from different cultural perspectives allows people from diverse cultural backgrounds to establish common ground. Indeed, as cultural boundaries become increasingly permeable and fuzzy, it is difficult to justify cutting up the cultural world with arbitrary boundaries into discrete and seemingly incommensurable meaning systems (Hermans & Kempen, 1998). Cultural boundaries of knowledge may be just as arbitrary.

In light of these arguments, we believe that although all human knowledge, including psychological knowledge, is suffused with cultural meanings, transcultural understanding is attainable. For this reason, we are optimistic about the prospect of developing a general model of cultural competence. We are also hopeful that the four components of cultural competence proposed in this chapter, namely, sensitivity to both inter- and intracultural variations in cultural meanings, use of context-appropriate cultural knowledge in intercultural interaction, flexibility in switching cultural frames for sense making, and use of cultural knowledge to foster creativity, will form the psychological foundation for transcultural understanding and multicultural competence.

NOTE

1. In this chapter, when group differences are described, collective nouns that denote a collectivity (e.g., "Westerners") refer to an average member (statistically speaking) of the collectivity (e.g., an average Westerner).

REFERENCES

Appadurai, A. (1996). *Modernity at large: Cultural dimensions of globalization*. Minneapolis: University of Minnesota Press.

Bandura, A. (2001). Social cognitive theory: An agentic perspective. In S. T. Fiske, D. L. Schacter, & C. Zahn-Waxler (Eds.), *Annual review of psychology* (Vol. 52, pp. 1–26). Palo Alto, CA: Annual Reviews.

Bandura, A. (2002). Social cognitive theory in cultural context. *Applied Psychology: An International Review, 51*, 269–290.

Barth, F. (2002). An anthropology of knowledge. *Current Anthropology, 43*, 1–18.

Bernal, M. E., & Castro, F. G. (1994). Are clinical psychologists prepared for service and research with ethnic minorities?: Report of a decade of progress. *American Psychologist, 49*, 797–805.

Blinco, P. M. (1992). A cross-cultural study of task persistence of young children in Japan and the United States. *Journal of Cross-Cultural Psychology, 23*, 407–415.

Briley, D. A., Morris, M. W., & Simonson, I. (2000). Reasons as carriers of culture: Dynamic versus dispositional models of cultural influence on decision-making. *Journal of Consumer Research, 27*, 157–178.

Brockner, J., & Chen, Y-r. (1996). The moderating roles of self-esteem and self-construal in reaction to a threat to the self: Evidence from the People's Republic of China and the United States. *Journal of Personality and Social Psychology, 71*, 603–615.

Brown, L. T., & Anthony, R. G. (1990). Continuing the search for social intelligence. *Personality and Individual Differences, 11*, 463–470.

Chang, W., Wong, W., & Teo, G. (2000). The socially oriented and individually oriented achievement motivation of Singaporean Chinese students. *Journal of Psychology in Chinese Societies, 1*, 39–63.

Chen, C., & Stevenson, H, W. (1995). Motivation and mathematics achievement: A comparative study of Asian-American, Caucasian-American, and East Asian high school students. *Child Development, 66*, 1215–1234.

Cheng, C., Chiu, C-y., Hong, Y-y., & Cheung, J. S. (2001). Discriminative facility and its role in the perceived quality of interactional experiences. *Journal of Personality, 69*, 765–786.

Chirkov, V., Kim, Y., Ryan, R. M., & Kaplan, U. (2003). Differentiating autonomy from individualism and independence: A self-determination theory perspective on internalization of cultural orientations and well-being. *Journal of Personality and Social Psychology, 84*, 97–110.

Chiu, C-y., & Chen, J. (2004). Symbols and interactions: Application of the CCC model to culture, language, and social identity. In S. H. Ng, C. Candlin, & C.-y. Chiu (Eds.), *Language matters: Communication, culture, and identity* (pp. 155–182). Hong Kong: City University of Hong Kong Press.

Chiu, C-y., Dweck, C. S., Tong, J. Y-y., & Fu, J. H-y. (1997). Implicit theories and conceptions of morality. *Journal of Personality and Social Psychology, 73*, 923–940.

Chiu, C-y., Hong, Y-y., & Dweck, C. S. (1997). Lay dispositionism and implicit theories of personality. *Journal of Personality and Social Psychology, 73*, 19–30.

Chiu, C-y., Hong, Y-y., Mischel, W., & Shoda, Y. (1995). Discriminative facility in social competence. *Social Cognition, 13*, 49–70.

Chiu, C-y., Morris, M. W., Hong, Y-y., & Menon, T.

(2000). Motivated cultural cognition: The impact of implicit cultural theories on dispositional attribution varies as a function of need for closure. *Journal of Personality and Social Psychology, 78,* 247–259.

Cunningham, P. B., Foster, S. L., Henggeler, S. W. (2002). The elusive concept of cultural competence. *Children's Services: Social Policy, Research and Practice, 5,* 231–243.

DiMaggio, D. (1997). Culture cognition. *Annual Review of Sociology, 23,* 263–287.

Dogra, N. (2001). The development and evaluation of a programme to teach cultural diversity to medical undergraduate students. *Medical Education, 35,* 232–241.

Dweck, C. S. (1999). *Self-theories: Their role in motivation, personality, and development.* Philadelphia: Psychology Press.

Dweck, C. S., Chiu, C-y., & Hong, Y-y. (1995). Implicit theories and their role in judgments and reactions: A world from two perspectives. *Psychological Inquiry, 6,* 267–285.

Dweck, C. S., Hong, Y-y., & Chiu, C-y. (1993). Implicit theories: Individual differences in the likelihood and meaning of dispositional inference. *Personality and Social Psychology Bulletin, 19,* 644–656.

Eaton, M. J., & Dembo, M. H. (2001). Differences in the motivational beliefs of Asian American and non-Asian students. *Journal of Educational Psychology, 89,* 433–440.

Elliot, A. J., Chirkov, V. I., Kim, Y., & Seldon, K. M. (2001). A cross-cultural analysis of avoidance (relative to approach) personal goals. *Psychological Science, 12,* 505–510.

Ford, M. E., & Tisak, M. S. (1983). A further search for social intelligence. *Journal of Educational Psychology, 75,* 196–206.

Friedman, J. (1994). *Cultural identity and global process.* London: Sage.

Gardner, W. L., Gabriel, S., & Lee, A. (1999). "I" value freedom, but "we" value relationships: Self-construal priming mirrors cultural differences in judgment. *Psychological Science, 10,* 321–326.

Gervey, B. M., Chiu, C-y., Hong, Y-y., & Dweck, C. S. (1999). Differential use of person information in decisions about guilt vs. innocence: The role of implicit theories. *Personality and Social Psychology Bulletin, 25,* 17–27.

Gjerde, P. F., & Onishi, M. (2000). Selves, cultures, and nations: The psychological imagination of the Japanese in the era of globalization. *Human Development, 43,* 216–226.

Grant, H., & Dweck, C. S. (2001). Cross-cultural response to failure: Considering outcome attributions with different goals. In F. Salili, C-y. Chiu, & Y-y. Hong (Eds.), *Student motivation: The culture and context of learning* (pp. 203–219). New York: Kluwer Academic/Plenum Press.

Greenberg, J., Solomon, S., & Pyszczynski, T. (1997).

Terror management theory of self-esteem and cultural worldview: Empirical assessments and conceptual refinements. In P. M. Zanna (Ed.), *Advances in experimental social psychology* (Vol. 29, pp. 61–141). San Diego: Academic Press.

Hampton, J. A. (1997). Emergent attributes in combined concepts. In T. B. Ward, S. M. Smith, & J. Vaid (Eds.), *Creative thought: An investigation of conceptual structures and processes* (pp. 83–110). Washington, DC: American Psychological Association.

Han, S.-P., & Shavitt, S. (1994). Persuasion and culture: Advertising appeals in individualistic and collectivistic societies. *Journal of Experimental Social Psychology, 30,* 326–350.

Hansen, N. D., Pepitone-Arreola-Rockwell, F., & Greene, A. F. (2000). Multicultural competence: Criteria and case examples. *Professional Psychology: Research and Practice, 31,* 652–660.

Heine, S. J., Kitayama, S., Lehman, D. R., Takata, T., Ide, E., Leung, C., et al. (2001). Divergent consequences of success and failure in Japan and North America: An investigation of self-improving motivations and malleable selves. *Journal of Personality and Social Psychology, 81,* 599–615.

Heine, S. J., & Lehman, D. R. (1997). Culture, dissonance, and self-affirmation. *Personality and Social Psychology Bulletin, 23,* 389–400.

Heine, S. J., Lehman, D. R., Markus, H. R., & Kitayama, S. (1999). Is there a universal need for positive self-regard? *Psychological Review, 106,* 766–794.

Heine, S. J., & Renshaw, K. (2002). Interjudge agreement, self-enhancement, and liking: Cross-cultural convergences. *Personality and Social Psychology Bulletin, 28,* 578–587.

Hermans, H. J. M., & Kempen, H. J. G. (1998). Moving cultures: The perilous problems of cultural dichotomies in a globalizing society. *American Psychologist, 53,* 1111–1120.

Hetts, J. J., Sakuma, M., & Pelham, B. W. (1999). Two roads to positive self-regard: Implicit and explicit self-evaluation and culture. *Journal of Experimental Social Psychology, 35,* 512–559.

Higgins, E. T. (1996). Knowledge activation: Accessibility, applicability and salience. In E. T. Higgins & A. E. Kruglanski (Eds.), *Social psychology: Handbook of basic principles* (pp. 133–168). New York: Guilford Press.

Higgins, E. T., Friedman, R. S., Harlow, R. E., Idson, L. C., Ayduk, O. N., & Taylor, A. (2001). Achievement orientations from subjective histories of success: Promotion pride versus prevention pride. *European Journal of Social Psychology, 31,* 3–23.

Ho, D. Y. F., & Chiu, C-y. (1994). Component ideas of individualism, collectivism, and social organization: An application in the study of Chinese culture. In U. Kim, H. C. Triandis, C. Kagitcibasi, G. Choi, & G. Yoon (Eds.), *Individualism and collectivism: Theory, method and applications* (pp. 137–156). Thousand Oaks, CA: Sage.

Hong, Y-y. (2001). Chinese students' and teachers' inferences of effort and ability. In F. Salili, C-y. Chiu, & Y-y. Hong (Eds.), *Student motivation: The culture and context of learning* (pp. 106–120). New York: Kluwer Academic/Plenum Press.

Hong, Y-y., Benet-Martinez, V., Chiu, C-y., & Morris, M. W. (2003). Boundaries of cultural influence: Construct activation as a mechanism for cultural differences in social perception. *Journal of Cross-Cultural Psychology, 34,* 453–464.

Hong, Y-y., & Chiu, C-y. (2001). Toward a paradigm shift: From cross-cultural differences in social-cognition to social-cognitive mediation of cultural differences. *Social Cognition, 19,* 181–196.

Hong, Y-y., Chiu, C-y., Dweck, C. S., Lin, D. M.-s., & Wan, W. (1999). Implicit theories, attributions, and coping: A meaning system approach. *Journal of Personality and Social Psychology, 77,* 588–599.

Hong, Y-y., Chiu, C-y., & Kung, T. M. (1997). Bringing culture out in front: Effects of cultural meaning system activation on social cognition. In K. Leung, Y. Kashima, U. Kim, & S. Yamaguchi (Eds.), *Progress in Asian social psychology* (Vol. 1, pp. 135–146). Singapore: Wiley.

Hong, Y-y., Ip, G., Chiu, C-y., Morris, M. W., & Menon, T. (2001). Cultural identity and dynamic construction of the self: Collective duties and individual rights in Chinese and American cultures. *Social Cognition, 19,* 251–269.

Hong, Y-y., & Mallorie, L. M. (2004). A dynamic constructivist approach to culture: Lessons learned from personality psychology. *Journal of Research in Personality, 38,* 59–67.

Hong, Y-y., Morris, M. W., Chiu, C-y., & Benet-Martinez, V. (2000). Multicultural minds: A dynamic constructivist approach to culture and cognition. *American Psychologist, 55,* 709–720.

Hui, C. H. (1988). Measurement of individualism–collectivism. *Journal of Research in Personality, 22,* 17–36.

Hume, D. (1894). *Essays: Literary, moral and political.* London: Routledge. (Original work published in 1784)

Ip, W-m., Chen, J., & Chiu, C-y. (2003). [Unpublished data.] University of Illinois, Urbana–Champaign.

Iyengar, S. S., & Lepper, M. R. (1999). Rethinking the value of choice: A cultural perspective on intrinsic motivation. *Journal of Personality and Social Psychology, 76,* 349–366.

Jellen, H. U., & Urban, K. (1989). Assessing creative potential worldwide: The first cross-cultural application of the Test for Creative Thinking—Drawing Production (TCT-DP). *Gifted Educational International, 6,* 78–86.

Jetten, J., Postmes, T., & Mcauliffe, B. (2002). "We're all individuals": Group norms of individualism and collectivism, levels of identification and identity threat. *European Journal of Social Psychology, 32,* 189–207.

Ji, L-j., Peng, K., & Nibsett, R. E. (2000). Culture, control, and perception of relationships in the environment. *Journal of Personality and Social Psychology, 78,* 943–955.

Kanagawa, C., Cross, S. E., & Markus, H. R. (2001). "Who am I?": The cultural psychology of the conceptual self. *Personality and Social Psychology Bulletin, 27,* 90–103.

Kashima, E. S., & Kashima, Y. (1998). Culture and language: The case of cultural dimensions and personal pronoun use. *Journal of Cross-Cultural Psychology, 29,* 461–486.

Kashima, Y., Woolcock, J., & Kashima, E. (2000). Group impressions as dynamic configurations: The tensor product model of group impression formation and change. *Psychological Review, 107,* 914–942.

Kelly, G. (1955). *A theory of personality: The psychology of personal constructs.* New York: Norton.

Kim, H. S., & Markus, H. R. (1999). Deviance or uniqueness, harmony or conformity?: A cultural analysis. *Journal of Personality and Social Psychology, 77,* 785–800.

Kitayama, S. (2002). Culture and basic psychological processes—toward a system view of culture: Comment on Oyserman et al. (2002). *Psychological Bulletin, 128,* 89–96.

Kitayama, S., Markus, H. R., Matsumoto, H., & Norasakkunkit, V. (1997). Individual and collective processes in the construction of the self: Self-enhancement in the United States and self-criticism in Japan. *Journal of Personality and Social Psychology, 72,* 1245–1267.

Knowles, E. D., Morris, M. W., Chiu, C-y., & Hong, Y-y. (2001). Culture and process of person perception: Evidence for automaticity among East Asians in correcting for situational influences on behavior. *Personality and Social Psychology Bulletin, 27,* 1344–1356.

Kurman, J. (2001). Self-enhancement: Is it restricted to individualistic cultures? *Personality and Social Psychology Bulletin, 27,* 1705–1716.

Kwan, V. S. Y., Bond, M. H., & Singelis, T. M. (1997). Pancultural explanations for life satisfaction: Adding relationship harmony to self-esteem. *Journal of Personality and Social Psychology, 73,* 1038–1051.

Lau, I. Y-m., Chiu, C-y., & Lee, S-l. (2001). Communication and shared reality: Implications for the psychological foundations of culture. *Social Cognition, 19,* 350–371.

Lau, I. Y-m., Lee, S-l., & Chiu, C-y. (2004). Language, cognition and reality: Constructing shared meanings through communication. In M. Schaller & C. Crandall (Eds.), *The psychological foundations of culture* (pp. 77–100). Mahwah, NJ: Erlbaum.

Lee, A. Y., Aaker, J. L., & Gardner, W. L. (2000). The pleasure and pains of distinct self-construals: The role of interdependence in regulatory focus. *Journal* of *Personality and Social Psychology, 78,* 1122–1134.

Lee, S-l. (2002). *Communication and shared representation: The role of knowledge estimation.* Unpublished doctoral dissertation: University of Hong Kong, Hong Kong.

Lehman, D., Chiu, C-y., & Schaller, M. (2004). Psychology and culture. In S. T. Fiske, D. L. Schacter, & C. Zahn-Waxler (Eds.), *Annual review of psychology* (pp. 689–714). Palo Alto, CA: Annual Reviews.

Leung, K-y. A., Chiu, C-y., & Hong, Y-y. (2004, January). *Bicultural individuals accommodate their interaction strategies to the projected distribution of promotion- and prevention-focused regulatory focus in interaction partner's cultural group.* Paper presented at the 5th Annual Meeting of the Society for Personality and Social Psychology, Austin, TX.

Li, Q., & Hong, Y-y. (2001). Intergroup perceptual accuracy predicts real-life intergroup interactions. *Group Processes and Intergroup Relations, 4,* 341–354.

Lyons, A., & Kashima, Y. (2001). The reproduction of culture: Communication processes tend to maintain cultural stereotypes. *Social Cognition, 19,* 372–394.

Menon, T., & Morris, M. W. (2001). Social structure in North American and Chinese cultures: Reciprocal influence between objective and subjective structures. *Journal of Psychology in Chinese Societies, 2,* 27–50.

Menon, T., Morris, M. W., Chiu, C-y., & Hong, Y-y. (1999). Culture and the construal of agency: Attribution to individual versus group dispositions. *Journal of Personality and Social Psychology, 76,* 701–717.

Morris, M. W., & Fu, H-y. (2001). How does culture influence conflict resolution?: A dynamic constructivist analysis. *Social Cognition, 19,* 324–349.

Nemeth, C., & Kwan, J. (1985). Originality of word associations as a function of majority versus minority influence. *Social Psychology Quarterly, 48,* 277–282.

Ng, S. H., & Bradac, J. (1993). *Power is language: Vernal communication and social influence.* Newbury Park, CA: Sage.

Niu, W., & Sternberg, R. J. (2002). Contemporary studies on the concept of creativity: The East and the West. *Journal of Creative Behavior, 36,* 269–288.

Norenzayan, A., Choi, I., & Nisbett, R. E. (2002). Cultural similarities and differences in social inference: Evidence from behavioral predictions and lay theories of behavior. *Personality and Social Psychology Bulletin, 28,* 109–120.

Norenzayan, A., Smith, E. E., Kim, B. J., & Nisbett, R. E. (2002). Cultural preferences for formal versus intuitive reasoning. *Cognitive Science, 26,* 653–684.

Oishi, S., & Diener, E. (2001). Goals, culture, and subjective well-being. *Personality and Social Psychology Bulletin, 27,* 1674–1682.

Oishi, S., Diener, E. F., Lucas, R. E., & Suh, E. M. (1999). Cross-cultural variations in predictors of life satisfaction: Perspectives from needs and values. *Personality and Social Psychology Bulletin, 25,* 980–990.

Oyserman, D., Coon, H. M., & Kemmelmeier, M. (2002). Rethinking individualism and collectivism: Evaluation of theoretical assumptions and meta-analyses. *Psychological Bulletin, 128,* 3–72.

Paulhus, D. (1984). Two component models of socially desirable responding. *Journal of Personality and Social Psychology, 46,* 598–609.

Rhee, E., Uleman, J. S., Lee, H. K., & Roman, R. J. (1995). Spontaneous self-descriptions and ethnic identities in individualistic and collectivistic cultures. *Journal of Personality and Social Psychology, 69,* 142–152.

Richter, L., & Kruglanski, A. W. (2004). Motivated closed mindedness and the emergence of culture. In M. Schaller & C. Crandall (Eds.), *The psychological foundations of culture* (pp. 101–121). Mahwah, NJ: Erlbaum.

Ross, M., Xun, W. Q. E., & Wilson, A. E. (2002). Language and the bicultural self. *Personality and Social Psychology Bulletin, 28,* 1040–1050.

Rudowicz, E., Lok, D., & Kitto, J. (1995). Use of the Torrance tests of creative thinking in an exploratory study of creativity in Hong Kong primary school children: A cross-cultural comparison. *International Journal of Psychology, 30,* 417–430.

Ryan, R. M., & Deci, E. L. (2000). Self-determination theory and the facilitation of intrinsic motivation, social development, and well-being. *American Psychologist, 55,* 68–78.

Salili, F., Chiu, C-y., & Lai, S. (2001). The influence of culture and context on student's motivational orientation and performance. In F. Salili, C-y. Chiu, & Y-y. Hong (Eds.), *Student motivation: The culture and context of learning* (pp. 221–247). New York: Kluwer Academic/Plenum Press.

Schimmack, U., Radhakrishnan, P., Oishi, S., & Dzokoto, V. (2002). Culture, personality, and subjective well-being: Integrating process models of life satisfaction. *Journal of Personality and Social Psychology, 82,* 582–593.

Sechrist, G. B., & Stangor, C. (2001). Perceived consensus influences intergroup behavior and stereotype accessibility. *Journal of Personality and Social Psychology, 80,* 645–654.

Sedikides, C., Gaertner, L., & Toguchi, Y. (2003). Pancultural self-enhancement. *Journal of Personality and Social Psychology, 84,* 60–79.

Shore, B. (1996). *Culture in mind: Cognition, culture, and the problem of meaning.* New York: Oxford University Press.

Shweder, R. A., & Sullivan, M. A. (1990). The semiotic subject of cultural psychology. In L. A. Pervin (Ed.), *Handbook of personality: Theory and research* (pp. 399–416). New York: Guilford Press.

Simonton, D. K. (1975). Sociocultural context of individual creativity: A transhistorical time–series analysis. *Journal of Personality and Social Psychology, 32,* 1119–1133.

Simonton, D. K. (1997). Foreign influence and national development: The impact of open milieus on Japanese civilization. *Journal of Personality and Social Psychology, 72,* 86–94.

Simonton, D. K. (2000). Creativity: Cognitive, personal, developmental, and social aspects. *American Psychologist, 55,* 151–158.

Sokefeld, M. (1999). Debating self, identity, and culture in anthropology. *Current Anthropology, 40,* 417–447.

Solomon, S., Greenberg, J., & Pyszczynski, T. (1991). A terror management theory of social behavior: The psychological functions of self-esteem and cultural worldview. In L. Berkowitz (Ed.), *Advances in experimental social psychology* (Vol. 24, pp. 93–159). San Diego: Academic Press.

Sparrow, L. M. (2000). Beyond multicultural man: Complexities of identity. *International Journal of Intercultural Relations, 24,* 173–201.

Sperber, D. (1996). *Explaining culture: A naturalistic approach.* Cambridge, MA: Blackwell.

Sternberg, R. J., & Smith, C. (1985). Social intelligence and decoding skills in nonverbal intelligence. *Social Cognition, 3,* 168–192.

Su, S. K., Chiu, C-y., Hong, Y-y., Leung, K., Peng, K., & Morris, M. W. (1999). Self organization and social organization: American and Chinese constructions. In T. R. Tyler, R. Kramer, & O. John (Eds.), *The psychology of the social self* (pp. 193–222). Mahwah, NJ: Erlbaum.

Sue, S. (1998). In search of cultural competence in psychotherapy and counseling. *American Psychologist, 53,* 440–448.

Suh, E. M. (2002). Culture, identity consistency, and subjective well-being. *Journal of Personality and Social Psychology, 83,* 1378–1391.

Suh, E. M., Diener, E., Oishi, S., & Triandis, H. C. (1998). The shifting basis of life satisfaction judgments across cultures: Emotions versus norms. *Journal of Personality and Social Psychology, 74,* 482–493.

Tafarodi, R. W., Lang, J. M., & Smith, A. J. (1999). Self-esteem and the cultural trade-off: Evidence for the role of individualism–collectivism. *Journal of Cross-Cultural Psychology, 30,* 620–640.

Tao, V., & Hong, Y. (2000). A meaning system approach to Chinese students' achievement goals. *Journal of Psychology in the Chinese Societies, 1,* 13–38.

Thorndike, E. L. (1920). Intelligence and its uses. *Harper's Magazine, 140,* 227–235.

Tong, Y-y., & Chiu, C-y. (2002). Lay theories and evaluation-based organization of impressions: An application of the memory search paradigm. *Personality and Social Psychology Bulletin, 28,* 1518–1527.

Trafimow, D., Silverman, E. S., Fan, R. M-t., & Law, J. S. F. (1997). The effects of language and priming on the relative accessibility of the private self and the collective self. *Journal of Cross-Cultural Psychology, 28,* 107–123.

Trafimow, D., Triandis, H. C., & Goto, S. G. (1991). Some tests of the distinction between the private self and the collective self. *Journal of Personality and Social Psychology, 60,* 649–655.

Verkuyten, M., & Pouliasi, K. (2002). Biculturalism among older children: Cultural frame switching, attributions, self-identification, and attitudes. *Journal of Cross-Cultural Psychology, 33,* 596–609.

Wan, W. W-n., & Chiu, C-y. (2002). Effects of novel conceptual combination on creativity. *Journal of Creative Behavior, 36,* 227–240.

Wang, Q. (2001). Culture effects on adults' earliest childhood recollection and self-description: Implications for the relation between memory and the self. *Journal of Personality and Social Psychology, 81,* 220–233.

Ward, C., Bochner, S., & Furnham, A. (2001). *The psychology of culture shock* (2nd ed.). New York: Routledge.

Ward, T. B., Patterson, M. J., Sifonis, C. M., Dodds, R. A., & Saunders, K. N. (2002). The role of graded category structure in imaginative thought. *Memory and Cognition, 30,* 199–216.

Wong, R. Y-m., Hong, Y-y (2003). Dynamic influences of culture on cooperation in the Prisoner's Dilemma. *Psychological Science.*

Yu, A-b., & Yang, K-s. (1994). The nature of achievement motivation in collectivist societies. In U. Kim, H. C. Triandis, C. Kagitcibasi, G. Choi, & G. Yoon (Eds.), *Individualism and collectivism: Theory, method and applications* (pp. 239–266). Thousand Oaks, CA: Sage.

PART VI

❧

Self-Regulatory Processes

CHAPTER 27

ଔ

The Hidden Dimension
of Personal Competence

Self-Regulated Learning and Practice

BARRY J. ZIMMERMAN
ANASTASIA KITSANTAS

As each generation traverses the path from childhood to adulthood, its sense of personal identity and esteem is determined by its perceived competence in diverse areas of functioning (Bandura, 1997). The importance of attaining academic competence is widely recognized (Covington, 1992), but other personal competencies also figure prominently in youths' sense of self—especially their athletic prowess (Horn & Hasbrook, 1987; Smoll, Smith, Barnett, & Everett, 1993). More than 50% of all American boys and girls participate in athletic programs between the age of 8 and 18, and millions more participate in interscholastic programs (Ewing & Seefeldt, 1995). But how do these youth acquire high levels of academic and athletic competence?

There is evidence that the attainment of peak levels of academic and athletic competence requires more than basic talent and high-quality instruction; it also involves self-belief, diligence, and self-discipline. The importance of this often hidden self-regulatory dimension of competence was stressed by Amby Burfoot (1997, p. 189), the 1986 Boston Marathon Champion: "I've always been one of those slow-but-steady runners. If I won a lot of races in my day, my success didn't come from any excess of athletic brilliance. It came from discipline and determination, from the fact that I stuck to my programs and goals no matter how slow and sometimes frustrating the progress." There are considerable empirical data to support Burfoot's observation about the importance of self-disciplined learning and practice. For example, Ericsson (1997) has found that high achievers in diverse fields, such as sport, dance, and music, started their learning and practiced at a younger age than lower achievers, and that their competence is directly related to the time they spent in these self-directed endeavors.

A social cognitive perspective regarding acquisition of academic and athletic competence focuses on the role of learners' social and self-regulatory processes during extensive study and practice. In this chapter, we describe self-regulation, explain the origins and inertia of self-empowering cycles of learning on individuals' academic and athletic competence, and describe how self-regulatory competence emerges from social modeling experiences in a series of levels.

DEFINING SELF-REGULATION AND DESCRIBING KEY SELF-REGULATORY PROCESSES

Although every student has some sense of what it means to self-regulate, most personal definitions involve vague beliefs about personal willpower. Although beliefs about self-regulation are important, social cognitive researchers also emphasize the role of specific self-initiated personal, behavioral, and environmental *processes* designed to attain personal goals cyclically (Zimmerman, 1989). Cyclical adjustments are necessary during the course of learning and performance, because individuals' personal, behavioral, and environmental factors are in constant flux and must be observed or monitored using three self-oriented feedback loops. Behavioral self-regulation involves self-observing and strategically adjusting performance processes, such as one's method of learning or performing, whereas environmental self-regulation refers to observing and adjusting environmental conditions or outcomes, such as one's place for studying or practicing. Covert self-regulation involves monitoring and adjusting cognitive and affective states, such as strategies for remembering or relaxing. To optimize their effectiveness, learners develop self-regulatory plans that involve all three triadic components (Bandura, 1986).

There is extensive evidence that successful students and academics, such as professional writers and athletes, use an array of self-regulatory processes to optimize their learning and performance (Zimmerman, 1998). For example, the key self-regulatory process of "goal setting" refers to specifying intended actions or ends (Locke & Latham (1990). The American baseball star, Steve Garvey, described the importance of goal setting in

the following terms, "You have to set goals that are almost out of reach. If you set a goal that is attainable without much work or thought you are stuck with something below your true talent and potential" (Anderson, 1997, p. 85). The American novelist William Faulkner put it similarly: "Always dream and shoot higher than you know you can do. Don't bother just to be better than your contemporaries or predecessors. Try to be better than yourself" (Cowley, 1959, p. 123). Novelists, such as Anthony Trollope and Ernest Hemingway, set daily or weekly page completion writing goals for themselves to guide their literary progress (Wallace & Pear, 1977).

Another key self-regulatory process is "task strategies," which refers to analyzing tasks and identifying specific, advantageous methods for learning or performing various components of a task. For example, the legendary golfer Sam Snead (1989) would purposely move his ball to the worst lie during practice rounds, because this strategy helped him "develop the shots you need to scramble out of trouble as well as teach you how much you can realistically afford to gamble when in a jam" (p. 160). Many professional writers intentionally end their daily efforts in midsentence, because they have discovered that this practice helps them subsequently to initiate writing (Murray, 1990).

The self-regulatory process of "imagery" refers to creating or recalling vivid mental images to assist learning (Pressley, 1977). One of the most successful golfers of all time, Jack Nicklaus (1992), regularly used visual images to guide his practice and competitive play. The Pulitzer Prize–winning writer Donald Murray (1990) also uses imagery to enhance his writing. "I see what I write and many times the focus of my writing is in my image" (p. 97). The self-regulatory process of "self-instruction" refers to overt or subvocal verbalization to guide performance (Meichenbaum, 1977). To help control their temper, athletes attending the Bolletieri Tennis Academy, where champions such as Monica Seles and Andre Agassi trained, are asked to express positive alternative statements, such as saying "Let it go" or "Come on" (p. 47) to focus or motivate themselves (Loehr, 1991). Professional writers also rely on listening to themselves develop their own personal voice. "As I draft, I write with my ear, hearing the language before it is on the page, following the beat, the melody, the phrasing that will reveal meaning to me" (Murray, 1990, p. 96).

The self-regulatory process of "time management" refers to estimating and budgeting use of time. Many elite athletes avoid burnout and stagnation by limiting their daily practice to approximately 4–5 hours, and by avoiding long practice episodes without periods of rest and sleep (Ericsson, 1997). Professional writers also manage their time by setting limits on daily writing efforts. The poet Philip Larkin cautioned, "I don't think you can write a poem for more than two hours. After that you're going round in circles, and it's much better to leave it for twenty-four hours. Some days it goes, and some days it doesn't go. But over weeks and months I am productive" (Murray, 1990, p. 16).

Another key form of self-regulation is "self-monitoring," which involves observing and tracking one's own performance and outcomes. Self-recording one's processes and outcomes can greatly assist self-monitoring, such as when students form lists of key terms and check them off as they memorize them for a forthcoming test. The legendary golfer Ben Hogan (1957, pp. 37–38) once wrote about self-monitoring and self-recording, "Golf also seems to bring out the scientist in the person. He soon discovers that unless he goes about observing and testing with an orderly method, he is simply complicating his problems." Writers also rely on self-recording to guide their creative efforts. "The process log or daybook will help you make the process yours, will give you a chance to see how you write when the writing goes well. If you are to keep improving your writing, you need to build on the procedures you used that have worked" (Murray, 1990, p. 14).

A closely related self-regulatory process is "self-evaluation," which refers to using standards to make self-judgments, such as when students compare their homework answers with those of other students. Standards need to be set appropriately, so that they are challenging but attainable. The poet William Safford warned that excessive self-evaluative standards are a major cause of writer's "block" (Murray, 1990). The famous golfer, Walter Hagen, prevented himself from re-

sponding negatively to errors by assuming beforehand that he would make three or four errors during each round (Nicklaus, 1992). This realistic self-evaluative standard enabled him to shrug off the frustration when an error occurred.

The self-regulatory process of "environmental structuring" involves selecting or creating effective physical settings for learning, such as when students seek out a quiet section of the home or dormitory to study more effectively. Athletes have often gone to special lengths to structure their training environments to increase their chances of success. To prepare himself to win the Tour de France in the mountainous sections of the racecourse, the American bicycle racer, Lance Armstrong, would sleep during training in a low-oxygen tent to adapt himself physiologically to high-altitude conditions ahead of time (Abt, 2001). The novelist William Faulkner humorously recommended a brothel as an ideal setting for writing, because "the place is quiet during the morning hours which is the best time of the day to work" (Cowley, 1959, p. 124).

The self-regulatory process of adaptive "help seeking" involves choosing models, teachers, or books to assist one to learn. Adaptive help seeking is distinguished from social dependence by three key characteristics: self-initiation, selective focus, and limited duration of help seeking. There is considerable evidence that students who are not self-regulated avoid asking for assistance because of concern about adverse social consequences of such requests (Newman, 1994). By contrast, self-regulated students seek help selectively by knowing who and what to ask. Getting social feedback on a selective basis is essential for high-level attainment among athletes, as well as students. For example, if Jack Nicklaus (1992) noticed that some bad habits had crept into his golf stroke, he would ask his former golf coach for assistance in identifying the errors and correcting them. "In my case, Jack Grout can get me back to fundamentals in minutes, whereas it might take me weeks of trial and error to iron out a basic fault on my own" (p. 136).

These anecdotal accounts illustrate the rich variety of self-regulatory processes that students and athletes use to achieve peak performance. The results of their personal experiences during many hours of self-directed learning and practice convinced them of the effectiveness of these techniques in acquiring and refining mastery of their field of endeavor. Although the ultimate effectiveness of a self-regulated learning process depends on the quality of its triadic match to the individual, environment, and behavioral task involved, there is growing evidence that students who use self-regulatory processes frequently enjoy greater success and are more motivated, as we discuss next.

ROLE OF SELF-REGULATORY PROCESSES IN ENHANCING MOTIVATION AND ACHIEVEMENT

To investigate the impact of self-regulatory processes in students' academic functioning, Zimmerman and Martinez-Pons (1986) developed a structured interview, the Self-Regulation Learning Interview Schedule (SRLIS), that involved asking students to respond to a series of common learning problems or contexts, such as "Most teachers give a test at the end of a marking period, and those tests greatly determine the final grade. Do you have a particular method for preparing for a test in classes like English or history?" The students' answers to these open-ended questions were coded into academic self-regulatory process categories, similar to those we described earlier, or a non-self-regulatory "other" category. The differences in the verbal protocols of students assigned to high- and regular-achievement tracks in school were significant in terms of both the quality and quantity of self-regulatory processes reported: High achievers surpassed regular achievers significantly in 13 of the 14 processes that were studied. High achievers not only reported greater use of personal self-regulatory processes, such as rehearsing and memorizing, but also social assistance processes, such as help seeking from teachers, classmates, and other adults. The other personal processes that were assessed included self-evaluation, organizing and transforming, seeking information, keeping records and monitoring, environmental structuring, providing self-consequences, and reviewing (e.g., tests, texts, and notes). It should be noted that students' reports of task strategies would be classified

within the organizing and transforming category of the SRLIS, and the self-verbalization and imagery processes would be classified within the rehearsing and memorizing category. Time management answers were classified within goal setting and planning or keeping records and monitoring categories of the SRLIS, depending on the details.

As a context-specific measure, the SRLIS assessed students' self-regulation during the course of typical academic assignments, such as reading, studying, and test preparation. However, students' statements that failed to indicate self-initiation (e.g., "I just do the assignment") or students' nonstrategic willpower statements (e.g., "I just try harder") were negatively related to achievement outcomes. Thus, students' responses to academic problems that were merely reactive to the prompts of others were associated with poorer learning. Although individual processes were assessed separately, it was expected that high-achieving students would use them in combination, which in fact was observed (Zimmerman & Martinez-Pons, 1986). As a result, the SRLIS was also analyzed as an omnibus measure of self-regulative functioning both in this study and in subsequent research. Students' combined use of self-regulatory processes accounted for 93% of the variance of their high school achievement track placement and was also highly predictive of their performance on a standardized test.

Ley and Young (1998) reported similar omnibus findings using the SRLIS to identify developmentally delayed students entering a community college. They found that these at-risk students were identified from regular students with 94% accuracy based on their reports of academic self-regulation. Purdie and Hattie (1996) used a questionnaire variant of the SRLIS (i.e., without an interviewer's probing) to study self-regulation by Australian and Japanese high school students, and found that high achievers surpassed medium and low achievers in using most of the self-regulated learning strategies.

In a subsequent study, Zimmerman and Martinez-Pons (1988) sought to validate the SRLIS against teachers' observations of their students' self-regulation in class. These teacher ratings of students dealt with overt manifestations of self-regulation in class, such as items referring to students who solicit additional information about tests (help seeking), display awareness concerning test performance before it is graded (self-monitoring and self-evaluation), complete assignments before deadlines (goal setting and attainment), and are prepared to participate in class (strategic planning). Because self-regulation involves self-initiation and perseverance, students' self-motivational beliefs are essential. Several indices of students' motivation were included in the teacher-completed scale: Does a student express interest in the course matter (intrinsic interest?) Does a student volunteer for special tasks related to the coursework (a learning goal orientation)? These researchers found that these teacher-derived measures of students' classroom functioning formed a single, large underlying self-regulation factor, and that the teacher-derived factor was highly correlated with the students' reports of using self-regulated learning strategies on the SRLIS. These researchers also discovered that the students' underlying self-regulation factor was distinctive from but significantly correlated with their scores on standardized tests of achievement. This indicated the divergent, as well as the convergent, validity of the teacher rating scale. Evidence that motivation measures loaded on the same factor as the self-regulatory process measures confirmed that self-regulation processes and motivation were closely associated.

Zimmerman and Martinez-Pons (1990) subsequently studied developmental differences in self-regulated learning strategy use with 5th-, 8th-, and 11th-grade students attending regular or gifted schools. Another key motivational belief was studied: *self-efficacy*, which refers to beliefs about personal capability to perform specific tasks at a designated level of proficiency. These researchers created a self-efficacy scale by selecting from a standardized test mathematical problems and verbal definition problems that ranged in difficulty from elementary school to high school levels. Students were asked to rate their confidence about answering each math or verbal item correctly. The researchers found significant developmental differences in use of self-regulated learning processes. Both regular and gifted students reported developmental increases in overall use of self-regulation processes, but gifted students surpassed regular students at each

grade level. These researchers also found that developmental increases in students' use of self-regulation processes corresponded to developmental increases in their verbal and mathematical self-efficacy. This indicates that use of self-regulatory processes is related closely to this form of motivation.

Two forms of self-efficacy beliefs have been studied to date: self-efficacy for *performance* or *learning* (including the use of self-regulation processes to learn). For example, self-efficacy for math performance involve judgments of capability to solve particular problems, whereas self-efficacy for learning involves a student's belief that he or she can learn the necessary processes to solve a particular problem (Schunk, 1989). There is evidence that self-efficacy for learning mathematical fraction problems is predictive of posttest self-efficacy for math problem-solving performance (Schunk, Hanson, & Cox, 1987). The former form of self-efficacy is particularly important when predicting students' motivation to learn an unfamiliar skill, such as a foreign language. Self-efficacy for self-regulated learning processes refers to self-beliefs about personal competence in using processes, such as goal setting, strategy use, and self-monitoring, to learn.

There is evidence that perceived efficacy for self-regulated learning processes is also predictive of perceived efficacy to perform. Zimmerman, Bandura, and Martinez-Pons (1992) investigated whether high school students' perceptions of self-efficacy regarding self-regulatory skill to learn were predictive of their self-efficacy for academic achievement performance. These researchers assessed self-efficacy for self-regulated learning through ratings of strategies similar to those assessed by the SRLIS, and they assessed self-efficacy for academic achievement using a range of academic subjects, such as math, science, and social studies. They found that self-efficacy for self-regulated learning was indeed linked to self-efficacy for academic achievement. The latter form of self-efficacy for performance, in turn, was predictive of the students' grade goals, as well as their final grades in social studies. Self-efficacy for academic achievement was also indirectly predictive of students' final grades through the goals they set. Interestingly, the self-efficacy and goal-setting measures (given in the fall) increased the prediction of the final grades in the spring by 31% compared to the students' social studies grade from the previous year. Clearly students' perceived efficacy to self-regulate learning was highly predictive of actual goal setting and academic success. Very similar findings were reported in a follow-up study with college students enrolled in an introductory writing course (Zimmerman & Bandura, 1994). Students' self-efficacy for self-regulation of learning to write was predictive of their self-efficacy for attaining high grades in the course. The latter form of self-efficacy was in turn predictive of the students' writing goals, as well as their final grade in the course.

Similarly, in athletic contexts, self-efficacy beliefs and self-regulatory processes, such as goal setting, have been highly predictive of personal effectiveness. Regarding self-efficacy, there is extensive evidence that athletes' self-efficacy beliefs are correlated positively with their levels of athletic performance (see Feltz, 1992, for a review). In a recent meta-analysis of 45 studies, Moritz, Feltz, Fahrbach, and Mack (2000) found that the average correlation between self-efficacy and sport performance was .38. Regarding the link between self-efficacy beliefs and self-regulation, athletes who report high self-efficacy beliefs regarding their performance are more likely to set challenging goals and devise strategies that will help them accomplish these goals. For example, Kane, Marks, Zaccaro, and Blair (1996) conducted a study to examine relations among measures of prior performance, self-efficacy, goals, and individual performance with 216 wrestlers competing at a wrestling camp. In general, findings showed that athletes' prior success in wrestling positively influenced their self-efficacy beliefs, which in turn affected the level of goals they set and, consequently, their performance. More interestingly, self-efficacy was found to be the only significant predictor of athletes' performance in overtime matches.

Goal setting has also received considerable attention in terms of its relevance in athletic motivation. Research indicates that proper establishment of goals plays an important role in an athlete's motivation, effort, and performance in sports (Roberts, 1992; Zimmerman & Kitsantas, 1996). Specifically, setting specific, difficult, yet attain-

able process goals has been associated with higher motivation and sport performance (Locke & Latham, 1990; Zimmerman & Kitsantas, 1996). Overall, goals not only direct athletes' attention to the task but also motivate them to search for effective strategies and strategically plan the next course of action.

Thus, there is compelling research evidence that self-regulated learning processes are predictive of both enhanced motivation and superior academic and athletic performance outcomes. However, how are these processes and motivational beliefs sustained by personal feedback, and how are they structurally linked to other sources of motivation? What leads successful student athletes to develop self-enhancing cycles of learning?

A CYCLICAL VIEW OF ACADEMIC AND ATHLETIC SELF-REGULATION OF LEARNING AND PERFORMANCE

To assess students' use of self-regulatory processes during ongoing efforts learn, social cognitive researchers (e.g., Zimmerman, 2000) have distinguished three cyclical self-regulatory phases: forethought, performance, and self-reflection (see Figure 27.1). Forethought phase processes and beliefs prepare individuals to learn. Performance phase processes influence attention, volition, and action, and self-reflection phase processes influence individuals' reactions to this learning. These self-reflective reactions cyclically influence forethought regarding subsequent learning efforts. Because of its cyclical nature, this model seeks to explain learning in informal contexts, where the goal is often a long-term continuing process of growth rather than a discrete outcome, such as when learning a foreign language or a life-long sport, such as golf, tennis, or skiing.

Forethought Phase

These self-regulatory processes and beliefs fall into two major categories: task analysis processes and self-motivation beliefs. In both academic and athletic fields of endeavor, highly self-regulatory individuals analyze the learning task prior to performance, whether it involves math problems or bas-

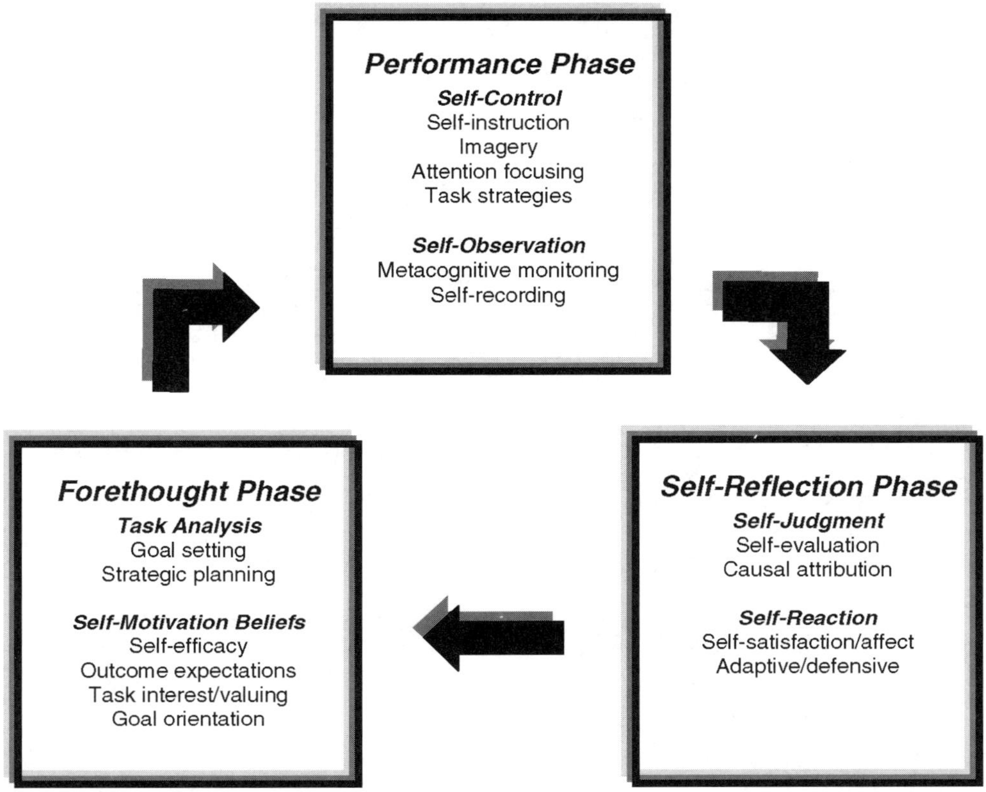

FIGURE 27.1. Phases and subprocesses of self-regulation. From Zimmerman and Campillo (2003, p. 239). Copyright 2003 by Cambridge University Press. Reprinted by permission.

ketball free throws. Highly self-regulated individuals break the task into component parts and *set goals* for learning the parts hierarchically, with subprocess and process goals linked to more distant outcome goals (Burfoot, 1997; Carver & Scheier, 2000), such as bending one's legs, positioning one's hands, and following through with one's arms during a basketball free throw). To reach these goals, highly self-regulated learners must *plan strategies* that are appropriate for the task and environmental setting (Weinstein & Mayer, 1986). For example, students may set subprocess goals in carrying out steps for solving math fractions and link them to the outcome goal of getting a higher grade on the next test (DeCorte, Verschaffel, & Op'T Eynde, 2000). The advantage of linking process goals to short- and long-term outcome goals in a hierarchical system is that it enables individuals to practice effectively by themselves for long

periods of time (Locke & Latham, 1990; Bandura, 1991).

The forethought processes of highly self-regulated learners depend on their advantageous self-motivational beliefs, namely, high perceptions of self-efficacy, outcome expectations, intrinsic interest, and learning goal orientation. As we noted, "self-efficacy" refers to personal beliefs about having the means to learn or perform effectively, and as we have already discussed, these beliefs are linked to students' motivation to initiate and sustain self-regulatory efforts (Bandura, 1997, Pajares, 1996). Don Murray (1990, p. 5) described the power of self-efficacy beliefs as follows: "Yet we also write best—just as we play tennis best—if we feel confident. We have to learn to write with confidence." A closely related source of motivation, "outcome expectation," refers to beliefs about the ultimate ends of performance (Bandura, 1997; Lens, Simons, & Dewitte, 2002). For example, self-efficacy refers to the belief that one can solve story problems on a math test or make a parallel turn on skis, whereas outcomes refer to expectations about the consequences these solutions will produce with their peers, such as receiving social acclaim. A "learning goal orientation" (Ames, 1992; Dweck, 1988; Harackiewicz, Barron, Pintrich, Elliot, & Thrash, 2002; Nicholls, 1984) refers to learners' intention to develop their competence rather than to achieve competitive success. This goal orientation was expressed by the tennis star, Monica Seles: "I really never enjoyed playing matches, even as a youngster. I just love to practice and drill and that stuff. I just hate the whole thought that one [player] is better than the other. It drives me nuts" (Vecsey, 1999, p. D1). Her statement reveals that the process of learning has supplanted achievement outcomes as a source of motivation.

"Intrinsic interest" refers to valuing a task for its inherent rather than its instrumental qualities in gaining other outcomes (Deci, 1975; Lepper & Hodell, 1989). The American actress Geena Davis took up archery just 3 years ago, but she has developed a high skill level by using powerful self-regulation techniques. She described how much she enjoys her solitary learning experiences and has described the feelings of intrinsic interest from practicing in the following way: "I guess I just got hooked. It is really fun to try to see how good you can get, and I don't know how good that is. I haven't maxed out. I haven't peaked. I'm trying to get better" (Litsky, 1999, p. D4). By contrast, poorly self-regulated learners perceive little efficacy, have low academic outcome expectations, are performance-oriented, and have little intrinsic interest in academic learning tasks.

Performance Phase

These phase processes have been grouped into two major classes: strategy use and self-observation. We have already discussed highly self-regulated learners' extensive use of strategic processes, such as self-instruction, imagery, and environmental structuring, whereas poorly self-regulated learners are not strategic in their approach to learning. Attention-focusing strategies are designed to improve one's concentration and screen out distracting events (Corno, 1993). Kuhl (1985) studied volitional methods of control, such as avoiding ruminating about past mistakes, and found them to be effective. The second major class of performance phase processes is "self-observation," which refers to metacognitive monitoring or physical record keeping of specific aspects of one's performance, the conditions that surround it, and the effects that it produces (Zimmerman & Paulsen, 1995). Because poorly self-regulated learners fail to set selective goals, they are often overwhelmed metacognitively by the amount of information that must be self-monitored, and they cannot adjust their strategies optimally. The legendary golfer Bobby Jones (Jones, 1966) put it this way: "But no human is able to think and at the same time execute the entire sequence of correct movements. The player must seek for a conception, or fix upon one or two movements, concentration on which will enable him to hit the ball" (p. 211). "Self-recording" of problem solution efforts can greatly increase the proximity, informativeness, accuracy, and valence of feedback (Zimmerman & Kitsantas, 1996), and there is evidence that highly self-regulated learners engage in more record keeping than do poorly self-regulated learners (Zimmerman & Martinez-Pons, 1986; 1988). Often professional writers record notes to guide their efforts to compose: "Process notes help me understand what I do when the writing goes well so I can look back and repeat it when the writing doesn't go well" (Murray, 1990, p. 21).

Self-Reflection Phase

Two major classes of self-reflection are self-judgments and self-reactions. "Self-judgments" involve self-evaluating one's learning performance and attributing causal significance to the outcomes. We have already discussed "self-evaluation" in terms of comparing self-monitored outcomes with a standard or goal. Highly regulated students self-evaluate more appropriately and more frequently than do poorly regulated students (Lan, 1998). Or, as one poorly regulated student put it, "I don't need no bad news!" Self-evaluative judgments are linked closely to *causal attributions* about the results of learning efforts, such as whether a failure is due to one's limited ability or to insufficient effort. Poorly regulated learners attribute their errors to uncontrollable variables such as fixed ability, whereas highly regulated ones attribute errors to controllable variables such as solution strategies. Attributions to uncontrollable variables discourage poorly regulated individuals from further learning efforts (Weiner, 1979), whereas attributions of errors to controllable variables sustain further efforts to learn (e.g., Zimmerman & Kitsantas, 1996, 1997). Similarly, elite golfers tend to disregard the possibility that factors outside their control play an important role (Kirschenbaum, O'Connor, & Owens, 1999) and instead attribute their performance to poor concentration, tenseness, and poor imagination and feel (McCaffrey & Orlick, 1989).

Two key forms of self-reactions to learning efforts have been studied to date: self-satisfaction and adaptive inferences. "Self-satisfaction" refers to perceptions of satisfaction or dissatisfaction and associated affect regarding one's performance. People will pursue courses of action that result in satisfaction and positive affect and avoid those courses that produce dissatisfaction and negative affect, such as anxiety (Bandura, 1991). Unlike poorly regulated learners, highly self-regulated ones condition their self-satisfaction on reaching their learning goals, which helps them direct their actions and persist in their efforts much better (Schunk, 1983). Although high achievers set higher evaluative standards for their self-satisfaction (Zimmerman & Bandura, 1994), all learners need to attain some level of personal satisfaction to sustain their motivation to continue their practice and play.

The other form of self-reactions involves "adaptive or defensive inferences," which are conclusions about how one needs to alter his or her approach during subsequent efforts to learn. Highly regulated learners make adaptive inferences, such as by choosing a more effective strategy (Butler, 1998; Winne, 1997), but poorly regulated ones resort to defensive inferences, which serve primarily to protect them from future dissatisfaction and aversive affect. Among the most insidious defensive self-reactions are helplessness, procrastination, task avoidance, cognitive disengagement, and apathy (Boekaerts & Niemivirta, 2000; Garcia &

Pintrich, 1994). Or as one hip inner-city student put it, "When it comes to school, I play defense!" After his bout with cancer, Lance Armstrong had to alter his bicycle training methods to minimize pedal resistance (which taxes leg strength), so he adapted by increasing pedal speed (which taxes aerobic capability). As he improved his aerobic capacity, this adaptation became a tremendous advantage over his competitors (Lehrer, 2001).

Because of the cyclical nature of self-regulation, self-reactions to learning efforts influence forethought processes regarding further solution efforts. For example, positive self-satisfaction reactions of highly regulated individuals strengthen their self-efficacy beliefs about eventually learning, enhance their learning goal orientations (Schunk, 1996), and increase their intrinsic interest in a task (Zimmerman & Kitsantas, 1997). These enhanced self-motivational beliefs are the source of highly regulated learners' greater sense of personal agency about continuing their cyclical self-regulatory efforts and eventually reaching a solution. The writer Murray (1990, p. 21) put it this way: "The affective—feelings—usually control the cognitive—thinking—in my life. It is important for me to know how I feel when I write well and what causes me to feel that way." A key implication of a cyclical model is that failures to engage in *proactive* forms of forethought, such as setting hierarchical goals and choosing a strategy, relegate learners to *reactive* forms of performance and self-reflection, such as unsystematic self-evaluation, attributions to uncontrollable causes, and dissatisfied self-reactions. Although the importance of the self-regulatory processes and beliefs has been widely recognized by academic and athletic experts, as we summarized earlier, the importance of cyclical interdependence is less well understood.

CYCLICAL RELATIONS AMONG SELF-REGULATORY PROCESSES AND SELF-MOTIVATIONAL BELIEFS

To examine the validity of a cyclical model of self-regulation, social cognitive researchers have adopted microanalytical research designs to reveal specific links between an individual's self-beliefs and use of self-regulatory processes during efforts to learn. A microanalytical methodology involves asking specific questions about important self-regulatory processes, such as self-efficacy and attribution beliefs, at key points during the act of learning and performing (Kitsantas & Zimerman, 2002). To test the descriptive accuracy of this model with high school athletes, Cleary and Zimmerman (2001) studied differences between expert and novice male basketball free-throw shooters in forethought and self-reflection phase processes among high school males who were basketball experts, nonexperts, or novices during a practice episode. *Experts* were boys who shot a high percentage of their free throws during varsity basketball games; *nonexperts* shot low percentage in those games, and *novices* had not played basketball on organized teams during high school. During individual practice sessions in a gymnasium, these adolescent boys were questioned regarding their forethought phase goals, strategy choices, self-efficacy beliefs, and intrinsic interest, as well as their self-reflection phase attributions and feelings of satisfaction as they practiced their free-throw shooting.

The experts and nonexperts were similar in age, practice time, playing experience, and basketball shooting, but there were significant differences in the use of goals and strategies among the three groups. Regarding forethought measures, experts adopted more specific process goals (i.e., focusing on shooting form) and selected more technique-oriented strategies (i.e., keeping one's elbow straight on the follow-through) than nonexperts or novices. Experts also reported higher self-efficacy perceptions and intrinsic interest in basketball shooting than novices. During the self-reflection phase, experts attributed their failures to strategy use and adjusted their strategies appropriately. By contrast, the nonexpert group members attributed their failure to successfully shoot a basket to general focus strategies, such as not being able to concentrate, and as a result, they made less effective strategy adjustments. Finally, it was found that although nonexperts' general knowledge of the skill was comparable to that of experts, the former did not utilize it in a self-regulated manner.

In another study examining differences in self-regulatory processes among experts, nonexperts, and novice female collegiate volleyball players, Kitsantas and Zimmerman (2002) found similar results. *Experts* were selected from the university's varsity volleyball team. The participants in the *nonexpert* group, selected from the university's volleyball club, had been on the club team for at least 3 years, and the *novices* were individuals who had not participated in volleyball as an organized sport but had played it informally. The volleyball players were studied individually while serving overhand during a practice episode. The overhand serve was selected because it is a difficult skill to master even for varsity volleyball players; thus, it represents a challenge for all expertise groups. Because the goal of the study was to discover differences in practice methods rather than in effects of differential knowledge of the overhand serve among the three expertise groups, all participants were given a modeled demonstration of this serve. A scoring procedure was created, wherein the opponents' court was divided into six designated target areas, with each area assigned a predetermined number of points written on the volleyball court.

It was shown that experts displayed better goals, planning, strategy use, self-monitoring, self-evaluation, attributions, and adaptation than either nonexperts or novices. Experts also displayed higher self-efficacy beliefs, perceived instrumentality, intrinsic interest, and self-satisfaction in volleyball serving than either nonexperts or novices. Interestingly, 94% of the accuracy in the girls' volleyball serving skill was explained by these self-regulation measures.

The additive effects of cyclical self-regulatory training in forethought, performance, and self-reflection phase processes during basketball free-throw shooting were studied with college students (Cleary, Zimmerman, & Keating, 2005). Participants were given three-phase training that involved forethought phase goal setting, performance phase self-recording, and self-reflection phase attributions and strategic adjustment processes. The two-phase group received identical training, with the omission of self-reflection processes (i.e., attributions, strategic adjustments), while the one-phase group received training only in goal setting. The results showed a positive linear trend between the number of self-regulatory phases in which the participants were trained and their free-throw shooting skill and shooting adaptation. The two- and three-phase training groups displayed significantly more accurate free throws and were able to self-correct following missed shots more frequently than the other groups. It should also be noted that the participants who received three-phase training displayed the most adaptive motivational profile, characterized by making strategic attributions and strategic adjustments, and using self-process criteria during self-evaluations.

In the academic realm, there is evidence that instructing students to self-monitor their learning more effectively can increase their other self-regulatory processes and beliefs, as well as their achievement. Lan (1996, 1998) used a written variant of the SRLIS as an outcome measure in a self-monitoring training study designed to improve college graduate students' self-regulation and achievement in a statistics course. Students were given a list of 75 statistical concepts that were goals of the course, along with a protocol for self-monitoring their study of each concept, as well as their self-efficacy about knowing it. This *self-monitoring* group was compared with an *instructor-monitoring* intervention, in which the students kept track of the teachers' coverage of the concepts, or with a no-treatment control group.

Students who self-monitored displayed significantly higher final course grades than students in the instructor-monitoring group and marginally significantly higher grades than students in the no-treatment control group. Compared to students in the other two experimental conditions, students in the self-monitoring group reported using self-evaluation and the planning, and use of the following self-regulatory strategies: environmental structuring, rehearsal and memorization, reviewing the textbook in preparation for a test, and reviewing previous tests in preparation for a test. The instructor-monitoring group reported seeking assistance from peers significantly more often than the self-monitoring group. Lan also discovered that students' use of self-evaluation, and the planning and use of five task strategies, were significantly correlated with their final course grades. These task strategies included seeking information, rehearsal and memori-

zation, seeking peers' assistance, reviewing the textbook, and reviewing previous tests in preparation for a test. Clearly, training in self-monitoring led students to increase their use of a range of self-regulatory strategies. The cyclical power of this self-monitoring intervention was particularly evident in one student's informal self-reflections: "It helped me to manage my studying time, and it helped me to determine when I felt comfortable with the material because I could rate my understanding while studying" (Lan, 1998, p. 99).

These studies revealed significant differences in the quality of self-regulation during personally directed learning efforts by high school and collegiate athletes of varying levels of expertise. Athletic experts were more focused in their goals, strategies, and attributions than nonexperts or novices, and they were more self-efficacious about their performance. Students who were trained in successive self-regulatory phase processes displayed not only higher levels of athletic and academic functioning but also superior motivational profiles. These studies indicate that self-regulatory training has important benefits. We now turn to the questions of how such training should be organized to be optimally effective.

ACQUIRING SELF-REGULATORY COMPETENCE AND MOTIVATION VIA SOCIAL COGNITIVE TRAINING

A social cognitive perspective (Schunk & Zimmerman, 1997; Zimmerman, 2000) envisions optimal self-regulatory training as initially social in form but becoming increasingly self-directed. What changes during the process of acquisition is a person's capability to self-regulate both internal processes and external forces *proactively* in specific areas of academic and athletic functioning, such as math or basketball playing.

Four signposts have been discerned on a social cognitive path to self-regulatory skill. When acquiring an academic or athletic skill at an *observational level*, learners must carefully watch a social model learn or perform (Rosenthal & Zimmerman, 1978; Zimmerman & Rosenthal, 1974). This first signpost involves discrimination of the correct form of the skill from a model's performance and descriptions, such as when a novice athlete can discern a difference between the golf swing of a professional and that of an amateur. Complete induction of a skill seldom emerges from a single exposure to a model's performance but usually requires repeated observation, especially across variations in task (Rosenthal & Zimmerman, 1976), such as seeing variations in golf swing based on the position of the ball and the club selected. A novice's motivation to learn at an observational level can be greatly enhanced by positive vicarious consequences to the model, such as an audience's applause for a golfer's fine play. Perceptions of personal similarity to a model increase the impact of consequences to that model vicariously on one's motivation (Brown & Inouye, 1978). In addition to conveying cognitive or motoric skill, expert models display implicit self-regulatory processes, such as adherence to performance standards, and motivational orientations and values (Schunk et al., 1987). For example, athletic models who self-correct their technique help observers to discriminate and rectify common errors. Such models also convey the high value placed on accurate speech and the need to persist in order to improve one's performance.

When acquiring a skill at an *emulation level*, the second signpost, a learner must duplicate the general form of a model's response on a correspondent task. Learners seldom copy the exact actions of the model; rather, they typically emulate the model's general pattern or style of functioning. Although learners can induce the major features of a complex skill from observation, they need performance experiences in order for the skill to become a behavioral reality. It is one thing to recognize the golf swing of a particular professional, but quite another thing to reproduce that swing oneself. Learners who emulate using a model's task can master basic response elements before contending with new task variations, which enhances their chances of a successful performance. Emulation can be improved through individualized modeling and social support. For example, during participant modeling (Bandura, 1986), a model repeats selected aspects of a skill based on a learner's emulative accuracy. As the learner acquires rudimentary aspects of a skill, the model will introduce more difficult compo-

nents. However, once an advanced level of mastery is attained, the model's support will be reduced. Although some critics have criticized modeling as a form of instruction, because of fears that it fosters response mimicry during emulation, these fears are largely unjustified because mimicry represents only a small part of emulative learning (Zimmerman & Rosenthal, 1974). Instead of duplicating a model's exact responses, observers primarily emulate the strategic features and blend them into their own repertoire of responses (Rosenthal, Zimmerman, & Durning, 1970).

When attaining a *self-controlled level* of self-regulatory skill, the third signpost, learners must practice it in structured settings outside the presence of models. To optimize learning at this level, learners should regulate their practice using representational standards (e.g., verbal recollections) of an expert model's pronunciation rather than direct observation of that model (Bandura & Jeffery, 1973). For example, students might rewrite a vague essay provided by their teacher using a model's strategy of inserting concrete examples for all abstract nouns. Learners' success in matching a covert standard during practice will determine the amount of self-reinforcement they will experience. Self-instruction, such as self-praise or self-critical statements, can help students encode and retrieve the strategy sequences during self-controlled learning (Meichenbaum & Beimiller, 1990), such as when the students reread their examples to judge their effectiveness. During third level practice sessions, learners who focus on fundamental processes or technique rather than on task outcomes are more successful in achieving *automaticity* (Zimmerman & Kitsantas, 1997, 1999), which is defined as the mastery of a model's technique. This automaticity is the most salient behavioral manifestation of the attainment of the third level of regulatory control. By focusing their practice goals on the strategic processes of proven models initially, novice learners can circumvent the frustrations of trial-and-error learning and can instead reinforce themselves for increasing motoric correspondence to this behavioral standard. By contrast, novices who focus on outcomes (e.g., the vagueness of an essay) before mastering fundamental techniques (e.g., the literary components of a compelling example) are expected to impair learning, because novices make ineffective process adjustments until they acquire self-evaluative expertise (Ellis & Zimmerman, 2001). Although regulation of a skill becomes covert at this level, it remains dependent on a representation of an external model's standard.

When acquiring a *self-regulated level* of task skill, the fourth signpost, learners should practice it in unstructured settings involving dynamic personal and contextual conditions. At this fourth level of skill, learners learn to make adjustments in their skill based on the outcomes of practice, such as whether an exemplification writing strategy reduces the vagueness of an essay. These mindful adaptations are made on the basis of self-monitored outcomes, such as the reaction of a reader, rather than on prior modeling experiences (Graham, Harris, & Troia, 1998). Learners' perceived efficacy in making these strategic adjustments influences their motivation to continue. At the fourth level, learners can practice with minimal process monitoring, and their attention can be shifted toward performance outcomes, without detrimental consequences, because the skill has become automatized at the prior level of self-regulation (LaBerge, 1981; Neves & Anderson, 1981). A self-regulated level of skill is acquired when learners can adapt their performance to changing personal conditions and outcomes. For learners to adapt their performance, they must discriminate key features of the transfer context, choose how to adapt their skill to that context, and monitor and evaluate the results. A behavioral manifestation of fourth level functioning is learners' development of their own distinctive styles of performing. Although social support is systematically reduced as learners acquire a self-regulatory level of skill, they continue to depend on social resources on a self-initiated basis, such as when they seek help from a coach (Murray, 1990). Because self-regulatory skill depends on context and outcomes, new performance tasks can uncover limitations in existing skills and require additional social learning experiences.

This multilevel formulation of self-regulation does not assume that learners must advance through the four levels in an invariant sequence, as developmental stage models assume, or that the fourth level is used universally once it is attained. Instead, a multilevel model assumes that individuals who master each skill level in sequence will learn more easily and effectively. We next turn to the issue of effectiveness of this formulation in both academic and athletic functioning.

EVIDENCE OF LEVELS IN ACQUISITION OF ACADEMIC AND ATHLETIC SKILL

To test the sequential validity of the first and second levels in the hierarchy, we compared the two primary sources of regulation for each level: modeling for the observation level, and performance and social feedback for the emulation level. In a study of writing revision (Zimmerman & Kitsantas, 2002), college students were asked to revise a series of sentences from commercially available sentence-combining workbooks. These exercises involved transforming a series of simple and often redundant sentences into a single, nonredundant sentence. For example, the sentences "It was a ball. The ball was striped. The ball rolled across the room" could be rewritten as "The striped ball rolled across the room." The mastery model performed flawlessly from the outset of the training, whereas the coping model initially made errors but gradually corrected them. Coping models are viewed as a qualitatively superior form of observational learning, because they convey self-regulatory actions, such as self-monitoring and self-correction, as well as writing revision skill. By contrast, mastery models portray primarily writing revision skill. Both modeling groups learned initially by observing an adult demonstrate a multistep-process writing revision strategy, whereas the no-modeling group learned only by hearing the multistep process described. Some members of each of the three experimental groups were given social feedback

Students in the two modeling groups that had the benefit of some form of observational learning significantly surpassed the revision skill of those who attempted to learn from only verbal description and performance outcomes. Students who observed the higher quality coping model outperformed students who observed the lower quality mastery model. In support of the theory, this writing study demonstrated that self-regulatory skills, such as self-monitoring and self-correcting actions of the coping model, were learned vicariously. As was hypothesized regarding enactive learning, social feedback improved writing skill for both forms of modeling. Once again, social feedback was insufficient for students in the no-modeling group to make up for their absence of vicarious experience. Finally, students exposed to both forms of modeling displayed higher levels of self-motivation, such as self-efficacy beliefs, than did students who relied on discovery and social feedback. These academic writing results confirmed the sequential advantages of engaging in observational learning before attempting enactive learning experiences.

In a similar study of athletic functioning of high school girls, Kitsantas, Zimmerman, and Cleary (2000) studied a high-quality coping modeling group, a lower quality mastery modeling group, and a no-modeling (enactive learning) group. The girls were taught a three-step strategy for throwing darts using coping or mastery models, or by verbal description and direct practice. Social feedback was given to some students in each experimental group. The results were supportive of a multilevel view of self-regulatory development. Adolescent girls in the two modeling groups significantly surpassed the dart-throwing skill of those who attempted to learn from only verbal description and performance outcomes. The coping model was significantly more effective than the mastery model, which indicates that the quality of the girls' observational learning experience influenced their development of athletic skill. During emulation, girls who received social feedback learned better than those who practiced on their own. However, the impact of this social feedback was insufficient in the no-modeling group to make up for the absence of vicarious experience. These results support the sequential advantage of engaging in observational learning before engaging in enactive learning experiences. Finally, girls exposed to observational learning from either form of modeling also showed higher levels of self-motivation, such as self-efficacy beliefs, than did students in the control group.

To test the sequentiality of the third and fourth levels of skill (i.e., self-control and

self-regulation) in the multilevel hierarchy, the two primary sources of regulation for these levels (i.e., process standards and outcomes) were compared. Recall that process goals are hypothesized to be optimal during acquisition at the self-control level, but outcome goals are expected to be superior during the acquisition at the self-regulation level. Zimmerman and Kitsantas (1999) tested the sequentiality of the third and fourth levels of the multi-level model with high school girls using the same writing revision task that was described above (Zimmerman & Kitsantas, 2002). These girls were initially taught the three steps of the revision strategy through observation and emulation (regulatory levels 1 and 2) that was described previously. During a practice session following training, girls in the process goal group focused on strategic steps for revising each writing task, whereas girls in the outcome goal group focused on decreasing the number of words in the revised passage. Some of the girls in each goal group were ask to self-record. The theoretically optimal group shifted from process goals to outcome goals when automaticity was achieved. Girls in the process-monitoring group recorded strategy steps they missed on each writing task, whereas girls in the outcome-monitoring group wrote down the number words used in each writing task. Girls in the shifting-goal group changed their method of self-monitoring when they shifted goals. Thus, the experiment compared the effects of process goals, outcome goals, and shifting goals, as well as self-recording during self-directed practice.

The results were consistent with a multilevel hierarchical view of goal setting: Girls who shifted goals from processes to outcomes after reaching level 4 (i.e., having achieved automaticity) surpassed the writing revision skill of girls who adhered exclusively to process goals or to outcome goals. Girls who focused on outcomes exclusively displayed the least writing skill, and self-recording enhanced writing acquisition for all goal-setting groups. In addition to their superior writing skill outcomes, girls who shifted their goals displayed advantageous forms of self-motivation, such as enhanced self-efficacy beliefs.

Zimmerman and Kitsantas (1997) used the same dart-throwing athletic task described earlier to examine the effectiveness of goal shifting during dart-throwing practice with high school girls. A process goal group focused on practicing the strategy steps for acquiring dart-throwing technique, whereas an outcome goal group focused on improving scores. The "bull's-eye" on the target had the highest numerical value, and the surrounding concentric circles gradually declined in value. The optimal goal-setting group from a multilevel perspective shifted from process goals to outcome goals when automaticity was achieved. Self-recording was taught to some girls in each goal group. Girls in the process-monitoring group recorded any strategy steps they may have missed on each practice throw, whereas girls in the outcome-monitoring group wrote down their target scores for each throw. Girls in the shifting-goal group changed their method of self-monitoring when they shifted goals. Before being asked to practice on their own, all of the high school girls were taught strategic components of the skill through observation and emulation (levels 1 and 2). The experiment compared the effects of process goals, outcome goals, and shifting goals, as well as self-recording during self-controlled practice. The results were supportive of a multilevel hierarchical view of goal setting: Girls who shifted goals developmentally from processes to outcomes surpassed classmates who adhered only to process goals or only outcome goals in posttest dart-throwing skill. Girls who focused on outcomes exclusively were the lowest in dart-throwing skill. Self-monitoring assisted learning for all goal-setting groups. In addition to their superior learning outcomes, students who shifted their goals displayed superior forms of self-motivation, such as self-efficacy beliefs.

CONCLUSIONS

Research on academic and athletic self-regulation reveals that an individual's development of optimal competence requires more than basic talent and high-quality instruction; it involves self-regulatory skill and accompanying self-motivational beliefs. This self-regulatory dimension of human competence, although often subtle, is pervasive in personal accounts of successful students, ex-

pert writers, and professional athletes. Donald Murray (1990) cautions novice writers about the hidden role of self-regulatory competence in successful writing: "Good writing does not reveal its making" (p. 5). "Getting writing done day in and day out, despite interruptions . . . is what separates the writer from the hope-to-be writer" (p. 15). In addition to anecdotal evidence from experts regarding the importance of key self-regulatory processes, there is extensive empirical evidence that learners' use of self-regulatory processes is highly predictive of their academic as well as athletic success. Furthermore, people's self-efficacy beliefs about their self-regulatory competence proved to be predictive of not only their use of self-regulatory processes but also their learning and performance outcomes.

The interrelation of various self-regulatory processes and self-motivational beliefs is explained in terms of three cyclical phases: forethought, performance, and self-reflection. Proactive learners, who engage in effective forethought, perform more effectively and experience more favorable self-reflections than reactive learners. Students' development of self-regulatory competence has been studied from a multilevel social cognitive perspective, and there is strong evidence that people who learn vicariously from self-regulatory models and adapt the model's techniques to their own personal functioning are more successful and better motivated than individuals who rely on asocial self-discovery. We believe this is vital information for the development of intervention programs designed to assist poorly motivated learners who are at academic and athletic risk.

ACKNOWLEDGMENT

We would like to thank Andrew J. Elliot and Carol S. Dweck for their helpful recommendations regarding a draft of this chapter.

REFERENCES

Abt, S. (July 29, 2001). Training, not racing, gives Armstrong his edge. *New York Times*, Section 8, pp. 1 and 7.

Ames, C. (1992). Achievement goals and the classroom motivational climate. In D. H. Schunk & J. L. Meece

(Eds.), *Student perceptions in the classroom* (pp. 327–348). Hillsdale, NJ: Erlbaum.

Anderson, P. (1997). *Great quotes from great sports heroes*. Franklin Lakes, NJ: Career Press.

Bandura, A. (1986). *Social foundations of thought and action: A social cognitive theory*. Englewood Cliffs, NJ: Prentice-Hall.

Bandura, A. (1991). Self-regulation of motivation through anticipatory and self-reactive mechanisms. In R. A. Dienstbier (Ed.), *Perspectives on motivation: Nebraska Symposium on Motivation* (Vol. 38, pp. 69–164). Lincoln: University of Nebraska Press.

Bandura, A. (1997). *Self-efficacy: The exercise of control*. New York: Freeman.

Bandura, A., & Jeffery, R. W. (1973). *Role* of symbolic coding and rehearsal processes in observational learning. *Journal of Personality and Social Psychology, 26,* 22–130.

Boerkaerts, M., & Niemivirta, M. (2000). Self-regulated learning: Finding a balance between learning goals and ego-protective goals. In M. Boekaerts, P. R. Pintrich, & M. Zeidner (Eds.), *Handbook of self-regulation* (pp. 417–451). San Diego: Academic Press.

Brown, I., Jr., & Inouye, D. K. (1978). Learned helplessness through modeling: The role of perceived similarity in competence. *Journal of Personality and Social Psychology, 36,* 900–908.

Burfoot, A. (1997). *Runner's World complete book of running*. Emmaus, PA: Rodale Press.

Butler, D. L. (1998). A strategic content learning approach to promoting self-regulated leaning by students with learning disabilities. In D. H. Schunk & B. J. Zimmerman (Eds.), *Self-regulated learning: From teaching to self-reflective practice* (pp. 160–183). New York: Guilford Press.

Carver, C., & Scheier, M. (2000). On the structure of behavioral self-regulation. In M. Boekaerts, P. Pintrich, & M. Zeidner (Eds.), *Self-regulation: Theory, research, and applications* (pp. 42–84). Orlando, FL: Academic Press.

Cleary, T., & Zimmerman, B. J. (2001). Self-regulation differences during athletic practice by experts, non-experts, and novices. *Journal of Applied Sport Psychology, 13,* 61–82.

Cleary, T. J., Zimmerman, B. J., & Keating, T. (2005). *Training novice athletes to self-regulate during basketball free-throw practice*. Manuscript submitted for publication.

Corno, L. (1993). The best-laid plans: Modern conceptions of volition and educational research. *Educational Researcher, 22*(2), 14–22.

Covington, M. (1992). *Making the grade: A self-worth perspective on motivation and school reform*. Cambridge, UK: Cambridge University Press.

Cowley, M. (1959). *Writers at work:* The Paris Review *interviews*. New York: Compass Books.

Deci, E. L. (1975). *Intrinsic motivation*. New York: Plenum Press.

De Corte, E., Verschaffel, L., & Op'T Eynde, P. (2000).

Self-regulation: A characteristic and a goal of mathematics education. In M. Boekaerts, P. R. Pintrich, & M. Zeidner (Eds.), *Handbook of self-regulation* (pp. 687–727). San Diego: Academic Press.

Dweck, C. S. (1988). Motivational processes affecting learning. *American Psychologist, 41,* 1040–1048.

Ellis, D., & Zimmerman, B. J. (2001). Enhancing self-monitoring during self-regulated learning of speech. In H. Hartman (Ed.), *Metacognition in teaching and learning* (pp. 205–228). New York: Kluwer Academic.

Ericsson, K. A. (1997). Deliberate practice and the acquisition of expert performance: An overview. In H. Jorgensen & A. C. Lehmann (Eds.), *Does practice make perfect?* (pp. 9–51). Stockholm: NIH Publikasjoner.

Ewing, M. E., & Seefeldt, V. (1995). Patterns of participation and attrition in American agency-sponsored youth sports. In F. L. Smoll & R. E. Smith (Eds.), *Children and youth in sport: A biopsychosocial perspective* (pp. 31–46). Dubuque, IA: Brown & Benchmark.

Feltz, D. L. (1992). Understanding motivation in sport: A self-efficacy perspective. In G. C. Roberts (Ed.), *Motivation in sport and exercise* (pp. 93–105). Champaign, IL: Human Kinetics.

Garcia, T., & Pintrich, P. R. (1994). Regulating motivation and cognition in the classroom: The role of self-schemas and self-regulatory strategies. In D. H. Schunk & B. J. Zimmerman (Eds.), *Self-regulation of learning and performance: Issues and educational applications* (p. 127–153). Hillsdale, NJ: Erlbaum.

Graham, S., Harris, K. R., & Troia, G. A. (1998). Writing and self-regulation: Cases from the self-regulated strategy development model. In D. H. Schunk & B. J. Zimmerman (Eds.), *Self-regulated learning: From teaching to self-reflective practice* (pp. 20–41). New York: Guilford Press.

Harackiewicz, J. M., Barron, K. E., Pintrich, P. R., Elliot, A. J., & Thrash, T. M. (2002). Revision of achievement goal theory: Necessary and illuminating. *Journal of Educational Psychology, 94,* 638–645.

Hogan, B., with Warren, H. (1957). *Five lessons: The modern fundamentals of golf*. New York: Simon & Schuster.

Horn, T. S., & Hasbrook, C. (1987). Psychological characteristics and the criteria children use for self-evaluation. *Journal of Sport Psychology, 9,* 208–221.

Jones, B. (1966). *Bobby Jones on golf*. Garden City, NY: Doubleday.

Kane, T. D., Marks, M. A., Zaccaro, S. J., & Blair, V. (1996). Self-efficacy, personal goals, and wrestlers' self-regulation. *Journal of Sport and Exercise Psychology, 18*(1), 36–48.

Kirchenbaum, D. S., O'Connor, E. A., & Owens, D. (1999). Positive illusions in golf: Empirical and conceptual analyses. *Journal of Applied Sport Psychology, 11,* 1–27.

Kitsantas, A., & Zimmerman, B. J. (2002). Comparing self-regulatory processes among novice, non-expert, and expert volleyball players: A microanalytic study. *Journal of Applied Sport Psychology, 14*, 91–105.

Kitsantas, A., Zimmerman, B. J., & Cleary, T. (2000). The role of observation and emulation in the development of athletic self-regulation. *Journal of Educational Psychology, 91*, 241–250.

Kuhl, J. (1985). Volitional mediators of cognitive behavior consistency: Self-regulatory processes and action versus state orientation. In J. Kuhl & J. Beckman (Eds.), *Action control* (pp. 101–128). New York: Springer.

LaBerge, D. (1981). Unitization and automaticity in perception. In J. H. Flowers (Ed.), *Nebraska Symposium on Motivation* (Vol. 28, pp. 53–71). Lincoln: University of Nebraska Press.

Lan, W. Y. (1996). The effects of self-monitoring on students' course performance, use of learning strategies, attitude, self-judgment ability and knowledge representation. *Journal of Experimental Education, 64*, 101–115.

Lan, W. Y. (1998). Teaching self-monitoring skills in statistics. In D. H. Schunk & B. J. Zimmerman (Eds.), *Self-regulated learning: From teaching to self-reflective practice* (pp. 86–105). New York: Guilford Press.

Lehrer, J. (2001, July 30). *The news hour with Jim Lehrer* [Televised program]. New York and Washington, DC: Public Broadcasting System.

Lens, W., Simons, J., & Dewitte, S. (2002). From duty to desire: The role of students' future time perspective and instrumentality perceptions for study motivation and self-regulation. In F. Pajares & T. Urdan (Eds.), *Academic motivation of adolescents* (Vol. 2, pp. 221–245). Greenwich, CT: Information Age.

Lepper, M. R., & Hodell, M. (1989). Intrinsic motivation in the classroom. In C. Ames & R. Ames (Eds.), *Research on motivation in education* (Vol. E, pp. 255–296). Hillsdale, NJ: Erlbaum.

Ley, K., & Young, D. B. (1998). Self-regulation behaviors in underprepared (developmental) and regular admission college students. *Contemporary Educational Psychology, 23*, 42–64.

Litsky, F. (August 6, 1999). Geena Davis zeros in with bow and arrows. *New York Times*, p. D4.

Locke, E. A., & Latham, G. P. (1990). *A theory of goal setting and task performance*. Englewood Cliffs, NJ: Prentice-Hall.

Loehr, J. E. (1991). *The mental game*. New York: Plume.

McCaffrey, N., & Orlick, T. (1989). Mental factors related to excellence among top professional golfers. *International Journal or Sports Psychology, 20*, 256–278.

Meichenbaum, D. (1977). *Cognitive-behavior modification: An integrative approach*. New York: Plenum Press.

Meichenbaum, D., & Beimiller, A. (1990, May). *In search of student expertise in the classroom: A meta-cognitive analysis*. Paper presented at the Conference on Cognitive Research for Instructional Innovation, University of Maryland, College Park, MD.

Moritz, S. E., Feltz, D. L., Fahrbach, K. R., & Mack, D. E. (2000). The relation of self-efficacy measures to sport performance: A meta-analytic review. *Research Quarterly for Exercise and Sport, 71*(3), 280–294.

Murray, D. M. (1990). *Write to learn* (3rd ed.). Fort Worth, TX: Holt, Rinehart & Winston.

Neves, D. M., & Anderson, J. R. (1981). Knowledge compilation: Mechanisms for the automatization of cognitive skills. In J. R. Anderson (Ed.), *Cognitive skills and their acquisitions* (pp. 463–562). Hillside, NJ: Erlbaum.

Newman, R. (1994). Academic help-seeking: A strategy of self-regulated learning. In D. H. Schunk & B. J. Zimmerman (Eds.), *Self-regulation of learning and performance: Issues and educational applications* (pp. 283–301). Hillsdale, NJ: Erlbaum.

Nicholls, J. (1984). Achievement motivation: Conceptions of ability, subjective experience, task choice, and performance. *Psychological Review, 91*, 328–346.

Nicklaus, J. (1992). *Jack Nicklaus' lesson tee*. New York: Simon & Schuster.

Pajares, F. (1996). Self-efficacy beliefs in achievement settings. *Review of Educational Research, 66*, 543–578.

Pressley, M. (1977). Imagery and children's learning: Putting the picture in developmental perspective. *Review of Educational Research, 47*, 586–622.

Purdie, N., & Hattie, J. (1996). Cultural differences in the use of strategies for self-regulated learning. *American Journal of Educational Research, 33*, 845–871.

Roberts, G. C. (1992). *Motivation in sport and exercise*. Champaign, IL: Human Kinetics.

Rosenthal, T. L., & Zimmerman, B. J. (1976). Organization and stability of transfer in vicarious concept attainment. *Child Development, 44*, 606–613.

Rosenthal, T. L., & Zimmerman, B. J. (1978). *Social learning and cognition*. New York: Academic Press.

Rosenthal, T. L., Zimmerman, B. J., & Durning, K. (1970). Observational induced changes in children's interrogative classes. *Journal of Personality and Social Psychology, 16*, 681–688.

Schunk, D. H. (1983). Progress self-monitoring: Effects on children's self-efficacy and achievement. *Journal of Experimental Education, 51*, 89–93.

Schunk, D. H. (1989). Social cognitive theory and self-regulated learning. In B. J. Zimmerman & D. H. Schunk (Eds.), *Self-regulated learning and academic achievement: Theory, research and practice* (pp. 137–159). Mahwah, NJ: Erlbaum.

Schunk, D. H. (1996). Goal and self-evaluative influences during children's cognitive skill learning. *American Educational Research Journal, 33*, 359–382.

Schunk, D. H., Hanson, A. R., & Cox, P. D. (1987). Peer model attributes and children's achievement behaviors. *Journal of Educational Psychology, 79,* 54–61.

Schunk, D. H., & Zimmerman, B. J. (1997). Social origins of self-regulatory competence. *Educational Psychologist, 32,* 195–208.

Smoll, F. L., Smith, R. E., Barnett, N. P., & Everett, J. J. (1993). Enhancement of children's self-esteem through social support training for youth sport coaches. *Journal of Applied Psychology, 78,* 602–610.

Snead, S., with Wade, D. (1989). *Better golf the Sam Snead way.* Chicago: Contemporary Books.

Vecsey, G. (September 3, 1999). Seles feels windy blast from past. *New York Times,* p. D1.

Wallace, I., & Pear, J. J. (1977). Self-control techniques of famous novelists. *Journal of Applied Behavior Analysis, 10,* 515–525.

Weiner, B. (1979). A theory of motivation for some classroom experiences. *Journal of Educational Psychology, 71,* 3–25.

Weinstein, C. E., & Mayer, R. E. (1986). The teaching of learning strategies. In M. C. Wittrock (Ed.), *Handbook of research on teaching* (3rd ed., pp. 315–327). New York: Macmillan.

Winne, P. H. (1997). Experimenting to bootstrap self-regulated learning. *Journal of Educational Psychology, 89,* 397–410.

Zimmerman, B. J. (1989). A social cognitive view of self-regulated academic learning. *Journal of Educational Psychology, 81,* 329–339.

Zimmerman, B. J. (1998). Academic studying and the development of personal skill: A self-regulatory perspective. *Educational Psychologist, 33,* 73–86.

Zimmerman, B. J. (2000). Attainment of self-regulation: A social cognitive perspective. In M. Boekaerts, P. Pintrich, & M. Zeidner (Eds.), *Self-regulation: Theory, research, and applications* (pp. 13–39). Orlando, FL: Academic Press.

Zimmerman, B. J., & Bandura, A. (1994). Impact of self-regulatory influences on writing course attainment. *American Educational Research Journal, 31,* 845–862.

Zimmerman, B. J., Bandura, A., & Martinez-Pons, M. (1992). Self-motivation for academic attainment: The role of self-efficacy beliefs and personal goal setting. *American Educational Research Journal, 29,* 663–676.

Zimmerman, B. J., & Campillo, M. (2003). Motivating self-regulated problem solvers. In J. E. Davidson & R. J. Sternberg (Eds.), *The nature of problem solving* (pp. 233–262). New York: Cambridge University Press.

Zimmerman, B. J., & Kitsantas, A. (1996). Self-regulated learning of a motoric skill: The role of goal setting and self-monitoring. *Journal of Applied Sport Psychology, 8,* 69–84.

Zimmerman, B. J., & Kitsantas, A. (1997). Developmental phases in self-regulation: Shifting from process to outcome goals. *Journal of Educational Psychology, 89,* 29–36.

Zimmerman, B. J., & Kitsantas, A. (1999). Acquiring writing revision skill: Shifting from process to outcome self-regulatory goals. *Journal of Educational, 91,* 1–10.

Zimmerman, B. J., & Kitsantas, A. (2002). Acquiring writing revision and self-regulatory skill through observation and emulation. *Journal of Educational Psychology, 94,* 660–668.

Zimmerman, B. J., & Martinez-Pons, M. (1986). Development of a structured interview for assessing students' use of self-regulated learning strategies. *American Educational Research Journal, 23,* 614–628.

Zimmerman, B. J., & Martinez-Pons, M. (1988). Construct validation of a strategy model of student self-regulated learning. *Journal of Educational Psychology, 80,* 284–290.

Zimmerman, B. J., & Martinez-Pons, M. (1990). Student differences in self-regulated learning: Relating grade, sex, and giftedness to self-efficacy and strategy use. *Journal of Educational Psychology, 82,* 51–59.

Zimmerman, B. J., & Paulsen, A. S. (1995). Self-monitoring during collegiate studying: An invaluable tool for academic self-regulation. In P. Pintrich (Ed.), *New directions in college teaching and learning: Understanding self-regulated learning* (No. 63, pp. 13–27). San Francisco: Jossey-Bass.

Zimmerman, B. J., & Rosenthal, T. L. (1974). Observational learning of rule governed behavior by children. *Psychological Bulletin, 81,* 29–42.

CHAPTER 28

☙

Engagement, Disengagement, Coping, and Catastrophe

CHARLES S. CARVER
MICHAEL F. SCHEIER

In 1992 Tom Pyszczynski and Jeff Greenberg published a book called *Hanging On and Letting Go*. That book was about processes behind depression. However, its title pointed to a fundamental and crucial division within human experience, with implications far broader than depression. On the one side of the division is a continuing engagement in the struggle to attain something desired, even when its attainment appears unlikely. It is easy to see this side as representing the exercise of motivation, a struggle for mastery in the short run, and for ever-greater competence in the long run. On the other side of the divide is giving up, ceasing the struggle, and releasing one's commitment to reaching the desired end.

Motivation, commitment, and the struggle for increased competence are a very important part of life. Little that is noteworthy has ever been accomplished without persistence in the face of setbacks, obstacles, and difficulties. Western society justifiably places great stock in hard work and the belief that diligence (along with ingenuity) can overcome whatever obstacles arise.

Yet holding on, continuing to try, is not *all* of life. Letting go is also important (Carver & Scheier, 2003; Wrosch, Scheier, Carver, & Schulz, 2003). People all need to give up sometimes. A key decision in life, which is made over and over in a wide variety of contexts, is when to hang on and when to let go. That decision is made with regard to very broad and important areas of life (e.g., whether to give up an unreachable career aspiration or a failed relationship), and it is also made on a much smaller scale (e.g., whether to keep trying for an A in a course, or whether to keep trying to solve a particular word puzzle). The ability to make these decisions wisely and well represents another sort of competence.

The divergence between these two orientations to a goal—engagement in its pursuit versus disengagement and abandonment of it—is the subject of this chapter. Our view is that these are both necessary parts of life, and that the forces inducing one or the other of these orientations are natural aspects of self-regulation. We begin with a brief overview of a broader conceptual framework within which we then address this distinction.

CONCEPTUAL OVERVIEW

We believe that intentional behavior is the attempt to make something occur in action that is already held in mind (Carver & Scheier, 1981, 1998). This view of behavior provides the basis for our use of the term "self-regulation." When we use this term, we intend to convey several things. One is that people's actions are purposive (even if the purpose is sometimes hard to identify by observers, or even by the actors themselves). Another is that self-corrective adjustments of the action occur as needed, to keep the action on track for the purpose being served. Yet another is that the corrective adjustments originate within the person. These ideas converge in the view that behavior is a continual process of moving toward (and sometimes away from) goal values, and that

this movement embodies the characteristics of feedback control.

Goals and Feedback Loops

This view converges in many respects with the interest in goal constructs in today's personality and social psychology (Austin & Vancouver, 1996; Elliott & Dweck, 1988; Emmons, 1986; Higgins, 1987, 1996; Markus & Nurius, 1986; Read & Miller, 1989; Pervin, 1982, 1989). Different theorists have their own distinct points of emphasis (for broader discussions, see Austin & Vancouver, 1996; Carver & Scheier, 1998, 1999a; Pervin, 1989), but they also have many similarities. All convey the sense that goals give direction to behavior, thus making the goal a key motivational concept. Indeed, in this view, the self is partly made up of the person's goals and the organization among them (cf. Mischel & Shoda, 1995).

How goals are used to produce behavior can be described in many ways. As indicated earlier, we think of the process in terms of feedback loops (Figure 28.1). A feedback loop (Miller, Galanter, & Pribram, 1960; MacKay, 1966; Powers, 1973; Wiener,

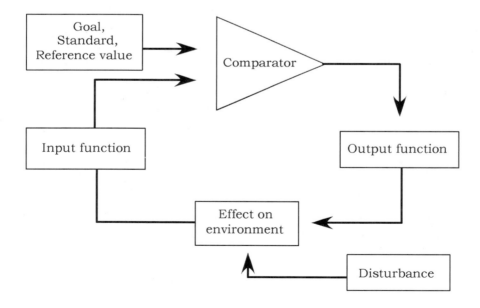

FIGURE 28.1. Schematic depiction of a feedback loop, the basic unit of cybernetic control. In a discrepancy-reducing loop, a sensed value is compared to a reference value or standard, and adjustments occur in an output function (if necessary) that shift the sensed value in the direction of the standard. In a discrepancy-enlarging loop, the output function moves the sensed value away from the standard.

1948) is an organization of four elements: an input function, a reference value, a comparator, and an output function. An input function (which we treat as equivalent to perception) brings information about an existing state into the system. A reference value is a second source of information, coming from within the system. We treat goals as a particular kind of reference value.

A comparator, the next element, is something that compares the input to the reference value. This yields one of two outcomes. Either the values being compared are discriminably different or they're not. (Either you're doing what you intended to do, or you're not.) The degree of discrepancy detected is sometimes referred to as an "error signal," with more error implying greater discrepancy. (The idea that error detection is fundamental to living systems is echoed in evidence that negative events [which imply discrepancies] draw attention; see Baumeister, Bratslavsky, Finkenauer, & Vohs, 2001.)

After the comparison comes an output function, which we treat as equivalent to behavior (though sometimes the behavior is internal). If the comparison yields "no difference," the output function remains as it was. If the comparison yields a judgment of "discrepancy," the output function changes. Change in the output changes the existing situation in some way. This in turn changes the input. The loop of information thus is closed, and the cycle continues.

There are two kinds of feedback loops, which differ in their overall function. In a *discrepancy-reducing* loop, the output function acts to reduce or eliminate any discrepancy noted between input and reference value. It keeps the error signal as low as possible. Such an effect is seen in human behavior in the attempt to attain a valued goal, or to conform to a standard. In a *discrepancy-enlarging* loop, the reference value is a value to avoid. It may be convenient to think of it as an "anti-goal." A discrepancy-enlarging loop senses existing conditions, compares them to the anti-goal, and acts to enlarge the discrepancy. Psychological examples of anti-goals are a feared or disliked possible self (Carver, Lawrence, & Scheier, 1999; Markus & Nurius, 1986; Ogilvie, 1987), interpersonal rejection, and a spoiled public image. Each of these is a condition to be avoided.

Enlarging a discrepancy thus is an avoidance process.

The action of discrepancy-enlarging processes in living systems is typically constrained by discrepancy-reducing processes. To put it differently, acts of avoidance often lead into compatible acts of approach (Figure 28.2). An avoidance loop tries to increase distance from an anti-goal. But there often is an approach goal (or even more than one) in nearby psychological space. If one is noticed and adopted, the tendency to escape from the anti-goal is joined by a tendency to move toward the goal. The approach loop pulls subsequent behavior into its orbit.

These two kinds of feedback processes have been found in many kinds of physical systems, ranging from physiological to social, ethological, and economic. The broad existence of such forces in multiple, diverse kinds of systems is one reason we have been drawn to the idea that the feedback concept has utility in thinking about behavior. For our present purposes, though, the main points are fairly simple. Discrepancy reduction is an approach process. Discrepancy enlargement is an avoidance process.

The idea that behavior is organized around approaching and avoiding is by no means novel. Approach and avoidance processes have been postulated on a variety of theoretical grounds over many years (cf. Miller, 1944; Miller & Dollard, 1941). These functions have recently come to the fore yet again, in a family of theories rooted in neuropsychology and conditioning. A system managing incentive motivation and approach has been postulated by a number of biologically oriented theorists, variously called the "Behavioral Activation System" (Cloninger, 1987; Fowles, 1980), the "Behavioral Approach System" (Gray, 1981, 1987, 1994), and the "Behavioral Facilitation System" (Depue & Collins, 1999). A system managing aversive motivation and withdrawal from or avoidance of aversive stimuli has been called the "Behavioral Inhibition System" (Cloninger, 1987; Gray, 1981, 1987, 1994), and "Withdrawal System" (Davidson, 1984, 1992a, 1992b, 1995).

These theories stand at a different level of abstraction than the ideas that were discussed just previously. These theories deal

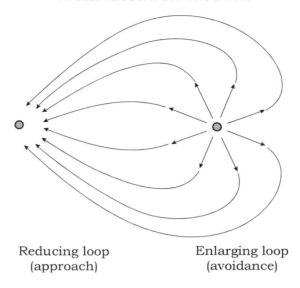

Reducing loop
(approach)

Enlarging loop
(avoidance)

FIGURE 28.2. The effects of discrepancy-enlarging feedback systems are often bounded or constrained by discrepancy-reducing systems. A value moves away from an undesired condition in a deviation-amplifying loop, and then comes under the influence of a discrepancy-reducing loop, moving toward its desired value. Adapted from Carver and Scheier (1998). Copyright 1998 by Cambridge University Press. Adapted by permission.

with neurobiological structures and how those structures may be involved in behavior. However, the two sets of ideas seem very compatible. The feedback loop is a more abstract construct. It might be viewed as being, in effect, a metatheory that is applicable to both neurobiology and other domains in which feedback influences occur.

Another comparison is also instructive. Most of the chapters in this volume are organized around the idea that people are motivated by the desire for increased competence. The authors of those chapters move from that starting assumption to consider some of the issues that follow from it. We, in contrast, are describing here a way of viewing the self-regulation of behavior *in general*. Some behaviors surely represent efforts to extend competence, but not all do, except in a limited sense. That is, we assume that the human organism continuously strives to make better predictions of events in the world (Carver & Scheier, 1999b). We assume that this is an operating characteristic of the organism, an aspect of the workings of our cognitive machinery. We believe (consistent with Piaget, 1963) that these tendencies result in greater elaboration, organization (integration of simple processes into a more complex whole), and adaptation. Do they therefore represent a striving for competence? Perhaps, but it is often an implicit rather than an explicit striving.

Affect

Overt behavior is important, but not all-important. Also important in human experience is affect. Just as behavior displays fundamental regularities, so does affect, or emotion. Affects serve as self-regulatory controls on what actions take place and with how much urgency (Carver & Scheier, 1990, 1998). Affect sometimes keeps people immersed in the actions they are now engaged in. Affect sometimes leads people to cease their actions.

What is affect, and where does it come from? It is widely held that affect pertains to one's desires and whether they are being met (e.g., Clore, 1994; Frijda, 1986, 1988; Ortony, Clore, & Collins, 1988). But what exactly is the internal process by which feelings arise? Answers to that question can also take any of several forms, ranging from neurobiological (e.g., Davidson 1984, 1992b, 1995) to cognitive (Ortony et al., 1988). We have suggested an answer (Carver & Scheier,

1990, 1998, 1999a, 1999b) that focuses on some of the functional properties of affect. Again we use feedback control as an organizing principle. But now the feedback control bears on a different quality than it did earlier.

We have suggested that feelings arise as a consequence of a feedback process that operates automatically, simultaneously with the behavior-guiding process, and in parallel to it. Perhaps the easiest way to convey what this second process is doing is to say that it's checking on how well the first process (the behavior loop) is doing *its* job. The input for this second loop thus is some representation of the *rate of discrepancy reduction in the action system over time* (we limit ourselves at first to discrepancy-reducing action loops).

Input by itself does not create affect (a given rate of progress has different affective effects in different circumstances). We believe that, as in any feedback system, this input is compared to a reference value (cf. Frijda, 1986, 1988). In this case, the reference is an acceptable or desired rate of behavioral discrepancy reduction. As in other feedback loops, the comparison checks for deviation from the standard. If there is a discrepancy, the output function changes.

We believe that the error signal in this loop is manifest phenomenologically as affect, a sense of positive or negative valence regarding the action taking place. If the rate of progress is below the criterion, negative affect arises. If the rate is high enough to exceed the criterion, positive affect arises. If the rate is not distinguishable from the criterion, no affect arises.

In essence, the argument is that positive feelings mean you are doing better at something than you intend to, and negative feelings mean you are doing worse than you intend to (for more detail, including a review of evidence on the link between this "velocity" function and affect, see Carver & Scheier, 1998, Chapters 8 and 9). One direct implication of this line of thought is that the affects that might potentially arise regarding any given action domain should fall along a bipolar dimension. That is, for a given action, affect can be positive, neutral, or negative, depending on how well or poorly the action is going.

Now consider discrepancy-enlarging action loops. The view just outlined rests on the idea that positive feelings occur when a behavioral system is making rapid progress in doing what it is organized to do. The systems considered thus far are organized to reduce discrepancies. There is no obvious reason, though, why the principle should not also apply to systems organized to enlarge discrepancies. If that kind of a system is doing well at what it is organized to do, there should be positive affect. If it is doing poorly, there should be negative affect.

The idea that affects of both valences can occur would seem applicable to both approach and avoidance systems. That is, both approach and avoidance have the potential to induce positive feelings (by doing well), and both have the potential to induce negative feelings (by doing poorly). But doing well at moving *toward an incentive* is not quite the same as doing well at moving *away from a threat*. Thus, the two positives may not be quite the same, nor the two negatives.

This line of thought, along with insights from Higgins (e.g., 1987, 1996) and his collaborators, has led us to argue for the existence of two bipolar affect dimensions (Carver, 2001; Carver & Scheier, 1998). One dimension relates to the system that manages the approach of incentives, the other to the system that manages the avoidance of, or withdrawal from, threat. The dimension pertaining to approach (in its "purest" form) includes affects such as elation, eagerness, and excitement on the positive side and frustration, sadness, and dejection on the negative side. The dimension related to avoidance (in its "purest" form) includes affects such as fear and anxiety on the negative side and relief, serenity, and contentment on the positive side.

The view we have taken implies a natural link between affect and action. If the input function of the affect loop is a sensed rate of progress in action, the output function must be a change in the rate of that action. Thus, the affect loop intrinsically has a direct influence on what occurs in the action loop. The latter controls what might be thought of as the person's "position," whereas the former controls what might be thought of as the person's "velocity." Action-managing loops handle the directional function of motivation (choosing specific actions from among many options, keeping the action on track). Affect-related loops handle the intensity function of motivation (the vigor, enthusiasm, effort, concentration, or thoroughness with which the action is pursued).

Two Aspects of Approach-Related Negative Affect

We said a little earlier that affect sometimes keeps people immersed in the actions they are now engaged in, and that affect sometimes leads people to cease their actions. What did we mean by that? In answering this question, we focus on negative affects (for discussion of positive affects see Carver, 2003). Furthermore, for the sake of clarity, we restrict ourselves here to *negative affects that are tied to goal-seeking efforts*—approach processes (a parallel line of argument applies to avoidance processes, but we do not talk about avoidance here).

Our argument is that falling behind in a goal-seeking effort creates negative affect. More specifically, this experience gives rise to feelings such as frustration, irritation, and even anger (Carver, 2004). The lagging of progress, or the affect thereby created, prompts an increase in exertion, an effort to catch up. Thus, these negative feelings (or the mechanism that underlies them) keep the person immersed in the ongoing action and engage the person's effort more fully (for findings that fit this view, see Harmon-Jones, Sigelman, Bohling, & Harmon-Jones, 2003; Lewis, Sullivan, Ramsay, & Allessandri, 1992; Mikulincer, 1988). Such effort often allows the person to increase movement toward the goal and make attaining the goal seem likely again. Consistent with this view, Frijda (1986, p. 429) has argued that anger as an emotion implies a hope that things can be set right (see also Harmon-Jones & Allen, 1998).

Sometimes, however, continued efforts do not have the desired effect. Indeed, if the situation involves loss, movement forward is precluded. When there is a loss, the goal is gone. These cases are more extreme than those described in the preceding paragraph. When failure seems assured or a loss has occurred, the negative affect has a different tone than in the case described in the preceding paragraph. Here, the feelings are sadness, depression, dejection, and grief (in-

deed, Finlay-Jones & Brown, 1981, and others have linked loss to clinical depression). Accompanying behaviors also differ. Rather than continue to struggle, the person tends to disengage from further effort toward the goal (Klinger, 1975; Wortman & Brehm, 1975; for supporting evidence, see Lewis et al., 1992; Mikulincer, 1988).

At least two studies have found patterns of affective responses that are consistent with this portrayal (Mikulincer, 1994; Pittman & Pittman, 1980). In these studies, participants had varying amounts of failure, and their emotional responses were assessed. In both studies, reports of anger were most intense after small amounts of failure and lower after larger amounts of failure. Reports of depression were low after small amounts of failure and intense after larger amounts of failure.

Thus, these two kinds of situations create two different kinds of negative feelings, which relate to opposite shifts in behavior. Although the behavioral shifts are opposite to each other, we believe they both have adaptive properties. In the first case (when the person falls behind but the goal is not seen as lost), feelings of frustration and anger yield an increase in effort, a struggle to gain the goal despite the setbacks. This struggle is adaptive (and the affect is adaptive) because that struggle can foster goal attainment.

In the second, more extreme situation, when effort is futile, feelings of sadness and grief yield *reduction* of effort. Sadness and despondency imply that things cannot be set right, that further effort is pointless. Reduction of effort in this circumstance also has adaptive functions (cf. Wrosch et al., 2003). It serves to conserve energy rather than waste it in futile pursuit of the unattainable (Nesse, 2000). If it also helps diminish commitment to the goal (Klinger, 1975), it eventually readies the person to take up pursuit of another incentive in place of this one.

Continued Effort and Giving Up

These two functions that we believe correspond to two kinds of approach-related negative affect take us to the heart of the theme of this chapter. The first class of affect (frustration, anger) is a precursor to (or a concomitant of) continued or even increased effort toward goal attainment. The second class of affect (sadness, despondency) is a precursor to (or a concomitant of) giving up.

Our interest in the tension between effort and giving up is reflected in this analysis of affect. It did not begin there, however. We were interested in this issue much earlier, before our analysis of affect had been developed. Some of our earliest work examined influences on people's responses to adversity when they worked on difficult laboratory tasks (Carver & Scheier, 1981). We found that sometimes when things are going poorly people keep trying, continue to struggle. Sometimes when things are going poorly they stop trying, reduce their efforts.

We have long held that this difference in behavioral response rests on a difference in *confidence versus doubt* about reaching the desired goal. Our view thus is one of a long tradition of expectancy–value theories (e.g., Atkinson, 1964; Bandura, 1997; Feather, 1982; Klinger, 1975; Kuhl, 1984; Kukla, 1972; Lewin, 1948; Shah & Higgins, 1997; Snyder, 1994; Vroom, 1964; Wright & Brehm, 1989). Given enough confidence, a person will continue to try, even in the face of obstacles and setbacks. Given enough doubt, the person will stop trying. It is clear that there is a link between affect and confidence—indeed, they may both reflect the same error signal. But we suspect that the link is less than perfect.

Interest in how this more cognitive sense of confidence or doubt influences behavior was what first led us to think about the contrast between engagement and disengagement. We examined both naturally occurring and experimentally manipulated expectancies. For example, in one study we subjected everyone to an initial failure experience, and then let them work on another task. We led some to expect to be able to make up for that failure on a second task, and led others to expect more failure. These manipulated expectancies were reflected in participants' subsequent persistence at what actually was an impossible task. Those expecting to be able to perform well tried longer than those expecting to perform more poorly. Other studies found that expectancies influenced actual performances on tasks and the seeking out of information about the tasks (Carver & Scheier, 1981, 1998). In all cases, greater confidence related to more en-

gagement, and doubt related to disengagement.

Our interest in confidence and engagement versus doubt and disengagement led us into several research literatures. We have explored this issue in focused domains, such as test anxiety, where some people have more difficulty than others performing in line with their wishes (Carver & Scheier, 1981). We found, for example, that people who are high in test anxiety are prone to disengage from their task efforts into off-task thinking, and therefore perform more poorly. They are also more likely to skip from item to item, in search of easy answers, and to be correspondingly less persistent at a given item. A similar pattern linking negative expectancies to decreases in effort has recently been found in university athletes (Hatzigeorgiadis & Biddle, 2001). We have also used the same line of reasoning to explore how people respond to health threats, in their coping efforts and their psychological well-being (Carver & Scheier, 2002; Scheier & Carver, 2003).

In this work on responses to health threats, we have also explored how this line of reasoning applies in people's broad orientation to the full range of life's experiences—their generalized sense of optimism versus pessimism (Scheier & Carver, 1992). Optimism and pessimism are confidence and doubt writ large, bearing on the person's entire life space. It appears that the same behavioral tendencies—engagement versus disengagement—flow from optimism and pessimism, just as they do from more focused confidence and doubt (Scheier & Carver, 2003; Scheier, Carver, & Bridges, 2001).

In particular, optimists appear to engage in coping responses that reflect a continued engagement with their goals, and with life more generally. A variety of research (reviewed in Scheier et al., 2001) has shown that people who are optimistic report more problem-focused coping (particularly when the situation is seen as potentially controllable), more acceptance of the reality of adverse circumstances, and more positive reframing of the situation, thereby maintaining their positive expectancies for being able to resolve the problems. In contrast, people who are more pessimistic report greater tendencies to deny the reality of the situation, as though they can somehow escape its existence by wishful thinking. They are more likely to do things that provide temporary distractions but don't help solve the problem. Sometimes they even report giving up trying to cope. All of these responses look very much like disengagement.

Giving Up and Avoidance

Effort and giving up create the potential for great complexity. However, reality is even more complex. Before continuing, we must make one more distinction to avoid confusion. Then, we place a limit on what is discussed in the rest of the chapter.

The distinction is between disengagement and avoidance. Earlier in the chapter, we described avoidance as an active effort to increase the distance between oneself and an anti-goal. We want to be clear that we regard that process as different from what occurs when a failure of approach leads to giving up. Giving up is a sinking away from effort. It is not an active attempt to distance oneself from a reference value. The surface topography of the physical actions that these processes induce can (in some circumstances) be very similar. The underlying processes, however, are not the same.

Thinking of approach and avoidance together gets very tricky in many areas of discussion, such as achievement. As we noted earlier (Figure 28.2), avoidance processes sometimes lead into compatible approach processes. For example, one way to avoid failure is to approach success (Atkinson, 1957). For that reason, a person who is motivated mostly by the desire to avoid failure at an achievement task may display strong effort when engaged in that task. That behavior can look a lot like the behavior of a person who is interested only in attaining success and is totally unconcerned with avoidance. But the motivational situations for the two people are not the same. The emotions they experience are likely to differ (Higgins, Shah, & Friedman, 1997, Study 4), and some of the strategies they use may also differ (Elliot & McGregor, 2001).

In truth, it is likely that most human behavior involves blends of approach and avoidance motivations. Analysis of how the two motivational bases for the same action lead to different experiences is potentially very important. However, that goal is beyond the scope of our undertaking here. For our present purposes, we disregard that complicating factor. Instead, from here onward, we focus exclusively on issues arising in approach processes.

Functions of Engagement and Giving Up

We said earlier that persistence in approach and giving up of approach are both important. Let us return to that assertion and expand upon it. It is easy to grasp that commitment, confidence, and persistence are keys to success. Expectancy–value motive models hold that people who are confident remain committed to their valued goals, remain engaged in attempts to move forward, even when effort thus far has been futile. Discussions framed in expectancy–value terms typically emphasize this idea: that continued effort can result in attainments.

That emphasis is quite reasonable, given that many of these theories have roots in analyses of achievement behavior. Much of the interest behind theories of achievement behavior is in the resulting achievement. Indeed, many who are interested in achievement behavior are interested more specifically in how achievement can be maximized. It is certainly true that a person who gives up whenever encountering difficulty will never accomplish anything. To accomplish things, people need to persist when confronting obstacles.

There are also reasons, however, why disengagement is sometimes a good idea. The simplest reason, described earlier, is that a person trying unsuccessfully to reach a goal experiences distress. This is true both in small-scale goal pursuit and in life's big picture (Wrosch et al., 2003). With respect to the big picture, lifespan development theorists point out that successful development inevitably requires people to make choices about which goals to continue pursuing and which to give up (Schulz & Heckhausen, 1996). A very basic reason why some goals should be abandoned concerns the biological resources available at different phases of the lifespan (Baltes, Cornelius, & Nesselroade, 1979; Heckhausen & Schulz, 1995). During early childhood, cognitive and physical abilities are limited. As the child grows, so do the abilities. The growth plateaus; then there is a decline in old age. This cycle of growth and decline limits what goals are within reach at any given point in the life course. If the resources are lacking, the goal cannot be attained. In the same way, goal attainment is sometimes limited by genetic potential. For example, to become a professional athlete is very unlikely for someone who lacks the physical attributes required by a particular sport. More simply, some goals are out of reach no matter how hard you try.

Another constraint is the limit placed by the time available in a person's life. Whatever is to be achieved or experienced in life must be done in a finite period of time. The acquisition of skills, knowledge, and expertise takes time (Ericsson & Charness, 1994). Thus, the person is constrained in the extent to which functioning can be maximized in multiple domains. To be committed to attaining excellence in many diverse life domains thus can be a set-up for distress, because there are only so many hours in a day, and so many days in a life.

In both the short term and the long term,

then, disengagement from certain goals plays an important function. Yet despite this, people sometimes keep struggling for things that seem unattainable. When something is important to them, people often will struggle well past the point where the goal has been lost. Why? In order to address that question properly, we need one more idea, the notion of hierarchicality.

Hierarchicality

Actions can take place at many different levels of abstraction (Powers, 1973; Vallacher & Wegner, 1987). You can try to be a successful person in your chosen profession, but you can also try to make a paragraph you are writing make sense (which entails the even more concrete attempt to hit the right keys on the computer with just the right amount of pressure). Thus, it is often said that actions (and the goals to which they relate) form a hierarchy (Carver & Scheier, 1998; Powers, 1973; Vallacher & Wegner, 1987). Abstract goals are attained by attaining the concrete goals that help define them (Figure 28.3).

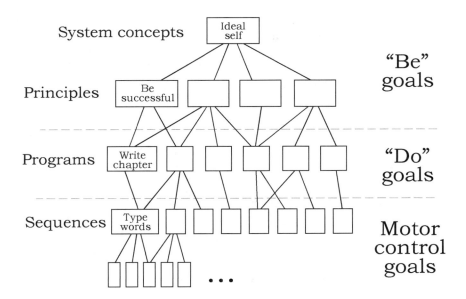

FIGURE 28.3. A hierarchy of goals (or of feedback loops). Lines indicate the contribution of lower level goals to specific higher level goals. They can also be read in the opposite direction, indicating that a given higher order goal specifies more concrete goals at the next lower level. The hierarchy described in text involves goals of "being" particular ways, which are attained by "doing" particular actions. Adapted from Carver and Scheier (1998). Copyright 1998 by Cambridge University Press. Adapted by permission.

What makes one goal matter more than another? Generally, the higher in the hierarchy a goal is, the more important it is—the more central to the overall sense of self. Concrete action goals (at lower levels) acquire importance from the fact that attaining them serves the attainment of broader, more abstract goals (Carver & Scheier, 1998, 1999a, 1999b; Powers, 1973; Vallacher & Wegner, 1985). The stronger the link between a given concrete goal and a deep value of the self, the more important is that concrete goal.

It is easy to disengage from unimportant goals. Important ones are hard to disengage from, for a very good reason. *Giving them up creates a disruption (an enlarging discrepancy) with respect to higher level core values of the self.* In light of the affect model described earlier, that disruption can be expected to create distress. Thus, if a concrete action goal is very important because of the nature of the self's organization, giving up on it is painful. For example, giving up the dream of becoming a surgeon after being unable to get into a medical school or being unable to do the required work successfully can shake one's self-image to its core. Indeed, giving up sometimes is even harder than that. Giving up the effort to combat a life-threatening illness means giving up on one's life.

It follows that one influence on engagement and persistence is likely to be the goal's importance. That is, all other things being equal, people are likely to struggle longer and harder to reach an important goal than to reach a goal that is less important. This greater persistence should occur despite the fact that the distress resulting from failing to approach an important goal should also be greater.

In some cases, it is possible to diminish the disruption that occurs at the higher level when giving up at a lower level, and thereby reduce the distress. This is because people often can satisfy the same higher order goal by engaging in diverse concrete activities. For an academic psychologist, many actions serve as pathways for making a contribution to one's profession, including doing and reporting original research, editing books that bring together several people's research, serving on committees in professional organizations, serving as a journal editor, serving

as a department chair, and writing textbooks.

The pathways to a given high order goal sometimes compensate for one another, so that if progress in one path is impeded, the person can shift efforts to a different one (Figure 28.4, Path 1). If one path is disrupted, another path may be taken instead, and indeed may become more important over time. By taking up an attainable alternative, the person remains engaged in progress toward the high-order goal. Although the process of switching pathways is not always free of distress, the end result is far less distress than if the person had remained committed to the initial pathway and been unable to move forward on it.

Sometimes people do not turn to alternative paths that are already in place. They step outside their existing framework and develop new paths, take up new activities they have never done before. There are many ways in which this can occur, but they may share a common element. We believe that the newly adopted activity is very likely to be one that contributes to the expression of some preexisting core aspect of the self (Carver & Scheier, 1999b). Thus, the effect of the new activity is to continue to foster the preexisting core value (Figure 28.4, Path 2).

Sometimes disengagement entails shifting from one concrete activity to another, but other times it involves something more subtle: scaling back from a lofty goal in a given domain to a less lofty one. This is a disengagement, in the sense that the person is giving up the first goal while adopting the lesser one (Figure 28.4, Path 3). It is more a limited disengagement than the cases already considered, in the sense that it does not entail leaving the behavioral domain. This shift keeps the person engaged in activity in the same domain that he or she had wanted to quit. By scaling back the goal (giving up in a small way), the person keeps trying to move ahead—thus *not* giving up, in a larger way. The person thereby retains the sense of purpose in activities in that domain.

It should be apparent from this discussion that some instances of specific goal disengagement serve the paradoxical function of helping the person to continue efforts toward higher order values. This is particularly obvious with regard to concrete goals for which disengagement has little or no cost: People remove themselves from blind alleys and wrong streets, give up plans that have been disrupted by unexpected events, and go away and come back later if the store is closed.

The same is also true, however, with regard to goals that are deeply connected to the self. Distress is lessened if one responds to the loss of a close relationship by letting it go (Field, Gal-Oz, & Bonanno, 2003; Orbuch, 1992; Stroebe, Stroebe, & Hansson, 1993), but especially if one has other ways to satisfy core relationship needs. Similarly, the adverse impact of a disrupted career path can be lessened if the person can isolate what made that career so appealing, and

find another career that also satisfies that desire. People need multiple paths to the core values of the self (cf. Linville, 1987; Showers & Ryff, 1996). That way, if one path becomes blocked or washed away, the person can jump to another one.

Not every disengagement serves this adaptive function, of course. In some cases, there appears to exist no alternative goal. In such a case, disengagement is not accompanied by a shift, because there is nothing to which to shift. This is the perhaps worst situation, where there is nothing to take the place of what is seen as unattainable. If the commitment to the unattainable goal wanes and there is no substitute, the result is simply emptiness (Figure 28.4, Path 4).

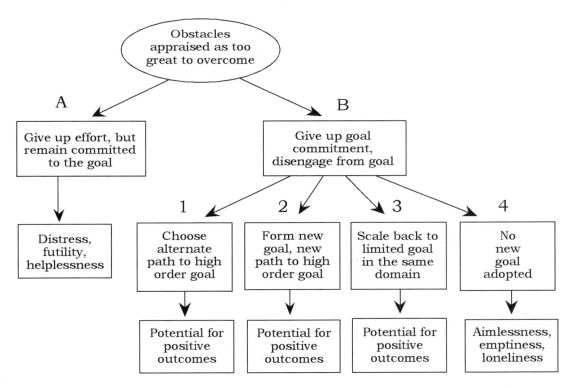

FIGURE 28.4. Responses to the perception that a goal is unattainable. The person (A) can remain committed to the goal and experience distress or (B) can dissolve the commitment and disengage from the goal. Disengagement has four potential patterns: (1) Choosing an alternative path to the same higher order value produces a situation in which positive outcomes and feelings are possible; (2) choosing a new goal yields a situation in which positive outcomes and feelings are possible; (3) scaling back aspirations while remaining in the same domain creates a situation in which positive outcomes and feelings are possible; (4) giving up commitment without turning to another goal, however, results in feelings of emptiness. From Carver and Scheier (2003). Copyright 2003 by the American Psychological Association. Reprinted by permission.

In general, disengagement appears to be an adaptive response *when it leads to—or is tied to—the taking up of other goals* (cf. Aspinwall & Richter, 1999; Wrosch, Scheier, Miller, Schulz, & Carver, 2003). By taking up an attainable alternative, the person remains engaged in activities that have meaning for the self, and life continues to have purpose.

Whenever one talks about disengagement and reengagement in a different pathway to a similar end, the issue of perceived competence emerges. People do not take up a particular pathway unless they feel they are competent to travel that path. Although there are many determinants of the choice of path, perceptions of the match between the demands of the path and the person's competencies play an important role. Thus, as an example, some psychologists serve their profession by serving as department heads, others by serving as editors.

GRADATIONS, BIFURCATIONS, AND CATASTROPHES

We turn now to a different issue. The dialectic between engagement and disengagement can be viewed in several different ways. The simplest way is to construe effort or even commitment as a linear continuum. In this view, task performance (or persistence, or effort) may be viewed as a reflection of the degree of the person's engagement with the task, with more engagement yielding better outcomes. This is the view that seems implicit, for example, in Bandura's model of the effects of self-efficacy (e.g., Bandura, 1997). People with a strong conviction that they can do something try harder at it than do people who lack that conviction, and the greater effort yields better outcomes. This linearly increasing view is readily applied to some contexts. However, there are also contexts in which it does not fit so well. In this section, we consider possibilities of greater complexity.

We have long held that there is a psychological watershed among responses to adversity—that is, that the responses diverge (Carver & Scheier, 1981) or (to use a currently more fashionable term) bifurcate, forming two categories. One class of responses reflects continued effort. The other

reflects disengagement of effort. Just as rainwater falling on a mountain ridge ultimately flows to one side of the ridge or the other, so do behaviors ultimately flow to one or the other of these classes. We took this position over two decades ago largely because of findings that self-focus has opposite effects on behavior as a function of confidence versus doubt. We are not the only ones to have emphasized a disjunction among these responses, however. Others have also done so, for reasons of their own.

One well-known model that bears on this issue is the integration between reactance and helplessness suggested by Wortman and Brehm (1975). Reactance and helplessness are virtual opposites. Both, however, appear to concern perceived problems with control. Wortman and Brehm argued that reactance and helplessness differ in the extent of the problem. Cases in which control is threatened, but not lost, are said to produce reactance and an attempt to reassert control. Perceptions that control is lost, in contrast, produce helplessless and giving up. Wortman and Brehm fit these ideas together by assuming a disjunction between two responses (reassertion and giving up) at the point where the perception of threat to control is becoming a perception that control is lost. This is a watershed model.

Brehm and his collaborators (Brehm & Self, 1989; Wright & Brehm, 1989) subsequently put forward an analysis of effort intensity, or task engagement, that appears to represent an extension or derivation from that earlier model. In this newer view, a person puts into behavior the effort that is needed to complete the behavior successfully. If a task is easy, thus requiring little effort, little effort will be expended. As the task becomes harder, more effort is needed to complete it, and more effort will be expended. In effect, the amount of effort expended grows to match the amount of effort needed.

At some point on the difficulty dimension, however, the person is exerting maximum effort. If the task gets any harder, the person will see it as beyond his or her capacity. At that point, the situation changes, and changes rather abruptly. There is no point in investing effort in an impossible task. Thus, at this point, the person stops trying. Once more, the result is an abrupt disjunction between two classes of response (see Wright, 1996, for a review of literature stemming from this theory). In simple terms, the principle behind this model is that you exert only as much effort as you need to succeed, and if no amount of effort will work, you quit.

As this brief sketch makes clear, there is at least some theoretical basis for the argument that there is a disjunction between two classes of response: effort and disengagement. The two responses do not necessarily shade gradually into one another. Rather, one appears to give way to the other, and in many cases, the giving way seems to entail some degree of abruptness.

Catastrophes

The idea that there is a disjunction between these two classes of response has resonances in other areas of thought (for a broader treatment, see Carver & Scheier, 1998). An example is what is called catastrophe theory. Catastrophe theory is a topological model that focuses on the creation of discontinuities, bifurcations, or splittings (Brown, 1995; Saunders, 1980; Stewart & Peregoy, 1983; Thom, 1975; van der Maas & Molenaar, 1992; Woodcock & Davis, 1978; Zeeman, 1976, 1977). A catastrophe occurs when a small change in one variable pro-

duces an abrupt (and usually large) change in another variable.

Many kinds of catastrophes exist (some of which are very difficult to visualize, because of the number of interacting variables involved). The kind that has been applied most frequently to human behavior is the *cusp catastrophe*, in which two control parameters (roughly equivalent to predictor variables) influence an outcome. Figure 28.5 portrays its three-dimensional surface. The control parameters here are x and z, and the outcome is y. Figure 28.6 displays three cross sections of this surface, slices made at three different values of variable z (moving from back to front of the surface in Figure 28.5). At low values of z, the surface of the catastrophe expresses a roughly linear relation between x and y. As x increases, so does y. As z increases, the relationship between x and y gradually becomes less linear, shifting toward something like a step function (Figure 28.6B). With yet further increase in z, the x–y relationship becomes even more discontinuous, with the upper and lower surfaces now overlapping (Figure 28.6C). Thus, changes in z cause a change in the way that x relates to y.

This overlap, called "hysteresis," is a particularly interesting feature of a catastrophe. There are several ways to characterize what this term measures and what it implies. The

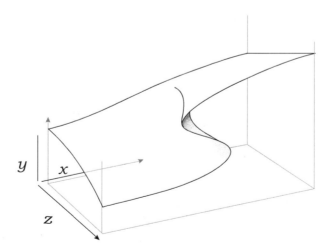

FIGURE 28.5. Three-dimensional depiction of a cusp catastrophe. Variables x and z are predictors; y is the system's "behavior," the dependent variable. From Carver and Scheier (1998). Copyright 1998 by Cambridge University Press. Reprinted by permission.

easiest way to start is to say is that at some range of z, there is a "foldover" in the middle of the x–y relationship. A region of x exists in which there is more than one value of y. This area is illustrated more precisely in Figure 28.7, which shows the same cross section as in Figure 28.6C.

Not all areas of the three-dimensional surface have the same properties. In particular, the dashed-line portion of Figure 28.7 that lies between values a and b on the x axis—the region where the fold is going "backward"—is different from the rest of the surface. It is generated by the mathematical function, but the behaving system that the function is modeling will never actually be there. The system will always be either at the surface above it or at the surface below it.

But which one? Interestingly, the behavior of the system that is being modeled depends on its recent history (Brown, 1995; Nowak & Lewenstein, 1994). Place yourself mentally on the surface (which you will recall is the outcome variable created by x and z). As you move into the range of variable x that lies between points a and b in Figure 28.7, a great deal depends on which side of the figure you are moving from. If the system (whatever it is) is moving from point c into the zone of hysteresis, it stays on the bottom surface until it reaches point b, where it shifts abruptly to the top surface. If it is moving from point d into the zone of hysteresis, it stays on the top surface until it reaches point a, where it shifts abruptly to the bottom surface. Thus, continuing move-

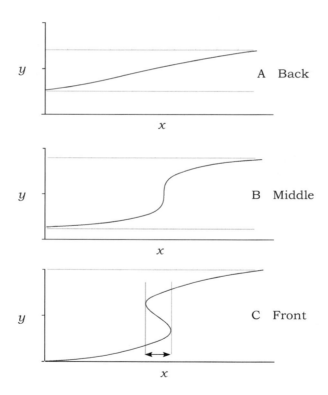

FIGURE 28.6. Three cross sections through a cusp catastrophe, illustrating relations between x and y from Figure 28.5: (A) Toward the back of the surface (relatively low values of z), the relation between x and y is relatively linear; (B) toward the middle of the surface (moderate values of z), the function spreads on the vertical axis and a nonlinear relation has begun to emerge between x and y, resembling a step function; (C) toward the front of the surface (larger values of z), the function spreads even farther on the vertical axis, and a region of overlap develops between upper and lower surfaces of the figure. From Carver and Scheier (1998). Copyright 1998 by Cambridge University Press. Reprinted by permission.

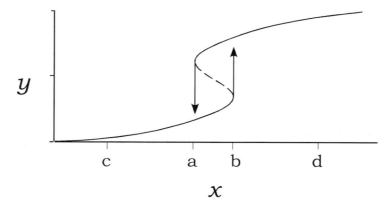

FIGURE 28.7. A cusp catastrophe exhibits a region of hysteresis (between values *a* and *b* on the *x* axis), in which *x* has two stable values of *y* (the solid lines) and one unstable value (the dotted line that cuts backward in the middle of the figure). Traversing the zone of hysteresis from the left of this figure results in an abrupt shift (at value *b* on the *x* axis) from the lower to the upper portion of the surface (right arrow). Traversing the zone of hysteresis from the right of this figure results in an abrupt shift (at value *a* on the *x* axis) from the upper to the lower portion of the surface (left arrow). Thus, the disjunction between portions of the surface occurs at two different values of *x*, depending on the starting point. From Carver and Scheier (1998). Copyright 1998 by Cambridge University Press. Reprinted by permission.

ment from either extreme of *x* toward the other extreme enters a region where either of two outcomes occurs, depending on the starting point.

How does catastrophe theory apply to human behavior? Several applications have been suggested (see Carver & Scheier, 1998, Chapter 15), one of which is of particular interest here: that confidence versus doubt as a partial determinant of effort versus disengagement may feed into a catastrophe (Figure 28.8). Thus, rather than always being linearly related to engagement, expectan-

cies may sometimes be involved in discontinuities in engagement. If there is actually a catastrophe here, there should be a region of hysteresis in the relation between expectancies and engagement.

We are unaware of behavioral evidence on this issue. There is, however, evidence that suggests a catastrophe in the perception of expectancies themselves. People's levels of confidence, once formed, tend to remain stable in the face of disconfirming evidence. A study making this point (though done for a different reason) was conducted some time

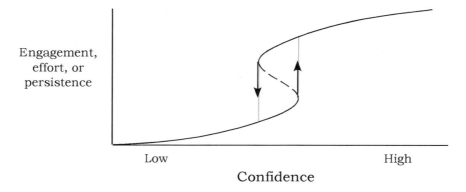

FIGURE 28.8. A catastrophe model of effort versus disengagement. From Carver and Scheier (1998). Copyright 1998 by Cambridge University Press. Reprinted by permission.

ago by Langer and Roth (1975). Participants received (or observed someone else receiving) false feedback of success or failure on each of 30 trials guessing (rigged) coin tosses. There were always 15 successes and 15 failures, but with different patterns. In one condition, the early part of the series was mostly failures, with a gradual shift to successes. In another condition, the early part of the series was mostly successes, with a gradual shift to failures (there was also a random condition that we ignore here).

After 30 trials, participants completed questionnaires, including items asking how often they (or the person they observed) had been correct on the 30 trials, and how many successes would have occurred if there had been 100 more trials. Participants who had started with mostly successes reported having more success than those who had started with mostly failures. A similar pattern, though weaker, emerged in expectations for the next 100 trials. Those with early success expected more success; those with early failure expected more failure. This pattern indicates that people tend to hold onto initial perceptions, even in the face of contradictory information.

In the same way, we suspect that a person who enters the region of hysteresis from the direction of high confidence (who starts out confident but confronts many contradictory cues) will continue to display efforts and engagement, even as the situational cues imply less and less basis for confidence (cf. Peterson et al., 2003). A person who enters that region from the direction of low confidence (who starts out doubtful but confronts contradictory cues) will continue to display little effort, even as the situational cues imply more and more basis for confidence.

This model helps indicate why it can be so difficult to get someone with strong and chronic doubts about success in some domain to exert real effort and engagement in that domain. It also provides a clearer sense of why a confident person is so rarely put off by encountering difficulties in the domain where the confidence lies. In terms of life in general, it helps show why optimists tend to stay optimistic and pessimists tend to stay pessimistic, even when their current circumstances are identical (i.e., are in the region of hysteresis; see also Aldwin, 1994, regarding divergent responses to stress).

The Wortman and Brehm (1975) model is reminiscent of the middle stage of the development of the catastrophe surface, where something resembling a step function has begun to emerge, but the region of hysteresis does not yet exist (Figure 28.6B). Does a region of hysteresis eventually develop? We suspect that there are cases in which a person who enters the situation with the strong belief of no control will continue to show little effort even when control begins to emerge. We also suspect that there are cases in which a person struggling with a threat to control will continue to struggle even when control disappears. Such effects of the person's behavioral history would yield hysteresis.

We think a case can be made for a region of hysteresis in the Brehm and Self (1989) model as well. A critical issue in this case may be the ambiguity of the situation the person faces. That theory tends to assume that the person knows the point at which maximum effort is required. But this will not always be true. A person who begins with a task that is far too hard to perform won't try seriously. If the task changes gradually, so that success is now possible, how will the person know, if only half-hearted effort is being exerted? Not knowing that success is now possible, why would the person try harder? A person who begins with a task that is challenging but attainable will exert strong effort. But how will this person know if the task demands increase to exceed his or her maximum potential effort, unless he or she continues to try? In short, it appears that there is good potential here for a region of hysteresis.

Two further points should be made here. First, we should be clear that however interesting these ideas are, evidence on them is lacking. Apparently the processes of effort and disengagement have not been studied in a parametric manner that would allow plotting effort across the full range of expectancies. The idea of a carryover as the task characteristics shift (i.e., a region of hysteresis) has not been around long, and it has not been the subject of any investigation of which we are aware.

A second point is that it is important to realize that catastrophe theory does not predict hysteresis all the time, but only under certain conditions. Farther back on the catastrophe surface, the relation of x to y looks more like a step function (Figure 28.6B). Farther back yet, it looks more like a linear function (Figure 28.6A). In order to see the hysteresis, it is critical to engage the control variable that is responsible for bringing out the bifurcation in the surface. If this variable is not at the appropriate level, the hysteresis would not emerge, even if the research procedures were otherwise suitable to observe it.

Inducing the Catastrophe

This raises an important question. What variable induces the bifurcation? We think that in the cases under discussion here, the variable is *importance*. Tesser (1980) pointed to social pressure as a potentially critical variable in another application of the catastrophe model. Our interpretation is that social pressure is only one of several forces that can make a behavior or a decision important. There are common threads among important events. In each case, the person preparing to act has something on the line. Important actions demand mental resources. We suspect that almost any strong pressure that demands resources (time pressure, self-imposed pressure, strong connection to a higher order value of the self) will induce similar bifurcating effects. When things are important, when there is a lot at stake, there seems to be a tendency toward polarization (see also Baron, Vandello, & Brunsman, 1996).

Earlier in the chapter, we suggested that people would continue their task efforts longer in the face of developing doubt when the goal was important than when it was not. Our argument there was based on the idea that it is hard to disengage from a value that is central to the self, because of the disruption it creates within the self. Thus, persistence should be greater for important than for unimportant goals.

It is of interest that the catastrophe principle makes the same point about persistence, and actually adds to it. The previous discussion implicitly assumed a behavioral history in which the person began with the belief that the goal was attainable. However, the catastrophe model adds the prediction that a person who begins with the belief that the goal is *not* attainable will stay in disengagement mode longer (as doubt fades) when the goal is important than when it is not.

These ideas are intriguing but untested. They seem to us to be worth exploring in some depth. Essentially the same principle is already under investigation in the context of close relationships (Gottman, Murray, Swanson, Tyson, & Swanson, 2002; Gottman, Swanson, & Swanson, 2002) and in the context of alcohol relapse (Hufford, Witkiewitz, Shields, Kodya, & Caruso, 2003). We hope to see it explored as well in the years to come with regard to other kinds of motives.

COMPETENCE, PERSISTENCE, AND DISENGAGEMENT

This volume contains a set of chapters that present differing perspectives on competence and motivation. In closing, we return to that overarching theme and reiterate what we regard as our contribution to it. People are engaged throughout their lives in a continuing process of both using and expanding their competencies. Engagement in effortful action is based in part on the perception that one has the competence needed to potentially succeed at attaining the goal. The competence in question might be a particular skill that is needed for the activity; alternatively, it might be the more general ability to acquire the skill needed to perform the activity (cf. Dweck, 1996). In either case, without the relevant sense of competence, effort will be minimal or brief.

For successful negotiation of the challenges life provides, however, we believe yet another kind of competence is also important: the ability to know when to continue the effort to reach a goal, and when to disengage and let it go. This is an important competence, because misapplication of either of these choices creates what many would hold to be adverse outcomes. Giving up a goal that is attainable at a reasonable cost results in what some would see as a stunted life, a life in which challenges go unmet and accomplishments within reach are foregone. On the other side, continued commitment to an unattainable goal produces continued distress.

Whether either of these outcomes is bad for the person is a value judgment that varies from one philosophical stance to another. For some people, there may be enough value in maintaining high aspirations to compensate for the negative feelings that result from the inability to move toward them adequately. For other people, there may be enough value in accommodating quickly to the intractability of a situation to compensate for the lost attainments that a demanding struggle might bring. For most people, however, the best path is somewhere between these two extremes. This intermediate path requires the competence to judge what kind of situation one is facing. Is this a situation where you should hang on, or a situation where you should let go?

ACKNOWLEDGMENTS

Preparation of this chapter was facilitated by support from the National Cancer Institute (Grant Nos. CA64710, CA64711, CA78995, and CA84944) and the National Heart, Lung, and Blood Institute (Grant Nos. HL65111 and HL 65112).

REFERENCES

Aldwin, C. M. (1994). *Stress, coping, and development: An integrative perspective.* New York: Guilford Press.

Aspinwall, L. G., & Richter, L. (1999). Optimism and self-mastery predict more rapid disengagement from unsolvable tasks in the presence of alternatives. *Motivation and Emotion, 23,* 221–245.

Atkinson, J. W. (1957). Motivational determinants of risk-taking behavior. *Psychological Review, 64,* 359–372.

Atkinson, J. W. (1964). *An introduction to motivation.* Princeton, NJ: Van Nostrand.

Austin, J. T., & Vancouver, J. B. (1996). Goal constructs in psychology: Structure, process, and content. *Psychological Bulletin, 120,* 338–375.

Baltes, P. B., Cornelius, S. W., & Nesselroade, J. R. (1979). Cohort effects in developmental psychology. In J. R. Nesselroade & P. B. Baltes (Eds.), *Longitudinal research in the study of behavior and development* (pp. 61–87). New York: Academic Press.

Bandura, A. (1997). *Self-efficacy: The exercise of control.* New York: Freeman.

Baron, R. S., Vandello, J. A., & Brunsman, B. (1996). The forgotten variable in conformity research: Impact of task importance on social influence. *Journal of Personality and Social Psychology, 71,* 915–927.

Baumeister, R. F., Bratslavsky, E., Finkenauer, C., &

Vohs, K. D. (2001). Bad is stronger than good. *Review of General Psychology, 5,* 323–370.

Brehm, J. W., & Self, E. A. (1989). The intensity of motivation. *Annual Review of Psychology, 40,* 109–131.

Brown, C. (1995). *Chaos and catastrophe theories* [Quantitative Applications in the Social Sciences, No. 107]. Thousand Oaks, CA: Sage.

Carver, C. S. (2001). Affect and the functional bases of behavior: On the dimensional structure of affective experience. *Personality and Social Psychology Review, 5,* 345–356.

Carver, C. S. (2003). Pleasure as a sign you can attend to something else: Placing positive feelings within a general model of affect. *Cognition and Emotion, 17,* 241–261.

Carver, C. S. (2004). Negative affects deriving from the behavioral approach system. *Emotion, 4,* 3–22.

Carver, C. S., Lawrence, J. W., & Scheier, M. F. (1999). Self-discrepancies and affect: Incorporating the role of feared selves. *Personality and Social Psychology Bulletin, 25,* 783–792.

Carver, C. S., & Scheier, M. F. (1981). *Attention and self-regulation: A control-theory approach to human behavior.* New York: Springer-Verlag.

Carver, C. S., & Scheier, M. F. (1990). Origins and functions of positive and negative affect: A control-process view. *Psychological Review, 97,* 19–35.

Carver, C. S., & Scheier, M. F. (1998). *On the self-regulation of behavior.* New York: Cambridge University Press.

Carver, C. S., & Scheier, M. F. (1999a). Themes and issues in the self-regulation of behavior. In R. S. Wyer, Jr. (Ed.), *Advances in social cognition* (Vol. 12, pp. 1–105). Mahwah, NJ: Erlbaum.

Carver, C. S., & Scheier, M. F. (1999b). Several more themes, a lot more issues: Commentary on the commentaries. In R. S. Wyer, Jr. (Ed.), *Advances in social cognition* (Vol. 12, pp. 261–302). Mahwah, NJ: Erlbaum.

Carver, C. S., & Scheier, M. F. (2002). Control processes and self-organization as complementary principles underlying behavior. *Personality and Social Psychology Review, 6,* 304–315.

Carver, C. S., & Scheier, M. F. (2003). Three human strengths. In L. G. Aspinwall & U. M. Staudinger (Eds.), *A psychology of human strengths: Fundamental questions and future directions for a positive psychology* (pp. 87–102). Washington, DC: American Psychological Association.

Cloninger, C. R. (1987). A systematic method for clinical description and classification of personality variants. *Archives of General Psychiatry, 44,* 573–588.

Clore, G. C. (1994). Why emotions are felt. In P. Ekman & R. J. Davidson (Eds.), *The nature of emotion: Fundamental questions* (pp. 103–111). New York: Oxford University Press.

Davidson, R. J. (1984). Affect, cognition, and hemispheric specialization. In C. E. Izard, J. Kagan, & R. Zajonc (Eds.), *Emotion, cognition, and behavior* (pp. 320–365). New York: Cambridge University Press.

Davidson, R. J. (1992a). Anterior cerebral asymmetry and the nature of emotion. *Brain and Cognition, 20,* 125–151.

Davidson, R. J. (1992b). Emotion and affective style: Hemispheric substrates. *Psychological Science, 3,* 39–43.

Davidson, R. J. (1995). Cerebral asymmetry, emotion, and affective style. In R. J. Davidson, & K. Hugdahl (Eds.), *Brain asymmetry* (pp. 361–387). Cambridge, MA: MIT Press.

Depue, R. A., & Collins, P. F. (1999). Neurobiology of the structure of personality: Dopamine, facilitation of incentive motivation, and extraversion. *Behavioral and Brain Sciences, 22,* 491–517.

Dweck, C. S. (1996). Implicit theories as organizers of goals and behavior. In P. M. Gollwitzer & J. A. Bargh (Eds.), *The psychology of action: Linking cognition and motivation to behavior* (pp. 69–90). New York: Guilford Press.

Elliot, A. J., & McGregor, H. A. (2001). A 2 × 2 achievement goal framework. *Journal of Personality and Social Psychology, 80,* 501–519.

Elliott, E. S., & Dweck, C. S. (1988). Goals: An approach to motivation and achievement. *Journal of Personality and Social Psychology, 54,* 5–12.

Emmons, R. A. (1986). Personal strivings: An approach to personality and subjective well being. *Journal of Personality and Social Psychology, 51,* 1058–1068.

Ericsson, K. A., & Charness, N. (1994). Expert performance: Its structure and acquisition. *American Psychologist, 49,* 725–747.

Feather, N. T. (Ed.). (1982). *Expectations and actions: Expectancy–value models in psychology.* Hillsdale, NJ: Erlbaum.

Field, N. P., Gal-Oz, E., & Bonanno, G. A. (2003). Continuing bonds and adjustment at 5 years after the death of a spouse. *Journal of Consulting and Clinical Psychology, 71,* 110–117.

Finlay-Jones, R., & Brown, G. W. (1981). Types of stressful life event and the onset of anxiety and depressive disorders. *Psychological Medicine, 11,* 803–815.

Fowles, D. C. (1980). The three arousal model: Implications of Gray's two-factor learning theory for heart rate, electrodermal activity, and psychopathy. *Psychophysiology, 17,* 87–104.

Frijda, N. H. (1986). *The emotions.* Cambridge, UK: Cambridge University Press.

Frijda, N. H. (1988). The laws of emotion. *American Psychologist, 43,* 349–358.

Gottman, J. M., Murray, J. D., Swanson, C. C., Tyson, R., & Swanson, K. R. (2002). *The mathematics of marriage: Dynamic nonlinear models.* Cambridge, MA: MIT Press.

Gottman, J. M., Swanson, C. C., & Swanson, K. R. (2002). A general systems theory of marriage: Nonlinear difference equation modeling of marital inter-

action. *Personality and Social Psychology Review, 6,* 326–340.

Gray, J. A. (1981). A critique of Eysenck's theory of personality. In H. J. Eysenck (Ed.), *A model for personality* (pp. 246–276). Berlin: Springer-Verlag.

Gray, J. A. (1987). Perspectives on anxiety and impulsivity: A commentary. *Journal of Research in Personality, 21,* 493–509.

Gray, J. A. (1994). Personality dimensions and emotion systems. In P. Ekman & R. J. Davidson (Eds.), *The nature of emotion: Fundamental questions* (pp. 329–331). New York: Oxford University Press.

Harmon-Jones, E., & Allen, J. J. B. (1998). Anger and frontal brain activity: Asymmetry consistent with approach motivation despite negative affective valence. *Journal of Personality and Social Psychology, 74,* 1310–1316.

Harmon-Jones, E., Sigelman, J. D., Bohling, A., & Harmon-Jones, C. (2003). Anger, coping, and frontal cortical activity: The effect of coping potential on anger-induced left frontal activity. *Cognition and Emotion, 17,* 1–24.

Hatzigeorgiadis, A., & Biddle, S. J. H. (2001). Athletes' perceptions of how cognitive interference during competition influences concentration and effort. *Anxiety, Stress, and Coping, 14,* 411–429.

Heckhausen, J., & Schulz, R. (1995). A life-span theory of control. *Psychological Review, 102,* 284–304.

Higgins, E. T. (1987). Self-discrepancy: A theory relating self and affect. *Psychological Review, 94,* 319–340.

Higgins, E. T. (1996). Ideals, oughts, and regulatory focus: Affect and motivation from distinct pains and pleasures. In P. M. Gollwitzer & J. A. Bargh (Eds.), *The psychology of action: Linking cognition and motivation to behavior* (pp. 91–114). New York: Guilford Press.

Higgins, E. T., Shah, J., & Friedman, R. (1997). Emotional responses to goal attainment: Strength of regulatory focus as moderator. *Journal of Personality and Social Psychology, 72,* 515–525.

Hufford, M. R., Witkiewitz, K., Shields, A. L., Kodya, S., & Caruso, J. C. (2003). Relapse as a nonlinear dynamic system: Application to patients with alcohol use disorders. *Journal of Consulting and Clinical Psychology, 112,* 219–227.

Klinger, E. (1975). Consequences of commitment to and disengagement from incentives. *Psychological Review, 82,* 1–25.

Kuhl, J. (1984). Volitional aspects of achievement motivation and learned helplessness: Toward a comprehensive theory of action control. In B. A. Maher (Ed.), *Progress in experimental personality research* (Vol. 13, pp. 99–170). New York: Academic Press.

Kukla, A. (1972). Foundations of an attributional theory of performance. *Psychological Review, 79,* 454–470.

Langer, E. J., & Roth, J. (1975). Heads I win, tails it's chance: The illusion of control as a function of the sequence of outcomes in a purely chance task. *Jour-*

nal of Personality and Social Psychology, 32, 951–955.

Lewin, K. (1948). Time perspective and morale. In G. W. Lewin (Ed.), Resolving social conflicts: Selected papers on group dynamics (pp. 103–124). New York: Harper.

Lewis, M., Sullivan, M. W., Ramsay, D. S., & Allessandri, S. M. (1992). Individual differences in anger and sad expressions during extinction: Antecedents and consequences. Infant Behavior and Development, 15, 443–452.

Linville, P. (1987). Self-complexity as a cognitive buffer against stress-related illness and depression. Journal of Personality and Social Psychology, 52, 663–676.

MacKay, D. M. (1966). Cerebral organization and the conscious control of action. In J. C. Eccles (Ed.), Brain and conscious experience (pp. 422–445). Berlin: Springer-Verlag.

Markus, H., & Nurius, P. (1986). Possible selves. American Psychologist, 41, 954–969.

Mikulincer, M. (1988). Reactance and helplessness following exposure to learned helplessness following exposure to unsolvable problems: The effects of attributional style. Journal of Personality and Social Psychology, 54, 679–686.

Mikulincer, M. (1994). Human learned helplessness: A coping perspective. New York: Plenum Press.

Miller, G. A., Galanter, E., & Pribram, K. H. (1960). Plans and the structure of behavior. New York: Holt, Rinehart & Winston.

Miller, N. E. (1944). Experimental studies of conflict. In J. McV. Hunt (Ed.), Personality and the behavior disorders (Vol. 1, pp. 431–465). New York: Ronald Press.

Miller, N. E., & Dollard, J. (1941). Social learning and imitation. New Haven, CT: Yale University Press.

Mischel, W., & Shoda, Y. (1995). A cognitive–affective system theory of personality: Reconceptualizing the invariances in personality and the role of situations. Psychological Review, 102, 246–268.

Nesse, R. M. (2000). Is depression an adaptation? Archives of General Psychiatry, 57, 14–20.

Nowak, A., & Lewenstein, M. (1994). Dynamical systems: A tool for social psychology. In R. R. Vallacher & A. Nowak (Eds.), Dynamical systems in social psychology (pp. 17–53). San Diego: Academic Press.

Ogilvie, D. M. (1987). The undesired self: A neglected variable in personality research. Journal of Personality and Social Psychology, 52, 379–385.

Orbuch, T. L. (Ed.). (1992). Close relationship loss: Theoretical approaches. New York: Springer-Verlag.

Ortony, A., Clore, G. L., & Collins, A. (1988). The cognitive structure of emotions. New York: Cambridge University Press.

Pervin, L. A. (1982). The stasis and flow of behavior: Toward a theory of goals. In M. M. Page & R. Dienstbier (Eds.), Nebraska Symposium on Motivation (Vol. 30, pp. 1–53). Lincoln: University of Nebraska Press.

Pervin, L. A. (Ed.). (1989). Goal concepts in personality and social psychology. Hillsdale, NJ: Erlbaum.

Peterson, J. B., DeYoung, C. G., Driver-Linn, E., Séguin, J. R., Higgins, D. M., Arseneault, L., et al. (2003). Self-deception and failure to modulate responses despite accruing evidence of error. Journal of Research in Personality, 37, 205–223.

Piaget, J. (1963). The child's conception of the world. Patterson, NJ: Littlefield, Adams.

Pittman, T. S., & Pittman, N. L. (1980). Deprivation of control and the attribution process. Journal of Personality and Social Psychology, 39, 377–389.

Powers, W. T. (1973). Behavior: The control of perception. Chicago: Aldine.

Pyszczynski, T., & Greenberg, J. (1992). Hanging on and letting go: Understanding the onset, progression, and remission of depression. New York: Springer-Verlag.

Read, S. J., & Miller, L. C. (1989). Inter-personalism: Toward a goal-based theory of persons in relationships. In L. Pervin (Ed.), Goal concepts in personality and social psychology (pp. 413–472). Hillsdale, NJ: Erlbaum.

Saunders, P. T. (1980). An introduction to catastrophe theory. Cambridge, UK: Cambridge University Press.

Scheier, M. F., & Carver, C. S. (1992). Effects of optimism on psychological and physical well-being: Theoretical overview and empirical update. Cognitive Therapy and Research, 16, 201–228.

Scheier, M. F., & Carver, C. S. (2003). Goals and confidence as self-regulatory elements underlying health and illness behavior. In L. D. Cameron & H. Leventhal (Eds.), The self-regulation of health and illness behavior (pp. 17–41). Reading, UK: Routledge.

Scheier, M. F., Carver, C. S., & Bridges, M. W. (2001). Optimism, pessimism, and psychological well-being. In E. C. Chang (Ed.), Optimism and pessimism: Implications for theory, research, and practice (pp. 189–216). Washington, DC: American Psychological Association.

Schulz, R., & Heckhausen, J. (1996). A life span model of successful aging. American Psychologist, 51, 702–714.

Shah, J., & Higgins, E. T. (1997). Expectancy × value effects: Regulatory focus as determinant of magnitude and direction. Journal of Personality and Social Psychology, 73, 447–458.

Showers, C. J., & Ryff, C. D. (1996). Self-differentiation and well being in a life transition. Personality and Social Psychology Bulletin, 22, 448–460.

Snyder, C. R. (1994). The psychology of hope. New York: Free Press.

Stewart, I. N., & Peregoy, P. L. (1983). Catastrophe theory modeling in psychology. Psychological Bulletin, 94, 336–362.

Stroebe, M. S., Stroebe, W., & Hansson, R. O. (Eds.). (1993). Handbook of bereavement: Theory, research, and intervention. Cambridge, UK: Cambridge University Press.

Tesser, A. (1980). When individual dispositions and social pressure conflict: A catastrophe. *Human Relations, 33,* 393–407.

Thom, R. (1975). *Structural stability and morphogenesis.* Reading, MA: Benjamin.

Vallacher, R. R., & Wegner, D. M. (1985). *A theory of action identification.* Hillsdale, NJ: Erlbaum.

Vallacher, R. R., & Wegner, D. M. (1987). What do people think they're doing?: Action identification and human behavior. *Psychological Review, 94,* 3–15.

van der Maas, H. L. J., & Molenaar, P. C. M. (1992). Stagewise cognitive development: An application of catastrophe theory. *Psychological Review, 99,* 395–417.

Vroom, V. H. (1964). *Work and motivation.* New York: Wiley.

Wiener, N. (1948). *Cybernetics: Control and communication in the animal and the machine.* Cambridge, MA: MIT Press.

Woodcock, A., & Davis, M. (1978). *Catastrophe theory.* New York: Dutton.

Wortman, C. B., & Brehm, J. W. (1975). Responses to uncontrollable outcomes: An integration of reactance theory and the learned helplessness model. In L. Berkowitz (Ed.), *Advances in experimental social psychology* (Vol. 8, pp. 277–336). New York: Academic Press.

Wright, R. A. (1996). Brehm's theory of motivation as a model of effort and cardiovascular response. In P. M. Gollwitzer & J. A. Bargh (Eds.), *The psychology of action: Linking cognition and motivation to behavior* (pp. 424–453). New York: Guilford Press.

Wright, R. A., & Brehm, J. W. (1989). Energization and goal attractiveness. In L. A. Pervin (Ed.), *Goal concepts in personality and social psychology* (pp. 169–210). Hillsdale, NJ: Erlbaum.

Wrosch, C., Scheier, M. F., Carver, C. S., & Schulz, R. (2003). The importance of goal disengagement in adaptive self-regulation: When giving up is beneficial. *Self and Identity, 2,* 1–20.

Wrosch, C., Scheier, M. F., Miller, G. E., Schulz, R., & Carver, C. S. (2003). Adaptive self-regulation of unattainable goals: Goal disengagement, goal re-engagement, and subjective well-being. *Personality and Social Psychology Bulletin, 29,* 1494–1508.

Zeeman, E. C. (1976). Catastrophe theory. *Scientific American, 234,* 65–83.

Zeeman, E. C. (1977). *Catastrophe theory: Selected papers 1972–1977.* Reading, MA: Benjamin.

CHAPTER 29

OR

Defensive Strategies, Motivation, and the Self

A Self-Regulatory Process View

FREDERICK RHODEWALT
KATHLEEN D. VOHS

"Who am I?" Most people respond to this question with a list of characteristics that includes dispositions, values, goals, and, most important, competencies. In fact, self-perceptions of competency touch on most every aspect of the self. A typical response to the "Who am I?" question might be, "I am charming (social competency), intuitive and insightful (intellectual competencies), and a golfer (athletic competency)." When asked about personal projects or goals, people report pursuing goals in which competency is either the means to, or the end state of goal attainment: "I am working on getting along better with people, learning to appreciate the Postimpressionists, and lowering my golf handicap."

It is not surprising then, that our senses of competency, agency, and effectiveness undergird our global self-esteem. In fact, Tafarodi and Swann (1995) have provided evidence that global self-esteem is composed of the somewhat independent dimensions of self-liking and self-competency. "Self-liking" refers to the extent to which people feel a sense of positive regard from others. "Self-competency," in contrast, reflects self-esteem derived from an evaluation of what one can do.[1]

Two implications of competency-based self-esteem are the focus of this chapter. First, because self-worth[2] is based, in part, on self-evaluations of competency in various domains, people should be highly motivated to display those competencies in relevant situations. The very definition of "competency" implies the *capacity* to produce effective, goal-directed behavior on demand. More specifically, given that their senses of competency are one critical basis of self-worth, people should be highly ego-involved in those situations in which their competency is on the line. The self-defined golfer should be more concerned about, and more emotionally involved in, a round of golf than should be the accidental hacker, who is out for an afternoon of fun in the sun with friends.

Second, because competency presumes the ability to produce desired consequences, performance feedback, successes, and failures imply something about the degree to which one possesses the competency in question. Therefore, performance outcomes become linked to one's self-worth via the diagnostic information that such outcomes provide about competency. None of this would be too complicated (1) if there were clear, objective, and unambiguous performance standards by which to measure competency; (2) if, relatedly, competency evaluation were not so often dependent on social comparison and interpersonal feedback; (3) if competencies, presumed to be a property of the individual, were not so context-dependent; and most important, (4) if people were always accurately confident about their skills, abilities, and capacities.

Unfortunately, for the purposes of clear and confident self-understanding, most competencies are defined socially and in circumscribed contexts. Consider, for example, intellectual competency. A young adult is believed to be intelligent based upon grades in college courses compared to other students who take the same courses at the same time. "Intelligence" in this case is defined as performance in specific contexts relative to others. However, our lay theories of competency in general and intelligence in particular assume generality across contexts and shifting comparison groups. The expectation is that the capable undergradate will also be a successful graduate student or an accomplished businessperson.

For many people, self-assessments of competency, and their related feelings of self-worth, are inferred from personal histories that include ambiguous, inconsistent, or overly circumscribed experiences (see Jones & Berglas, 1978, for a similar argument). Although they may believe that they possess desired competencies, they are not confident in these assessments. This is not a problem so long as they are not called upon to perform or to provide evidence of their competency in a novel context, or for a new audience. It is only then that they are confronted with the possibility of disconfirmation, disrespect, or rejection. The stakes are high for these people. In addition to issues of competency, their self-esteem, because it is linked to competency, is also under siege.

In this chapter, we are concerned with what people do when they are threatened with the disconfirmation of a desired competency self-image. Specifically, we focus on the defensive cognitive, emotional, and behavioral responses that are in the service of competency-related self-image protection. We take the perspective that most defensive strategies can be understood in terms of self-regulatory processes that are internally coherent and, at least in the short term, adaptive or successful. Self-handicapping behavior (Jones & Berglas, 1978; Rhodewalt & Tragakis, 2002) is used to illustrate the self-regulatory processing approach to defensive strategies. Other defensive strategies are then interpreted in terms of our model. We conclude the chapter with a discussion of defensive behavior and accurate self-assessment of ability, competency, and self-worth.

Although we assume that all people's self-esteem is anchored, in part, by their senses of competency and efficacy, there are broad individual differences in conceptions of competency, thresholds for experiencing threat, and the preferred strategies employed in response to threat. Consider two college seniors, both of whom believe that they are academically talented but who have yet to prove that talent in graduate school. For both students, the upcoming Graduate Record Examination (GRE) poses a potential threat to their competency and esteem. The night before the exam, one senior gets in some light studying, has a good meal, and gets a full night's sleep, while the other stays out until very late, gets quite drunk, and wakes 30 minutes before the exam starts. The former set of behaviors would be nondefensive, since this student is approaching the upcoming threatening situation diligently, with behaviors clearly aimed at achieving the goal of doing well on the test. The latter behaviors are defensive, because they potentially mask the extent to which performance indicates the student's "true" abilities (see the later section on self-handicapping). In the course of describing our model, we also address the psychological units and processes that give rise to these individual differences in the frequency of use and the preferred modes of defensive behavior.

CONCEPT OF DEFENSE WITHIN
THE PROCESS OF SELF-REGULATION

Our core assumption is that people possess desired or valued self-images, including competency images. Moreover, they are motivated to produce outcomes that verify these competencies. Such confirmation sustains or boosts self-esteem, while confirmation failure threatens or damages self-esteem. There is wide agreement in the social-psychological literature that people are motivated to view themselves positively (Leary & Downs, 1995; Sedikides & Strube, 1995) and to have others view them in a way that is consistent with their self-views (Swann, 1983, 1985). Given the importance of competency to feelings of self-worth, it follows that people would develop ways of defending these self-views in the face of challenges to their veracity.

What is meant by defense? The concept of defense has had a long and often controversial history in psychology, in part because of its principal residency within psychodynamic psychology (see Paulus, Fridhandler, & Hayes, 1997, for a recent review). Paulus et al. (1997) noted that, traditionally, "psychological defense" has been defined as "the process of regulating painful emotions such as anxiety, depression, and self-esteem" (p. 543) and "defense mechanisms" have been viewed as "mental processes that operate unconsciously to reduce some painful emotion" (p. 543). Typically, these terms have been used to connote indirect, implicit, or otherwise unhealthy means of alleviating negative emotions.

Our approach to the discussion of defense is both narrower and broader than traditional conceptions of the construct. In our view, psychological defense reflects efforts to maintain desired self-images, including beliefs about one's competency in the face of threatening feedback. These defensive acts may be cognitively, affectively, behaviorally, or interpersonally based behaviors—or some combination—enacted by the individual in anticipation of, or as a reaction to threats to the self. Although the defenses differ in function, they share the common element of defending the self by changing or altering the interpretation of "psychological reality." Whether these defensive strategies are conscious or unconscious, automatic or controlled, is not the main focus of this perspec-

tive. Undoubtedly, self-deception is at that heart of most defensive behavior but, as we argue in a later section, individuals have some implicit or explicit awareness of their strategic behavior.

From this perspective, psychological defense is a special case of self-regulation. In our view, the maintenance and protection of competency self-images embody the constructs and processes described in the social intelligence model of personality (Cantor & Kihlstrom, 1987; see also Cantor, 1990, 1994). The social intelligence perspective is that people bring their social intelligence (self-conceptions, autobiographical memories, constructs, decision rules, and if–then contingencies) to bear on the problems that they are currently trying to solve. People set goals, define challenges to be met and problems to be solved, and then choose and shape situations in order to meet these goals and solve these problems. With specific reference to defensive acts, at the most abstract level of generalization, the problem to be solved is one of maintaining coherence between self-beliefs about competency and external contexts that may challenge those beliefs. The way that people define these beliefs, perceive threats, and select strategic responses to blunt or redirect those threats constitutes the essence of the defensive problem-solving cycle.

Figure 29.1 displays the competency–defense self-regulation cycle. The cycle includes both individual difference characteristics (distal motives) and situational factors, including transient goal states (proximal motives). Motivation in this model reflects chronic or acute orientations to protect competency images from threat or disconfirmation.

With regard to distal motivation, people may have had competency-related learning histories that were capricious and inconsistent, so that although they believe that they possess high ability or skill, confidence in these assessments is uncertain. People also differ in their contingencies of self-worth (Crocker & Wolfe, 2001). Some are more convinced than others that the display of competency is linked to love and acceptance by significant others. In addition, people's naive theories about the extent to which competencies are modifiable (Dweck, 1999; Dweck & Leggett, 1988) contribute to distal defensive motivation. Finally, people vary in

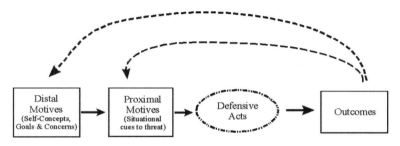

FIGURE 29.1. Competency/defense self-regulation cycle.

how central any given competency is to their sense of self-worth. Self-defining competencies are more vulnerable to threat than are more peripheral self-views. In short, distal defensive motivation is high when people's senses of competency are high but fragile, when the competency forms an important basis of self-worth, and when people believe that the competency in question is stable and unmodifiable. It is low to the extent that people are confident in their ability, view the competency as less important to self-worth, or believe that the competency can be modified through factors such as effort, practice, and instruction.

Proximal defensive motivation reflects current demands on the individual. Current demands take meaning in the context of chronic distal motives and concerns. For example, being called upon to demonstrate business acumen with a new corporate partner is more threatening for individuals who are unclear about the causes of their past successes than for those who are certain of their abilities in this domain. The primary contextual trigger is the demand to produce an ability-related outcome. However, other situational factors can exacerbate threat to one's competency beliefs. Situations that differ from past competency-relevant arenas contribute to the individual's uncertainty about displaying the ability or skill in the new context. For instance, graduate school provides a test of intellectual competency that calls upon similar competencies that produced success in college. Nonetheless, it is not clear that competencies that were sufficient for success in college will be equally sufficient for success in graduate school. Thus, the proximal situation presents a potential threat that should be experienced more intensely by those who possess chronic

defensive motivation than in those who do not. People have a vast array of defensive responses available that encompass both intrapersonal and interpersonal tactics. In general, people use these strategies to regulate emotions and thoughts about self-beliefs. The examples provided here are by no means exhaustive; rather, they provide a sample of the types of responses people enlist in defense of the self. The distinction between intra- and interpersonal defensive strategies is also somewhat arbitrary, in that many strategies are both. For instance, self-handicapping behavior is a defensive strategy that enables individuals to dismiss incompetence as an explanation for poor performance (an intrapersonal outcome) and also protect their self-images in the eyes of others (an interpersonal consequence).

Defensive strategies are intrapersonally based to the extent that they arise and proceed primarily within the head of the person, and involve interpretations and distortions of meaning. The purpose of these tactics is to allow interpretations of self and situation that preserve desired competency images. Defensive strategies are interpersonally based to the extent that the defensive person uses other people to bolster feelings and thoughts about the self. These strategies allow people to modify their thoughts or feelings about others, to alter perceived relationship closeness, or to use others as an audience that serves to verify the self, or at least the self as displayed for public consumption.

Intrapersonal Strategies

People's self-protective cognitive gymnastics can be quite remarkable. They have an uncanny ability to take self-relevant but threatening information about the self (or the anticipation thereof) and turn it into something more benign. Attribution processes are perhaps the most fundamental and widely used intrapersonal defensive strategy; they are the "duct tape" in the defensive strategy toolbox. Greenwald's (1980) influential article on the totalitarian ego brought to light the point that people are generally biased to see themselves as good and competent. In this review of the literature, Greenwald coined the term "beneffectance," a word that is a combination of the words "beneficence" (meaning to do good) and "effectance" (meaning to be competent), to reflect people's tendency to view themselves as producers of good but not bad outcomes. The self-serving attribution bias is one manifestation of *beneffectance*. People persistently offer internal attributions for success and external attributions for failure (Miller & Ross, 1975; Weary, 1978).

Most important to this discussion, self-serving attributions are triggered or exacerbated by threats to the self. Self-serving attributions take the form of crediting the self for good outcomes but blaming others or the situation for bad outcomes. For instance, if a golfer has a particularly good round during a day on the course, he may think that the modification he made to his swing is to credit. Conversely, if on the next round, he has a particularly terrible score, he may blame the other people with whom he golfed for being too distracting during his shots.

Support for the idea that self-serving attributions are pronounced under conditions of threat is found in the Campbell and Sedikides (1999) meta-analysis of data from approximately 7,000 participants. The data revealed that self-threat exercised a considerable influence on the magnitude of self-serving attribution biases. More pertinent to this discussion, the association between self-threat and the self-serving bias was a function of not only the presence of threat-related situational factors (e.g., status differences) but also motivation-related individual differences (e.g., achievement motivation). Thus, from the perspectives of beneffectance and the self-serving bias, people defensively call upon tried-and-true attributional defenses in times of threat, in order to alter their causal interpretations and protect the self.

A different intrapersonal defensive strategy involves selective recall and editing of autobiographical memories. This work builds on Michael Ross's pioneering work on biased recall of personal histories (for a review, see Ross, 1989). This research has been termed "revising what you had to get what you want" (see Conway & Ross, 1984), which is an apt descriptor of what people do when they are motivated to justify or accommodate their current circumstances. There is evidence that such revisionist history can be called upon in response to threats the self. Ybarra (1999) provided participants with positive feedback, negative feedback, or no feedback about their performance on an analogies test, then also provided positive and negative information about a target person. Results from an incidental recall task for the target's behaviors revealed that negative-feedback participants showed the misanthropy effect by recalling more negative than positive target behaviors. Although not directly tested, the implication of these findings is that memory distortions may result from the need for self-esteem protection. Rhodewalt and Eddings (2002) provide a more direct test of the self-esteem protection hypothesis in their study of narcissism and autobiographical memory distortion. High- and low-narcissistic men were interviewed by a woman, purportedly for the purposes of a possible date, and also reported their romantic histories. A week later, they learned that the woman had chosen or rejected them as her dating partner. Participants again recalled their history of romantic relationships. Narcissistic men who were rejected reported dating histories that were significantly more self-aggrandizing than the histories that they had reported prior to the rejection. Moreover, the more they inflated their romantic pasts, the more their self-esteem was protected from the effects of the rejection.

In summary, people construct and reinterpret their understandings of past events, as well as their personal attributes, feelings, and experiences, in order to bolster current self-views and self-beliefs. Whether they are cognitive gymnasts, totalitarian rulers, or reconstructive historians, people find a way to regulate intrapersonally relevant self- and social knowledge so as to preserve desired self-beliefs about who they were to aid them in thinking about who they are.

Interpersonal Strategies

The interpersonal arena also affords venues for defensive behavior, in that most defensive strategies involve public behaviors, social interactions, or interpersonal relationships. It stands to reason that if other individuals are often sources of threat, then they should also be potential implements in diffusing these threats. It is a special feature of *interpersonal* defensive behaviors that they create or manipulate the reactions of other individuals, or that the behaviors have clear and direct implications for the nature of an interpersonal relationship. The reactions of others, which are often not the ones intended by the actor, thus intensify rather than ameliorate the threat, requiring additional defensive reactions from the threatened individual.

Perhaps the best illustration of interpersonal defensive behavior may be found in research inspired by Tesser's self-evaluation maintenance theory (SEM; 1988). In essence, SEM involves manipulating interpersonal closeness for the purpose of self-esteem protection or enhancement. For instance, people feel threatened when someone close to them, such as a good friend, has outperformed them on a domain that is important and relevant to their self-concept.[3] According to Tesser, the state of "comparison threat" triggers a number of possible self-evaluation maintenance responses. A person experiencing comparison threat from a close other may attempt to reduce the threat by decreasing either the perceived (or actual) closeness of the relationship or the relevance of the domain to the self-concept. In our framework, the former response would be interpersonal, and the latter would be intrapersonal. There is an abundance of findings supporting the SEM model. For example, Tesser demonstrated that the when siblings were outperformed by a brother or sister close in age (i.e., relevance of the comparison is high), participants decreased the closeness of the relationship by lowering the extent to which they identified with that sibling. Another SEM strategy is to sabotage the threatening individual, so that he or she is less likely to do well in the future. For example, students failed to give a friend the best help (as measured by the quality of hints that were given to the friend by the

participant to help him or her on a verbal test) when the friend had outperformed them on an earlier verbal test (Pemberton & Sedikides, 2001).

Consistent with an SEM perspective, interpersonal reactions of anger and hostility are frequent defensive reactions exhibited when people encounter a threat to their competencies. Along with anger and hostility, people also alter their views of others to become more denigrating (Morf & Rhodewalt, 1993). High self-esteem people may be particularly prone to this type of defensive response. For instance, high self-esteem people who are threatened by negative competency feedback respond by derogating others, namely, they decrease how favorably they rate generalized others and even personal friends (Brown, 1986; Brown & Gallagher, 1992). In another example, Fein and Spencer (1997) reported that high self-esteem people threatened by negative feedback about their intellectual competencies derogated outgroup members to a greater extent than did threatened low self-esteem participants. Furthermore, derogating others seemed to have served a compensatory function, in that those participants who played the derogation card also experienced a boost in self-esteem.

Strategic self-presentations are frequently used for interpersonal defensive purposes. For example, people respond with self-aggrandizing presentations when they feel threatened, and with approval seeking when they feel rejected. In one investigation, Baumeister and Jones (1978) found that people who believed that their interaction partner saw a "personality profile" of theirs that contained negative information about their abilities, responded with compensatory self-enhancement. Specifically, they evaluated more positively their skills in other, unrelated domains. A qualification to this finding is that it occurred primarily among high self-esteem people for whom negative feedback threatens a positive self-perception of abilities more so than for people with low self-esteem.

One question that is pertinent throughout this discussion of defensive behavior: Do these strategies work? The answer to this question within the domain of defensive self-presentations is complex, because self-presentational strategies rely on the responses of others. Thus, their success may be considered in terms of interpersonal costs and benefits. In general these costs should be high given that threatened individuals (particularly those with high self-esteem) make more self-aggrandizing statements (Baumeister, 1982) and derogate the source of threat (Morf & Rhodewalt, 1993). Because of these characteristic responses to threat, Vohs and Heatherton (2003; Heatherton & Vohs, 2000) hypothesized that high self-esteem people would be seen as less likable after receiving information that their intellectual abilities are below average. This prediction was supported by the finding that threatened high self-esteem people received lower likeability ratings from previously unacquainted interaction partners (who had been given no information about the person's intellectual abilities and was thus unthreatened). Low self-esteem people, conversely, were liked more after being told that they possessed subpar intellectual abilities, a topic we discuss more fully when we consider individual differences in rejection sensitivity as a defensive strategy. Threatened high self-esteem participants were seen by their partners as arrogant, unfriendly, rude, uncooperative, and insincere. Apparently, they self-enhanced to their partners during the course of the interaction and, as a consequence, were less appealing. Additional studies showed there to be an explicit social comparison dimension to this effect, such that high self-esteem people who were told that their intellectual abilities were poor responded by boosting judgments of themselves relative to their interaction partner and generalized others (Vohs & Heatherton, 2003).

Research on self-verification processes (Swann, 1985) also supports the notion that people respond to threat with strategic self-presentations. When people engage in self-verification, they are choosing or eliciting from the environment feedback that conforms to their preestablished views of self. This desire to receive feedback consistent with self-beliefs has been found to hold across self-esteem levels and other personality traits. The purpose of self-verification is to increase control and predictability of outcomes in an uncertain world (Swann, Stein-Seroussi, & Giesler, 1992). There are two types of self- and other-perception discrepancies that threaten one's competencies: one

in which others' perceptions are more positive than one's self-view, and the other, in which one's self-perceptions are more positive than others' perceptions. In the former case, threat arises from the idea that others may be expecting better performance or outcomes than one can actually produce. In the latter, threat arises from the idea that others are underestimating one's likely performance. Both can therefore be problematic, because they set the stage for perceptions of one's abilities that will not match up to actual performance.

In this section, we have provided an overview of the cognitive, behavioral, and interpersonal responses that can be summoned in response to threats to the self. Each strategy was characterized as being primarily intra- or interpersonal, and research demonstrating their defensive nature was reviewed. This selective list is offered only to illustrate the wide range of responses that can be enlisted in the service of preserving one's self-concept and sense of competency. We return now to the competency/defense self-regulation model by providing examples of how specific defensive strategies form the nucleus of a cycle of behavior that we characterize as defensive styles.

DEFENSIVE STYLES

People differ in the learning histories upon which their competency self-conceptions are built. Moreover, they vary in the extent to which competency defines self-worth, and they diverge in their theories about the underlying causes of competency. All of these factors, we have argued, underlie distal defensive motivation. The combination of these elements also shapes problem definition, so that challenges to competency images take on different meanings and suggest different solutions (defensive reactions) for different people. One conclusion of this reasoning is that there should be consistent individual differences in the employment of preferred defensive strategies; that is, there should be defensive styles. Self-handicapping behavior provides an excellent example of the competency/defense self-regulation cycle as manifested in a unique defensive style.

"Self-handicapping" is a defensive strategy in which people create, or at least claim, obstacles to successful performances when they harbor doubts about their ability to be successful, and when failure would confirm that the ability is lacking (Jones & Berglas, 1978). According to Jones and Berglas, the person who arrives late for a job interview or who gets drunk the night before taking the bar examination to enter legal practice is manipulating in a self-serving way the attributions that one may draw about the actor's ability or competency. Tardiness and inebriation not only decrease the likelihood of receiving an offer of employment or passing the examination, but they also protect one's belief that he or she has the ability to do well. Jones and Berglas argued that the self-handicapper is capitalizing on the attributional principles of *discounting* and *augmentation* (Kelley, 1972); that is, conclusions about lack of ability are *discounted*, or downplayed, because the handicap offers an equally plausible explanation for the rejection or failure. In the unlikely event of success, attributions to ability are *augmented*, or accorded greater causal importance, because the good performance happened despite the handicap. The self-handicapper then is willing to trade the increased likelihood of failure for the opportunity to protect a desired self-image. It is important to point out that self-handicappers are willing to accept the label of slacker or drunkard in order to preserve a more central belief that they are competent. The label implied by the

handicap is almost always applied to a quality that is external to the individual or is believed to be under the individual's control, while the attribute that is being protected is believed to be fixed and unmodifiable, a point to which we return momentarily.

Over the past quarter-century, self-handicapping behavior has been extensively investigated (for reviews, see Arkin & Oleson, 1998; Rhodewalt & Tragakis, 2002). Collectively, this work illustrates the competency–defense model outlined in Figure 29.1. Research findings can be grouped into categories representing the distal and proximal antecedents of self-handicapping, the strategic behaviors enlisted in the service of self-handicapping, and the consequences of these behaviors for the individual. Figure 29.2 provides a schematic of this model for self-handicapping behavior. As in the generic Figure 29.1, self-handicapping is recursive in the sense that the consequences of self-handicapping feed back into the process and reinforce self-handicapping acts, while maintaining, or perhaps exacerbating, antecedent motives and concerns.

Distal Motives

In their original theoretical statement, Jones and Berglas (1978) proposed that self-handicapping is motivated by a desire to protect a positive but insecurely held competency im-

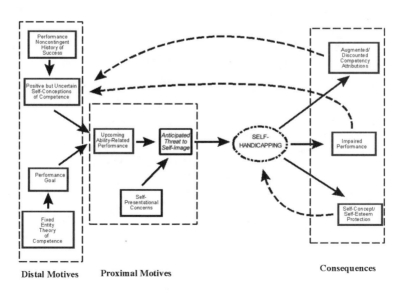

FIGURE 29.2. Self-handicapping self-regulation cycle. Adapted from Rhodewalt and Tragakis (2002). Copyright 2002. Reproduced by permission of Routledge/Taylor & Francis Books, Inc.

age. In fact, the standard experimental paradigm employed to elicit self-handicapping behavior in the laboratory provides participants with response-noncontingent success feedback on an important competency such as intellectual ability. This experimental manipulation is thought to mimic real-world situations in which people are uncertain of what they did to produce the success that is being attributed to their competency. For example, publication of scholarly papers in prestigious journals is evidence of the brilliance of the researcher. The introspective researcher need only think of all of the serendipity that went into the production of that scientific publication to be uncertain that he or she can replicate that brilliance in the future. The experimental evidence consistently shows that compared to individuals who receive response-contingent success feedback, participants who receive response-noncontingent success feedback subsequently opt to self-handicap prior to taking a second ability test. This experimental analogue is thought to reflect the real-world circumstance of people who have experienced success in the past and attributed that success to their ability, but are uncertain that the attribution is correct. In summary, one distal motivation to engage in self-handicapping behavior involves competency self-images derived from a capricious history of success. Consider two entering college freshmen who both wish to believe that they are academically gifted but differ in the past events that would support such a claim. One student may have attained an almost perfect high school grade point average (GPA), been a National Merit scholar, and earned an academic scholarship. This student studied conscientiously but did not spend every waking minute hitting the books. The second student may also have an almost perfect high school GPA, but here the comparison with the first student ends. The second student's mother was the high school principal; this student played sports and in fact had been awarded an athletic scholarship to college. This student studied very hard and at several times throughout high school received tutoring. Both students want to interpret their high grades as evidence of superb academic ability, but the former student should be more confident in this judgment than the latter, because this student experienced more ability-contingent academic successes than the

second student. The second student also experienced academic success, but it was unclear because of other plausible explanations whether these successes were attributable to ability. How much did the mother's power over the teachers, the teachers' concerns about the student's athletic eligibility, or extraordinary effort and exceptional preparation contribute to this student's high grades?

Both students in the foregoing example should be equally comfortable until called upon to produce evidence of their academic ability. It is at this point that the student who is uncertain might be drawn to self-handicap. However, not all individuals who harbor concerns about their competency self-handicap when entering evaluative situations. There is a second set of distal factors that promote self-handicapping as the logical response. Past research has shown that people differ in their naive theories about the causes of ability. Specifically, Carol Dweck and her colleagues (Dweck, 1999; Dweck & Leggett, 1988; Elliot & Dweck, 1988) have discussed these "self-theories" with regard to mastery-oriented versus helpless behaviors in achievement contexts. According to this perspective, people fall into one of two camps with regard to their beliefs about the causes of ability and competency. "Fixed entity" theorists believe that ability is a fixed trait. Whatever one's capacity, it is relatively fixed and unmodifiable. In contrast, "incremental" theorists assume that ability can be cultivated through learning, that one's capacities are malleable. It is probably more accurate to say that most people entertain both theories and differ in the extent to which they favor one over the other as the predominant explanation for ability. Dweck also contends that "fixed-entity" and "incremental" self-theories are associated with different goals in achievement contexts. The "fixed entity" theorist pursues performance goals, that is, goals of receiving positive feedback and outcomes, such as a high grade or praise from the teacher. The "incremental" theorist, in contrast, pursues learning goals, characterized by learning something new or improving upon an existing skill.

We believe that the Dweck framework extends to an understanding of self-handicapping behavior. If individuals enter achievement settings with different beliefs about the nature of their abilities, then competency feedback has different implications for self-worth. Our model specifies that the combination of a "fixed entity" view of competency and the pursuit of performance goals should also promote the tendency to self-handicap when the individual anticipates negative feedback about the "fixed entity." Returning to our college freshman who is uncertain about his or her academic ability, consider this student's possible reactions to the first set of course exams. If our hypothetical student embraces an "incremental theory/learning goal" orientation, this is clearly an unsettling situation. The evaluation is important, and the outcome is uncertain. However, the meaning of that outcome, while potentially disappointing, is not damning. A negative evaluation signals that more training and preparation are required before the student can move on. But what if our hypothetical student holds a "fixed entity theory/performance goal" orientation? Failure for this student does not mean that more preparation is required. Rather, it signals that ability is lacking, and this is a devastating message, because, according to the fixed-entity view, there is not much one can do to remedy the deficit. Thus, when situations require the demonstration of a certain competence, the performance goals and focus on ability of those who hold fixed theories of competence may also motivate strategic defensive behavior, especially self-handicapping.

Returning to Figure 29.2, one can see that the use of self-handicapping strategies is the product of two learning histories (Rhodewalt, 1994). First, the self-handicapper has had a set of socialization experiences that instill the belief that competency is fixed and can only be demonstrated rather than improved. Second, this person possesses ability self-conceptions that are based on a causally ambiguous and shaky history of success. Thus, self-handicappers enter many evaluative situations with the goal of demonstrating an ability of which they are uncertain. It is the confluence of these two learning histories and the more immediate performance demands that set the stage for self-handicapping. Evaluative situations that pose the threat of negative feedback about the self are to be avoided, because their implications are so damaging. In these contexts, people will embrace self-handicaps, because the trade-off of increased risk of failure for the protection of an ability self-conception seems like a bargain.

Is it the case that people who display a tendency to self-handicap also hold "fixed entity" views of competency and pursue performance goals? This important question has not been extensively investigated, but existing data suggest that the answer is "yes." Rhodewalt (1994) devised several measures to probe respondents about their naive theories of competency. For example, individuals provided responses to a set of open-ended questions, such as "What does it mean to be intelligent (athletic, socially skilled)?"; "What does it mean to be unintelligent (unathletic, not socially skilled)?"; and "What could one do, if anything, to become more intelligent (athletic, socially skilled)?" A second measure required respondents to read a vignette about a bright and accomplished college student who had been accepted to medical school. They rated the person in the vignette for intelligence and then apportioned 100 points among possible causes of her academic achievement, including the factors "innate intelligence," "effort," and "privileged background." With respect to goals in achievement contexts, participants completed a measure of goals in school (Nicholls, 1984) that assessed both performance and learning goals.

Participants also completed the Self-Handicapping Scale (SHS; Jones & Rhodewalt, 1982). The SHS is a face-valid, self-report measure of people's tendencies to make excuses and use self-handicaps. In support of the hypothesis, the tendency to self-handicap was significantly related to the endorsement of fixed-entity theories of ability across both measures of assessment and all ability domains (intelligence, athleticism, and social skills). Also, as hypothesized, self-handicapping was associated with the pursuit of performance goals in academic settings. More recently, Elliot and Church (2003) conducted a motivational analysis of self-handicapping and reported that self-handicapping tendencies were positively related to performance approach goals and performance avoidance goals (avoidance of failure), and negatively related to mastery goals.

There are two points that merit mention at this point in our discussion. The first concerns the issue of defensive strategies and regulatory coherence. We have argued that defensive behavior can be understood in terms of a logical problem-solving cycle. The relation between the distal motives and self-handicapping strategies illustrates this point. Given the underlying competency beliefs and concerns held by these individuals, self-handicapping makes sense, because it defends against the threat to competency as it is defined by the individual. Second, as we have noted elsewhere (Rhodewalt & Tragakis, 2002), although self-theories and their related goals form one branch of distal motivation, and positive but uncertain self-conceptions form a separate branch, as depicted Figure 29.2, the two factors are probably embedded in the same developmental history. They may connect at a developmental level that involves understanding of the contingencies between behavior and outcomes. Jones and Berglas (1978) argued that the self-handicapper simply does not understand the connection between past success and personal attributes. We suggest that the same sort of ambiguous understanding of ability is more compatible with a fixed-entity view than with an incremental view of competency; that is, an incremental theory implies an understanding of the contingencies among effort, practice, preparation, and performance. A fixed entity view of ability requires less attention to contextual and motivational influences on performance. Future research may reveal that the same developmental experiences that contribute to a positive but confused self-image also foster fixed entity beliefs about the characteristics of that self-image.

We would be remiss if we did not mention one additional distal factor. This factor is highlighted by our example of students about to enter college. For both students, academic ability is important to their self-worth. It is only those domains of competency that are important to the individual's self-esteem that comprise part of the distal constellation of self-handicapping motives.

Proximal Motives

Proximal motives are engendered by features of the situation that pose a potential threat to the individual's self-image of competency. The most frequent and immediate threat is being called upon to exhibit the valued attribute or competency. It is the fear that one cannot produce evidence of a competence, skill, ability, or attribute that elicits acts of self-handicapping. This was the central focus of the Jones and Berglas (1978) formulation of self-handicapping; however, Snyder and Smith (1982) have argued more broadly that self-handicapping is a response to anticipated threats to the self. Thus, self-handicaps can be used both to hide feelings of inferiority and to protect a shaky self-concept. While some may object to this characterization of self-handicapping (Berglas, 1988), it does capture the wide array of research findings in the literature. Clearly, having a desired self-conception debunked by a poor performance is a threat to the self.

Because most acts of self-handicapping are enacted before an audience, a second set of proximal motives becomes relevant. Self-handicapping could be motivated by the desire to preserve competency images in the eyes of others (i.e., self-presentation motive), or it could be in the service of protecting the self from the realization that one is not as competent as one desires to be (i.e., self-deception motive). A number of researchers have examined this issue without providing conclusive results. Berglas and Jones (1978) attempted to address this question in their initial demonstration of self-handicapping by varying whether the experimenter would know of the participant's choice to self-handicap. Whether or not the experimenter was allegedly aware of the self-handicap did not make a difference, leading Berglas and Jones to conclude that self-handicapping was for self-protection. Others (see Kolditz & Arkin, 1982) have produced evidence that self-presentational concerns can increase the likelihood of self-handicapping. Rhodewalt and Fairfield (1991) found that self-handicappers who anticipated doing poorly on an IQ test stated that they were not going to try on the upcoming test (and actually withdrew effort) even when these response were ostensibly anonymous and could serve no self-presentational purpose. Certainly, both motives could be operating, and the pursuit of one does not preclude the other.

Consequences of Self-Handicapping

Much of our work has focused on the outcomes of self-handicapping behavior. Does it work? And if so, what are the costs to the self-handicapper? The view that self-handicapping is an example of defensive self-regulation would suggest that, to some extent, the strategy accomplishes the goal of preserving self-perceived competency, and in the short term, it does. The right side of Figure 29.1 illustrates the hypothesized direct effects of self-handicapping. Self-handicapping should have direct effects on the quality of the performance. It should also influence attributions for that performance. And it should buffer competency images and self-worth from the implications of failure.

Discounting and Augmentation of Competency Attributions

There is clear and consistent evidence that self-handicaps are recruited into the explanations people offer for their successes and failures. In both laboratory and field studies of self-handicapping, participants discount attributions to ability when the failure occurs in the presence of a handicap. On some occasions, they will augment attributions to ability following success when that success occurred despite the presence of a self-handicap. For example, there have been a number of "classroom studies" of the effects of self-handicapping on attributional responses to success and failure (Feick & Rhodewalt, 1998; McCrea & Hirt, 2001; Rhodewalt & Hill, 1995). The procedure was similar in all investigations. In our work, students reported their expected class performance and were assessed for individual differences in self-handicapping (SHS) and self-esteem at the beginning of the academic term. Prior to the first exam, they reported any "handicaps" they were undergoing that might affect their performance on the upcoming exam. As expected, high SHS students claimed more handicaps than did low SHS students. When the graded exams were returned, students were asked to make attributions for their performance and to report their state self-esteem at that moment. In the Rhodewalt and Hill study (1995), all students received exam grades that were one-third of a grade lower than the highest grade they said would dissatisfy them. In the Feick and Rhodewalt (1988) investigation, we categorized students' performances by comparing their grades on the exam with their grade expectations reported at the beginning of the term. Students were grouped into those who performed worse than they ex-

pected (failure), equal to their expectations (expected success), or better than their expectations (unexpected success). In both studies (and also in McCrea & Hirt, 2001), students who received failing grades, and who also had claimed handicaps prior to the test, discounted attributions to lack of ability; that is, students who failed reported that they possessed significantly higher ability if they had previously handicapped than if they had not. In fact, in the Feick and Rhodewalt (1988) study, the ability attributions of failing self-handicappers were no different that the ability attributions of students who had performed up to their expectations—clear evidence of discounting. Students who performed better than they expected claimed augmented ability if they achieved this success in the presence of a handicap. These students reported levels of ability that were significantly higher than those of students who had performed unexpectedly well but had not handicapped. McCrea and Hirt (2001) also found evidence of augmentation among those students who had self-handicapped and subsequently performed well on the exam. Collectively, these studies provide clear support for the attributional component of the model.

Competency and Self-Worth

Our main argument is that people employ defensive behavior in order to protect competency images, because our senses of competency form a cornerstone of our self-worth. Evidence from laboratory as well as field studies consistently documents that failure in the presence of a self-handicap preserves the self-handicapper's feelings of competency and self-worth. For example, Rhodewalt, Morf, Hazlett, and Fairfield (1991, Study 2) led participants to believe that they had performed well on an intelligence test and then administered a second form of the same test. Half of the students received feedback that they continued to be successful on the second test, and half received feedback that they were now failing. Independent of this feedback was the presence or absence of an experimenter-imposed handicap. Those students who failed but had a handicap reported levels of ability and self-esteem equal to those who succeeded on both tests. In contrast, students who failed and did not have a handicap concluded that they had low ability and displayed lowered self-esteem.

Naturalistic studies described earlier also document the competency- and esteem-buffering effects of self-handicapping (Feick & Rhodewalt, 1998; McCrea & Hirt, 2001; Rhodewalt & Hill, 1995). All of these investigations found that students' claimed handicaps buffered perceptions of ability and self-esteem from the effects of failure—although this, too, was more consistently true for men than for women (McCrea & Hirt, 2001; Rhodewalt & Hill, 1995). Most important, these studies showed that the self-esteem of self-handicappers who failed was not significantly different from that of successful students and significantly higher than that of failing non-self-handicappers.

These findings return us to the question of motives. Specifically, are self-handicappers mainly concerned with self-protection or self-enhancement? Some findings suggest that high self-esteem individuals may self-handicap to seek opportunities to augment anticipated success (Rhodewalt et al., 1991; Tice, 1991). Our reading of the research suggests that most acts of self-handicapping are primarily in the service of self-concept protection. Although it is true that certain individuals, particularly high self-esteem, high self-handicappers, are quick to understand and accept augmented ability attributions, self-enhancement is unlikely to be the primary reason for their self-handicapping behavior. These individuals self-handicap only when they are uncertain about their ability. If the goal of self-handicapping for high self-esteem individuals were self-enhancement, then one would observe self-handicapping among individuals who are certain of their ability. There is no evidence to support this argument.

Self-Handicapping and Performance

The question of whether self-handicapping affects performance is complicated by the wide range of ways in which people can self-handicap. It appears obvious that behavioral handicaps such as drinking alcohol or failing to prepare should harm performance more than should claimed handicaps, such as reports of illness or effort withdrawal. The data are not so clear in this regard. For ex-

ample, in one study in our laboratory, we (Rhodewalt & Fairfield, 1991) asked students to state privately how hard they were going to try on an upcoming test of intelligence (with lack of effort being a claimed self-handicap). Unknown to the students, we had manipulated the difficulty of a set of practice items, so that half of the students expected to do well and half expected to do poorly. Students who were suspicious that they would not do well on the IQ test *claimed* prior to taking it that they did not intended to put forth as much effort as did students who expected to do well. All students were then administered the same test. What is striking about this experiment is that students who made the claim of low intended effort actually performed significantly worse than did students who did not make the claim. Given that the test was the same for everyone, we assume that stating that they were not going to try led them to try less hard, which accounted for their poorer performance. In the McCrea and Hirt (2001) "classroom study," prior to the exam, high self-handicapping men reported putting less effort and time into preparation than did all other groups of students. These students who reported poor preparation performed poorly on the test, averaging 71% compared to 79% averaged by their classmates. Nonetheless, as already reported, these self-handicapping students made nonability attributions for their poor performance and maintained high estimates of ability and self-esteem. Clearly, the relation between the mode of self-handicap and performance is complex and warrants additional research.

A second way to address the self-handicapping and performance question is to examine the long-term effects of self-handicapping. To the extent that an individual chronically self-handicaps, one would expect that there would be deleterious effects on achievement and accomplishment. We have evidence suggesting that this is true. We created an index of over- and underachievement by using students' Scholastic Aptitude Test (SAT) and American College Test (ACT) scores as a measure of aptitude, and their GPAs as a measure of achievement (Rhodewalt & Saltzman, reported in Rhodewalt, 1990). In samples from two different universities, the over- and underachievement index correlated negatively with scores on the SHS; that is, the more a student was a chronic self-handicapper, as evidenced by his or her SHS score, the less likely his or her grades were as high as what would be expected from his or her SAT/ACT scores.

Zuckerman, Kieffer, and Knee (1998) provided a follow-up examination of the relation between chronic self-handicapping and academic performance. In two studies, these researchers found that individual differences in self-handicapping, as measured by the SHS, were related to lower academic performance, as indexed by GPA. Moreover, the negative relation between the SHS and GPA was independent of verbal and quantitative SAT, and level of self-esteem. Zuckerman et al. also measured study habits and found that poor exam preparation seemed to drive the relationship between individual differences in the tendency to use self-handicaps and poor performance.

Recursive Effects of Self-Handicapping

Self-handicapping behavior also illustrates the cyclical aspect of our competency/defense self-regulation model. As depicted in Figure 29.2, short-term "positive" outcomes, such as preserved competency images and protected self-esteem, should reinforce the use of self-handicapping in the future. However, there are longer term consequences as well. The strategy works in the short-term, because it creates ambiguity about the causes of poor performance. If, as we have argued, uncertainty about competency is a distal motive, this uncertainty should be perpetuated, if not exacerbated, by a strategy that preserves or creates additional uncertainty. In addition, to the extent that self-handicapping actually undermines performance, self-handicappers should experience a higher base rate of competency-threatening outcomes. This last influence is compounded by the audience's willingness to give more harsh feedback to self-handicappers than to non-self-handicappers (Rhodewalt, Sanbonmatsu, Tschanz, Feick, & Waller, 1995). In brief, the self-handicapping cycle is self-perpetuating, because it maintains the positive but insecure competency images that motivated the defensive strategy in the first place.

Other Defensive Styles

Although most of our work on the competency/defense self-regulation model has focused on the antecedents and consequences of self-handicapping behavior, we believe our analysis may be expanded to other "defensive styles" as well. We illustrate this claim with the examples of defensive pessimism (Norem & Cantor, 1986) and rejection sensitivity (Downey & Feldman, 1996). According to Norem and Cantor (1986) certain people employ *defensive pessimism* as a motivational tool in competency-relevant situations. In their view, defensive pessimists have a demonstrated history of achievement in competency-relevant domains, yet harbor expectations of failure in the future. For these individuals, the demonstration of competency is very important, and much anxiety and negative affect is associated with such evaluative events. However, rather than being debilitated by anxiety, these individuals draw on it as a source of strength to prepare for the anticipated evaluation. Defensive pessimists set low expectations for themselves and play through negative (and oftentimes low base rate) possible outcomes for the future event. Defensive pessimists are often contrasted with optimists, who set high expectations for themselves and pursue promotion-focused strategies for achievement goal attainment. In terms of actual competency, however, the two groups do not differ in performance or achievement. The notion that defensive pessimism is strategic is evidenced by the fact that when blocked from being pessimistic by being provided with encouragement, these individuals perform poorly (Norem & Cantor, 1986). Defensive pessimism is cast as a motivational strategy designed to maximize performance in achievement settings. In Cantor's (1990) terms, defensive pessimism is an example of social intelligence, in that it is a functional and adaptive strategy employed by some individuals in achievement contexts. Although we have no empirical documentation, we suggest that defensive pessimists bring to achievement contexts concerns about their competencies (distal motives) that prime them to view situational demands to demonstrate competency as potentially threatening to the self. In this regard, we view defensive pessimists as being quite similar to self-handicappers in their motivation to manage others' impressions of their abilities. Dwelling on the possibility of failure and expressing these self-doubts to others, defensive pessimists reduce others' expectations of them. In addition, by suggesting that failure, if it occurs, was the result of elevated emotional distress and not because of poor ability, they have established a self-protective attribution for the anticipated but unwanted outcome (cf. Smith, Snyder, & Handlesman, 1982). Consistent with this notion, Elliot and Church (2003) reported a significant positive correlation between defensive pessimism and self-handicapping. The distal motive of seeking to preserve a competent and able self-view is enabled by the strategy of defensive pessimism.

Relationship Defenses

There has been considerable recent interest in the extent to which one's significant relationships form a part of the self (Andersen & Chen, 2002). Importantly, a person's self-views and feelings when in particular significant relationships can be activated by current interaction partners (Hinkley & Andersen, 1996). Given the importance of significant interpersonal relationships to the self, it follows that responses from relationship partners can threaten the self. The threat of rejection, abandonment, exclusion, or ridicule not only threatens the self but also calls into question the person's competency and value as a relationship partner. Threats to one's sense of interpersonal competency should initiate defensive behaviors. Are there then relationship-specific individual differences in the way that people respond to potential interpersonal difficulties and the threats to the self that they imply? According to Downey and Feldman (1996), *rejection-sensitive* people are chronically anxious and expect to be rejected by their significant others. High rejection-sensitive people are more likely to respond to ambiguous behaviors by another as signaling rejection, and to perceive hurtful intentions from their partner, whereas low rejection sensitive people do not. Downey and Feldman also found that rejection-sensitive people have partners who are more dissatisfied with the relationship. Moreover, Downey, Freitas, Michaelis, and Khouri (1998) observed that

rejection-sensitive women were likely to turn their expectations into reality, such that their relationships were more likely to dissolve than relationships among women who were low in rejection sensitivity. Importantly, rejection-sensitive women's conflict-engendering interpersonal style was found to be a precipitating cause of the breakups. On the surface, rejection sensitivity appears to be self-defeating, in that it precipitates the unwanted outcome, rejection and relationship dissolution, that was feared in the first place. However, by conceiving of rejection sensitivity within the competency/defense self-regulation framework, such responses make sense. Rejection-sensitive people bring to relationships concerns about their attractiveness as a relationship partner and their abilities to maintain the relationship and avoid rejection. These distal concerns and motives make rejection-sensitive people vigilant for signs that their partners are losing interest or are discovering their weaknesses and negative characteristics. Perceived evidence of impending rejection serves as the proximal motivation to initiate the set of defensive interpersonal strategies characteristic of the style. Although the defensive strategies spawn rejection, they also allow individuals to preserve a sense of relationship competency and to guard their fragile self-esteem. After all, it was the partner who could not accept the truth about his or her flaws and shortcomings, and who lacked commitment to stay with the relationship. It is also likely that rejection sensitivity–related interpersonal strategies have the self-perpetuating effect of enhancing the person's sense of predictability in the social environment and fueling fears of rejection in future relationships.

Another form of rejection sensitivity is suggested by Sandra Murray and her colleagues (Murray, Rose, Bellavia, Holmes, & Kusche, 2002), one that clearly links such strategic behavior to the self. Murray et al. reported that self-esteem moderates the reactions to perceived rejection within close relationships. In a series of experiments, people with high and low self-esteem were made to believe that their partners complained about their faults or would dislike a "secret" aspect of their personality. After receiving this threat to their relationship value, low—but not high—self-esteem people overreacted to their partner's response by seeing themselves as lacking in worth and believing that their partners were pulling away from the relationship. In response to this threat to their relationship competencies, low self-esteem people derogated the partner's traits and reported less closeness to the partner. In contrast, threatened high self-esteem people did not derogate the partner or suspect the partner's intentions with regard to the relationship; rather, they affirmed the partner in the face of possible acceptance threats. Despite their anxieties and differences in defensive (among low self-esteem people) or reaffirming (among high self-esteem people) responses, relationships partners viewed their threatened high and low self-esteem partners equally positively. As was the case with high rejection-sensitive women, the vulnerable self-concepts and doubtful feelings of acceptance among low self-esteem people may paradoxically set up relationship failures through their capriciousness and ill-behaved responses to a partner's (largely ambiguous) behavior. Relational insecurities thus produce a set of deleterious behaviors that allow the relationship to unfold as expected, thus preserving a limited sense of relationship competency for low self-esteem individuals.

No doubt there are any number of interpersonal orientations that embody interpersonal competency concerns and prescribe a set of defensive self-regulatory responses. Our intention here is not provide an exhaustive list but to suggest that the self- and competency concerns are embedded in our interpersonal relationships and, as a consequence, relationships provide threats to the self that, in turn, elicit strategic defensive reactions.

CONCLUSIONS

People embrace their self-perceived competencies as integral components of their self-concept and as cornerstones of their self-esteem. To the extent that people's competency images are positive and central to self-worth but also insecure, and to the extent that they believe that competence is stable and unmodifiable, competency/defense motivation will be chronically high. It is a unique feature of our competencies that they are frequently put to the test. It is in such circumstances that the insecure individual will be threatened and respond with defensive behaviors intended to protect the competency self-image. Competency and defensive behavior are linked through their relation to the self. In this chapter, we have proposed the competency/defense self-regulation model to give coherence and meaning to defensive behaviors and illustrated our model with research on self-handicapping behavior. It is our position that defensive behavior can best be understood when it is placed within the context of self-regulatory processes. In this view, defensive strategies are neither illogical nor mysterious; rather, they are tools wielded by individuals whose sense of competency is in question. We suspect that many paradoxical behaviors will lend themselves to analysis within the competency/defense self-regulation framework.

NOTES

1. Throughout the chapter, we use the terms "self-esteem" and "self-worth" interchangeably.
2. Any discussion of self-esteem raises the issue of whether self-esteem is contingent (Crocker & Wolfe, 2001) or "optimal" (Kernis, 2003) or "true" (Deci & Ryan, 1995). Our interest is somewhat orthogonal to this concern; global self-esteem, in our view, is a composite of self-evaluations across personally important competencies and social relationships. In this sense, all self-esteem is contingent. Less relevant to our focus is the extent to which self-evaluations are contingent on the values and desires of others or the self, which is the crux of the more general debate.
3. When the topic is low in relevance to person's self-concept, the corresponding effect is that of feeling better about the self. We do not discuss this "reflection" process, because it is not central to the concept of self-defense, as is the former "comparison" process.

REFERENCES

Andersen, S. M., & Chen, S. (2002). The relational self: An interpersonal social-cognitive theory. *Psychological Review, 109,* 619–645.

Arkin, R. M., & Oleson, K. C. (1998). Self-handicapping. In J. Darley & J. Cooper (Eds.), *Attribution and social interaction: The legacy of Edward E. Jones* (pp. 313–348). Washington, DC: American Psychological Association.

Baumeister, R. F. (1982). A self-presentational view of social phenomena. *Psychological Bulletin, 91,* 3–26.

Baumeister, R. F., & Jones, E. E. (1978). When self-presentation is constrained by the target's knowledge: Consistency and compensation. *Journal of Personality and Social Psychology, 36,* 608–618.

Berglas, S. (1988). The three faces of self-handicapping: Protective self-presentation, a strategy for self-esteem enhancement, and a character disorder. In R. Hogan (Ed.), *Perspectives in personality* (Vol. 1, pp. 235–270). Greenwich, CT: JAI Press.

Berglas, S., & Jones, E. E. (1978). Drug choice as a self-handicapping strategy in response to non-contingent success. *Journal of Personality and Social Psychology, 36,* 405–417.

Brown, J. D. (1986). Evaluations of self and others: Self-enhancement biases in social judgment. *Social Cognition, 4,* 353–376.

Brown, J. D., & Gallagher, F. M. (1992). Coming to terms with failure: Private self-enhancement and public self-effacement. *Journal of Experimental Social Psychology, 28,* 3–22.

Campbell, W. K., & Sedikides, C. (1999). Self-threat magnifies the self-serving bias: A meta-analytic integration. *Review of General Psychology, 3,* 23–43.

Cantor, N. (1990). From thought to behavior: "Having" and "doing" in the study of personality and cognition. *American Psychologist, 45,* 735–750.

Cantor, N. (1994). Life task problem solving: Situational affordances and personal needs. *Personality and Social Psychology Bulletin, 20,* 235–243.

Cantor, N., & Kihlstrom, J. (1987). *Personality and social intelligence.* Englewood, NJ: Prentice-Hall.

Conway, M., & Ross, M. (1984). Getting what you want by revising what you had. *Journal of Personality and Social Psychology, 47,* 738–748.

Crocker, J., & Wolfe, C. T. (2001). Contingencies of self-worth. *Psychological Review, 108,* 593–623.

Deci, E. M., & Ryan, R. M. (1995). Human autonomy: the basis of true self-esteem. In M. H. Kernis (Ed.), *Efficacy, agency, and self-esteem* (pp. 31–39). New York: Plenum Press.

Downey, G., & Feldman, S. I. (1996). Implications of rejection sensitivity for intimate relationships. *Journal of Personality and Social Psychology, 70,* 1327–1343.

Downey, G., Freitas, A. L., Michaelis, B., & Khouri, H. (1998). The self-fulfilling prophecy in close relationships: Rejection sensitivity and rejection by romantic partners. *Journal of Personality and Social Psychology, 75,* 545–560.

Dweck, C. S. (1999). *Self-theories: Their role in motivation, personality and development.* Philadelphia: Psychology Press.

Dweck, C. S., & Leggett, E. L. (1988). A social-cognitive approach to motivation and personality. *Psychological Review, 95,* 256–273.

Elliot, A. J., & Church, M. A. (2003). A motivational analysis of defensive pessimism and self-handicapping. *Journal of Personality, 71,* 369–396.

Elliot, E. S., & Dweck, C. S. (1988). Goals: An approach to motivation and achievement. *Journal of Personality and Social Psychology, 54,* 5–12.

Feick, D. L., & Rhodewalt, F. (1998). The double-edged sword of self-handicapping: Discounting, augmentation, and the protection and enhancement of self-esteem. *Motivation and Emotion, 21,* 147–163.

Fein, S., & Spencer, S. J. (1997). Prejudice as self-image maintenance: Affirming the self through derogating others. *Journal of Personality and Social Psychology, 73,* 31–44.

Greenwald, A. G. (1980). The totalitarian ego: Fabrication and revision of personal history. *American Psychologist, 35,* 603–618.

Heatherton, T. F., & Vohs, K. D. (2000). Interpersonal evaluations following threats to self: Role of self-esteem. *Journal of Personality and Social Psychology, 78,* 725–736.

Hinkley, K., & Andersen, S. M. (1996). The working self-concept in transference: Significant other activation and self-change. *Journal of Personality and Social Psychology, 71,* 1279–1295.

Jones, E. E., & Berglas, S. (1978). Control of attributions about the self through self-handicapping strategies: The appeal of alcohol and the role of underachievement. *Personality and Social Psychology Bulletin, 4,* 200–206.

Jones, E. E., & Rhodewalt, F. (1982). *The Self-Handicapping Scale.* Available from F. Rhodewalt, Department of Psychology, University of Utah, Salt Lake City, UT.

Kelley, H. H. (1972). Attribution in social interaction. In E. E. Jones, D. F. Kanouse, H. H. Kelley, R. E. Nisbett, S. Valins, & B. Weiner (Eds.), *Attribution: Perceiving the causes of behavior* (pp. 1–26). Morristown, NJ: General Learning Press.

Kernis, M. H. (2003). Toward a conceptualization of optimal self-esteem. *Psychological Inquiry, 14,* 1–26.

Kolditz, T. A., & Arkin, R. M. (1982). An impression management interpretation of the self-handicapping strategy. *Journal of Personality and Social Psychology, 43,* 492–502.

Leary, M. R., & Downs, D. L. (1995). Interpersonal functions of the self-esteem motive: The self-esteem system as a sociometer. In M. H. Kernis (Ed.), *Efficacy, agency, and self-esteem* (pp. 123–144). Plenum series in social/clinical psychology. New York: Plenum Press.

McCrea, S. M., & Hirt, E. R. (2001). The role of ability judgments in self-handicapping. *Personality and Social Psychology Bulletin, 27,* 1378–1389.

Miller, D. T., & Ross, M. (1975). Self-serving biases in the attribution of causality: Fact or fiction? *Psychological Bulletin, 82,* 213–225.

Morf, C. C., & Rhodewalt, F. (1993). Narcissism and self-evaluation maintenance: Explorations in object relations. *Personality and Social Psychology Bulletin, 19,* 668–676.

Murray, S. L., Rose, P., Bellavia, G. M., Holmes, J. G.,

& Kusche, A. G. (2002). When rejection stings: How self-esteem constrains relationship-enhancement processes. *Journal of Personality and Social Psychology, 83,* 556–573.

Nicholls, J. G. (1984). Achievement motivation: Conceptions of ability, subjective experience, task choice, and performance. *Psychological Review, 91,* 328–346.

Norem, J. K., & Cantor, N. (1986). Defensive pessimism: "Harnessing" anxiety as motivation. *Journal of Personality and Social Psychology, 52,* 1208–1217.

Paulus, D. L., Fridhandler, B., & Hayes, S. (1997). Psychological defense: contemporary theory and research. In R. Hogan, J. Johnson, & S. Briggs (Eds.), *Handbook of personality psychology* (pp. 543–579). San Diego: Academic Press.

Pemberton, M., & Sedikides, C. (2001). When do individuals help close others improve?: The role of information diagnosticity. *Journal of Personality and Social Psychology, 81,* 234–246.

Rhodewalt, F. (1990). Self-handicappers: Individual differences in the preference for anticipatory self-protective acts. In R. Higgins, C. R. Snyder, & S. Berglas (Eds.), *Self-handicapping: The paradox that isn't* (pp. 69–106). New York: Plenum Press.

Rhodewalt, F. (1994). Conceptions of ability, achievement goals and individual differences in self-handicapping behavior: On the application of implicit theories. *Journal of Personality, 62,* 67–85.

Rhodewalt, F., & Eddings, S. K. (2002). Narcissus reflects: Memory distortion in response to ego relevant feedback in high and low narcissistic men. *Journal of Research in Personality, 36,* 97–106.

Rhodewalt, F., & Fairfield, M. (1991). Claimed self-handicaps and the self-handicapper: The relation of reduction in intended effort to performance. *Journal of Research in Personality, 25,* 402–417.

Rhodewalt, F., & Hill, S. K. (1995). Self-handicapping in the classroom: The effects of claimed self-handicaps in responses to academic failure. *Journal of Personality and Social Psychology, 16,* 397–416.

Rhodewalt, F., Morf, C., Hazlett, S., & Fairfield, M. (1991). Self-handicapping: The role of discounting and augmentation in the preservation of self-esteem. *Journal of Personality and Social Psychology, 61,* 121–131.

Rhodewalt, F., Sanbonmatsu, D. M., Tschanz, B. T., Feick, D. L., & Waller, A. (1995). Self-handicapping and interpersonal trade-offs. *Personality and Social Psychology Bulletin, 21,* 1042–1050.

Rhodewalt, F., & Tragakis, M. (2002). Self-handicapping and the social self: The costs and rewards of interpersonal self-construction. In J. P. Forgas & K. D. Williams (Eds.), *The social self: Cognitive, interper-* sonal, and intergroup perspectives (pp. 121–140). New York: Psychology Press.

Ross, M. (1989). Relation of implicit theories to the construction of personal histories. *Psychological Review, 96,* 341–357.

Sedikides, C., & Strube, M. (1995). The multiply motivated self. *Personality and Social Psychology Bulletin, 21,* 1330–1335.

Smith, T. W., Snyder, C. R., & Handelsman, M. M. (1982). On the self-serving function of an academic wooden leg: Test anxiety as a self-handicapping strategy. *Journal of Personality and Social Psychology, 48,* 970–980.

Snyder, C. R., & Smith, T. W. (1982). Symptoms as self-handicapping strategies: The virtues of old wine in a new bottle. In G. Weary & H. L. Mirels (Eds.), *Integration of clinical and social psychology* (pp. 104–127). New York: Oxford University Press.

Swann, W. B. (1983). Self-verification: Bringing social reality into harmony with the self. In J. Suls & A. Greenwald (Eds.), *Psychological perspectives on the self* (Vol. 2, pp. 33–66). Hillsdale, NJ: Erlbaum.

Swann, W. B. (1985). The self as architect of social reality. In B. Schlenker (Ed.), *The self and social life* (pp. 100–125). New York: McGraw-Hill.

Swann, W. B., Stein-Seroussi, A., & Giesler, R. B. (1992). Why people self-verify. *Journal of Personality and Social Psychology 62,* 392–401.

Tafarodi, R. W., & Swann, W. B., Jr. (1995). Self-liking and self-competence as dimensions of global self-esteem: Initial validation of a measure. *Journal of Personality Assessment, 65,* 322–342.

Tesser, A. (1988). Toward a self-evaluation maintenance model of social behavior. In L. Berkowitz (Ed.), *Advances in experimental social psychology* (Vol. 21, pp. 181–227). New York: Academic Press.

Tice, D. (1991). Esteem protection or enhancement?: Self-handicapping motives and attributions differ by trait self-esteem. *Journal of Personality and Social Psychology, 60,* 711–725.

Vohs, K., & Heatherton, T. F. (2003). The effects of self-esteem and ego threat on interpersonal appraisals of men and women: A naturalistic study. *Personality and Social Psychology Bulletin, 29,* 1407–1420.

Weary, G. B. (1978). Self-serving biases in the attribution process: A re-examination of the fact or fiction question. *Journal of Personality and Social Psychology, 36,* 56–71.

Ybarra, O. (1999). Misanthropic person memory when the need to self-enhance is absent. *Personality and Social Psychology Bulletin, 25,* 261–269.

Zuckerman, M., Kiefer, S., & Knee, C. R. (1998). Consequences of self-handicapping: Effects on coping, academic performance, and adjustment. *Journal of Personality and Social Psychology, 74,* 1619–1628.

CHAPTER 30

☙

Social Comparison and Self-Evaluations of Competence

LADD WHEELER
JERRY SULS

Festinger (1954a, 1954b) was the first to advance a systematic formulation of the role of social comparisons on self-evaluations and behavior. His social comparison theory was cast in the form of nine hypotheses, eight corollaries, and eight derivations. For our purposes here, it can be reduced to the following: We need to have accurate appraisals of our opinions and abilities, and when we cannot get these appraisals through objective means, we try to get them through comparison with similar others (the similarity hypothesis). In the case of abilities, there is a unidirectional drive upward, so that we want to be slightly better than others.

Festinger did not specify clearly what he meant by "similarity." Early researchers (e.g., Wheeler, 1966) took it to mean similarity on the dimension of comparison. There is circularity involved in this, however, because one must have already compared with someone to know that he or she is similar. Wheeler neatly avoided this problem by giving participants information

about their position in a rank order. Thus, they knew that they were more similar to some people than to others, but they did not know *how* similar (in terms of scores) they were to anyone. The general result of this line of "rank-order paradigm" research was that participants compared themselves to those adjacent to them in the ranking, and much more with the person just better than themselves than with the person just worse than themselves. Thus, the research supported both the unidirectional drive upward and the similarity hypothesis.

An interesting exception to the usual results occurred when no information was given about the highest score in the group. In that case, most participants compared with the highest ranking person, a case of the unidirectional drive upward completely overwhelming the desire for a similar comparison other.

Goethals and Darley (1977) proposed the related attributes hypothesis (see Wheeler & Zuckerman, 1977), in which similarity was based upon characteristics related to and predictive of the trait to be evaluated. If one swims better than a man of his age, physical condition, and swimming experience, then he is a good swimmer (better than he ought to be based on related attributes). It is easy to imagine a situation in which similarity on the attribute to be evaluated is distinct from similarity on related attributes. For example, a comparison target might have a score similar to that of another on the ability (attribute to be evaluated), and a different comparison target might have the same amount of practice (the related attribute) on the ability. When that occurs, both types of similarity influence choice of a comparison other (Wheeler, Koestner, & Driver, 1982).

Research beginning in the 1980s showed that people who feel the need for self-enhancement make comparisons resulting in affective and motivational outcomes that are different from those of people motivated by self-evaluation or the need for accurate evaluations of one's abilities. For example, a breast cancer patient might make predominantly downward comparisons in order to make herself feel better about her own state. See Wills (1981) and Wood, Taylor, and Lichtman (1985) for theory and research on self-enhancement. However, in everyday life, the line between self-evaluation and self-enhancement probably is fuzzy, because people should want both to acquire information about their standing (so they can make informed decisions about what things they can do) and to feel good about themselves (or at least not feel poorly). The question we consider in this chapter is how social comparisons contribute to an individual's personal sense of competence. For a greater breadth and depth of information about social comparison processes, see Suls and Wheeler (2000).

It is strange that social comparison theory has not been better integrated into the achievement motivation literature. Much of Festinger's work prior to social comparison was on level of aspiration (LOA), and that work was integral to the achievement motivation literature and clearly influenced social comparison theory. His first publication, based on undergraduate research done at City College of New York, dealt with social factors affecting LOA (Hertzman & Festinger, 1940), as did his Master's thesis done under Kurt Lewin (Festinger, 1942a,

1942b). The research showed that participants raised their LOA if they scored below other group members (particularly if they were high school students and therefore of lower status than the college participants), and lowered their LOA if they scored above others (particularly if these others were graduate students and therefore of higher status than the participants). Here, we see clear evidence for what was later to be called the related attributes hypothesis (Goethals & Darley, 1977): The college student participants felt that they *ought* to score higher than high school students and lower than graduate students because of the related attributes of age and education.

Tamara Dembo (1931) introduced the concept of LOA in her 1930 PhD thesis in Berlin, and the first experiment was published that same year (Hoppe, 1930), both influenced by Lewin. Throughout the 1930s and early 1940s, LOA was a thriving area for research and theory, including work by researchers such as Hilgard, R.R. Sears, P. Sears, and Rotter. Festinger went to Iowa to study with Lewin because he wanted to work on tension systems, boundaries, satiation, force fields, and related issues, but found that Lewin was by then interested more in practical social problems. The classic theoretical and review chapter, "Level of Aspiration" (Lewin, Dembo, Festinger, & Sears, 1944), which marks the end of this period of research and theory, was developed by Dembo, P. Sears, and Festinger from Lewin's conceptual system (see Patnoe, 1988). They followed the "resultant valence theory," presented by Escalona (1940) and elaborated by Festinger (1942b).

A fundamental puzzle with regard to LOA (and achievement motivation in general) is the apparent inconsistency between setting up higher and higher goals, and the notion that life appears to be governed by the tendency to avoid unnecessary effort. Looking at the psychological situation that individuals face as they make up their minds about the next goal can solve this problem. Experimental results have shown that with increasing difficulty level, the valence of success increases, and the valence of failure decreases. Therefore, given two levels of difficulty, the valence will always be greater at the higher level of difficulty (Valence = Valence of Success − Valence of Failure). The situation is complicated by the necessity to take into account both the probability as well as the valence of future events. If success at the highest level of difficulty has very positive valence, but the probability of achieving success is zero, then there will be little resultant motivation to attempt that level of difficulty. The "weighted" valence of success is the product of the valence and of the probability of success. Motivation will tend to be highest at that level of difficulty at which there is a subjective 50–50 probability of success and failure.

All decisions about valence and the probability of success are made within existing frames or scales of reference. There are usually many coexisting frames of reference for a level of aspiration (e.g., task-referential, past-referential, and other-referential; Elliot, McGregor, & Thrash, 2002). One reference scale based, for example, upon the individual's past achievement might lead to one LOA, while another reference scale, based upon group standards, might lead to a different LOA. These two reference scales are combined according to the relative weight or "potency" of the two frames of reference. There are also different types of group standards. Given a college standard of a "Gentleman's C," the resultant valence is maximum at "C" and falls off rapidly in both directions. In other cases, the group standard might set a minimum level, and anything above that would have much success valence and little failure valence. Standards set from outside do not have to be related to another group but may come from a significant individual (friend, teacher, etc.) or from requirements of law or society. Lewin et al. (1944) also stressed that there are great differences between people in their relative tendencies to seek success and to avoid failure, so that the valence of success and failure will certainly not be the same for all people in the same situation (Elliot & Church, 1997).

The Lewin et al. (1944) paper had a major impact on the development of the achievement motivation literature. It also presaged much of social comparison theory. The unidirectional drive upward of social comparison theory comes directly from the resultant valence theory of Lewin et al., which also provides the basis for (McClelland, Atkinson, Clark, & Lowell (1953) influential achievement motivation framework.

Our task in the remainder of this chapter is to discuss how social comparison may influence achievement motivation and perceptions of competence.

PROXIES AND PERFORMANCE PREDICTION

There are many tasks that one might not want to attempt without prior knowledge that one has a very good chance of succeeding. Examples include swimming across a bay, pursuing graduate study, rebuilding a car engine, and getting married. Wheeler, Martin, and Suls (1997) proposed a proxy model of social comparison to deal with the issue of predicting one's own competence (see also Martin, 2000).

How would a woman know whether she might succeed in graduate school? She might extrapolate from her undergraduate performance. To the extent that she did well as an undergraduate, she should do well as a graduate student. However, she knows that all graduate students have done well as undergraduates, and that not all of them succeed as graduate students. She needs something more. She might well talk to another woman who attended her undergraduate school and subsequently succeeded brilliantly in graduate school. If she found that this proxy performed the same as she did as an undergraduate and that graduate school had not been a terrible challenge, she would feel more confident that she was competent enough to work toward her PhD; that is, on Task 1 (undergraduate education), she was similar to the proxy, so she should be similar to the proxy on Task 2 (graduate school). There is one complication to this, however. It is possible that the proxy exerted very little effort on Task 1. Perhaps she was a party girl, the social chairperson of her sorority, a member of the golf team, and a frequent visitor to tropical islands and European capitols. Our comparer, on the other hand, had to work hard for similar grades. The comparer and the proxy are quite different, then, on effort, a related attribute (Goethals & Darley, 1977), and it is unlikely that the proxy's performance on Task 1 was indicative of her maximal effort or true competence. Therefore, in this case, the comparer should not expect similar Task 2 performance.

Related attributes are important only when the proxy's Task 1 performance may not indicate maximal effort. If we know that the proxy exerted maximal effort, then the prediction from Task 1 performance to Task 2 performance is straightforward.

There is empirical support for the basic premises of the proxy model, using both physical strength and intellectual problem-solving tasks (Martin, Suls, & Wheeler, 2002). For example, when predicting performance on a grip strength task, participants paid attention to the related attribute, hand size, but only when the proxy's performance on Task 1 may not have been maximal. Participants' predictions factored in relative hand size in deciding whether they would perform better, worse, or the same as the proxy had. When the proxy's performance on Task 1 was clearly the best that the proxy could do, participants ignored hand size in predicting their own performance on the grip strength task. In this case, participants predicted that they would perform as well as the proxy had.

The Wheeler et al. (1997) theoretical paper argued that one of the most important questions that might be answered through social comparison is "Can I do X?" That question may be answered through comparison with a similar proxy who has already attempted X. If the similar proxy can do it, so, probably, can you. There is not a direct connection to motivation beyond the fact that knowing you *can* do something may indeed motivate you to do it. Basically, however, the proxy model assumes prior motivation. In the next section, we examine a similar line of research (Lockwood & Kunda [1997] on superstars) in which self-views and motivation rather than prediction are the major dependent variables. The superstar and proxy arguments are similar in one important way. In both cases, the comparer is comparing him- or herself to a target that has already had a chance to demonstrate competence. The comparer is not in direct competition with the target, as in many social comparison situations, because the comparer is about to undertake a task that the target has already performed and from which he or she has now moved away. Rather than competing with the target, the comparer is using the target as a source of information and/or inspiration.

SUPERSTARS AND SUPERFLOPS

In the original superstar research (Lockwood & Kunda, 1997), first-year and fourth-year accounting students were exposed to an article about an outstanding graduating student in accounting or to a no-target control. Participants then rated themselves on adjectives relevant to general career success. First-year students rated themselves considerably higher after exposure to the superstar, whereas fourth-year students rated themselves insignificantly lower. The superstar's success was attainable for the first-year students but not for the fourth-year students. First-year students rated the target as a more relevant comparison than did fourth-year students, and in open-ended explanations of their relevance ratings, often mentioned that the superstar inspired them, and that they were similar to the superstar on dimensions other than intended occupation. In a follow-up study, first-year students with a malleable view of intelligence gave higher self-ratings after exposure to a fourth-year superstar, but those with a fixed view of intelligence did not, again supporting the view that attainability is crucial.

The dependent variable in this research was self-ratings on adjectives generally related to career success (e.g., bright, competent, ambitious, intelligent), essentially a measure of self-esteem. In their next research, Lockwood and Kunda (1999) also included measures of motivation. One measure was objective estimates of how much time participants would devote to six activities that were related to areas in which the target excelled (e.g., "Next week I plan to spend _____ hours studying," "This year I plan to spend about _____ hours on volunteer work or charity-related activities." In the second measure, participants were asked to estimate the likelihood that they would engage in eight activities (e.g., making a special effort to study hard for exams, volunteering to do more community work). Each item on the two scales was standardized, and all items were combined to form a single index of motivation.

The purpose of the Lockwood and Kunda (1999) research was to demonstrate that increasing the salience of people's best selves would undermine the inspiration created by a superstar. The researchers increased the salience of participants' best selves (Study 1) by asking them, before exposure to the superstar, to describe a peak academic experience that had made them feel especially proud, or (Study 2) by asking them to describe the academic and career achievement they hoped to accomplish over the next 10 years. Both of these "success primes" were expected to ground participants in reality, thus reducing the inspirational impact of the superstar, both as measured by adjective self-ratings and by the motivation scale. However, this prediction was correct only for adjective self-ratings. For the motivation index, the only significant effect was a reduction in motivation in Study 1 by the addition of the superstar model in the success prime conditions. Neither the superstar nor the success prime in either study increased motivation.

So far, we have examined only superstars, or highly successful role models. It could be, however, that failing models, or "superflops" (our term) would increase motivation to avoid sharing their fate. Lockwood (2002) exposed first-year participants to a poorly coping, recent university graduate who could get a job only in a fast-food outlet. Participants in a simulation condition were asked to describe a realistic scenario about how they might become like the superflop, whereas students in a no-simulation condition described their typical daily activities. There was also a no-target control condition. Only when asked to simulate did the participants show any effect of being exposed to a superflop. It is important to note that when the comparison target is a superstar, participants readily assimilate to the target, but when the target is a superflop, participants require the stronger manipulation of being asked to describe how it could happen to them. Otherwise, they just shrug it off.

In a follow-up study in which all participants were asked to simulate, adjective self-ratings were lower in the superflop condition than in a control condition; in other words, participants assimilated their self-views to the superflop. A measure of avoidance goals was higher in the superflop condition, but a measure of approach goals was not lower in the superflop condition. A new motivation scale was added for this study (e.g., "I plan to spend more time at the li-brary," "I plan to stop myself from procrastinating"). This scale showed motivation to be highest in the superflop condition. Moreover, motivation was correlated with avoidance goals but not with approach goals.

In summary, a superflop comparison target decreased adjective self-ratings but increased motivational plans and avoidance goals. Having seen that both superstars and superflops can have motivational effects, a reasonable question to ask is whether situationally induced approach and avoidance goals will determine whether superstars or superflops have the greater influence on motivation. The prediction is that superstars will be more effective when approach goals are induced, whereas superflops will be more effective at increasing motivation when avoidance goals are induced. Lockwood, Jordan, and Kunda (2002) investigated this question.

In two studies, approach and avoidance goals were primed in different ways. Participants then read about a recent graduate of their own academic program who was either a superstar or superflop. There was also a no-target control group. The dependent variable was the motivation scale described earlier. In both studies, participants were more motivated by a comparison target consistent with their primed motivation: approach-primed participants responded with greater motivation to a superstar, and avoidance-primed participants responded with greater motivation to a superflop. In Study 2 only, a target incongruent with the primed motivation actually decreased motivation (e.g., a superflop target with approach-primed participants). In a third study, participants completed new approach–avoidance scales containing items such as "I frequently imagine how I will achieve my hopes and aspirations," and "I frequently think about how I can prevent failures in my life," and then generated an example of a person whose success or failure had motivated them in the past. Participants with relatively higher approach scores were more likely to recall positive role models.

Lockwood and Kunda's research shows that exposure to a superstar can increase self-esteem and motivation, if the star is not a competitor. The achievements of the role model should appear attainable, however. Furthermore, learning about superflops does not undermine personal self-esteem, unless people are encouraged to think about how it could happen to them. As others have suggested, comparison direction is not intrinsically tied to a particular affective outcome (Buunk, Collins, Taylor, Van Yperen, & Dakoff, 1990). Although there are conditions in which a comparison might be demoralizing, people have considerable flexibility under most circumstances to protect themselves from the undesirable implications of comparisons and perhaps gain a greater sense of competence or inspiration, even when the comparison is with someone who is exceptional. Exposure to people who fail might undermine self-concept (at least momentarily), but simultaneously strengthen an individual's resolve to avoid the state of the superflop.

UPWARD COMPARISON AND HIGHER GRADES

Researchers in educational environments have used different methods but further substantiate the importance of role models and comparisons as sources of motivation and information concerning perceived competence. Blanton, Buunk, Gibbons, and Kuyper (1999) conducted a longitudinal investigation of the effects of comparison on academic performance among ninth-grade students in the Netherlands. In each of seven different courses, participants nominated the student with whom they typically compared their exam grades. The grade of that nominated person was used to determine whether the comparison was an upward or a downward comparison, and how similar it was. That was in turn related to the participant's subsequent performance in the course.

The average comparison target was slightly upward, as predicted by Festinger (1954a) and as demonstrated by Wheeler (1966) and many subsequent researchers. The most important result, however, was that, controlling for prior grades, upward comparison predicted higher grades both cross-sectionally and longitudinally.

Huguet, Dumas, Monteil, and Genestoux (2001) replicated this research with ninth-grade students in French public schools, and several potential psychological moderators were also measured: (1) importance of the

academic domain; (2) closeness to the target, in terms of frequency of talking; (3) identification with the target, in terms of believing that grades will become more similar to those of the target; and (4) perceptions of academic control, in terms of believing that grades can be increased by increasing effort.

Consistent with Blanton et al. (1999), upward comparison predicted higher grades. Identification was increased by upward comparison, closeness, and perception of control. Unfortunately, none of the moderators interacted with comparison choice in predicting grades. The authors expected perceptions of control to moderate the effect of comparison choice on grades (e.g., Major, Testa, & Blysma, 1991). Upward comparison should not be motivating, unless there is a perception of control over the outcome. Similarly, the authors expected identification to moderate the effect of comparison choice on grades (e.g., Berger, 1977; Buunk & Ybema, 1997). Upward comparison should be motivating only to the extent that a person believes he or she will become more like the comparison target. What we are really left with, then, in the absence of interactions with these moderators, is the fact that students who report upward comparisons get better grades. We do not know why. It could easily be that a third variable, perhaps need for achievement, influences both comparison and grades independently. Or it could be, as the authors of these papers argue, that the actual upward comparison improves grades by giving information about how to improve, or by increasing motivation to improve. The lack of a moderation effect is not necessarily a problem for this explanation, because students may make upward comparisons *only if* they think they have academic control and/or identify with the comparison target.

In both the Blanton et al. (1999) and the Huguet et al. (2001) papers, another social comparison variable in addition to comparison direction was featured. It was "comparative evaluation" and refers to the evaluation of one's ability relative to others. It was measured by asking participants to rate how good they were "compared to most of your classmates" in each of the academic domains on a scale ranging from "much worse" to "much better." The expectation was that people with a high comparative evaluation have a high sense of self-efficacy and performance expectation, which should lead to higher performance. Thus, the prediction of both Blanton et al. (1999) and Huguet et al. (2001) was that both upward comparison and high comparative evaluation would independently lead to better performance. There is a potential problem here, however, because upward comparison should lead logically to lower comparative evaluation. If individuals are comparing with people better than themselves, they should be less likely to claim that they are better than their peers. We return to this later.

Blanton et al. (1999) and Huguet et al. (2001) did indeed find that high comparative evaluation predicted high performance, independent of comparison choice and with prior grades controlled. They also found that comparative evaluation was not influenced by comparison choice but was influenced by participants' own grades; that is, comparing upward did not lower comparative evaluation, but having higher grades raised comparative evaluation. Again, however, comparative evaluation did not interact consistently with the moderator variables in Huguet et al. (2001), and we are left with the somewhat unsatisfactory conclusion that higher comparative evaluation increases performance regardless of moderators such as perceived academic control. Once again, however, it may be that higher comparative evaluation is based on a perception of academic control; thus, moderation would not be exhibited.

One possible psychological inconsistency found in both studies was that students compared upward (mentioning a student who had slightly better grades) but maintained that they were just as good as other people (on the comparative evaluation measure). This inconsistency may be more apparent than real, however. Comparing oneself with an individual who has slightly better grades does not preclude thinking that one is just as good as *most* of one's classmates; in fact, if the student identifies with a slightly superior peer, this may lead to the inference that one is better off than most students. Collins (2000) reviewed a considerable amount of research showing that people intentionally compare themselves with superior targets (e.g., Suls & Tesch, 1978; Wheeler, 1966),

and that such comparisons produce more favorable self-estimates (e.g., Pelham & Wachsmuth, 1995). Because people want and believe that they possess positive attributes, they perceive similarity with upward targets and conclude they are "almost as good as the very good ones" (Wheeler, 1966, p. 30). A similar kind of assimilation was also found in Lockwood and Kunda's research, and the expectation that one will perform like the proxy also is suggestive of assimilation (Wheeler et al., 1997).

SMALL FISH AND BIG PONDS

The focus of the contemporary social comparison literature has been on how people learn about their capabilities and maintain or enhance feelings of self-esteem and self-competence through the strategic selection and construal of upward and downward comparison targets. The general consensus of researchers is that people have the flexibility to select consciously or to construct comparison targets, so as to maximize various goals. But there are situations in which social comparisons are imposed and lasting negative or positive effects on self-concept result (Diener & Fujita, 1977; Marsh, Kong, & Hau, 2000). Research on the "small fish in a big pond effect" (SFBPE) illustrates this point. The SFBPE refers to a phenomenon in which a person acquires a negative self-concept as a function of being among high-ability peers—a result that appears to be the opposite of what Lockwood and Kunda (1997) found after exposure to superstars and the results of Blanton et al. (1999) and Huguet et al. (2001). Earlier, we emphasized the ways that self-evaluations can be displaced toward the comparison target (i.e., assimilation). In the SFBPE, we see that evaluations also can be displaced away from the target (i.e., a contrast). After we review SFBPE research and its implications for perceived competence, we attempt to identify why the SFBPE situation produces lower perceived competence, whereas the Lockwood–Kunda situation produces the opposite outcome. Identifying the variables responsible for inspiration or deflation of expectations is important for not only understanding sources of perceived competence but also evaluating educational practices.

The SFBPE

In a seminal study of the career aspirations of college men, Davis (1966) was the first to refer to the so-called "frog pond" phenomenon. He wanted to understand why the academic quality of a college apparently had little effect on career aspirations. He proposed that attending a high-ability college ("a big pond") would result in a poorer grade point average (GPA), independent of individual academic ability, because academic standards should be more stringent in elite institutions than in a less selective institution (i.e., "a small pond"). Lower GPAs would lead to students' lower self-evaluations of academic competence and, in turn, less ambitious career aspirations. Based on analysis of survey data, Davis concluded, "The aphorism, 'It is better to be a big frog in a small pond than a small frog in a big pond' is not perfect advice, but it is not trivial" (p. 31).

Marsh and his colleagues have produced some of the strongest evidence for the SFBPE from studies of grade school and high school students. The basic idea is that schools place great emphasis on social comparison and achievement levels of classmates. Schools also differ in average ability level, so that each school sets a particular frame of reference for academic achievement. This means that equally able students who attend schools in which school-average achievement differs will use correspondingly different frames of reference in evaluating their academic accomplishments, and this process will affect academic self-concept and subsequent academic outcomes. A consistent finding from several studies is an SFBPE in which equally able students have lower academic self-concepts when the average achievement level is higher than those in schools where the average achievement level is lower.

In a representative study, Marsh and Parker (1984) surveyed grade school classes from high and low socioeconomic status neighborhoods in the same geographical area. There were substantial differences in reading achievement and IQ scores between the two kinds of neighborhoods. When individual ability level was controlled, the correlation between school-average ability and academic self-concept was negative; that is, being enrolled in a high average-ability school (vs. a low average-ability school) was associated with lower academic self-concept.

Marsh (1987) also reanalyzed data from the longitudinal Youth in Transition Study, which included standardized tests of academic aptitude, GPA, socioeconomic status, and academic self-concept (e.g., How intelligent do you think you are, compared with others your age?) in a large sample of high school students. Both at Time 1 and Time 2 (a year later), the association between school-average ability and academic self-concept was negative (−.23), consistent with the negative SFBPE. School-average ability also was negatively associated with GPA, which was positively associated with academic self-concept.

The SFBPE seems to result from two separate processes: Any given student in a low-ability school generally finds him- or herself with less able students, which leads to higher academic self-concept. Students in low-ability schools also should earn higher grades than equally able students in high-ability schools, and this, too, contributes to higher academic self-concepts. Path analysis also used Time 1 measures to predict Time 2 measures. Attending a high-ability school produced lower academic self-concept at Time 1, which produced poorer grades at Time 2. It also is worth noting that global self-esteem was measured in this sample, but there was no SFBPE for self-esteem or general self-concept. The effect was specific to academic self-concept.

In a subsequent study, Marsh (1991) assessed whether the negative effects of school-average ability extended to other academic outcomes. This is important, because educators and parents assume that selective schools (i.e., high average ability) provide academic benefits to their students; the SFBPE, however, suggests that this assumption is incorrect. Marsh measured academic self-concept, selection of advanced course work, and educational and occupational aspirations while the student attended high school and college, and occupational aspirations 2 years after high school graduation. Attending higher ability high schools appeared to have negative effects on almost all outcomes. Furthermore, these effects were mediated by the negative SFBPE on academic self-concept.

Apparently, if students compare their accomplishments with those of their classmates in academically selective schools, then their academic self-concept declines. As mentioned earlier, the SFBPE is based on a contrast effect. Of course, for students enrolled in an unselective or low average-ability school, the state of affairs is the opposite of that for students in an unselective school: The frame of reference will be lower (than in a high-ability school), so academic self-concept of students actually will be enhanced in an unselective school environment ("the big fish in the small pond effect").

Until recently, SFBPE research focused almost entirely on negative contrast effects; however, Marsh et al. (2000) noted that the effect is actually the net effect of two opposing forces: the negative contrast effects, described earlier, and positive reflected glory, or assimilation effects. The latter refers to a well-documented effect in which self-concept is enhanced by people associating with successful others (Cialdini et al., 1976; Tesser, 1988) or joining valued groups. For example, in the school context, students might gain more positive academic self-concepts merely by being enrolled in a highly selective program. Essentially, the student thinks, "If I am a student here I must be smart." If the positive assimilation effect conferred by reflected glory is as strong as the negative contrast effect, then there should be no net effect of school context or SFBPE. However, the consistency of the SFBPE found in prior research suggests that the contrast effect tends to be stronger than the assimilation effect.

Marsh et al. (2000) studied both the SFBPE and reflected glory in a large cohort of high schools in Hong Kong. Two characteristics of this school system are notable: It is one of the most highly achievement-segregated systems in the world—a feature that should heighten the contrast effect that forms the basis of the SFBPE. However, Hong Kong is a collectivistic society; one's reputation is of special concern in Chinese culture, and admission to a prestigious high school should represent a gain in status for the student and his or her family, resulting in a reflected glory effect, or assimilation. This naturalistic experiment permitted the researchers to evaluate whether the highly achievement-segregated system would in-

crease the negative contrast, or whether the cultural differences would reduce the contrast and magnify the reflected glory/assimilation effects.

Marsh et al. (2000) analyzed pretest achievement test scores (prior to start of high school), achievement scores during secondary school, and academic self-concept in a sample of nearly 8,000 secondary school students in Hong Kong. In addition, each student completed some questionnaire items to gauge perception of their school's status to test the effects of reflected glory. Consistent with previous research, students who attended schools with higher school-average achievement scores had lower academic self-concepts than predicted on the basis of their high levels of pretest achievement, *and* lower self-concepts than students with similar abilities in schools with lower school-average achievement scores. Hence, the SFBPE was replicated. However, when perceived school status was included in the statistical model, there was a positive, albeit weaker, effect of school status on academic self-concept, indicative of a reflected glory/assimilation effect: Students who rated their school higher in status tended to have higher academic self-concept.

Marsh et al. (2000) concluded:

> The results imply that attending a school where school-average is high—particularly in Hong Kong—simultaneously results in a more demanding basis of comparison for students within the school to compare their accomplishments (the basis of the negative social comparison effect) and a source of pride for students within the school (the basis of the positive reflected glory effects). (p. 347)

The implication is that the negative contrast effect (SFBPE) would be even stronger if students' affiliation with the school did not serve as a source of pride.

EXPLAINING THE DISCREPANCY

We have seen from Lockwood and Kunda's (1997) research that superstars can be inspiring and buoy estimates of self-competence. Furthermore, naturalistic studies (Blanton et al., 1999; Huguet et al., 2001) demonstrate that upward comparison choices appear to enhance academic performance and motivation. However, SFBPE research indicates that being in a selective school with smarter classmates, where there should be many upward comparisons, seems to have a negative effect on perceived competence. What accounts for the difference in results?

Although it is not possible to identify a single cause, there are some key differences in the situations examined by these researchers. Lockwood and Kunda (1997) demonstrated that it is essential that the superstar not be at the same stage in his or her career as the participants. In contrast, the students in the SFBPE studies were exposed to the academic accomplishments of their classmates (same-age peers). Lockwood and Kunda's subjects still have time, and can hope and strive to match the superstar, but Marsh's grade school or secondary school students were already aware that they had not attained the success of their classmates.

This argument does not appear to apply, however, to the studies by Blanton et al. (1999) and Huguet et al. (2001). The people with whom the ninth graders compared exam grades were same-age peers. But the results showed that upward comparisons were motivating. The important difference might be that students nominated a classmate with *slightly better* grades as a comparison target, and therefore attainable accomplishments, and not a superstar, whose accomplishments might be seen as unattainable. Unfortunately, a direct comparison between the SFBPE studies and Blanton et al. (1999) and Huguet et al. (2001) studies is impossible, because the latter researchers did not compare high- and low average-ability schools.

What may be happening is this: Some students in both low- and high-ability schools compare themselves with those who have slightly higher grades, and as a result do better, either by being more highly motivated, or by learning how to make better grades. Thus, assimilation is occurring for some students, as shown by Blanton et al. (1999) and Huguet et al. (2001), and these slightly upward comparisons should be encouraged. Simultaneously, and in opposition to the effects of slightly upward comparisons, students in high-ability schools are doing less well than students in low-ability schools (holding aptitude constant) and thus suffer a decline in academic self-concept. Students in the high-ability schools are also involuntarily exposed to superstars, who are age peers and therefore evoke a contrasting academic self-concept. The net result of these factors is a lower academic self-concept in the high-ability schools.

This outcome might be avoided if students had the flexibility and cognitive manipulation of comparison information that has been demonstrated in some laboratory and field research (Wood et al., 1985). However, these devices are probably severely limited in the school environment. Marsh et al. (2000, p. 339) noted, "The school is a total environment in that there are so many inherent constraints and a natural emphasis on social comparison of achievement levels in a school setting." Under such circumstances, in which competition for grades is an integral element, it is scarcely surprising that negative contrast tends to be the dominant element.

MODELS AND MELODRAMA

In this chapter, we have focused on the role of comparisons for achievement and perceptions of personal competence. Another form of social comparison—the use of social models in drama—is being used to create large-scale social change. Population Communications International is a nonprofit organization specializing in "entertainment–education" radio and television programs created to bring social change (Smith, 2002). Miguel Sabido pioneered the technique in Mexico in the 1970s in his efforts to promote adult literacy and family planning.

Programs are now aimed at reducing unwanted pregnancies, reducing the spread of HIV, promoting literacy, and empowering women, and there are offices in China, Egypt, India, Kenya, Mexico, and Pakistan. The long-term radio–television programs are deliberately melodramatic, showing a clash between positive and negative values in an exaggerated way. Great care in taken with character development and the use of tension and conflict, cliffhangers, music, and various plots and subplots. The melodramas feature ordinary people who are positive role models, negative role models, or transitional models, who start out negatively but turn into positive models over time. It is particularly important that the transitional models be very similar to the viewers, so that the viewers can see themselves changing in the same way. The melodrama should increase self-efficacy—the belief that one can change one's behavior and improve one's life. Rewards and punishments are always the natural outgrowth of the characters' behavioral choices; that is, someone with a drinking problem would be punished with a car accident but not by contracting cancer.

At the end of some episodes, someone, often a celebrity, summarizes the lessons and tells viewers where they can get further information or help. These programs are often more popular than the pure entertainment programs, and evaluation data show that they have strong effects on behavior. The technique has even been used with American soap operas. Two episodes of *The Bold and the Beautiful*, dealing with HIV and giving a number to call for more information, increased the number of calls by 16-fold over the normal volume.

The primary inspiration for the efforts of Population Communications International was Bandura's (1977) social learning theory. However, social comparison is a component of social learning theory and social cognitive theory (Bandura, 1986), and is, we believe, the most important part of the dynamics involved in the large-scale social change efforts. Seeing others obtain valued outcomes as a result of their efforts can instill a belief in observers that they, too, can obtain the valued outcomes, and thus motivates them to do so. Observers must believe that they have the efficacy to produce the modeled performances, and that similar behavior will bring them similar outcomes. People compare themselves with others to learn what they can and want to accomplish. Although such social comparisons do not constitute the sole source of information that underlies personal competence. They seem to be important.

CONCLUSIONS

Perceptions of competence and motivation are strongly influenced by social comparisons. However, as we have described, social comparison can produce assimilative and contrastive effects (Mussweiler, 2001; Stapel & Koomen, 2000). We have described how superstars and persons (proxies) who have attempted tasks that we are contemplating can serve as role models, allowing us to identify or assimilate to them. Their successes can be an important source of knowledge and motivation, because they are not our direct competitors. These role models, however, do need to have some similarities (in related attributes) with us, as social comparison theory stipulates, to be meaningful and allow us to identify or assimilate with them.

Comparisons also can produce contrastive outcomes. Being exposed to a superflop may lower self-evaluations if people are forced to think about how the same thing could happen to them (assimilation), but it also prompts action to help them avoid such an outcome (contrast). In the school environment, the presence of many high-ability peers can reduce academic self-concept and academic aspirations via a contrast effect. We think that the contrast effect exceeds any effect of pride of identification with being in a selective school because of the inherent competition with same-age peers. However, in our view assimilation and contrast are not all-or-none outcomes. Probably every social comparison creates both the pull of assimilation and the push of contrast. Which process predominates depends on the person's degree of freedom and flexibility to make strategic comparisons. As we learn more about how social environments expand or constrain this comparison flexibility, we may be able to provide educators, developmentalists, and policymakers with tangible suggestions about how a person can acquire a sense of personal competence that strikes a balance between realistic appraisal and confidence.

ACKNOWLEDGMENT

Preparation of this chapter was facilitated by National Science Foundation Grant No. BCS-99-10592, awarded to Jerry Suls.

REFERENCES

Bandura, A. (1977). *Social learning theory*. Englewood Cliffs, NJ: Prentice-Hall.
Bandura, A. (1986). *Social foundations of thought and*

action: A social cognitive theory. Englewood Cliffs, NJ: Prentice-Hall.

Berger, S. M. (1977). Social comparison, modeling, and perseverance. In J. Suls & R. Miller (Eds.), *Social comparison processes* (pp. 209–234). Washington, DC: Hemisphere.

Blanton, H., Buunk, B. P., Gibbons, F. X., & Kuyper, H. (1999). When better-than-others compare upward: Choice of comparison and comparative evaluation as independent predictors of academic performance. *Journal of Personality and Social Psychology,76,* 420–430.

Buunk, B., Collins, R., Taylor, S., Van Yperen, N., & Dakoff, G. (1990). The affective consequences of social comparison: Either direction has its ups and downs. *Journal of Personality and Social Psychology, 59,* 1238–1249.

Buunk, B. P., & Ybema, J. F. (1997). Social comparison and occupational stress: The identification–contrast model. In B. P. Buunk & F. X. Gibbons (Eds.), *Health, coping, and well-being: Perspectives from social comparison theory* (pp. 359–388). Hillsdale, NJ: Erlbaum.

Cialdini, R., Borden, R. J., Thorne, A., Walker, M. R., Freeman, S., & Sloan, L. R. (1976). Basking in reflected glory: Three (football) field studies. *Journal of Personality and Social Psychology, 34,* 366–375.

Collins, R. (2000). Among the better ones: Upward assimilation in social comparison. In J. Suls & L. Wheeler (Eds.), *Handbook of social comparison* (pp. 159–172). New York: Kluwer/Plenum Press.

Davis, J. (1966). The campus as frog pond: An application of theory of relative deprivation to career decisions for college men. *American Journal of Sociology, 72,* 17–31.

Dembo, T. (1931). Der Arger als dynmisches Problem [Anger as a dynamic problem]. (Untersuchungen zur Handlukngs- und Affektpsychologie. X. Ed. by Kurt Lewin). *Psychologische Forschung, 15,* 1–144.

Diener, E., & Fujita, F. (1997). Social comparison and subjective being. In B. Buunk & F. X. Gibbons (Eds.), *Health, coping and well-being: Perspectives from social comparison theory* (pp. 329–358). Mahwah, NJ: Erlbaum.

Elliot, A. J., & Church, M. (1997). A hierarchical model of approach and avoidance achievement motivation. *Journal of Personality and Social Psychology, 72,* 218–232.

Elliot, A. J., McGregor, H. A., & Thrash, T. M. (2002). The need for competence. In E. Deci & R. Ryan (Eds.), *Handbook of self-determination research* (pp. 362–387). Rochester, NY: University of Rochester Press.

Escalona, S. K. (1940). The effect of success and failure upon the level of aspiration and behavior in manic-depressive psychoses. *University of Iowa Studies in Child Welfare, 16*(3), 199–302.

Festinger, L. (1942a). Wish, expectation and group standards as factors influencing level of aspiration. *Journal of Abnormal and Social Psychology, 37,* 184–200.

Festinger, L. (1942b). A theoretical interpretation of shifts in level of aspiration. *Psychological Review, 57,* 271–282.

Festinger, L. (1954a). A theory of social comparison processes. *Human Relations, 7,* 117–140.

Festinger, L. (1954b). Motivation leading to social behavior. In M.R. Jones (Ed.), *Nebraska Symposium on Motivation* (Vol. 2, pp. 191–218). Lincoln: University of Nebraska Press.

Goethals, G., & Darley, J. (1977). Social comparison theory: An attributional approach. In J. Suls & R. Miller (Eds.), *Social comparison processes: Theoretical and empirical processes* (pp. 259–278). Washington, DC: Hemisphere.

Hertzman, M., & Festinger, L. (1940). Shifts in explicit goals in a level of aspiration experiment. *Journal of Experimental Psychology, 27,* 439–452.

Hoppe, F. (1930). Erfolg und Misserfolg [Success and failure]. (Untersuchungen zur Handlukngs- und Affektpsychologie. IX. Ed. by Kurt Lewin). *Psychologische Forschung, 14,* 1–62.

Huguet, P., Dumas, F., Monteil, J. M., & Genestoux, N. (2001). Social comparison choices in the classroom: Further evidence for students' upward comparison tendency and its beneficial impact on performance. *European Journal of Social Psychology, 31,* 557–578.

Lewin, K., Dembo, T., Festinger, L., & Sears, P. (1944). Level of aspiration. In J. McV. Hunt (Ed.), *Personality and the behavior disorders* (pp 333–378). New York: Ronald Press.

Lockwood, P. (2002). Could it happen to you?: Predicting the impact of downward comparisons on the self. *Journal of Personality and Social Psychology, 82*(3), 343–358.

Lockwood, P., Jordan, C. H., & Kunda, Z. (2002). Motivation by positive or negative role models: Regulatory focus determines who will best inspire us. *Journal of Personality and Social Psychology, 83*(4), 854–864.

Lockwood, P., & Kunda, Z. (1997). Superstars and me: Predicting the impact of role models on the self. *Journal of Personality and Social Psychology, 73,* 91–103.

Lockwood, P., & Kunda, Z. (1999). Increasing the salience of one's best selves can undermine inspiration by outstanding role models. *Journal of Personality and Social Psychology, 76,* 214–228.

Major, B., Testa, M., & Bylsma, W. H. (1991). Responses of upward and downward social comparison: The impact of esteem-relevance and perceived control. In J. Suls & T. A. Wills (Eds.), *Social comparison: Classic and contemporary perspectives* (pp. 237–257). Hillsdale, NJ: Erlbaum.

Marsh, H. (1987). The big-fish-little-pond effect on academic self-concept. *Journal of Educational Psychology, 79,* 280–295.

Marsh, H. (1991). The failure of high-ability high schools to deliver academic benefits: The importance of academic self-concept and educational aspirations. *American Educational Research Journal, 28,* 445–480.

Marsh, H., Kong, C.-K., & Hau, K.-T. (2000). Longitudinal multilevel models of the big-fish-little-pond effect on academic self-concept: Counterbalancing contrast and reflected glory-effects in Hong Kong schools. *Journal of Personality and Social Psychology*, *78*, 337–349.

Marsh, H., & Parker, J. (1984). Determinants of student self-concept: Is it better to be a relatively large fish in a small pond even if you don't learn to swim as well? *Journal of Personality and Social Psychology*, *47*, 213–231.

Martin, R. (2000). "Can I do X?": Using the proxy model to predict performance. In J. Suls & L. Wheeler (Eds.), *The handbook of social comparison: Theory and research* (pp. 67–80). New York: Kluwer/Plenum Press.

Martin, R., Suls, J., & Wheeler, L. (2002). Ability evaluation by proxy: Role of maximum performance and related attributes in social comparison. *Journal of Personality and Social Psychology*, *82*, 781–791.

McClelland, D. C., Atkinson, J. W., Clark, R. A., & Lowell, E. L. (1953). *The achievement motive*. New York: Appleton–Century–Crofts.

Mussweiler, T. (2001). "Seek and ye shall find": Antecedents of assimilation and contrast in social comparison. *European Journal of Social Psychology*, *31*, 499–509.

Patnoe, S. (1988). *A narrative history of experimental social psychology: The Lewin tradition*. New York: Springer-Verlag.

Pelham, B., & Wachsmuth, J. (1995). The waxing and waning of the social self: Assimilation and contrast in social comparison. *Journal of Personality and Social Psychology*, *69*, 825–838.

Smith, D. (2002). The theory heard 'round the world. *Monitor on Psychology*, *33*, 30–32.

Stapel, D. A., & Koomen, W. (2000). Distinctness of others and malleability of selves: Their impact on social comparison effects. *Journal of Personality and Social Psychology*, *79*, 1068–1087.

Suls, J., & Tesch, F. (1978). Students' preferences for information about their test performance: A social comparison study. *Journal of Applied Social Psychology*, *8*, 189–197.

Suls, J., & Wheeler, L. (Eds.). (2000). *Handbook of social comparison*. New York: Kluwer/Plenum Press.

Tesser, A. (1988). Toward a self-evaluation maintenance model of social behavior. In L. Berkowitz (Ed.), *Advances in experimental social psychology* (Vol. 21, pp. 181–227). New York: Academic Press.

Wheeler, L. (1966). Motivation as a determinant of upward comparison. *Journal of Experimental Social Psychology*, (Suppl. 1), *2*, 27–31.

Wheeler, L., Koestner, R., & Driver, R. E. (1982). Related attributes in the choice of comparison others: It's there, but it isn't all there is. *Journal of Experimental Social Psychology*, *18*, 489–500.

Wheeler, L., Martin, R., & Suls, J. (1997). The proxy social comparison model for self-assessment of ability. *Personality and Social Psychology Review*, *1*, 54–61.

Wheeler, L., & Zuckerman, M. (1977). Commentary. In J. Suls & R. Miller (Eds.), *Social comparison processes* (pp. 335–357). Washington, DC: Hemisphere.

Wills, T. (1981). Downward comparison principles in social psychology. *Psychological Bulletin*, *90*, 245–271.

Wood, J., Taylor, S., & Lichtman, R. (1985). Social comparison in adjustment to breast cancer. *Journal of Personality and Social Psychology*, *49*, 1169–1183.

CHAPTER 31

◌ଛ

The Concept of Competence

A Starting Place for Understanding Intrinsic Motivation
and Self-Determined Extrinsic Motivation

EDWARD L. DECI
ARLEN C. MOLLER

During the first half of the 20th century, within both the empirical and the psychoanalytic approaches to psychology, the dominant theories of motivation focused on physiological drives as the source of energy for *all* motivated behavior. In both traditions, it had become clear by the 1950s that drive-based approaches could not provide adequate explanations for a wide range of phenomena, including exploration, achievement, and healthy development. Accordingly, a new motivational psychology emerged that uses cognitive concepts, differentiates intrinsic and extrinsic motivation, and views the innate psychological needs for competence, autonomy, and relatedness as an essential concept for understanding human behavior in social contexts.

In this chapter, we begin by briefly reviewing the early work that led to the emergence of this new approach. Then we focus on one strand of that new work by reviewing concepts and research on intrin-

sic motivation, arguing that a differentiated analysis of extrinsic motivation is also essential. Finally, we discuss the importance of innate psychological needs for integrating the research on intrinsic and extrinsic motivation.

WITHIN THE EMPIRICAL APPROACH

The most prominent early empirical theory of motivation was Hull's (1943) drive theory, which posited that the motivation for all behaviors—learning, interacting with others, and performing in a game or concert—is reducible to a small set of drives (i.e., physiological deficit needs), namely, hunger, thirst, sex, and the avoidance of pain. According to the theory, behavior is regulated or directed by associative bonds, which involve a behavior being linked to an internal or external stimulus through either primary or secondary reinforcement. Primary reinforcement occurs when a behavior results in the direct reduction of one of the four drives in the presence of a stimulus, thus linking the behavior to the stimulus. Secondary reinforcement requires an initially neutral object to be paired with the reduction of one of the four drives, so that the neutral object will take on secondary reinforcing properties. Then an associative bond between a stimulus and behavior can develop when the behavior leads to the secondary reinforcer in the presence of the stimulus. Primary and secondary reinforcement are the mechanisms that, taken together, were said to explain how drives underlie all motivated behaviors.

Studies of exploration and play proved highly problematic within this tradition, because they contradicted a basic premise of drive theory. Animals were observed to engage in exploratory behaviors that induced rather than reduced drives. For example, Dashiell (1925) reported that rats who had not eaten would, under some conditions, forego food in order to explore novel territory. Furthermore, Nissen (1930) reported the even more problematic phenomenon of rats crossing an electrified grid, thus enduring pain, in order to explore novel territory on the other side of the grid. According to drive theory, rats that had not eaten should have been more enticed by the food than by the opportunity to explore, and rats should not have behaved in a manner that induced pain rather than avoided it. In short, these behaviors were in stark opposition to the predictions of the physiological drive reduction premise.

Subsequent studies demonstrated that opportunities to explore (Butler, 1953; Butler & Harlow, 1957; Montgomery, 1954; Myers & Miller, 1954; Zimbardo & Miller, 1958) and to manipulate novel objects (Harlow, 1950; Harlow, Harlow, & Meyer, 1950; Hill, 1956; Kagan & Berkun, 1954) could function as "reinforcers" to produce learning in both rats and monkeys, yet neither exploration nor manipulation reduced drives. Furthermore, there was no evidence of extinction after numerous trials, even if the exploration or manipulation had not been repaired with food or other primary reinforcers, which would have been required for exploration and manipulation to be second-

ary reinforcers. Thus, it appeared that these play-like behaviors acted as if they were primary reinforcers, even though they had no relation to drive reduction.

WITHIN THE PSYCHOANALYTIC APPROACH

In a manner parallel to Hullian theory, Freud's (1915/1925) theory of psychosexual development was built on the assertion that *all* behaviors are reducible to primary instincts, namely, sex and aggression, with sex being the more important. Operating largely unconsciously, the instincts (or drives) were theorized to become associated with objects in the environment through the process of cathexis, which in turn forms the basis for the regulation or direction of behavior. The process of neutralization is the means through which the energy of the instincts (based in the id) can be commandeered for the functions of the ego, such that behaviors that do not appear to be motivated by sex or aggression can nonetheless be considered derivative of those instincts.

In this approach, as in the empirical approach, careful consideration of developmentally important behaviors such as exploration and play led theorists to conclude that although an analysis of the libidinal instinct during the first three stages of psychosexual development provided a possible account of the development of neuroses, it did not work well as a basis for understanding healthy development (e.g., Hartmann, 1939/1958). Within the theory, normal development would require satisfactory resolution of the oral, anal, and phallic conflicts, yet the theory is structured in a way that makes that impossible (White, 1960). Specifically, the theory involves a set of conflicts between a child's libido and demands of the socializing agent that the child be weaned, toilet trained, and unsuccessful in his (or her) oedipal (or electra) desires. Socializing agents will, of course, ensure that children are weaned and toilet trained, and that they not win the desired parent, so the children will invariably lose each conflict. This would imply that no child would develop in a healthy way because no conflict could be satisfactorily resolved for the child, if one in fact assumed, as the theory suggests, that the child is motivated only by the libido.

ATTEMPTS TO EXPLAIN EXPLORATION AND PLAY

Within both the empirical and psychoanalytic traditions, theorists attempted, with minimal change of orthodoxy, to explain the phenomenon of interested engagement with growth promoting activities. For example, empiricists proposed that exploration was motivated by the drive to avoid pain, arguing essentially that novelty produces anxiety, and exploration is the means for reducing the pain of anxiety. Fenichel (1945), a psychoanalytic theorist, similarly argued that the motivation of activities promoting normal development is based to a significant degree in managing anxiety. Yet such explanations were not satisfactory because, if novelty promotes anxiety, the likely response would be to flee the novelty rather than to charge headstrong into it. Furthermore, rats and humans alike frequently appeared to be experiencing excitement and joy rather than anxiety when playfully exploring new stimuli. As another approach to try to resolve the problem, writers within each tradition proposed new drives (or instincts) that would encompass playful or exploratory behaviors—for example, the exploratory drive within the empirical tradition (Montgomery, 1954) and the instinct to master within the psychoanalytic tradition (Hendrick, 1942)—yet these new "drives" did not fit the formal definition of a "drive" or "instinct" (e.g., they did not reduce a tissue deficit), so their use would have required a major change in the nature of the theories. As such, they did not represent a satisfactory solution to the problem of explaining the kinds of exploratory or playful behaviors that are necessary for normal development.

It thus seemed clear that for a meaningful motivational explanation of normal development, positing some other type of primary, though non-drive-based, motivation was essential. White (1959) was the first to make a definitive proposal for this new type of innate or primary motivation that would operate in addition to that based in the basic drives.

WHITE'S PROPOSAL

White (1959) used the term "competence" to connote people's capacity to interact effectively with the environment—to understand the effects they can have on the environment and the effects the environment has on them. According to White, to develop is to attain greater competence. Thus, he suggested that competence is attained over time and requires directed, selective, and persistent activity. Exploration and manipulation—the behaviors that were the most problematic for Hullian drive theory—fall under the rubric of competence-related behaviors, as do a wide array of other behaviors that underlie development.

White (1959) further proposed that competence must be thought of as a concept encompassing motivation, as well as capacity. He labeled this energizing force "effectance motivation" (although other writers frequently call it "competence motivation"), and he said that the subjective side of competence is the feeling of efficacy. This feeling is what provides "the reward" for behaviors that are energized by effectance motivation. Thus, competence refers to the structures through which effectance motivation operates, and the feeling of efficacy is the result. Simply stated, as people develop, they experience efficacy.

White (1959) emphasized that effectance motivation is not drive-derivative, that it is in no sense a deficit motivation. Rather, it is neurogenic; its energies are inherent to the living cells of the nervous system. He further stated that competence-promoting behavior "satisfies an intrinsic need to deal with the environment" (p. 318). Thus, White was proposing a new type of motivation, a motivation that is innate but not drive-based, that is persistent and "occupies the spare waking time between episodes of homeostatic crisis" (p. 321), that is the basis of healthy development, and that supplements the basic drives, which are essential for understanding consummatory behavior. This new motivation provided a solution to the problems encountered within the Hullian and Freudian approaches. It would clearly motivate exploration, manipulation, achievement, and play, which the empirical theories were unable to explain satisfactorily. Further, having this new type of motivation allowed for the possibility that children could engage weaning, toilet training, and oedipal wishes as developmental challenges to be mastered, with effectance motivation providing the energy to do so. Thus, the children could "win" the conflict—or rather, their egos could win even though their ids did not—so healthy development could occur.

There are four important issues concerning White's formulation that require further discussion in order to present a more complete characterization of this new type of motivation. The first concerns the concept of "need."

A Need for Competence?

In his discussion of competence, White (1959) did not refer to a "need" for competence (or effectance). Rather, he referred simply to effectance motivation. Only once did he use the term "need" in discussing the concept, and that was in his comment about satisfying "an intrinsic need to deal with the environment" (p. 318). It is likely that the reason White tended to avoid the term "need" is that its most common usage in motivational psychology to that point had been to refer to the physiological needs that underlie drive, and one of White's central aims was to show the importance of a motivational concept that did not have deficit needs as its basis. White was talking about a motivation (a *need*, if you will) that was psychological, and that was based in the central nervous system rather than in non-nervous-system tissue deficits, so using the concept of need to describe it might have seemed to him to be too confusing. Furthermore, the concept of psychological needs, as it was being used at that time in personality psychology by Murray (1938) and by McClelland, Atkinson, Clark, and Lowell (1953), treated needs as learned, and thus as individual differences. White (1959), on the other hand, was referring to what might be called a *universal need*. In other words, he was not concerned with individual differences in people's effectance motivation, but was instead concerned with everyone's motivation to be effective in dealing with the environment.

Still, it is clear that White's (1959) conception of effectance motivation would satisfy the definition of an innate psychological need (Deci & Ryan, 2000; Elliot, McGregor, & Thrash, 2002); that is, he described it as innate to all human beings, as directed and persistent, and as essential to health and well-being. Indeed, it was being proposed as the motivational basis of healthy development. Thus, had White referred to a need for competence, as subsequent researchers have done (e.g., Deci & Ryan, 1980), it would have been consistent with the criteria for a universal need, namely, a persistent motivator that, if satisfied, promotes health and, if thwarted, results in ill-being. In short, White was introducing the concept of a need for effectance (or competence) without using the term.

Intrinsic Motivation

The second issue requiring clarification concerns the concept of intrinsic motivation. White did not use the term "intrinsic motivation." As far as we know, that term had been introduced by Harlow (1950), when he discussed the fact that monkeys displayed great resistance to the extinction of manipulation behaviors, thus implying that the behaviors were intrinsically motivated and did not represent an instance of secondary reinforcement. It is nonetheless clear that the idea of effectance motivation, as described by White (1959), did indeed represent what Deci (1975) and others have referred to as intrinsic motivation. Specifically, it is not deficit-based, and it motivates activities in which the sole rewards are the spontaneous feelings of interest and enjoyment that occur when one engages in the activities.

The Goal of Effectance Motivation

The third issue concerns the goal of competence-promoting behaviors. White (1959) emphasized that play—for example, the behaviors of exploration and manipulation that were so problematic for drive theory—is serious business for children and, presumably, for adults as well, albeit to a lesser extent. However, he further stated that for children, play "is merely something that is interesting and fun to do" (p. 321). In other words, although children are busy building competencies, their goal is *not* to become more competent, it is to do what they find interesting and fun. Competence is essentially a by-product in terms of people's intentions; it develops as they do what they find interesting and fun. Of course, developing greater competence could be the goal of behaviors that are energized by effectance motivation, such as when a high-school girl is interested in practicing free throws in order to improve her basketball game. But it is extremely important to note that in the conception of what has come to be called intrinsically motivated behaviors, although based at least in part in effectance motivation, one need not have the goal of becoming more competent. The goal may simply be to do an activity that one finds interesting.

Competence and Self-Determination

The fourth issue concerns the relation of competence to self-determination or autonomy. In White's (1959) discussion, he reviewed the work of Angyal (1941), who emphasized the fact that living organisms assimilate aspects of the environment, transforming them into aspects of the self. In other words, over time, organisms internalize and integrate aspects of their environment as part of the process of mastering that environment. This trend, Angyal argued and White concurred, is toward greater autonomy or self-determination. Organisms, by their nature, attempt to subordinate heteronomous forces of the environment in the service of their own developing autonomy. Throughout his writings, White steadfastly focused on effectance or competence, and he gave relatively little attention to autonomy or self-determination, but he was essentially saying that effectance-motivated behavior would have the characteristic of being autonomous. Thus, White was essentially including autonomy or self-determination within the purview of effectance motivation.

In a subsequent discussion, deCharms (1968) stated that "Man's primary motivational propensity is to be effective in producing changes in his environment. Man strives to be a causal agent, .. to experience personal causation" (p. 269). Here we see the same two ideas—to be competent in dealing with the environment and to be personally causative or self-determined. However, deCharms's work, in contrast to White's,

emphasized personal causation or self-determination and essentially viewed competence as an aspect of personal causation. Thus, these two seminal thinkers focused on the same two elements, namely, competence and self-determination, but they placed different emphases on which was the more primary.

In line with White (1959) and deCharms (1968), who essentially treated the two needs as one, Deci (1971, 1975) referred to the human need to be "competent and self-determining." It was not until 1980 that Deci and Ryan made clear that these are two separate needs. They argued that it was essential to propose two universal psychological needs—one for competence and one for autonomy—in order to provide a meaningful interpretation of all the experimental findings that had emerged in the study of intrinsic motivation during the 1970s.

BASIC PSYCHOLOGICAL NEEDS AND INTRINSIC MOTIVATION

One of the most important reasons for postulating innate psychological needs is that they provide the basis for making predictions about the effects of social-contextual forces on natural, growth-oriented processes and psychological well-being. According to self-determination theory (Deci & Ryan, 1985, 2000), basic psychological needs are defined in terms of the nutrients that are essential for healthy development. Thus, those contextual factors that might be expected to satisfy psychological needs would be predicted to facilitate natural processes and psychological health, whereas those factors that might be expected to thwart psychological needs would be predicted to have negative consequences. For example, specifying a basic need for competence allows one to predict that the aspects of the social environment that promote competence would facilitate well-being, whereas those that undermine competence would diminish well-being.

Intrinsic motivation is posited to be a natural psychological process (Deci, 1975). It is a manifestation of the proactivity inherent in the nature of human life. When people are not blocked or discouraged from doing so, they engage their physical and social environments, doing what interests them and attempting to master aspects of their world. This motivation is so persistent that, at times, it is more prepotent than drive-based motivation. According to self-determination theory, there are three innate psychological needs, those for competence, autonomy, and relatedness, but competence and autonomy are the more central for intrinsic motivation. Thus, the theory proposes that the needs for competence and autonomy must be satisfied for intrinsic motivation to be promoted and maintained, and a considerable amount of research has examined the question of whether satisfying these two needs is in fact positively related to the flourishing of natural processes and well-being, whereas thwarting the needs is negatively related to those outcomes. We turn now to a review of that experimental work, which concerns social-contextual influences on intrinsic motivation, and to the interpretation of the results based on the concept of basic psychological needs.

SOCIAL CONTEXTS AND INTRINSIC MOTIVATION

The study of social-contextual influences began with an exploration of the effects of extrinsic rewards on intrinsic motivation. Expectancy–valence theories (e.g., Porter & Lawler, 1968) had proposed that intrinsic and extrinsic motivation are additive, yielding total motivation. This led to the suggestion that activities (learning, work, etc.) should be designed to be as interesting as possible to stimulate intrinsic motivation, and that social contexts should be organized to provide extrinsic rewards that are contingent upon effective performance at the activities. That way, there would be maximal motivation, consisting of the sum of the intrinsic motivation from the interesting activities and the extrinsic motivation from the contingent rewards.

Attribution theory made a different prediction, however. deCharms (1968) suggested that when people perceive the locus of causality for their behavior to be within themselves, they tend to be intrinsically motivated, but when they perceive the locus of causality to be external, they tend to be extrinsically motivated. In line with Heider (1958) and Kelley (1967), deCharms further

suggested that when extrinsic motivators are present, there is a tendency to attribute the cause of a behavior to an external factor (e.g., a reward) and to discount the internal factor (i.e., intrinsic motivation). Thus, the addition of an extrinsic motivator to intrinsic motivation would produce a negative interaction, resulting in the diminishment of intrinsic motivation.

Effects of Extrinsic Rewards on Intrinsic Motivation

Initial experiments testing this reasoning involved participants' working on an interesting target activity within one of two groups. Participants in one group received a reward, whereas those in the other did not, and the subsequent level of intrinsic motivation of the two groups was assessed. The primary measure was the so-called "free-choice" behavioral measure, in which participants were provided a period of free play, when they could choose the target activity or alternatives, and the amount of time they spent with the target activity represented their intrinsic motivation for that activity. The secondary measure was participants' reports of how interesting they found the target activity.

Deci (1971) did the first of these experiments. In it, college students in one group received monetary rewards for working on interesting spatial-relations puzzles, and those in the other group did the same puzzles without rewards. Results indicated that participants in the reward condition showed decrements in intrinsic motivation relative to participants in the no-reward control group. A study by Lepper, Greene, and Nisbett (1973) found comparable results when preschool children doing an art activity were given good player awards, and dozens of subsequent studies have replicated the general result (see Deci, Koestner, & Ryan, 1999a).

It appears then that the addition of a tangible extrinsic reward does tend to undermine intrinsic motivation by shifting the perceived locus of causality from internal to external. However, Deci and Ryan (1985) argued that an attributional explanation does not provide a full account of this undermining. Although people might perceive the locus of causality to become more external when they begin to receive a reward for doing an interesting activity, it is not clear why that alone should diminish people's interest, energy, and desire to do the activity. The authors argued, however, that if people have an innate need to be self-determining, to feel like the initiators of their own activities, then the addition of the external reward might leave them feeling controlled by the reward, thus thwarting their experience of autonomy or self-determination and resulting in the diminishment of the natural process of intrinsic motivation.

Positive Feedback (aka Verbal Rewards)

Along with the early studies of tangible rewards on intrinsic motivation were studies that examined the effects of positive feedback (referred to by some as "verbal rewards") on intrinsic motivation. These studies found that whereas tangible rewards tended to undermine intrinsic motivation, positive feedback tended to enhance it (Deci, 1971). Deci and Ryan (1980) argued that the positive feedback enhanced intrinsic motivation by satisfying participants' need for competence, and mediational analyses showed that perceived competence did in fact account for the changes in intrinsic motivation following feedback (Elliot et al., 2000; Vallerand & Reid, 1984). Thus, these various studies suggested that whereas tangible rewards undermine intrinsic motivation by thwarting people's need for autonomy, positive feedback enhances intrinsic motivation by supporting their need for competence.

The Rewards Controversy

The finding that extrinsic rewards undermine intrinsic motivation was controversial from the time it first appeared in the literature (e.g., Calder & Staw, 1975; Scott, 1975), and it continues to be so. For example, Eisenberger and Cameron (1996) discussed a meta-analysis that had been done by Cameron and Pierce (1994), concluding that there is no evidence for the undermining of intrinsic motivation by extrinsic rewards. However, it turned out that, as detailed by Deci et al. (1999a), the meta-analysis by Cameron and Pierce (1994) was fatally flawed, and the conclusions were wholly in-

valid. Subsequently, Eisenberger, Pierce, and Cameron (1999) argued, citing the work of investigators such as Harackiewicz and Manderlink (1984), that at least performance-contingent rewards do not undermine intrinsic motivation but instead enhance it. Performance-contingent rewards are those given for doing well at an activity—that is, for meeting or surpassing some standard. Again, it turned out that the claim by the Eisenberger group (1999) was invalid (see Deci, Koestner, & Ryan, 1999b). In fact, the meta-analysis showed quite clearly that, on average, performance-contingent rewards undermined intrinsic motivation, assessed with the behavioral measure, and did not affect enjoyment of the activity (Deci et al., 1999a). Thus, across all performance-contingent reward studies, there was no evidence for enhancement either of intrinsic motivation or enjoyment.

Performance-contingent rewards are more complexly related to intrinsic motivation than are most other reward contingencies because, like all tangible expected rewards, they not only have a strong controlling component but they also convey positive competence information to those who receive them; that is, the rewards tend to thwart the need for autonomy, while satisfying the need for competence. Ryan, Mims, and Koestner (1983) thus argued that the effects of performance-contingent rewards would depend on how they were administered—that is, whether they were administered so that the controlling component is more salient or the positive competence information is more salient. These investigators found that if the style of administration provided support for autonomy and emphasized the positive information, the rewards enhanced intrinsic motivation relative to a no-reward/no-feedback comparison group; however, they still undermined intrinsic motivation relative to a no-reward group that got positive competence information comparable to the information conveyed by the performance-contingent reward. It thus appears that although, on average, performance-contingent rewards decrease intrinsic motivation, if the style of administration is autonomy-supportive, performance-contingent rewards can enhance intrinsic motivation for the people who get them relative to no rewards and no feedback. This, presumably, is because they increase perceived competence. However, positive feedback is even more effective at enhancing intrinsic motivation relative to no rewards and no feedback than are performance-contingent rewards. Furthermore, for people who attempt to obtain performance-contingent rewards and fail to do so, the reward contingency is likely to be highly detrimental, because it diminishes feelings of both competence and autonomy.

Effects of Other External Factors on Intrinsic Motivation

If the general undermining of intrinsic motivation by tangible extrinsic rewards is really a function of its thwarting the need for autonomy, then other external motivators that might be expected to control behavior ought also to undermine intrinsic motivation. To test this, Deci and Cascio (1972) did a study in which participants in one group learned that they would receive an aversive event (a loud buzzer) if they did not solve puzzles within the allotted time. Comparison-group participants did the same puzzles with the same time allotments, but they had no expectation of a punishment if they failed to complete the puzzles in the allotted time. Results of this experiment showed that trying to solve the puzzles under the condition of avoiding a punishment decreased people's intrinsic motivation for the target activity relative to the comparison group. Thus, it appears that working to avoid a punishment decreased participants' intrinsic motivation relative to that of the participants not working under conditions of threat. Complementary findings by Elliot and Harackiewicz (1996) indicated that having the goal of trying to avoid failure in order to prove one's competence relative to others also undermined intrinsic motivation.

Additional studies showed that deadlines (Amabile, DeJong, & Lepper, 1976; Reader & Dollinger, 1982), surveillance (Lepper & Greene, 1975; Pittman, Davey, Alafat, Wetherill, & Kramer, 1980; Plant & Ryan, 1985), evaluations (Church, Elliot, & Gable, 2001; Smith, 1975), imposed goals (Mossholder, 1980), and competition (Deci, Betley, Kahle, Abrams, & Porac, 1981) can all undermine intrinsic motivation. These external factors are frequently used by one person to try "to motivate" others, so it is reasonable to think that those others might experience these external factors as controls—that is, as pressures from someone else to think, feel, or behavior in particular ways. Thus, presumably, the undermining of intrinsic motivation by these external events would have been due to a thwarting of the people's need for autonomy.

Enhancing Autonomy and Intrinsic Motivation

To the extent that external events such as rewards and deadlines undermine intrinsic motivation because they thwart satisfaction of the autonomy need, events that facilitate satisfaction of the need for autonomy should enhance intrinsic motivation. Zuckerman, Porac, Lathin, Smith, and Deci (1978) reasoned that providing participants choice about which of a set of puzzles to work on and how long to spend on each should allow them to feel more autonomous, thus enhancing their intrinsic motivation relative to participants who are assigned the puzzles and time allotments chosen by others. Indeed, the results did support this reasoning. Subsequent studies (e.g., Cordova & Lepper, 1996; Iyengar & Lepper, 1999) have shown that providing participants with choice rather than having the experimenter make choices for them enhanced intrinsic motivation, a result that was found for both European Americans and Asian Americans.

Koestner, Ryan, Bernieri, and Holt (1984) suggested that acknowledging people's perspectives—that is, relating to them from their internal frame of reference, while communicating with them—should also leave people feeling more self-initiating and volitional and should thus enhance their intrinsic motivation. An experiment by these researchers using late elementary school children as participants confirmed their reasoning. Participants whose feelings were acknowledged displayed greater intrinsic motivation for a task than those whose feelings were not acknowledged.

Competence and Intrinsic Motivation

Intrinsic motivation for an activity involves engaging it out of interest, and theorists (Csikszentmihalyi, 1975; Deci, 1975) have suggested that one important feature of activities that will be intrinsically motivating is that they represent an optimal challenge given the person's capacities. Danner and Lonky (1981) did a study in which children were free to choose from various activities that differed in terms of difficulty. The researchers had pretested the children for cognitive ability relevant to the task, and they found that when the children were free to select which tasks to work on, they went to the ones that were somewhat more difficult than their pretested skill levels. These tasks were also rated by the children as most interesting.

Additional studies (e.g., Shapira, 1976) found comparable results emphasizing the importance of optimal challenge for intrinsic motivation. It makes sense that intrinsic motivation, which is a manifestation of the natural growth tendency within humans, would be facilitated by exposure to tasks that are optimally challenging, because these are the ones that could provide stimulation for developing greater competence, thus satisfying the basic human need for competence.

As mentioned earlier in the chapter, research (e.g., Deci, 1971) has found that positive feedback for doing well at an activity tends to enhance intrinsic motivation for interesting activities, and, as also noted, this was interpreted as indicating that the positive feedback promoted satisfaction of people's need for competence. In line with this interpretation, Deci, Cascio, and Krusell (1973) found that negative feedback decreased people's intrinsic motivation, presumably because it thwarted satisfaction of their need for competence (see also Vallerand & Reid, 1984). However, studies have shown that in order for positive feedback to have a positive effect on intrinsic motivation, the positive feedback must be experienced within a context of support for autonomy (Fisher, 1978; Ryan, 1982). Positive feedback statements such as "Good, you did just as you should on that one" were experienced as pressuring and controlling, thus thwarting the need for autonomy, and did not have a positive effect on intrinsic motivation even though they provided positive competence feedback (Ryan, 1982). Complementary results from Ryan, Koestner, and Deci (1991) showed that when people were ego-involved, thus being controlled rather than autonomous, positive feedback did not enhance their intrinsic motivation.

Two additional findings about positive feedback are worth noting. First, studies by Deci, Cascio, and Krusell (1975) and Kast and Connor (1988) showed that although positive feedback enhanced the intrinsic motivation of male participants, it decreased the intrinsic motivation of females. To interpret this, Deci et al. (1975) used the distinction between the informational and controlling aspects of feedback. Whereas the informational aspect signifies competence, the controlling aspect pressures people to behave in ways that will yield further positive feedback. The researchers suggested that, for the males, the informational aspect was more salient, so they experienced the feedback as affirmation of their competence, whereas, for females, the controlling aspect was more salient, so they came to believe that they did the behavior in order to get the feedback. This, the authors speculated, could be a function of socialization, which traditionally has emphasized independent achievement for males and interpersonal sensitivity for females. Although several other studies of positive feedback did not report any sex differences, the results of the two studies do imply that females may be more susceptible than males to being controlled by positive feedback.

The second additional finding is that in a meta-analysis, Deci et al. (1999a) found that, across more than 30 studies, although positive feedback enhanced intrinsic motivation for college student participants, it did not have an enhancing effect on intrinsic motivation for children. It appears that, for children, the controlling aspect of positive feedback was salient enough to offset the competence affirmation, leaving no enhancement of intrinsic motivation. Presumably, with their greater cognitive capacity and independence, college students were more able to focus on the informational aspect of the positive feedback without feeling controlled by it.

To summarize, competence is an important element for intrinsic motivation. People need to develop competencies, and engagement with optimally challenging activities is the basis through which this occurs. Furthermore, feedback affects intrinsic motivation by affecting people's experience of satisfaction versus thwarting of the need for competence. Positive feedback tends to increase intrinsic motivation by enhancing perceived competence, and negative feedback tends to decrease intrinsic motivation by diminishing perceived competence. However, for the positive feedback to promote intrinsic motivation, the feedback must be presented in a way that allows the person to feel volition in doing the activity and ownership of the performance. Furthermore the likelihood that positive feedback will have a positive effect on intrinsic motivation is less for women than for men and less for children than for adults.

Interpersonal Contexts and Intrinsic Motivation

Several studies have examined the general climate or ambience of a situation (e.g., a classroom) as it affects the intrinsic motivation of people in it. In one study, for example, Deci, Schwartz, Sheinman, and Ryan (1981) studied teachers in fourth- through sixth-grade classrooms, examining their relative endorsements of the ideas of controlling students' behavior versus supporting students' autonomy. Controlling behavior involves pressuring the students to think, feel, or behave in particular ways; whereas supporting autonomy involves understanding the students' perspective, providing choice, and encouraging self-initiation. The reasoning was that teachers who were oriented toward controlling behavior would tend to create a controlling climate in their classrooms, which would undermine intrinsic motivation, whereas those oriented toward supporting autonomy would create a more open and informational climate that would enhance intrinsic motivation. Results of the research supported this reasoning; within the first 2 months of a school year, students in the autonomy-supportive classrooms gained in perceived competence and intrinsic motivation relative to students in the controlling classrooms.

Ryan and colleagues (e.g., Ryan, 1982; Ryan et al., 1983) did a set of laboratory experiments in which they created an autonomy-supportive versus controlling climate within the laboratory and examined whether specific external events such as rewards or positive feedback would have different ef-

fects on intrinsic motivation, depending on the interpersonal climate within which they were administered. They found that, although tangible rewards that convey positive competence information tend to undermine intrinsic motivation in general, they maintain or enhance intrinsic motivation when administered in an autonomy-supportive context (Ryan et al., 1983). Furthermore, positive feedback, which tends, on average, to increase intrinsic motivation by enhancing perceived competence, had a negative effect on intrinsic motivation when administered in a controlling context (Ryan, 1982). Finally, competition, which tends to undermine intrinsic motivation, can also provide competence affirmation (Elliot & Moller, 2003). Reeve and Deci (1996) found that when the interpersonal context surrounding competition is less pressuring and controlling, the competition is less detrimental to intrinsic motivation. Thus, both the interpersonal context and the specific external events administered within them affect people's intrinsic motivation.

INTERNALIZATION OF MOTIVATION

When people are experiencing satisfaction of their basic psychological needs, they tend to do what interests them. In other words, they tend to be intrinsically motivated. Thus, intrinsic motivation requires experiencing an activity as interesting, while also feeling some support for one's basic needs. The fact that interest is so central to intrinsic motivation implies, of course, that if an individual did not find an activity interesting, he or she would not be intrinsically motivated for it. Under such circumstances, for the person to do the activity at all would require some type of extrinsic motivation—"extrinsic motivation" being defined as doing an activity for some operationally separable consequence.

The bulk of the research examining the relation of extrinsic to intrinsic motivation seemed to show that extrinsic and intrinsic motivation were negatively interactive, therefore suggesting that to be extrinsically motivated is to be controlled and thus not autonomous or self-determined. However, in most of the studies reviewed earlier, the extrinsic motivation involved a specific extrinsic contingency linking behavior to a tangible outcome that was implemented by one individual to motivate another.

Internalization

According to self-determination theory (Deci & Ryan, 1985), those external contingencies represent only one type of extrinsic motivation. Other types could be more autonomous, while also satisfying the needs for competence and relatedness. The theory maintains that this occurs through internalization of a regulatory process and the value implicit in it. However, self-determination theory uses a differentiated conception of internalization. Specifically, whereas many theories (e.g., Bandura, 1977; Mead, 1934) view internalization as a unitary concept, that is, a regulatory process and value are either external or they have been internalized, self-determination theory maintains that people can internalize behaviors and values to differing degrees, ranging from taking them in but not accepting them as their own, to internalizing them and integrating them into their sense of self (Ryan, Connell, & Deci, 1985).

Self-determination theory proposes that internalization is an active process through which people engage their social world, gradually transforming socially sanctioned mores or requests into personally endorsed values and self-regulations. When internalization processes function optimally, people identify with the value of an activity or regulation and make that an aspect of their integrated self. If, however, the internalization process is not adequately supported, so that identification does not occur, the regulation will be internalized but not integrated. According to self-determination theory, four distinct types of regulation are associated with extrinsic motivation, resulting from differing degrees to which the regulation and value have been internalized. Ranging from least to most internalized, the types of regulation are external, introjected, identified, and integrated.

External Regulation

When people's behavior is controlled by specific external contingencies, the regulation is said to be external. People behave with the intent to attain a desired reward or to avoid a threatened punishment. This is the type of extrinsic motivation that has been extensively examined and found to undermine intrinsic motivation (Deci et al., 1999a). Within self-determination theory, externally regulated behaviors are considered contingency-dependent, and these behaviors tend not to persist once the contingency has been terminated (Deci & Ryan, 1985).

Introjection

When people take in an external regulation without making it their own, the regulation is said to be introjected. Behaviors are then controlled by internal contingencies—that is, by sanctions people administer to themselves. Prototypical examples of introjection are contingent self-worth and threats of guilt and shame, as well as ego involvement (Ryan, 1982) and public self-consciousness (Plant & Ryan, 1985). Introjection is a particularly interesting type of regulation, because it is internal to the person but is relatively external to the person's integrated self.

Identification

When people recognize and accept the underlying value of a behavior, they are said to have identified with it. This process is a much fuller type of internalization than is introjection, because identification indicates that the people have, to a substantial degree, made the regulation their own. As such, they will be relatively autonomous in carrying out the behavior. Still, the behavior will be extrinsically motivated, because it is instrumental to a separable outcome rather than being intrinsically motivated, which would require its being done solely as a source of spontaneous interest and enjoyment.

Integration

Finally, within the self-determination theory conceptualization of internalization, integration represents the fullest, most mature form of extrinsic motivation. It involves not only identifying with the importance of a behavior but also integrating that identification with other aspects of one's self. When the identification has been integrated, what had initially been an external regulation will have been fully transformed into autonomous self-regulation.

Interpersonal Contexts and Internalization

Like the ongoing functioning of intrinsic motivation, internalization and integration are natural, growth-oriented processes that are inherent to the nature of life. Within people's nature is the tendency to internalize and integrate into themselves aspects of their world, and these processes allow people to be more effective in dealing with that world. Yet like all natural, human processes, these require nutriments to function effectively. From the perspective of self-determination theory, the essential nutriments are satisfaction of the basic psychological needs for competence, relatedness, and autonomy.

Internalization and Need Satisfaction

We mentioned earlier that the needs for competence and autonomy are the most important for maintaining and enhancing intrinsic motivation, and that the influence of relatedness is more distal. In other words, people can remain intrinsically motivated without having immediate satisfaction of the relatedness need while doing the activity, but people must experience satisfaction of the needs for competence and autonomy while doing the activity in order to remain intrinsically motivated. With the process of internalization, however, the need for relatedness (see, e.g., Baumeister & Leary, 1995) plays a more central role than it does with intrinsic motivation.

Specifically, self-determination theory proposes that people's tendency to internalize regulations is energized by their needs for relatedness and competence; that is, people's desires to belong within the social world and to be effective in negotiating that world prompt them to take in the regulation of activities that are not interesting in their own right. It is thus because of people's desires to maintain and enhance interpersonal relationships and to feel effective in doing a wide range of behaviors that they will both internalize ambient values, mores, behaviors, and attitudes, and learn to do things that are not interesting but are important for succeeding within society. However, although the needs for competence and relatedness are important motivators for internalization, satisfaction of these needs does not determine whether the internalizations will be merely introjected or more fully integrated. It is satisfaction of the autonomy need with respect to a target behavior that is necessary to promote integration. Thus, although feelings of competence and relatedness are necessary contributors toward integration, they are not sufficient to promote it. Satisfaction of all three needs is necessary. Thus, failure to satisfy the basic needs for competence, relatedness, and autonomy will interfere with full internalization. Chaotic and rejecting environments (i.e., those that thwart satisfaction of competence and relatedness) are likely to interfere with any internalization, and excessive pressure is likely to interfere with identification and integration, forestalling internalization at the level of introjection.

Studies of Internalization

Empirical support for this analysis of internalization has been provided by both field studies and laboratory experiments. In one study, Grolnick and Ryan (1989) did extensive interviews with the parents of fourth- through sixth-grade children. These interviews focused on the parents' approach to dealing with their children in regard to homework and chores around the house. The responses were used to characterize the parents in terms of the degree to which they (1) were involved with their children concerning these issues, (2) provided an optimal amount of structure for the children in relation to these activities, and (3) were autonomy supportive rather than controlling in these realms. Subsequently, the children's motivation was assessed by questionnaires in their regular classrooms. Results indicated that parents who were more involved, provided more optimal structure, and were more autonomy supportive had children who not only were more intrinsically motivated for schoolwork but had also internalized behavioral regulations and values more fully. These motivational factors were in turn positively associated with teachers' ratings of the children's competence, standardized achievement, and well-being. A follow-up study by Grolnick, Ryan, and Deci (1991) assessed children's perceptions of their parents' autonomy support and involvement, and found that the children's perceptions were also related to greater internalization.

A field study done in two medical schools provided additional evidence concerning this issue (Williams & Deci, 1996). The course was for second-year students who were learning to interview patients. The investigators found that the instructors who were more autonomy supportive (vs. controlling) had students who more fully internalized the values and regulations emphasized in the course, and whose interviewing of patients done 6 months after the course ended was rated as more effective.

Deci, Eghrari, Patrick, and Leone (1994) did a laboratory experiment that focused on three specific external factors that were hypothesized to allow satisfaction of the basic needs and thus facilitate internalization. The factors were (1) a meaningful rationale that conveys why it is important to do the activity effectively, (2) acknowledgment of people's feelings about the activity, and (3) use of language that conveyed choice rather than control. Results showed that these three factors did facilitate internalization. Even more importantly, results indicated that when at least two of the facilitating factors were present, internalization tended to be integrated, as indexed by significant *positive* correlations between subsequent behavior and self-reports of valuing the activity and feeling free while doing it. In contrast, in conditions with at most one facilitating factor present, internalization was only introjected as reflected by *negative* correlations between subsequent behavior and the self-report variables. When there were fewer facilitating factors, people who did display more subsequent behavior felt less free and enjoyed the activity less. In short, conditions that promote greater satisfaction of the psychological needs tend not only to promote more internalization but also to ensure that the internalization will be more integrated.

A study by Assor, Roth, and Deci (2004) examined internalization under conditions in which parents create conflict within their children about being able to satisfy their needs. Specifically, the researchers assessed whether parents had provided conditional acceptance and regard to their children, dependent upon the children displaying competence in particular domains such as schoolwork and sports. In other words, the parents provided attention and affection (thus satisfying relatedness) for the children's successes (thus satisfying competence), but by making their love contingent, they were undermining their children's autonomy. Results indicated that contingent regard from parents led the children to introject the regulations—that is, they subsequently engaged in the behaviors, but they felt a sense of inner compulsion to do it. Along with these feelings of inner compulsion, the children displayed contingent self-esteem, short-lived satisfaction after successes, shame and guilt after failures, and resentment of their parents. This, then, supports the hypothesis that satisfaction of the needs for competence and relatedness will facilitate internalization, but it will take the form of introjection, not integration, if support for autonomy is not also present.

Competence Valuation

Intrinsic motivation and integrated extrinsic motivation represent the two forms of self-determined behavior. Intrinsic motivation is based in people's interest in the activity itself, while integrated extrinsic motivation is based in the importance of the activity for people's self-selected goals. When people understand and accept the value of a behavior, they will internalize its regulation. Self-determination theory maintains, however, that internalizing an extrinsic motivation does not typically transform it into an intrinsic motivation, because intrinsic motivation is about interest in the activity, whereas extrinsic motivation is about the activity's instrumental value.

"Competence valuation" means that being competent at an activity is very important for people. Harackiewicz and Sansone (2000) proposed that when the value of being competent at an activity is emphasized, people will become more intrinsically motivated for the activity. The self-determination theory perspective maintains, however, that if the importance of doing a behavior well is emphasized, people may be more likely to identify with the activity and thus be more autonomous in their extrinsic motivation for it, but they will not be more intrinsically motivated. Intrinsic motivation is based in interest rather than value, and there is little reason to expect that competence valuation will enhance intrinsic motivation for the behavior, although it could promote identification.

Summary

Internalization is the means through which people can deal with uninteresting behaviors in a way that allows satisfaction of their basic psychological needs. We have argued that the needs for competence and relatedness provide energy for internalizing behavioral regulations, and that the need for autonomy is the motivational basis for integrating, rather than just introjecting, behavioral regulations. The concept of basic needs for competence, relatedness, and autonomy has thus proven useful for interpreting results of research not only on intrinsic motivation but also on the internalization of extrinsic motivation.

HUMAN NEEDS AS UNIVERSALS

The fact that the concept of basic human needs has had great utility for interpreting a range of empirical phenomena has provided some support for the proposition that humans do indeed have these fundamental needs. However, additional lines of research have focused more directly on verifying that these are universal needs. There are two primary strands to this work. First, because needs are defined as essential nutriments, evidence that satisfaction of the needs is associated with well-being and that thwarting of the needs is associated with ill-being would represent important support for the postulate. Second, because the needs are assumed to be universal, comparability of phenomena across cultures would also provide critical evidence. Thus, we now review some relevant studies.

Relation of Need Satisfaction to Well-Being

"Well-being" concerns the experiences of psychological and physical health and life satisfaction. It has been variously defined, with emotional positivity being a central element in most definitions. Self-determination

theory emphasizes, however, that the concept of well-being must include a full sense of organismic functioning and wellness (Ryan & Frederick, 1997; Ryan, Deci, & Grolnick, 1995). Thus, for example, feeling negative emotions can be important and restorative under certain circumstances. Self-determination theory further proposes that need satisfaction over time will affect well-being at the level of individual differences, and also that fluctuations in need satisfaction will directly predict fluctuations in well-being over short periods of time.

Two studies have tested the relation of need satisfaction to well-being over time using a diary procedure that assessed both need satisfaction and well-being on a daily basis. The use of multilevel modeling with these data allowed examination of both between-person and within-person associations of experienced need satisfaction to indicators of well-being. Sheldon, Ryan, and Reis (1996) examined daily variations in people's experiences of autonomy and competence over a 2-week period. They found that at the between-person level, individual differences in perceived autonomy and perceived competence correlated significantly with 2-week aggregates of well-being indicators such as positive affect, vitality, and the inverse of negative affect and physical symptoms. Then, after removing between-person variance, daily fluctuations in satisfaction of needs for autonomy and competence were found to predict daily fluctuations in well-being. On days when people felt autonomous and competent, they reported feeling happy and well.

In the second study, Reis, Sheldon, Gable, Roscoe, and Ryan (2000) examined the three basic psychological needs for competence, autonomy, and relatedness. At the between-person level, they found that measures of autonomy, competence, and relatedness were all associated with aggregate indices of well-being, thus confirming the between-person predictions. As in the Sheldon et al. (1996) study, after person-level variance was removed, daily variability in satisfaction of the three needs independently predicted daily variability in well-being. Thus, the two studies showed a clear linkage between need satisfaction and well-being at both within-person and between-person levels of analysis. Furthermore, they showed independent contributions from satisfaction of each basic need for each day's well-being.

Other studies have focused within domains to examine the relation of need satisfaction to well-being. In one such study, Ilardi, Leone, Kasser, and Ryan (1993) found that the reports of factory workers about the satisfaction of their autonomy, competence, and relatedness needs in the workplace were related to their self-esteem and general health. Another study in a banking company related satisfaction of the basic needs to vitality and to the inverse of both anxiety and somatization (Baard, Deci, & Ryan, 2004). Studies by Kasser and Ryan (1999) and by Vallerand and O'Connor (1989) showed that ongoing need satisfaction in the lives of aged residents in institutional settings predicted their well-being and perceived health.

To summarize, after determining that the postulate of three basic psychological needs served a very useful function in providing a meaningful integration of experimental results concerning intrinsic motivation and the internalization of extrinsic motivation, subsequent research showed that the experienced satisfaction of these three needs was directly related to psychological health and well-being among a range of participants in varied settings.

Need Satisfaction across Cultures

Several recent studies have examined the importance of basic need satisfaction in various cultures, in part to provide evidence consistent with the self-determination theory hypothesis that the needs for competence, autonomy, and relatedness are universal. For example, in one study of workers in America and Bulgaria, Deci et al. (2001) related managers' styles to employees' experiences of need satisfaction on the job and, in turn, to well-being. The Bulgarian workers were from state-owned companies that operated primarily by central planning principles, whereas the American workers were recruited from a privately owned data management company that operated by market–economy principles. Analyses revealed that the various constructs being examined were comparable across the two cultures and, importantly that, in both cultures, managers'

being more autonomy supportive predicted greater satisfaction of the competence, autonomy, and relatedness needs among employees, which in turn predicted greater vitality, less anxiety, and fewer physical symptoms in the employees. These results thus complemented those reviewed earlier from the studies by Baard et al., (2004) and Ilardi et al. (1993). In short, in these two disparate cultures with different economic systems, social-contextual supports predicted satisfaction of the basic needs, which in turn predicted greater psychological and physical adjustment.

A study by Chirkov, Ryan, Kim, and Kaplan (2003), involving data from Turkey, South Korea, Russia, and the United States, concerned internalization of the values of individualism (a strongly endorsed Western value) and collectivism (a strongly endorsed Eastern value). As we have seen, internalization functions most effectively under conditions of satisfaction of all three basic needs and, as would therefore be expected, the degree of integration of the values for participants across the four cultures did predict enhanced psychological health and well-being.

SUMMARY AND CONCLUSIONS

During the 1950s, psychology was still focused primarily on drives such as hunger and sex as the energizing basis for all motivated behaviors. White (1959) argued, however, that a set of phenomena had been identified with humans, as well as with rats and monkeys, that vitiate this claim. Specifically, people and other animals were observed engaging in behaviors such as play and exploration that did not appear to reduce drives; indeed, they appeared to induce them. White thus proposed a new type of motivation that would supplement the drives as an energizing force. Maintaining that it is implicit in the natural tendency to master people's internal and external environments, White named it "effectance motivation" and posited that its effective functioning is the basis for healthy development. White's description of effectance motivation fit the definition of a "need for competence" (Deci & Ryan, 1980), although he refrained from using that term.

deCharms (1968), in discussing this new type of motivation, emphasized that people strive to master their environment and thus to feel like causal agents. In making this statement, deCharms was emphasizing what has come to be called the "need for autonomy or self-determination" as an important motivational force.

The idea of fundamental psychological needs for competence and self-determination (Deci & Ryan, 1980) proved useful in interpreting the results of experiments on intrinsic motivation. For example, social-contextual conditions, such as optimal challenge and positive feedback, tended to enhance intrinsic motivation by promoting perceived competence. Similarly, rewards tended to decrease intrinsic motivation, and choice tended to enhance it, because the former left people feeling controlled, while the latter left them feeling more autonomous. Research on the internalization of extrinsic motivation made clear that, while satisfaction of the needs for competence and autonomy are important for internalization, the basic need for relatedness is also critical for this process. In part, people are inclined to internalize the behaviors and values in their social environment in order to feel both a sense of belonging within that environment and a sense of competence and autonomy. Thus, the concept of the three basic psychological needs proved essential for integrating research results related to both intrinsic and extrinsic motivation.

Subsequent research has been more directly concerned with providing evidence that the new type of motivation is indeed based in psychological needs. For example, studies have shown that when people experience satisfaction of the basic needs, they also evidence greater well-being, whereas when satisfaction of the needs is thwarted, there are negative psychological consequences. Finally, studies in several cultures have now yielded results indicating that satisfaction of the needs for competence, autonomy, and relatedness is associated with greater psychological health—results that are consistent with the assertion in self-determination theory that competence, autonomy, and relatedness are universal psychological needs. Thus, the theorizing begun by White (1959), and supplemented by Harlow (1958) and deCharms (1968), has provided a founda-

tion for our contemporary understanding of people's motivation for functioning competently in their social and physical environments.

REFERENCES

Amabile, T. M., DeJong, W., & Lepper, M. R. (1976). Effects of externally imposed deadlines on subsequent intrinsic motivation. *Journal of Personality and Social Psychology, 34*, 92–98.

Angyal, A. (1941). *Foundations for a science of personality.* New York: Commonwealth Fund.

Assor, A., Roth, G., & Deci, E. L. (2004). The emotional costs of parents' conditional regard: A self-determination theory analysis. *Journal of Personality, 72*, 47–89.

Baard, P. P., Deci, E. L., & Ryan, R. M. (2004). Intrinsic need satisfaction: A motivational basis of performance and well-being in two work settings. *Journal of Applied Social Psychology, 34*, 2045–2068.

Bandura, A. (1977). *Social learning theory.* Englewood Cliffs, NJ: Prentice-Hall.

Baumeister, R., & Leary, M. R. (1995). The need to belong: Desire for interpersonal attachments as a fundamental human motivation. *Psychological Bulletin, 117*, 497–529.

Butler, R. A. (1953). Discrimination learning by rhesus monkeys to visual exploration motivation. *Journal of Comparative and Physiological Psychology, 46*, 95–98.

Butler, R. A., & Harlow, H. F. (1957). Discrimination learning and learning sets to visual exploration incentives. *Journal of General Psychology, 57*, 257–264.

Calder, B. J., & Staw, B. M. (1975). The interaction of intrinsic and extrinsic motivations: Some methodological notes. *Journal of Personality and Social Psychology, 31*, 76–80.

Cameron, J., & Pierce, W. D. (1994). Reinforcement, reward, and intrinsic motivation: A meta-analysis. *Review of Educational Research, 64*, 363–423.

Chirkov, V., Ryan, R. M., Kim, Y., & Kaplan, U. (2003). Differentiating autonomy from individualism and independence: A self-determination theory perspective on internalization of cultural orientations and well-being. *Journal of Personality and Social Psychology, 84*, 97–110.

Church, M. A., Elliot, A. J., & Gable, S. L. (2001). Perceptions of classroom environment, achievement goals, and achievement outcomes. *Journal of Educational Psychology, 9*, 43–54.

Cordova, D. I., & Lepper, M. R. (1996). Intrinsic motivation and the process of learning: Beneficial effects of contextualization, personalization, and choice. *Journal of Educational Psychology, 88*, 715–730.

Csikszentmihalyi, M. (1975). *Beyond boredom and anxiety.* San Francisco: Jossey-Bass.

Danner, F. W., & Lonky, E. (1981). A cognitive-developmental approach to the effects of rewards on intrinsic motivation. *Child Development, 52,* 1043–1052.

Dashiell, J. F. (1925). A quantitative demonstration of animal drive. *Journal of Comparative Psychology, 5,* 205–208.

deCharms, R. (1968). *Personal causation: The internal affective determinants of behavior.* New York: Academic Press.

Deci, E. L. (1971). Effects of externally mediated rewards on intrinsic motivation. *Journal of Personality and Social Psychology, 18,* 105–115.

Deci, E. L. (1975). *Intrinsic motivation.* New York: Plenum Press.

Deci, E. L., Betley, G., Kahle, J., Abrams, L., & Porac, J. (1981). When trying to win: Competition and intrinsic motivation. *Personality and Social Psychology Bulletin, 7,* 79–83.

Deci, E. L., & Cascio, W. F. (1972, April). *Changes in intrinsic motivation as a function of negative feedback and threats.* Paper presented at the meeting of the Eastern Psychological Association, Boston, MA.

Deci, E. L., Cascio, W. F., & Krusell, J. (1973, May). *Sex differences, verbal reinforcement, and intrinsic motivation.* Paper presented at the meeting of the Eastern Psychological Association, Washington, DC.

Deci, E. L., Cascio, W. F., & Krusell, J. (1975). Cognitive evaluation theory and some comments on the Calder and Staw critique. *Journal of Personality and Social Psychology, 31,* 81–85.

Deci, E. L., Eghrari, H., Patrick, B. C., & Leone, D. R. (1994). Facilitating internalization: The self-determination theory perspective. *Journal of Personality, 62,* 119–142.

Deci, E. L., Koestner, R., & Ryan, R. M. (1999a). A meta-analytic review of experiments examining the effects of extrinsic rewards on intrinsic motivation. *Psychological Bulletin, 125,* 627–668.

Deci, E. L., Koestner, R., & Ryan, R. M. (1999b). The undermining effect is a reality after all: Extrinsic rewards, task interest, and self-determination. *Psychological Bulletin, 125,* 692–700.

Deci, E. L., & Ryan, R. M. (1980). The empirical exploration of intrinsic motivational processes. In L. Berkowitz (Ed.), *Advances in experimental social psychology* (Vol. 13, pp. 39–80). New York: Academic Press.

Deci, E. L., & Ryan, R. M. (1985). *Intrinsic motivation and self-determination in human behavior.* New York: Plenum Press.

Deci, E. L., & Ryan, R. M. (2000). The "what" and the "why" of goal pursuits: Human needs and the self-determination of behavior. *Psychological Inquiry, 11,* 227–268.

Deci, E. L., Ryan, R. M., Gagné, M., Leone, D. R., Usunov, J., & Kornazheva, B. P. (2001). Need satisfaction, motivation, and well-being in the work organizations of a former Eastern bloc country. *Personality and Social Psychology Bulletin, 27,* 930–942.

Deci, E. L., Schwartz, A. J., Sheinman, L., & Ryan, R. M. (1981). An instrument to assess adults' orientations toward control versus autonomy with children: Reflections on intrinsic motivation and perceived competence. *Journal of Educational Psychology, 73,* 642–650.

Eisenberger, R., & Cameron, J. (1996). Detrimental effects of reward: Reality of myth? *American Psychologist, 51,* 1153–1166.

Eisenberger, R., Pierce, W. D., & Cameron, J. (1999). Effects of reward on intrinsic motivation—negative, neutral, and positive: Comment on Deci, Koestner, and Ryan (1999). *Psychological Bulletin, 125,* 677–691.

Elliot, A. J., Faler, J., McGregor, H. A., Campbell, W. K., Sedikies, C., & Harackiewicz, J. M. (2000). Competence valuation as a strategic intrinsic motivational process. *Personality and Social Psychology Bulletin, 26,* 780–794.

Elliot, A. J., & Harackiewicz, J. M. (1996). Approach and avoidance achievement goals and intrinsic motivation: A mediational analysis. *Journal of Personality and Social Psychology, 70,* 461–475.

Elliot, A. J., McGregor, H. A., & Thrash, T. M. (2002). The need for competence. In E. L. Deci & R. M. Ryan (Eds.), *Handbook of self-determination research* (pp. 361–387). Rochester, NY: University of Rochester Press.

Elliot, A. J., & Moller, A. C. (2003). Performance-approach goals: Good or bad forms of regulation? *International Journal of Educational Research, 39,* 339–356.

Fenichel, O. (1945). *The psychoanalytic theory of neurosis.* New York: Norton.

Fisher, C. D. (1978). The effects of personal control, competence, and extrinsic reward systems on intrinsic motivation. *Organizational Behavior and Human Performance, 21,* 273–288.

Freud, S. (1925). Instincts and their vicissitudes. In *Collected Papers* (Vol. 4, pp. 60–83). London: Hogarth. (Original work published in 1915)

Grolnick, W. S., & Ryan, R. M. (1989). Parent styles associated with children's self-regulation and competence in school. *Journal of Educational Psychology, 81,* 143–154.

Grolnick, W. S., Ryan, R. M., & Deci, E. L. (1991). The inner resources for school achievement: Motivational mediators of children's perceptions of their parents. *Journal of Educational Psychology, 83,* 508–517.

Harackiewicz, J. M., & Manderlink, G. (1984). A process analysis of the effects of performance-contingent rewards on intrinsic motivation. *Journal of Experimental Social Psychology, 20,* 531–551.

Harackiewicz, J. M., & Sansone, C. (2000). Rewarding competence: The importance of goals in the study of intrinsic motivation. In C. Sansone & J. M. Harackiewicz (Eds.), *Intrinsic and extrinsic motivation: The search for optimal motivation and performance* (pp. 79–103). San Diego: Academic Press.

Harlow, H. F. (1950). Learning and satiation of response in intrinsically motivated complex puzzle performance by monkeys. *Journal of Comparative and Physiological Psychology, 43,* 289–294.

Harlow, H. F. (1958). The nature of love. *American Psychologist, 13,* 673–685.

Harlow, H. F., Harlow, M. K., & Meyer, D. R. (1950). Learning motivated by a manipulation drive. *Journal of Experimental Psychology, 40,* 228–234.

Hartmann, H. (1958). *Ego psychology and the problem of adaptation.* New York: International Universities Press. (Original published in 1939)

Heider, F. (1958). *The psychology of interpersonal relations.* New York: Wiley.

Hendrick, I. (1942). Instinct and the ego during infancy. *Psychoanalytic Quarterly, 11,* 33–58.

Hill, W. F. (1956). Activity as an autonomous drive. *Journal of Comparative and Physiological Psychology, 49,* 15–19.

Hull, C. L. (1943). *Principles of behavior: An introduction to behavior theory.* New York: Appleton–Century–Crofts.

Ilardi, B. C., Leone, D., Kasser, T., & Ryan, R. M. (1993). Employee and supervisor ratings of motivation: Main effects and discrepancies associated with job satisfaction and adjustment in a factory setting. *Journal of Applied Social Psychology, 23,* 1789–1805.

Iyengar, S. S., & Lepper, M. R. (1999). Rethinking the value of choice: A cultural perspective on intrinsic motivation. *Journal of Personality and Social Psychology, 76,* 349–366.

Kagan, J., & Berkun, M. (1954). The reward value of running activity. *Journal of Comparative and Physiological Psychology, 47,* 108.

Kasser, V. G., & Ryan, R. M. (1999). The relation of psychological needs for autonomy and relatedness to vitality, well-being, and mortality in a nursing home. *Journal of Applied Social Psychology, 29,* 935–954.

Kast, A., & Connor, K. (1988). Sex and age differences in response to informational and controlling feedback. *Personality and Social Psychology Bulletin, 14,* 514–523.

Kelley, H. H. (1967). Attribution theory in social psychology. In D. Levine (Ed.), *Nebraska Symposium on Motivation* (Vol. 15, pp. 192–238). Lincoln: University of Nebraska Press.

Koestner, R., Ryan, R. M., Bernieri, F., & Holt, K. (1984). Setting limits on children's behavior: The differential effects of controlling versus informational styles on intrinsic motivation and creativity. *Journal of Personality, 52,* 233–248.

Lepper, M. R., & Greene, D. (1975). Turning play into work: Effects of adult surveillance and extrinsic rewards on children's intrinsic motivation. *Journal of Personality and Social Psychology, 31,* 479–486.

Lepper, M. R., Greene, D., & Nisbett, R. E. (1973). Undermining children's intrinsic interest with extrinsic rewards: A test of the "overjustification" hypothesis. *Journal of Personality and Social Psychology, 28,* 129–137.

McClelland, D. C., Atkinson, J. W., Clark, R. W., & Lowell, E. L. (1953). *The achievement motive.* New York: Appleton–Century–Croft.

Mead, G. H. (1934). *Mind, self, and society.* Chicago: University of Chicago Press.

Montgomery, K. C. (1954). The role of exploratory drive in learning. *Journal of Comparative and Physiological Psychology, 47,* 60–64.

Mossholder, K. W. (1980). Effects of externally mediated goal setting on intrinsic motivation: A laboratory experiment. *Journal of Applied Psychology, 65,* 202–210.

Murray, H. A. (1938). *Explorations in personality.* New York: Oxford University Press.

Myers, A. K., & Miller, N. E. (1954). Failure to find a learned drive based on hunger: Evidence for learning motivated by "exploration." *Journal of Comparative and Physiological Psychology, 47,* 428–436.

Nissen, H. W. (1930). A study of exploratory behavior in the white rat by means of the obstruction method. *Journal of Genetic Psychology, 37,* 361–376.

Pittman, T. S., Davey, M. E., Alafat, K. A., Wetherill, K. V., & Kramer, N. A. (1980). Informational versus controlling verbal rewards. *Personality and Social Psychology Bulletin, 6,* 228–233.

Plant, R., & Ryan, R. M. (1985). Intrinsic motivation and the effects of self-consciousness, self-awareness, and ego-involvement: An investigation of internally controlling styles. *Journal of Personality, 53,* 435–449.

Porter, L. W., & Lawler, E. E. (1968). *Managerial attitudes and performance.* Homewood, IL: Irwin-Dorsey.

Reader, M. H., & Dollinger, S. J. (1982). Deadlines, self-perceptions, and intrinsic motivation. *Personality and Social Psychology Bulletin, 8,* 742–747.

Reeve, J., & Deci, E. L. (1996). Elements within the competitive situation that affect intrinsic motivation. *Personality and Social Psychology Bulletin, 22,* 24–33.

Reis, H. T., Sheldon, K. M., Gable, S. L., Roscoe, J., & Ryan, R. M. (2000). Daily well-being: The role of autonomy, competence, and relatedness. *Personality and Social Psychology Bulletin, 26,* 419–435.

Ryan, R. M. (1982). Control and information in the intrapersonal sphere: An extension of cognitive evaluation theory. *Journal of Personality and Social Psychology, 43,* 450–461.

Ryan, R. M., Connell, J. P., & Deci, E. L. (1985). A motivational analysis of self-determination and self-regulation in education. In C. Ames & R. E. Ames (Eds.), *Research on motivation in education: The classroom milieu* (pp. 13–51). New York: Academic Press.

Ryan, R. M., Deci, E. L., & Grolnick, W. S. (1995). Autonomy, relatedness, and the self: Their relation to development and psychopathology. In D. Cicchetti & D. J. Cohen (Eds.), *Developmental psychopathology: Vol. 1. Theory and methods* (pp. 618–655). New York: Wiley.

Ryan, R. M., & Frederick, C. M. (1997). On energy, personality, and health: Subjective vitality as a dynamic reflection of well-being. *Journal of Personality, 65,* 529–565.

Ryan, R. M., Koestner, R., & Deci, E. L. (1991). Varied forms of persistence: When free-choice behavior is not intrinsically motivated. *Motivation and Emotion, 15,* 185–205.

Ryan, R. M., Mims, V., & Koestner, R. (1983). Relation of reward contingency and interpersonal context to intrinsic motivation: A review and test using cognitive evaluation theory. *Journal of Personality and Social Psychology, 45,* 736–750.

Scott, W. E. (1975). The effects of extrinsic rewards on "intrinsic motivation": A critique. *Organizational Behavior and Human Performance, 14,* 117–129.

Shapira, Z. (1976). Expectancy determinants of intrinsically motivated behavior. *Journal of Personality and Social Psychology, 34,* 1235–1244.

Sheldon, K. M., Ryan, R. M., & Reis, H. T. (1996). What makes for a good day?: Competence and autonomy in the day and in the person. *Personality and Social Psychology Bulletin, 22,* 1270–1279.

Smith, W. E. (1975). *The effect of anticipated vs. unanticipated social reward on subsequent intrinsic motivation.* Unpublished doctoral dissertation, Cornell University, Ithaca, NY.

Vallerand, R. J., & O'Connor, B. P. (1989). Motivation in the elderly: A theoretical framework and some promising findings. *Canadian Psychology, 30,* 538–550.

Vallerand, R. J., & Reid, G. (1984). On the causal effects of perceived competence on intrinsic motivation: A test of cognitive evaluation theory. *Journal of Sport Psychology, 6,* 94–102.

White, R. W. (1959). Motivation reconsidered: The concept of competence. *Psychological Review, 66,* 297–333.

White, R. W. (1960). Competence and the psychosexual stages of development. In M. R. Jones (Ed.), *Nebraska Symposium on Motivation* (Vol. 8, pp. 97–141). Lincoln: University of Nebraska Press.

Williams, G. C., & Deci, E. L. (1996). Internalization of biopsychosocial values by medical students: A test of self-determination theory. *Journal of Personality and Social Psychology, 70,* 767–779.

Zimbardo, P. G., & Miller, N. E. (1958). Facilitation of exploration by hunger in rats. *Journal of Comparative and Physiological Psychology, 51,* 43–46.

Zuckerman, M., Porac, J., Lathin, D., Smith, R., & Deci, E. L. (1978). On the importance of self-determination for intrinsically motivated behavior. *Personality and Social Psychology Bulletin, 4,* 443–446.

CHAPTER 32

ભ

Flow

MIHALY CSIKSZENTMIHALYI
SAMI ABUHAMDEH
JEANNE NAKAMURA

A GENERAL CONTEXT FOR A CONCEPT OF MASTERY MOTIVATION

What makes people want to go on with the effort required from life? Every epistemology of behavior must sooner or later cope with this basic question. The question is not so mysterious for nonhuman organisms, which presumably have built-in genetic programs instructing them to live as long as their physical machinery is able to function. But our species has a choice: With the development of consciousness, we have the ability to second-guess and occasionally override the instructions coded in our chromosomes. This evolutionary development has added a great deal of flexibility to the human repertoire of behaviors. But the freedom gained has its downside—too many possibilities can have a paralyzing effect on action (Schwartz, 2000). Among the options we are able to entertain is that of ending our lives; thus, as the existential philosophers remarked, the question of

why one should not commit suicide is fundamental to the understanding of human life.

In fact, most attempts at a general psychology also start with the assumption that human beings have a "need" or a "drive" for self-preservation, and that all other motivations, if not reducible to, are then at least based on such a need. For example Maslow's hierarchy assumes that survival takes precedence over all other considerations, and no other need becomes active until survival is reasonably assured.

But where is this will to live located? Is it nothing but a variation of the survival instincts all living organisms share, chemically etched into our genes? The last try for a comprehensive human psychology, that of Sigmund Freud, posited *Eros* as the source of all behavior—a force akin to the *élan vital* of the French philosopher Henri Bergson (1931/1944) and to similar concepts of life energy proposed by a long list of thinkers going back to the beginnings of speculative thought.

Eros, which originally referred to the need of the organism to fulfill its physical potential, was soon reduced in Freud's writings, and even more so in those of his followers, to the libidinal pleasure that through natural selection has become attached to the sexual reproductive act and to the organs implicated in it. Thus, "erotic" eventually became synonymous with "sexual."

This reduction of the concept of vitality to the reproductive function rested on a reasonably sound logic. The Darwinian revolution highlighted the role of sexual selection in evolution; thus, it made sense to see sexuality as the master-need from which all other interests and motives derive. A species survives as long as its members reproduce. If the drive to reproduce became well entrenched in a species, its survival would be enhanced. Following Ockham's principle of parsimony, one might expect that as long as sexual drives are well established, other motives become secondary. Whatever men and women do, from making songs to mapping the heavens, is just a disguised expression of Eros, a manifestation of the reproductive drive.

On closer examination, however, this single causality seems much less convincing. A species needs to take care of many other priorities besides reproduction in order to survive. At the human stage of evolution, where adaptation and survival depend increasingly on flexible responses mediated by conscious thought, members of the species had to learn how to master and control a hostile and changing environment. It makes sense to assume that natural selection favored those individuals, and their descendants, who enjoyed acts of mastery and control—just as survival was enhanced when other acts necessary for survival, such as eating and sex, became experienced as pleasurable.

The various behaviors associated with control and mastery—such as curiosity, interest, exploration; the pursuit of skills, the relishing of challenges—need not be seen as derivatives of thwarted libidinal sexuality. They are just as much a part of human nature, just as necessary for our survival, as the drive to reproduce. The ancients understood this when they coined the aphorism *Libri aut liberi*: "Books or sons." As humans, we have the option of leaving a trace of our existence by writing books (or shaping tools,

raising buildings, writing songs, etc.) and thus leaving a cultural legacy, as well as leaving our genes to our progeny. The two are not reducible to each other, but are equally important motives that have become ingrained in our natures.

The idea that the ability to operate effectively in the environment fulfills a primary need is not new in psychology. In Germany, Karl Groos (1901) and Karl Bühler (1930) elaborated the concept of *Funktionlust*, or "activity pleasure," which Jean Piaget (1952) included in the earliest stages of sensorimotor development as the "pleasure of being a cause" that drove infants to experiment. In more recent psychological thought, Hebb (1955) and Berlyne (1960) focused on the nervous system's need for optimal levels of stimulation to explain exploratory behavior and the seeking of novelty, while White (1959) and deCharms (1968) focused on people's need to feel in control, to be the causal agents of their actions. Later Deci and Ryan (Deci, 1971; Deci & Ryan, 1985) elaborated on this line of argument by suggesting that both competence and autonomy were innate psychological needs that must be satisfied for psychological growth and well-being.

Theories that provide explanations for why people are motivated to master and control tend to be *distal*. In other words, they provide sensible explanations, typically based on an evolutionary framework, for why such behaviors should have become established over many generations, in order to support the reproductive success of the individual. However, for an activity pattern to become established in a species' repertoire, it has to be experienced as enjoyable by the individual. To explain how this happens, a *proximal* theory of motivation is needed.

Such a theory must rely on at least four complementary lines of explanation. In the first place, it is likely that mastery-related behavior has become personally rewarding because it has evolved, through literally millions of years of trial and error, as an effective strategy to achieve other goals, such as mates and material resources. Overcoming challenges and excelling is therefore adaptive and increases chances for reproductive success.

Second, one may adopt a more Freudian line and see mastery-related behavior as an internalized drive that could serve either the purposes of the id (in the case of tyrants or robber barons) or of the superego (in the case of creative, prosocial individuals). In this, as in the previous case, the behavior does not serve an independent function but is a disguised manifestation of other forces seeking their own aims.

Third, the person may seek out such behaviors because of innate or learned psychological needs, such as competence and autonomy. According to this explanation, the enjoyment one experiences during intrinsically motivated behavior is largely a result of the satisfaction of these basic psychological needs.

This chapter deals with a fourth kind of explanation, which we call the "phenomenological account." It tries to look very closely at what people actually experience when they are involved in activities that involve mastery, control, and autonomous behavior, without prejudging the reasons for why such experiences exist. This line of explanation assumes that the human organism is a system in its own right, not reducible to lower levels of complexity, such as stimulus–response pathways, unconscious processes, or neurological structures.

These four kinds of explanations are not incompatible with each other. In fact, they are likely to be all implicated in the genesis and maintenance of mastery behavior at the individual level. Quite often, they support each other, driving the organism in the same direction. But it is also often the case that the genetically programmed instructions may come into conflict with the learned ones, or that the unconscious forces press in a direction contrary to what the phenomenological reality suggests.

THE NATURE OF FLOW

The fourth of these lines of explanation, focused on events occurring in the consciousness of the individual, is the one here identified with the study of the flow experience. This experience emerged over a quarter-century ago as a result of a series of studies of what were initially called *autotelic activities*; that is, things people seem to do for the activity's own sake.

Why do people perform time-consuming,

difficult, and often dangerous activities for which they receive no discernible extrinsic rewards? This was the question that originally prompted one of us into a program of research that involved extensive interviews with hundreds of rock climbers, chess players, athletes, and artists (Csikszentmihalyi, 1975; Nakamura & Csikszentmihalyi, 2002). The basic conclusion was that, in all the various groups studied, the respondents reported a very similar subjective experience that they enjoyed so much that they were willing to go to great lengths to experience it again. This we eventually called the "flow experience," because in describing how it felt when the activity was going well, several respondents used the metaphor of a current that carried them along effortlessly.

Flow is a subjective state that people report when they are completely involved in something to the point of forgetting time, fatigue, and everything else but the activity itself. It is what we feel when we read a well-crafted novel or play a good game of squash, or take part in a stimulating conversation. The defining feature of flow is intense experiential involvement in moment-to-moment activity. Attention is fully invested in the task at hand, and the person functions at his or her fullest capacity. Mark Strand, former Poet Laureate of the United States, in one of our interviews, described this state while writing as follows:

> You're right in the work, you lose your sense of time, you're completely enraptured, you're completely caught up in what you are doing. . . . When you are working on something and you are working well, you have the feeling that there's no other way of saying what you're saying. (in Csikszentmihalyi, 1996, p. 121)

The intense experiential involvement of flow is responsible for three additional subjective characteristics commonly reported: the merging of action and awareness, a sense of control, and an altered sense of time.

The Merging of Action and Awareness

The default option of consciousness is a chaotic review of things that one fears or desires, resulting in a phenomenological state we have elsewhere labeled "psychic entropy" (Csikszentmihalyi & Csikszentmihalyi,

1988). During flow, however, attentional resources are fully invested in the task at hand, so that objects beyond the immediate interaction generally fail to enter awareness.

One such object is the self. Respondents frequently describe a loss of self-consciousness during flow. Without the required attentional resources, the self-reflective processes that often intrude into awareness and cause attention to be diverted from what needs to be done are silenced, and the usual dualism between actor and action disappears. In the terms that George Herbert Mead introduced (1934/1970), the "me" disappears during flow, and the "I" takes over. A rock climber in an early study of flow put it this way:

> You're so involved in what you're doing you aren't thinking about yourself as separate from the immediate activity. You're no longer a participant observer, only a participant. You're moving in harmony with something else you're part of. (in Csikszentmihalyi, 1975, p. 86)

A Sense of Control

During flow, we typically experience a sense of control—or, more precisely, a lack of anxiety about losing control that is typical of many situations in normal life. This sense of control is also reported in activities that involve serious risks, such as hang gliding, rock climbing, and race car driving—activities that to an outsider would seem to be much more potentially dangerous than the affairs of everyday life. Yet these activities are structured to provide the participant with the means to reduce the margin of error to as close to zero as possible. Rock climbers, for example, insist that their hair-raising exploits are safer than crossing a busy street in Chicago, because, on the rock face, they can foresee every eventuality, whereas when crossing the street, they are at the mercy of fate. The sense of control respondents describe thus reflects the possibility, rather than the actuality, of control.

Worrying about whether we can succeed at what we are doing—on the job, in relationships, even in crossing a busy street—is one of the major sources of psychic entropy in everyday life, and its reduction during flow is one of the reasons such an experience becomes enjoyable and thus rewarding.

Altered Sense of Time

William James (1890, Ch. 15, Sec. 4) noted that boredom seems to increase when "we grow attentive to the passage of time itself." During flow, attention is so fully invested in moment-to-moment activity that there is little left over to devote toward the mental processes that contribute to the experience of duration (Friedman, 1990). As a result, persons deeply immersed in an activity typically report time passing quickly (Conti, 2001).

Exceptions occur in certain sports or jobs that require precise knowledge of time, but these are exceptions that prove the rule: Basketball players must learn not to dribble the ball in their own side of the court for more than 10 seconds; football players must learn to "manage the clock" in a close game. Awareness of time in these situations is not extraneous information signifying boredom, but a challenge that the person has to overcome in order to perform well.

THE CONDITIONS OF FLOW

Flow experiences are relatively rare in everyday life, but almost everything—work, study or religious ritual—is able to produce them, provided certain conditions are met. Past research suggests three conditions of key importance. First, flow tends to occur when the activity one engages in contains a *clear set of goals*. These goals serve to add direction and purpose to behavior. Their value lies in their capacity to structure experience by channeling attention rather than being ends in themselves.

A second precondition for flow is *a balance between perceived challenges and perceived skills*. This condition is reminiscent of the concept of "optimal arousal" (Berlyne, 1960; Hunt, 1965), but differs from it in highlighting the fact that what counts at the phenomenological level is the *perception* of the demands and abilities, not necessarily their objective presence.

When perceived challenges and skills are well matched, as in a close game of tennis or a satisfying musical performance, attention is completely absorbed. This balance, however, is intrinsically fragile. If challenges begin to exceed skills, one typically becomes anxious; if skills begin to exceed challenges, one relaxes and then becomes bored. These subjective states provide feedback about the shifting relationship to the environment and press the individual to adjust behavior in order to escape the more aversive subjective state and reenter flow.

Finally, flow is dependent on the presence of *clear and immediate feedback*. The individual needs to negotiate the continually changing environmental demands that are part of all experientially involving activity (Reser & Scherl, 1988). Immediate feedback serves this purpose: It informs the individual how well he or she is progressing in the activity, and dictates whether to adjust or maintain the present course of action. It leaves the individual with little doubt about what to do next.

Because flow takes place at a high level of challenge, the feedback one receives during the course of an activity will inevitably include "negative" performance feedback. From a phenomenological viewpoint, this negative feedback will not necessarily be detrimental to task involvement. Provided the individual perceives that he or she possesses the skills to take on the challenges of the activity, the valence of the feedback is of less consequence for activity enjoyment than the usefulness of the feedback in suggesting appropriate corrective measures. Indeed, it is not difficult to think of situations in which we intentionally elicit negative feedback in order to direct attention and behavior (e.g., a pianist practicing with a metronome).

To summarize, clear goals, optimal challenges, and clear, immediate feedback are all necessary features of activities that promote the intrinsically rewarding experiential involvement that characterizes flow. Of course, this is not to say that these are the only factors that affect the degree to which one becomes involved in an activity. Research on task involvement suggests that the importance an individual places on doing well in an activity (i.e., "competence valuation") predicts the individual's involvement in that activity (Greenwald, 1982; Harackiewicz & Elliot, 1998; Harackiewicz & Manderlink, 1984), as does the congruence between task-specific, behaviorally based goals (e.g., "I want to attach a flag to my car's antenna") and higher level, more abstract goals (e.g., "I want to show my pa-

triotism"), with greater congruence leading to greater involvement (Harackiewicz & Elliot, 1998; Rathunde, 1989; Sansone, Sachau, & Weir, 1989). Furthermore, the personal implications an individual attributes to success or failure at an activity can affect his or her interpretation of performance feedback, which in turn has consequences for task involvement (Mueller & Dweck, 1998). With respect to individual differences, Wong (2000) found that autonomy orientation (Deci & Ryan, 1985) was positively related to involvement in school-related activities; absorption (Tellegen & Atkinson, 1974), a trait construct used to measure hypnotic susceptibility, and conceptually related to openness to experience, has been shown to be positively associated with experiential involvement (Glisky, Tataryn, Tobias, Kihlstrom, & McConkey, 1991; Levin & Fireman, 2001; Wild, Kuiken, & Schopflocher, 1995).

FLOW AND MOTIVATION

Theories of motivation generally neglect the phenomenology of the person to whom motivation is being attributed. They explain the reason for action in functional terms, that is, by considering outcomes rather than processes (Sansone & Harackiewicz, 1996). How the person feels while acting tends to be ignored. Yet individuals constantly evaluate their quality of experience and often will decide to continue or terminate a given behavioral sequence based on their evaluations. Our research suggests that the phenomenological experience of flow is a powerful motivating force. When individuals are fully involved in an activity, they tend to find the activity enjoyable and intrinsically rewarding. Whatever the original motivation for playing chess or playing the stock market, or going out with a friend, such activities will not continue unless they are enjoyable—or unless people are motivated by extrinsic rewards.

Flow and Competence Motivation

Perceived competence has traditionally played a central part in theories of motivation (Bandura, 1982; Deci, 1975; Harter, 1978; White, 1959). These theories generally argue that intrinsic motivation is promoted by feelings of competence and efficacy. In support of this, several researchers have found that positive competence feedback is positively related to subsequent motivation to perform an activity (Deci, 1971; Elliot et al., 2000; Fisher, 1978; Harackiewicz, 1979; Ryan, 1982; Vallerand & Reid, 1984).

These findings are consistent with past research on flow. Our studies have found that actors who perceive that they lack the skills to take on effectively the challenges presented by the activity in which they are participating experience anxiety or boredom, depending on how much they value doing well in the activity (Csikszentmihalyi & LeFevre, 1989; Csikszentmihalyi & Nakamura, 1989; Csikszentmihalyi, Rathunde, & Whalen, 1993). Simply put, if an actor feels incompetent in a given situation, he or she will tend not be motivated. However, our research also suggests that although perceived competence seems to be an important precondition for intrinsic motivation, it is often not a predominating characteristic of the phenomenological experience associated with intrinsically motivated behavior. More specifically, much of the reward of intrinsically motivated behavior is derived from the experience of absorption and interest, the epitome of which is flow.

Consider the following example: A person picks up a novel to read. As she begins reading it, she senses that her abilities are not up to the task, that the material is too complex for her to appreciate fully. Feeling unable to take on the challenges of the book because her skills are lacking, she will experience anxiety or boredom, and will probably opt for a less demanding novel or activity. However, if she feels that the complexities of the book are within her capacities and is able to digest the material, her decision either to continue reading the novel or to put it down will be based primarily on her quality of experience while reading the book, namely, the extent to which she finds the book involving and interesting.

Emergent Motivation

The phenomenology of flow further suggests that we may enjoy a particular activity because of something discovered through the interaction. It is commonly reported, for instance, that a person is at first indifferent or bored by a certain activity, such as listening to classical music or using a computer. Then, when the opportunities for action become clearer or the individual's skills improve, the activity begins to be interesting and, finally, enjoyable. It is in this sense that the rewards of these types of intrinsically motivating activities are "emergent" or a priori unpredictable.

The phenomenon of *emergent motivation* means that we can *come to* experience a new or previously unengaging activity as intrinsically rewarding, if we find flow in it. The motivation to persist in or return to the activity arises out of the experience itself. What happens next is responsive to what happened immediately before, within the interaction, rather than being dictated by a preexisting intentional structure located within either the person (e.g., a goal or drive) or the environment (e.g., a tradition, script, or set of rules). The flow experience is thus a force for expansion in relation to the individual's goal and interest structure, as well as for the growth of skills in relation to an existing interest (Csikszentmihalyi & Nakamura, 1999).

Certain technologies become successful at least in part because they provide flow, thus motivating people to use them. A good example is the Internet, developed with funds made available by the U.S. Department of Defense for purposes of national security. This technology has been adapted to all sorts of unexpected uses and has made possible an enormous variety of unpredicted experiences. It partly accounts, for instance, for the spectacular success of the Linux open system software, where tens of thousands of amateur and professional programmers work hard to come up with new software for the sheer delight of solving a problem, and for being appreciated by respected peers. In the process, Linux has been making headway against much more formidable competitors, such as Microsoft, who have to pay their programmers to write software—a clear example of emergent intrinsic rewards actually trumping extrinsic rewards.

In summary, quality of experience is the proximal cause of intrinsically motivated behavior. When an individual begins, continues, or ends an activity that is not motivated by extrinsic rewards, such decisions are based primarily on the current or anticipated enjoyment accompanying the activity. In this context, both motivation and goals are emergent, in the sense that they are determined by the actor's moment-to-moment experience.

Is deep experiential involvement a prerequisite for intrinsically motivated behavior? Clearly, it is not. As past research on the structure of affect has demonstrated, positive affect can be in the form of both high- and low-activation positive affect (Tellegen, Watson, & Clark, 1999). Whereas flow represents a state of high-activation positive affect, it contrasts sharply with low-activation positive affect, which is associated with states such as relaxation and contentment. It is consistent with current understandings of evolution to suppose that both of these strategies for coping with the environment, one conservative and the other expansive, were selected over time as important components of the human behavioral repertoire, even though they motivate different—in some sense, opposite—behaviors. Yet because it is only during states of high activation that we are pushed to expand our existing capacities, flow is particularly important to understand given the implications it has for personal growth.

FLOW AND COMPETENCE-RELEVANT OUTCOMES

High levels of both mental and physical performance usually depend on goal-directed attention produced by specific challenges and clear feedback (Locke, Shaw, Saari, & Latham, 1981). It is therefore not surprising that a host of studies have found a strong positive relationship between flow and performance. For example, flow is positively associated with artistic and scientific creativity (e.g., Perry, 1999; Sawyer, 1992), effective teaching (Csikszentmihalyi, 1996), learning (Csikszentmihalyi et al., 1993), and peak performance in sports (Jackson, Thomas, Marsh, & Smethurst, 2002; Stein, Kimiecik, Daniels, & Jackson, 1995).

Perhaps more compelling than situationally based positive outcomes, however, are the developmental implications of the flow

model. As individuals master challenges in an activity, they develop greater levels of skill, and the activity ceases to be as involving as before. To continue experiencing flow, they must identify increasingly greater challenges. Thus, over time, the balance between challenges and skills enhances competence. Experiential goals thus introduce a principle of selection into psychological functioning that fosters growth and stretches a person's existing capacities (cf. Vygotsky, 1978).

This positive relationship between flow and skill development has been demonstrated in a number of studies that have used the experience sampling method (Csikszentmihalyi & Larson, 1984) to examine the phenomenological experience of students within school settings. In longitudinal research with talented adolescents, students still committed to pursuing their talent area at age 17 were compared to peers who had already disengaged. Four years earlier, those who were still committed had experienced more flow and less anxiety than their peers while engaged in school-related activities; they were also more likely to have identified their talent area as a source of flow (Csikszentmihalyi et al., 1993). In a longitudinal study of students talented in mathematics, Heine (1996) showed that those who experienced flow in the first part of the course performed better in the second half, controlling for their initial abilities and grade point average (GPA). Also controlling for initial abilities, Wong and Csikszentmihalyi (1991) found that immediate, experience-based motivation was a better predictor of the difficulty level of classes that students subsequently chose than their motivation to achieve long-term academic goals.

Longitudinal research on resilience suggests that, in addition to enhancing positive outcomes, a subjectively optimal matching of challenge and skill in daily life may protect against negative outcomes (Schmidt, 1999). In a national sample of American adolescents, teenagers who had experienced high adversity at home and/or at school but had access to extracurricular and other challenging activities, and who were involved in these activities and felt successful when engaged in them, were much less likely to have problems years later.

FLOW AND SPECIES-LEVEL DEVELOPMENT

Flow and the Evolution of Consciousness

Consciousness is the complex system that has evolved in humans for selecting, processing, and storing the profusion of information provided by the senses. Consciousness gives us a measure of control, freeing us from complete subservience to the dictates of genes and culture, by representing alternative courses of action in awareness, thereby introducing the alternative of rejecting rather than enacting them. It thus serves as a clutch between programmed instructions and adaptive behaviors (Csikszentmihalyi & Csikszentmihalyi, 1988). Alongside the genetic and cultural guides to action, it establishes a *teleonomy of the self*, a set of goals that have been freely chosen by the individual (cf. Brandstadter, 1998; Csikszentmihalyi & Massimini, 1985; Deci & Ryan, 1985). It might, of course, prove dangerous to disengage our behavior from direct control by the genetic and cultural instructions that have evolved over millennia of adapting to the environment. On the other hand, doing so may increase the chances for adaptive fit with the present environment, particularly under conditions of radical or rapid change.

In order for consciousness to be used for such positive ends, however, a person must learn to enjoy being conscious. People value in principle but seldom resort to free choice, reflection, and the weighing of alternatives. As Dostoevsky eloquently described in his tale of the Grand Inquisitor, it is much easier to act in terms of habit and convention, relying on genetic and cultural programs, than to decide in terms of one's own experience. This is in part due to the fact that the skills for being conscious need to be cultivated, or the task will seem too daunting and thus produce anxiety.

Our schools are geared to teach cognitive skills, but these do not necessarily develop the skill for being conscious. A young person needs to exercise freedom in the allocation of attention, the pursuit of interests, and the mastering of challenges; only then will he or she begin to enjoy being conscious. This opportunity is rarely present in the normal school environment—or even

earlier, in the family environment of the young child. But unless we learn to enjoy using the mind freely, yet in an orderly fashion, the evolution of consciousness is going to be hampered.

Flow and the Evolution of Culture

Flow is not only an important mechanism in the development of the person, but it also plays an important role in the development of culture. As we mentioned earlier in discussing the successful spread of the Linux open software system, new technologies, beliefs, lifestyles—and even political systems—are often adopted or rejected on the basis of whether they enhance or diminish the probability of producing flow.

Professor Fausto Massimini of the University of Milan was the first scholar to realize the potential of flow to explain the selection of new cultural artifacts, or "memes" (Csikszentmihalyi & Massimini, 1985; Inghilleri, 1999; Massimini, Csikszentmihalyi, & Delle Fave, 1988). Essentially, the likelihood that a new idea, product, or process will survive over time is a function of the attention it attracts. A song, a scientific theory, or a religious system will be remembered and transmitted to the next generation only if some people pay attention to it. And people will pay attention in large part because the new meme provides an enjoyable challenge.

This is clearly the case in the advancement of science. Thomas Kuhn (1970) describes how by focusing attention upon a small range of relatively esoteric problems, scientists are able to delve in greater depth and detail into their investigations, and thereby advance their field. Yet such focused attention cannot be sustained unless there are interesting problems that challenge the scientist. If there are none, the paradigm becomes boring, and the field disappears for lack of young recruits who are attracted to a different field by more interesting problems.

The same holds true for art, according to Collingwood (1938) and Martindale (1990). More generally, any field of creative accomplishment requires concentrated attention, to the exclusion of all other stimuli, which temporarily become irrelevant (Csikszentmihalyi, 1975; Getzels & Csikszentmihalyi,

1976; Nakamura & Csikszentmihalyi, 2001). Yet one does not need to look at great accomplishments to realize this basic function of attention. More mundane work is just as dependent on it. In describing the workers that made industrialization possible at the dawn of capitalism, Max Weber (1930, p. 71) commented on the relationship between puritanical religious beliefs and training on the one hand, and productivity on the other: "The ability of mental concentration . . . is here most often combined with . . . a cool self-control and frugality which enormously increase performance. This creates the most favorable foundation for the conception of labor as an end in itself."

The late Roman Empire, the last decades of Byzantium, and the French court in the second half of the 18th century are only a few of the most notorious examples of what can happen when large segments of society fail to find enjoyment in productive life. To provide such experiences, the rulers of society had to resort to increasingly elaborate and expensive means of control and repression, or else artificial stimulations—circuses, chariot races, balls, and hunts—that drain the attention of a passive population without leaving any useful residue. Whenever a society is unable to provide flow experiences in productive activities, its members will find flow in activities that are either wasteful or actually disruptive.

CONCLUSIONS

The ability to enjoy challenges and then master them is a fundamental metaskill that is essential to individual development and to cultural evolution. Yet many obstacles prevent individuals from experiencing flow. These range from inherited genetic malfunctions to forms of social oppression that reduce personal freedom and prevent the acquisition of skills.

But even in the most benign situations, flow may be difficult to attain. For instance, in our society at present, most parents are determined to provide the best conditions for their children's future happiness. They work hard, so that they can buy a nice home in the suburbs, get all the consumer goods they can afford, and send the children to the best schools possible. Unfortunately, none of this guarantees that the children will get what they need to learn in order to enjoy life. In fact, a growing number of studies suggests that excessive concern for safety, comfort, and material well-being is detrimental to optimal development (Csikszentmihalyi & Hunter, 2003; Kasser & Ryan, 1993; Schmuck & Sheldon, 2001). The sterile surroundings of our living arrangements, the absence of working parents and other adults who could initiate young people into the joys of living, the addictive nature of passive entertainment and the reliance on material rewards, and the excessive concern of schools with testing and with disembodied knowledge all militate against learning to enjoy mastering the challenges that life inevitably presents.

Thus, understanding how flow works is essential for social scientists interested in improving the quality of life at either the subjective or objective level. Transforming this knowledge into effective action is not easy. But the challenges this presents promise almost infinite opportunities for enjoyment to those who are willing to develop the skills necessary to master them.

REFERENCES

Bandura, A. (1982). Self-efficacy mechanism in human agency. *American Psychologist, 37,* 122–147.

Bergson, H. (1944). *Creative evolution.* New York: The Modern Library. (Original published in 1931)

Berlyne, D. (1960). *Conflict, arousal, and curiosity.* New York: McGraw-Hill.

Brandstadter, J. (1998). Action perspectives in human development. In R. M. Lerner (Ed.), *Handbook of child psychology* (Vol. 1, pp. 807–863). New York: Wiley.

Bühler, C. (1930). Die geistige Entwicklung des Kindes [The mental development of children]. Jena, Germany: G. Fischer.

Collingwood, R. G. (1938). *The principles of art.* Oxford, UK: Oxford University Press.

Conti, R. (2001). Time flies: Investigating the connection between intrinsic motivation and the experience of time. *Journal of Personality, 69*(1), 1–26.

Csikszentmihalyi, M. (1975). *Beyond boredom and anxiety.* San Francisco: Jossey-Bass.

Csikszentmihalyi, M. (1996). *Creativity: Flow and the psychology of discovery and invention.* New York: HarperCollins.

Csikszentmihalyi, M., & Csikszentmihalyi, I. (Eds.). (1988). *Optimal experience: Psychological studies of flow in consciousness.* New York: Cambridge University Press.

Csikszentmihalyi, M., & Hunter, J. (2003). Happiness in everyday life: The uses of experience sampling. *Journal of Happiness Studies, 4*(2), 1–15.

Csikszentmihalyi, M., & Larson, R. (1984). *Being adolescent*. New York: Basic Books.

Csikszentmihalyi, M., & LeFevre, J. (1989). Optimal experience in work and leisure. *Journal of Personality and Social Psychology, 56*(5), 815–822.

Csikszentmihalyi, M., & Massimini, F. (1985). On the psychological selection of bio-cultural information. *New Ideas in Psychology, 3*(2), 115–138.

Csikszentmihalyi, M., & Nakamura, J. (1989). The dynamics of intrinsic motivation: A study of adolescents. In R. Ames & C. Ames (Eds.), *Research on motivation in education: Goals and cognitions* (pp. 45–71). New York: Academic Press.

Csikszentmihalyi, M., & Nakamura, J. (1999). Emerging goals and the self-regulation of behavior. In R. S. Wyer (Ed.), *Advances in social cognition: Vol. 12. Perspectives on behavioral self-regulation* (pp. 107–118). Mahwah, NJ: Erlbaum.

Csikszentmihalyi, M., Rathunde, K., & Whalen, S. (1993). *Talented teenagers*. Cambridge, UK: Cambridge University Press.

deCharms, R. (1968). *Personal causation*. New York: Academic Press.

Deci, E. (1971). Effects of externally mediated rewards on intrinsic motivation. *Journal of Personality and Social Psychology, 18*(1), 105–115.

Deci, E. L. (1975). *Intrinsic motivation*. New York: Plenum Press.

Deci, E., & Ryan, R. (1985). *Intrinsic motivation and self-determination in human behavior*. New York: Plenum Press.

Elliot, A. J., Faler, J., McGregor, H. A., Campbell, W. K., Sedikides, C., & Harackiewicz, J. (2000). Competence valuation as a strategic intrinsic motivation process. *Personality and Social Psychology Bulletin, 26*(7), 780–794.

Elliot, A. J., & Harackiewicz, J. (1994). Goal setting, achievement orientation, and intrinsic motivation: A mediational analysis. *Journal of Personality and Social Psychology, 66*(5), 968–980.

Fisher, C. D. (1978). The effects of personal control, competence, and extrinsic reward systems on intrinsic motivation. *Organizational Behavior and Human Performance, 21*, 273–288.

Friedman, W. J. (1990). *About time: Inventing the fourth dimension*. Cambridge, MA: MIT Press.

Getzels, J. W., & Csikszentmihalyi, M. (1976). *The creative vision*. New York: Wiley.

Glisky, M. L., Tataryn, D. J., Tobias, B. A., Kihlstrom, J. F., & McConkey, K. M. (1991). Absorption, openness to experience, and hypnotizability. *Journal of Personality and Social Psychology, 60*(2), 263–272.

Greenwald, A. (1982). Ego task analysis: An integration of research on ego-involvement and self-awareness. In A. H. Hastorf & A. M. Isen (Eds.), *Cognitive social psychology* (pp. 109–147). New York: Elsevier/North Holland.

Groos, K. (1901). *The play of man*. New York: Appleton.

Harackiewicz, J. M. (1979). The effects of reward contingency and performance feedback on intrinsic motivation. *Journal of Personality and Social Psychology, 37*, 1352–1363.

Harackiewicz, J. M., & Elliot, A. J. (1998). The joint effects of target and purpose goals on intrinsic motivation: A mediational analysis. *Personality and Social Psychology Bulletin, 24*(7), 675–689.

Harackiewicz, J. M., & Manderlink, G. (1984). A process analysis of the effects of performance-contingent rewards on intrinsic motivation. *Journal of Experimental Social Psychology, 20*, 531–551.

Harackiewicz, J. M., Sansone, C., & Manderlink, G. (1985). Competence, achievement orientation, and intrinsic motivation: A process analysis. *Journal of Personality and Social Psychology, 48*(2), 493–508.

Harter, S. (1978). Effectance motivation reconsidered: Toward a developmental model. *Human Development, 2*(1), 34–64.

Hebb, D. O. (1955). Drive and the CNS. *Psychological Review, 62*, 243–252.

Heine, C. (1996). *Flow and achievement in mathematics*. Unpublished doctoral dissertation, University of Chicago, Chicago, IL.

Hunt, J. (1965). Intrinsic motivation and its role in development. In *Nebraska Symposium on Motivation* (Vol. 12, pp. 189–282). Lincoln: University of Nebraska Press.

Inghilleri, P. (1999). *From subjective experience to cultural change*. Cambridge, UK: Cambridge University Press.

Jackson, S. A., Thomas, P. R., Marsh, H. W., & Smethurst, C. J. (2002). Relationships between flow, self-concept, psychological skills, and performance. *Journal of Applied Sport Psychology, 13*(2), 129–153.

James, W. (1890). *The principles of psychology*. New York: Holt.

Kasser, T., & Ryan, R. (1993). A dark side of the American dream: Correlates of financial success as a central life aspiration. *Journal of Personality and Social Psychology, 65*, 410–422.

Kuhn, T. S. (1970). *The structure of scientific revolutions*. Chicago: University of Chicago Press.

Levin, R., & Fireman, G. (2001). The relation of fantasy proneness, psychological absorption, and imaginative involvement to nightmare prevalence and nightmare distress. *Imagination, Cognition and Personality, 21*(2), 111–129.

Locke, E. A., Shaw, K. N., Saari, L. M., & Latham, G. P. (1981). Goal setting and task performance: 1969–1980. *Psychological Bulletin, 90*(1), 125–152.

Martindale, C. (1990). *The clockwork muse: The predictability of artistic change*. New York: Basic Books.

Massimini, F., Csikszentmihalyi, M., & Delle Fave, A. D. (1988). Flow and biocultural evolution. In M. Csikszentmihalyi & I. S. Csikszentmihalyi (Eds.), *Optimal experience: Psychological studies of flow in consciousness* (pp. 60–81). New York: Cambridge University Press.

Mead, G. H. (1970). *Mind, self and society.* Chicago: University of Chicago Press. (Original published in 1934)

Mueller, C. M., & Dweck, C. S. (1998). Praise for intelligence can undermine children's motivation and performance. *Journal of Personality and Social Psychology, 75,* 33–52.

Nakamura, J., & Csikszentmihalyi, M. (2001). Catalytic creativity: The case of Linus Pauling. *American Psychologist, 56*(4), 337–341.

Nakamura, J., & Csikszentmihalyi, M. (2002). The concept of flow. In C. R. Snyder & S. J. Lopez (Eds.), *Handbook of positive psychology* (pp. 89–105). New York: Oxford University Press.

Perry, S. K. (1999). *Writing in flow.* Cincinnati: Writer's Digest Books.

Piaget, J. (1952). *The origins of intelligence in children.* New York: International Universities Press.

Rathunde, K. (1989). The context of optimal experience: An exploratory model of the family. *New Ideas in Psychology, 7*(1), 91–97.

Reser, J. P., & Scherl, L. M. (1988). Clear and unambiguous feedback: A transactional and motivational analysis of environmental challenge and self-encounter. *Journal of Environmental Psychology, 8*(4), 269–286.

Ryan, R. M. (1982). Control and information in the intrapersonal sphere: An extension of cognitive evaluation theory. *Journal of Personality and Social Psychology, 43,* 450–461.

Sansone, C., & Harackiewicz, J. M. (1996). "I don't feel like it": The function of interest in self-regulation. In L. L. Martin & A. Tesser (Eds.), *Striving and feeling: Interactions among goals, affect, and self-regulation* (pp. 203–228). Mahwah, NJ: Erlbaum.

Sansone, C., Sachau, D. A., & Weir, C. (1989). Effects of instruction on intrinsic interest: The importance of context. *Journal of Personality and Social Psychology, 57*(5), 819–829.

Sawyer, K. (1992). Improvisational creativity: An analysis of jazz performance. *Creativity Research Journal, 5*(3), 253–263.

Schmidt, J. A. (1999). Overcoming challenges: Exploring the role of action, experience, and opportunity in fostering resilience among adolescents. *Dissertation Abstracts International: Section B: Sciences and Engineering, 59*(11-B), 6095.

Schmuck, P., & Sheldon, K. M. (Eds.). (2001). *Life goals and well-being: Towards a positive psychology of human striving.* Seattle: Hogrefe & Huber.

Schwartz, B. (2000). Self-determination: The tyranny of freedom. *American Psychologist, 55*(1), 79–88.

Stein, G. L., Kimiecik, J. C., Daniels, J., & Jackson, S. A. (1995). Psychological antecedents of flow in recreational sport. *Personality and Social Psychology Bulletin, 21*(2), 125–135.

Tellegen, A., & Atkinson, G. (1974). Openness to absorbing and self-altering experiences ("absorption"), a trait related to hypnotic susceptibility. *Journal of Abnormal Psychology, 83*(3), 268–277.

Tellegen, A., Watson, D., & Clark, L. A. (1999). On the dimensional and hierarchical structure of affect. *Psychological Science, 10,* 297–303.

Vallerand, R. J., & Reid, G. (1984). On the causal effects of perceived competence on intrinsic motivation: A test of cognitive evaluation theory. *Journal of Sport Psychology, 6*(1), 94–102.

Vygotsky, L. (1978). *Mind in society.* Cambridge, MA: Harvard University Press.

Weber, M. J. (1930). *The Protestant ethic and the spirit of capitalism.* New York: Scribner.

White, R. (1959). Motivation reconsidered: The concept of competence. *Psychological Review, 66,* 297–333.

Wild, T. C., Kuiken, D., & Schopflocher, D. (1995). The role of absorption in experiential involvement. *Journal of Personality and Social Psychology, 69*(3), 569–579.

Wong, M. (2000). The relations among causality orientations, academic experience, academic performance, and academic commitment. *Personality and Social Psychology Bulletin, 26*(3), 315–326.

Wong, M., & Csikszentmihalyi, M. (1991). Motivation and academic achievement: The effects of personality traits and the quality of experience. *Journal of Personality, 59*(3), 539–574.

CHAPTER 33

℘

Motivation, Competence, and Creativity

MARK A. RUNCO

Creative potential is one of the most important forms of human capital. The benefits for both individuals and societies are easy to see. It contributes to advances in science and technology, for instance, and provides us with many kinds of pleasure and satisfaction (e.g., the arts and entertainment). *Creativity* is, however, a slippery concept. It takes different forms in different domains, for example, and at different points in the lifespan. It appears that different paths can each lead to creative work; none of them is always necessary or always guarantees creative results. Those studying creativity capture these variations by defining creativity as a "complex" or syndrome (MacKinnon, 1965; Mumford & Gustafson, 1988; Runco & Albert, 1990). But briefly, creativity is a blend of cognitive, metacognitive, emotional, and motivational components.

Motivation is recognized in virtually all contemporary definitions of creativity. In fact, it has long been recognized: Galton (1869) emphasized the incredible persistence of the geniuses he studied, as did Cox (1926). Creativity does differ in some ways

in the arts and sciences, and in various other domains, but motivation is a factor in each. Creative potential is not be fulfilled unless the individual (and his or her social support) is motivated to do so, and creative solutions are not found unless the individual is motivated to apply his or her skills.

This chapter explores the role of motivation in creative efforts. This is in some ways not only a review of the literature on motivation and creativity but also an examination of how competence can play a role in creative work, and how creative competence may differ from the motivations that characterize most other human behaviors. Many human behaviors—and especially those of older and mature individuals—are directed toward the conservation of resources (e.g., energy) and, thus, toward efficiency. We develop routines, for example, to make our lives easier. Creative behavior is typically very different. Frequently, creative inventions make our lives easier, but the discovery of the necessary technologies may require a huge amount of effort and avoidance of routine. Creative behavior is not necessarily efficient behavior, nor is it even always adaptive (Richards, 1990; Runco, 1994a), and the motivations to act in a creative fashion or develop competencies for creative work are similarly unique.

WHAT MOTIVATES THE CREATIVE PERSON?

What motivates the creative person? Certainly it depends to some extent on the person, the context, and the domain in which the person is interested and perhaps working. There is some evidence that extrinsic incentives can influence creative work. That influence can work both ways, sometimes encouraging creative efforts, and sometimes undermining them. Useful research on extrinsic factors is summarized in the next section of this chapter. After that, the research on intrinsic motives is reviewed, along with the theories that take both intrinsic and extrinsic factors into account. Throughout the discussion, connections to the achievement motivation and competence are explored.

EXTRINSIC INCENTIVES AND REWARDS

Operant theorists have addressed the question of motivation and creativity, and they emphasize extrinsic and environmental factors. They also insist on operationalizing the terms such that everything is overt and highly objective. Creativity per se is not the typical target here, for it is not entirely objective, so the focus is usually on related behaviors, such as novelty or variation, or perhaps insight (Epstein, 1990; Skinner, 1939). Each of these is indeed clearly related to originality and creativity, so the results are interesting and pertinent. The emphasis is on the environment; it is the environment that motivates (or at least elicits and controls) creative behavior.

It may be difficult to see how creative and original things can be controlled, in part because the target behavior must change. After all, if one specific behavior is targeted, it will not be original for very long! It will only be original the first time it is displayed. For this reason, these efforts use shaping and contingencies and target behavioral *variation*

(Ryan & Winston, 1978; Stokes, in press; Stokes & Balsam, in press). The organism is thus reinforced only when it emits a behavior that has not been displayed previously. The organisms in this research are not always humans. Pryor, Hoag, and O'Reilly (1969), for example, reinforced the leaping and swimming of porpoises. They targeted responses that were novel for any one particular training session. Findings indicated that the porpoises emitted novel behaviors in each new session, and did so earlier and earlier in the session. Goetz and Baer (1973; Holman, Goetz, & Baer, 1977) used analogous procedures with children. The work of Holman et al. (1977) demonstrated that novel behaviors can not only be controlled with extrinsic consequences but also that they generalize across tasks.

Epstein (1990) held a similar perspective but was interested in new insights rather than continued variation. Seemingly creative solutions to problems are often labeled "insightful," the idea being that trial and error was not used, and that the individual seemed to have jumped all at once to a solution—the "Aha!" or insight (Gruber, 1981). Epstein (1990) demonstrated that insightful problem solving can be shaped. The shaping focuses on specific and discrete behaviors, and when the organism is placed in the problem situation, it tends to "integrate spontaneously" the previously learned discrete behaviors, the result being a new composite that may appear to be insightful.

In this line of work, the behavior is emitted in order to (1) earn a reinforcer or to (2) avoid a punisher. The implication is that some behaviors, including insightful and creative, may be efforts to approach a goal or reinforcer, and some may be efforts to avoid an aversive situation or punisher (Elliot, 1997). I have more to say later about the distinction between approach and avoidance behaviors. First it is useful to consider the psychoeconomic theory of creativity and motivation, because it in some ways parallels the operant view.

Rubenson and Runco (1992, 1995) relied on the concept of investments in their explanation of why creative persons work to develop competencies. Many creative persons invest heavily in their creative potentials and competencies, with some investing in traditional competencies, and others investing in competencies that no one else will notice or appreciate. If creative talent is defined such that it depends on original contributions to a field, then it is likely that traditional competencies have been developed, perhaps in addition to creative competencies. This applies to some fields—especially the highly technical ones—more than others. It explains why we do not see prodigies in some fields, such as physics, but we do see them regularly in others (e.g., music). If traditional competencies must be mastered before high-level performance is possible, and if the field has a large amount of material to be mastered, it is impossible for there to be prodigies. Time is necessary to develop the relevant competencies, and after that time has been invested, the individual is no longer a child (thus, not a prodigy).

Investments in traditional competencies can facilitate creative work. Most eminent creators have invested huge amounts of time and energy in their fields, and as a result, are able to see where gaps exist and to know a good problem or creative solution when they see one. Hayes (1978) went so far as to estimate that 10,000 hours must be invested to develop *expertise* (also see Simon & Chase, 1973). The 10,000-hour estimate may not apply to all domains, however; in fact, it certainly is a generalization. Importantly, expertise does not guarantee creative performance, and sometimes experts actually become rigid and inflexible, thus losing the capacity for creativity. They are competent in a traditional fashion but not in a creative fashion. Such is the cost of expertise. (A parallel with the operant view is apparent: Behavior in the psychoeconomic perspective responds to costs and benefits; much operant behavior responds to reinforcers and punishers.)

Significantly, the more the individual has invested, the more he or she has to lose. If an individual invests a dollar in something, and then loses it, it may not seem very tragic. If, on the other hand, a million dollars is invested instead of one dollar, the individual will certainly feel more strongly about the investment. A loss would be much more costly. Similarly, if an individual invests a few hours in developing a competence but that competence becomes obsolete, not much will have been lost. But when one's entire career is devoted to (invested in) some specific expertise or field, losses are extremely costly, and strong resistance to criticisms of that field or competence are likely. This would apply to the scientist who devotes (invests) all of his or her career into one topic. If people criticize it after the scientist has invested 30 years, the scientist is likely to resist suggestions of an alternative perspective. This is very relevant, because resistance implies a lack of flexibility, and flexibility is characteristic of creative work (Hofstadter, 1986; Runco, 1995). Many individuals do indeed become more rigid and less flexible as they get older (Chown, 1961).

The most interesting implication of this psychoeconomic theory is that individuals who have invested greatly in one style or perspective (e.g., a scientist who has spent years developing one theory or model) will be motivated to justify its usage. If his or her pet model were replaced, the scientist's investment (temporal and psychical) would depreciate. Note that it is essentially linear: the greater the investment, the higher the motivation to avoid depreciation. Experts would thus be highly motivated in a particular fashion, as would anyone who has devoted years to a topic or model or perspective. Note also that this prediction about experts' motives is not necessarily consistent with the idea of competence. The expert may reject new data or opportunities, or anything that is contrary to his or her investment, even if objectively they seem to lead in a useful direction.

The inflexibility of some older adults makes it very difficult for them perform in a creative manner. Not all older adults become rigid, however. As a matter of fact, many famous creative individuals have demonstrated outstanding flexibility late in life. The "old-age style" of certain famous painters, for example, involves flexibility, in that the painter changes his or her painting technique, often repeatedly. As a result, there are dramatic changes in the work, and often renewed creativity. Very likely these changes reflect a change not only in perspective but also in competence. New competencies are no doubt required each time the painter changes his or her technique.

CREATIVE WORK
AND PERSONAL STANDARDS

It is critical to distinguish between personal and traditional competencies, or between competencies that reflect personal versus social standards. As Elliot (1999) wrote:

> Competence must be evaluated according to a standard, and three primary standards may be identified: an absolute standard inherent in a task, skill, or characteristic; an intrapersonal standard implicating a pattern observed in the past or that could be observed in the future; and an interpersonal standard implicating normative comparison. (p. 183)

Sometimes a conflict in standards occurs. Apparently the standards encouraged in the school, for instance, conflict with those (intrapersonal standards) held by the student. Creative children do not share many traits with what teachers tend to consider "the ideal student" (Raina & Raina, 1971; Torrance, 1963). The conflict may be between the standards encouraged in the home and those required in the schools (Roe, 1963). Sadly, traditional education does often encourage noncreative competencies. Rubenson and Runco (1995) explained this in terms of the different manifest benefits of the different competencies. Suppose an employer interviews someone who has a Master's degree in the most relevant field. That employer will have a pretty good idea about what that job applicant knows and can do. There would be a fairly certain "return" if that applicant were hired. What if the applicant had invested the same amount of time as that required for a Master's degree in the study and practice of creative skills? In many fields, creativity is appreciated, but the return on the investment is much less certain. The interviewer may not be willing to take a risk on this applicant, and the risk would be greater. It is not unlike the risks that characterize "guaranteed interest" stocks versus, say, "aggressive stocks." This difference can in turn influence what decisions will be made by applicants and students. They know there is a likely payoff if they stay in school. They do not know what the payoff will be if they invest instead in any sort of creativity development program. Rubenson and Runco (1995) concluded that the United

States is very likely underinvesting in the creative competencies of its students.

INTRINSIC MOTIVATION
FOR CREATIVE EFFORT

Most theories of creativity emphasize intrinsic rather than extrinsic motivation. This in part reflects a tendency in the creativity literature to focus on the individual. The preponderance of theories of creativity assumes that creativity is a result of individual effort. There are theories that also acknowledge, or even emphasize, social and historical context (e.g., Amabile, 1990; Csikszentmihalyi, 1990; Montuori & Purser, 1999; Simonton, 1984), and in fact this may be a trend in the creativity literature toward social and contextual theories. But for most of its history as a scientific field, the focus in creativity literature has been on the individual.

The more precise focus is usually personality. Barron (1972, 1995) and MacKinnon (1960/1983, 1970), for instance, administered a number of personality (and intelligence) tests to several different samples of creative individuals (including writers and architects); they identified intrinsic motivation as what is now often called a "core characteristic" of creative people. Not long ago Dudek and Hall (1991) reported results from a longitudinal study involving many of the same research participants who had been involved 40 years earlier. Dudek and Hall used the Adjective Checklist and also found that intrinsic motivation characterizes the more creative individuals.

Amabile and her colleagues (1990; Amabile, Goldfarb, & Brackfield, 1990; Hennessey, 1969) examined the relationship between intrinsic motivation and creativity using more experimental procedures and looking more at actual performance rather than at personality traits. They reported both (1) value in allowing individuals to rely on intrinsic motivation and (2) an inhibitive effect of extrinsic rewards. The inhibitive factors included evaluations by others and expected evaluations by others. They took the next logical step and identified the means to "immunize" individuals to the "deleterious effect of extrinsic incentives." Obviously, this line of research is of huge practical value.

Amabile (1990) defined "intrinsic motivation" as "the motivation to do an activity for its own sake, because it was intrinsically interesting, enjoyable, or satisfying. In contrast "extrinsic motivation" was defined as "the motivation to do an activity primarily to achieve some extrinsic goal, such as a reward" (p. 62). Intrinsic motivation comes from within the individual; extrinsic motivation is imposed or offered by the environment. The latter may include rewards, reinforcers, punishers, incentives, feedback, and so on.

In Amabile's (1990) words,

> Intrinsic motivation is conducive to creativity, but extrinsic motivation is detrimental. In other words people will be most creative when they feel motivated primarily by the interest, enjoyment, satisfaction, and challenge of the work itself—and not by external pressures. (p. 67)

Amabile supported this conclusion in various ways, including examination of biographies, autobiographies, interviews, journals, and personal letters (e.g., Gertrude Stein, Isaac Asimov, John Irving, Albert Einstein, James Watson, Mozart, Pablo Casals, Ansel Adams, Margaret Mead, Woody Allen, Anne Sexton, Sylvia Plath, D. H. Lawrence, Joyce Carol Oates, and Thomas Wolfe). Her experimental evidence was most impressive. Here, she cited earlier research on "overjustification." Overjustification occurs when individuals who are initially intrinsically motivated lose that intrinsic interest when given an extrinsic reason for behaving in a particular fashion or performing in a particular way. It is as though the individuals stop attributing interest to the task and start attributing their activity to the incentives and the rewards. Again, by way of a conclusion, Amabile felt that her research as a whole supported the following conclusions: Expected evaluation is detrimental to creativity; actual evaluation is detrimental to creativity; surveillance is detrimental to creativity; reward, or what she called "contracted for" reward, is detrimental to creativity; bonus rewards, which are not contracted for, have a positive influence on creativity; competition has a detrimental effect on creativity; and a restricted choice, particularly about how to proceed with an activity, has a detrimental affect on creativity. Notice that these factors are social in nature. Amabile's work has a connection to and clear implications for a social psychology of creativity.

In one early study, Amabile (1990) presented research participants with a questionnaire that led half of the sample to think about the intrinsic reasons for a particular task. The other half of the sample received a questionnaire that led them to think of the extrinsic reasons. The questionnaire was used for a kind of priming. Participants each had experience and interest in creative writing. Most of them were graduate and undergraduate students in the Boston area. Apparently none were professional writers, or at least the self-reported amount of time spent each week writing only ranged from 3 to 18 hours. This is an important point, because the biographical evidence for intrinsic motivation, mentioned briefly earlier, dealt with well-known and professional individuals. The evidence would add to the credibility and validity of the intrinsic motivation principle if it were also found to characterize the creativity of noneminent and nonprofessional individuals. Participants who received the questionnaire that emphasized intrinsic interest were later asked to write a haiku-style poem. The poems were subsequently judged, using a consensual assessment technique, to be much more creative than those written by a control group. (The control group had not received a questionnaire; they had simply written the haiku.) This difference apparently was not statistically significant. The dramatic finding was between the experimental group, who had received the intrinsic interest questionnaire, and the participants who had received the questionnaire that emphasized extrinsic motives and goals, including selling their work, making money, and public recognition. The haikus of this group were significantly less creative than those of the experimental or control group. In addition to demonstrating that intrinsic motivation is important for nonprofessionals, this study is noteworthy in that the manipulation is quite simple. Apparently, the questionnaire, though quite brief, was sufficient to change the quality of the subjects' haikus.

Amabile (1990) suggested that the value of intrinsic motivation depends on the task at hand. Consider her distinction between algorithmic and heuristic tasks. Algorithmic tasks have clear solution procedures (the algorithms), which, if used, always lead to a correct solution. Heuristic tasks allow exploration. Sometimes that exploration does not lead to the correct solution. Because there is opportunity for individual input, exploration, and creativity in a heuristic task, intrinsic motivation plays a larger role than it does in algorithmic tasks.

Amabile (1990) also cited Csikszentmihalyi's (1975) work on enjoyment as influencing her thinking about creativity and intrinsic motivation. Csikszentmihalyi also found that individuals became highly involved in creative tasks. He described the experience of flow as a kind of peak involvement. When experiencing flow, an individual would not be thinking about rewards, objectives, or anything extrinsic. It is a very intrinsically meaningful experience. Individuals can experience flow in a variety of settings, although some—rock climbing for example—are more conducive to flow than others. These ideas about flow are entirely consistent with other reports of the psychic underpinnings of creative moments (e.g., Hoppe & Kyle, 1991), though flow is a description of peak experiences and not necessarily tied to creativity.

Still, data from both personality and laboratory experimental research support the importance of intrinsic motivation in the creative process. There is also a cogent logic behind this perspective. It is easy to see how creativity, by its very nature, would depend on intrinsic motivation, and how it can be adversely influenced by extrinsic factors. Put briefly, creativity depends on originality. Creative behaviors and products are always original; originality is necessary but not sufficient. It is not sufficient because sometimes original endeavors are bizarre, inappropriate, and do not solve the problem at hand (if the creative work is an attempt to solve a problem). Sometimes endeavors are original precisely because they are inappropriate! Creative behaviors and products (including works of art, publications, performances, or simply ideas) are both original and useful. They fit, sometimes in the sense of solving a problem, but other times in the sense of their aesthetic appeal.

Originality is the key here, because it is the only aspect of creativity on which every-one agrees. It also ties creativity to intrinsic motivation, that is because original things are different, unique, unusual, or novel. And being unique, unusual, or novel in turn assumes that the individual is capable, or even interested in, being unconventional. As a matter of fact, creative persons are often described as unconventional (Runco, 1993a), oppositional (Ludwig, 1995), nonconforming (Crutchfield, 1962), eccentric (Weeks & James, 1995), or contrarian (Runco, 1993a). Each of these suggests an independence of thought and motivation.

Creative individuals do seem to be highly motivated, and some are interested in some sorts of extrinsic goals. Moreover, creative persons do sometimes achieve great things, and achievement can be a powerful goal and influence motivation. Yet the term "achievement motivation" is not very often found in the creativity literature. This may reflect the typical conception of "achievement" as tied to public recognition (or at least recognition in some overt way). Achievement motivation defined in that fashion has not contributed much to the understanding of creative efforts, which tend to be *intrinsically motivated* instead (Amabile, 1990; MacKinnon, 1970; Runco, 1994a). The creative individual very likely is motivated more by intrapersonal standards than by social achievement. Creative persons are notorious for ignoring the social implications of their actions or work; many of them are rebellious, nonconforming, eccentric, contrarian, or at least unconventional. Some blatantly ignore acclaim, success, or any sort of objective or public result. There is not much on creativity and achievement motivation in the research literature; but a great deal can be found if "achievement" is defined in intrapersonal terms. Achievement implies the attainment of some goal or goals, but those goals may be intrinsic rather than extrinsic. Similarly, achievement may be gauged against certain standards, but these may be personal rather than social standards.

This is actually quite consistent with current views of competence and motivation. Elliot and McGregor (2001), for example, raised the possibility that achievement motivation can sometimes be best understood in terms of task-based intrapersonal and intrapersonal goals. This definitely applies to creativity. Elliot and McGregor (2001) further distinguished between task-based/ "self-defining" intrapersonal accomplishment and normative accomplishment. This helps bring creativity under the umbrella of behaviors that might be tied to certain achievement motivations. The research on creativity indicates that we must allow for self-defined goals. Creative work is rarely directed to normative accomplishments.

At least one empirical study of creative talent distinguished between social and individual achievement motivation. Albert and Runco (in press) studied exceptionally gifted boys and their parents. One of the ways that the participants in this research—both the boys and the parents—differed from norms was in "achievement through independence." Actually, the boys and their parents had much higher scores than are usual on the "achievement through independence" scale of the California Psychological Inventory (CPI), and they had significantly lower scores than the normative groups in terms of "achievement though conformity." This fits extremely well with the creativity literature, for creative persons are usually independent. It is difficult to be creative without being independent, because creativity requires originality, and originality can be found through independent thoughts and actions. Originality cannot be found through conformity. As a matter of fact, originality is just about the opposite of the normative. This research demonstrates that we can identify the motivational characteristics of talented persons, but we should focus on the kind of motivation that is required for creative behavior. At the very least, we need to distinguish between achievement through independence and achievement through conformity. Additional support for this was given by Gough and Bradley (1999), who found that achievement through independence scores correlated with Barron Welsh Art Scale scores.

DOMAINS OF PERFORMANCE

Here, I must revisit the concept of domains. Differences among domains have been recognized in the creativity literature for as long as it has existed. Patrick (1935, 1937), for example, studied poets, and earlier in this chapter, Barron (1972, 1995), Mac-

Kinnon (1960/1983, 1970), and the research with writers and architects were each cited. More recently Albert (1980) and Runco (1987) identified domain differences among gifted children, and, at this point, researchers are looking not only at general domains but also subdomains (e.g., writers of fiction vs. journalists, composers vs. performers). There is a minor controversy about domains (Baer, 1991; Plucker, 2000), with some believing that there is a general capacity that applies to all expressions of creativity, across all domains, and others (the majority) believing that creative skills vary from one domain to the next.

Elliot and Dweck (Chapter 1, this volume, p. 4) addressed the domain issue when they described how

> most research in the achievement motivation literature has emerged from Western, individualistic societies. . . . As a result, more often than not, research in the achievement motivation literature has focused on individual, self-defining, normative accomplishment in the domains of school, sports, and work.

Creativity often occurs outside of the prototypical domains. The achievement motivation of a creative person, then, may be directed at goals in some marginal domain, or in some domain that is not popular or conventional.

This makes it difficult to judge competence. Similarly, it may be a competence that has value only to the individual. Others may see neither the value nor the creativity. Creativity is frequently difficult to judge, and errors in judgment abound (Runco, 1999a). Decca Records apparently refused to sign the Beatles in 1963; Capitol Records did the same in 1964. Alfred Harcourt, of Harcourt Brace Jovanavich, told the publisher of *The Sound and the Fury* that he was "the only damn fool in New York that would publish it" (Cerf & Navasky, 1984, p. 160). The author, William Faulker, won a Nobel Prize for literature in 1949. Jan Lievens and Adrien va der Werff were much more respected than Rembrandt in their era. Picasso's painting was described in 1907 as "the work of a madman" by Vollard, a highly reputable art dealer. The list of misjudgments is extensive (see Runco, 1999a) and it has even been said that truly creative things, be they works of music, the visual arts, or science, can never be recognized at first. They are creative, and thus original and difficult to judge. There are no standards if something is new.

Again, quoting Elliot and Dweck (2004):

> Competence is a flexible construct that may be conceptualized at different levels (e.g., specific outcomes, patterns of skills or abilities), using different standards (intrapersonal, interpersonal), with different loci (individual, collective), and in relation to different domains (e.g., academic, athletic).

This works well for creativity, with the recognition of the intrapersonal and individual standards and loci, and the allowance for domain differences. Creative people, for example, sometimes focus on one topic or technique, producing a series of very similar works. These works may even appear to be identical to observers, the revisions are so subtle. Gruber (1988) referred to this as "deviation amplification" and described the benefits to the creative person. The point is that a creative individual could spend years refining his or her ability at capturing "reflections on a pond" in watercolor—and only feel competent once that particular skill was perfected (to his or her own liking). In summary, the skill in question, or the topic and project in question, or even the domain that determines the creative person's sense of competence may not be appreciated by anyone else, at least at first.

PRODUCT VERSUS PROCESS

This description of the intrapersonal nature of competence is consistent with existing assumptions in the field of creative studies. If the last phrase in the previous section, "at least at first," were omitted, on the other hand, the description would be very controversial. Studies of creativity have become extremely objective and product-oriented, and the more rigorous theories do not label personal efforts "creative." They reserve that for actual products that have impressed some qualified audience.

There are problems with this product-oriented perspective, and implications for theories of creative motivation. Process-oriented perspectives of creativity and the recent theory of "personal creativity" are much more amenable to the view of achievement motivation, which allows individualistic goals.

The most influential theory of the creative process is an old one. In this theory, the creative process begins with a *preparation* stage, then moves to *incubation*, *illumination*, and *verification* stages. Although quite old by the standards of behavioral science, this theory has been supported and is still very widely used (see Runco, 1994b). It does not, however, include any extracognitive influences on creative work. Runco and Chand (1995) presented a somewhat different theory of the creative process that does include motivational influences. This has been called a "componential model," of which there are several in the creativity literature (Amabile, 1990; Chand & Runco, 1992; Runco & Chand, 1995; Sternberg, 2000). Runco and Chand (1995), for example, outlined what they call a two-tiered model. On the first tier are three primary components involved in the creative process. The first of these involves what is commonly called "problem finding," which is a general label for several subprocesses. Of particular importance are problem identification and problem definition. Problem *identification* is involved when an individual simply recognizes that there is a challenge, hurdle, or problem at hand. Problem *definition* occurs later and involves actually changing or altering the problem to make it workable. It is often obvious when someone has a problem, but the problem is not in a form that allows solution. That is where problem definition (and redefinition) comes in.

These skills—problem identification and problem definition—could easily interact with various kinds of motivation. A problem might motivate an individual, or an individual might be disturbed, even in an ambiguous "free floating" fashion, and be motivated to identify exactly what the problem is or be motivated to define the problem in such a way as to facilitate its solution. This is the most important aspect of problem finding: It sets the stage for problem solving. It has been said a number of times that a high-quality and creative solution depends upon a high-quality problem. Empirical demonstrations of the distinctiveness of problem finding from problem solving and individual differences in problem finding were summarized by Runco (1994b).

The second primary component in the two-tiered model involves ideation. Here again, it is important to subdivide: Ideation can vary in terms of fluency, originality, flexibility, and apparently in several other ways as well (Runco 1991, 2003). Fluency, originality, and flexibility are the most commonly used indices of ideation. "Fluency" is defined in terms of productivity; high ideational fluency indicates that the individual generates many ideas. These ideas frequently represent the options and alternatives that are involved in problem solving. The ideas may represent alternative definitions of the problem, for example, or they may represent possible solutions. "Originality" is operationally defined in terms of the unusualness or uniqueness of ideas. Here, again, there are clear individual differences, and, of course, ideational originality would be the part of this model that is most directly related to creativity per se. This is because originality is a prerequisite for creativity. Creative things are often much more than original; they tend to be somehow fitting or aesthetically appealing; but originality is necessary for creativity even if it is not sufficient in and of itself. Motivation is necessary in that only a motivated individual will persist with a problem or problem-solving efforts. This is sometimes vital, especially when the problem solving efforts are *protracted* and extend over a long period of time (Gruber, 1988).

As noted earlier in this chapter, originality is necessary but not sufficient for creativity. This is because original ideas may not be creative. They may be bizarre and irrelevant to the task at hand. In this case they are original, yet are not solutions, and they will certainly lack aesthetic appeal. What else is necessary for creativity besides originality? Again, aesthetic appeal and some sort of fit and appropriateness help, but this just begs the question. Where and why does an individual invest the effort in finding ideas and solutions that are both original and fitting? One answer to this question is given in the two-tiered componential model, and, in particular, in the third primary component. It involves a kind of judgment, evaluation, or appraisal. It is this skill that works with ide-

ation to ensure that ideas are both original and fitting. This skill can be expressed in several ways, so it is not really one skill, but, again, that was true of problem finding and ideation, and would be no surprise here. One relevant kind of judgment involves evaluation and is probably closest to traditional forms of critical thinking. But too often this kind of judgment leads an individual to unoriginal ideas. The critical thinking is directed at criticism per se, and the focus is on what is wrong with an idea and how it is inadequate as a solution to a given problem. Creative thinking sometimes requires valuation rather than evaluation. This is because original ideas are appreciated. But because they are original, they may be surprising, or their adequacy and fit may be initially difficult to determine. The easy judgment would be to conclude that the ideas are inappropriate, but with persistent valuation, an individual may determine that the ideas are useful, or at least have potential. If they have potential, the individual might persist with the individual ideational path and eventually find highly creative ideas. Note again that all of this assumes that the individual is motivated to persist. Research suggests that the judgmental and valuative processes involved in creative thinking are distinct from traditional forms of critical thinking, as well as from IQ and similar measures of traditional intelligence (Runco & Smith, 1992). This same research demonstrates clearly that IQ and traditional intelligence are by no means synonymous with creative thinking skills (Runco & Albert, 1986).

The two-tiered componential model of the creative process posits motivation as an influence on creative thinking and problems solving. Both intrinsic and extrinsic motivation are included. The other secondary component in this model is knowledge. Knowledge can be declarative, which is conceptual and factual, or it can be procedural, which is strategic and tactical. Knowledge, of course, interacts with each of the other components. When generating ideas, for example, an individual often draw from long-term memory and his or her knowledge base, although the ideas may be generated though associative processes as well. Knowledge interacts with motivation in several ways. Motivated individuals may be interested in learning new procedures, as well as new factual information, especially if they realize that they need to be better informed in order to solve a problem. The interaction works the other way as well: An individual's work may lead to the recognition that there is some sort of deficiency or gap, and this gap in turn motivates the person to learn something new or think creatively.

PERSONAL CREATIVITY AND INTENTIONS

A second process view suggests an even closer relationship between achievement motivation and creativity. This is the recent theory of "personal creativity." Like componential theory, extracognitive influences are recognized. More specifically, the theory of personal creativity emphasizes the *intentions* of the creative person. Intentions represent one of the three parts of personal creativity, the other two being transformational capacity and discretion.

Transformations are key in the sense that objective experience is interpreted by the individual, and, as is the case with all interpretations, there is a difference between subjective and objective experience. Objective experience is assimilated, or transformed, into something that is meaningful to the individual, which is why two individuals may have entirely different interpretations of one shared (objective) experience. Motivation may actually result from this process. This does represent yet another controversy: It is possible that understanding of experience is developed only if the individual is motivated to attend to details and assimilate the relevant information, but it is also possible that motivation is a result of a cognitive "appraisal" (Lazarus, 1991a, 1991b; Runco, 1994a; Zajonc, 1990). The controversy, then, is over which comes first, motivation or cognition (understanding). Piaget (1970, 1976) offered a very reasonable perspective and concluded that individuals are intrinsically motivated by the need to understand their experience. In other words, when we have an experience we do not understand, we are motivated to do something about it, and we often put effort into formulating a new interpretation or reinterpreting the experience, until we understand. Note that this occurs on a personal, individual basis. It is,

then, intrinsic motivation. This is a critical point, because it means that the theory that uses transformation and interpretation is consistent with the various, numerous empirical demonstrations of the role of intrinsic motivation in creative work (Amabile, 1990; Barron, 1972, 1995; Runco, 1993b, 1994a).

Personal creativity also emphasizes intentions. The definition of "intention" assumed here is exactly the same as is implied by the expression, "I intend to mow the lawn." It is intentions that distinguish between creative accomplishments that are original and original things that are not creative. Originality is necessary but not sufficient for creativity, and sometimes things are original but lacking, unappealing, and uncreative. Psychotic individuals can be highly original, but they are rarely, if ever, truly creative in the sense of producing worthwhile ideas (Eysenck, 1999). Their originality is unintentional. The view that intentions play a role in creative work is also compatible with the corpus of research showing that creative individuals are highly strategic and tactical (Root-Bernstein, 1988; Runco, 1999b). The individual will not employ some tactic unless he or she is trying to (i.e., intending to) accomplish something. Tactics are by definition intentional.

Not everyone agrees that intentions are important. Hofstadter (1986), for example, argued that creators can "exploit serendipity," but that most of the action is beyond control. In this view, intentions do not account for much. All an individual can do is "playfully explore a serendipitious connection" (p. 252). The connections themselves are out of the individual's control. Díaz de Chumaceiro (in press) has also described serendipity as a part of creative work. Intentions are also inconsistent with theories of creativity that emphasize the workings of the unconscious and the impact of psychic tension, conflict, trauma, or discontent (reviewed by Runco, 1994a, 1999c). This takes us to the role of psychological need.

CREATIVITY AND PSYCHOLOGICAL NEED

The theory of personal creativity just outlined assumes that we are intrinsically motivated to understand our experience. We construct interpretations of our experiences, and sometimes these may lead to creative solutions and insights. And, again, we put the effort into constructing interpretations, because it is adaptive to do so. Piaget (1970, 1976) suggested that understanding is a universal need. There may also be a psychological need to create, to behave in an autonomous and original fashion, and to express oneself. Indeed, Maslow (1971) and Rogers (1961) both reported that self-actualized individuals are creative, as well as spontaneous and self-accepting. In fact, toward the end of their careers, they both gave up trying to separate self-actualization from creativity. Maslow concluded that the two might be "inextricable." Runco, Ebersole, and Mraz (1991) reported correlational support for this view to complement the observational and clinical observations of Rogers and Maslow.

Creative self-expression is also strongly related to physical health. Pennebaker, Kiecolt-Glaser, and Glaser (1997), for instance, found that the immune efficiency of student who were required to write several times each week (as part of a college course), and asked to write about their own lives, improved significantly (also see Eisenman, 1997). Members of a control group was also allowed to write, but they were given mundane assignments that precluded self-expression, or what Pennebaker et al. (1997) called "disclosure." The immune efficiency of the control group did not improve.

There are, then, data that show that creative persons are healthy, both psychologically and physically. There are also data that suggest that creative persons have a tendency toward affective disorder and even suicide (Andreasen, 1997; Jamison, 1997). Perhaps there is one causal pathway leading from ill-health to creativity, and a second pathway leading from creativity to health. The former apparently can occur when there is excessive openness to preconscious material that frightens or depresses the person but at the same time provides him or her with original insights (Rothenberg, 1990). The latter may occur when creative insights and projects result from self-expression, and such self-expression provides the vent or catharsis that maintains health (Pennebaker et al., 1997). If it is cathartic, the motivation may be a result of trauma experienced early

in life. Csikszentmihalyi (1988) described this as "cathartic originality." He also described "abreactive creativity," which is the result of traumatic experiences from childhood. It can thus be difficult to ascertain what actually motivates creative work, because the result may be symbolic and temporally far removed from the cause. Even artists who are experiencing this abreactive creativity may themselves be uncertain of their motives (Jones, Runco, Dorinan, & Freeland, 1997). The creative person may appear to be motivated by competence per se, but may actually be motivated to develop that competence in order to deal effectively with the trauma. Competence in this light is not an end in and of itself, but is instead a means to an ends.

The kind of creativity that is self-expressive is functionally tied to both psychological and physical health (Pennebaker et al., 1997; Runco et al., 1991). Perhaps there is a need for creative expression that represents a basic human need, and when this need is unfulfilled, problems of various sorts (e.g., health) may result. That need for expression can lead to competence, but it is not a need for competence; it may instead be a need for expression. This is not too far from what Maslow (1971) and Rogers (1961) said about human need, self-actualization, and creativity.

CONCLUSIONS

Elliot and Dweck (Chapter 1, this volume, p. 6) proposed that "the need for competence . . . [is] a fundamental motivation [in all individuals] that serves the evolutionary role of helping people develop and adapt to their environment." I would add that adaptations and meaningful evolution will be especially likely if it is motivation specifically for creativity. Creativity provides the variations that are necessary for cultural evolution (Campbell, 1960; Simonton, 1988; Runco, in press). The motivation specifically for creativity may be among the most useful for humans, at least in terms of evolution, progress, and adaptability.[1]

I have also suggested that the "motivation specifically for creativity" is indeed specific. It probably differs from "achievement through conformance," for example, and from similar motives that are directed toward socially acknowledged accomplishment. Along the same lines, there seem to be different motives that can each lead to creative effort. Creativity may be tied to the motivation to express oneself, to maintain or improve health, to construct meaningful interpretations of experience, or to retain a sense of autonomy and rely on one's own (intrinsic) standards and goals.

When the focus is on creative *accomplishment* (and not just creative effort), there may be a need to recognize motivation independent of competence—or at least as an antecedent to competence. Admittedly, models such as the two-tiered componential one (Chand & Runco, 1992) suggest that the greatest benefit results when the person is both motivated and competent. There is also the possibility that competence is so highly developed that it takes the form of an expertise that can inhibit the individual (Rubenson & Runco, 1995). Earlier, I described this as rigidity or inflexibility of thought. Still, many creative achievements do require competence and skill. Motivation may be an antecedent of this, though, of course, it can sometimes take time for the skill to develop. The Wright brothers, just to name one example, were highly motivated to fly but did not succeed until their persistence paid dividends in the form of technical skill and competence.

Great care should be taken if parents, educators, or organizational specialists attempt to manipulate the goals and incentives that motivate children's creative efforts. Recall that incentives and other extrinsic contingencies may actually undermine the autonomous thinking that is a part of the creative process. Additionally, goals are as difficult as problems to operationalize. Consider the issues surrounding the definitions of "problem." Many creative insights are the result of a problem-solving effort (Mumford, Baughman, & Sager, 2003; Runco, 1994b), and some people view creativity as one kind of problem solving. The assumption is that all creativity is an effort to solve a problem. This view is frequently criticized, however, for many creative efforts seem to be more self-expressive and playful, and not reactions to a problem. The complication arises because it may be that self-expression is an effort to solve the problem of how best to

express something. An artist might say, "No, I am not painting to solve any problem; I am simply trying to find the best way to capture that starry night." What if the artist then adds, "I just can't decide if this method is best, or that one." That artist has a problem: Which method is best? Goals may similarly depend on one's perspective. The Wright brothers may have persisted because they wanted fly, but someone else might have said that their goal was to build an airplane.

At the very least, parents, and teachers, or managers and supervisors in an organizational setting, should take great care with the expectations they hold for their charges. It would be inappropriate for any of these individuals to expect a moderately skilled individual to, through enhanced motivation, perform beyond the limits of his or her capacities. Motivation does not compensate for deficient skills, but instead allows the individual to fulfill his or her potential and to perform at the highest level. Not all of us have what it takes to develop a new method for flying, like the Wrights, but each of us has creative potential, and a better understanding of motivation will allow each of us to best use our creative talents.

NOTE

1. Additionally, creativity can be proactive, and this means that problems do not even need to be encountered (Heinzen, 1994). Problems can be avoided, and not merely solved, if we are creative. We may not even need to experience the problems. To be proactive, however, requires that there be an interest in monitoring and maintaining the status quo. This is very different from the motivation to solve problems, which is reactive rather than proactive.

REFERENCES

Albert, R. S. (1980). Exceptionally gifted boys and their parents: Basic educational, cognitive, and creative similarities. *Gifted Child Quarterly, 24,* 174–179.

Albert, R. S., & Runco, M. A. (in press). Parents' personality and the creative potential of exceptionally gifted boys. *Creativity Research Journal.*

Amabile, T. M. (1990). Within you, without you: Towards a social psychology of creativity and beyond. In M. A. Runco & R. S. Albert (Eds.), *Theories of creativity* (pp. 61–91). Newbury Park, CA: Sage.

Amabile, T. M., Goldfarb, P., & Brackfield, S. C.

(1990). Social influences on creativity: Evaluation, coaction, and surveillance. *Creativity Research Journal, 3,* 6–21.

Andreasen, N. (1997). Creativity and mental illness: Prevalence rates in writers and their first-degree relatives. In M. A. Runco & R. Richards (Eds.), *Eminent creativity, everyday creativity, and health* (pp. 7–18). Norwood, NJ: Ablex.

Barron, F. (1972). *Artists in the making.* New York: Seminar Press.

Baer, J. (1991). Generality of creativity across performance domains. *Creativity Research Journal, 4,* 23–40.

Barron, F. (1995). *No rootless flower: An ecology of creativity.* Cresskill, NJ: Hampton Press.

Campbell, D. (1960). Blind variation and selective retention in creative thought as in other knowledge processes. *Psychological Review, 67,* 380–400.

Cerf, C., & Navasky, V. (1984). *The experts speak: The definitive compendium of authoritative misinformation.* New York: Pantheon.

Chand, I., & Runco, M. A. (1992). Problem finding skills as components in the creative process. *Personality and Individual Differences, 14,* 155–162.

Chown, S. M. (1961). Age and the rigidities. *Journal of Gerontology, 16,* 353–362.

Cox, C. M. (1926). *Genetic studies of genius. Vol. 2: The early mental traits of three hundred geniuses.* Stanford, CA: Stanford University Press.

Crutchfield, R. S. (1962). Conformity and creative thinking. In H. E. Gruber, G. Terrell, & M. Wertheimer (Eds.), *Contemporary approaches to creative thinking* (pp. 120–140). New York: Atherton.

Csikszentmihalyi, M. (1975). *Beyond boredom and anxiety.* San Francisco: Jossey-Bass.

Csikszentmihalyi, M. (1988). The dangers of originality: Creativity and the artistic process. In M. M. Gedo (Ed.), *Psychoanalytic perspectives on art* (pp. 213–224). Hillsdale, NJ: Analytic Press.

Csikszentmihalyi, M. (1990). The domain of creativity. In M. A. Runco & R. S. Albert (Eds.), *Theories of creativity* (pp. 190–212). Newbury Park, CA: Sage.

Díaz de Chumaceiro, C. L. (in press). Serendipity and pseudo-serendipity in career paths of successful women: Orchestra conductors. *Creativity Research Journal.*

Dudek S. Z., & Hall, W. (1991). Personality consistency: Eminent architects 25 years later. *Creativity Research Journal, 4,* 213–232.

Eisenman, R. (1997). Creativity, preference for complexity, and physical and mental health. In M. A. Runco & R. Richards (Eds.), *Eminent creativity, everyday creativity, and health* (pp. 99–106) Norwood, NJ: Ablex.

Elliot, A. J. (1997). Integrating "classic" and "contemporary" approaches to achievement motivation: A hierarchical model of approach and avoidance achievement motivation. In P. Pintrich & M. Maehr

(Eds.), *Advances in motivation and achievement* (Vol. 10, pp. 143–179). Greenwich, CT: JAI Press.

Elliot, A. J. (1999). Approach and avoidance motivation and achievement goals. *Educational Psychologist, 34,* 149–169.

Elliot, A. J., & Dweck, C. S. (2004). *Competence and motivation: Competence as the core of the achievement motivation literature.* Manuscript draft.

Elliot, A. J., & McGregor, H. A. (2001). A 2 × 2 achievement goal framework. *Journal of Personality and Social Psychology, 80,* 501–519.

Epstein, R. (1990). Generativity theory as a theory of creativity. In M. A. Runco & R. S. Albert (Eds.), *Theories of creativity* (pp. 116–140). Newbury Park, CA: Sage.

Eysenck, H. J. (1999). Personality and creativity. In M. A. Runco (Ed.), *Creativity research handbook.* Cresskill, NJ: Hampton Press.

Galton, F. (1869). *Hereditary genius.* New York: Macmillan.

Goetz, E. M., & Baer, D. M. (1973). Social control of form diversity and the emergence of new forms in children's blockbuilding. *Journal of Applied Behavior Analysis, 6,* 209–217.

Gough, H. G., & Bradley, P. (1999). In A. Montuori (Ed.), *Create to be free: Essays in honor of Frank Barron.* Cresskill, NJ: Hampton Press.

Gruber, H. E. (1981). On the relation between "aha" experiences and the construction of ideas. *History of Science, 19,* 41–59.

Gruber, H. E. (1988). The evolving systems approach to creative work. *Creativity Research Journal, 1,* 27–51.

Hayes, J. R. (1978). *Cognitive psychology.* Homewood, IL: Dorsey.

Heinzen, T. (1994). Situational affect: Proactive and reactive creativity. In M. A. Runco & M. Shaw (Eds.), *Creativity and affect* (pp. 127–146). Norwood, NJ: Ablex.

Hennessey, B. A. (1989). The effect of extrinsic constraint on children's creativity when using a computer. *Creativity Research Journal, 2,* 151–168.

Hofstadter, D. (1986). *Metamagical themas.* New York: Basic Books.

Holman, J., Goetz, E. M., & Baer, D. M. (1977). The training of creativity as an operant and an examination of its generalization characteristics. In B. C. Etzel, J. M. LeBlanc, & D. M. Baer (Eds.), *New directions for behavioral research* (pp. 441–472). Hillsdale, NJ: Erlbaum.

Hoppe, K., & Kyle, N. (1991). Dual brain, creativity, and health. *Creativity Research Journal, 3,* 150–157.

Jamison, K. (1997). Mood disorders and patterns of creativity in British writers and artists. In M. A. Runco & Richards, R. (Eds.), *Eminent creativity, everyday creativity, and health* (pp. 19–32). Norwood, NJ: Ablex.

Jones, K., Runco, M. A., Dorinan, C., & Freeland, D. C. (1997). Influential factors in artists' lives and themes in their art work. *Creativity Research Journal*, *10*, 221–228.

Lazarus, R. S. (1991a). Cognition and motivation in emotion. *American Psychologist*, *46*, 352–367.

Lazarus, R. S. (1991b). Progress on a cognitive–motivational–relational theory of emotion. *American Psychologist*, *46*, 819–834.

Ludwig, A. (1995). *The price of greatness*. New York: Guilford Press.

MacKinnon, D. W. (1965). Personality and the realization of creative potential. *American Psychologist*, *20*, 273–281.

MacKinnon, D. W. (1970). The personality correlates of creativity: A study of American architects. In P. E. Vernon (Ed.), *Creativity* (pp. 289–311). Harmondsworth, UK: Penguin.

MacKinnon, D. (1983). The highly effective individual. In R. S. Albert (Ed.), *Genius and eminence: A social psychology of creativity and exceptional achievement* (pp. 114–127). Oxford: UK. (Original work published in 1960)

Maslow, A. H. (1971). *The farther reaches for human nature*. New York: Viking Press.

Montuori, A., & Purser, R. (Eds.). (1999). *Social creativity* (Vol. 1). Cresskill, NJ: Hampton Press.

Mumford, M. D., Baughman, W., & Sager, C. E. (2003). Picking the right material: Cognitive processing skills and their role in creative thought. In M. A. Runco (Ed.), *Critical creative processes* (pp. 19–68). Cresskill, NJ: Hampton Press.

Mumford, M. D., & Gustafson, S. B. (1988). Creativity syndrome: Integration, application, and innovation. *Psychological Bulletin*, *103*, 27–43.

Patrick, C. (1935). Creative thought in poets. *Archives of Psychology*, *26*, 1–74.

Patrick, C. (1937). Creative thought in artists. *Journal of Psychology*, *4*, 35–73.

Pennebaker, J. W., Kiecolt-Glaser, J. K., & Glaser, R. (1997). Disclosure of traumas and immune function: Health implications for psychotherapy. In M. A. Runco & R. Richards (Eds.), *Eminent creativity, everyday creativity, and health* (pp. 287–392). Norwood, NJ: Ablex.

Piaget, J. (1970). Piaget's theory. In P. H. Mussen (Ed.), *Carmichael's handbook of child psychology* (3rd ed., pp. 703–732). New York: Wiley.

Piaget, J. (1976). *To understand is to invent*. New York: Penguin.

Plucker, J. (2000). Beware of hasty, simple conclusions: The case for the content generality of creativity. *Creativity Research Journal*, *11*, 179–182.

Pryor, K. W., Hoag, R., & O'Reilly, J. (1969). The creative porpoise: Training for novel behavior. *Journal of the Experimental Analysis of Behavior*, *12*, 653–662.

Raina, T. N., & Raina, M. K. (1971). Perception of teacher–educators in India about the ideal pupil. *Journal of Educational Research*, *64*, 303–306.

Richards, R. (1990). Everyday creativity, eminent creativity, and health: Afterview for CRJ issues on creativity and health. *Creativity Research Journal*, *3*, 300–326.

Roe, A. (1963). Personal problems and science. In C. W. Taylor & F. Barron (Eds.), *Scientific creativity: Its recognition and development* (pp. 132–138). New York: Wiley.

Rogers, C. R. (1961). *On becoming a person*. Boston, MA: Houghton Mifflin.

Root-Bernstein, R. (1988). *Discovering*. New York: Cambridge University Press.

Rothenberg, A. (1990). Creativity, mental health, and alcoholism. *Creativity Research Journal*, *3*, 179–201.

Rubenson, D. L., & Runco, M. A. (1992). The psychoeconomic approach to creativity. *New Ideas in Psychology*, *10*, 131–147.

Rubenson, D. L., & Runco, M. A. (1995). The psychoeconomic view of creative work in groups and organizations. *Creativity and Innovation Management*, *4*, 232–241.

Runco M. A. (1987). The generality of creative performance in gifted and nongifted children. *Gifted Child Quarterly*, *31*, 121–125.

Runco, M. A. (Ed.). (1991). *Divergent thinking*. Norwood, NJ: Ablex.

Runco, M. A. (1993a). Moral creativity: Intentional and unconventional. *Creativity Research Journal*, *6*, 17–28.

Runco, M. A. (1993b). Operant theories of insight, originality, and creativity. *American Behavioral Scientist*, *37*, 59–74.

Runco, M. A. (1994a). Creativity and its discontents. In M. P. Shaw & M. A. Runco (Eds.), *Creativity and affect* (pp. 102–123). Norwood, NJ: Ablex.

Runco, M. A. (Ed.). (1994b). *Problem finding, problem solving, and creativity*. Norwood, NJ: Ablex.

Runco, M. A. (1995). Insight for creativity, expression for impact. *Creativity Research Journal*, *8*, 377–390.

Runco, M. A. (1999a). Misjudgment of creativity. In M. A. Runco & S. Pritzker (Eds.), *Encyclopedia of creativity* (pp. 235–240). San Diego, CA: Academic Press.

Runco, M. A. (1999b). Tactics and strategies for creativity. In M. A. Runco & S. Pritzker (Eds.), *Encyclopedia of creativity* (pp. 611–615). San Diego: Academic Press.

Runco, M. A. (1999c). Tension, adaptability, and creativity. In S. W. Russ (Ed.), *Affect, creative experience, and psychological adjustment* (pp. 165–194). Philadelphia: Taylor & Francis.

Runco, M. A. (2003). Creativity, cognition, and their educational implications. In J. C. Houtz (Ed.), *The educational psychology of creativity* (pp. 25–56). Cresskill, NJ: Hampton Press.

Runco, M. A. (in press). Creative giftedness. In R. S. Sternberg & J. E. Davidson (Eds.), *Conceptions of giftedness* (Rev. ed.). New York: Cambridge University Press.

Runco, M. A., & Albert, R. S. (1986). The threshold hypothesis regarding creativity and intelligence: An

empirical test with gifted and nongifted children. *Creative Child and Adult Quarterly, 11*, 212–218.

Runco, M. A., & Albert, R. S. (Eds.). (1990). *Theories of creativity.* Newbury Park: Sage.

Runco, M. A., & Chand, I. (1995). Cognition and creativity. *Educational Psychology Review, 7*, 243–267.

Runco, M. A., Ebersole, P., & Mraz, W. (1991). Self-actualization and creativity. *Journal of Social Behavior and Personality, 6*, 161–167.

Runco, M. A., & Smith, W. R. (1992). Interpersonal and intrapersonal evaluations of creative ideas. *Personality and Individual Differences, 13*, 295–302.

Ryan, B. A., & Winston, A. S. (1978). Dimensions of creativity in children's drawings. *Journal of Educational Psychology, 70*, 651–656.

Simon, H. A., & Chase, W. (1973). Skill in chess. *American Scientist, 61*, 394–403.

Simonton, D. K. (1984). *Genius, creativity, and leadership.* Cambridge, MA: Harvard Univesity Press.

Simonton, D. K. (1988). *Scientific genius.* New York: Cambridge University Press.

Skinner, B. F. (1939). The alliteration in Skakespeare's sonnets: A study in literary behavior. *Psychological Record, 3*, 186–192.

Sternberg, R. (2000). *Handbook of creativity.* New York: Cambridge University Press.

Stokes, P. D. (in press). Creativity and operant research: Selection and reorganization of responses. In M. A. Runco (Ed.), *Creativity research handbook* (Vol. 3). Cresskill, NJ: Hampton Press.

Stokes, P. D., & Balsam, P. (in press). Effects of early strategic hints on sustained variability levels. *Creativity Research Journal.*

Torrance, E. P. (1963). The creative personality and the ideal pupil. *Teachers College Record, 65*, 220–227.

Weeks, D., & James, J. (1995). *Eccentrics.* London: Weidenfeld & Nicolson.

Zajonc, R. B. (1990). Feeling and thinking: Preferences need no inferences. *American Psychologist, 35*, 151–175.

CHAPTER 34

☙

Automaticity in Goal Pursuit

PETER M. GOLLWITZER
JOHN A. BARGH

The intersection of competence and motivation involves the ability to attain one's goals, to accomplish what one sets out to do. Both modern and classic theory and research on goal pursuit have focused mainly on the conscious and deliberate ways that people strive toward desired end states. In this chapter, we focus on the role played by automatic or unconscious motivations in the competent pursuit of one's important goals. How can such unconscious goal pursuit add to a person's competencies in a given domain? We show that unconsciously pursued goals are especially effective in keeping a person "on task" and moving in thought and action toward the desired goal, even when the conscious mind is distracted or focused elsewhere. Automatic or unconscious motivations respond immediately and effortlessly to environmental conditions (triggers) that promote or support the goal in question, such as in recognizing and acting upon opportunities that otherwise might have been missed. And the efficient nature of unconscious motivation makes it an especially effective means of goal pursuit in complex and busy social environments in which conscious attention is divided and in short supply.

Two main forms of unconscious goal pursuit have been featured in our research: one (automatic motivations) a long-term, chronic form that develops out of extended experience; the other (implementation intentions) a temporary and strategic form by which one sets up intended actions in advance, so that they later unfold in an automatic fashion. Before describing these two lines of research, we begin with some historical background on the concept of unconscious motivation as it has come and gone within psychology over the past century.

HISTORY OF THE UNCONSCIOUS MOTIVATION CONCEPT

The unconscious has had a long and bumpy ride through the history of psychology. Few, if any, other psychological concepts have instigated this much contention and polarization of opinion. William James considered it "a tumbling ground for whimsies," and Jean-Paul Sartre railed against it as a way to abdicate personal responsibility for one's actions. Sigmund Freud, of course, championed the unconscious as a causal force in human thought and behavior, yet his medical and therapeutic perspective led him to focus as well on the unconscious's negative effects. Many modern-day motivational psychologists continue to hold this negative opinion (Bandura 1986; Locke & Latham, 1990; Mischel, Cantor, & Feldman, 1996). In their treatments, unconscious influences are characterized as rigid, undesirable habits of thought or behavior that must be overcome by conscious acts of will.

Freud's dynamic unconscious was primarily motivational in nature, driving behavior to express and fulfill deep-seated needs and wishes, and guarding and defending conscious experience from unpleasant memories of the past or threatening stimuli of the present. Following Freud's lead, the early work on unconscious influences within experimental psychology also focused on the motivational properties of the unconscious. This was the classic "New Look" perception research by Bruner and Postman and their colleagues (see reviews by Allport, 1955; Bruner, 1957; Erdelyi, 1974). The idea of perceptual defense involved motivational influences on the initial perception and awareness of environmental stimuli. Many studies showed, for example, that significantly longer tachistoscopic presentation times were needed for a participant to recognize taboo words or other stimuli (e.g., swastikas, spiders) likely to produce negative emotional reactions, compared to the recognition of emotionally neutral or positive stimuli.

But the New Look ideas concerning motivational influences on perceptual recognition and identification had difficulty gaining acceptance into the then-mainstream of psychological science. Erdelyi's (1974) historical analysis and review of the New Look indicates that 1950s psychology was just not ready for the idea of preconscious influences on stimulus recognition. But this all changed with the so-called "cognitive revolution" in psychology of the 1960s. Neisser's (1967) influential book, *Cognitive Psychology*, for example, reviewed experimental evidence of preattentive or preconscious perceptual analysis (e.g., pattern recognition, figural synthesis). Most notably, the classic research and theory on attention allocation of Broadbent, Treisman, Norman, and others, which showed how stimuli could be analyzed for meaning prior to the person's conscious awareness of them, made the idea of early motivational screening of environmental stimuli much more plausible than it had been in the 1950s (see review by Lachman, Lachman, & Butterfield, 1979).

Thus, the idea of unconscious influences on perception gained a great deal of traction from the cognitive revolution and soon flourished in social and clinical psychology as well. It is now completely uncontroversial in mainstream psychology. But what happened to the concept of unconscious motivation? It did not reap the benefits of the cognitive revolution; rather, within social psychology, one of the consequences of that revolution was an attempt to eliminate motivational explanations for as many phenomena as possible (e.g., Nisbett & Ross, 1980).

Unconscious motivation, as a scientific concept within social psychology, thus had to overcome two separate historical resistances—the long-standing one to the unconscious as an explanatory variable, and the more recent one to motivational explanations as well. But just as research on the unconscious snuck back into respectability through the sheep's clothing of "attention research" (Broadbent, 1958), motivation research made its comeback under the cover of "task goals" (Srull & Wyer, 1986; Anderson & Pichert, 1978). Social cognition researchers had shown that the outcome of information-processing activities—such as organization of material in memory and ease of retrieval—varied as a function of the particular task goals assigned to participants (e.g., memorizing behavioral information vs. forming an impression based on it; Hamilton, Katz, & Leirer, 1980).

Accordingly, by about 1990, it had become clear that any complete model of social cognition had to take into account the individual's task or processing goals. The goal concept began to be included in social cognition models, mainly by assuming that goals were represented mentally in a similar way as was known for other classes of social stimuli, such as types of social behavior, roles, and groups (Bargh, 1990; Kruglanski, 1996). The auto-motive model (Bargh, 1990; see below) grew out of this idea: If goals were represented mentally just like other varieties of social concepts (e.g., stereotypes), then the same properties that had been found to hold for other social representations—such as the capability of becoming activated outside of conscious awareness—should hold for goals as well. And so the concept of unconscious motivation made its return to scientific psychology: It was "unconscious" because it was automatic in the sense of being triggered and guided by external stimuli instead of an act of conscious choice and subsequent conscious control (Bargh, 1994), and it was "motivation" because goal representations were the particular cognitive concepts being automatically activated.

AUTO-MOTIVE THEORY: AUTOMATIC ACTIVATION AND PURSUIT OF PERSONAL GOALS

The auto-motive model of unconscious social motivations built upon the research of the 1970s, and especially the 1980s, that demonstrated the automatic activation capability of social mental representations, such as trait concepts (e.g., honest, aggressive), attitudes, and group stereotypes (see reviews by Bargh, 1989; Brewer, 1988; Wegner & Bargh, 1997). This research showed that frequently used mental representations will, over time, become active upon the mere presence of relevant information in the person's environment. For stereotypes, this would be easily identifiable group features such as skin color, gender, speech accent, and so on. For attitudes, the environmental trigger would be the mere presence of the attitude object in the environment (Fazio, 1986). For trait concepts, it would be features of observed social behaviors corresponding to the trait in question (Uleman, Newman, & Moskowitz, 1996).

The principle underlying all of these cases of automatic process development was that automatic associations are formed between the representations of environmental features (e.g., attitude objects, or common situations and settings) and other representations (e.g., evaluations or stereotypes, respectively) to the extent that they are consistently active in memory at the same time (Hebb, 1948). If one repeatedly and consistently thinks of members of a particular social group in stereotypical ways, for in-

stance, then the stereotype eventually would become active automatically upon the mere presence in the environment of a member of that group (Bargh, 1989; Brewer, 1988).

Under the assumption that goals, too, are represented mentally, and become automatically activated by the same principles, then goal representations should be capable of automatic activation by features of the contexts in which those goals have been pursued often and consistently in the past. If a given individual always competed with his or her siblings, then the goal of competition should become automatically activated upon just the mere presence of a sibling. In other words, it should become active even though the person may not intentionally and consciously choose to compete at that time and in that situation.

The auto-motive model further assumes that, once activated in this unconscious manner, the goal representation would then operate in the same way as when it is consciously and intentionally activated; that is, the model predicts that an automatically activated goal would have the same effects on thought and behavior as when the person consciously pursues that same goal (i.e., as when the goal is activated by an act of conscious will). In essence, then, the original auto-motive model (Bargh, 1990) derived the historical notion of unconscious motivation from the basic principles of modern-day cognitive psychology.

Such theoretical derivations are all well and good, but more was needed to establish the mundane reality of unconscious motivations in social life than logical or theoretical arguments. Accordingly, experimental research was conducted to test the model empirically. This research focused on three main questions: Can we observe goal attainment effects on thoughts, feelings, and behaviors by implicitly activated (primes) goals? Once activated, can unconscious goals keep operating outside of conscious awareness? And is automatic goal pursuit characterized by the same features as is conscious goal pursuit?

Goal Attainment Effects of Implicitly Activated Goals (Goal Priming)

The first question to be addressed was whether goals could be activated outside of conscious awareness. The standard method used within social cognition research to test such a hypothesis is the priming or unrelated-studies paradigm (Bargh & Chartrand, 2000). In this design, the concept under study is first primed by causing the participant to think about or use it in some way that is unrelated to the focal task that comes next in the experiment. For example, to prime or passively activate the concept of honesty, the participant might be exposed to some synonyms of honesty in the course of working on a sentence construction task, such as the scrambled sentence test developed by Srull and Wyer (1979). The use of the concept in this first task should cause the concept to become activated. It is assumed that such activation persists for some time after the use of the concept, even though participants do not realize it (Higgins, Bargh, & Lombardi, 1985). Thus, the still-active concept can have an influence on information processing in the next experimental task (e.g., forming an impression of a target person), without the person being aware of this influence.

Chartrand and Bargh (1996) used this paradigm to test whether goal representations could be primed in the same manner. In one study, participants completed a scrambled sentence test that contained either some words related to the goal of impression formation (e.g., "judge," "evaluate") or to the goal of memorization (e.g., "retain," "absorb"). When this task had been completed, participants were given a second, ostensibly unrelated task to complete: to read each of a series of 16 behaviors performed by a target person and then answer some questions about them. After participants had read all of the behaviors, they were given a surprise recall task.

Previous research (Hamilton et al., 1980) had used the same procedure, but with explicit (conscious) instructions to participants either to memorize the presented information, or to form an impression of the person based on the behaviors. That study had found significantly better recall, and also greater thematic organization of the behavioral information in memory, for participants in the impression-formation condition. But in our study, no such explicit instructions were given; instead, all participants were given the same (generic) instructions about answering some questions later on. Nonetheless, the results were the same as

those in the previous study: participants in the impression-formation goal-priming condition both recalled more behaviors and showed greater thematic organization of them in memory compared to those in the memorization–goal-priming condition.

These findings suggest that goals can indeed be primed, and then produce the same outcomes as when consciously pursued. Subsequent studies found similar effects with a variety of other goals. For example, priming the goal of achievement (i.e., to perform well) causes participants to score higher on verbal tasks than do control group participants (Bargh & Gollwitzer, 1994; Bargh, Gollwitzer, Lee-Chai, Barndollar, & Trötschel, 2001), and priming the goal of cooperation causes them to make more cooperative responses in a negotiation task in which they were free to compete or cooperate (Bargh et al., 2001, Study 2).

Although these studies primed goal concepts rather directly, by presenting participants with words synonymous with the goal, goals can also become automatically activated indirectly, through their strong association with certain situational features that are primed instead. Indeed, this is closer to the way that the auto-motive model assumes that goals become automatically activated in the real world—that is, by the presence of situational features within which the goal has been frequently pursued in the past. Situational power is one such feature: priming the concept of power causes participants with sexual harassment tendencies to become more attracted to a female confederate than they otherwise would have been (Bargh, Raymond, Pryor, & Strack, 1995). It also causes people to behave more in line with their own self-interest, and against the interests of their fellow experimental participants (Chen, Lee-Chai, & Bargh, 2001). These findings support the model's assumption that strong, automatic associations develop between situational and goal representations, to the extent that the goal is pursued frequently and consistently within that situation.

Another important and common situational trigger for goal pursuit is the presence of a significant other. These are people such as our parents, siblings, children, dating partners, or spouses, friends, and close colleagues—people whom we think about a lot, and interactions with whom yield outcomes that substantially impact on our moods and life satisfaction. Fitzsimons and Bargh (2003) assumed that our mental representations of these close others contain within them the goals that we frequently and consistently pursue when with them. For instance, a person might have the chronic and long-standing goals of making her mother proud of her, competing with her brother, and relaxing and having fun when with her best friend. Even though there may by people who share such goals with respect to these significant others, other people may want to avoid their mothers, to have fun with their brothers, and to look up to and emulate their best friends. Thus, there should be not only commonalities in goal pursuit across people but also some degree of individual variation in goals, given the same significant other (e.g., one's mother). This was confirmed in a preliminary survey of college undergraduates, in which they were asked to list the goals they pursued with five different types of significant others.

Next, in several laboratory experiments and one field experiment, participants' mental representations of a given type of significant other (e.g., a best friend) were primed without their awareness, and then participants were given an opportunity to pursue the goal chronically associated with that partner. In every case, participants did behave in line with this goal, even though their significant other was not, of course, physically present in the experimental situation. For instance, in participants who usually try to make their mothers proud of them, priming the representation of the mother caused them to outperform control participants on measures of verbal ability. In line with the auto-motive model's predictions, priming the mother had no effect on the verbal ability task performance of participants who pursued other goals with their mothers (e.g., friendship, helping her). Also, those who did have the goal of making their mothers proud, but who were not primed with the mother, did not perform any better than did the control group. Both ingredients were necessary: the priming or preactivation of the representation of one's mother, and the chronic, automatic association of one's mother with the goal of high performance. In practice, then, thinking about or being reminded of a certain significant other—which

can be prompted easily and innocently by merely glancing at their photograph on our wall or desk—is sufficient to put into motion those goals one chronically pursues when with that person. So even when they are not present, one starts to behave as if he or she were in their company.

A further real-life, implicit activation of goals may occur when we observe the goal-directed actions of others, even nonsignificant others. By perceiving other people's goal pursuits, the respective mental goal representations should become activated in ourselves, with the effect that we start to act on them as well. This goal-contagion hypothesis, according to which individuals automatically take on a goal that is implied by another's behavior, has recently been examined in a series of studies (Aarts, Gollwitzer, & Hassin, 2004). Participants were briefly exposed to behavioral information about another person, implying a specific goal (e.g., making money), and were then given the opportunity to act on this goal in a different way and context. Participants' own actions started to serve the same goal, and they acquired features of goal-directedness in the sense that they were affected by goal strength (i.e., were in line with the participants' personal need for money), showed persistence over time, and were more readily engaged when the given situation clearly lent itself to meeting the goal at hand. Most interestingly, participants were immune against the automatic adoption of the goals of others if these were pursued in an inappropriate, socially unacceptable way. Apparently, goal contagion will not occur if the observed goal pursuits of others are perceived to be unattractive and undesirable.

Unconscious Operation of Primed Goals

It is one thing to claim that goals can be activated automatically, but quite another to argue that once activated, goals continue to operate outside of conscious awareness. But this is indeed the strong form of the auto-motive model, and there is now evidence consistent with this claim. For one thing, in all such automatic goal studies, participants are carefully questioned and debriefed following the experiment, to make sure they were not aware of pursuing that goal during the experimental task. Very few if any participants show this awareness (the data of those who do are removed prior to analyses); most are surprised, if not skeptical, that we, the experimenters, had caused them to pursue a goal without their knowledge. For example, in the Chartrand and Bargh (1996) study, impression-primed participants were no more likely to report having tried to form an impression of the target person than were memorization-primed participants, who in turn were no more likely to report having tried to memorize the information than were the impression-primed participants. More than that, very few participants reported having pursued either goal while reading the target's behaviors. In the Fitzsimons and Bargh (2003) research, participants in the field experiment at a major international airport, who were approached to participate while waiting for their flight to depart, largely did not believe the experimenter's explanation that they had been induced to volunteer to help the experimenter (or not) by first answering some questions about their friend (vs. coworker). People's personal theories about what causes them to do things just do not include the idea (and thus allow for the possibility) of unconscious motivations or causes (Wilson & Brekke, 1994).

Perhaps stronger evidence as to the unconscious operation of goals is furnished by Experiment 2 of Bargh et al. (2001), in which people were either primed (or not) to cooperate with their opponent in a negotiation task, or were told explicitly (or not) by the experimenter to cooperate. These two factors were crossed in the design of the study, in order to compare the conscious versus unconscious operation of the same goal. As in the other goal-priming studies, those who were primed to cooperate did so more than did nonprimed participants. Also, not surprisingly, those who were explicitly (consciously) told to cooperate did so more than those who were not. After the experimental task had been completed, all participants were then asked to rate how much they had tried to cooperate while performing the negotiation task with their opponent.

For each participant, then, we could compare these ratings of how much they had consciously tried to cooperate with their actual cooperative behavior during the negotiation (measured in terms of the relative numbers of cooperative moves they had made during the task). For those in the explicit, conscious cooperation condition, these ratings correlated significantly with actual behavior: Those who had reported having tried harder to cooperate actually had cooperated more than other participants. In other words, self-reports accurately reflected the actual behavior. But for those in the unconscious (primed) cooperation condition, self-reports of how much they had tried to cooperate did not correspond at all (correlations near zero) with how much cooperation actually occurred. This is our strongest evidence to date that, for automatically activated goals, people are not consciously aware of the operation of these goals, even while they are successfully pursuing them.

Similarities of Unconscious to Conscious Goal Pursuits

Thus far, the evidence shows that unconscious goal pursuit produces the same effects (in terms of goal attainment) on thought, memory, and behavior as are known for conscious goal pursuit. Whether the goal has to do with how incoming social information is to be processed, how well an intellectual task is to be performed, or how one is to interact with another person, significant performance differences emerge between groups primed to unconsciously pursue different goals, just as they did in previous studies between groups explicitly told (or not) to pursue such goals. As Bargh and Chartrand (1999) noted, exactly how a given goal is put into play (i.e., consciously or unconsciously) does not seem to matter with respect to goal attainment. Regardless of how it became activated, the active goal operates on the available information that is relevant to its purposes, and guides thought and behavior toward the desired end state.

Thus, on outcome measures (i.e., how well the person attains the goal), the findings to date show high similarity between conscious and unconscious goal pursuit. However, the classic literature on conscious goal pursuit has also documented various content-free features of conscious goal pursuit; thus, one wonders whether unconscious goal pursuits also carry these features.

Consequences of Goal Attainment

Whenever goals are attained, people are said to experience positive self-evaluative consequences (e.g., succeeding on a given goal leads to feelings of pride, expecting to be praised by others; Atkinson, 1957; Heckhausen, 1977) that should put them in a positive mood. Moreover, succeeding on a given goal is said to lead to striving for more challenging goals (i.e., proactive goal striving; Bandura, 1997). To test whether the similarity of conscious and unconscious goal operation extends to these aftereffects of goal attainment, Chartrand (1999; Chartrand & Bargh, 2002) conducted several studies in which participants were induced to unconsciously pursue a goal (via a priming manipulation), which they then succeeded on or failed to meet. In one experiment, for example, a high-achievement goal was primed or not, and then all participants were given a set of anagrams to solve. Critically, the anagrams were either very easy to solve or impossible to solve. In this way, Chartrand manipulated whether participants succeeded or failed at their unconscious goal to perform well. Following the anagram task, participants completed either a mood measure or a test of verbal ability. The mood measure was intended to tap the predicted emotional consequences of a positive self-evaluation following goal attainment; the verbal ability test was intended to tap the predicted proactive goal striving.

The results confirmed that unconscious goal pursuit is characterized by the same goal attainment effects as have been found for conscious goal pursuit. Take first the findings in the no-goal condition, in which no high-achievement goal had been primed; whether the anagram task was easy or difficult made no difference to mood or performance on the verbal ability test. This was expected, because participants in the no-goal condition had no high-achievement goal activated on which they could succeed or fail.

For participants in the unconscious high-achievement goal condition, however, their moods and subsequent task performance were markedly affected by whether they had just completed the easy versus difficult anagram task. On the mood measure, those in the easy anagram condition were significantly happier than were participants who

had just worked on the difficult anagrams; and the easy anagram participants also outperformed the difficult anagram participants on the subsequent verbal ability test. Because the high-achievement goal was unconscious, and operating without the participant's awareness, these findings indicate that one's mood and also subsequent pursuit of relevant, more challenging goals can be affected by whether one succeeds or fails at a goal one does not even know one has. Chartrand's findings therefore suggest that unconscious goal striving leads to goal attainment consequences (positive self-evaluations; proactive goal striving) similar to those of conscious goal pursuit.

Goal Projection

It has always been assumed that people project not only their traits but also their goals onto others. Holmes (1978) referred to more than just traits when he defined "projection" as a "process by which persons attribute personality traits, characteristics, or motivations to other persons as a function of their own personality traits, characteristics, or motivations" (p. 677). He even suggested that projection should be more easily observed with motivational impulses than with traits (Holmes, 1968). Accordingly, we recently tested whether the projection effects postulated for explicit goals also hold true for implicit goals (Kawada, Oettingen, Gollwitzer, & Bargh, 2004).

In one study, the experimenter explicitly assigned the goal to compete to some participants (i.e., explicit goal condition) and then asked them to rate the competitive orientation of a presumed partner participant, with whom they expected to play a Prisoner's Dilemma game. In the implicit goal condition, the goal to compete was activated using a scrambled sentence technique that exposed participants to words such as "compete," "win," and "succeed." Compared to control participants, who entered the presumed Prisoner's Dilemma game without any assigned or activated competition goal, both implicit and explicit competition participants expected the presumed partner to act more competitively throughout the game. These results indicate that goal projection occurs regardless of whether the goal is unconscious or consciously held.

In a follow-up experiment, the goal to compete was implicitly activated by subliminally presenting competition-related words; in the explicit goal condition, participants were again asked to take a competitive stand in the upcoming Prisoner's Dilemma game. Moreover, the experimenters weakened the goal to compete by allowing some participants to meet this goal in an alternative competition task (Wicklund & Gollwitzer, 1982), prior to performing the Prisoner's Dilemma game. First, we could replicate the goal projection effect (as compared to a no-goal control group) with implicit and explicit competition goal participants whose goals had not been weakened. Second, however, when the goal to compete had been weakened, goal projection effects were no longer observed in both the implicit and the explicit goal condition. This finding supports the claim that it was indeed the participants' goal to compete that was being projected onto others, and not just the trait concept of competitiveness. Moreover, it demonstrates that implicitly activated (primed) goals and explicitly assigned goals are both readily projected onto others, and that both seem to have the property of losing strength after having been served successfully.

Motivational Qualities: Sustained Goal Activation, Persistence, and Resumption

Since the time of Kurt Lewin, motivational states and processes have classically been distinguished by features and qualities different from those of nonmotivational, purely cognitive processes. These qualities include behavioral features, such as persisting in attempting to reach the goal when facing difficulties and returning to the goal activity after being disrupted, as opposed to giving up at the first obstacle or walking away from the interrupted activity (Lewin, 1935). Atkinson and Birch (1970) identified a further signature of motivational states: the tendency to stay activated or even increase in activation strength over time, until the desired outcome is reached or one has gone through an active, effortful process of disengagement from wanting to attain it. Cognitive (nonmotivational) representations, in contrast, tend to decrease quickly in activation strength over time since last use (e.g., Higgins et al., 1985).

Because much of the research that has tested and supported the auto-motive model has relied on the same priming techniques and manipulations as those previously used to study unconscious social perception and cognition (Bargh, 1989; Bargh & Chartrand, 2000), the following question arises: Could the same perceptual, nonmotivational social representations (e.g., trait concepts) that had been primed in those previous studies be responsible for the so-called "motivational effects" described earlier? Why should the same or very similar priming manipulations be said to produce perceptual or nonmotivational effects in some studies, but motivational effects in others?

This is an important and complex question for which we do not yet have a complete answer, but some additional findings shed light on what that answer might eventually be. At present, it appears that the same priming manipulation can activate qualitatively different concepts or processes at the same time (Bargh, 1997). Thus, stimuli related to the concept of achievement activate or prime the perceptual construct of achievement, the category used to identify achievement behavior in someone else, as well as the motivational or goal representation of achievement, which is used to energize and guide our own strivings for high performance on a task.

The best evidence to date for this proposition comes from Study 3 by Bargh et al. (2001), in which participants were first primed (or not) with achievement-related stimuli. Next, there was either a 5-minute delay before the participant worked on the next task, or he or she worked on it right away, with no interpolated delay. The final factor in the design was the type of task participants worked on: They either read a story about a target person who behaved in a somewhat ambiguous achievement-oriented manner (the social perception task), or they worked on a verbal task, in which they tried to find as many different words as they could in a set of Scrabble letter tiles (the performance task). Note that the achievement-priming manipulation was the same for all participants in that condition, whether they subsequently worked on the social judgment or the verbal performance task.

The expected priming effects were obtained on both tasks in the no-delay condition, with those primed with achievement-related stimuli either judging the target person as more achievement-oriented (in the judgment task condition), or finding significantly more words (in the verbal performance task condition), than did the nonprimed participants. However, as predicted, the time delay differentially impacted the priming effect on the perceptual versus the motivational task. On the perceptual task, the significant priming observed under no-delay condition disappeared after the 5-minute delay; this is consistent with previous studies of the time course of priming effects on social–perceptual tasks (Higgins et al., 1985). But on the motivational word-search task, the priming effect actually increased significantly in strength over the 5-minute delay. This is what would be expected, following Atkinson and Birch's (1970) dynamic theory of action, if a motivational state were driving the verbal task performance.

These findings help to establish that our goal-priming manipulations are indeed activating a motivational state, as opposed to the same perceptual and nonmotivational constructs as in prior research. Other recent experiments provide additional supportive evidence. In another experiment by Bargh et al. (2001, Study 4), participants' goal of achievement or high performance was primed (or not), and they then worked on the same Scrabble word-search task. The experimenter told participants that she had to see to another study in a different room but would give them the signal to stop working on the task over an intercom when the time came. Unknown to the participants, a hidden video camera recorded their behavior when and after the stop signal had been given. The dependent variable was whether the participant would keep working on the word-search task, trying for even higher scores, after the experimenter gave the stop signal, or whether they would stop working when faced with this obstacle to better performance. The results were clear: Over 50% of the participants in the achievement-primed condition continued to search for words after the stop signal had been given, compared to just over 20% of the nonprimed participants.

Thus, when one places an obstacle in the way of an unconsciously motivated person, a hindrance to attaining the goal (in this case) of the highest possible score on the task, the person will act to remove or bypass that obstacle if at all possible. Experimental participants for whom this unconscious goal is not operating show much less of a tendency to keep working on the task; for them, it is just an experiment, and not a very involving task at that. It is the activation and operation of the unconscious high-achievement goal in this experiment that makes participants care enough about their performance to persistently strive for an ever-higher score, even though they have to do so secretly and surreptitiously (they believe) after the stop signal has been given.

We have also tested goal-primed participants' motivational tendency to resume an interrupted goal, even in the face of more attractive behavioral options. In this study (Bargh et al., 2001, Study 5), participants were told that they would complete two different tasks. Participants were first primed (or not) to activate the achievement goal, and then all participants worked on a word-search task. Halfway through that task, a staged power outage forced everyone to stop work. After a 5-minute delay, the power was restored, but now (as the experimenter informed participants) there was no longer enough time during the session for them to complete both of the tasks. They were given the option of going back to the first task, or moving on to the second task, in which they would rate each of a series of cartoons as to how funny they were. Pretesting had shown that this cartoon-rating task was greatly preferred over the word-search task.

The dependent variable was the percentages of participants in the goal-primed versus not-primed conditions who went back and completed the word-search task, forgoing the opportunity to view and rate the cartoons. As would be expected if our goal-priming manipulation had produced a strong motivational state, significantly more participants in the goal-primed condition (66%) returned to the incomplete first task, compared to 35% of the no-goal participants.

Summary of Goal Priming Research

Our research has demonstrated, first, that goals can be triggered without an act of will or conscious choice on the part of the individual, simply by the presence of relevant situational cues. Moreover, once activated, the goal continues to operate in an unconscious fashion, with people unable to report or recognize immediately afterward that they have just pursued that goal, even though they have given every indication (on our dependent measures) of having done so. On several different types of commonly held goals—achievement, cooperation, impression formation, and memorization, the unconscious operation of the goal produced the same effects that others have observed when that goal is pursued with full conscious awareness and intent. These effects are not restricted to the outcome of the goal pursuit, but extend to content-free characteristics, such as self-evaluation, proactive goal striving, projection, sustained goal activation, persistence, and resumption. It appears, then, that successful goal pursuit does not require consciously held goals and conscious instigation and monitoring of respective goal striving. Rather, goals can be pursued and attained regardless of their status in consciousness.

STRATEGIC AUTOMATION OF GOAL PURSUIT: IMPLEMENTATION INTENTIONS

Classic theories of motivation (e.g., Atkinson, 1957, Fishbein & Ajzen, 1975; Heckhausen, 1977, McClelland, 1985; see reviews by Gollwitzer, 1990; Gollwitzer & Moskowitz, 1996; Oettingen & Gollwitzer, 2001) see the implementation of consciously set goals in direct relation to the strength of the goal, which in turn is a product of expected utility (desirability) of goal attainment and the likelihood that the goal can be attained (feasibility). However, even though (self-set or assigned) goals to do more good and less bad have been found to be reliably associated with actual efforts in the intended directions (Ajzen, 1991; Godin & Kok, 1996; Sheeran, 2002), these intention–behavior relations are modest. This is largely due to the fact that people, despite having formed strong intentions on the basis of high desirability and feasibility beliefs, fail to act on them (i.e., people are inclined but still abstain; Orbell & Sheeran, 1998).

The gap between intentions and behavior is largely due to the fact that the successful translation of goals (intention) into respective behaviors requires solving numerous problems of self-regulation, many of them having to do with being burdened by thoughts, feelings, and actions that are irrelevant to the goal pursuit at hand (Gollwitzer, 1996). In order to meet their goals, people often have to seize quickly viable opportunities to initiate relevant actions, a task that becomes particularly difficult when attention is directed elsewhere (e.g., when one is absorbed by competing goal pursuits, wrapped up in ruminations, gripped by intense emotional experiences, or simply tired). But even if the person has successfully started to act on a set goal, the ongoing goal pursuit needs to be shielded from getting derailed by negative influences from outside (e.g., temptations, distractions) and inside (e.g., self-doubts).

With all of these problems of goal pursuit, automatic control of goal-directed action should come in handy, because established routines linked to a relevant context would release the critical goal-directed behavior immediately, efficiently, and without a conscious intent. Often, however, such routines are not established, and the goal-directed behavior is not yet part of an everyday routine. Research on implementation intentions (Gollwitzer, 1993, 1999) suggests that—as a substitute—ad hoc automatic action control can be achieved by forming implementation intentions that take the format, "If Situation X is encountered, then I will perform Behavior Y!" In an implementation intention, a mental link is created between an anticipated future situational cue and an intended instrumental goal-directed response.

Implementation intentions need to be distinguished from goals or goal intentions. Goal intentions have the format ("I intend to reach Z!"), whereby Z may relate to a certain outcome or behavior to which the individual feels committed. Both goal intentions and implementation intentions are acts of willing, wherein the first specifies an intention to meet a goal, and the second refers to an intention to perform a plan. Commonly, implementation intentions are formed in the service of goal intentions, because they specify the when, where, and how of goal-directed responses. For instance, a possible implementation intention in the service of meeting the health goal of eating vegetarian food would link a suitable situational cue (e.g., one's order is taken at a restaurant) to an appropriate goal-directed behavior (e.g., asking for a vegetarian meal).

The mental if–then links created by implementation intentions are expected to facilitate goal attainment on the basis of various psychological processes that relate to both the anticipated situation and the linked behavior (Gollwitzer, 1999). Because forming implementation intentions implies the selection of a critical future internal or external cue (i.e., a viable opportunity), it is assumed that the mental representation of this situation becomes highly activated, hence more accessible. This heightened accessibility should make it easier to detect the critical situation in the surrounding environment and to attend readily to it even when one is busy with other things. Moreover, once the critical cue is encountered, the response specified in the then part of the implementation intention should be triggered in an automatic fashion that is immediate, efficient, and without necessitating a conscious intent. In summary, the formation of implementation intentions is a strategy of regulating goal pursuit that switches conscious control of goal-directed action to automatic control.

Research on action control via implementation intentions to date has focused on the following three questions: Are implementation intentions of help in overcoming the various problems of goal pursuit? Do implementation intentions indeed allow for the automatic control of goal-directed action? And what kind of price do people pay when self-regulating their goal pursuits by forming if–then plans?

Implementation Intentions Help Overcome Classic Problems of Conscious Goal Pursuit

The conscious self-regulation of goal pursuit often runs aground. This is true, whether the problems at hand are related to getting started, staying on track in the face of internal or external disturbances, keeping up motivation in the face of difficulties, or switching from ineffective to more effective means. However, research on the effects of forming implementation intentions on translating goal intentions into behavior shows that all of these problems benefit from the strategic automation of goal pursuit provided by implementation intentions.

Getting Started

This problem of goal pursuit embraces three different issues, each of which militates against effectively getting started on one's goals. The first has to do with remembering one's goal intention (Einstein & McDaniel, 1996). When acting on a given goal is not part of one's routine, or when one has to postpone acting on it until a suitable opportunity presents itself, one can easily forget to do so. Dealing with many things at once, or becoming preoccupied by a particular task, can make this even more likely, especially when the given goal is new or unfamiliar. Empirical support of this reason for the intention–behavior gap comes from retrospective reports by inclined abstainers. For example, 70% of participants who had intended to perform a breast self-examination but failed to do so offered forgetting as their reason for nonperformance (Milne, Orbell, & Sheeran, 2002; Orbell, Hodgkins, & Sheeran, 1997). Also, meta-analysis has shown that the longer the time interval between measures of goal intentions and goal achievement, the less likely it is that intentions are realized (Sheeran & Orbell, 1998). These findings suggest that remembering one's goal intentions does not come easy to people.

But even if one remembers what one is supposed to do, there is another problem that may need to be resolved, namely, seizing the opportunity to act. This problem is likely to be especially acute when there is a deadline for performing the behavior, or when the opportunity to act is presented only briefly. In these circumstances, people may fail to initiate goal-directed responses because they fail to notice that a good time to get started has arrived, they are unsure how they should act when the moment presents itself, or they simply procrastinate. Oettingen, Hönig, and Gollwitzer (2000, Study 3) showed that considerable slippage can occur even when people have formed strong goal intentions to perform a behavior at a particular time. Participants were provided with diskettes containing four concentration tasks and formed goal intentions to perform these tasks on their computers at a particular time each Wednesday morning for the next 4 weeks. The program on the diskette recorded the time that participants started to work on the task from the clock on participants' computers. Findings indicated that the mean deviation from the intended start time was 8 hours, that is, a discrepancy of 2 hours on average for each specified opportunity. Similar findings were obtained by Dholakia and Bagozzi (2003, Study 2) when participants' task was to evaluate a website that could be accessed only during a short time window. Here, only 37% of participants who formed a respective goal intention were successful at accomplishing the task. In summary, people may not get started with goal pursuit, because they fail to seize good opportunities to act.

There are also many instances in which people remember their goal intentions (e.g., to order a low-fat meal) and recognize that an opportune moment is upon them (e.g., it is lunchtime at one's usual restaurant) but nonetheless fail to initiate goal-directed behaviors, because they start to reflect anew on the desirability of the goal intention (i.e., start to have second thoughts). This problem has to do with overcoming an initial reluctance to act that is likely to arise when people have decided to pursue a goal that involves a trade-off between attractive long-term consequences versus less attractive short-term consequences (Mischel, 1996). For example, a strong goal intention to order low-fat meals is commonly formed on the basis of long-term deliberative thinking, according to which eating low-fat food is perceived as highly desirable; however, once the critical situation is confronted, short-term desirability considerations are triggered that occupy cognitive resources at the moment of action (e.g., the low-fat meal is perceived as tasteless at the critical juncture). Such dilemmas between the head and the heart should thus also get in the way of readily acting on the respective goal in the face of good opportunities (Loewenstein, Weber, Hsee, & Welch, 2001; Metcalfe & Mischel, 1999; Trafimow & Sheeran, in press).

So the question arises: Does forming implementation intentions that plan out in ad-vance when, where, and how one wants to move toward goal attainment ameliorate the problems of action initiation spelled out earlier. Various studies on the effects of implementation intentions on the rate of goal attainment suggest a positive answer to this question given the type of goals that have been found to benefit from forming implementation intentions. For instance, Gollwitzer and Brandstätter (1997) analyzed a goal intention (i.e., writing a report about how one spent Christmas Eve) that had to be performed at a time (i.e., during the subsequent Christmas holiday) when people were commonly busy with other things. Similarly, Oettingen et al. (2000, Study 3) observed that implementation intentions help people to act on their task goals (i.e., taking a concentration test) on time (e.g., at 10 A.M. in the morning of every Wednesday over the next 4 weeks). Other studies have examined the effects of implementation intentions on goal attainment rates with goal intentions that are somewhat unpleasant to perform. For instance, the goal intentions to perform regular breast examinations (Orbell et al., 1997), cervical cancer screenings (Sheeran & Orbell, 2000), resumption of functional activity after joint replacement surgery (Orbell & Sheeran, 2000), and engaging in physical exercise (Milne et al., 2002), were all more frequently acted on when people had furnished these goals with implementation intentions. Moreover, implementation intentions were found to facilitate the attainment of goal intentions when it is easy to forget to act on them (e.g., regular intake of vitamin pills, Sheeran & Orbell, 1999; the signing of work sheets with the elderly, Chasteen, Park, & Schwarz, 2001).

The results of these studies suggest that implementation intentions indeed facilitate the initiation of goal-directed behaviors by simplifying this process (i.e., making it less effortful). This conclusion is also supported by the finding that the beneficial effects of implementation intentions are commonly more apparent with difficult-to-implement goals compared to easy goals. For instance, implementation intentions were more effective in helping people to complete difficult, compared to easy, personal projects during Christmas break (Gollwitzer & Brandstätter, 1997, Study 1). And forming implementation intention was more beneficial to frontal lobe patients, who typically have severe problems with executive control, than to college students (Lengfelder & Gollwitzer, 2001, Study 2).

Staying on Track

Many goals cannot be accomplished by simple, discrete, one-shot actions but require continuous striving and repeated complex behavioral performances to be attained. Once a person has initiated these more complex goal pursuits, bringing them to a successful ending may be very difficult when certain internal (e.g., being anxious, tired, overburdened) or external stimuli (e.g., temptations, distractions) are not conducive to goal realization but instead generate interferences that could potentially derail the ongoing goal pursuit. Thus, one wonders whether implementation intentions can facilitate the shielding of such goal pursuits from the negative influences of interferences from inside and outside the person.

There are two major strategies in which implementation intentions can be used to shield an ongoing goal pursuit: (1) directing one's implementation intentions toward the suppression of negative influences, and (2) directing one's implementation intentions toward spelling out the ongoing goal pursuit, so that it becomes sheltered from these negative influences. For example, in the realm of social competence: If a person wants to avoid being unfriendly to a friend who is known to make outrageous requests, she can protect herself from showing the unwanted unfriendly response by forming suppression-oriented implementation intentions. Suppression-oriented implementation intentions can take different formats. The person may focus on reducing the intensity of the unwanted response by intending not to show the unwanted response: "And if my friend approaches me with an outrageous request, then I will not respond in an unfriendly manner!" But the person may also try to reduce the intensity of the unwanted response by specifying the initiation of the respective antagonistic response: "And if my friend approaches me with an outrageous request, then I will respond in a friendly manner!" Finally, suppression-oriented implementation intentions may even focus a person away from the critical stimulus: "And if my friend approaches me with an outrageous request, then I'll ignore it!"

Two sets of experiments analyzed the effects of suppression-oriented implementation intentions. The first looked at the control of unwanted spontaneous attention to tempting distractions (Gollwitzer & Schaal, 1998). Participants had to perform a boring task (i.e., a series of simple arithmetic tasks) while being bombarded with attractive distracting stimuli (e.g., video clips of award-winning commercials). Whereas control participants were asked to form a mere goal intention ("I will not let myself get distracted!"), experimental participants in addition formed one of two implementation intentions: "And if a distraction arises, then I'll ignore it!" or "And if a distraction arises, then I will increase my effort at the task at hand!" The ignore implementation intention always helped participants to ward off the distractions (as assessed by their task performance), regardless of whether the motivation to perform the tedious task (assessed at the beginning of the task) was low or high. The effort-increase implementation intention, in contrast, was effective only when motivation to perform the tedious task was low. Apparently, when motivation is high to begin with, effort-increase implementation intentions may create overmotivation that hampers task performance. It seems appropriate therefore to advise motivated individuals who suffer from being distracted (e.g., ambitious students doing their homework) to resort to ignore implementation intentions rather than to implementation intentions that focus on the strengthening of effort.

The second set of experiments analyzing suppression-oriented implementation intentions studied the control of the automatic activation of stereotypical beliefs and prejudicial evaluations (Gollwitzer & Schaal, 1998). In various priming studies, with short stimulus-onset asynchronies of less than 300 ms between primes (presentations of members of stigmatized groups) and targets (adjectives describing relevant stereotypical attributes or neutral positive–negative adjectives), implementation intentions helped to inhibit both the automatic activation of stereotypical beliefs and the prejudicial evaluations relative to women, the elderly, and the homeless. These implementation intentions (i.e., if–then plans) specified being confronted with a member of the critical group in the if part, and either "Then I won't stereotype" (respectively, "Then I won't evaluate negatively") or "Then I will ignore the group membership" in the then part. Regardless of which then parts were used, both types of suppression-oriented implementation intentions were effective.

The research presented in the preceding two paragraphs used implementation intentions that specified a potential interference in the if part. The specified interference was linked to a then part that described an attempt at suppressing the unwanted negative influence of this interference on one's goal pursuit. Self-regulation by this type of implementation intention implies that one has to be in a position to anticipate these potential interferences on the way to the goal; one even needs to know what kind of unwanted responses these interferences elicit, if one prefers to specify not showing this response in the then part of the implementation intention (rather than showing a goal-directed response or simply ignoring the interfering event). Fortunately, a simpler way to use implementation intentions to protect an ongoing goal pursuit from getting derailed is also available. Instead of gearing one's implementation intentions toward anticipated potential interferences and the disruptive responses they trigger, one may form implementation intentions geared at stabilizing the ongoing goal pursuit at hand. We again use the example of a tired person who is approached by her friend with an outrageous request, and who will likely respond in an unfriendly manner: If this person has stipulated in advance in an implementation intention what she will converse about with her friend, the critical interaction may simply run off as planned, and being tired should thus fail to affect the person's relating to her friend. As is evident from this example, the present self-regulatory strategy should be of special value whenever the influence of detrimental self-states (e.g., being tired, irritated, anxious) on derailing one's goal-directed behavior has to be controlled. This should be true whether or not such self-states and/or their negative influences on one's goal-directed behavior reside in consciousness.

Gollwitzer and Bayer (2000; Gollwitzer, Bayer, & McCulloch, 2005) tested this hypothesis in a series of experiments in which participants were asked (or not) to make if–then plans regarding the implementation of an assigned task goal. Prior to beginning work on the task, participants' self-states were manipulated, so that the task at hand became more difficult (e.g., a state of self-definitional incompleteness prior to a task that required perspective taking; Gollwitzer & Wicklund, 1985; a good mood prior to a task that required evaluation of others nonstereotypically; Bless & Fiedler, 1995; and a state of ego-depletion prior to solving difficult anagrams; Baumeister, 2000; Muraven, Tice, & Baumeister, 1998). The induced critical self-states negatively affected task performance only for those participants who had not planned out in advance how they wanted to perform the task at hand (i.e., had only set themselves the goal to come up with a great performance). Implementation intention participants were effectively protected from the negative influences associated with the induced detrimental self-states.

This research provides a new perspective on the psychology of self-regulation. Commonly, effective self-regulation (Baumeister, Heatherton, & Tice, 1994) is understood in terms of strengthening the self, so that the self can meet the challenge of being a powerful executive agent. Therefore, most research on goal-directed self-regulation focuses on strengthening the self in such a way that threats and irritations become less likely, or on restoring an already threatened or irritated self. All of these maneuvers are targeted in the end on changing the self, so that the self becomes a better executive. Instead, the findings of Gollwitzer and Bayer (2000) suggest a perspective on goal-directed self-regulation that gets around changing the self by facilitating action control via linking it to situational cues.

People's goal pursuits, however, are threatened not only by detrimental self-states but also by adverse situational conditions. Many situations have negative effects on goal attainment, unbeknownst to the person who is striving for the goal. A prime example is the social loafing phenomenon, in which people show reduced effort in the face of work settings that produce a reduction of accountability (i.e., performance outcomes can no longer be checked at an individual level). Because people are commonly not aware of this phenomenon, they cannot form implementation intentions that specify a social loafing situation as a critical situation, thereby rendering an implementation intention that focuses on suppressing the social loafing response as an unviable self-regulatory strategy. As an alternative, people may again resort to forming implementation intentions that stipulate how the intended task is to be performed, thus effectively blocking any negative situational influences.

Supporting this contention, when Endress (2001) performed a social loafing experiment that used a brainstorming task (i.e., participants had to find as many different uses for a common knife as possible), she observed that implementation intentions ("And if I have found one solution, then I will immediately try to find a different solution!"), but not goal intentions ("I will try to find as many different solutions as possible!"), protected participants from social loafing effects. Findings reported by Trötschel and Gollwitzer (2004) also support the notion that goal pursuits planned by forming implementation intentions become invulnerable to adverse situational influences. In their experiments on the self-regulation of negotiation behavior, loss-framed negotiation settings failed to unfold their negative effects on fair and cooperative negotiation outcomes when the negotiators had in advance planned out their goal intentions to be fair and cooperative, with if–then plans. Finally, in further experiments, Gollwitzer (1998) observed that competing goal intentions activated outside of a person's awareness (by using goal-priming procedures described in the first part of this chapter) failed to affect a person's ongoing goal pursuit, if this goal pursuit was planned out in advance via implementation intentions.

It appears, then, that the self-regulatory strategy of planning out goal pursuits in advance via implementation intentions allows the person to reap the desired positive outcomes, without having to change the environment from an adverse to a facilitative one. This is very convenient, because such environmental change is often very cumbersome (e.g., it takes the costly interventions of mediators to change the loss frames adopted by conflicting parties into gain frames), or not under the person's control. Moreover, people are often not aware of the adverse influences of the current environment (e.g., a deindividuated work setting or a loss-framed negotiation setting), or they do not know what alternative kind of environmental setting is actually facilitative (e.g., an individualized work setting or a gain-framed negotiation setting). In such performance situations, the self-regulatory strategy of specifying critical situations in the if part of an implementation intention and linking them to a coping response in the then part does not qualify as a viable alternative self-regulatory strategy. Rather, people need to resort to the strategy of planning out their goal pursuits in advance via implementation intentions, thereby protecting them from adverse situational influences.

Motivation Control

Ideally, people set themselves goals in line with their beliefs that the goal can actually be attained (i.e., goal strength reflects perceived feasibility; Oettingen, 2000; Oettingen, Pak, & Schnetter, 2001). Such beliefs may take the form of high-outcome expectations or more specific high self-efficacy expectations (i.e., beliefs that one possesses what it takes to reach the goal; Bandura, 1997). In any case, a person who has decided to strive for a certain goal on the basis of high expectations should be highly motivated to strive for the chosen goal. Still, one wonders what happens when people run into difficulties in trying to implement the goal. Will they simply adjust their outcome expectations and self-efficacy beliefs downwards, thus losing motivation to strive for the goal? As Kuhl (1984) has pointed out, people can and do push back by keeping up their motivation to pursue the goal at hand (i.e., they engage in motivation control).

Because overcoming the self-doubts originating from difficulties and failures is a rather complex affair for which some people may be better equipped than others (Dweck, 1999; Elliot & Thrash, 2002), Gollwitzer and Bayer (2004) wondered whether the self-regulatory strategy of forming implementation intentions could be used to facilitate such motivation control. In a first experiment, high school students were asked to perform a very challenging math test composed of 10 individual problems. In the mere goal intention condition, the students had to take the test with the assigned goal of excelling on it (i.e., correctly solve a very large number of problems). In the implementation intention condition, participants had to furnish this goal intention with the following if–then plan: "And as soon as I start to work on a new problem, then I tell myself: I can do it!" Even though the mean number of problems solved was very low in the whole sample (i.e., 3.5 problems), implementation intention participants solved significantly more problems (4.3 problems) than mere goal intention participants (2.8 problems). Apparently, the simple plan of assuring themselves of their high self-efficacy when taking on a new, individual problem helped participants to perform well.

In a follow-up experiment, we asked college students to solve a series of Raven Matrices that became increasingly more difficult. We again established a mere goal intention group (i.e., correctly solve a very large number of matrices) and an implementation intention group (i.e., "As soon as I start working on a new matrix, I'll tell myself that I can do it"). In addition, there was also a group of goal intention participants who had to tell themselves right after having received the goal intention instruction that they could meet this goal (i.e., "I can do it!"). As it turned out, only the implementation intention group achieved a superior performance on the test. This finding suggests that again, implementation intentions allow for effective motivation control, and that this is achieved by linking self-assuring statements to distinct critical cues.

Switching to More Effective Means

There is a further self-regulatory problem with successfully moving toward goal attainment: switching to better means when the chosen means turn out to be unproductive (Carver & Scheier, 1999; Gollwitzer, 1990). People often fail readily to disengage from a chosen failing strategy or means because of a strong self-justification motive (Brockner, 1992). Such escalation effects should be reduced effectively, however, by the use of implementation intentions that specify exactly when to switch to a different strategy or means, because action control is then delegated to this specified cue. The self-regulatory strategy of simply setting goals (e.g., to avoid the escalation of commitment by always pursuing the best strategy) should be comparatively less effective, because it demands effortful deliberation of the instrumentality of the chosen strategy or means *in situ* (i.e., when failure experiences are mounting), which—to make things worse—will likely be biased by self-defensiveness.

Henderson, Gollwitzer, and Oettingen (2004, Study 1) tested the hypothesis that furnishing disengagement goals with implementation intentions should help people to relinquish a failing strategy of goal pursuit more effectively. For this purpose, a classic paradigm was used that creates a strong escalation tendency (Bobocel & Meyer, 1994): Participants had to choose and subsequently justify their choice among four different strategies of performing an assigned test measuring an important aptitude (i.e., general academic knowledge). Prior to working on the test with the chosen strategy, participants in the mere goal intention condition repeated the statement, "I will always pursue the best strategy!" Participants in the implementation intention condition repeated this goal intention to themselves, along with the plan, "And if I receive disappointing feedback, then I'll switch to a different strategy!" In line with our expectations that implementation intentions facilitate switching to a different strategy, 19 out of 29 participants (66%) in the goal intention group, and 27 out of 29 participants (93%) in the implementation intention group, disengaged from their initial strategy when false failure feedback was given on participants' quality of test performance.

The Psychological Mechanisms Underlying Implementation Intention Effects

It is assumed (Gollwitzer, 1993) that implementation intentions manage to switch the conscious and effortful mode of the control of goal-directed action to the automatic mode of action control (i.e., direct control by specified internal or external cues). To empirically test such a shift, it does not suffice to show that many of the problems of goal pursuit that are difficult to master by conscious and effortful self-regulation are more easily mastered by forming implementation intentions (as has been extensively demonstrated in the studies reported earlier). One would also like to see experiments that more directly assess whether the action control achieved by implementation intentions does indeed carry features of automaticity: immediate, efficient, and not requiring conscious intent.

Implementation Intentions: The Specified Situation

Swift and efficient responding to the critical situation specified in the if part of an implementation intention implies that this situation is readily attended to and easily detected (Gollwitzer, Bayer, Steller, & Bargh, 2002). One study, using a dichotic-listening paradigm, demonstrated that words describing the anticipated critical situation were highly disruptive to focused attention in implementation intention participants compared to goal intention participants (i.e., the shadowing performance of the focused attention materials decreased). In another study using an embedded figures test (Gottschaldt, 1926), where smaller a-figures are hidden within larger b-figures, enhanced detection of the hidden a-figures was observed with participants who had specified the a-figure in the if part of an implementation intention (i.e., had made plans on how to create a traffic sign from the a-figure). Similarly, Aarts, Dijksterhuis, and Midden (1999) used a lexical decision task and found that the formation of implementation intentions led to subjects' faster lexical decisions for those words that described the critical situation.

Implementation Intentions: The Specified Goal-Directed Behavior

The postulated automation of action initiation has also been supported by the results of various experiments that tested immediacy, efficiency, and the presence–absence of conscious intent. Gollwitzer and Brandstätter (1997, Study 3) demonstrated the immediacy of action initiation in a study in which participants had been induced to form implementation intentions that speci-

fied viable opportunities for presenting counterarguments to a series of racist remarks made by a confederate. Participants with implementation intentions initiated counterarguments sooner than did participants who had formed the mere goal intention to counterargue.

The efficiency of action initiation was further explored in two experiments using a go–no-go task embedded as a secondary task in a dual-task paradigm (Brandtstätter, Lengfelder, & Gollwitzer, 2001, Studies 3 and 4). Participants formed the goal intention to press a button as fast as possible if numbers appeared on the computer screen, but not if letters were presented. Participants in the implementation intention condition additionally made the plan to press the response button particularly fast if the number three was presented. Implementation intention participants showed a substantial increase in speed of responding to the number three compared to the control group, regardless of whether the simultaneously demanded primary task (a memorization task in Study 3 and a tracking task in Study 4) was either easy or difficult to perform. Apparently, the immediacy of responding induced by implementation intentions is also efficient, in the sense that it does not require much in the way of cognitive resources (i.e., can be performed even when demanding dual tasks have to be performed at the same time).

Two experiments by Bayer, Moskowitz, and Gollwitzer (2002) tested whether implementation intentions lead to action initiation even in the absence of conscious intent. In these experiments, the critical situation was presented subliminally, and immediacy of initiation of the goal-directed response was assessed. Results indicated that subliminal presentation of the critical situation led to a speed-up in responding in implementation participants but not in goal intention participants. These effects suggest that, when planned via implementation intentions, the initiation of goal-directed behavior becomes triggered by the presence of the critical situational cue, without the need for further conscious intent.

Additional process mechanisms underlying the effects of implementation intentions on action control have been explored. For instance, furnishing goals with implementation intentions might produce an increase in goal commitment, which in turn cause heightened goal attainment. However, this hypothesis has not received any empirical support. For instance, when Brandstätter et al. (2001, Study 1) analyzed whether heroin addicts suffering from withdrawal would benefit from forming implementation intentions to submit a newly composed curriculum vitae before the end of the day, they also measured participants' commitment to do so. While the majority of the implementation intention participants succeeded in handing in the curriculum vitae in time, none of the goal intention participants succeeded in this task. These two groups, however, did not differ in terms of their goal commitment ("I feel committed to compose a curriculum vitae" and "I have to complete this task") measured after the goal intention and implementation intention instructions had been administered. This finding was replicated with young adults who participated in a professional development workshop (Oettingen et al., 2000, Study 2), and analogous results were reported in research on the effects of implementation intentions on meeting health promotion and disease prevention goals (e.g., Orbell et al., 1997).

Potential Costs of Action Control via Implementation Intentions

Given the many benefits of forming implementation intentions, a question of any possible costs arises. Two issues have been analyzed empirically so far: First, forming implementation intentions may be a very costly self-regulatory strategy if it produces a high degree of ego depletion and consequently handicaps needed self-regulatory resources. Second, even though implementation intentions can successfully suppress unwanted thoughts, feelings, and actions in a given context, these very thoughts, feelings, and actions may rebound in a temporally subsequent, different context.

The assumption that implementation intentions subject behavior to the direct control of situational cues (Gollwitzer, 1993) implies that the self is not implicated when behavior is controlled via implementation intentions. As a consequence, the self should not become depleted when task performance is regulated by implementation intentions.

Indeed, using different ego-depletion paradigms, research participants who used implementation intentions to self-regulate in one task did not show reduced self-regulatory capacity in a subsequent task. Whether the initial self-regulation task was controlling emotions while watching a humorous movie (Gollwitzer & Bayer, 2000) or performing a Stroop task (Webb & Sheeran, 2003, Study 1), implementation intentions successfully preserved self-regulatory resources, as demonstrated by greater persistence on subsequent difficult or unsolvable tasks.

To test whether suppression-oriented implementation intentions create rebound effects, Gollwitzer, Trötschel, and Sumner (2004) ran two experiments using research paradigms developed by Macrae, Bodenhausen, and Jetten (1994). In both studies, participants first had to suppress the expression of stereotypes in a first-impression formation task that focused on a particular member of a stereotyped group (i.e., homeless people). Rebound was measured in terms of either subsequent expression of stereotypes in a task that demanded the evaluation of the group of homeless people in general (Study 1), or a lexical decision task that assessed the accessibility of homeless stereotypes (Study 2). Participants who had been assigned the mere goal of controlling stereotypical thoughts while forming an impression of the given homeless person were more stereotypical in their judgments of homeless people in general (Study 1) and showed a higher accessibility of homeless stereotypes (Study 2) than participants who had been asked to furnish this lofty goal with relevant if–then plans. Rather than causing rebound effects, implementation intentions appear to be effective in preventing them.

Although implementation intentions seem to achieve their effects without much cost, this does not mean that the regulation of goal pursuit via implementation intentions is foolproof. In everyday life, people may not succeed in forming effective implementation intentions for various reasons. For instance, in the if part of an implementation intention, a person may specify an opportunity that hardly ever arises. Or in the then part of an implementation intention, people may falsely specify behaviors that have zero instrumentality with respect to reaching the goal, or behaviors that turn out to be out-side of people's control.

There is also the question of how con-cretely people should specify the if and then parts in their implementation intentions. If the goal is to perform well on a given task goal, one can form an implementation inten-tion that holds either this very behavior in the then part or a more concrete operation-alization of it. The latter seems appropriate whenever a whole array of specific opera-tionalizations is possible, because planning in advance which type of goal-directed behavior is to be executed, once the situa-tion specified in the if part of the implemen-tation intention is encountered, prevents dis-ruptive deliberation *in situ* (with respect to choosing one behavioral strategy over an-other). An analogous argument applies to the specification of situations in the if part of an implementation intention. People should specify the situation in the if part to such a degree that a given situation will no longer raise the question of whether it quali-fies as the critical situation. Finally, simply concretizing a goal intention by putting more context-related information into the description of the desired behavior (e.g., "I will solve math problems at my desk each Wednesday at 10 P.M.!") will not achieve the same beneficial action control effects as a goal intention ("I will solve math prob-lems!") that is furnished with a implementa-tion intention ("And if it is 10 P.M. on Wednesday, then I will sit down at my desk!"; Oettingen et al., Study 3).

Summary of Research on Automating Goal Pursuit by Forming Implementation Intentions

The benefits of the self-regulation strategy of forming implementation intentions is evi-dent in the numerous studies documenting the effects of implementation intentions in helping people overcome the various problems of goal pursuit. Whether getting started, staying on track in the face of interferences, holding up motivation, or switching to more effective means, research participants who formed implementation in-tentions were better in solving these prob-lems than research participants who oper-ated on the basis of mere goal intentions. This research also indicates that people may

want to adjust the type of implementation intention formed to the self-regulation prob-lem at hand. For instance, while suppres-sion-oriented implementation intentions are viable when certain distractions, tempta-tions, and unwanted responses are antici-pated, plans that bolster the ongoing goal pursuit are needed in situations in which goal pursuit is threatened by detrimental self-states and adverse situational influences of which the individual is not aware.

Research on the potential costs of using implementation intentions indicates that they do not drain self-regulatory resources (i.e., produce ego depletion), and suppres-sion-oriented implementation intentions are not associated with rebound. Thus, forming implementation intentions suggests itself as an effective and quite cost-free self-regula-tory strategy of goal pursuit; people can achieve strong effects by making simple plans.

CONCLUSIONS

The idea of unconscious motivation has a long intellectual history but has only re-cently become integrated into mainstream psychological science. Theoretical advances in cognitive psychology over the past quar-ter-century have made the notion of uncon-scious motivation much more plausible than before, enabling researchers to generate models of unconscious motivational influ-ences that are in harmony with basic cogni-tive principles. By thinking about goals as another form of mental representation, sub-ject to the same rules and principles as are known to hold for other mental representa-tions, researchers have established the effects of unconsciously operating information-pro-cessing, achievement, and interpersonal goals. And by testing the effects of making if–then plans (i.e., forming implementation intentions that specify an anticipated critical situation and link it to an instrumental goal-directed response) on overcoming classic problems of goal pursuit, researchers have discovered that people may strategically (i.e., by a conscious act of will) automate their goal pursuits by setting up action plans in advance.

All of this implies that competent perfor-mances may come about not only by conscious goal setting and conscious guidance of the respective goal pursuits but also by relying on the automatic activation and pursuit of goals one has been striving for in the past. And if people cannot fall back on such positive past experiences, there is still the option of automating goal pursuit strategically by preparing it ahead of time in the form of making if–then plans.

ACKNOWLEDGMENTS

Preparation of this chapter was supported by National Institutes of Health Grant No. R01-60767 to John A. Bargh and National Institutes of Health Grant No. R01-67100 to Peter M. Gollwitzer. The collaboration of the two authors was facilitated by the Interdisciplinary Center for Research on Intentions and Intentionality at the University of Konstanz.

REFERENCES

Aarts, H., Dijksterhuis, A., & Midden, C. (1999). To plan or not to plan? Goal achievement or interrupting the performance of mundane behaviors. *European Journal of Social Psychology, 29,* 971–979.

Aarts, H., Gollwitzer, P. M., & Hassin, R. R. (2004). Goal contagion: Perceiving is for pursuing. *Journal of Personality and Social Psychology, 87,* 23–37.

Ajzen, I. (1991). The theory of planned behavior. *Organizational Behavior and Human Decision Processes, 50,* 179–211.

Allport, G. W. (1955). *The nature of prejudice.* Cambridge, MA: Addison-Wesley.

Anderson, R. C., & Pichert, J. W. (1978). Recall of uncontrollable information following a shift in perspective. *Journal of Verbal Learning and Verbal Behavior, 17,* 1–12.

Atkinson, J. W. (1957). Motivational determinants of risk-taking behavior. *Psychological Review, 64,* 359–372.

Atkinson, J. W., & Birch, D. (1970). *A dynamic theory of action.* Cambridge, MA: Harvard University Press.

Bandura, A. (1986). *Social foundation of thought and action: A social cognitive theory.* Englewood Cliffs, NJ: Prentice-Hall.

Bandura, A. (1997). *Self-efficacy: The exercise of control.* New York: Freeman.

Bargh, J. A. (1989). Conditional automaticity: Varieties of automatic influence in social perception and cognition. In J. S. Uleman & J. A. Bargh (Eds.), *Unintended thought* (pp. 3–51). New York: Guilford Press.

Bargh, J. A. (1990). Auto-motives: Preconscious determinants of social interaction. In E. T. Higgins & R.

M. Sorrentino (Eds.), *Handbook of motivation and cognition* (Vol. 2, pp. 93–130). New York: Guilford Press.

Bargh, J. A. (1994). The four horseman of automaticity: Awareness, efficiency, intention, and control in social cognition. In R. S. Wyer, Jr. & T. K. Srull (Eds.), *Handbook of social cognition* (2nd ed., pp. 1–40). Hillsdale, NJ: Erlbaum.

Bargh, J. A. (1997). The automaticity of everyday life. In R. S. Wyer, Jr. (Ed.), *The automaticity of everyday life: Advances in social cognition* (Vol. 10, pp. 1–61). Mahwah, NJ: Erlbaum.

Bargh, J. A., & Chartrand, T. L. (1999). The unbearable automaticity of being. *American Psychologist, 54,* 462–479.

Bargh, J. A., & Chartrand, T. L. (2000). The mind in the middle: A practical guide to priming and automaticity research. In H. T. Reis & C. M. Judd (Eds.), *Handbook of research methods in social and personality psychology* (pp. 253–285). New York: Cambridge University Press.

Bargh, J. A., & Gollwitzer, P. M. (1994). Environmental control of goal-directed action: Automatic and strategic contingencies between situations and behavior. In W. Spaulding (Ed.), *Nebraska Symposium on Motivation* (Vol. 41, pp. 71–124). Lincoln: University of Nebraska Press.

Bargh, J. A., Gollwitzer, P. M., Lee-Chai, A., Barndollar, K., & Trötschel, R. (2001). The automated will: Nonconscious activation and pursuit of behavioral goals. *Journal of Personality and Social Psychology, 81,* 1014–1027.

Bargh, J. A., Raymond, P., Pryor, J., & Strack, F. (1995). Attractiveness of the underling: An automatic power–sex association and its consequences for sexual harassment and aggression. *Journal of Personality and Social Psychology, 68,* 768–781.

Baumeister, R. F. (2000). Ego-depletion and the self's executive function. In A. Tesser, R. B. Felson, & J. M. Suls (Eds.), *Psychological perspectives on self and identity* (pp. 9–33). Washington, DC: American Psychological Association.

Baumeister, R. F., Heatherton, T. F., & Tice, D. M. (1994). *Losing control: How and why people fail at self-regulation.* San Diego: Academic Press.

Bayer, U. C., Moskowitz, G. B., & Gollwitzer, P. M. (2002). *Implementation intentions and action initiation without conscious intent.* Unpublished manuscript, University of Konstanz, Germany.

Bless, H., & Fiedler, K. (1995). Affective states and the influence of activated general knowledge. *Personality and Social Psychology Bulletin, 21,* 766–778.

Bobocel, R. D., & Meyer, J. P. (1994). Escalating commitment to a failing course of action: Separating the roles of choice and justification. *Journal of Applied Psychology, 79,* 360–363.

Brandstätter, V., Lengfelder, A., & Gollwitzer, P. M. (2001). Implementation intentions and efficient action initiation. *Journal of Personality and Social Psychology, 81,* 946–960.

Brewer, M. (1988). A dual process theory of impression formation. In T. K. Srull & R. S. Wyer (Eds.), *Advances in social cognition* (Vol. 1, pp. 1–36). Hillsdale, NJ: Erlbaum.

Broadbent, D. (1958). *Perception and communication.* London: Pergamon Press.

Brockner, J. (1992). The escalation of commitment to a failing course of action: Toward theoretical progress. *Academy of Management Review, 17,* 39–61.

Bruner, J. S. (1957). On perceptual readiness. *Psychological Review, 64,* 123–152.

Carver, C. S., & Scheier, M. F. (1999). Themes and issues in the self-regulation of behavior. In R. S. Wyer, Jr. (Ed.), *Advances in social cognition* (Vol. 12, pp. 1–105). Mahwah, NJ: Erlbaum.

Chartrand, T. L. (1999). *Mystery moods and perplexing performance: Consequences of succeeding and failing at a nonconscious goal.* Unpublished dissertation, New York University, New York City.

Chartrand, T. L., & Bargh, J. A. (1996). Automatic activation of impression formation and memorization goals: Nonconscious goal priming reproduces effects of explicit task instructions. *Journal of Personality and Social Psychology, 71,* 464–478.

Chartrand, T. L., & Bargh, J. A. (2002). Nonconscious motivations: Their activation, operation, and consequences. In A. Tesser, D. Stapel, & J. Wood (Eds.), *Self and motivation: Emerging psychological perspectives* (pp. 13–41). Washington, DC: American Psychological Association Press.

Chasteen, A. L., Park, D. C., & Schwarz, N. (2001). Implementation intentions and facilitation of prospective memory. *Psychological Science, 12,* 457–461.

Chen, S., Lee-Chai, A. Y., & Bargh, J. A. (2001). Relationship orientation as a moderator of the effects of social power. *Journal of Personality and Social Psychology, 80,* 173–187.

Dholakia, U. M., & Bagozzi, R. P. (2003). As time goes by: How goal and implementation intentions influence enactment of short-fuse behaviors. *Journal of Applied Social Psychology, 33,* 889–922.

Dweck, C. S. (1999). *Self-theories: Their role in motivation, personality, and development.* Philadelphia: Psychology Press.

Einstein, G. O., & McDaniel, M. A. (1996). Retrieval processes in prospective memory: Theoretical approaches and some new empirical findings. In M. Bradimonte, G. O. Einstein, & M. A. McDaniel (Eds.), *Prospective memory: Theory and applications* (pp. 115–141). Mahwah, NJ: Erlbaum.

Elliot, A. J., & Thrash, T. M. (2002). Approach–avoidance motivation in personality: Approach–avoidance temperaments and goals. *Journal of Personality and Social Psychology, 82,* 804–818.

Endress, H. (2001). *Die Wirksamkeit von Vorsätzen auf Gruppenleistungen. Eine empirische Untersuchung anhand von brainstorming* [Implementation intentions and the reduction of social loafing in a brainstorming task]. Unpublished MA thesis, University of Konstanz, Germany.

Erdelyi, M. H. (1974). A new look at the New Look: Perceptual defense and vigilance. *Psychological Review, 81,* 1–25.

Fazio, R. H. (1986). How do attitudes guide behavior? In R. M. Sorrentino & E. T. Higgins (Eds.), *Handbook of motivation and social cognition* (Vol. 1, pp. 204–243). New York: Guilford Press.

Fishbein, M., & Ajzen, I. (1975). *Belief, attitude, intention, and behavior: An introduction to theory and research.* Reading, MA: Addison-Wesley.

Fitzsimons, G. M., & Bargh, J. A. (2003). Thinking of you: Nonconscious pursuit of interpersonal goals associated with relationship partners. *Journal of Personality and Social Psychology, 84,* 148–164.

Godin, G., & Kok, G. (1996). The theory of planned behavior: A review of its applications in health-related behaviors. *American Journal of Health Promotion, 11,* 87–98.

Gollwitzer, P. M. (1990). Action phases and mind-sets. In E. T. Higgins & R. M. Sorrentino (Eds.), *The handbook of motivation and cognition* (Vol. 2, pp. 53–92). New York: Guilford Press.

Gollwitzer, P. M. (1993). Goal achievement: The role of intentions. *European Review of Social Psychology, 4,* 141–185.

Gollwitzer, P. M. (1996). The volitional benefits of planning. In P. M. Gollwitzer & J. A. Bargh (Eds.), *The psychology of action: Linking cognition and motivation to behavior* (pp. 287–312). New York: Guilford Press.

Gollwitzer, P. M. (1998, October). *Implicit and explicit processes in goal pursuit.* Paper presented at the Symposium, Implicit vs. Explicit Processes, at the Annual Meeting of the Society of Experimental Social Psychology. Atlanta, GA.

Gollwitzer, P. M. (1999). Implementation intentions: Strong effects of simple plans. *American Psychologist, 54,* 493–503.

Gollwitzer, P. M., & Bayer, U. C. (2000, October). *Becoming a better person without changing the self.* Paper presented at the Self and Identity Preconference of the Annual Meeting of the Society of Experimental Social Psychology, Atlanta, GA.

Gollwitzer, P. M., & Bayer, U. C. (2004). *Reducing self-doubts by implementation intentions.* Unpublished manuscript, University of Konstanz, Germany.

Gollwitzer, P. M., Bayer, U. C., & McCulloch, K. C. (2005). The control of the unwanted. In R. Hassin, J. Uleman, & J. A. Baugh (Eds.), *The new unconscious* (pp. 485–515). Oxford: Oxford University Press.

Gollwitzer, P. M., Bayer, U. C., Steller, B., & Bargh, J. A. (2002). *Delegating control to the environment: Perception, attention, and memory for pre-selected behavioral cues.* Unpublished manuscript, University of Konstanz, Germany.

Gollwitzer, P. M., & Brandstätter, V. (1997). Implementation intentions and effective goal pursuit. *Journal of Personality and Social Psychology, 73,* 186–199.

Gollwitzer, P. M., & Moskowitz, G. B. (1996). Goal effects on action and cognition. In E. T. Higgins & A. W. Kruglanski (Eds.), *Social psychology: Handbook of basic principles* (pp. 361–399). New York: Guilford Press.

Gollwitzer, P. M., & Schaal, B. (1998). Metacognition in action: The importance of implementation intentions. *Personality and Social Psychology Review, 2,* 124–136.

Gollwitzer, P. M., Trötschel, R., & Sumner, M. (2004). *Mental control via implementation intentions is void of rebound effects.* Unpublished manuscript, University of Konstanz, Germany.

Gollwitzer, P. M., & Wicklund, R. A. (1985). Self-symbolizing and the neglect of others' perspectives. *Journal of Personality and Social Psychology, 56,* 531–715.

Gottschaldt, K. (1926). Über den Einfluß der Erfahrung auf die Wahrnehmung von Figuren [On the effects of familiarity on the perception of figures]. *Psychologische Forschung, 8,* 261–317.

Hamilton, D. L., Katz, L. B., & Leirer, V. O. (1980). Organizational processes in impression formation. In R. Hastie, T. M. Ostrom, E. B. Ebbesen, R. S. Wyer, D. L. Hamilton, & D. E. Carlston (Eds.), *Person memory: The cognitive biases of social perception* (pp. 121–153). Hillsdale, NJ: Erlbaum.

Hebb, D. O. (1948). *Organization of behavior.* New York: Wiley.

Heckhausen, H. (1977). Achievement motivation and its constructs: A cognitive model. *Motivation and Emotion, 4,* 283–329.

Henderson, M. D., Gollwitzer, P. M., & Oettingen, G. (2004). *Implementation intentions and disengagement from a failing course of action.* Manuscript submitted for publication.

Higgins, E. T., Bargh, J. A., & Lombardi, W. (1985). The nature of priming effects on categorization. *Journal of Experimental Psychology: Learning, Memory, and Cognition, 11,* 59–69.

Holmes, D. S. (1968). Dimensions of projection. *Psychological Bulletin, 69,* 248–268.

Holmes, D. S. (1978). Projection as a defense mechanism. *Psychological Bulletin, 85,* 677–688.

Kawada, C. L. K., Oettingen, G., Gollwitzer, P. M., & Bargh, J. A. (2004). The projection of implicit and explicit goals. *Journal of Personality and Social Psychology, 86,* 545–559.

Kruglanski, A. W. (1996). Goals as knowledge structures. In P. M. Gollwitzer & J. A. Bargh (Eds.), *The psychology of action* (pp. 599–618). New York: Guilford Press.

Kuhl, J. (1984). Volitional aspects of achievement motivation and learned helplessness: Toward a comprehensive theory of action control. In B. A. Maher & W. A. Maher (Eds.), *Progress in experimental personality research* (Vol. 13, pp. 99–171). New York: Academic Press.

Lachman, R., Lachman, J., & Butterfield, E. C. (1979). *Cognitive psychology and information processing: An introduction.* Hillsdale, NJ: Erlbaum.

Lengfelder, A., & Gollwitzer, P. M. (2001). Reflective and reflexive action control in patients with frontal brain lesions. *Neuropsychology, 15,* 80–100.

Lewin, K. (1935). *A dynamic theory of personality.* New York: McGraw-Hill.

Locke, E. A., & Latham, G. P. (1990). *A theory of goal setting and task performance.* Englewood Cliffs, NJ: Prentice-Hall.

Loewenstein, G. F., Weber, E. U., Hsee, C. K., & Welch, N. (2001). Risks as feelings. *Psychological Bulletin, 127,* 267–286.

Macrae, C. N., Bodenhausen, G. V., Milne, A. B., & Jetten, J. (1994). Out of mind but back in sight: Stereotypes on the rebound. *Journal of Personality and Social Psychology, 67,* 808–817.

McClelland, D. C. (1985). How motives, skills, and values determine what people do. *American Psychologist, 41,* 812–825.

Metcalfe, J., & Mischel, W. (1999). A hot/cool-system analysis of delay of gratification: Dynamics of willpower. *Psychological Bulletin, 106,* 3–19.

Milne, S., Orbell, S., & Sheeran, P. (2002). Combining motivational and volitional interventions to promote exercise participation: Protection motivation theory and implementation intentions. *British Journal of Health Psychology, 7,* 163–184.

Mischel, W. (1996). From good intentions to willpower. In P. M. Gollwitzer & J. A. Bargh (Eds.), *The psychology of action* (pp. 197–218). New York: Guilford Press.

Mischel, W., Cantor, N., & Feldman, S. (1996). Goal-directed self-regulation. In E. T. Higgins & A. W. Kruglanski (Eds.), *Social psychology: Handbook of basic principles* (pp. 329–360). New York: Guilford Press.

Muraven, M., Tice, D. M., & Baumeister, R. F. (1998). Self-control as a limited resource: Regulatory depletion pattern. *Journal of Personality and Social Psychology, 74,* 774–789.

Neisser, U. (1967). *Cognitive psychology.* New York: Appleton–Century–Crofts.

Nisbett, R. E., & Ross, L. (1980). *Human inference: Strategies and shortcomings of social judgment.* Englewood Cliffs, NJ: Prentice-Hall.

Oettingen, G. (2000). Expectancy effects on behavior depend on self-regulatory thought. *Social Cognition, 18,* 101–129.

Oettingen, G., & Gollwitzer, P. M. (2001). Goal setting and goal striving. In M. Hewstone & M. Brewer (Editors-in-chief) A. Tesser & N. Schwarz (Eds.), *Blackwell handbook in social psychology: Vol. 1. Intraindividual processes* (pp. 329–347). Oxford: Blackwell.

Oettingen, G., Hönig, G., & Gollwitzer, P. M. (2000). Effective self-regulation of goal attainment. *International Journal of Educational Research, 33,* 705–732.

Oettingen, G., Pak, H., & Schnetter, K. (2001). Self-regulation of goal setting: Turning free fantasies about the future into binding goals. *Journal of Personality and Social Psychology, 80,* 736–753.

Orbell, S., Hodgkins, S., & Sheeran, P. (1997). Implementation intentions and the theory of planned behavior. *Personality and Social Psychology Bulletin, 23*, 945–954.

Orbell, S., & Sheeran, P. (1998). "Inclined abstainers": A problem for predicting health-related behavior. *British Journal of Social Psychology, 37*, 151–165.

Orbell, S., & Sheeran, P. (2000). Motivational and volitional processes in action initiation: A field study of the role of implementation intentions. *Journal of Applied Social Psychology, 30*, 780–797.

Sheeran, P. (2002). Intention-behavior relations: A conceptual and empirical review. *European Review of Social Psychology, 12*, 1–30.

Sheeran, P., & Orbell, S. (1998). Do intentions predict condom use?: A meta-analysis and examination of six moderator variables. *British Journal of Social Psychology, 37*, 231–250.

Sheeran, P., & Orbell, S. (1999). Implementation intentions and repeated behavior: Augmenting the predictive validity of the theory of planned behavior. *European Journal of Social Psychology, 29*, 349–369.

Sheeran, P., & Orbell, S. (2000). Using implementation intentions to increase attendance for cervical cancer screening. *Health Psychology, 19*, 283–289.

Srull, T. K., & Wyer, R. S., Jr. (1979). The role of category accessibility in the interpretation of information about persons: Some determinants and implications. *Journal of Personality and Social Psychology, 37*, 1660–1672.

Srull, T. K., & Wyer, R. S., Jr. (1986). The role of chronic and temporary goals in social information processing. In R. M. Sorrentino & E. T. Higgins (Eds.), *Handbook of motivation and cognition* (Vol. 1, pp. 503–549). New York: Guilford Press.

Trafimow, D., & Sheeran, P. (in press). A theory of the translation of cognition into affect and behavior. In G. Haddock & G. R. O. Maio (Eds.), *Perspectives on attitudes for the 121st century: The Cardiff Symposium*. London: Psychology Press.

Trötschel, R., & Gollwitzer, P. M. (2004). *Implementation intentions and the control of framing effects in negotiations*. Manuscript submitted for publication.

Uleman, J. S., Newman, L. S., & Moskowitz, G. B. (1996). People as spontaneous interpreters: Evidence and issues from spontaneous trait inference. In M. P. Zanna (Ed.), *Advances in experimental social psychology* (Vol. 28, pp. 211–279). San Diego: Academic Press.

Webb, T. L., & Sheeran, P. (2003). Can implementation intentions help to overcome ego-depletion? *Journal of Experimental Social Psychology, 39*, 279–286.

Wegner, D. M., & Bargh, J. A. (1997). Control and automaticity in social life. In D. Gilbert, S. Fiske, & G. Lindzey (Eds.), *Handbook of social psychology* (4th ed., Vol. I, pp. 446–496). Boston: McGraw-Hill.

Wicklund, R. A., & Gollwitzer, P. M. (1982). *Symbolic self-completion*. Hillsdale, NJ: Erlbaum.

Wilson, T. D., & Brekke, N. C. (1994). Mental contamination and mental correction: Unwanted influences on judgments and evaluation. *Psychological Bulletin, 116*, 117–142.

CHAPTER 35

Cℛ

Fantasies and the Self-Regulation of Competence

GABRIELE OETTINGEN
MEIKE HAGENAH

Competence may be studied not only in terms of whether people behave in competent ways when solving certain problems (e.g., academic, professional, and social), but also in terms of how they think and feel about their competencies. Such subjective or perceived competence has predominantly been conceptualized as beliefs or expectations. Examples are efficacy expectations (Bandura, 1977, 1997), competence expectancies (Elliot & Church, 1997), agency beliefs (Little, Oettingen, Stetsenko, & Baltes, 1995; Oettingen, Little, Lindenberger, & Baltes, 1994; Skinner, Chapman, & Baltes, 1988), control beliefs (Skinner, Wellborn, & Connell, 1990), perceived control (Skinner, 1996), and control appraisals (Jensen & Karoly, 1991). Construing perceived competence as beliefs or expectations, however, ignores that people conceive of their competencies also in other forms of thought. In this chapter, we focus on such other forms of thought in the form of fantasies and daydreams about the future, in which people

mentally depict themselves solving given problems in a competent way. We investigate people's daydreams and fantasies about how wonderful it will be to have realized their competencies, and how gloriously they will behave on the way to attaining such positive outcomes.

Fantasies about future competencies should have different motivational consequences than competence beliefs and expectations. In the first part of the chapter, we analyze perceived competence in terms of expectations of the future on the one hand, and in terms of daydreams and fantasies about the future on the other. We show that the motivational impact of competence expectations dramatically differs from that of competence fantasies. Specifically, competence expectations facilitate motivation and successful performance, whereas competence fantasies turn out to be an impediment. However, competence fantasies do not always hurt motivation. When they are mentally contrasted with the reality that stands in the way of attaining them, they merge with competence expectations to result in binding competence goals with subsequent goal striving and goal attainment. Experimental studies support these ideas in various life domains (academic, professional, and interpersonal). They also attest to the benefits of the mental contrasting procedure under critical conditions, such as when people are confronted with strong negative feedback or need to perform in front of a highly evaluative audience.

SUBJECTIVE COMPETENCE: EXPECTATIONS VERSUS FANTASIES

Competence Expectations

Subjective competence has been conceptualized as competence beliefs or competence expectations. These are judgments about one's present or future competencies that are based on past behavior. Expectations are thus informed by one's experiences and thereby represent a person's performance history (Bandura, 1977, 1997; Mischel, 1973; Mischel, Cantor, & Feldman, 1996; Olson, Roese, & Zanna, 1996). Observed performances of others, persuasive messages received by respected others, and experienced levels of arousal during performance are also known to influence expectations (Bandura, 1977, 1997; Bandura & Locke, 2003).

The content of competence beliefs and expectations depends on the content of the objective competence on which the person is focusing. Objective competence in turn may be described by successful learning (Schunk, 1989), by achieving high grades and test scores, or simply by demonstrating a strong performance on a given task (Elliot & McGregor, 2001; Pajares & Miller, 1994; Shell, Colvin, & Bruning, 1995). Finally, both subjective and objective competence may be conceived in terms of how they are anchored (i.e., defined in absolute, intrapersonal, or normative standards; Butler, 1998; Elliot & McGregor, 2001; Rheinberg, 1998; Ruble & Frey, 1991), their regulatory focus (i.e., promotion vs. prevention; Higgins, 1997), their valence and means by which they are approached (i.e., framed as success vs. failure and as approach vs. avoid-

ance; Atkinson, 1957; Elliot & McGregor, 2001; Elliot & Thrash, 2002; McClelland, 1980; Murray, 1938), and in terms of the strategies used to achieve them (eager vs. vigilant strategies; Higgins, Idson, Freitas, Spiegel, & Molden, 2003).

Because high-competence beliefs are based on successful performance in the past, on observational learning, and on persuasion by informed sources, they can be taken as a valid signal that behavioral investment will pay off in the future. Thus, it comes as no surprise that investigations of the predictive value of high-subjective competence in the form of beliefs or expectations have yielded a large number of findings consistently pointing in the same direction: High-subjective competence predicts strong behavioral investment and, thus, the accumulation of objective competence. These findings hold true (Lent, Brown, & Hackett, 1994; see meta-analysis by Multon, Brown, & Lent, 1991) whether competence expectations are operationalized as self-efficacy beliefs (beliefs on whether one can implement a specific behavior necessary for a specified desired outcome; Bandura, 1997; Pietsch, Walker, & Chapman, 2003; Schunk, 1989) or as more global agency or control beliefs (beliefs on whether one generally behaves in a way that leads to desired outcomes; Little et al., 1995; Oettingen et al., 1994; Skinner et al., 1988). Strongest relations between subjective and objective competence have been observed when both variables match in level of specificity (Lent, Brown, & Gore, 1997).

Findings that attest to the predictive power of competence expectations not just amass for academic and professional achievement. Positive competence expectations predict objective competence also in the athletic and in the health domains (McAuley, 1985, 1993). High-competence expectations facilitate the initiation and maintenance of health-promoting and disease-preventing behaviors (McAuley, 1993; Wilcox & Storandt, 1996), warding off health damaging and risky activities (O'Leary, 2001), and recovery after surgery (Scheier et al., 2003). In addition, by increasing objective competence, competence expectations have benefited further variables such as mental health (Bandura, Pastorelli,

Barbaranelli, & Carprara, 1999) and well-being (Christensen, Stephens, & Townsend, 1998; Lachman & Weaver, 1998).

Competence Fantasies

Subjective competence, however, does not need to be conceptualized in the form of beliefs or expectations. As noted earlier, competence might occupy our thoughts also in the form of mental images or fantasies. Beliefs and images were first distinguished by William James (1890/1950, Vol. I): "Everyone knows the difference between imagining a thing and believing in its existence, between supposing a proposition and acquiescing in its truth" (p. 283). James's differentiation between believing and imagining pertains to events of the past and present. Following his reasoning, we differentiate two kinds of thinking about the future: expectancy judgments (beliefs) that assess the probability of occurrence of future events (behaviors and outcomes), and fantasies (images) that depict such future events per se. Consequently, positive competence expectations are beliefs that a desired competence is likely to be reached; positive competence fantasies about the future, to the contrary, are positively experienced images of future competencies that emerge in the stream of thought.

In such fantasies about the future, people can embellish events and scenarios regarding their own competencies regardless of their past behavior and performance, and regardless of how likely it is that they will ever attain these competencies. People might see themselves as Harry Potter on the broom, as elegant figure skaters spinning pirouettes and getting ready for high jumps, as speaking Chinese fluently, or as being celebrated for having authored a brilliant play. People usually know very well that these fantasies are disconnected from what they believe will come true, and that the chances of successfully obtaining these futures are minute.

Glorious competence fantasies, however, might not necessarily come in the form of such *Zauberdenken* (i.e., thoughts depicting actions and events that violate natural laws or social norms; Lewin, 1926; Mahler, 1933). People also fantasize about not yet realized but principally possible competen-

cies. For example, they may fantasize of their competence to combine work and family life, to attain a longed for job, to regularly practice health behavior, or to shake off the squeeze of time. In this sense, fantasies are similar to daydreams (i.e., thoughts pertaining to immediate or delayed desires, including instrumental activities to attain the desired outcomes; Klinger, 1971). However, even if daydreams or fantasies about one's future competencies obey natural and social laws, they still can be disconnected from expectations or probabilities of successfully reaching these competencies, due to the fact that daydreams and fantasies are not constrained by the cognitive mechanisms that make people appraise factual information (Klinger, 1971, 1990; Singer, 1966). In short, people can experience future blessings in their fantasies, without considering the probabilities that these blessings will actually occur.

THE MOTIVATIONAL FUNCTION OF SUBJECTIVE COMPETENCE: EXPECTATIONS VERSUS FANTASIES

Competence expectations, by applying past facts to predict future events (Bandura, 1977; Mischel, 1973), promise that future investment is worthwhile. To the contrary, competence fantasies fail to be a valid signpost for action. Rather, they tempt the person to mentally enjoy desired competencies in the present moment, concealing the necessity to still realize them in actuality. Therefore, fantasizing about one's future competencies should trigger little motivation to actually attain the mentally enjoyed abilities. Moreover, fantasies about a trouble-free path to accumulate competencies should hinder the preparation for upcoming obstacles and the hammering out of effective plans specifying how to overcome such obstacles. Lacking preparatory action and careful planning should further compromise motivation and attaining objective competence.

Positive competence fantasies may focus on having successfully achieved competence, moving smoothly toward achieving it, or both. Regardless of whether such competence fantasies are outcome- or process-based, they should produce little motivation and weak performance. If, however, individuals question a future of unlimited competence and its smooth attainment, the desired future should no longer be experienced as merely enjoyable but as something to be achieved in actuality. People can now lay out the road to achieving competence successfully, prepare for setbacks and hindrances, exert effort, and show persistence. In summary, whereas positive expectations about future competence should predict effortful action and the achievement of objective competence, positive fantasies should predict the reverse.

The following two studies test this idea of a differential relation between competence expectations and competence fantasies, and actually achieved competence. In each study, we assessed competence expectations and competence fantasies at least 1 week before we measured effort and success in building objective competence. We operationalized competence expectations by the perceived probability of building competence, and we measured competence fantasies by using idiographic techniques tapping participants' thoughts and images about their achieving respective competencies in the future.

Building Academic Competence

Right before their midterm examination, college students enrolled in an introductory psychology class were asked to indicate the grade they would like to obtain in the course. To measure expectations, we asked participants to indicate the likelihood that they would actually receive this course grade (Oettingen & Mayer, 2002; Study 3). We then assessed their course grade-related fantasies. Participants completed a scenario in writing that depicted them as already having taken all the exams and being on their way to the building in which the course grades are posted. Immediately thereafter, participants rated the experienced positivity–negativity of the reported thoughts and images. Objectively achieved competence was measured by the change of course grades from the midterm (when expectations and fantasies were assessed) to the final exam.

Previous research has amply documented that high competence expectations build ac-

ademic competence. This is true for students of different ages and educational backgrounds, and with respect to a variety of indicators (e.g., standardized tests, course grades, solving intellectual tasks, application of learning strategies; Lent et al., 1997; Schunk, 1982, 1989; Zimmerman & Martinez-Pons, 1992; see summaries by Bandura, 1997; Multon et al., 1991). The predictive power of positive fantasies for achieving academic competence, however, has not been analyzed. Following the ideas presented earlier, we hypothesized and observed that students entertaining positive competence expectations put in much study effort and achieved comparatively well, while students entertaining positive competence fantasies failed to study hard and achieved comparatively low course grades from the midterm to the final exam.

The predictive relation between positive fantasy and low performance was mediated by a lack of effort, as measured by the number of hours students had spent studying, by their reported study effort, and by the amount of extracredit work they had been handing in between their midterm and their final exam. Thus, positive fantasies led to less studying than more negatively toned fantasies, and this in turn produced lower levels of objective competence, as measured by course grades.

This study investigated the role of expectations versus fantasies in building intellectual competence. In the next study, we addressed the role of the two ways of thinking about the future in building physical competence (Oettingen & Mayer, 2002, Study 4). The building of physical competence becomes a particularly pressing concern when frailty sets in, that is, in older adulthood.

Building Physical Competence

Participants in our study were older adults admitted to a hospital to undergo total-hip-replacement surgery, which is a commonly performed surgery in patients with osteoarthritis of the hip, the most frequent joint disorder and a particular problem in the elderly (Gogia, Christensen, & Schmidt, 1994). In surgery, affected bone and cartilage are removed and replaced with an artificial joint made from metal and plastic. Functional disability and pain in the absence of primary and secondary preventive measures are the two predominant indications for total-hip-replacement surgery (Verbrugge, 1990).

The day before surgery, we assessed participants' expectations and fantasies regarding their future physical competence. Two exemplary items measured expectations: "How likely do you think it is, that 2 weeks after surgery you will be able to go for a brief walk using an assistive cane?" and "How functionally able do you think will you be 3 months after surgery?" To assess competence fantasies, we asked participants to imagine in writing five scenarios to their completion, and then to rate their own thoughts and images. The scenarios pertained to various points in time after surgery (i.e., immediately after, end of hospital stay, and 3 months later). For example, one of the scenarios read: "At the end of your hospital stay, you want to buy a newspaper in the hospital's newspaper stand. As you are getting out of bed . . . " After imagining a story to completion and writing down the respective thoughts and images, participants indicated how positively and how negatively they had experienced their thoughts and images. As a response to the scenario just described, one participant fantasized: "I am walking on the stairways without help, and I walk easily and quickly to the newspaper stand." However, another participant imagined herself as less competent: "I am trying to walk to the door first, using my cane. But how shall I open the door? Uh, and then walking to the elevator? How will I ever get there?"

Two weeks after surgery, while participants were still in the hospital, each physical therapist mainly responsible for a particular patient indicated the functional status of that patient's hip (Gogia et al., 1994). Physical therapists used classic indicators, such as degree of hip joint motion (i.e., abduction, extension, and flexion) and competence to walk on stairs (Dekker, Boot, van der Woude, & Bijlsma, 1992). In addition, they evaluated patients' general recovery (e.g., in terms of muscular strength and degree of pain).

Competence expectations and competence fantasies differentially predicted actually achieved competence also in the physical domain. While competence expectations were precursors of objective competence, competence fantasies were a hindrance, and this was true whether patients' physical competence was measured via specific criteria (i.e., hip joint motion or walking on stairs) or via more general measures (i.e., general recovery). These findings stayed unchanged after controlling for presurgery hip condition (as assessed by the doctors), weight (70% of the sample was overweight), and gender.

Subsequent content analyses of the patients' fantasies revealed that participants had idealized their future physical competence with respect to both outcome (they imagined possessing or having achieved competence) and process (they imagined an easy and effortless way to achieve competence). Though idealization of outcome was more frequent than idealization of process, both were positively related to the subjective measure of the positivity of competence fantasies. Thus, positively experienced fantasies contain both outcome and process in its idealized form, that is, the possession of high competence, as well as effortless and unencumbered progress toward attaining competence. Most importantly, however, it was the subjectively experienced competence fantasies rather than the expressed idealization, as picked up by the raters, that predicted low objective competence (i.e., functional status of the hip and successful recovery). This finding implies that the personal affective involvement in the created fantasies produces their motivational and performance consequences.

Process Simulations and Illusory Optimism

The previous studies support the notion that positive fantasies about future competencies, whether pertaining to the achieved outcome or to the process leading there, are a motivational burden, because they reduce effort to build competence and conceal the steps that are needed to develop it. Thus, this research differs from research on outcome versus process simulations (Taylor, Pham, Rivkin, & Armor, 1998). Taylor and colleagues found that process simulations (rehearsing the cumbersome steps needed to reach a set goal; e.g., getting an A) lead to more effort and superior performance than outcome simulations (rehearsing the enjoyment of reaching the goal) via reduced anxiety and heightened planning. This approach, to the contrary, focuses on the experienced affective tone of fantasies about the future and postulates that positive competence fantasies (both outcome and process) are a motivational hindrance.

Furthermore, positive competence fantasies need to be distinguished from illusory optimism (Schneider, 2001; Taylor & Brown, 1988; Taylor, Kemeny, Reed, Bower, & Gruenewald, 2000). Because competence fantasies do not pertain to facts or likelihoods of occurrence, they cannot be taken as an indicator of illusory optimism. Only competence expectations can be illusory-optimistic, because they assess the future events' reality. This assessment of reality, then, can be more or less realistic (accurate) or illusory (inaccurate).

Summary

Subjective competence, depending on how it is conceptualized, predicts objective competence in differential ways. Assessed by expectancy judgments, subjective competence positively predicts improvement of objective competence, whereas, measured by affective tone of fantasies, it negatively predicts the development of objective competence. Effort and persistence mediate the negative relation between positive competence fantasies and the building of objective competence.

We replicated this pattern of results in further areas of the health domain (e.g., chronic illness, Oettingen & Mayer, 2003, Study 4; weight loss, Oettingen & Wadden, 1991), as well as in different life domains such as the interpersonal domain (e.g., starting a romantic relationship, Oettingen & Mayer, 2002, Study 2) and the professional domain (e.g., obtaining a desired job, Oettingen & Mayer, 2002, Study 1). In all of these studies, expectations and fantasies were measured long before we assessed the final measure of actual competence (up to 4 years).

Given the results of these studies, positive fantasies about future competencies appear to be problematic when it comes to the motivational question of realizing these fantasies in actuality. However, positive compe-

tence fantasies have a beneficial function, when it comes to the setting of goals. Specifically, they produce binding goals that are based on high competence expectations. For this purpose, competence fantasies about the future need to be contrasted with reflections on impediments of present reality.

MERGING EXPECTATIONS AND FANTASIES INTO COMPETENCE GOALS: MENTAL CONTRASTING

In his theory on proactive goal setting, Bandura (1991) argues that people who have successfully attained a goal will set themselves an even more aspiring goal due to their strengthened efficacy expectations. Social cognitive theory thus postulates two self-regulatory systems in attaining competence: A proactive discrepancy production system and a discrepancy reduction system (Bandura & Locke, 2003). Arguing that humans are motivated by foresight relative to where they want to be, rather than only by hindsight relative to what they did wrong, Bandura and Locke posed the following question:

> Discrepancy reduction is only half of the story and not necessarily the more interesting half. The greater challenge is to explain why people inflict on themselves high standards that demand hard work and beget a lot of stress, disappointments, and failures along the way rather than to explain why they should seek tranquility by matching a standard. (p. 91)

Bandura and Locke maintain that people whose efficacy expectations have been strengthened by previous goal attainment will set themselves more aspiring goals. However, not every heightened efficacy expectation will be turned into a challenging goal. Thus, the question remains as to how people whose efficacy has been strengthened manage to set themselves binding goals. We provide an answer to this question by referring to the model of fantasy realization (Oettingen, 2000; Oettingen, Pak, & Schnetter, 2001), which specifies how fantasies about the future can be used to turn high expectations into aspiring goals that in turn lead to persistent goal striving and effective goal attainment.

The Model of Fantasy Realization

The model of fantasy realization specifies three routes to goal setting that result from how people deal with their fantasies about a desired future (Oettingen, 1999, 2000; Oettingen et al., 2001). The first route to goal setting originates from solely fantasizing about a desired future. The second entails merely reflecting on the negative reality standing in the way of attaining these fantasies. The third route, finally, entails contrasting one's fantasies about the desired future with reflections on the negative impeding status quo.

Three Routes to Goal Setting: Proposed Mechanisms

The first route to goal setting is based on indulging in thoughts, fantasies, daydreams, and images about a desired future (e.g., becoming a lawyer, excelling in math, learning a language). Such fantasizing seduces a person into mentally enjoying the positive future in the here and now, because no reflections on reality point to the impediments of attaining the desired future. Therefore, goal commitment to realize the desired future (i.e., determination and effort to reach the goal, and persistence in pursuing it over time; Locke & Latham, 1990) should solely result from the implicit pull triggered by the positivity of the imagined future events.

The second route to goal setting is based on dwelling on negative aspects of present reality that stand in the way of realizing the desired future (e.g., having not yet graduated, being distracted, and feeling lazy, respectively). Such reflections remain recurring ruminations, because no fantasies about the future designate the direction in which to act. Therefore, goal commitment to realize the desired future should solely reflect the implicit push triggered by the negativity of the reality events about which the person is thinking.

The third route to goal setting entails mentally contrasting the desired future with negative aspects of impeding reality, such as contrasting thoughts of excelling in math with thoughts about being distracted from working on math improvement. Such mental contrast between a positive future and negative reality instigates a more complex goal-setting mechanism. Conjoint mental elaboration of the desired future and the present reality creates heightened simultaneous accessibility of cognition about both the desired future and the negative reality. In addition, the negative reality is viewed as an obstacle, or as "standing in the way" of realizing the desired future, thereby emphasizing a necessity to attain the desired future. This necessity to attain the future activates expectations, which then will be applied in goal setting. Thus, individuals engaging in mental contrasting should display flexible and strategic behavior, in that they refrain from setting themselves binding goals when expectations of success are low, but fully commit themselves to the attainment of the desired future when expectations of success are high.

Because a necessity to attain the desired future only emerges after mental contrasting, but not after indulging or dwelling, indulging and dwelling should not activate relevant expectations. Thus, indulging and dwelling will make people fail to draw on expectations when setting themselves goals. The implicit pull and push should lead to moderate goal commitment that is independent of perceived chances of success.

A series of experiments studying goal setting via the different modes of thought support these hypotheses. In the following sections we present two exemplary studies that pertain to attaining high competence in the academic and health domains. Specifically, the two studies investigate the role of indulging, dwelling, and mental contrasting in setting goals to attain competence in mathematics and in reducing cigarette consumption.

Setting Competence Goals in the Academic Domain

The fantasy theme of the study was excelling in mathematics (Oettingen et al., 2001; Study 4). Participants were male adolescents, freshmen enrolled in two vocational schools for computer programming. The curriculum entailed full-day training to become media or computer specialists, and mathematics was the critical subject in the first year of studies. Thus, accumulating competence in math was a most important desire in the lives of these adolescents concerned about their professional education.

We first measured participants' expectations to improve their competence in mathematics, and then asked them to name four positive aspects of improving in math and four negative aspects that impeded their improvement in math. We then established the three experimental groups, a fantasy–reality contrast (mental contrast) group, a fantasy-only (indulging) group, and a reality-only (dwelling) group. In the fantasy–reality contrast group, participants had to mentally elaborate in writing two positive aspects of improving their competence in math, and two negative aspects of impeding reality in alternating order, beginning with a positive aspect of the future. In the fantasy-only group, participants only had to mentally elaborate four aspects of improving in math, and in the reality-only group, participants only had to mentally elaborate four aspects of impeding reality.

Directly following these mental exercises, all participants reported how energized they felt (e.g., energetic, active, eventful). Moreover 2 weeks after the experiment, we asked teachers to evaluate each student's effort for the past fortnight (e.g., how much persistent effort the student showed in studying math, and how intrinsically interested he or she was). In addition, to measure actual achieved competence, we asked teachers to give a course grade to each student.

In mental contrast participants, we noted that feelings of energization, exerted effort, and achieved grades were more in line with competence expectations than in the indulging and dwelling participants. High-expectancy participants in the mental contrast group felt most energized, exerted most effort, and were given the highest course grades by their teachers. Low-expectancy participants, however, felt least energized, exerted least effort, and achieved the lowest course grades. To the contrary, indulging and dwelling participants felt moderately energized, independent of their expectations. Similarly, teachers rated them as showing moderate effort and gave them mediocre course grades, whether the students believed in their own competence or not.

For the participating adolescents who are beginning their vocational training and still have career options available, mental contrasting seems beneficial. Those who have high chances to excel invest their time and effort in a promising career, while those with minor chances to excel do not invest in vain and thus can move on and use their energies otherwise (Carver & Scheier, 1998). The pattern of goal commitment for indulging and dwelling participants seems less beneficial. Being implicitly pulled by the future or pushed by the reality, respectively, those with high expectations do not invest enough and thus suffer from failing to realize their potential. Those with low expectations, on the other hand, invest too much and thus waste their energies in a lost case; that is, both indulging and dwelling put people at risk in terms of being out of touch with their potential.

Setting Competence Goals in the Health Domain

The previous study described how expectations and fantasies can be merged to set goals geared at building academic competence. We now turn to an experiment that describes how mental contrasting can be used to set goals geared toward improving competence in the health domain (Oettingen, Mayer, & Thorpe, 2005a). Students who smoked were asked for their expectations relative to reducing their cigarette consumption or to stop smoking. Thereafter, all participants were asked to name four positive aspects of a future in which they had reduced their cigarette consumption and four aspects of impeding reality. As desirable aspects of the future, participants named, for example, physical fitness, self-respect, and pretty skin. As impeding aspects of present reality, they named stress, partying, and peer pressure. We then established the three experimental groups in the same way as in the experiment on developing math competence. Specifically, in the mental contrast group, participants had to elaborate two aspects of a future with fewer cigarettes and two aspects of impeding reality, in alternating order, beginning with a positive future aspect; in the positive future (indulging) group, participants elaborated four aspects of the positive future, and in the negative reality (dwelling) group, four aspects of negative reality. Thereafter, participants received a 14-day diary, in which they were to record in writing every cigarette they had smoked. Finally, 2 weeks after the experiment, we asked participants to indicate the exact date when they had actually started to reduce their cigarette consumption.

Participants in the mental contrast group reduced their cigarette consumption in line with their competence expectations, while those in the indulging and dwelling groups acted independently of their expectations to successfully resist cigarettes. In light of high expectations, contrasting participants tried to reduce their smoking right after the experiment, and tended to light fewer cigarettes per day than those in the indulging and dwelling groups, while the reverse was true for participants with low expectations.

Summary

Mental contrasting translated adolescents' high competence expectations into good mathematics grades and built competence even in participants showing addictive behaviors (smoking). For participants with low competence expectations, it prevented the setting of respective goals. Indulging and dwelling, to the contrary, led to goal setting that is disconnected from competence expectations, and thus from participants' past performance and experience.

We replicated these results in further studies. In the academic domain, for example, experiments pertained to studying abroad (Oettingen et al., 2001, Study 2), to combining work and family life (Oettingen, 2000, Study 2), and to acquiring a second language (Oettingen, Hönig, & Gollwitzer, 2000, Study 1). In the interpersonal domain, experiments focused on solving interpersonal conflicts (Oettingen et al., 2001, Studies 1 and 2), on getting to know an attractive stranger (Oettingen, 2000, Study 1), and on successfully seeking help (Oettingen et al., 2005b, Study 3).

In most of these studies, we used the salience paradigm described earlier; that is, participants rated their expectations of achieving the competence in question, generated positive aspects of having reached that competence and negative aspects potentially impeding such an achievement, then (depending upon condition) either mentally elaborated both future and reality, future only, or reality only. Another paradigm based on ignoring either reality (indulging), future (dwelling), or neither future nor reality (mental contrasting)

by reinterpreting the reality and the future through minimizing or maximizing their validity, respectively, generated the same pattern of results (Oettingen, 2000, Study 2; Oettingen, Mayer, Thorpe, Janetzke, & Lorenz, in press, Study 1).

The results hold for goal commitment assessed by cognitive, affective, and behavioral indicators (e.g., planning, anticipated disappointment in case of failure, financial investment) via self-report and observations, measured directly after the experiment or weeks later, and for samples of different cultural contexts (Europe and the United States). Mental contrasting turned out to be an easy to apply self-regulatory tool to increase objective competence, because the described effects were obtained even when participants elaborated the future and the reality only very briefly (i.e., were asked to imagine only one positive aspect of the desired future and one obstacle standing in the way of realizing the desired future; Oettingen et al., 2000, Study 1).

Taken together, these findings indicate that perceiving the acquisition of competence as desirable (positive attitude or high incentive value; i.e., the person values mastery and competence) and feasible (perceived control or efficacy expectations; i.e., the person sees a high likelihood of achieving objective competence) is an important prerequisite for the emergence of strong goal commitments to excel (Ajzen & Fishbein, 1980; Ajzen & Madden, 1986). To create binding goals to excel in competence, however, people need to mentally contrast fantasies about the desired future with impeding reality; only then will high expectations be translated into respective goal commitments.

So far we have shown that positive fantasies contrasted with negative reality help people to translate their high expectations into binding goal commitments geared toward achieving competence. In the study reported below, we explored whether negative fantasies contrasted with positive aspects of reality instigate goals that are geared toward avoiding incompetence.

SETTING COMPETENCE GOALS: APPROACH VERSUS AVOIDANCE

The distinctions between approach motivation and hope for success versus avoidance motivation and fear of failure have long been considered critical for decision making and action (Atkinson, 1957; Heckhausen, 1963; McClelland, 1980, Murray, 1938). In addition, Elliot and Thrash (2002) have pointed out that approach and avoidance temperaments meaningfully correlate to different types of achievement goals. Furthermore, there are life domains in which people have a hard time generating positive fantasies about the future and should thus be reluctant to form approach goals. For example, people who adhere to health-damaging behavior (e.g., excessive alcohol consumption) might not readily generate positive fantasies about stopping such behavior. Thus, it is important to ask whether mental contrasting can also regulate the setting of avoidance goals.

To create relevant avoidance goals, we took advantage of the fearful images and daydreams that befall people when thinking about undesirable futures. Specifically, we made people generate fantasies about their continued giving in to behaviors known to be detrimental to their future health. Such fearful fantasies about a future of incompetence that are mentally contrasted with a positive reality potentially endangered by such incompetence (e.g., fantasies about failing to reduce cigarette consumption contrasted with reflections on one's current healthy body) should produce goals directed at avoiding this incompetence.

The previously described study on smoking reduction tested these ideas by containing three further conditions that referred to negative fantasies about a feared future. Participants in these three conditions, instead of listing positive aspects of a future of reduced smoking and negative aspects of impeding reality, listed negative aspects of a future in which they continued to smoke at the present level (e.g., participants listed getting cancer, being a bad model for children, and lifelong addiction), then named positive aspects of present reality that they might lose if they continued to smoke at the present level (e.g., participants listed healthy lungs, pretty skin, physical endurance). We then established the three experimental groups. In the negative future–positive reality contrast group, participants alternated in their mental elaborations between negative fantasies about con-

tinued smoking and positive aspects of reality that they might lose if they continued smoking at the present level. In the negative future group, participants only fantasized about the negative future of continued smoking. Finally, in the positive reality group, participants only reflected on positive aspects of the endangered reality. As described earlier, dependent variables included the number of cigarettes smoked, as recorded in the subsequent 14-day diary, and the immediacy of trying to reduce cigarette consumption (in days after the experiment).

Participants in the negative fantasy–positive reality contrast group acted according to their competence expectations. High-expectation participants tended to smoke fewer cigarettes and started earlier to exert respective effort, while the reverse was true for low- expectation participants. To the contrary, those who indulged in their fearful fantasies and those who dwelled on their still-healthy body did not use their expectations as a guide for reducing their cigarette consumption. Only after mental contrasting did participants with high expectations form the goal to avoid the feared future of continued smoking.

Summary

Future fantasies, be they positive or negative, merge with competence expectations to form approach and avoidance goals, respectively. They only need to be contrasted with the relevant reality (i.e., with the negative reality when creating approach goals, and with the positive reality when creating avoidance goals). Indulging in the future, or dwelling on reality, whether the future and reality images are positive or negative, lead to the setting of goals that are independent of competence expectations.

Because mental contrasting in light of high competence expectations produces the strong goal commitments we have observed (e.g., promoting course grades across a period of weeks and months; Oettingen et al., 2000, 2001), the question arises whether mental contrasting not only fosters goal setting but also benefits processes of goal striving. Critical processes of goal striving pertain to how people respond to negative feedback that they encounter on their way to successful goal attainment. Furthermore, in her work on implicit theories about the nature of intelligence and the emergence of respective achievement goals, Carol Dweck and her colleagues have repeatedly pointed out that the pivotal issue in achieving competence is how people respond to negative feedback (Dweck, 1999; Dweck & Leggett, 1988; Grant & Dweck, 2003). Therefore, in the following section, we investigate how the three routes to goal setting influence responses to negative feedback.

MENTAL CONTRASTING AND GOAL STRIVING: RESPONDING TO NEGATIVE FEEDBACK

Mental contrasting in light of high expectations should foster the effective processing of negative feedback, because such negative feedback provides relevant clues on how best to achieve the desired competence (Gollwitzer, 1996; Gollwitzer & Bayer, 1999). Appraising negative feedback as useful information for goal striving rather than as a sign of incompetence should, in addition, guarantee that it does not diminish one's self-view of competence (Dweck, 1999; Dweck & Leggett, 1988). Therefore, mental contrasting in light of high expectations should allow for effective processing of goal-relevant information, as well as for maintaining a robust self-view of competence, even after obtaining strong negative feedback. In two studies using the same paradigm, we tested whether mental contrasting would indeed serve such a dual purpose when it comes to responding to negative feedback.

Mental Contrasting and the Processing of Negative Feedback

In a simple cued recall experiment, we investigated whether mental contrasting in light of high expectations facilitates the processing of relevant negative feedback (Pak, 2002, Study 1). Students participated in two supposedly independent experiments. In the first experiment, which used a procedure similar to that in the experiments described earlier, students first named their most important current interpersonal concern. They

listed, for example, "to get to know someone," "to solve the problems with my partner," and "to get along with my roommate." Then they indicated their expectations of competently solving their concern, and listed four positive aspects of having solved it, as well as four aspects that might impede their solving this concern.

As part of the second experiment, participants were asked to complete two different competence tests, one of which supposedly measured social competence. In the social competence test, students were asked to study a variety of art portraits and then to fill out semantic differential-type questionnaires about their impressions of the people depicted in these paintings. Finally, participants received 12 statements providing feedback; among them, the following three statements contained negative feedback relevant to their social competence: "In socially challenging situations, you are *tense*," "When communicating with other people, you are *reserved*, " and "In stressful social situations, you react *impulsively*." Thereafter, the three experimental groups were established: the mental contrast group, the indulging group, and the dwelling group, as in the experiments described earlier. Finally, participants had to report on the feedback they had received using a cued recall procedure.

Recall performance was best in the high-expectancy mental contrast group, while the worst recall was observed in the low-expectancy mental contrast group. Indulging and dwelling participants recalled a medium number of words, independent of their competence expectations. This pattern of data implies that only mental contrasting participants with high competence expectations were eager to process information that was relevant to achieving the desired future competence; mental contrasting participants with low competence expectations failed to process the bothersome information that they did not deem important anymore. Finally, indulging and dwelling participants processed the negative feedback independently of their competence expectations. Whether they perceived their chances of solving the interpersonal problem as high or low (thus, whether the information was valuable or not), they always processed the same medium amount of negative feedback.

Apparently, the three modes of self-regulatory thought not only differentially affect goal setting but also impact goal striving. Processing negative information with respect to one's goal pursuit should only be beneficial, however, if it does not create insecurities that undermine using the negative information to improve one's moving toward the goal. Accordingly, we wondered whether mental contrasting in light of high competence expectations protects a person from experiencing such insecurities due to negative feedback. Negative feedback should not force these individuals to diminish their relevant positive self-view of competence.

Mental Contrasting and Self-View of Competence after Negative Feedback

In this experiment (Pak, 2002, Study 2), using the same paradigm and design as the previous experiment, we measured change in self-view of social competence as a dependent variable. Specifically, participants again named an interpersonal concern, and indicated expectations of competently solving the concern. For a baseline measure regarding self-view of social competence, we asked the following two questions: "How would you estimate your social competence?" and "How would you estimate your interpersonal intelligence?" Participants then listed four positive future aspects of competently solving their interpersonal concern, and four negative reality aspects that stand in its way. Thereafter, in a supposed second experiment, they took a social competence test, similar to the test in the last experiment.

We had established the three groups: mental contrasting fantasies of competently solving the interpersonal problem, indulging in those fantasies, and dwelling on impeding reality. In subsequent false-negative feedback, we told participants that their performance on the social competence test was very weak (i.e., they only had achieved 18 out of 60 points, which they were told was a very low performance in their age group), and that people with such test results would be plagued by conflicted and disharmonious relationships.

While high-expectancy mental contrasting participants remained unaffected by this detrimental personal feedback, low-expectancy mental contrasting participants suffered from a dramatic loss in their self-view of social competence. Again, participants in the indulging and dwelling groups fared in between, independent of their expectations. It appears, then, that mental contrasting protects participants with high competence expectations from having their self-view shattered by negative feedback.

Summary

The findings so far suggest that mental contrasting influences objective competence by two different mechanisms. First, it causes people to set themselves feasible goals, and second, it facilitates goal striving through beneficial responses to negative feedback. These beneficial responses encompass processing goal-relevant negative feedback (thereby unveiling clues for effective goal striving) and preserving a stable positive self-view of competence even in the face of massive negative feedback (norm-oriented and person-oriented; Elliot & McGregor, 2001; Kamins & Dweck, 1999). People profit in their goal striving from both processing negative feedback (Bandura & Cervone, 1983; Carver & Scheier, 1998; Dweck, 1999; Dweck & Leggett, 1988) and holding a positive self-view of competence (even illusory positive; Gollwitzer & Kinney, 1989; Taylor & Brown, 1988; Taylor & Gollwitzer, 1995; Taylor, Lerner, Sherman, Sage, & McDowell, 2003). Accordingly, these findings suggest that mental contrasting provides access to the major tools of successful goal striving and goal attainment.

By allowing appraisal of one's weaknesses, along with keeping a strong sense of overall competence in the face of offensive feedback, mental contrasting equips people for stressful situations. However, mental contrasting might also shelter people from stressful situations by other mechanisms. It might be even used to form goals explicitly geared toward competently coping with stress.

MENTAL CONTRASTING AND SETTING GOALS TO COPE WITH STRESS

Coping with stress has been widely studied in psychology. The literature largely considers coping as emerging from an interaction between the environment and the individual. For example, Lazarus and Folkman (1984) conceptualize the coping process as consisting of primary appraisal, in which the individual appraises the features of the situation, and secondary appraisal, in which the individual appraises the resources available for dealing with the situation. The kinds and number of resources that people possess for altering or overcoming the stressor at hand are critical.

We argue that individuals who have set themselves binding goals to deal with a stressful situation will more effectively maximize their resources (e.g., plan, exert effort, and persist) than individuals who are less committed to such goals. Indeed, Lazarus (1993) conceives of coping as a goal-directed process in which people direct their thoughts and actions toward the goal of mastering the stressor. Carver, Scheier, and Weintraub (1989), based on the model of behavioral self-regulation (Carver & Scheier, 1981), also have conceptualized effective coping with stress in terms of goal pursuit. In the COPE Inventory, they specified various scales capturing successful coping, some of which are synchronous with aspects of successful goal pursuit (e.g., planning, shielding against distractions, delay of gratification, and persistence; Carver et al., 1989). These goal-related scales predict effective coping (Carver et al., 1989), as do scales in further questionnaires that also focus on goal-related features (see summary by Compas, Connor-Smith, Saltzman, Thompsen, & Wadsworth, 2001). Accordingly, we hypothesized that setting binding goals to change or overcome a stressor should be an effective way to maximize one's coping resources, and to guarantee effective coping with stress.

Mental contrasting should be a beneficial strategy to form goals geared at overcoming a stressor. When competence expectations to overcome the stressor are high (i.e., resources are plentiful), mental contrasting should translate these expectations into binding coping goals, with subsequent mastery of the stressor. When competence expectations to overcome the stressor are low, however, mental contrasting should lead people to turn their back to this stressor, thus conserving their resources for mastering less overwhelming stressors. Three exemplary studies that tested these hypotheses are now described.

Mental Contrasting and Coping with Chronic Stress

In a pilot study, pediatric intensive care nurses indicated that their most disturbing and troublesome chronic everyday stressor was communication with patients' relatives. Therefore, we chose this aspect of the pediatric nurses' patient–provider communication as the topic of our experiment (Oettingen et al., 2005b, Study 1). Participants first indicated their competence expectations of being able to improve communication with patients' relatives. Subsequently, they listed aspects of a future in which they had competently mastered this stressor, and aspects of the negative reality that potentially impeded successful coping. The three experimental conditions were established in the same way as described earlier. In the mental contrast group, nurses had to generate both fantasies of effectively coping with the stressor and reflections on impeding obstacles, while in the indulging and dwelling groups, they had to come up with only future fantasies or only reality reflections, respectively. Two weeks later, as indicators of commitment to improve the relationship to the patients' relatives, we assessed respective effort (in number of steps taken; Oettingen et al., 2001), and willingness to take remedial action (readiness to participate in a workshop providing relevant information; Hong, Chiu, Dweck, Lin, & Wan, 1999).

In light of high competence expectations (i.e., to be able to improve communication with patients' relatives), nurses in the mental contrast group showed the greatest effort to improve the relationship with patients' relatives and the greatest willingness to take remedial action, whereas the opposite held true for those whose competence expectations were low. Nurses who indulged or dwelled showed a moderate amount of effort and remedial action, irrespective of their beliefs in how much they could do for the patients' relatives. Thus, we have shown that mental contrasting influences coping with chronic stress. In the next study, we analyzed the role of mental contrasting in setting goals to cope with acute stress.

Mental Contrasting and Coping with Acute Stress

Economics students were told that they were participating in a study trying out a new recruitment tool for senior students entering the job market (Oettingen et al., 2005b, Study 2). Therefore, they had to give a presentation in front of a video camera, so that their talk could be evaluated by a group of human resources experts. Giving a presentation in front of a camera has been frequently used as an acute stressor (e.g., Britt, Cohen, Collins, & Cohen, 2001). Because the stressor is standardized and applied in the laboratory, it allows us to measure participants' appraisal of the stressor, as well as their *in situ* persistence and coping performance.

Participants first noted how well they wanted to do in their presentations. To measure their competence expectations, we asked them how likely they thought it would be that they actually achieved their desired performance. As in the previous studies, participants named positive aspects of doing well (e.g., participants listed "Feeling good about myself," "Knowing I can cope with an interview situation," "Becoming confident about the application process") and negative aspect of impeding reality (e.g., participants listed "Not having enough time for preparation," "Feeling shy," "The stupid camera"). Finally, we established a mental contrast and an indulging condition (due to the complexity of the data collection, we did not include a dwelling condition) in the same manner as described in the previous studies.

We observed a stronger link between competence expectations and coping effort (measured by length of presentation), as well as the quality of coping performance (assessed by independent raters blind to conditions), in the mental contrast condition than in the indulging condition. Thus, mental contrasting can be seen as a self-regulatory tool that makes people adjust their immediate coping responses to their available resources. In addition, mental contrasting and indulging predictably affected how participants appraised the impending stressor, how they felt about the stressor in the aftermath, and how well they considered themselves to be coping.

These findings are important, because prospective appraisal of a situation has been found to influence the coping strategies people use (Carver & Scheier, 1994; Lazarus & Folkman, 1984). Moreover, retrospective appraisal of a stressor, as well as positive self-evaluations of one's coping efforts, will benefit appraisal of and responses to future stressors. Thus, by creating competence-based coping goals, mental contrasting fosters not only active and constructive coping responses toward the current stressor but also benefits coping responses toward similar stressors in the future. In summary, the results show the usefulness of mental contrasting for mastering acute stress and demonstrate its role for both coping cognition (i.e., appraisal and self-evaluation) and coping behavior (persistence and actual coping performance).

The previous two studies suggest that mental contrasting in light of high competence expectations creates strong goals to cope with chronic and acute stress; in light of low competence expectations, it leads people to abstain from setting coping goals and to save resources for more promising coping endeavours. In other words, mental contrasting reveals which stressors one should overcome or change, and which stressors one should avoid. These considerations suggest that inducing mental contrasting as a metacognitive strategy that can be applied to diverse everyday problems should facilitate making up one's mind and effectively managing precious resources (e.g., time and money), thereby alleviating the accumulation of chronic and acute stress.

Inducing Mental Contrasting as a Metacognitive Strategy

To test the idea that mental contrasting taught as a metacognitive strategy prevents stress by improved decision making and superior resource management, one group of health care managers was instructed in mental contrasting, while a control group of managers was taught to fantasize positively only (Oettingen et al., 2005b, Study 4). The interventionist then explained to participants in both groups how to apply these strategies to their most cumbersome everyday problems or stressors.

Specifically, depending on condition, we first asked participants to do the mental contrasting versus indulging exercise in writing with respect to their current most important problem. In order to practice further the respective procedures of mental elaboration (i.e., mental contrasting vs. indulging), participants were then asked to imagine as many pressing professional and personal everyday stressors and problems as possible that were relatively controllable but made them feel clearly uneasy (e.g., participants named "Being assertive in a staff meeting," "Visiting my mother," "Terminating the job contract of a coworker," "Inviting people for dinner"). Depending on experimental condition, either mental contrasting or indulging procedures were then used for the first six of the named problems. Finally, all participants received a 14-day diary and were asked to do their mental exercise in writing with respect to the stressor that made them feel most uneasy on a given day. They were encouraged also to use the mental exercise with respect to any other problem or concern that would appear during the day, and to apply the exercise whenever they felt there was a good opportunity to do so (e.g., while waiting for the bus).

Two weeks after the intervention, we asked participants how they fared in their daily decision making and time management since the intervention. In comparison with participants in the indulging group, those in the mental contrast group reported having experienced greater ease in their decision making and having organized their time in a more efficient way. Moreover, they were more successful both in completing some projects and in relinquishing others. Apparently, mental contrasting can be successfully taught and readily applied in self-instructions to the various professional and private problems and stressors people face in their daily life. Furthermore, mental contrasting can be seen as a self-regulatory strategy that guides people to improve their ease in decision making, their time management, and their readiness to relinquish some projects in favor of completing others.

Based on the findings of our past studies that mental contrasting leads to setting strong coping goals in light of high competence expectations but to relinquishing coping goals in light of low competence expectations, we speculate that by applying mental contrasting, participants relinquish those projects and stressors in which they felt they had little competence or resources available, thus avoiding psychological distress stemming from pursuing pointless endeavors. To the contrary, when competence expectations were high, mental contrasting should have led people to pursue vigorously and complete ongoing projects. Teaching how to apply mental contrasting to everyday problems and stressors rather than indulging in their successful solution helped the managers to deal with their daily lives in a way that prevented the cumulative stress of having to deal with unpromising and too many projects.

Summary

We have observed the benefits of experimentally induced mental contrasting for coping with chronic and acute stressors. The findings also suggest that mental contrasting, taught as a metacognitive strategy in a simple intervention and applied to various daily problems (e.g., organizing a dinner party, being assertive in meetings), prevents long-standing stress by fostering the completion of feasible tasks and by refraining from tackling unfeasible ones. Indulging, on the other hand, causes people to be halfheartedly engaged in too many, often unpromising projects.

Our findings are in line with the literature on denial and wishful thinking, in which these ways of thinking are observed to impede effective coping with stress, especially when the stressors do not dissolve by themselves but require attention and effortful action to be overcome (Carver et al., 1989). Based on these considerations, we speculate that even though the present studies show that the consequences of indulging are maladaptive when the individual has a choice to face or not to face the stressor at hand, indulging may be beneficial for coping with stressors that are characterized as being inescapable, in the sense that they can neither be mastered nor relinquished. For example, elementary school children with low competence expectations of excelling in math should benefit from indulging in future fantasies about their math successes. Mental contrasting, in this case, would only focus them on their low competence, thus, leading them to relinquish efforts to improve in math. Indulging, to the contrary, should prevent them from taking their bleak prospects into consideration, thus fostering at least moderate problem-focused coping and thereby development of unnoticed resources and potentials. In addition, while students are kept moderately engaged through indulging, the teacher can strengthen their efficacy expectations. Once efficacy expectations are strong (Bandura, 1977, 1997; Bandura & Schunk, 1981), mental contrasting procedures can be fruitfully applied.

CONCLUSIONS

Based on William James's (1890/1950) distinction between beliefs and images, we observed that thinking about the future in terms of competence expectations fosters motivation and objective competence, while thinking about the future in terms of competence fantasies is detrimental to motivation and performance. Competence fantasies, however, can be merged with high competence expectations to form binding competence goals. They only need to be contrasted with reflections on impeding reality. This simple procedure of mental contrasting also benefits goal striving: It guarantees that critical feedback is processed in terms of valuable information instead of self-damaging criticism. Moreover, mental contrasting can be used to create goals geared at coping with chronic and acute stress, and when taught as a metacognitive strategy, to prevent long-term stress by fostering ease of decision making and effective resource management.

"The person who is aware of the past knows about the future!" This slogan captures the benefits of mental contrasting, because mental contrasting fosters action according to experiences of the past. The slogan also alludes to the conditions in which mental contrasting is beneficial: whenever one needs to be aware of one's past performance in order to predict the future.

The findings may also be interpreted from a sociocultural perspective. For example, it might be argued that in modern, rather than in more traditional societies, past experience needs to inform future action, because myths and norm-oriented rituals are fading in modern societies and thus cannot guide action anymore. Few norm-oriented rituals

provide assurance and boundaries for acting (by determining who interacts with whom, when, where, and how; Boesch, 1982). What, then, provides the basis for action in modern societies? We suggest that in modern societies, expectations are taking over the function of norms and rituals (Oettingen, 1997). Specifically, by reflecting experiential histories, expectations provide the necessary assurance to act and show the boundaries of acting.

As expectations gain a pivotal role in guiding action, and mental contrasting activates expectations, self-regulatory thought in terms of mental contrasting should be important in modern societies, allowing us to be agents of our own development and change (Bandura, 1989; Brandtstädter & Lerner, 1999). In traditional cultures, to the contrary, where normative rituals rather than expectations guide action, there is less need for mental contrasting. Hence, indulging in the future and dwelling on reality can flourish. Indulging in a desired future has the additional advantage that it helps people to overlook pessimistic expectations about continued hardships of normative constraint, thus providing hope for a better future. Engaging in such hopeful pessimism will prevent disengagement and should yield more positive affect and well-being than mental contrasting.

Although we have pointed at the perils of indulging in a desired future and of dwelling on negative reality throughout this chapter, the latter considerations imply that the benefits of mental contrasting versus indulging and dwelling are context-dependent. Only when expectations need to guide action, and the person can be the agent of his or her own development, should mental contrasting be the beneficial strategy. Under normative constraints, to the contrary, indulging in positive fantasies may well prove to be the more comforting solution.

REFERENCES

Ajzen, I., & Fishbein, M. (1980). *Understanding attitudes and predicting social behavior.* Englewood Cliffs, NJ: Prentice-Hall.
Ajzen, I., & Madden, T. J. (1986). Prediction of goal-directed behavior: Attitudes, intentions, and perceived behavioral control. *Journal of Experimental Social Psychology, 22,* 453–474.

Atkinson, J. W. (1957). Motivational determinants of risk-taking behavior. *Psychological Review, 64*, 359–372.

Bandura, A. (1977). Self-efficacy: Toward a unifying theory of behavioral change. *Psychological Review, 84*, 191–215.

Bandura, A. (1989). Human agency in social cognitive thinking. *American Psychologist, 44*, 1175–1184.

Bandura, A. (1991). Self-regulation of motivation through anticipatory and self-reactive mechanisms. In R. A. Dienstbier (Ed.), *Nebraska Symposium on Motivation: Vol. 38. Perspectives on motivation* (pp. 69–163). Lincoln: University of Nebraska Press.

Bandura, A. (1997). *Self-efficacy: The exercise of control.* New York: Freeman.

Bandura, A., & Cervone, D. (1983). Self-evaluative and self-efficacy mechanisms governing the motivational effects of goal systems. *Journal of Personality and Social Psychology, 45*, 1017–1028.

Bandura, A., & Locke, E. A. (2003). Negative self-efficacy and goal effects revisited. *Journal of Applied Psychology, 88*, 87–99.

Bandura, A., Pastorelli, C., Barbaranelli, C., & Caprara, G. V. (1999). Self-efficacy pathways to childhood depression. *Journal of Personality and Social Psychology, 76*, 258–269.

Bandura, A., & Schunk, D. H. (1981). Cultivating competence, self-efficacy and intrinsic interest through proximal self-motivation. *Journal of Personality and Social Psychology, 41*, 586–598.

Boesch, E. E. (1982). Ritual und Psychotherapie [Ritual and psychotherapy]. *Zeitschrift für Klinische Psychologie und Psychotherapie, 30*, 214–234.

Brandtstädter, J., & Lerner, R. M. (1999). *Action and self-development: Theory and research through the life span.* London: Sage.

Britt, D. M., Cohen, L. M., Collins, F. L., & Cohen, M. L. (2001). Cigarette smoking and chewing gum response to a laboratory-induced stressor. *Health Psychology, 20*, 361–368.

Butler, R. (1998). Determinants of help seeking: Relations between perceived reasons for classroom help-avoidance and help-seeking behaviors in an experimental context. *Journal of Educational Psychology, 90*, 630–643.

Carver, C. S., & Scheier, M. F. (1981). *Attention and self-regulation: A control-theory approach to human behavior.* New York: Springer.

Carver, C. S., & Scheier, M. F. (1994). Situational coping and coping dispositions in a stressful transaction. *Journal of Personality and Social Psychology, 66*, 184–195.

Carver, C. S., & Scheier, M. F. (1998). *On the self-regulation of behavior.* New York: Cambridge University Press.

Carver, C. S., Scheier, M. F., & Weintraub, J. K. (1989). Assessing coping strategies: A theoretically based approach. *Journal of Personality and Social Psychology, 56*, 267–283.

Christensen, K. A., Stephens, M. A. P., & Townsend, A. L. (1998). Mastery in women's multiple roles and well-being: Adult daughters providing care to impaired parents. *Health Psychology, 17*, 163–171.

Compas, B. E., Connor-Smith, J. K., Saltzman, H., Thomsen, A. H., & Wadsworth, M. E. (2001). Coping with stress during childhood and adolescence: Problems, progress, and potential in theory and research. *Psychological Bulletin, 127*, 87–127.

Dekker, J., Boot, B., van der Woude, L. H., & Bijlsma, J. W. (1992). Pain and disability in osteoarthritis: A review of biobehavioral mechanisms. *Journal of Behavioral Medicine, 15*, 189–214.

Dweck, C. S. (1999). *Self-theories: Their role in motivation, personality, and development.* Philadelphia: Psychology Press.

Dweck, C. S., & Leggett, E. L. (1988). A social-cognitive approach to motivation and personality. *Psychological Review, 95*, 256–273.

Elliot, A. J., & Church, M. A. (1997). A hierarchical model of approach and avoidance achievement motivation. *Journal of Personality and Social Psychology, 72*, 218–232.

Elliot, A. J., & McGregor, H. A. (2001). A 2 × 2 achievement goal framework. *Journal of Personality and Social Psychology, 80*, 501–519.

Elliot, A. J., & Thrash, T. M. (2002). Approach–avoidance motivation in personality: Approach and avoidance temperaments and goals. *Journal of Personality and Social Psychology, 82*, 804–818.

Gogia, P. P., Christensen, C. M., & Schmidt, C. (1994). Total hip replacement in patients with osteoarthritis of the hip: Improvement in pain and functional status. *Orthopedics, 17*, 145–150.

Gollwitzer, P. M. (1996). The volitional benefits of planning. In P. M. Gollwitzer & J. A. Bargh (Eds.), *The psychology of action* (pp. 287–312). New York: Guilford Press.

Gollwitzer, P. M., & Bayer, U. (1999). Deliberative versus implemental mind-sets in the control of action. In S. Chaiken & Y. Trope (Eds.), *Dual-process theories in social psychology* (pp. 403–422). New York: Guilford Press.

Gollwitzer, P. M., & Kinney, R. F. (1989). Effects of deliberative and implemental mind-sets on the illusion of control. *Journal of Personality and Social Psychology, 56*, 531–542.

Grant, H., & Dweck, C. S. (2003). Clarifying achievement goals and their impact. *Journal of Personality and Social Psychology, 85*, 541–553.

Heckhausen, H. (1963). *Hoffnung und Furcht in der Leistungsmotivation* [Hope and fear in achievement motivation]. Meisenheim/Glan: Hain.

Higgins, E. T. (1997). Beyond pleasure and pain. *American Psychologist, 52*, 1280–1300.

Higgins, E. T., Idson, L. C., Freitas, A. L., Spiegel, S., & Molden, D. C. (2003). Transfer of value from fit. *Journal of Personality and Social Psychology, 84*, 1140–1153.

Hong, Y., Chiu, C., Dweck, C. S., Lin, D. M.-S., &

Wan, W. (1999). Implicit theories, attributions, and coping: A meaning system approach. *Journal of Personality and Social Psychology, 77,* 588–599.

James, W. (1950). *The principles of psychology* (2 vols.). New York: Dover. (Original work published in 1890)

Jensen, M. P., & Karoly, P. (1991). Control beliefs, coping efforts, and adjustment to chronic pain. *Journal of Consulting and Clinical Psychology, 59,* 431–438.

Kamins, M., & Dweck, C. S. (1999). Person versus process praise and criticism: Implications for contingent self-worth and coping. *Developmental Psychology, 35,* 835–847.

Klinger, E. (1971). *Structure and functions of fantasy.* New York: Wiley.

Klinger, E. (1990). *Daydreaming: Using waking fantasy and imagery for self-knowledge and creativity.* Los Angeles: Tarcher.

Lachman, M. E., & Weaver, S. L. (1998). The sense of control as a moderator of social class differences in health and well-being. *Journal of Personality and Social Psychology, 74,* 763–773.

Lazarus, R. S. (1993). Coping theory and research: Past, present and future. *Psychosomatic Medicine, 55,* 2324–2347.

Lazarus, R. S., & Folkman, S. (1984). *Stress, appraisal and coping.* New York: Springer.

Lent, R. W., Brown, S. D., & Gore, P. A., Jr. (1997). Discriminant and predictive validity of academic self-concept, academic self-efficacy, and mathematics-specific self-efficacy. *Journal of Counseling Psychology, 44,* 307–315.

Lent, R. W., Brown, S. D., & Hackett, G. (1994). Toward a unifying social cognitive theory of career and academic interest, choice, and performance. *Journal of Vocational Behavior, 45,* 79–122.

Lewin, K. (1926). Vorsatz, Wille und Bedürfnis [Intention, will, and need]. *Psychologische Forschung, 7,* 330–385.

Little, T. D., Oettingen, G., Stetsenko, A., & Baltes, P. B. (1995). Children's action–control beliefs about school performance: How do American children compare to German and Russian children? *Journal of Personality and Social Psychology, 69,* 686–700.

Locke, E. A., & Latham, G. P. (1990). *A theory of goal setting and task performance.* Englewood Cliffs, NJ: Prentice-Hall.

Mahler, W. (1933). Ersatzhandlungen verschiedenen Realitätsgrades [Compensatory action based on different degrees of reality]. *Psychologische Forschung, 18,* 27–89.

McAuley, E. (1985). Modeling and self-efficacy: A test of Bandura's model. *Journal of Sport Psychology, 7,* 283–295.

McAuley, E. (1993). Self-efficacy and the maintenance of exercise participation in older adults. *Journal of Behavioral Medicine, 16,* 103–113.

McClelland, D. C. (1980). Motive dispositions: The merits of operant and respondent measures. In L.

Wheeler (Ed.), *Review of personality and social psychology* (Vol. 1, pp. 10–41). Beverly Hills, CA: Sage.

Mischel, W. (1973). Toward a cognitive social learning reconceptualization of personality. *Psychological Review, 80,* 252–283.

Mischel, W., Cantor, N., & Feldman, S. (1996). Principles of self-regulation: The nature of willpower and self-control. In E. T. Higgins & A. W. Kruglanski (Eds.), *Social psychology: Handbook of basic principles* (pp. 329–360). New York: Guilford Press.

Multon, K. D., Brown, S. D., & Lent, R. W. (1991). Relation of self-efficacy beliefs to academic outcomes: A meta-analytic investigation. *Journal of Counseling Psychology, 38,* 30–38.

Murray, H. A. (1938). *Explorations in personality.* New York: Oxford University Press.

Oettingen, G. (1997). Culture and future thought. *Culture and Psychology, 3,* 353–381.

Oettingen, G. (1999). Free fantasies about the future and the emergence of developmental goals. In J. Brandtstädter & R. M. Lerner (Eds.), *Action and self-development: Theory and research through the life span* (pp. 315–342). Thousand Oaks, CA: Sage.

Oettingen, G. (2000). Expectancy effects on behavior depend on self-regulator thought. *Social Cognition, 18,* 101–129.

Oettingen, G., Hagenah, M., Mayer, D., Brinkmann, J., Schmidt, L., & Pak, H. (2005b). *Fantasies and the self-regulation of goal setting in everyday life.* Manuscript submitted for publication.

Oettingen, G., Hönig, G., & Gollwitzer, P. M. (2000). Effective self-regulation of goal attainment. *International Journal of Educational Research, 33,* 705–732.

Oettingen, G., Little, T. D., Lindenberger, U., & Baltes, P. B. (1994). Causality, agency, and control beliefs in East versus West Berlin children: A natural experiment on the role of context. *Journal of Personality and Social Psychology, 66,* 579–595.

Oettingen, G., & Mayer, D. (2002).The motivating function of thinking about the future: Expectations versus fantasies. *Journal of Personality and Social Psychology, 83,* 1198–1212.

Oettingen, G., & Mayer, D. (2003). *Mastering the consequences of chronic illness: Expectations versus fantasies.* Unpublished manuscript, University of Hamburg, Hamburg, Germany.

Oettingen, G., Mayer, D., & Thorpe, J. S. (2005a). *Self-regulation of approach and avoidance goals: The role of mental contrasting.* Manuscript submitted for publication.

Oettingen, G., Mayer, D., Thorpe, J. S., Janetzke, H., & Lorenz, S. (in press). Turning fantasies about positive and negative futures into self-improvement goals. *Motivation and Emotion.*

Oettingen, G., Pak, H., & Schnetter, K. (2001). Self-Regulation of goal setting: Turning free fantasies about the future into binding goals. *Journal of Personality and Social Psychology, 80,* 736–753.

Oettingen, G., & Wadden, T. A. (1991). Expectation,

fantasy, and weight loss: Is the impact of positive thinking always positive? *Cognitive Therapy and Research*, *15*, 167–175.

O'Leary, A. (2001). Social-cognitive theory mediators of behavior change in the National Institute of Mental Health Multisite HIV Prevention Trial: The National Institute of Mental Health Multisite HIV Prevention Trial Group. *Health Psychology*, *20*, 369–376.

Olson, J. M., Roese, N. J., & Zanna, M. P. (1996). Expectancies. In E. T. Higgins & A. W. Kruglanski (Eds.), *Social psychology: Handbook of basic principles* (pp. 211–238). New York: Guilford Press.

Pajares, F., & Miller, M. D. (1994). Role of self-efficacy and self-concept beliefs in mathematical problem solving: A path analysis. *Journal of Educational Psychology*, *86*, 193–203.

Pak, H. (2002). *Mentale Kontrastierung und die Verarbeitung rückgemeldeter Informationen* [Mental contrasting and the processing of feedback]. Doctoral dissertation, University of Konstanz, Konstanz, Germany.

Pietsch, J., Walker, R., & Chapman, E. (2003). The relationship among self-concept, self-efficacy, and performance in mathematics during secondary school. *Journal of Educational Psychology*, *95*, 589–603.

Rheinberg, F. (1998). Theory of interest and research on motivation to learn. In L. Hoffmann, K. A Renninger, & J. Baumert (Eds.), *Interest and learning: Proceedings of the Seeon Conference on Interest and Gender* (pp. 126–145). Kiel, Germany: IPN.

Ruble, D. N., & Frey, K. S. (1991). Changing patterns of comparative behavior as skills are acquired: A functional model of self-evaluation. In J. Suls & T. A. Wills (Eds.), *Social comparison: Contemporary theory and research.* (pp. 79–113). Hillsdale, NJ: Erlbaum.

Scheier, M. F., Matthews, K. A., Owens, J. F., Magovern, G. J., Sr., Lefebvre, R. C., Abbott, R. A., et al. (2003). Dispositonal optimism and recovery from coronary artery bypass surgery: The beneficial effects on physical and psychological well-being. In P. Salovey & A. J. Rothman (Eds.), *Social psychology of health: Key readings in social psychology* (pp. 342–361). New York: Psychology Press.

Schneider, S. L. (2001). In search of realistic optimism: Meaning, knowledge, and warm fuzziness. *American Psychologist*, *56*, 250–263.

Schunk, D. H. (1982). Effects of effort attributional feedback on children's perceived self-efficacy and achievement. *Journal of Educational Psychology*, *74*, 548–556.

Schunk, D. H. (1989). Self-efficacy and cognitive skill

learning. In C. Ames & R. Ames (Eds.), *Research on motivation in education: Goals and cognitions* (Vol. 3, pp. 13–44). San Diego: Academic Press.

Shell, D. F., Colvin, C., & Bruning, R. H. (1995). Self-efficacy, attribution, and outcome expectancy mechanisms in reading and writing achievement: Grade-level and achievement-level differences. *Journal of Educational Psychology*, *87*, 386–398.

Singer, J. L. (1966). *Daydreaming.* New York: Random House.

Skinner, E. A. (1996). A guide to constructs of control. *Journal of Personality and Social Psychology*, *71*, 549–570.

Skinner, E. A., Chapman, M., & Baltes, P. B. (1988). Control, means–ends, and agency beliefs: A new conceptualization and its measurement during childhood. *Journal of Personality and Social Psychology*, *54*, 117–133.

Skinner, E. A., Wellborn, J. G., & Connell, J. P. (1990). What it takes to do well in school and whether I've got it: A process model of perceived control and children's engagement and achievement in school. *Journal of Educational Psychology*, *82*, 22–32.

Taylor, S. E., & Brown, J. D. (1988). Illusion and well-being: A social psychological perspective on mental health. *Psychological Bulletin*, *103*, 193–210.

Taylor, S. E., & Gollwitzer, P. M. (1995). Effects of mindset on positive illusions. *Journal of Personality and Social Psychology*, *69*, 213–226.

Taylor, S. E., Kemeny, M. E., Reed, G. M., Bower, J. E., & Gruenewald, T. L. (2000). Psychological resources, positive illusions, and health. *American Psychologist*, *55*, 99–109.

Taylor, S. E., Lerner, J. S., Sherman, D. K., Sage, R. M., & McDowell, N. K. (2003). Are self-enhancing cognitions associated with healthy or unhealthy biological profiles? *Journal of Personality and Social Psychology*, *85*, 605–615.

Taylor, S. E., Pham, L. B., Rivkin, I. D., & Armor, D. A. (1998). Harnessing the imagination: Mental stimulation, self-regulation, and coping. *American Psychologist*, *53*, 429–439.

Verbrugge, L. M. (1990). Disability. *Rheumatic Disease Clinic*, *16*, 741–761.

Wilcox, S., & Storandt, M. (1996). Relations among age, exercise, and psychological variables in a community sample of women. *Health Psychology*, *15*, 110–113.

Zimmerman, B. J., & Martinez-Pons, M. (1992) Perceptions of efficacy and strategy use in the self-regulation of learning. In D. H. Schunk & J. L. Meece (Eds.), *Student perceptions in the classroom: Causes and consequences* (pp. 185–207). Hillsdale, NJ: Erlbaum.

Author Index

670 Author Index

Csikszentmihalyi, M., 111, 193,
586, 600, 603, 604, 605, 606,
612, 614, 619
Cummings, L. L., 63
Cunningham, J., 204
Cunningham, P. B., 489
Curhan, K. B., 465
Curnow, C., 241
Currie, J. M., 416
Cury, F., 64, 138, 324, 325, 326,
327, 328, 329

Dabul, A. J., 81, 386
d'Ailly, H., 263
Da Fonseca, A., 327
Da Fonseca, D., 64, 138, 327, 328
Dakoff, G., 571
Daleiden, E. L., 153, 175
Daly, J. A., 144
Damon, W., 203
D'Andrade, R., 41, 42, 265, 408
Daniels, D., 209
Daniels, J., 604
Danner, F. W., 587
Darcis, C., 443
Dardis, G. J., 213
Darley, J. M., 439, 444, 566, 567,
568
Darling, N., 262, 263, 269
Darling-Hammond, L., 369, 425
Darwin, C., 187
Das, J. P., 462
Dashiell, J. F., 580
Datnow, A., 402
Dauber, S. L., 118
Dauenheimer, D., 381
Dave, P. N., 43, 44
Davey, M. E., 586
Davidson, D. H., 457
Davidson, L. L., 424
Davidson, R. J., 169, 529, 530
Davies, D. R., 250
Davies, P. G., 381, 440, 447, 451
Davis, A., 437, 448
Davis, J., 573
Davis, M., 539
Davis-Kean, P., 222
Dearing, E., 419
Deary, I. J., 145, 160
Deater-Deckard, K., 425
Deaux, K., 194, 376, 384, 448
Debacker, T. K., 380
Debus, R., 215, 230, 362
deCharms, R., 34, 35, 43, 44, 46,
114, 260, 305, 362, 473, 478,
583, 584, 593, 594, 599
Deci, E. L., 6, 10, 91, 108, 109,
112, 113, 114, 115, 225, 260,
262, 263, 301, 303, 304, 305,
327, 355, 359, 360, 361, 362,

363, 473, 478, 491, 492, 516,
563, 582, 583, 584, 585, 586,
587, 588, 589, 590, 591, 592,
593, 594, 599, 602, 603, 605
DeCorte, E., 515
DeCourcey, W., 263
De Groot, E. V., 93
DeJong, W., 586
Dekker, J., 651
Delgado-Gaitan, C., 475
Delle Fave, A. D., 605
DelVecchio, W. F., 349
Dembo, M. H., 476, 492
Dembo, T., 59, 90, 567
Depner, C., 7, 384
Deprès, G., 445
Depue, R. A., 169, 529
Derryberry, D., 168, 169, 171,
175, 178
Desai, K. A., 474
Désert, M., 443
DesForges, C., 311
Deshon, R. P., 64
de Tocqueville, A., 469
Devaney, B. L., 416
DeVet, K., 192
Devine, P. G., 396, 399, 438
De Vos, G. A., 474
Dew, K. M. H., 145
Dewey, J., 360
Dewitte, S., 515
DeZolt, D., 379
Dholakia, U. M., 635
Diamond, A., 178
Diaz, R. M., 263
Díaz de Chumaceiro, C. L., 618
Diener, C. I., 53, 206
Diener, E., 80, 476, 493, 572
Dijksterhuis, A., 640
DiMaggio, D., 491
Dittman-Kohli, F., 242
Dodds, R. A., 499
Dodge, K. A., 270, 272, 281, 286,
290, 292
Dodson, N., 403
Dogra, N., 490
Dollard, J., 529
Dollinger, S. J., 586
Dong, Q., 271, 426
Donnell, C., 153
Dooley, D., 249
Dorinan, C., 619
Dornbusch, S. M., 94, 223, 234,
263, 271, 476
Douvan, E., 7, 384
Dovidio, J. F., 400
Downey, D., 402
Downey, G., 422, 448, 561, 562
Downs, D. L., 550
Doyle, W., 311

Draper, D. C., 282, 283
Dretzke, B. J., 94
Drew, K. D., 180
Driscoll, D., 398
Driver, R. E., 263, 567
Dubiner, K., 173
Dubow, E. F., 289
Duckett, E., 266
Duda, J. L., 56, 57, 58, 63, 64,
318, 319, 320, 321, 322, 323,
324, 325, 326, 328, 329, 330,
331
Dudek, S. Z., 612
Duffy, J., 381
Dumas, F., 571
Dumas, T., 394
Dumas-Hines, F., 133
Duncan, G. J., 414, 415, 417, 419,
420, 421, 422
Dunifon, R., 417, 423, 428
Dunlap, K. G., 262
Dunn, J. D. H., 147
Dunning, D., 213
Dunton, B. C., 439
Durkheim, E., 242
Durkin, M. S., 424
Durning, K., 520
Dutrévis, M., 439, 443, 449
Dweck, C. S., 4, 6, 7, 19, 53, 54,
55, 56, 58, 62, 64, 65, 66,
79, 96, 110, 115, 122, 123,
124, 126, 127, 129, 130, 131,
133, 134, 135, 137, 188, 190,
191, 192, 193, 194, 195, 196,
202, 204, 205, 206, 210, 211,
215, 217, 218, 226, 259, 260,
264, 265, 281, 298, 305, 318,
319, 320, 322, 324, 326, 327,
329, 330, 331, 363, 364, 368,
379, 385, 398, 414, 436, 437,
439, 452, 461, 466, 477, 496,
497, 516, 523, 528, 543, 550,
556, 602, 638, 657, 658, 659
Dzokoto, V., 493

Eagly, A. H., 376
Earl, R. W., 43
Earls, F. J., 424, 426
Eaton, M. J., 8, 476, 492
Eaton, M. M., 262, 269, 272, 273
Ebbeck, V., 321
Ebersole, P., 619
Eccles, J. S., 90, 94, 96, 105, 108,
109, 110, 112, 113, 116, 117,
118, 119, 222, 224, 225, 226,
227, 228, 229, 231, 232, 259,
260, 265, 266, 269, 273, 290,
302, 303, 318, 376, 378, 380,
381, 398, 407, 439
Eccles-Parsons, J., 376

Author Index

Subject Index

"f" following a page number indicates a figure; "t" following a page number indicates a table.